Apheresis: Principles and Practice
3rd Edition

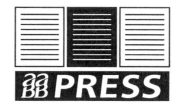

Other related publications from the AABB:

Apheresis: Principles and Practice, 3rd edition (CD-ROM)
Edited by Bruce C. McLeod, MD; Zbigniew (Ziggy) M. Szczepiorkowski, MD, PhD, FCAP; Robert Weinstein, MD; and Jeffrey L. Winters, MD

Therapeutic Apheresis: A Physician's Handbook, 3rd edition
Edited by Jeffrey L. Winters, MD

Look This Up, Too! (A Quick Reference in Apheresis)
By Mark E. Brecher, MD; Shauna Hay, MT(ASCP), MPH; and Beth Shaz, MD

To purchase books or to inquire about other book services, including chapter reprints and large-quantity sales, please contact our sales department:
- 866.222.2498 (within the United States)
- +1 301.215.6499 (outside the United States)
- +1 301.951.7150 (fax)
- www.aabb.org>Bookstore

AABB customer service representatives are available by telephone from 8:30 am to 5:00 pm ET, Monday through Friday, excluding holidays.

Apheresis: Principles and Practice
3rd Edition

Editors

Bruce C. McLeod, MD
Rush Medical College
Rush University Medical Center
Chicago, Illinois

Zbigniew (Ziggy) M. Szczepiorkowski, MD, PhD, FCAP
Dartmouth Medical School
Dartmouth-Hitchcock Medical Center
Lebanon, New Hampshire

Robert Weinstein, MD
University of Massachusetts Medical School
UMass Memorial Medical Center
Worcester, Massachusetts

Jeffrey L. Winters, MD
Mayo Clinic
Mayo Clinic College of Medicine
Rochester, Minnesota

AABB Press
Bethesda, Maryland
2010

AABB
8101 Glenbrook Road
Bethesda, Maryland 20814-2749

ISBN NO. 978-1-56395-305-7
Printed in the United States

Library of Congress Cataloging-in-Publication Data

Apheresis : principles and practice / editors, Bruce C. McLeod ... [et al.]. — 3rd ed.
p. ; cm.
Includes bibliographical references and index.
ISBN 978-1-56395-305-7
1. Hemapheresis. I. McLeod, Bruce C. II. AABB.
[DNLM: 1. Blood Component Removal—methods. WH 460]
RM173.A64 2010
615'.39—dc22

2010030205

Dedication

This book is dedicated to the memory of

Allen Latham, Jr.

who gave us an instrument for collecting platelets, and

Scott Murphy, MD

who taught us so much about how to store them.

Contributors

Christina Anderson, RN, BSN, HP(ASCP)
Carter BloodCare
Dallas, Texas

Joseph H. Antin, MD
Harvard Medical School
Dana-Farber Cancer Institute/Brigham
and Women's Hospital
Boston, Massachusetts

Nicholas Bandarenko, MD
Duke University Medical Center
Durham, North Carolina

P. Dayanand Borge, Jr, MD, PhD
Warren Grant Magnuson Clinical Center
National Institutes of Health
Bethesda, Maryland

Mark E. Brecher, MD
Laboratory Corporation of America
Burlington, North Carolina
University of North Carolina
Chapel Hill, North Carolina

Randy Brown, MD
University of Florida College of Medicine
Gainesville, Florida

Edwin Burgstaler, MT, HP(ASCP)
Mayo Clinic
Rochester, Minnesota

Kathryn M. Bushnell, MT(ASCP)
Dartmouth-Hitchcock Medical Center
Lebanon, New Hampshire

Vishesh Chhibber, MD
UMass Memorial Medical Center
University of Massachusetts Medical School
Worcester, Massachusetts

Jaehyuk Choi, MD, PhD
Yale School of Medicine
New Haven, Connecticut

Christopher Chun, MT(ASCP)HP
American Red Cross Biomedical Services
Salt Lake City, Utah

Kendall P. Crookston, MD, PhD
University of New Mexico School of Medicine
TriCore Reference Laboratories
Albuquerque, New Mexico

Jillian Ferschke, BS
UMass Memorial Medical Center
Worcester, Massachusetts

Francine M. Foss, MD
Yale School of Medicine
New Haven, Connecticut

Richard O. Francis, MD, PhD
Columbia University Medical Center
New York Presbyterian Hospital
New York, New York

Andre A. Kaplan, MD, FACP, FASN
University of Connecticut Health Center
Farmington, Connecticut

Haiwon C. Kim, MD
The Children's Hospital of Philadelphia
University of Pennsylvania School of Medicine
Philadelphia, Pennsylvania

Karen E. King, MD
Johns Hopkins Medical Institutions
Baltimore, Maryland

Joseph E. Kiss, MD
University of Pittsburgh
Pittsburgh, Pennsylvania

Harvey G. Klein, MD
National Institutes of Health
Bethesda, Maryland

Sara C. Koenig, MD
University of North Carolina
Chapel Hill, North Carolina

Wanda B. Koetz, RN, HP(ASCP)
American Red Cross Biomedical Services
Washington, District of Columbia

Daniela S. Krause, MD, PhD
Massachusetts General Hospital
Boston, Massachusetts

Michael L. Linenberger, MD, FACP
University of Washington
Seattle Cancer Care Alliance
Seattle, Washington

Evelyn Lockhart, MD
Duke University Medical Center
Durham, North Carolina

Marisa B. Marques, MD
University of Alabama at Birmingham
University Hospital Transfusion Services
Birmingham, Alabama

Janice G. McFarland, MD
BloodCenter of Wisconsin, Inc.
Milwaukee, Wisconsin

Bruce C. McLeod, MD
Rush Medical College
Rush University Medical Center
Chicago, Illinois

Deborah J. Novak, MD
University of New Mexico School of Medicine
United Blood Services of New Mexico
Albuquerque, New Mexico

David W. O'Neill, MD
New York University School of Medicine
New York University Cancer Institute Vaccine
and Cell Therapy Core Facility
New York, New York

Anand Padmanabhan, MD, PhD
University of Pittsburgh
Pittsburgh, Pennsylvania

Yara A. Park, MD
University of North Carolina
Chapel Hill, North Carolina

David L. Porter, MD
University of Pennsylvania
University of Pennsylvania Medical Center
Philadelphia, Pennsylvania

Thomas H. Price, MD
Puget Sound Blood Center
University of Washington
Seattle, Washington

David T. Scadden, MD
Harvard University
Massachusetts General Hospital
Boston, Massachusetts

Joseph Schwartz, MD
Columbia University Medical Center
New York Presbyterian Hospital
New York, New York

Beth H. Shaz, MD
Emory University
Atlanta, Georgia

James W. Smith, MD, PhD
Oklahoma Blood Institute
Oklahoma City, Oklahoma

Ronald G. Strauss, MD
University of Iowa College of Medicine
Iowa City, Iowa

Zbigniew (Ziggy) M. Szczepiorkowski, MD, PhD, FCAP
Dartmouth Medical School
Dartmouth-Hitchcock Medical Center
Lebanon, New Hampshire

Edwin G. Taft, MD
Albany Medical College
Albany, New York

Ralph R. Vassallo, Jr, MD, FACP
American Red Cross Blood Services
Penn-Jersey Region
Philadelphia, Pennsylvania

Michelle A. Vauthrin, MT(ASCP)SBB
UMass Memorial Medical Center
Worcester, Massachusetts

Robert Weinstein, MD
University of Massachusetts Medical School
UMass Memorial Medical Center
Worcester, Massachusetts

John R. Wingard, MD
University of Florida College of Medicine
Gainesville, Florida

Jeffrey L. Winters, MD
Mayo Clinic
Mayo Clinic College of Medicine
Rochester, Minnesota

Baldeep Wirk, MD
University of Florida College of Medicine
Gainesville, Florida

Table of Contents

17. Therapeutic Plasma Exchange for Renal and Rheumatic Diseases. 349

Andre A. Kaplan, MD, FACP, FASN

18. Apheresis in Solid Organ Transplantation 371

Marisa B. Marques, MD

19. Red Cell Exchange and Other Therapeutic Alterations of Red Cell Mass 391

Beth H. Shaz, MD

20. Selective Extraction of Plasma Constituents 411

Jeffrey L. Winters, MD

Table of Contents

Preface

APHERESIS IS A WELL-ESTAB-
lished specialty discipline, with its
most complete and coherent
expression found in the broader
area of transfusion medicine.
National societies, such as the
American Society for Apheresis (ASFA) and
similar organizations in Europe, Japan, South
America, and elsewhere hold regular meetings
for individuals interested in apheresis. International societies, such as the World Apheresis
Association, also meet regularly. Apheresis has
been the subject of countless presentations and
publications; indeed, several biomedical journals are devoted primarily to this field. Before
publication of the first edition of this book,
however, there had not been a reference text
on apheresis.

The editors believe this volume will continue to fill that need. Like its predecessors, the
third edition provides a comprehensive account
of the scientific, technical, and practical aspects
of most of the uses thus far found for apheresis
instruments. The list of chapter authors is again
eclectic and, like the list of editors, contains
several new names. It includes engineers and
inventors who have developed apheresis instruments, physicians with expertise in the science
of apheresis and the treatment of diseases for
which apheresis products or procedures are
important therapeutically, nurses and technologists who work with apheresis instruments on a
daily basis and understand how to care for
donors and patients during procedures, and
individuals with expertise in regulatory and
managerial issues pertaining to apheresis. The
book is intended for health-care professionals
working in any branch of apheresis donation or
therapy; it should be useful for individuals at all
levels in the transfusion medicine and blood
banking communities, as well as for physicians
and other medical professionals who care for
patients needing apheresis products or procedures.

The third edition retains the format of 32
chapters grouped into six sections. Section I is
introductory. The first two chapters are historical and cover apheresis instruments and applications, respectively. The senior authors of
these chapters were all active participants in
the early era of apheresis and played important
roles in the definition and growth of the specialty. Chapter 1 is virtually unchanged from
the first edition, while Chapter 2 is a new chapter covering the history of both donor and
patient apheresis from the standpoint of Dr.
Edwin Taft, the archivist of ASFA. The remaining two chapters in this section cover fundamental current knowledge that is relevant to
most of the succeeding chapters. Chapter 3 presents physiologic concepts pertinent to apheresis, including adverse reactions, particularly
those related to hypovolemia and ionized
hypocalcemia. Chapter 4, which describes the
state of the art in apheresis instrumentation,
contains descriptions of new instruments
intended for multiple component donations
and a new device for photopheresis.

Component donation is covered in Section
II. This is the purpose for which apheresis

instruments were originally intended, and the one that still accounts for the majority of apheresis procedures performed in the United States and elsewhere. Chapter 5 describes the assessment and care of apheresis donors. The next six chapters are devoted to various aspects of transfusable components obtained by apheresis, including production, storage, leukocyte content, bacterial contamination, matching, and clinical use.

Section III covers direct therapeutic applications of apheresis—the modern incarnations of the medieval practice of "bloodletting" to remove evil humors. It provides the reader with scientific background and practical recommendations on therapeutic apheresis and the diseases treated with it. Chapter 12 presents an overview of the approach to patients requiring apheresis therapy. Therapeutic removal of platelets and leukocytes is covered in Chapter 13, while in Chapter 14 the reader will find mathematical and metabolic principles of blood component exchanges and plasma replacement solutions. Chapters 15 through 17 focus on the role of therapeutic plasma exchange in specific disorders, grouped by organ system. Chapter 18 is a new chapter, devoted to therapeutic apheresis in the context of organ transplantation. The section concludes with chapters on the exchange, removal, and transfusion of red cells by apheresis; the selective extraction of specific plasma components for therapeutic purposes; and the application of therapeutic apheresis to pediatric patients. Each chapter has been fully updated with the results of relevant clinical studies published since the second edition was released. We are particularly pleased that we have been able to provide the latest ASFA indication category assignments as they appear in the special issue of the *Journal of Clinical Apheresis* published in 2010.

Section IV, which is devoted to stem cell transplantation, has been considerably expanded in this edition. All the chapter authors are new, and the scope of most of the chapters has been broadened. The opening chapter discusses clinical stem cell transplantation from its beginning to the current state of the art, including the prevalent use of hematopoietic progenitor cells collected with apheresis instruments. The next chapter focuses mobilization and collection of progenitor cells. It covers new and experimental mobilizing agents, including their mechanisms of action, instruments and methods for collection, and developing regulations applicable to these activities. The following chapter combines material previously covered in two separate chapters into a single, integrated discussion of stem cell processing, from receipt in the laboratory through issue for transplantation. The final chapter in this section is devoted to the new field of regenerative medicine, which is a topic that should be of interest to many readers of this work because of its many areas of overlap with apheresis and blood stem cell processing.

Section V explores the use of mononuclear cells collected by apheresis, including T lymphocytes and dendritic cells, to modulate immunity, particularly in patients with malignant or infectious diseases. Treatment strategies range from straightforward transfer of unmodified cells to elaborate protocols that include ex-vivo activation, immunization, or gene insertion, sometimes coupled with expansion in culture before infusion. The chapter on photopheresis includes the latest guidelines for clinical use of this presumably immunomodulatory technique. The last chapter in this section covers gene transfer, which, in addition to its potential immunomodulatory effects, can correct some inherited deficiency disorders.

Section VI deals with regulatory and quality management aspects of apheresis. We asked authors who have experience in management of regulatory affairs and quality assurance programs to discuss these areas as they relate to the operation of an apheresis unit. One chapter describes regulatory agencies that oversee apheresis and summarizes their most pertinent documents and requirements. Another presents quality management concepts and their application to apheresis facilities and equipment. The concluding chapter is devoted to quality management of the personnel who work in apheresis facilities. All these chapters have been updated with the latest concepts and regulatory requirements.

In editing chapters we have not tried to eliminate all instances of duplication of content. We expect that most readers will consult individual chapters as needs arise rather than moving steadily from cover to cover. We have therefore preferred that each chapter contain enough information to stand alone and have purposely retained some repetition of fundamental concepts for that purpose.

As editors, we could not close without acknowledging the invaluable assistance we received in the course of bringing this new edition to completion. We cannot possibly name all the persons who deserve our gratitude, but the list would include all the chapter authors and the highly professional editorial staff at AABB Press.

Astute readers may note that several important uses of apheresis instruments have been omitted, either because they do not ordinarily occur in the transfusion medicine arena or because they have been well-covered in other texts. These uses include red cell washing and deglycerolization and intraoperative blood recovery. We again chose not to describe several excellent apheresis instruments that are not available in the United States. With these exceptions, however, we strove for the most comprehensive possible coverage. We expect that anyone with a specific question about any area of apheresis will be able to find the answer with this book, either in the references cited or, in most cases, in the text itself.

Bruce C. McLeod, MD
Zbigniew (Ziggy) M. Szczepiorkowski, MD, PhD
Robert Weinstein, MD
Jeffrey L. Winters, MD
Editors

About the Editors

 Bruce C. McLeod, MD, has been affiliated with the Rush University Medical Center and its predecessor organizations in Chicago since 1969. He is currently the director of the Blood Center and oversees therapeutic apheresis, stem cell collection, and stem cell processing as well as the donor center and transfusion service. Dr. McLeod is also professor of medicine and pathology at the Rush Medical College.

Dr. McLeod received his medical degree from the Harvard Medical School in Boston in 1969. He completed a residency in internal medicine at Rush in 1972 and a fellowship in immunology at Rush and the Royal Post-Graduate Medical School in London in 1974. He is board certified in internal medicine and rheumatology.

Dr. McLeod's early publications dealt with the complement system, including its interactions with infusible agents, plastic tubing, and plasma separator membranes used in various apheresis instruments. He subsequently devised several new apheresis procedures, including a plasma exchange donation that allows selective collection of cryoprecipitate. His current scholarly interests include both the evidential basis for therapeutic apheresis and the support of stem cell and solid organ transplantation. He is a past president of the American Society for Apheresis (ASFA), having served two terms on its board of directors, and a past chairperson of the AABB Hemapheresis Committee. Dr. McLeod has served on the editorial boards of

TRANSFUSION, the *Journal of Clinical Apheresis,* and *AABB Press.*

Zbigniew (Ziggy) M. Szczepiorkowski, MD, PhD, FCAP, has been affiliated with the Dartmouth-Hitchcock Medical Center in Lebanon, NH, since 2003. He is currently associate professor of pathology and of medicine at Dartmouth Medical School, and he is the medical director of the Transfusion Medicine Service and Center for Transfusion Medicine Research and director of the Cellular Therapy Center at Dartmouth-Hitchcock Medical Center. He is also an investigator at Norris Cotton Cancer Center (National Cancer Institute Comprehensive Cancer Center at Dartmouth) and a consultant in pathology services at the Massachusetts General Hospital (Boston, MA).

Dr. Szczepiorkowski graduated from the Medical University of Warsaw, Poland, in 1991. He was an intern in Mokotowski Hospital in Warsaw, after which he pursued a postdoctoral fellowship at Massachusetts General Hospital/ Harvard Medical School. He obtained his PhD in medicine at the Medical Center for Postgraduate Education in Warsaw in 1997. He was the chief resident in clinical pathology at Massachusetts General Hospital, where he also completed a Grove Rasmussen fellowship in transfusion medicine and subsequently served as an attending physician for 5 years. He is board certified in clinical pathology and blood banking/transfusion medicine.

Dr. Szczepiorkowski is the immediate past president of ASFA. He is also a member of the Board of Directors of the AABB and National

Marrow Donor Program (NMDP) and is a coleader of the Cellular Therapy Team of the Biomedical Excellence for Safer Transfusion (BEST) Collaborative. He has served as a member of the executive and advisory committee of the Center for International Blood and Marrow Transplantation Research, as well as having served on the National Heart, Lung, and Blood Institute Small Business Innovation Research Grant Program; National Institutes of Health ad hoc panels; and various committees of the AABB, ASFA, College of American Pathologists, Foundation for the Accreditation of Cellular Therapy, and the NMDP. Serving on the editorial boards of the *Journal of Clinical Apheresis* and the *Journal of Transfusion Medicine* (Warsaw, Poland), he has also published in the fields of laboratory medicine, cellular therapy, apheresis, and transfusion medicine.

Robert Weinstein, MD, is chief of the Division of Transfusion Medicine at UMass Memorial Medical Center and professor of medicine and pathology at the University of Massachusetts Medical School in Worcester, MA, where he serves as chairman of the Faculty Council.

After obtaining his doctor of medicine degree from the New York University School of Medicine in 1975, Dr. Weinstein completed a residency in internal medicine at the University of Miami Affiliated Hospitals in 1978. He then moved to Boston for fellowship training in hematology at the Beth Israel Hospital, Harvard Medical School, where he became assistant professor of medicine in 1981. He served as chief of hematology and transfusion medicine at Caritas St. Elizabeth's Medical Center (Brighton, MA) from 1985 to 2006 and then joined the faculty at the University of Massachusetts.

Dr. Weinstein joined ASFA in 1991. He has served as chairman of its Awards, Membership, and Advocacy and Public Affairs committees and is a past president of the society. He is currently serving as president of the World Apheresis Association. His major interests include adverse effects of apheresis, therapeutic apheresis in neurologic disorders, and vascular access.

Jeffrey L. Winters, MD, graduated with high distinction from the University of Kentucky College of Medicine in Lexington, KY, in 1993. His postgraduate training consisted of an anatomic/clinical pathology residency in the Department of Pathology and Laboratory Medicine at the University of Kentucky and a transfusion medicine/blood banking fellowship in the Division of Transfusion Medicine at the Mayo Clinic in Rochester, MN. He is certified by the American Board of Pathology in anatomic pathology, clinical pathology, and blood banking/transfusion medicine.

Following the completion of his training in 1999, Dr. Winters served as the associate director of the blood bank at the University of Kentucky Chandler Medical Center, the director of the blood bank at the Cooper Drive Division of the Veteran's Affairs Medical Center, and the associate medical director of the Central Kentucky Blood Center (all in Lexington).

In 2001, Dr. Winters returned to the Mayo Clinic in Rochester, MN, as a physician in the Department of Laboratory Medicine and Pathology. He is currently an associate professor of laboratory medicine and pathology in the Mayo College of Medicine and is the medical director of the Mayo Clinic Therapeutic Apheresis Treatment Unit, a fifteen-bed unit performing approximately 3000 therapeutic apheresis procedures annually. In addition to his apheresis responsibilities, he is an attending physician on the transfusion service.

Since 2004, he has served as the director of Mayo Clinic's transfusion medicine training programs for residents and fellows. In 2005 and 2009, Dr. Winters was recognized as the Mayo Fellow's Association Clinical Pathology Teacher of the Year.

Dr. Winters is the president of ASFA for 2010-2011. He has served on numerous ASFA committees, including the Apheresis Applications Committees responsible for the 2000, 2007, and 2010 special editions of the *Journal of Clinical Apheresis,* for which he is currently an associate editor. In 2002, he received the Junior Investigator Award from ASFA.

In: McLeod BC, Szczepiorkowski ZM, Weinstein R, Winters JL, eds.
Apheresis: Principles and Practice, 3rd edition
Bethesda, MD: AABB Press, 2010

1

Development of Apheresis Instrumentation

Frank Corbin; Herbert M. Cullis; Emil J. Freireich, MD, DSc (Hon.); Yoichiro Ito, MD; Robert M. Kellogg, PhD; Allen Latham, Jr.; and Bruce C. McLeod, MD

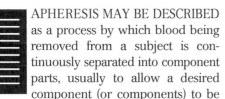

APHERESIS MAY BE DESCRIBED as a process by which blood being removed from a subject is continuously separated into component parts, usually to allow a desired component (or components) to be retained while the remainder is returned to the subject. Apheresis depends on instrumentation, and many advances in the practice of apheresis have been linked to advances in instrumentation. This chapter contains accounts of the early history of apheresis devices related by individual authors who helped to make that history. It covers the efforts and events underlying development of all the major families of instruments available today.

Every general-purpose blood cell separator device released to date has relied on centrifugation to separate blood into component parts on the basis of differences in density. Apheresis instruments use one of the two versions of continuous flow centrifugation: either continuous processing or batch processing, the latter having been termed intermittent (or, sometimes, discontinuous) flow centrifugation in the apheresis field. Either allows blood to be processed in increments small enough that their temporary loss into the instrument is well tolerated by the subject. In this way, it is possible to process total quantities of blood that equal or exceed the subject's blood volume.

The earliest continuous flow centrifugation device to find widespread commercial success was the hand-cranked cream separator invented in Sweden in 1877 by Dr. Carl Gustav Patrik De Laval, and patented in the United States in

Reprinted from the first edition.

1881.[1] Subsequent devices are to some extent conceptually related to this technological breakthrough. Continuous flow centrifugation has since found many applications in addition to blood separation, having been used in the petroleum industry to remove particulate impurities from lubricating oil, in the nuclear fuel industry to separate uranium isotopes, and in waste management to separate solid and liquid wastes from a mixed stream, to name just a few. In addition, it is still used in the dairy industry.[2]

A structural feature common to many such devices is a means to join rotary and stationary components so that unseparated material can be fed into the centrifuge and separated components can be retrieved from it. Blood separation imposes unique constraints on this module, which must remain cool to avoid denaturation of biologic molecules and must preserve sterility. The rotary seal is one solution that has found numerous applications. Alternatively, sealless centrifuges have been devised, extending a concept originally introduced as a way to maintain electrical contacts in a rotating antenna.

Cohn Centrifuge

Much of the earliest work on continuous flow centrifugation for the separation of blood components was done in the early 1950s in the laboratories of Edwin J. Cohn, PhD, at Harvard Medical School. Dr. Cohn had devised a biochemical fractionation scheme for plasma and was the central figure in a huge wartime effort to provide albumin for battlefield management of shock. By the late 1940s, concern for the national blood resource had broadened to include cellular components that might be needed in the event of nuclear war. In January 1949, Dr. Cohn convened the first meeting of the Formed Elements Group to begin to address these new concerns, and part of the ensuing effort was directed at the separation of cellular components. Early in 1951, while vacationing briefly in Arizona, Dr. Cohn envisioned a device for the immediate, on-line separation of whole blood into components during the donation process itself, and he soon set about to develop the "biomechanical equipment" that would accomplish this (DM Surgenor, personal communication).

With help from mechanical experts such as Charles Gordon, Fred Gilchrist, and Robert Tinch, Dr. Cohn quickly designed and constructed instruments[3-5] in which citrated or decalcified whole blood flowed upward under pressure into the conical upper portion of a separation chamber rotating at about 2000 rpm (Fig 1-1).[6] As blood in the rotating chamber flowed downward under the influence of gravity, lighter components (eg, plasma) were separated from heavier components (eg, red cells). When the upper chamber became full, a dynamic (ie, opened by centrifugal force) valve mechanism near the axis of rotation allowed egress of plasma into a lower chamber, from which it fell free into the peripheral zone of a stationary collecting cup (Fig 1-2),[6] and from there into a storage bag. Meanwhile, red cells continued to accumulate in the upper chamber, which was sized so that it filled with cells when about 500 mL of whole blood of normal hema-

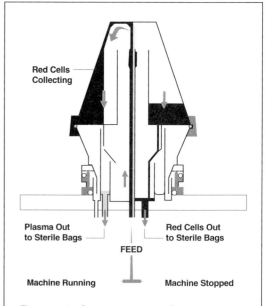

Figure 1-1. Cross section of Cohn centrifuge bowl. See text for structural and operational details. (Used with permission from Tullis et al.[6])

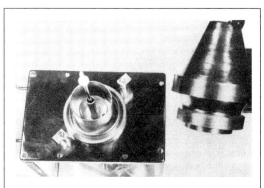

Figure 1-2. Collecting cup for Cohn centrifuge with bowl removed. See text for structural and operational details. (Used with permission from Tullis et al.[6])

tocrit had been withdrawn. At this point the centrifuge motor was stopped. The dynamic valve consequently closed, and the red cells flowed by gravity into the central zone of the collecting cup and thence to either another separation stage or a separate collection bag. Variations on this basic theme were designed with a view to separate platelets and leukocytes as well. Yet another application explored at that time was the gradual removal of glycerol from Red Blood Cell (RBC) units that had been stored in the frozen state. The performance of these instruments and their effects on blood and blood components were studied by teams of investigators under the direction of James L. Tullis, MD, and Douglas M. Surgenor, PhD, among others.[5,6]

The original instruments had outer rotating seals comprising stainless steel rings, fabricated in Harvard's machine shop, which met graphite rings, adapted from their intended use in automotive transmissions, under spring tension to join the fixed and rotating portions. The centrifuge drive mechanism was applied externally to the conical bowls so that the separation and collection elements could be preassembled and sterilized as a unit, allowing blood to be processed in a sterile closed system. However, the centrifuge bowls and seals had to be reused and therefore required disassembly, thorough cleaning, and reassembly between uses.

Two manufacturers, the American Optical Company[4] and Arthur D. Little, Inc,[6] developed versions of this device for research use. The latter device (the Cohn ADL Centrifuge) had some success as a means for processing frozen RBCs; indeed, more than a third of RBC units transfused at the Chelsea Naval Hospital in the late 1950s were prepared in this way.[7] However, the inherent limitations of the device, as well as simultaneous advances in processing individual citrated units in plastic bags soon after donation, precluded widespread clinical use. Nevertheless, the concept of immediate, on-line separation of donated blood into what might be called "component donations" held considerable appeal and served as a stimulus for further development. Most subsequent work on component separation continued to use centrifugation, although eventually membrane separation, which depends solely on particle size, was also investigated and proved to be suitable for some tasks, particularly the primary separation of plasma from formed elements.

Haemonetics Instruments and the Latham Bowl

Allen Latham, Jr., Founder, Haemonetics Corporation, Braintree, Massachusetts

The key event leading to development of the Latham bowl and the Haemonetics line of apheresis devices was a request by Dr. Cohn at Harvard Medical School for help in solving a bearing problem in connection with his development of a novel centrifuge. This request was made to Arthur D. Little, Inc, in 1952 and was assigned to me as head of the engineering group. Failures of this bearing were severely retarding progress in the use of glycerol to prevent destructive crystal formation during long-term frozen storage of RBCs. My brief analysis revealed that many of the principles of bearing application had been disregarded. One of my engineers quickly completed a redesign and supervised construction of a trial machine, which was rushed over to Dr. Cohn's laboratory for a preliminary "show and tell" evaluation. Dr.

Cohn's assistants insisted on putting this machine to immediate use without our taking time to embellish it with a fine external finish.

In lieu of payment for doing this work, Dr. Cohn agreed to let us sell similar machines to other laboratories. As it turned out, there was enough demand for these machines to justify forming an independent business. Initially, I was urged to make no change in the bowl design and to correct only the bearing failure problem. However, after we had sold 16 machines and about 100 of the Cohn bowls, I initiated a complete redesign of the drive mechanism and the bowls, primarily to establish a basis for the ultimate advance to a disposable bowl. The 4-inch-diameter rotary seal in the Cohn bowl obviously was not acceptable for use in a disposable version. Nor was the arrangement of exposed outlet streams from the bottom of the bowl desirable. The redesigned bowl used a relatively small rotary seal at the top, where it also incorporated both inlet and outlet connections. The outlet used a double-disk form of fluid pickup, which had been applied in Scandinavian milk centrifuges many years earlier.

To verify the acceptability of this design before tooling up for manufacturing, I made a few trial bowls by machining the large body parts from extruded polycarbonate bar stock. These experimental bowls functioned very well, and the blood processed in them was found to be satisfactory for human use. In fact, for the first time it was easy to harvest substantial quantities of platelets with the equipment we had designed for RBC washing. By connecting a donor to the machine and passing blood through the bowl one unit at a time, it was readily practical to collect a full therapeutic quantity of platelets by retaining just the platelets and returning the other fractions to the donor in a multicycle run. A cross-sectional diagram of the bowl is shown in Fig 1-3. Later, we also designed a simplified bowl for the commercial collection of plasma. Throughout the early years of centrifuge bowl development, Dr. Tullis provided invaluable support by critically reviewing our plans. Robert Tinch, a senior technician in Dr. Tullis's laboratory, was partic-

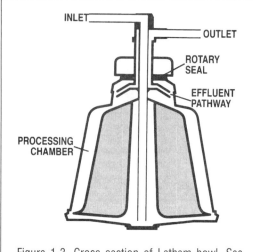

Figure 1-3. Cross section of Latham bowl. See text for structural and operational details. (Courtesy of Haemonetics Corporation.)

ularly helpful in conducting initial trials of the experimental bowls.

Rather than raise the substantial amount of capital needed to establish both the manufacture and the marketing of blood-processing bowls, I chose to set up a license with a company already serving the blood-processing equipment market. Abbott Laboratories accepted a license for this purpose, invested in the necessary molding dies, and initiated the sale of sterile, disposable bowls. About 3 years later, however, they suffered a forced recall of their line of sterile solutions, which was one of their most important products. Under the stress of reestablishing their sterile solution business, they withdrew from our license.

With the help of a small venture capital firm called Breck, McNeish, and Nagel, about 35 private investors were persuaded to put in enough capital for us to form Haemonetics Corporation and purchase the molding tools and a modest inventory of bowls from Abbott. At about the same time I persuaded Gordon Kingsley to help develop Haemonetics into a profitable, growing business. Haemonetics was then located in one of the rental buildings at the East Natick Industrial Park. Within a few years we were renting seven of its buildings. A few years later we moved to a single large building in Braintree.

Having read about the success another laboratory equipment manufacturer had gained by sponsoring professional meetings of its customers, I inaugurated similar meetings for our customers. There, they described other applications for our equipment, such as leukocyte collection, plasma exchange, and partial red cell exchange. These meetings were popular with our customers, who eventually formed their own associations for conducting such meetings both domestically and overseas. Editors note: References 3-15 constitute a bibliography for Mr. Latham's portion of the chapter.

NCI-IBM Blood Cell Separator

Emil J. Freireich, MD, DSc (Hon.), Director, Adult Leukemia Research Program, M. D. Anderson Cancer Center, Houston, Texas

My interest in blood cell separation arose from the observation that fresh whole blood containing viable platelets could reduce hemorrhage in thrombocytopenic patients.[16] This observation led to the development of a manual procedure for collecting platelets from 2 to 4 units of platelet-rich plasma (PRP) from a single donor. This could be accomplished weekly using a two-plastic bag closed system with commercial centrifuges.[17] This primitive plateletpheresis procedure provided a highly effective platelet replacement program that substantially decreased morbidity and mortality from hemorrhage in patients with leukemia and other malignant diseases.[18]

The availability of platelet transfusions resulted in a dramatic shift in morbidity and mortality from hemorrhage to infection. Because the infections were associated with severe neutropenia, we considered the possibility that an intermittent apheresis procedure to provide granulocyte replacement might have an equally dramatic effect on the occurrence of infection. Unfortunately, the physiology of the granulocyte made this technical feat virtually impossible because the half-life of the granulocyte in

the circulation is short and the concentration of granulocytes in donor blood is low. We estimated that even if we were able to collect all the granulocytes in the total peripheral blood of a volunteer donor, we would have only enough cells to temporarily increase the granulocyte level in recipients for about 6 to 12 hours. We made several attempts to accomplish this with plastic bags and intermittent collection, but failed.

Then we conceived of collecting granulocytes from donors with untreated benignphase chronic myelocytic leukemia (CML), whose circulating granulocyte levels could be 100-fold higher than those of normal donors. In 1962, we reported the first transfusions of granulocytes from CML donors into neutropenic children with acute leukemia, and the data were subsequently published in 1964.[19] In these studies, we confirmed that an increase in cell dose could allow meaningful granulocyte replacement. Transfusions of 10^{11} granulocytes could normalize granulocyte concentrations for periods of up to 24 hours and were therapeutically effective in children with septicemia.

While I was working on developing a technique for separating granulocytes from whole blood, an unusual event occurred. George Judson, an engineer from International Business Machines (IBM-Endicott), appeared in my laboratory on April 15, 1962, and told me that his 17-year-old son had developed CML. His son had been referred to the National Cancer Institute (NCI) and was being cared for by Jerome Block, MD. When Mr. Judson recognized the investigative climate at the Clinical Center, it occurred to him that, as an engineer, he might make some contribution to the treatment of leukemia and specifically to his son's care. He asked Dr. Block about this, who replied that he was familiar with my effort to develop equipment to separate white cells and that perhaps an engineer could be helpful to me. Mr. Judson proved to be a really extraordinary person. First, he was able to convince IBM management that by working on this project he would enhance IBM's product line. Second, he convinced IBM management and the NCI administration that it would be possible to have a collaboration on a voluntary basis. In a period of less than 2 months, we obtained all the necessary approvals from IBM and the NCI for Mr. Judson to begin working officially as a collaborator in my laboratory.

At our first session, we set down the following objectives: 1) Leukocytes should be separated from whole blood at reasonable efficiency by sedimentation in a centrifuge. 2) Operation should be conducted on a continuous flow basis to allow large quantities of blood to be processed at optimal speed and efficiency. 3) A vein-to-vein procedure should be used to avoid arterial puncture. 4) An anticoagulant should be used that did not require anticoagulation of the donor with its associated risks. 5) The loss of platelets, red cells, and plasma should be minimal to allow the processing of large volumes of blood from a single donor. 6) The system should be completely closed, needle-to-needle, and without any air-blood interface, to obviate the dangers of air injection and bacterial contamination. 7) The entire system should contain a volume of blood less than 500 mL at all times. 8) The system should be easily cleaned, mostly disposable, and sufficiently automated to be operated by a single nonprofessional operator.

The project proceeded with a collection of "junk parts" from the IBM instrumentation shops and with nuts, bolts, and screws that we could purchase at a hardware store. For these laboratory studies, we used donated blood that was unacceptable for transfusion because of hepatitis or syphilis contamination. We had many problems maintaining a blood path, and blood was often spattered throughout the laboratory. In retrospect, it was miraculous that no one working in the laboratory became infected from handling this material. The equipment we were using was separating blood, and we were able to collect buffy coats. However, our major problem was the juncture between the moving and stationary parts of the centrifuge. Mr. Judson learned that a centrifuge had been developed at Oak Ridge Laboratories with an innovative seal that he was able to incorporate into our instrument. In November 1962, we were sufficiently encouraged by the early laboratory studies that we turned to the NCI for funding to support further development of an instrument. After 5 months of intensive review by many different evaluating bodies, we obtained a grant of $13,000 to produce the first instrument used for patient studies. On April 8, 1963, we studied our first patient.

We first had to convince the review and surveillance bodies in the Clinical Center that this was a reasonable strategy without going through an animal test. The scientific basis for this was the evidence in vitro and in vivo that the blood of any animal we might study would have flow and separation characteristics quite different from those of human blood. We felt that because we had demonstrated safety with human blood in vitro, the move to in-vivo studies could be cautiously undertaken. In the first patient, we ran only 250 cc of blood through the instrument and returned it to the donor. I chose patient-donors with benign-phase CML who had already volunteered to donate by the manual two-bag leukapheresis procedure and who now volunteered to assist in evaluating this instrument. Within 4 months, we had demonstrated that we could process 11 L of blood on a continuous flow basis using this primitive equipment.[20]

On the strength of these preliminary results we were able to convince the NCI to initiate a formal contract for more than $300,000 to cover a period of 18 months, during which time IBM would deliver a prototype instrument for further clinical study. The first version of the instrument was tested at the end of January 1964. Studies in three cancer patients with normal hematologic values revealed substantial engineering weaknesses: specifically, the peristaltic blood pumps were inefficient and traumatic to the red cells, the seals allowed leakage across the seal faces so that separated components were contaminated during the collection procedure, and the safety devices for preventing air injection were inadequate. It was therefore back to the drawing boards for IBM to deliver a functional instrument before June 1965.

In 1964, there were major changes in the Clinical Center. Emil Frei, III, MD, who was the chief of our section, decided to go to M. D. Anderson Hospital in Houston, and he recruited me to join him there in 1965. The continuing development of the blood cell separator then came under the leadership of Seymour Perry, MD; Dean Buckner, MD; Robert Eisel; and Robert Graw, MD. On their part, IBM found three spectacular engineers—Bob Kellogg, Vic Kruger, and Alan Jones—who completed the development of the instrument.[21,22] Cross-sectional diagrams of the bowl and seal are shown in Fig 1-4.[21]

In November 1965, after being at M. D. Anderson for only 5 months, I received a call from IBM management indicating that an instrument had been delivered to the NCI to complete their contractual obligations. However, IBM felt that evaluation of the instrument only in Bethesda would be an inadequate field trial. They had decided to manufacture, at their own expense, three additional instruments to place at other sites. This began a period of negotiation between M. D. Anderson and IBM, which ultimately resulted in our receiving an

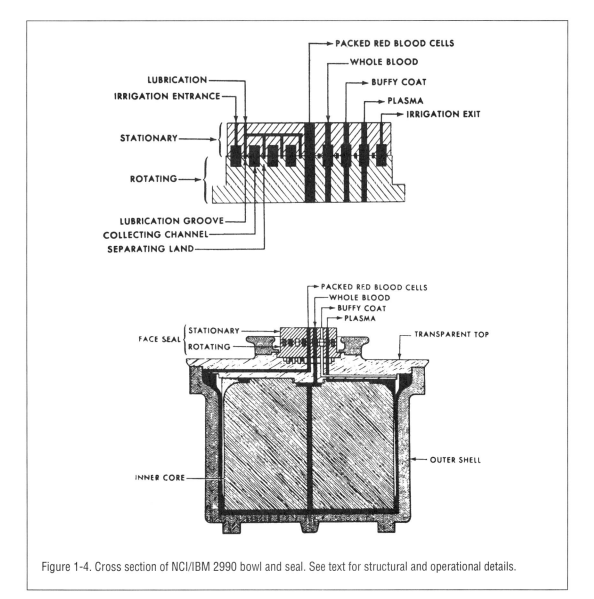

Figure 1-4. Cross section of NCI/IBM 2990 bowl and seal. See text for structural and operational details.

instrument, now officially designated "2990," ready for testing on December 5, 1966. We immediately began in-vitro studies with human blood and discovered that the peristaltic pump problem had been resolved. The seals had also been substantially improved so that leakage across the seal faces was minimal. I can recall how we assembled, by hand, the complex plastic tubing setups necessary to operate the instrument, and gas sterilized them within our institution for our first clinical studies.

We initiated clinical studies in patients with chronic lymphocytic leukemia because we had previously learned that lymphocytes were more efficiently separated than granulocytes, which tended to blend into the red cell layer, resulting in poor separation efficiencies. I can recall vividly our first clinical study. The instrument was primed and made ready in the laboratory. We then rolled it on castors to the patient's bedside, where we would perform the venipunctures and conduct the procedure. Fortunately, there was no blood spewing about the room, and the

first studies, beginning with low volumes, were highly successful. However, we convinced our administration to allow us to use an abandoned hospital-ward kitchen to study patients in a more isolated environment, where we would not disturb the nursing personnel and other patients on the nursing unit (Fig 1-5). A major advance occurred during these early trials when Bob Kellogg conceived of making channels on the metal half of the face seals; this allowed continuous injection of saline across the face seals and totally eliminated cross-contamination of adjacent collection channels. By September 1969, we requested a second instrument and began to study the blood cell separation process further. Kenneth McCredie, MD, who had joined our team in August 1969, assumed a leadership role in developing the 2990 to its practical utility. Our initial studies were conducted with lymphocytes, and we were able to demonstrate the adoptive transfer of immunity from immune donors to non-immune recipients.[23]

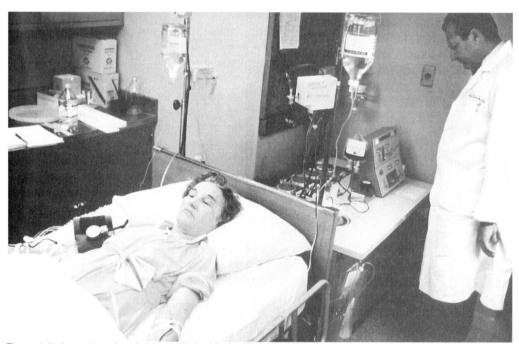

Figure 1-5. An early patient being studied with the IBM 2990 blood cell separator. The operator is the author. Note the small pressure gauge (purchased in a hardware store!) that was used to ensure that the separate peristaltic pump maintained an adequate pressure for injecting saline across the face seals.

We were still frustrated by our inability to collect a sufficient number of granulocytes from a normal donor to accomplish transfusion, and we set about to find an agent for increasing red cell sedimentation. Human fibrinogen (Cohn Fraction 1) might have worked, but it was often contaminated with hepatitis virus. We ran across a 1962 publication by Dr. W. L. Thompson relating to starch derivatives as volume expanders. I contacted Dr. Thompson and we obtained several samples. We found that hydroxyethyl starch was an excellent agent for inducing red cell rouleaux and greatly increased our ability to extract granulocytes with the blood cell separator. We also tried to increase the concentration of granulocytes in the donors. In our first efforts, we used etiocholanolone, a naturally occurring steroid. It had unpleasant side effects such as fever and chills, but it approximately doubled the concentration of circulating granulocytes. By combining these two changes to the procedure, we were able to collect 1 to 2 $\times$ 10^{10} granulocytes from normal donors on a regular basis, and we began to study the effectiveness of such granulocytes in patients.[24] Another major advance was the discovery that, with the blood cell separator, cells capable of forming hematopoietic colonies in soft agar could be isolated from the peripheral blood and a granulocyte donation collected a sufficient number of peripheral stem cells to be potentially capable of serving as donor cells for an allograft.[25]

By 1977, the NCI-IBM 2990 and the Aminco Celltrifuge, a conceptually similar instrument that had an identical centrifuge bowl, were being used worldwide for plasma exchange, platelet collection, granulocyte collection, lymphocyte collection, red cell depletion, and protein depletion. However, a major technical problem remained in that the blood path was still not completely disposable. The plastic tubing sets came presterilized, but the centrifuge bowl itself had to be disassembled with screwdrivers, cleaned thoroughly to remove pyrogens, reassembled, and gas sterilized for each use. These deficiencies made it necessary to completely rethink the design of the centrifuge and the technique for collecting the separated blood components from the centrifuge. The torch was now passed to Jeane P. Hester, MD, who had joined our group to work with Dr. McCredie and myself, and back to IBM, whose team of engineers successfully realized many improvements with the development of the IBM 2997.

Like the Model T Ford, the NCI-IBM 2990 is now history, but it initiated the era of continuous flow blood cell separation, a procedure whose full potential has yet to be realized.

Sealless Continuous Flow Centrifuge

Yoichiro Ito, MD, Laboratory of Biophysical Chemistry, National Heart, Lung and Blood Institute, Bethesda, Maryland

For many decades it was assumed that a continuous flow centrifuge for particle separation would require a rotary seal, typically consisting of a pair of discoid structures, one of which moves with the rotor while the other remains stationary. Rotary seals have been satisfactorily used in various techniques, including countercurrent elutriation, field-flow fractionation, zonal centrifugation, and so on. However, when the Celltrifuge, a commercial blood centrifuge equipped with a rotary seal, was used for long-term plasmapheresis of sheep, severe loss of the circulating platelets was observed. This prompted Jacques Suaudeau, MD, et al, working in the Laboratory of Technical Development at the National Institutes of Health, Heart, Lung, and Blood Institute, to write the following statements:

An efficient procedure for continuous plasmapheresis in long-term extracorporeal circulation has not yet been developed. This technique could be important in plasma exchange or cross-exchange and in artificial organ support if it could be accomplished safely using heparin as the anticoagulant. When sheep were connected to the Celltrifuge for 23 hours and administered 150 units/kg per hour of heparin anticoagulant, we found gross platelet clumping in separated plasma and a 60% fall in platelet count. When 120,000 units of heparin were directly injected into the centrifuge bowl at the onset of the centrifugation followed by hourly heparin administration at 500 units/kg, there was no platelet clumping but the platelet count fell to 52%.[26]

Meanwhile, the American Instrument Company (Aminco) in Silver Spring, MD, was pursuing a project to design a seal-free continuous flow centrifuge to replace the Celltrifuge with its rotary seal. The company first tried to adapt a device reported by Adams,[27] which can avoid twisting the tube leading from a rotating platform. In this design, the tube starts upwards from the center of the platform, gradually arches toward the periphery, and then makes a loop downward to reach the bottom of the rotary device. This orientation, however, is not easily adaptable to the flow-through centrifuge. About this time, I was developing a series of rotary-seal-free coil planet centrifuge schemes[28] for performing countercurrent chromatography at the Laboratory of Technical Development. Modification of one of these centrifuge schemes led to construction of the first prototype of the seal-free continuous flow centrifuge, and this was successfully applied to long-term plasmapheresis of sheep without the aforementioned complications.

The mechanisms of several flow-through centrifuge schemes free of rotary seals are diagrammatically illustrated in Fig 1-6.[28] Each diagram indicates the orientation and motion of the cylindrical coil holder with a bundle of flow tubes tightly supported at the stationary point (marked by a black circle on the central axis). These schemes are divided into planetary and nonplanetary, as indicated at the top of the diagram. In the planetary series, rotation and revolution of the holder are synchronized in such a way that one revolution (around the central axis of the apparatus) gives exactly one rotation (around its own axis) of the holder. In the nonplanetary series, rotation and revolution share a common axis, resulting in either no rotation or a single rotation around the central axis of the apparatus, as in the conventional system.

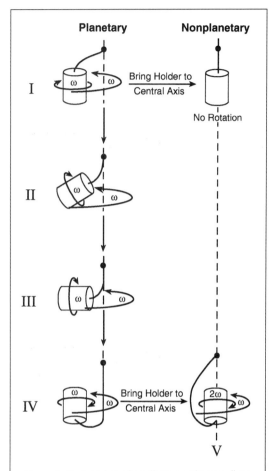

Figure 1-6. A series of sealless continuous flow centrifuge schemes developed for performing countercurrent chromatography. (Used with permission from Ito.[28])

Scheme I in the planetary series has an upright holder, which counterrotates about its own axis while revolving around the central axis of the centrifuge. This counterrotation of the holder automatically unwinds the twist of the flow tubes during each revolution, thus eliminating the need for the rotary seal. The resulting circular motion of the holder is as simple as, and equivalent to, that of a beaker when a chemist mixes its contents with his hand. This seal-free mechanism works equally well in tilted (Scheme II), horizontal (Scheme III), and even inverted (Scheme IV) orientations of the holder. In the inverted scheme, the holder undergoes a synchronous planetary motion in which its revolution and rotation are both in the same direction and at the same angular velocity, ω

If the holder of Scheme I is shifted to the centrifuge axis, it becomes stationary because its synchronous counterrotation cancels out the revolution effect (nonplanetary, top). However, if this same procedure is applied to the holder of Scheme IV, the holder is transformed into an ideal seal-free centrifuge system (nonplanetary, bottom, Scheme V). Because the rotation and revolution of the holder are in the same direction, as described above, this transposition of the holder results in summation of the rates of rotation and revolution. Consequently, the holder rotates at the doubled speed of 2ω around the central axis. This shift also causes relocation of the flow tubes from the central axis toward the periphery, where they revolve around the central axis at an angular velocity, ω as indicated in the diagram. It should be noted here that, in retrospect, the present system is equivalent to the device reported by Wrench,[29] and also to the inverted Adams device.[27]

The first prototype of the seal-free continuous flow centrifuge is illustrated in Fig 1-7, which shows the orientation and motion of the centrifuge bowl and the flow tubes (A)[30] essential for avoiding twisting as described above, and the centrifuge designs (B and C)[30,31] that meet all these requirements. The original sketch for the design of the seal-free centrifuge (B) was made in October 1973, as indicated, but it was improved in the first prototype centrifuge (C), which was fabricated at our machine shop sometime during 1974 when requested by Dr. Suaudeau and Theodore Kolobow, MD, of our laboratory's Pulmonary and Cardiac Assist Devices Section.

In the first prototype, shown in Fig 1-7(C), the frame of the centrifuge body consists of three horizontal plates that hold three rotary structures: the centrifuge bowl, the countershaft (right), and the tube-supporting hollow shaft (left). The coupling of the lower pulley of the countershaft to the stationary pulley on the motor housing causes the countershaft to counterrotate with respect to the rotating frame.

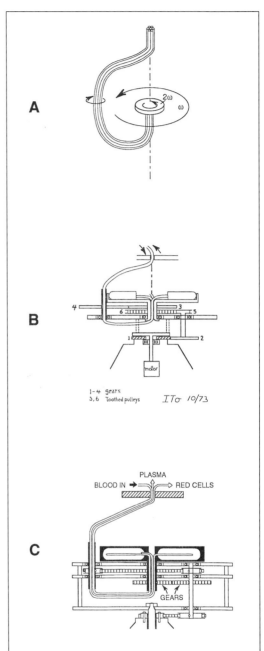

Figure 1-7. The principle and designs of sealless continuous flow centrifuge: (A) motions of centrifuge bowl and flow tubes required for the sealless continuous flow centrifuge system; (B) the original sketch for the sealless continuous flow centrifuge; and (C) the improved design for the first prototype of the sealless continuous flow centrifuge. [(A) and (C) used with permission from Ito et al.[30]]

This motion is then conveyed to the central bowl by 1:1 gearing to double the angular velocity of the bowl. The motion of the countershaft is also transferred to the tube-supporting hollow shaft by means of the 1:1 ratio pulley coupling. Thus, the system satisfies all the requirements indicated in Fig 1-7(A).

This first prototype seal-free centrifuge was successfully applied to long-term plasmapheresis by Suaudeau et al.[26] The performance of our prototype with a ringshaped chamber made of blood-compatible silicon rubber sheet was compared with that of the Celltrifuge. The results are indicated in Fig 1-8,[26] in which sheep platelet count (percentage of the initial count) during plasmapheresis is plotted against time (hours) using the Celltrifuge (A) and our seal-free continuous flow centrifuge (B). With

the Celltrifuge device, the blood platelet count steadily fell and finally reached 40% of the original level after 23 hours of plasmapheresis. When a similar study was performed with our seal-free continuous flow centrifuge, the platelet count showed no change during the same period.[26]

This severe platelet loss observed in the Celltrifuge system may be partly attributed to various thrombogenic surfaces in the system, including polycarbonate, Teflon, ceramic, stainless steel, polyvinyl chloride, and conventional silicone rubber, whereas in our prototype, blood fractions contact only silica-free silicon rubber known to be hypothrombogenic.[32] However, other systems using these thrombogenic materials do not appear to suffer from this problem. Therefore, we consider that the

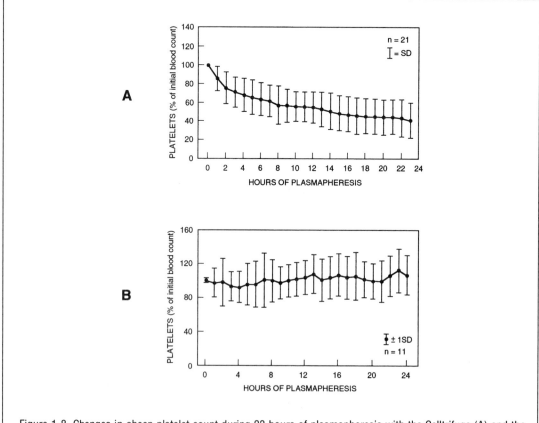

Figure 1-8. Changes in sheep platelet count during 23 hours of plasmapheresis with the Celltrifuge (A) and the Ito flow-through centrifuge (B). (Used with permission from Suaudeau et al.[26])

absence of a rotary seal in our system prevented platelet deterioration in long-term plasmapheresis.

Aminco Celltrifuge II and Fenwal CS3000

Herbert M. Cullis, President, American Fluoroseal Corporation, Gaithersburg, Maryland

Aminco began marketing the original Celltrifuge (I) in 1969. IBM had ceased marketing the NCI-IBM (2990) centrifuge the year before, and the Celltrifuge was then the only apheresis device marketed. The Baxter-Travenol Corporation bought Aminco in 1970.

Sealless Blood Processor

The concept for the sealless blood-processing centrifuge that was eventually used in the CS3000 and the Celltrifuge II began in January 1973 when I read an article by Dale Adams describing a nonrotating electrical connection technique. It occurred to me that the Adams technique could be applied to blood centrifuges to eliminate the troublesome rotating seal. I intended to apply the Adams principle to the Fenwal Elutramatic blood washer and the Aminco Celltrifuge. I called this the "jump rope" technique.

During early 1973, I discussed this concept and the potential advantages of a closed system with directors of the Aminco and Fenwal divisions of Baxter. A model of the mechanism was constructed to illustrate the concept (Fig 1-9) and a written proposal was submitted to the Fenwal Division on September 27, 1973. Fenwal approved and funded the jump rope centrifuge on November 29, 1973. The first centrifugation with a sealless centrifuge (Fig 1-10) was demonstrated on May 10, 1974. Aminco pursued both sealless blood washers and sealless blood separators in parallel. By 1976, both washers and separators were under laboratory testing. The blood washer project was dropped but the blood separator project continued and the jump rope principle was

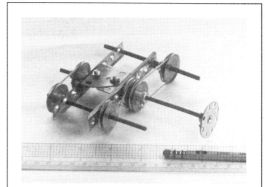

Figure 1-9. Erector set model of sealless centrifuge mechanism.

applied to both the Celltrifuge II and the CS3000. These were the first sealless apheresis devices to be sold.

Celltrifuge II

The Celltrifuge II used the sealless jump rope principle with a disposable bowl that had the same general operating characteristics and appearance as the reusable bowl of the IBM 2990 and the Celltrifuge. One of the accomplishments in designing the Celltrifuge II was the development of a disposable bowl that could be manufactured economically and would maintain the close mechanical tolerances required for the bowl to separate blood

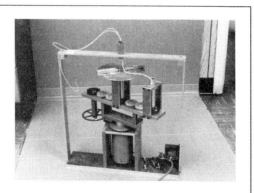

Figure 1-10. Jump rope demonstration centrifuge.

efficiently. In addition to the sealless connection and disposable blood path, the Celltrifuge II included an optical sensor for monitoring the collected product and automatically adjusting the pump speeds to maintain efficient separation without constant operator attention. The optical control system minimized operator attention, but the system required aseptic connections at the time of use, and the Celltrifuge II did not become a fully closed system. It was sold until the early 1980s.

CS3000

While the Celltrifuge collected blood components effectively, it required a skilled operator for high-efficiency separations. Under Fenwal funding, I continued to develop a machine that did not depend on the skill of the operator. Microprocessor chips were becoming available that could relieve the operator from making the tedious decisions of controlling the machine. These 8080 microprocessors directed routines to prime and test the tubing and mechanical parts of the machine before each apheresis. The microprocessor also responded to signals from an optical monitor to direct the separation with great efficiency. These microprocessors proved to be very reliable.

The blood separation development produced two different separation techniques. I first developed a flexible multistage belt separation chamber in which separation occurred in an annular channel. Aspects of this multistage belt design are incorporated in the Fenwal Amicus blood separator that was introduced in the 1990s. But in 1976, this belt proved difficult to manufacture in a plant that was devoted to manufacturing bags. So many belts leaked in early testing that I was encouraged to use conventional blood bags as the separation chambers.

In 1976, the two-bag separation system of the CS3000 that has remained in use for more than 25 years was developed. The CS3000 employs two bags and replaceable bag holders to form centrifuge chambers. The bags have specific shapes imposed on them by the rigid bag holders. Whole blood enters the first bag chamber for separation of component-rich plasma from red cells. The plasma and the components in it are passed through an optical monitor and directed to the second bag chamber. Components are collected in the second chamber and the remainder joins the red cells to return to the donor. The system has a constant volume. The pump flow rates—and, thereby, the component collection—are controlled by the microprocessor in response to the optical monitor. The combination of replaceable bag holders to give different types of separation and the programmability of the microprocessor chips has permitted the CS3000 to be adapted for granulocyte, lymphocyte, and peripheral blood progenitor cell collections as well as for the production of platelet concentrates with reduced leukocyte content.

When introduced in 1979, the CS3000 was the first sealless, computer-controlled centrifuge. Its automation reduced operator training time and its fully closed system of tubing and solutions extended storage time for apheresis products from 24 hours to many days. At this writing, this machine is still in worldwide use.

IBM 2997/COBE Spectra

Robert M. Kellogg, PhD, Abingdon, Maryland

IBM 2997

In 1973, our group at the IBM Development Laboratory in Endicott, NY, began design work on a second-generation continuous flow blood cell separator. We felt we had learned much from almost 10 years' experience with the 2990 and its forerunners. For example, we were painfully aware that the entire blood path needed to be disposable. In addition, the centrifuge bowl was an axial flow separator; that is, blood flowed parallel to the axis of rotation during separation, with the separated elements accumulating at the top of the bowl where they were extracted continuously. This configuration had (at least) two perceived limitations. First, it had a very large interfacial area upon which the buffy coat formed. This resulted in thin buffy coats that were difficult to extract. Some operators could position the cell layers appropriately, but others apparently could not. Second, it was geometrically complicated and not well suited for disposability. With this background we quickly established these goals for our redesign efforts: 1) a completely disposable blood path, including the rotating seal; 2) reduced operator involvement in the collection of the separated elements; 3) improved separation efficiency to decrease run times; and 4) improved safety monitoring.

After considerable thought and analysis, we decided that a circumferential flow geometry would address the limitations identified for the axial flow bowl. In this configuration, blood flow during separation would be around the axis of rotation, either with or against it (or in both directions, for that matter). In fact, the circumferential geometry seemed to offer almost complete flexibility in channel design; for example, multistage, multiwrap configurations were possible.[33]

Next came implementation. Our group had recently finished development of the 2991 Blood Cell Processor, a batch washer using a bag laminated from flat stock as the processing chamber. It seemed natural to consider this approach first. Scaling studies[34] were performed to guide fabrication of a "floppy bag" (Fig 1-11), into which was laminated a channel that looked much like a cross section of the

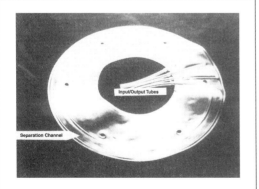

Figure 1-11. IBM "floppy bag" centrifuge fluid container. See text for structural and operational details.

channel in the 2990 bowl, which had been wrapped in an arc around the center of rotation. Preliminary evaluation of this structure indicated that acceptable plasma separation could be attained with it. Differential cell separation, however, was abysmal, or at least impractical, in that acceptable results could be obtained only at whole blood flow rates of less than 10 mL per minute. These experiences led us to select a rectangular cross-section channel having a height (parallel to the axis of rotation) much greater than its radial width. We further decided on a two-stage channel for the preparation of platelet concentrates, which would replicate the manual technique by first producing platelet-rich plasma and then concentrating platelets from it. All other procedures would be performed in a single-stage channel.

We next considered how to automate the cell collection process—that is, how to automatically position the red cell interface at some predetermined radial location within the channel. Note that we were not attempting to automate the entire apheresis process, only the collection step. Several optical approaches were examined and discarded as being too expensive, too complicated, or too unreliable. For example, an optical system that monitors the collection tube is not activated until the tube contains unwanted material, which must be cleared before collection can resume. This further complicates both tubing set fabrication and system operation. These considerations suggested that an ideal control scheme should operate directly on the interface and would most likely be based on the behavior of the separated components in a centrifugal field. This realization, together with the observation that the red cell interface is circular (ie, it has the same radial location everywhere), led us to the "autoport" method of interface control for the single-stage channel, which is described in detail below. Unfortunately, we were frustrated in all attempts to apply this method to the collection of two-stage platelets. Their collection remained under the direct control of the operator, albeit at a less demanding level: now the operator would be required only to maintain the red cell/plasma interface within the first stage and not to position platelets precisely at a collection port.

The final challenge in attaining a completely disposable blood path was the rotating seal. This complicated structure appeared, at first, to be just too expensive to discard after only one use. However, after much brainstorming and consultation, we arrived at a design that used relatively inexpensive molded parts to achieve the required complexity. One machining step was required to finish the ceramic seal faces to optical flatness. This machining and the final assembly were the only "hands-on" processes in seal fabrication, and they resulted in costs low enough for disposability. To this day, though, we all feel that throwing a seal away is like dropping a diamond down the drain.

With the preliminaries behind us, we were ready to start clinical evaluation of the 2997 concepts in late 1975. We asked Emil Freireich, MD, whether the University of Texas M. D. Anderson Cancer Center would be interested in doing the evaluations. We were doubly fortunate: his reply was yes, and his colleague Dr. Hester agreed to directly supervise and, more often than not, perform the evaluations. We had modified a 2990 to accept the much larger diameter centrifuge bowl required by the circumferential flow channels. This approach was taken so that differences, if any, could be attributed directly to the new channels and seals, and not to changes in the rest of the system. We experienced no anomalies during initial evaluations, so the modified 2990 was replaced by a prototype 2997, and system characterization began in earnest.

Single-Stage Channel

The single-stage channel that resulted from this intense collaborative effort is shown in Fig 1-12, together with a detail of the collection chamber. The channel has a rectangular cross-section with an aspect ratio (height to width) of about 5. It is formed into a loop whose circumference exceeds 20 inches; however, blood cannot flow around its entire periphery because the inlet and collection regions are not connected. Whole blood enters the channel

through a single port and is separated by centrifugal force as it flows once around the channel and into the collection chamber. Therein, the separated flow encounters a partial (in radial extent) barrier, which forces plasma to flow around its radially innermost side while red cells flow around its outermost side. Circumferential flow at the interface stagnates against the barrier, forcing buffy coat to accumulate there while a plasma/red cell interface that is free of buffy coat forms behind (downstream from) the barrier.

Extraction ports are positioned in the collection chamber as follows: Buffy coat is collected through a port located adjacent to the upstream side of the barrier, near the center (both radially and top to bottom) of the rectangular separation channel. The autoport has essentially the same location relative to the channel walls but is on the downstream side of the barrier. Initially, we supposed that these two ports would suffice, in the following manner: As whole blood entered the chamber, saline and then plasma would be withdrawn from the autoport as red cells accumulated in the channel. When the interface reached the radial position of the autoport, both red cells and plasma should automatically be withdrawn at rates appropriate for the donor's hematocrit and the interface should stabilize at the ideal position within the collection chamber. If the interface moved (radially) inward, more red cells than plasma would be removed, forcing the interface outward; conversely, if the interface moved outward, more plasma would be removed, bringing the interface inward. Because, as was noted earlier, the red cell/plasma interface attains the same radial location throughout the entire channel, it would then be "automatically" positioned at the buffy coat collection port on the upstream side of the barrier.

In trials, a single-stage channel of this design did function as described early in a procedure; as the run progressed, however, the upstream interface was found to drift radially inward with respect to the downstream interface. This behavior was traced to uneven red cell packing; that is, red cells in the upstream part of the chamber were packed slightly less than those

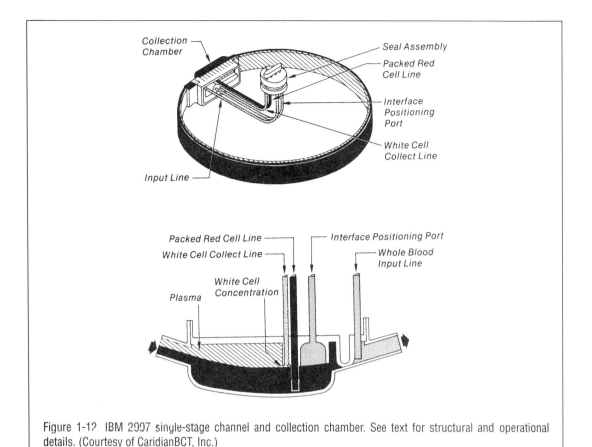

Figure 1-12. IBM 2997 single-stage channel and collection chamber. See text for structural and operational details. (Courtesy of CaridianBCT, Inc.)

downstream. This was ultimately controlled by adding a third collection port, which extended almost to the outer wall downstream from the barrier, to extract the most densely packed red cells. This minimized the radial offset of the interfaces, making it much easier to attain stable interface positioning and buffy coat collection. Operating conditions and collection performance of the single-stage channel have been published.[35,36]

Dual-Stage Channel

The problems we encountered in the design and evaluation of the single-stage channel paled in comparison to those confronting us for the dual-stage channel. Previously, the continuous flow collection of platelets had involved their extraction off the top of a buffy coat, where they were surrounded by other blood cells. We now proposed to continuously separate, concentrate, and collect platelets from a plastic surface. The two-step manual procedure suggested that it would be possible to continuously prepare a platelet concentrate if we were willing to accumulate (ie, "plaster") platelets against a surface in a portion of the separation channel. However, this would have required a final manual resuspension step, which we hoped to avoid, along with the detrimental effects that mechanical agitation and prolonged exposure to high *g*'s might entail.

Although our direction was determined, we still encountered both mechanical and physiological problems. One problem that proved to be the most challenging spanned both areas: the determination of the optimal slope for the outer wall of the second stage. Our concept required that separated platelets be able to "slide" down this wall into a collection well.

Much trial and error on our part (ie, the "channel of the month" phase), along with Herculean efforts by Dr. Hester and her staff, resulted in a design and procedure that allowed continuous collection of platelets at concentrations of several million per microliter. This breakthrough depended on precise acidification of the processed blood, so that platelet activation and aggregation were temporarily blocked and platelet function was maintained while total anticoagulant dose was limited to minimize donor side effects.

The resulting dual-stage channel is shown in Fig 1-13. The first (semicircular) stage produces platelet-rich plasma by separating and removing red and white cells. The second region has an increasing radius and terminates in a well; it separates and collects both cell-free plasma and concentrated platelets. The geometric center of the first stage is offset slightly from the axis of rotation. As a result, red and white cells packed against the outer wall beyond the red cell removal port experience a centrifugal impetus to flow back "upstream" to it. This "bidirectional flow," plus a sharp decrease in radius at the transition between the two stages, impedes red/white cell entry into the second stage. The bidirectional flow approach was taken in this design to simplify manufacturing, as all ports could then be located in only two molded parts. However, the concept had far-reaching implications, allowing truly significant improvement in a later dual-stage design, as discussed further on. Operating conditions and collection performance of the dual-stage channel have been published.[37]

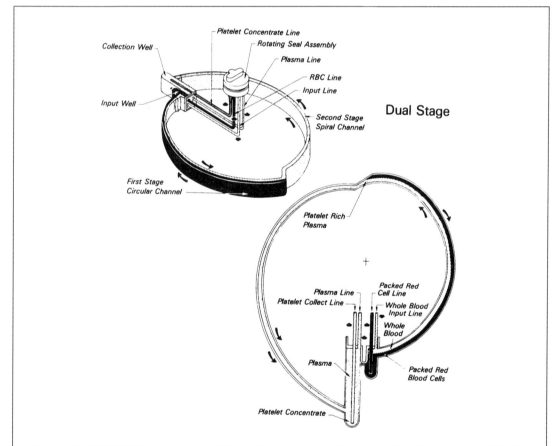

Figure 1-13. IBM 2997 dual-stage channel. See text for structural and operational details. (Courtesy of Caridian-BCT, Inc.)

The 2997 became available in 1977, first with only the single-stage channel and then, several months later, with the dual-stage channel. It found broad use as the field of apheresis matured.

COBE Spectra

In 1982, the growing demand for extended life, single-donor platelets prompted our group to begin work on a third-generation instrument to replace the 2997. For this effort our goals were to 1) replace the rotating seals with sealless technology, 2) automate the collection phase of dual-stage platelets, and 3) fully automate the entire apheresis procedure using control and yield predictive algorithms. In 1984, IBM withdrew from the biomedical market and sold its interests in the blood-processing area to COBE Laboratories. At that point, our group had successfully implemented sealless technology using a bearing-guided loop that greatly reduced loop strain and heating. Work on process automation had started, but much remained to be done there as well as with overall machine design and layout.

Dual-Stage Channel

Our most significant accomplishment, however, had been to finally automate the collection of dual-stage platelets. In a flash of brilliance, Alfred P. Mulzet, PhD, of our group came up with the idea of using a modification of the autoport concept along with bidirectional cell flow in the first stage. He connected the end of the second stage, which contains cell-free plasma, to the first stage. Because this creates a continuous fluid path around the entire channel, the inner wall must be moved radially inward at the point of interconnection to keep plasma from flowing back into the first stage. In effect, this change in radius acts like a partial barrier, but this time allows only red and white cells to flow around it. The first stage remains essentially circular, with its center still displaced from the axis of rotation, but now platelet-rich plasma flows out of one end into the second stage while red and white cells flow toward the

other end for removal from the channel. The whole blood inlet was moved to a more central location in the first stage so as not to interfere with the exiting flows at each end. The second stage was also modified with the collection well moved nearer the point where platelet-rich plasma exits the first stage. This has the effect of producing a bidirectional flow of platelets in the second stage and decreases the distance they must slide along the walls. Concentrated platelets are removed from the well as before; most of the cell-free plasma is removed through a port located opposite the first stage, which is considered to be the end of the second stage, although the channel is continuous as described.

Red and white cells and the remaining plasma are removed through two ports, located on the plasma side of the radial barrier, which are joined external to the channel. In addition to component removal, the radial positions of these coacting ports provide stable interface positioning with resultant automatic channel operation. This is accomplished with the use of tubes that differ significantly in diameter. The larger tube, which removes the bulk of the red and white cell flow, reaches almost to the outer wall. The smaller, "control" tube ends at the desired radial location of the interface. Because these tubes join together, their combined flow is constant, set by the controlling pump rates. When the rate of plasma removal is slightly less than its incoming flow rate, the interface moves radially outward and eventually the control port is in the plasma layer. When this happens, flow through the control port increases because plasma is much less viscous than packed cells. This increasing plasma flow and (because combined flow is constant) consequent decreased cell flow through the large port force the interface inward until a stable position is obtained over the entire first stage. This improved dual-stage channel is shown in Fig 1-14.

Other Spectra Innovations

In 1987, COBE announced the Spectra, which incorporated our accomplishments together with a large body of COBE's own innovations. This device is fully automated by means of con-

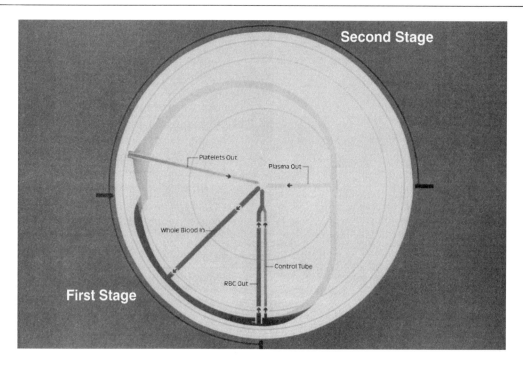

Figure 1-14. COBE Spectra dual-stage channel. See text for structural and operational details. (Courtesy of CaridianBCT Inc.)

trolling algorithms for all the most common procedures. In addition to the dual-stage channel described above, it can use improved single-stage channels tailored for collection, depletion, or exchange procedures. Improvements include simplified porting for exchange channels and a totally new collection chamber for white cells. The latter uses the control port concept for interface positioning and is significantly smaller in size, thereby minimizing red cell packing effects and channel volume. Operation and performance of the Spectra have also been published.[38,39]

Membrane Plasma Separation

Frank Corbin, Director, Research and Development, COBE (Gambro) BCT, Lakewood, Colorado

During the 1960s and 1970s, COBE Laboratories had become an established supplier of extracorporeal systems for hemodialysis and cardiopulmonary bypass. In the 1970s, therapeutic plasma exchange (TPE) was being evaluated for the treatment of a wide range of immunologically mediated diseases but, compared with hemodialysis, was relatively difficult to accomplish with existing equipment. We reasoned that TPE could become more widely practiced if there were an instrument that allowed it to be performed as easily as a hemodialysis procedure. We had considerable expertise in making flat membrane dialysers, and the availability of hollow fiber membranes with appropriate pore size was limited at that time. COBE therefore began development of a flat membrane plasma separation system, which would eventually be known as the Centry TPE system.

Membrane devices for plasma separation offer several potential advantages. They do not need rotating seals or "one-omega/two-omega" loops to get blood in and out of a rotating centrifuge chamber in a sterile fashion; they require a relatively simple monitor/control system; they are smaller and more transportable than most centrifuges; and they produce cell-free plasma. Early attempts to use membrane separators were plagued by problems such as hemolysis, lower than expected plasma removal rates, and significant performance degradation over time. The following paragraphs describe some of the key principles that were found to apply to the separation of plasma using mem-

branes and the ways in which these principles were applied to development of the Centry TPE.

The first objective of membrane plasma separation is to select a membrane that is biocompatible and has a pore size that will allow the passage of all plasma constituents, including electrolytes, albumin, fibrinogen, immunoglobulins, and immune complexes, while retaining red cells, white cells, and platelets. The performance of a membrane with respect to any

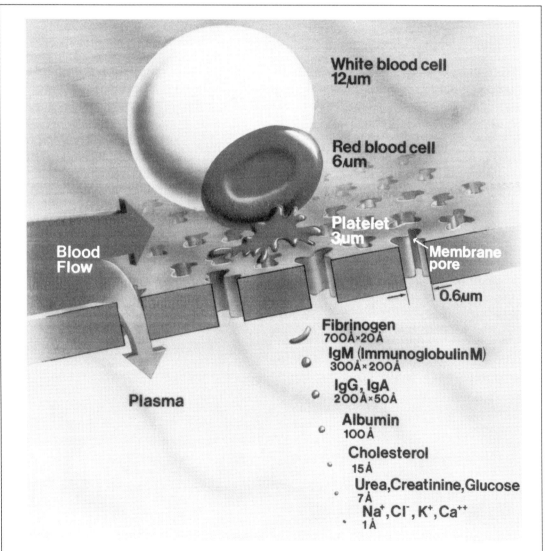

Figure 1-15. Comparative sizes of blood components. Note the large size difference between the largest plasma constituent and the smallest cellular elements. (Courtesy of CaridianBCT, Inc.)

plasma constituent can be measured and expressed as the Sieving Coefficient (SC): SC = Cf/Ci, where Cf is the concentration of the constituent of interest in the filtrate and Ci is its concentration in the inlet blood.[40] Membranes having pore sizes in the range of 0.1 to 0.6 μ are typical and achieve SCs of greater than 0.95 for all the constituents of plasma while retaining virtually all cellular components.[41] Figure 1-15 depicts the relative sizes of key blood constituents.

After an appropriate membrane is selected, the next objective is to put it into a geometry that will provide appropriate flow conditions for the blood. An important aspect of this effort is to ensure that the shear rate of the blood is sufficiently high to keep cellular components from being drawn to the surface of the membrane as plasma leaves the blood channel

through it. If cellular components become coated onto the membrane, they block the pores, thereby causing unfavorable changes in SCs and plasma flux. Three basic geometries have appeared in workable membrane devices. In hollow fiber geometries, cellular coating is prevented by selecting the appropriate combination of fiber diameter, fiber length, and fiber count for the desired range of blood flow rates. Thus, different filter configurations are required for different blood flow rate ranges. A second basic geometry is one that uses a drum-shaped membrane rotating inside a cylinder to provide the requisite blood shear rate. It was G. Delbert Antwiler at COBE who recognized that the third basic geometry, a flat membrane, could be adapted to control blood shear rate by adjusting the thickness of the blood channels as the blood flow rate changed. At low blood flow

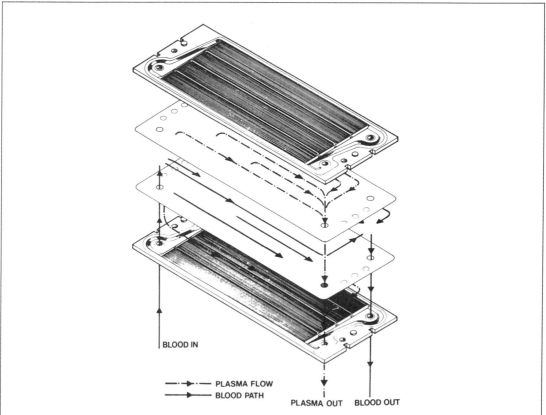

BLOOD IN

– ▶ · – PLASMA FLOW
——▶—— BLOOD PATH

PLASMA OUT   BLOOD OUT

Figure 1-16. Flat plate membrane plasma separator with adjustable thickness blood channel as used in the COBE Centry TPE system. See text for structural and operational details. (Courtesy of CaridianBCT, Inc.)

rates an automatic clamp squeezes on the separator, causing the blood channels to become thinner. At high blood flow rates the clamp relaxes, allowing the channels to become thicker. This results in control of the shear rate within appropriate ranges. Figure 1-16 shows a single layer of the separator and its fluid flow paths. The complete device comprised a stack of six such layers.

To ensure safe and effective performance, the device managing a membrane plasma separator must control several important operating parameters in addition to those routinely required for extracorporeal blood circulation. The first parameter is transmembrane pressure, which is the difference in pressure between the blood and the filtrate sides of the membrane. This difference should typically be less than 50 mm Hg to avoid lysis of red cells that contact the membrane surface, as well as to avoid plugging of membrane pores, with a resultant decrease in SCs.[42] The second parameter is the hematocrit in the red cell fraction. As blood proceeds along the length of a plasma filter, plasma is continuously lost and the hematocrit therefore rises. The removal of plasma should be limited such that a certain critical hematocrit is not exceeded while blood is in the filter. This prevents excessive deposition of cells on the membrane and the resultant degradation of performance; it also avoids the effects of excessive whole blood viscosity associated with a high hematocrit. Finally, it is important for membrane separators to be primed and operated conservatively early in a run to allow a protein layer to be laid down on the membrane without excessive cell layering. This protein layer can also help to reduce subsequent cellular damage.

Along with these principles of membrane plasma separation, the Centry TPE system incorporated the features of automated replacement fluid balance and integral replacement fluid warming. The system was introduced in the US market in 1982 as the first membrane plasma exchange system to receive the approval of the Food and Drug Administration. However, while the Centry TPE was a very real technical achievement and gained significant market share, the therapy did not prove to be effective in high-incidence diseases. As a result, marketing of the system was discontinued in 1995.

Conclusion

Almost 60 years have passed since Cohn envisioned biomechanical equipment for the immediate separation of blood components, a vision that gradually evolved into the concept of apheresis. The advances in instrumentation described in this chapter were essential prerequisites for this evolution, but were also responses to needs perceived by medical personnel using earlier devices. The interaction between clinic and machine shop—between physicians and instrument operators on the one hand, and inventors and engineers on the other—is a recurring theme in the ensuing essays. The following chapter covers the early history of the use of apheresis instruments, both to collect blood components from donors and to manipulate patient blood for therapeutic purposes. The remainder of the book then describes the state of the art as apheresis enters the seventh decade since its inception. Surely the early workers in this field would be gratified to know that an entire textbook can be devoted to the ramifications of their original ideas. Dr. Cohn, in particular, would surely be pleased to learn that some of the most recent developments in donor apheresis, described in Chapter 6, represent a return to his original vision of on-line donation of multiple blood components.

References

1. De Laval CGP, Inventor. US Patent 247,804. 1881.
2. Hsu H-W. Separations by centrifugal phenomena. Vol XVI. In: Perry ES, ed. Techniques of Chemistry. New York: John Wiley & Sons, 1981:1-7.
3. Cohn EJ, Tullis JL, Surgenor DM, et al. Biochemistry and biomechanics of blood collection, processing and analysis. Abstract of paper

presented at the National Academy of Sciences, New Haven, CT, November 5-7, 1951. Science 1951;114:479.

4. Tullis JL. Newer techniques for the separation and fractionation of whole blood. N Y State J Med 1953;53:525-7.

5. Surgenor DM. Blood. The red fluid of the human body is a rich mixture of cells and molecules. New methods of fractionation and preserving these many constituents increase their usefulness to medicine. Sci Am 1954;190:54-62.

6. Tullis JL, Surgenor DM, Tinch RJ, et al. New principle of closed system centrifugation. Science 1956;124:792-7.

7. Haynes LL, Tullis JL, Pyle HM, et al. Clinical use of glycerolized frozen blood. JAMA 1960; 173:1657-63.

8. Cohn EJ. Blood collection and preservation. Proceedings, Fourth Annual Meeting, American Association of Blood Banks, October 22, 1951, Minneapolis, MN.

9. Tullis JL, Rochows EE. Non-wettable surfaces. Blood 1952;7:850-5.

10. Cohn EJ, Surgenor DM, Schmid K, et al. Development of metal protein complexes, metal buffer, specific ion exchange resins and biomechanical equipment. Abstract presented at the second International Biochemical Congress, Paris, July 21-27, 1952.

11. Tullis JL. Principles involved in glycerolization and deglycerolization of red cells using the Cohn fractionator. Proceedings of a Conference on Plasma Proteins and Cellular Elements of the Blood, November 15, 1954. Cambridge, MA: Protein Foundation, Inc. and the Commission on Plasma Fractionation and Related Processes, 1954:17-8.

12. Driscoll S. Use of Cohn fractionator in connection with the preservation of red cells in glycerol. Proceedings of a Conference on Plasma Proteins and Cellular Elements of the Blood, November 15, 1954. Cambridge, MA: Protein Foundation, Inc. and the Commission on Plasma Fractionation and Related Processes, 1954:19-21.

13. Ketchel MM, Tinch RJ. Use of Cohn fractionator in connection with the preservation of red cells in glycerol. Proceedings of a Conference on Plasma Proteins and Cellular Elements of the Blood, November 15, 1954. Cambridge, MA: Protein Foundation, Inc. and the Commission on Plasma Fractionation and Related Processes, 1954:22-4.

14. Tullis JL. Use of Cohn fractionator in connection with the preservation of red cells in glycerol. Proceedings of a Conference on Plasma Proteins and Cellular Elements of the Blood, November 15, 1954. Cambridge, MA: Protein Foundation, Inc. and the Commission on Plasma Fractionation and Related Processes, 1954:25-6.

15. Tullis JL, Tinch RJ, Baudanza P, et al. Plateletpheresis in a disposable system. Transfusion 1971;11:368-77.

16. Freireich EJ, Schmidt PJ, Schneiderman MA, Frei E III. A comparative study of the effect of transfusion of fresh and preserved whole blood on bleeding in patients with acute leukemia. N Engl J Med 1959;260:6-11.

17. Kliman A, Gaydos LA, Schroeder LR, Freireich EJ. Repeated plasmapheresis of blood donors as a source of platelets. Blood 1961;18:303-9.

18. Freireich EJ, Kliman A, Gaydos LA, et al. Response to repeated platelet transfusions from the same donor. Ann Intern Med 1963; 59:277-87.

19. Freireich EJ, Levin RH, Whang J, et al. The function and fate of transfused leukocytes from donors with chronic myelocytic leukemia in leukopenic recipients. Ann N Y Acad Sci 1964; 113:1081-9.

20. Freireich EJ, Judson G, Levin RH. Separation and collection of leukocytes. Cancer Res 1965; 25:1516-20.

21. Judson G, Jones A, Kellogg R, et al. Closed continuous-flow centrifuge. Nature 1968;217: 816-8.

22. Jones AL. The IBM blood cell separator and blood cell processor: A personal perspective. J Clin Apheresis 1988;4:171-82.

23. Curtis JE, Hersh EM, Freireich EJ. Antigen specific immunity in recipients with leukocyte transfusions from immune donors. Cancer Res 1970;30:2921-9.

24. McCredie KB, Freireich EJ, Hester JP, Vallejos C. Increased granulocyte collection with the blood cell separator and the addition of etiocholanolone and hydroxyethyl starch. Transfusion 1974;14:357-64.

25. McCredie KB, Hersh EM, Freireich EJ. Cells capable of colony formation in the peripheral blood of man. Science 1971;171:293-4.

26. Suaudeau J, Kolobow T, Vaillancourt R, et al. The Ito "flow-through" centrifuge: A new device for long-term (24 hours) plasmapheresis without platelet deterioration. Transfusion 1978;18:312-9.

27. Adams DA, Inventor. Apparatus for providing energy communication between a moving and a stationary terminal. US Patent 3,586,413, June 22, 1971.

28. Ito Y. Countercurrent chromatography (mini-review). J Biochem Biophys Methods 1981;5: 105-29.

29. Wrench EH, Inventor. Coupling. US Patent 3,358,072, December 12, 1967.

30. Ito Y, Suaudeau J, Bowman RL. New flow-through centrifuge without rotating seals applied to plasmapheresis. Science 1975; 189:999-1000.

31. Ito Y, Inventor. Flow-through centrifuge free of rotating seals particularly for plasmapheresis. U.S. Patent 4,425,112, January 10, 1984. (The patent application was filed on February 25, 1976 based on the publication of Ito et al,[30] but its issuance was delayed because of the patent interference lawsuit between the US government and Aminco, which lasted for 8 years.)

32. Kolobow T, Stool EW, Weathersby PK, et al. Superior blood compatibility of silicone rubber free of silica filler in the membrane lung. Trans Am Soc Artif Intern Organs 1974;20A:269.

33. Kellogg RM, Kruger VR, Inventors. Centrifuge fluid container. US Patent 4,010,894 and US Patent 4,007,871, 1977.

34. Hester JP, Kellogg RM, Mulzet AP, et al. Principles of continuous flow cell separation in a circumferential flow disposable channel. In: Catsimpooolas N, ed. Biological separations. Methods of cell separation. Vol 3. New York: Plenum Press, 1980:101-13.

35. Hester JP, Kellogg RM, Mulzet AP, et al. Principles of blood separation and component extraction in a disposable continuous-flow single-stage channel. Blood 1979;54:254-67.

36. Hester JP, Kellogg RM, Freireich EJ. Mononuclear cell (MNC) collection by continuous-flow centrifugation (CFC). J Clin Apheresis 1983;1:197-201.

37. Hester JP, Kellogg RM, Mulzet AP, et al. Continuous-flow techniques for platelet concentrate collection: A step toward standardization and yield predictability. J Clin Apheresis 1985;2:224-30.

38. Hester JP, Ventura GH, Boucher T. Platelet concentrate collection in a dual-stage channel using computer-generated algorithms for collection and prediction of yield. Plasma Ther Transfus Technol 1987;8:377-85.

39. Hester JP, Ventura J. Mathematic modeling for apheresis procedures: Advantages and limitations. In: Sibinga CT, Das PC, Högman CF, eds. Automation in blood transfusion. Boston: Kluwer Academic Publishers, 1988:121-7.

40. Colton CK, Henderson LW, Ford CA, Lysaght MJ. Kinetics of hemodiafiltration, I: In vitro transport characteristics of a hollow fiber blood ultrafilter. J Lab Clin Med 1975;85:355-71.

41. Smith JW, Malchesky PS, Nose Y. Membrane plasmapheresis and the developing technology of plasma therapy. Cleve Clin Q 1984;51:135-42.

42. Malchesky PS, Sueoka A, Matsubara S, et al. Membrane plasma separation. In: Nose Y, Malchesky PS, Smith JW, Krakauer R, eds. Plasmapheresis: Therapeutic applications and new techniques. New York: Raven Press, 1983:81-92.

In: McLeod BC, Szczepiorkowski ZM, Weinstein R, Winters JL, eds.
Apheresis: Principles and Practice, 3rd edition
Bethesda, MD: AABB Press, 2010

2

Applications History

Edwin G. Taft, MD

APPLICATION OF APHERESIS technology to blood donors arose as part of a general movement toward blood component therapy, which in turn evolved from a wish to obtain a specific blood fraction to address a corresponding deficiency in intended recipients. Therapeutic apheresis arose from the perception that the ability to separate blood into its components rapidly and on line could permit reconfiguration of patient blood in ways that could favorably affect some disease processes. The generally accepted origin of the term "apheresis" is a 1914 paper by Abel, Rowntree, and Turner[1] in which the term "plasmaphaeresis" was applied to a procedure (performed in phlebotomized dogs) that separated the plasma from red cells and afterwards reinfused the latter. The return of red cells was observed to counteract the deleterious effects of bleeding. They suggested that "in the preparation of antitoxic sera, great economy might be effected in the use of horses" by substituting plasmapheresis for near exsanguination as the means to harvest antiserum, thereby preserving the horse for subsequent bleedings to harvest more antiserum. Greater economy in the use of horses was eventually achieved about 60 years later,[2] with the application of an early semiautomated blood cell separator to the harvesting of equine plasma.

Manual Plasmapheresis and Plateletpheresis

Plasma has been routinely separated from red cells from single units of whole blood as a donor product since the World War II era. The beginning of therapeutic apheresis is usually attributed to Skoog and Adams, who described manual plasmapheresis for Waldenström macroglobulinemia in a 1959 abstract.[3] There is, however, an earlier report[4] as well as a belated report[5] of therapeutic plasmapheresis occurring before 1959. Harvesting concentrates of plate-

Edwin G. Taft, MD, Clinical Associate Professor, Albany Medical College, Albany, New York
The author has disclosed no conflicts of interest.

lets from platelet-rich plasma obtained by manual plasmapheresis was described by Kliman et al,[6] beginning the trend toward use of apheresis platelets. Colman[7] was the first to use plateletpheresis therapeutically for platelet depletion in a patient with myeloproliferative thrombocytosis.

Donor Plasmapheresis and Plateletpheresis by Blood Cell Separator

All centrifugal apheresis instruments owe a technological debt to the continuous-flow cream separator invented in 1877 by deLaval. This includes the Cohn-ADL (for Arthur D. Little) fractionator that was the basic platform from which James L. Tullis[8-10] developed much of blood component preparation as we know it today. Allen "Jack" Latham established the Haemonetics family of apheresis instruments (Haemonetics Corp, Braintree, MA), inspired by the Cohn fractionator. The Haemonetics Model 10, in part conceived for deglycerolizing frozen red cells, was applied to harvest platelets for transfusion. It was succeeded by the Model 30, which was used mainly for plateletpheresis but was also adapted for collection of other blood components, including plasma and granulocytes. Later models, much smaller and more portable, are capable of rapidly harvesting 2 units of plasma or a double Red Blood Cell (RBC) unit from a single donor. The historical aspects of automated apheresis equipment are discussed in Chapter 1 and have also been described by Millward and Hoeltge.[11]

Pooled Platelets from Whole Blood vs Single-Donor Plateletpheresis

The availability of apheresis platelets raised the question of whether they were "better," in some meaningful way, than platelets derived from individual pints of whole blood. HLA matching for platelet transfusion to alloimmunized recipients was shown to be advantageous in 1969.[12] Collection by apheresis has a clear advantage in such cases because it produces a much larger platelet dose from a matched donor. Another issue concerns sensitization of recipients to donor HLA antigens. The question is whether a large "dose" of the limited number of HLA antigens in a "single-donor" preparation of apheresis platelets is more or less likely to immunize a recipient than the smaller "dose" of a larger number of HLA antigens present in a pool of platelet units derived from several donors. Several attempts to answer this question have been reported, but interpretation has been complicated by differences in methodology and yields, by patient differences (in responses to transfusion), and by nonmedical issues. Pooled platelet transfusions may contain the platelets from as few as 4 to as many as 10 units of whole blood; the customary dose may vary from region to region, as well as between hospitals in a single region, making multicenter comparisons difficult. An early study of equivalent doses of apheresis vs pooled platelets seemed to favor apheresis platelets; however, some of the pooled platelet transfusions were older (nearer their outdate) than the apheresis units, so the comparison was not entirely valid.[13]

A related question—whether selection of HLA-matched platelets early in a patient's course of transfusions could delay or prevent HLA-sensitization—remained unclear in 1980.[14] Dutcher et al[15] then observed that many recipients of multiple platelet transfusions never become alloimmunized, even with pooled-platelet transfusions, which implied that many patients had nothing to gain from the extra effort and expense required for preemptive HLA matching. Leukocyte reduction of platelet concentrates was later shown to lower the frequency and rapidity of alloimmunization by platelet transfusions.[16] By 1997 it was clear that leukocyte reduction techniques obviated any advantage of apheresis platelets in preventing alloimmunization.[17]

Further complicating comparisons of apheresis vs whole-blood-derived platelets were the increasing yields of the latter obtained with refinements in technique.[18] These came at the same time that the practice of "splitting" apheresis platelet collections into two or three transfusions, each of which carries a charge equivalent to or higher than a pooled platelet transfusion, became prevalent. This practice eliminates any platelet dose advantage for apheresis platelets, which may therefore not be considered as *cost*-effective in comparison to pooled whole-blood-derived platelet transfusions.[19]

There has been a divergence in platelet usage patterns between the United States (US) and the European Union (EU) countries.[20,21] Differences in the method of preparing platelets from whole blood (eg, from platelet-rich plasma in the US vs buffy coat in the EU) and in the percentage of apheresis preparations being used (higher in the US than in the EU) have further complicated identification of the "best" platelets. Thus the question of the relative clinical efficacy of apheresis-derived vs pooled whole-blood-derived platelets remains unresolved.[22] The popularity of apheresis platelets in the US is based partly on advantages concerning convenience for producers and transfusion services, as described in Chapter 8.

Continuous-Flow Centrifuge

While the Cohn-ADL and Haemonetics cell separators lacked a continuous-flow mode, the NCI-IBM (National Cancer Institute collaborating with IBM Corporation) cell separator [and its copy, the Aminco (Silver Spring, MD) Celltrifuge I] incorporated continuous-flow operation.[23] That instrument was intended specifically to deplete and harvest granulocytes, and it eventually did produce concentrated granulocytes,[24] although its relatively modest yields from normal donors (1 to 2×10^{10}) were likely insufficient to confer clear-cut therapeutic benefit to neutropenic patients, except in limited situations. The instrument was also capable of concentrating platelets, but clumping of the platelets after passage through the rotational-stationary interface, particularly when heparin was used as an anticoagulant, made it less desirable than its intermittent-flow counterparts for obtaining donor platelet concentrates.

Therapeutic Plateletpheresis

Instruments developed for semiautomated platelet collection have also functioned therapeutically to acutely reduce platelet levels in patients with underlying myeloproliferative disorders who have either secondary bleeding or threatened/actual thrombotic complications. Both intermittent- and continuous-flow instruments are capable of rapidly lowering platelet counts, because there is no downside to clumping in the "product." Miller et al[25] published an early description of therapeutic plateletpheresis by continuous-flow centrifugation. This topic is covered further in Chapter 13.

Granulocyte Apheresis

The procurement and transfusion of granulocytes has a long history—attempts date from at least 1950[26-28]—but the goal of obtaining a suitable number of cells from a normal donor to favorably alter the course of bacterial or fungal infection in a neutropenic patient still remains elusive. Although a suitable dose for granulocytes is in the same order of magnitude as that for a platelet transfusion (10^{11}), harvesting granulocytes in such quantities has been problematic.[29] Processing of multiple donor blood volumes is theoretically required to obtain a suitable number of granulocytes, compared to less than one blood volume for platelets. Because of the difficulty in obtaining a transfusable quantity of granulocytes from a normal donor, some early attempts used leukemic granulocytes from patients with chronic granulocytic leukemia, as described later in this chapter.

Collection of granulocytes from normal donors by apheresis can be divided into two eras, which differed in the preparation of the donor and the treatment of the recipient. Sedimenting agents such as hydroxyethyl starch (or related starches)[30] have been used to enhance separation of granulocytes from red cells to improve yields in both eras. In the initial period, c. 1966-1990, donors were either unstimulated or stimulated to have a moderate leukocytosis with steroids.[31] Granulocyte recipients in that era received anti-infective agents that were relatively ineffective by current standards. Since the 1990s, granulocyte colony-stimulating factor (G-CSF) has become available as a more effective agent to stimulate a donor leukocytosis and improve yields.[32] Beginning in the 1990s, the currently preferred antibiotics became available; use of these agents alone has decreased infection-related mortality in granulocytopenic patients, without granulocyte transfusions. The antifungal agent amphotericin has been superseded by newer antifungal agents (the "azoles") that lack significant toxicities associated with amphotericin (eg, hypokalemia, renal insufficiency). This has led to more widespread use of antifungal therapy in neutropenic patients. Also, many in the current generation of senior hematologists and oncologists were trained in the 1970-1990 era, when most studies of granulocyte transfusions reported, at best, relatively equivocal benefits,[33-35] and these physicians may not request granulocyte transfusions for that reason.

Administration of drugs to normal donors to stimulate a leukocytosis has always been controversial. Steroids can result in side effects in donors.[36] A single dose of G-CSF has relatively few immediate side effects, though it occasionally results in bone pain; however, repeated administration for serial donations is not well studied. The logistics of getting the steroid and/or G-CSF dose to the prospective granulocyte donor on the day before donation are challenging, especially in comparison to the single visit required for plateletpheresis. Also, the exposure of donors to hydroxyethyl starch, with its demonstrated persistence in donor tissues,[37,38] has never been comfortably accepted by some in the transfusion community. Granulocyte collection and transfusion are covered in detail in Chapter 11.

Filtration Leukapheresis

Granulocyte concentrates can be obtained by filtration leukapheresis, which takes advantage of selective adherence of the cells to nylon-wool filters. This was described by Djerassi et al in 1970,[39] and filter sets became commercially available within a few years. Early studies[40,41] disclosed granulocyte functional abnormalities and diminished posttransfusion recovery.[42] Additionally, a transient donor neutropenia during collection was noted,[43,44] and morphologic changes (degranulation)[45] and diminished viability[46] were reported in the harvested cells. Some of these changes were linked to complement activation by the nylon fibers.[47,48] Worrisome donor reactions were reported in the late 1970s, including abdominal/pelvic pain in female donors[49] and priapism in male donors.[50] These donor safety issues soon led to filtration leukapheresis being abandoned as a donor procedure. This history is possibly relevant to newer procedures, available outside the US, for depleting granulocytes (and monocytes) by absorption. A cellulose acetate adsorptive column [Adacolumn (JIMRO, Takasaki, Japan)] is being used for inflammatory bowel disease.[51] No significant adverse effects among the treated patients have been reported as yet.

Other Normal-Cell Leukapheresis

More recently, leukapheresis has been employed to harvest other types of leukocytes, mostly mononuclear cells such as lymphocytes and circulating hematopoietic stem cells, either unmodified or modified for specific purposes. These products differ from earlier apheresis products in that they are transfused or transplanted to restore functional defects in the recipient rather than to simply replace a numerically deficient cell population. Such products are discussed further in Chapters 22 to 29.

Peripheral Blood Stem Cell Collection

The most widely applied procedure is peripheral blood stem cell (PBSC) collection, which was begun experimentally in the mid-1970s. At that time, hematopoietic stem cells for clinical use were harvested from marrow, which required aspiration of several hundred milliliters under general anesthesia and often required additional processing (including the use of cell separators in some cases). The feasibility of recovering sufficient stem cells from peripheral blood was suggested by the recovery of lethally irradiated dogs given autologous peripheral blood leukocytes.[52] Immunophenotyping by flow cytometry to identify and count stem cells was not then possible. Rather, cells capable of hematopoietic reconstitution of a myeloablated recipient were identified by growth in culture. The number of colony-forming units (CFUs) reflected the number of hematopoietic stem cells present in the sample. Chronic myelogenous leukemia (CML) patients were found to have increased numbers of CFUs in the peripheral blood,[53] and these could be harvested by leukapheresis.[54] Richman et al described an increase in circulating stem cells during recovery from chemotherapy of solid tumors.[55] Subsequently, Lasky et al[56] demonstrated the collection of apparently adequate numbers of stem cells by apheresis of normal donors, and To et al[57] demonstrated recovery of high numbers of stem cells from patients with acute myeloid leukemia entering remission. Kessinger et al[58] then demonstrated engraftment of PBSCs to speed recovery from chemotherapy in breast cancer patients. Barlogie, using autologous marrow transplantation,[59] was able to administer otherwise supra-lethal radiation and chemotherapy to myeloma patients with resistant disease. PBSC support[60] subsequently replaced the marrow transplant, and high-dose therapy with autologous stem cell rescue has become commonplace in the treatment of multiple myeloma and lymphomas. It is used infrequently in acute leukemias because of a high relapse rate, but it is still occasionally recommended for chronic lymphocytic leukemia (CLL) when the disease is aggressive and the patient fairly young. A similar transplant-based approach, either autologous or allogeneic, was recommended for chronic granulocytic leukemia until the mid-1990s; however, tyrosine kinase inhibitors (imatinib and its analogs) have become the preferred therapy. Transplantation is now reserved for patients who fail tyrosine kinase inhibitor therapy.

Lymphocytes and Dendritic Cells

Lymphocytes have been used in a minimally manipulated state as an immunologic adjunct to allogeneic hematopoietic stem cell transplantation and as a "donor lymphocyte infusion," either to augment hematopoietic function for threatened late rejection or to potentiate a graft-vs-tumor effect.[61] More recently, natural killer cells have been suggested for situations in which donor lymphocyte infusions may increase the risk of graft-vs-host disease, but their preparation in adequate numbers remains difficult.[62]

In the late 1980s, the use of lymphokine-activated killer cells for a direct antitumor effect was reported.[63-65] Autologous lymphocytes were harvested by leukapheresis, subjected to in-vitro activation regimens, and reinfused along with interleukin-2 infusions. Unfortunately, the clinical results have not yet justified the massive effort and expense required for widespread application to patient care.

Dendritic cells have been prepared from monocytes, autologous leukemic blasts, and CD34+ hematopoietic progenitor cells in hopes of generating antitumor activity, frequently as antitumor "vaccines." Harvesting techniques have been described[66,67] and limited clinical trials have been reported,[68] but at the current time these protocols are not in widespread use.

Leukapheresis of Pathologic Leukocytes

Removal of leukemic leukocytes was among the earliest applications of cell separators.[69,70] Patients with CLL and CML were among the first to be subjected to therapeutic leukapheresis, with the leukapheresis products from CML patients used for transfusion to neutropenic patients.[71]

Hyperleukocytosis [generally defined as white cell (WBC) count $>100,000/\mu L$] with leukostasis in acute leukemia remains an indication for urgent leukapheresis. A high mortality rate is associated with hyperleukocytosis,[72-77] and there are several reports of therapeutic leukapheresis in this setting.[78-80] There is, however, a difference between actual leukostasis and threatened leukostasis in the presence of a high WBC count; the former is rated a "Category I" (standard and acceptable) indication for leukapheresis, while the latter is rated a "Category III" indication (suggestion of benefit) by the American Society for Apheresis (ASFA) in its 4th "Clinical Applications" issue published in 2007.[81] Nevertheless, leukapheresis is not a "cure" for the morbidity and mortality associated with hyperleukocytic acute leukemia, as these patients may die from central nervous system bleeds or respiratory failure despite a "successful" leukapheresis procedure that lowers the WBC count to a "safe" level.

Although it is possible to remove considerable numbers of cells from patients with CML, CLL, or prolymphocytic leukemia by leukapheresis, this does not seem to confer any clinical benefit.[82,83] For CML, the only current indication for leukapheresis is presentation with an extremely high WBC count (eg, 300,000 to 500,000/μL) and symptoms of leukostasis. Leukapheresis has also been reported for "hairy cell" leukemia (leukemic reticuloendotheliosis, or LRE),[84] but current chemotherapy with 2-chlorodeoxyadenosine (also known as cladribine or 2-CDA) and other agents is quite effective and preferable. There is a single case report[85] of repeated leukaphereses in the *pancytopenic* phase of LRE; only modest numbers of leukocytes were removed (average = 4×10^9), but improvement in peripheral counts occurred nevertheless.

Similarly, older reports described clinical benefit from leukapheresis in leukemic cutaneous T-cell lymphomas (eg, Sézary syndrome).[86,87] Currently, however, photopheresis would be considered the treatment of choice.[88]

Sporadic reports have described leukapheresis, with or without therapeutic plasma exchange (TPE), for hypereosinophilic syndromes.[89,90] The density of eosinophils is similar to that of granulocytes and young erythrocytes, so that effective separation and removal in centrifugal systems is technically difficult. Alternative therapies as simple as oral hydroxyurea may be equally effective, so that leukapheresis of eosinophils cannot be recommended currently. Therapeutic leukocyte depletion is covered in more detail in Chapter 13.

Red Cell Exchange and Related Procedures

Centifugal cell separators can remove red cells while replacing colloid or saline. This capability has been used to collect 2 "units" of red cells at a single apheresis donation.[91] The same technique can rapidly remove several "units" of red cells from a severely polycythemic patient at risk for thrombosis[92] or from a hemochromatosis patient.[93] Rapid removal of abnormal red cells and replacement with normal donor red cells (red cell exchange) has been an obvious strategy for treatment of complications of sickle cell anemia[94-97] or methemoglobinemia.[98] Removal of a large volume of infected red cells from a malaria patient[99,100] or babesosis patient[101] with a high degree of parasitemia can be life saving. Therapeutic red cell exchange is discussed in greater detail in Chapter 19.

A more subtle form of red cell exchange, the neocyte-gerocyte exchange (ie, removal of denser, "old" patient red cells and replacement with a population of less dense, "young" or reticulocyte-rich donor red cells previously collected by apheresis), could theoretically extend the interval between RBC transfusions and decrease the number of units required per unit of time.[102,103] This strategy received considerable attention in the late 1970s and early 1980s but seems to have fallen into disuse, probably because of the considerable effort required for relatively small benefit.[104] Thalassemia major and similar transfusion-dependent congenital anemias were the main targets for neocyte-gerocyte exchanges, in part to decrease iron loading. Iron-chelating agents, particularly the oral agents that have become available in the past decade, now fill this therapeutic niche.

Therapeutic Plasma Exchange

Beginning in the late 1970s, there was a rapid increase in the number of conditions reported to have been treated with and potentially responding to TPE, and there have been several attempts, including those by various insurers/payors, to separate illnesses in which TPE is truly effective from less obviously responsive conditions. Only 12 disorders are rated by ASFA as Category I, meaning diseases for which therapeutic apheresis is "standard and acceptable" either as a primary therapy or a valuable adjunct to other therapy.[81] The Category I indications for TPE will be addressed individually in the text to follow. Table 2-1 summarizes these as well as many of the more numerous non-Category-I indications, including the year and initial reference reporting benefit from TPE, with limited commentary. A more detailed discussion of most of these diseases can be found in Chapters 15, 16, 17, 18, 20, or 21. The conditions reported to benefit from TPE involve many medical subspecialties, and publications on TPE may appear in many specialty journals as well as the transfusion and apheresis literature. The author of the current chapter has attempted to identify the most relevant literature but cheerfully concedes that not every possibly applicable paper is cited herein.

Category I Indications for Therapeutic Plasma Exchange

Hyperviscosity

Symptoms of hyperviscosity in Waldenström macroglobulinemia were the indication for the first therapeutic use of plasmapheresis[3] and were again the targeted clinical manifestation in the 1960 Schwab and Fahey paper.[165] Hyperviscosity may also occur in IgA, IgG or IgE myelomas and rarely in disorders not associated with plasma cell dyscrasias. Paraproteins

occasionally express a pathogenetic antibody specificity; in such cases, resultant symptoms may provide a rationale for TPE.[105,166]

Goodpasture Syndrome

Goodpasture syndrome is a progressive pulmonary-renal syndrome. Linear deposits of IgG demonstrated by immunofluorescence microscopy strongly suggested that an autoantibody is central to its pathogenesis. It was therefore a logical target for TPE. The first successes with TPE were reported by Lockwood and colleagues in the mid-1970s.[106] Goodpasture syndrome remains a Category I indication for TPE. Experience has taught that early diagnosis is essential to successful treatment. If the diagnosis is delayed until anuria and renal failure have ensued, TPE and immunosuppressive drug therapy may not reverse the renal lesion.

Homozygous Familial Hypercholesterolemia

Subcutaneous xanthomas in young patients with homozygous familial hypercholesterolemia were reported by the mid-1970s to regress with TPE.[107] By the mid-1990s selective lipid-absorbing procedures were shown to be similarly effective.[167]

Myasthenia Gravis

Myasthenia gravis is mediated by an autoantibody to the acetylcholine receptor on the motor end plate at the neuromuscular junction. It was therefore another promising target for TPE. The 1975 paper by Pinching et al was the first to show that a neurologic condition could be responsive to TPE,[108] and myasthenia remains a frequently-treated condition in many apheresis units.

Thrombotic Thrombocytopenic Purpura

Thrombotic thrombocytopenic purpura (TTP) was found empirically to respond to TPE by Bukowski et al, who published their findings in 1977.[109] Unlike most other conditions respon-

Table 2-1. History of Conditions Treated by TPE

Year of Initial Report	Condition	Reference	Comments
	Category I Indications[81]:		
1959	Waldenström macroglobulinemia*	3	Initial reports did not comment on viscosity
1960	Hyperviscosity	165	First report to mention viscosity
1975	Goodpasture syndrome	106	
1975	Homozygous familial hypercholesterolemia	107	TPE has been superseded by affinity columns to spare HDL
1976	Myasthenia gravis	108	
1977	Thrombotic thrombocytopenic purpura	109	Preceded by whole blood exchange
1978	Guillain-Barré syndrome	110	Largely superseded by IVIG
1979	CIDP	111	
1980	Cryoglobulinemia	112	
1991	Paraproteinemic polyneuropathy	114	
1996	Sydenham chorea	115	
1999	PANDAS	175	
	Non-Category-I Indications:		
1952	Myeloma	4	
1966	Coagulation-factor deficiency	116	
1967	Acute liver failure	117	
1968	Rh alloimmunization in pregnancy	118	
1970	Thyrotoxicosis	119	
1972	Refsum disease	120	
1973	Factor VIII inhibitor (with hemophilia)	121	

1973	Idiopathic thrombocytopenic purpura	122	Largely superseded by IVIG, others
1974	Posttransfusion purpura	123	Largely superseded by IVIG, others
1975	Painful bruising syndrome	124	
1976	Systemic lupus erythematosus	125	
1976	Cancer	126	Stimulus for protein-A columns
1977	ABO-incompatible marrow transplant	127	
1977	Cold agglutinin hemolytic anemia	128	
1977	Immune complex crescentic GN	129	
1977	Pyoderma gangrenosum	130	
1978	ANCA-associated GN (Wegener)	131	
1978	Hypertriglyceridemic pancreatitis	132	
1978	Pemphigus vulgaris	133	
1978	Renal transplant antibody-mediated rejection	134	
1978	Scleroderma	135	Superseded by photopheresis
1979	Warm autoimmune hemolytic anemia	136	
1979	Hemolytic uremic syndrome	137	
1979	Lambert-Eaton myasthenic syndrome	138	
1979	Rheumatoid arthritis	139	
1979	Meningococcemia with DIC	140	
1979	Henoch-Schonlein purpura	141	
1979	Psoriasis	142	
1980	Herpes gestationis	143	
1980	Leukocytoclastic vasculitis	144	
1980	Necrotizing (cutaneous) vasculitis	145	
1980	Polymyositis and dermatomyositis	146	

(Continued)

Table 2-1. History of Conditions Treated by TPE (Continued)

Year of Initial Report	Condition	Reference	Comments
1981	Pruritus of hyperbilirubinemia	147	Affinity columns preceded TPE
1981	Pure red cell aplasia	148	
1982	Paroxysmal nocturnal hemoglobinuria	149	
1982	Dermatitis herpetiformis	150	
1983	Aplastic anemia	151	
1983	Porphyria cutanea tarda	152	
1984	Quinidine-induced thrombocytopenia	153	
1984	Leprosy reversal reaction	154	
1985	Focal segmental glomerulosclerosis	155	Terminology has changed over past three decades
1986	Factor XI deficiency	156	
1986	Platelet alloimmunization	157	
1987	Anti-P	158	
1989	Stiff person syndrome	159	
1990	Delayed hemolytic transfusion reaction	160	
1990	Paraneoplastic neurologic syndromes	161	
1992	Wilson disease	162	
1997	Factor X inhibitor (with amyloid)	163	
1998	Factor X inhibitor (non-amyloid)	164	

*A 1981 report described plasmapheresis for Waldenström macroglobulinemia occurring in 1956.[5]
TPE = therapeutic plasma exchange; HDL = high-density lipoprotein; IVIG = intravenous immunoglobulin; CIDP = chronic inflammatory demyelinating polyneuropathy; PANDAS = pediatric autoimmune neuropsychiatric disorders associated with streptococcus; GN = glomerulonephritis; ANCA = antineutrophil cytoplasmic antibodies; DIC = disseminated intravascular coagulation.

sive to TPE, TTP requires donor plasma as the replacement medium. An early explanation offered for the plasma requirement was the finding that normal plasma decreased a platelet-aggregating capability of TTP plasma.[168] More recently the pathogenesis of TTP has been attributed to autoantibody-induced ADAMTS-13 (a disintegrin and metalloproteinase with thrombospondin motifs) deficiency and platelet interaction with the resulting ultra-large von Willebrand multimers. Several publications suggest that the effect of plasma is to replace deficient ADAMTS-13,[169,170] in addition to the "usual" TPE effect of removing the autoantibody. No one has proposed an adequate explanation for the finding that TTP patients may recover clinically yet still have ADAMTS-13 deficiency and measurable inhibitor levels. Recently, treatment of TTP with an anti-von Willebrand factor aptamer has been reported, but this seems to neither affect the underlying ADAMTS-13 inhibitor nor alter the overall disease course.[171]

Guillain-Barré Syndrome

Guillain-Barré syndrome (acute inflammatory demyelinating polyneuropathy, or AIDP) can be reproduced in animals with serum from patients, suggesting that an autoantibody to myelin is involved in pathogenesis. AIDP was first reported to respond to TPE by Brettle et al in 1978,[110] and by 1985 a multicenter controlled trial had firmly established that TPE hastened recovery.[172] In 1992 a Dutch study reported that AIDP was also responsive to intravenous immunoglobulin therapy (IVIG), with the observed magnitude of the IVIG effect slightly greater than that of TPE.[173] Use of TPE for AIDP has subsequently decreased, as neurologists can administer IVIG without the need for large-bore central catheter placement.

Chronic Inflammatory Demyelinating Polyneuropathy

Antimyelin antibodies can also be found in some patients with chronic inflammatory demyelinat-ing polyneuropathy (CIDP), which was first reported to respond to TPE by Server et al in 1979.[111] The responsiveness of this disorder seems more heterogeneous than that of AIDP; some patients respond dramatically, while others with a similar history and findings do not seem to respond.

Cryoglobulinemia

Cryoglobulinemia is a heterogeneous disorder with many case reports of successful treatment by TPE. Berkman and Orlin described good responses as early as 1980.[112] Cryoglobulins can be completely removed from patient plasma by centrifugation following refrigeration. Cryoglobulinemia therefore presents a unique opportunity to diminish the cost of plasma replacement by returning cryoglobulin-depleted autologous plasma in a series of exchanges.[174] Although a Category I indication, cryoglobulinemia is relatively uncommon and very few series of patients are reported.

Neuropathy with Monoclonal Gammopathy

A monoclonal gammopathy is found more commonly in patients with the CIDP syndrome than in the general population. Moreover, such a neuropathy is more frequent in patients with monoclonal gammopathy than in the general population.[113] These epidemiologic features suggest a possible causal role for the paraprotein. Dyck et al conducted a randomized, sham-controlled trial of TPE in patients with monoclonal gammapathy and the clinical picture of CIDP, and the findings supported the conclusion that TPE is beneficial in this context.[114]

Sydenham Chorea

Sydenham chorea, which may follow a streptococcal infection, has been associated with circulating antibodies. Garvey et al showed in a randomized controlled trial that both TPE and IVIG can reduce the duration and/or severity of an episode of poststreptococcal chorea,[115] resulting in a Category I assignment.

PANDAS

Childhood tic disorders and obsessive-compulsive disorder may occur in the course of Sydenham chorea but may also be recognized following streptococcal infection in children who do not have chorea. The acronym PANDAS, for pediatric autoimmune neuropsychiatric disorders associated with streptococcal infection, was coined to describe such patients. Perlmutter et al showed in a randomized controlled trial that both TPE and IVIG could ameliorate symptoms in these patients as well,[175] which again resulted in assignment to Category I.

Non-Category-I Indications for TPE

Non-Category-I indications account for a substantial fraction of TPE activity in many facilities. Category III indications especially tend to be disorders that do not respond well to "conventional" medical therapy and for which there are one or several reports in the literature of improvement following TPE. (Again, see Table 2-1.)

Conclusion

The development of apheresis techniques for blood component separation over the past half century have contributed greatly to transfusion therapy as we know it today. Therapeutic applications of apheresis devices and techniques have improved the medical management of many disorders and also contributed markedly to our understanding of their pathophysiology.

References

1. Abel JJ, Rowntree LG, Turner BB. Plasma removal with return of corpuscles (plasmaphaeresis). J Pharmacol Exp Therapy 1913-1914;5:625-41.
2. Poonawalla C, Namjoshi AC. Large-scale plasmapheresis in equines adapting an IBM continuous-flow cell separator. Plasma Therapy and Transfusion Technology 1987;8:177-83.
3. Skoog WA, Adams WS. Plasmapheresis in a case of Waldenström's macroglobulinemia. Clin Res 1959;7:96.
4. Adams WS, Blahd WH, Bassett SH. A method of human plasmapheresis. Proc Soc Exp Biol Med 1952;80:377-9.
5. Reynolds WA. Late report of the first case of plasmapheresis for Waldenström's macroglobulinemia. JAMA 1981;245:606-7.
6. Kliman A, Gaydos LA, Schroeder LR, Freireich E. Repeated plasmapheresis of blood donors as a source of platelets. Blood 1961;18:303-9.
7. Colman RW, Sievers CA, Pugh RP. Thrombocytapheresis: A rapid and effective approach to symptomatic thrombocytosis. J Lab Clin Med 1966;68:389-99.
8. Tullis JL, Surgenor DM, Tinch RJ, et al. New principle of closed system centrifugation. Science 1956;124:792-4.
9. Tullis JL, Surgenor DM, Baudanza P. Preserved platelets: Their preparation, storage and clinical use. Blood 1959;14:456-75.
10. Tullis JL, Tinch RJ, Gibson JG, Baudanza P. A simplified centrifuge for the separation and processing of blood cells. Transfusion 1967;7:232-42.
11. Millward BL, Hoeltge GA. The historical development of automated apheresis. J Clin Apher 1982;1:25-32.
12. Yankee RA, Grumet FC, Rogentine GN. Platelet transfusion therapy. The selection of compatible platelet donors for refractory patients by lymphocyte HL-A typing. N Engl J Med 1969;281:1208-12.
13. Patel IP, Ambinder E, Holland JF, Aledort LM. In vitro and in vivo comparison of single-donor platelets and multiple-donor pooled platelets transfusions in leukemia patients. Transfusion 1978;18:116-19.
14. Slichter SJ. Controversies in platelet transfusion therapy. Ann Rev Med 1980;31:509-40.
15. Dutcher JP, Schiffer CA, Aisner J, Wiernik PH. Alloimmunization following platelet transfusion: The absence of a dose-response relationship. Blood 1981;57:395-8.
16. Schiffer CA, Dutcher JP, Aisner J. A randomized trial of leukocyte-depleted platelet transfusion to modify alloimmunization in patients with leukemia. Blood 1983;62:815-20.
17. Slichter SJ. Leukocyte reduction and ultraviolet B irradiation of platelets to prevent allo-immu-

nization and refractoriness to platelet transfusions. N Engl J Med 1997;337:1861-9.

18. Kelley DL, Fegan RL, Ng AT. High-yield platelet concentrates attainable by continuous quality improvement reduce platelet transfusion cost and donor exposure. Transfusion 1987; 37:482-6.

19. Lopez-Plaza I, Weissfeld J, Triulzi DJ. The cost-effectiveness of reducing donor exposures with single-donor versus pooled random-donor platelets. Transfusion 1999;39:925-32.

20. Murphy S (for BEST collaborative). Platelets from pooled buffy coats: An update. Transfusion 2005;45:634-9.

21. Vassallo RR, Murphy S. A critical comparison of platelet preparation methods. Curr Opin Hematol 2006;13:323-30.

22. Pietersz RNI. Pooled platelet concentrates: An alternative to single donor apheresis platelets? Transfus Apher Sci 2009;41:115-19.

23. Judson G, Jones A, Kellogg R, et al. Closed continuous-flow centrifuge. Nature 1968;217:816-18.

24. Freireich EJ, Judson G, Levin RH. Separation and collection of leukocytes. Cancer Res 1965; 25:1516-20.

25. Miller DS, Rundles RW, Silver CD. Rapid plateletpheresis by continuous flow blood cell separation (abstract). Clin Res 1971;19:646.

26. Lanman JT, Bierman HR, Byron RL. Transfusion of leukemic leukocytes in man. Blood 1950;5:1099-113.

27. Hirsch EO, Gardner FH. The transfusion of human blood platelets with a note on the transfusion of granulocytes. J Lab Clin Med 1952;39:556-69.

28. Brecher G, Wilbur KM, Cronkite EP. Transfusion of separated leukocytes into irradiated dogs with aplastic marrows. Proc Soc Exp Biol Med 1953;84:54-6.

29. Henderson ES, Graw RG, Anderson RM, et al. Obstacles to routine transfusion support of myelosuppressive patients. Cancer Chemother Rep 1973;4:51-9.

30. Mishler JM, Hadlock DC, Fortuny IE, et al. Increased efficiency of leukocyte collection by the addition of hydroxyethyl starch to the continuous flow centrifuge. Blood 1974;44:571-81.

31. Shoji M, Vogler WR. Effects of hydrocortisone on the yield and bactericidal function of granulocytes collected by continuous-flow centrifugation. Blood 1974;44:435-43.

32. Strauss RG. Neutrophil (granulocyte) transfusions in the new millenium (editorial). Transfusion 1998;38:710-12.

33. Graw RG, Herzig G, Perry S, Henderson ES. Normal granulocyte transfusion therapy. N Engl J Med 1972;287:367-71.

34. McCredie KB, Freireich EJ, Hester JP, Vallejos C. Leukocyte transfusion therapy for patients with host-defense failure. Transplant Proc 1973;5:1285-7.

35. Fortuny IE, Bloomfield CD, Hadlock DC, et al. Granulocyte transfusion: A controlled study in patients with acute nonlymphocytic leukemia. Transfusion 1975;15:548-58.

36. Strauss RG. Glucocorticoid stimulation of neutrophil donors: A medical, scientific, and ethical dilemma (editorial). Transfusion 2005;45: 1697-9.

37. Rock G, Wise P. Plasma expansion during granulocyte procurement: Cumulative effects of hydroxyethyl starch. Blood 1979;53:1156-63.

38. Strauss RG, Koepke JA. Chemistry, pharmacology and donor effects of hydroxyethyl starch as used during leukapheresis. Plasma Therapy 1980;1:35-44.

39. Djcrassi I, Kim JS, Mitrakul C, et al. Filtration leukopheresis for separation and concentration of transfusable amounts of normal human granulocytes. J Med 1970;1:358-64.

40. Debelak KM, Epstein RB, Andersen BR. Granulocyte transfusions in leucopenia dogs: In vivo and in vitro function of granulocytes obtained by continuous-flow filtration leukopheresis. Blood 1974;43:757-66.

41. Wright DG, Kauffmann JC, Chusid MJ, et al. Functional abnormalities of human neutrophils collected by continuous flow filtration leukapheresis. Blood 1975;46:901-11.

42. Price TH, Dale DC. Neutrophil transfusion: Effect of storage and of collection method on neutrophil blood kinetics. Blood 1978;51:789-98.

43. Schiffer CA, Aisner J, Wiernik P. Transient neutropenia during continuous flow filtration leukapheresis. In: Goldman JM, Lowenthal RM, eds. Leucocytes: Separation, collection, and transfusion. London: Academic Press, 1975: 160-7.

44. Rubins JM, MacPherson JL, Nusbacher J, Wiltbank T. Granulocyte kinetics in donors undergoing filtration leukapheresis. Transfusion 1976;16:56-62.

45. Klock JC, Bainton DF. Degranulation and abnormal bactericidal function of granulocytes

procured by reversible adhesion to nylon wool. Blood 1976;48:149-61.

46. Roy AJ, Yankee RA, Brivkalns A, Fitch M. Viability of granulocytes obtained by filtration leukapheresis. Transfusion 1975;15:539-47.

47. Nusbacher J, Rosenfeld SI, MacPherson JL, et al. Nylon fiber leukapheresis-associated complement component changes and granulocytopenia. Blood 1978;51:359-65.

48. Hammerschmidt DE, Craddock PR, McCullough J, et al. Complement activation and pulmonary leukostasis during nylon fiber filtration leukapheresis. Blood 1978;51:721-30.

49. Wiltbank TB, Nusbacher J, Higby DJ, MacPherson JL. Abdominal pain in donors during filtration leukapheresis. Transfusion 1977;17:159-62.

50. Dahlke MB, Shah SL, Sherwood WC, et al. Priapism during filtration leukapheresis. Transfusion 1979;19:482-6.

51. Saniabadi AR, Hanai H, Fukunaga K et al. Therapeutic leukacytapheresis for inflammatory bowel disease. Transfus Apher Sci 2007; 37:191-200.

52. Cavins JA, Scheer SC, Thomas ED, Ferrebee JW. The recovery of lethally irradiated dogs given infusions of autologous leukocytes preserved at −80 C. Blood 1964;23:38-43.

53. Goldman JM, Th'ng KH, Lowenthal RM. In vitro colony forming cells and colony stimulating factor in chronic granulocytic leukemia. Brit J Cancer 1974;30:1-12.

54. Goldman JM, Lowenthal RM, Buskard NA, et al. Chronic granulocytic leukemia—selective removal of immature granulocytic cells by leukapheresis. Ser Haematol 1975;8:28-40.

55. Richman CM, Weiner RS, Yankee RA. Increase in circulating stem cells following chemotherapy in man. Blood 1976;47:1031-9.

56. Lasky LC, Ash RC, Kersey JH, et al. Collection of pluripotential hematopoietic stem cells by cytapheresis. Blood 1982;59:822-7.

57. To LB, Haylock DN, Kimber RJ, Juttner CA. High levels of circulating haematopoietic stem cells in very early remission from acute non-lymphoblastic leukaemia and their collection and cryopreservation. Br J Haematol 1984;58:399-410.

58. Kessinger A, Armitage JO, Landmark JD, Weisenburger DD. Reconstitution of human hematopoietic function with autologous cryopreserved circulating stem cells. Exp Hematol 1986;14:192-6.

59. Barlogie B, Alexanian R, Dicke KA, et al. High-dose chemoradiotherapy and autologous bone marrow transplantation for resistant multiple myeloma. Blood 1987;70:869-72.

60. Jagannath S, Vesole DH, Glenn L, et al. Low risk intensive therapy for multiple myeloma with combined autologous bone marrow and blood stem cell support. Blood 1992;80:1666-72.

61. Kolb HJ, Mittermuller J, Clemm C, et al. Donor leukocyte transfusions for treatment of recurrent chronic myelogenous leukemia in marrow transplant patients. Blood 1990;76:2462-5.

62. Meyer-Monard S, Passweg J, Siegler U, et al. Clinical-grade purification of natural killer cells in haploidentical hematopoietic stem cell transplantation. Transfusion 2009;49:362-71.

63. Lotze MT, Grimm EA, Mazumder A, et al. Lysis of fresh and cultured autologous tumor by human lymphocytes cultured in T-cell growth factor. Cancer Res 1981;41:4420-5.

64. Rosenberg SA, Lotze MT, Muul LM, et al. Observations on the systemic administration of autologous lymphokine-activated killer cells and recombinant interleukin-2 to patients with metastatic cancer. N Engl J Med 1985;313:1485-92.

65. Klein HG. Adoptive immunotherapy: Novel applications of blood cell separators. J Clin Apher 1988;4:198-202.

66. Elias M, vanZanten J, Hospers GAP, et al. Closed system generation of dendritic cells from a single blood volume for clinical application in immunotherapy. J Clin Apher 2005; 20:197-207.

67. Chen Y, Hoecker P, Zeng J, Dettke M. Combination of COBE AutoPBSC and Gambro Elutra as a platform for monocyte enrichment in dendritic cell (DC) therapy: Clinical study. J Clin Apher 2008;23:157-62.

68. Stevenson HC, Lacerna LV, Sugarbaker PH. Ex vivo activation of killer monocytes (KM) and their application to the treatment of human cancer. J Clin Apher 1988;4:118-21.

69. Bierman HR, Marshall GJ, Kelly KH, Byron RL. Leukapheresis in man. III. Hematologic observations in patients with leukemia and myeloid metaplasia. Blood 1963;21:164-82.

70. Perry S, Judson G, Vogel J. Studies with the NCI-IBM cell separator. Exp Hematol 1966;9:38-44.

71. Morse EE, Freireich EJ, Carbone PP, et al. The transfusion of leukocytes from donors with

chronic myelocytic leukemia to patients with leukopenia. Transfusion 1966;16:183-92.

72. Vaughan WP, Kimball AW, Karp JE, et al. Factors affecting survival of patients with acute myelocytic leukemia presenting with high WBC counts. Cancer Chemother Rep 1981; 65:1007-13.

73. Hug V, Keating M, McCredie K, et al. Clinical course and response to treatment of patients with acute myelogenous leukemia presenting with a high leukocyte count. Cancer 1983;52: 773-9.

74. Lester TJ, Johnson JW, Cuttner J. Pulmonary leukostasis as the single worst prognostic factor in patients with acute myelocytic leukemia and hyperleukocytosis. Am J Med 1985;79:43-8.

75. Creutzig U, Ritter J, Budde M, et al. Early deaths due to hemorrhage and leukostasis in childhood acute myelogenous leukemia. Associations with hyperleukocytosis and acute monocytic leukemia. Cancer 1987;60:3071-9.

76. Dutcher JP, Schiffer CA, Wiernik PH. Hyperleukocytosis in adult acute nonlymphocytic leukemia: Impact on remission rate and duration, and survival. J Clin Oncol 1987;5:1364-72.

77. Ventura GJ, Hester JP, Smith TL, Keating MJ. Acute myeloblastic leukemia with hyperleukocytosis: Risk factors for early mortality in induction. Am J Hematol 1988;27:34-7.

78. Lane TA. Continuous-flow leukapheresis for rapid cytoreduction in leukemia. Transfusion 1980;20:455-7.

79. Taft EG, Sullivan SA. Leukapheresis in acute leukemia—is it necessary? In: Vogler WR, ed. Cytapheresis and Plasma Exchange. Clinical Indications. New York: Alan R. Liss, 1982:189-205.

80. Novotny JR, Muller-Beibenhirtz H, Herget-Rosenthal S, et al. Grading of symptoms in hyperleukocytic leukaemia: A clinical model for the role of different blast types and promyelocytes in the development of leukostasis syndrome. Eur J Haematol 2005;74:501-10.

81. Szczepiorkowski ZM, Shaz BH, Bandarenko N, Winters JL. The new approach to assignment of ASFA categories—introduction to the fourth special issue: Clinical applications of therapeutic apheresis. J Clin Apher 2007;22:96-105.

82. Hocker P, Pittermann E, Gobets M, Stacher A. Treatment of patients with chronic myeloid leukaemia (CML) and chronic lymphocytic leukaemia (CLL) by leucapheresis with a continuous flow blood cell separator. In: Goldman JM,

Lowenthal RM, eds. Leucocytes: Separation, collection, and transfusion. London: Academic Press, 1975:510-18.

83. Buskard NA, Lowenthal RM, Goldman JM, Galton DAG. Treatment of prolymphocytic leukaemia by leucapheresis. In: Goldman JM, Lowenthal RM, eds. Leucocytes: Separation, collection, and transfusion. London: Academic Press, 1975:543-7.

84. Fay JW, Moore JO, Logue GL, Huang AT. Leukopheresis therapy of leukemic reticuloendotheliosis (hairy cell leukemia). Blood 1979;54: 747-9.

85. Choudhury AM, Bhoopalam NB, Hoffstadter LK. Effects of intense leukocytapheresis in pancytopenic phase of hairy cell leukemia. Transfusion 1983;23:526-9.

86. Edelson R, Facktor M, Andrews A, et al. Successful management of the Sézary syndrome. Mobilization and removal of extravascular neoplastic cells by leukapheresis. N Engl J Med 1974;291:293-4.

87. Bongiovanni MB, Katz RS, Tomaszewski JE, et al. Cytapheresis in a patient with Sézary syndrome. Transfusion 1981;21:332-4.

88. Edelson R, Berger C, Gasparro F, et al. Treatment of cutaneous T-cell lymphoma by extracorporeal photochemotherapy. N Engl J Med 1987;316:297-303.

89. Ellman L, Miller L, Rappeport J. Leukapheresis therapy of a hypereosinophilic disorder. JAMA 1974;230:1004-5.

90. Davies J, Spry C. Plasma exchange or leukapheresis in the hypereosinophilic syndrome (letter). Ann Intern Med 1982;96:791.

91. Meyer D, Bolgiano DC, Sayers M, et al. Red cell collection by apheresis technology. Transfusion 1993;33:819-24.

92. Spengel FA, Zoller WG. Erythrocytapheresis: A new effective tool for treatment of central venous thrombosis of the eye. Plasma Ther Transfus Technol 1986;7:139-42.

93. Muncunill J, Vacquer P, Galmes A, et al. In hereditary hemochromatosis, red cell apheresis removes excess iron twice as fast as manual whole blood phlebotomy. J Clin Apher 2002; 17:88-92.

94. Kernoff LM, Botha MC, Jacobs P. Exchange transfusion in sickle cell disease using a continuous-flow blood cell separator. Transfusion 1977;17:269-71.

95. Rifkind S, Waisman J, Thompson R, Goldfinger D. RBC exchange pheresis for priapism in sickle cell disease. JAMA 1979;242:2317-18.

96. Sheehy TW, Law DE, Wade BH. Exchange transfusion for sickle cell intrahepatic homeostasis. Arch Intern Med 1980;140:1364-6.

97. Miller DM, Winslow RM, Klein HG, et al. Improved exercise performance after exchange transfusion in subjects with sickle cell anemia. Blood 1980;56:1127-31.

98. Golden PJ, Weinstein R. Treatment of high-risk, refractory acquired methemoglobinemia with automated red blood cell exchange. J Clin Apher 1998;13:28-31.

99. Yarrish RL, Janas JS, Nosanchuk JS, et al. Transfusion malaria. Treatment with exchange transfusion after delayed diagnosis. Arch Intern Med 1982;142:187-8.

100. Files JC, Case CJ, Morrison FS. Automated erythrocyte exchange in fulminant falciparum malaria. Ann Intern Med 1984;100:396.

101. Cahill KM, Benach JL, Reich LM, et al. Red cell exchange: Treatment of babesiosis in a splenectomized patient. Transfusion 1981;21:193-8.

102. Klein HG. Neocytopheresis: Collection, preparation and clinical results. In: Proceedings, Apheresis symposium: Current concepts and future trends. Chicago: American Red Cross Blood Sevices (Mid-America Region)/Michael Reese Research Foundation/University of Illinois Blood Bank, 1979:88-95.

103. Klein HG. Selective isolation of young red cells for chronic transfusion. Plasma Therapy 1981; 2:175-80.

104. Montoya AF. Neocyte transfusion: A current perspective. Transfus Sci 1993;14:147-56.

105. Dighiero G, Guilbert B, Fermand J-P et al. Thirty-six human monoclonal immunoglobulins with antibody activity against cytoskeleton proteins, thyroglobulin, and native DNA: Immunologic studies and clinical correlations. Blood 1983;62:264-70.

106. Lockwood CM, Boulton-Jones JM, Lowenthal RM, et al. Recovery from Goodpasture's syndrome after immunosuppressive treatment and plasmapheresis. Br Med J 1975;2:252-4.

107. Thompson GR, Lowenthal R, Myant NB. Plasma exchange in the management of homozygous familial hypercholesterolemia. Lancet 1975;2:1208-11.

108. 108. Pinching AJ, Peters DK. Remission of myasthenia gravis following plasma-exchange. Lancet 1976;2:1373-6.

109. Bukowski RM, King JW, Hewlett JS. Plasmapheresis in the treatment of thrombotic thrombocytopenic purpura. Blood 1977;50:413-17.

110. Brettle RP, Gross M, Legg NJ, et al. Treatment of acute polyneuropathy by plasma exchange (letter). Lancet 1978;2:1100.

111. Server AC, Lefkowith J, Braine H, McKhann G. Treatment of chronic relapsing inflammatory polyradiculoneuropathy by plasma exchange. Ann Neurol 1979;6:258-61.

112. Berkman EM, Orlin JB. Use of plasmapheresis and partial plasma exchange in the management of patients with cryoglobulinemia. Transfusion 1980;20:171-8.

113. Kyle RA. Monoclonal proteins in neuropathy. Neurol Clin 1992;10:713-34.

114. Dyck PJ, Low PA, Windebank AJ, et al. Plasma exchange in polyneuropathy associated with monoclonal gammopathy of undetermined significance. N Engl J Med 1991;325:1482-6.

115. Garvey MA, Swedo SE, Shapiro MB, et al. Intravenous immunoglobulin and plasmapheresis as effective treatments of Sydenham's chorea (abstract). Neurology 1996;46:A147.

116. Perkins HA. Plasmapheresis of the patient as a method for achieving effective levels of coagulation factors using fresh frozen plasma. Transfusion 1966;6:293-301.

117. Lepore MJ, Martel AJ. Plasmapheresis in hepatic coma. Lancet 1967;2:771-2.

118. Powell LC. Intense plasmapheresis in the pregnant Rh-sensitized woman. Am J Obstet Gynecol 1968;101:153-70.

119. Ashkar FS, Katims RB, Smoak WM, Gilson AJ. Thyroid storm treatment with blood exchange and plasmapheresis. JAMA 1970;214:1275-9.

120. Lundberg A, Lilja LG, Lundberg PO, Try K. Heredopathia atactica polyneuritiformis (Refsum's disease). Eur Neurol 1972;8:309-24.

121. Edson JR, McArthur JR, Branda RF, et al. Successful management of a subdural hematoma in a hemophiliac with an anti-FVIII antibody. Blood 1973;41:113-22.

122. McCullough J, Fortuny IE, Kennedy BJ, et al. Rapid plasma exchange with the continuous flow centrifuge. Transfusion 1973;13:94-9.

123. Abramson N, Eisenberg PD, Aster RH. Posttransfusion purpura: Immunologic aspects and therapy. N Engl J Med 1974;291:1163-6.

124. Lockwood M, Pearson T. Use of plasma exchange in treatment of allergic diseases. Haemonetics Advanced Component Seminar. Boston: HRI, 1975:1-8.

125. Verrier Jones J, Cumming RH, Bucknall RC, et al. Plasmapheresis in the management of acute systemic lupus erythematosus. Lancet 1976;1:709-11.

126. Hersey P, Isbister J, Edwards A, et al. Antibody-dependent, cell-mediated cytotoxicity against melanoma cells induced by plasmapheresis. Lancet 1976;1:825-7.

127. Gale RP, Feig S, Ho W, et al. ABO blood group system and bone marrow transplantation. Blood 1977;50:185-94.

128. Taft EG, Propp RP, Sullivan SA. Plasma exchange for cold agglutinin hemolytic anemia. Transfusion 1977;17:173-6.

129. Lockwood CM, Rees AJ, Pinching AJ, et al. Plasma-exchange and immunosuppression in the treatment of fulminating immune-complex crescentic nephritis. Lancet 1977;1:63-7.

130. Clayton R, Feiwel M, Valdimarsson H. Pyoderma gangrenosum with cellular immunity defect and red cell aplasia. Proc R Soc Med 1977;70:571-2.

131. Lockwood CM, Worlledge S, Nicholas A et al. Reversal of impaired splenic function in patients with nephritis or vasculitis (or both) by plasma exchange. N Engl J Med 1978;300:524-30.

132. Betteridge DJ, Bakowski M, Taylor KG, et al. Treatment of severe diabetic hypertriglyceridaemia by plasma exchange. Lancet 1978;1:1368.

133. Ruocco V, Rossi A, Argenziano G, et al. Pathogenicity of the intercellular antibodies of pemphigus and their periodic removal by plasmapheresis. Br J Dermatol 1978;98:237-41.

134. Cardella CJ, Sutton DMC, Folk JA, et al. Effect of intensive plasma exchange on renal transplant rejection and serum cytotoxic antibody. Transplant Proc 1978;10:617-19.

135. Talpos G, Horrocks M, White JM, et al. Plasmapheresis in Raynaud's disease. Lancet 1978;1:416-17.

136. Ruberto G, Gulinati L, Pellegrino S, Ascari E. Plasmapheresis in the treatment of autoimmune hemolytic anemia. Haematologia 1979;64:759-65.

137. Remuzzi G, Misiani R, Marchesi D, et al. Treatment of hemolytic uremic syndrome with plasma. Clin Nephrol 1979;12:279-84.

138. Dau PC, Lindstrom JM, Denys EH. Plasmapheresis in neurologic disorders. In: Nemo GJ, Taswell H, US Department of Health and Human Services (PHS/NIH). Proceedings of the workshop on therapeutic plasmapheresis and cytapheresis, Mayo Clinic, Rochester, MN, April 25-26, 1979. NIH publication no. 82-1665. Bethesda, MD: NIH, 1981:169-98.

139. Wallace DJ, Goldfinger D, Gatti R, et al. Plasmapheresis and lymphoplasmapheresis in the management of rheumatoid arthritis. Arthritis Rheum 1979;22:703-10.

140. Scharfman W, Tillotson J, Taft E. Plasmapheresis for meningococcemia with DIC (letter). N Engl J Med 1979;300:1277.

141. MacKenzie PE, Taylor AE, Woodroffe AJ, et al. Plasmapheresis in glomerulonephritis. Clin Nephrol 1979;12:97-108.

142. Dau PC. Resolution of psoriasis during plasmapheresis therapy (letter). Arch Dermatol 1979;115:1179.

143. van de Wiel A, Hart AC, Flinterman J, et al. Plasma exchange in herpes gestationis. Br Med J 1980;281:1041-2.

144. Cohen J, Lockwood CM, Calnan CD. Plasma exchange in treatment of leukocytoclastic vasculitis. J R Soc Med 1980;73:457-61.

145. Valbonesi M, Garelli S, Mosconi L, et al. Plasma exchange in the management of a patient with diffuse necrotizing cutaneous vasculitis. Vox Sang 1980;39:241-5.

146. Brewer EJ, Giannini EH, Rossen RD, et al. Plasma exchange therapy of a childhood onset dermatomyositis patient. Arthritis Rheum 1980;23:509-13.

147. Levy VG, Julien PE. Traitement de la cholestase par la plasmapherese. Presse Med 1981;10:2588.

148. Messner HA, Fauser AA, Curtis JE, Dotten D. Control of antibody-mediated pure red cell aplasia by plasmapheresis. N Engl J Med 1981;304:1334-8.

149. Szymanski IO, Snyder LM. Treatment of life-threatening anemia with plasmapheresis in a patient with paroxysmal nocturnal hemoglobinuria. Plasma Therapy 1982;3:51-6.

150. Wexler D, Clark W. Plasma exchange and dermatitis herpetiformis (letter). Arch Dermatol 1982;118:141-2.

151. Young NS, Klein HG, Griffith P, Nienhuis AW. A trial of immunotherapy in aplastic anemia and pure red cell aplasia. J Clin Apher 1983;1:95-103.

152. Miyauchi S, Shiraishi S, Miki Y. Small volume plasmapheresis in the management of porphyria cutanea tarda. Arch Dermatol 1983;119:752-6.

153. Guthrie TH, Pallas CW, Squires JE. Quinidine-induced thrombocytopenia successfully treated with plasma exchange. Plasma Therapy Transfusion Technology 1984;5:361-3.

154. Lucht F, Rifle G, Portier H, et al. Successful plasma exchange in type I leprosy reversal reaction. Br Med J (Clin Res Ed) 1984;289:1647-8.

155. Zimmerman SW. Plasmapheresis and dipyridamole for recurrent glomerular sclerosis. Nephron 1985;40:241-5.

156. Novakova IRO, vanGinneken CAM, Verbruggen HW, Haanen C. Factor XI kinetics after plasma exchange in severe Factor XI deficiency. Haemostasis 1986;16:51-6.

157. Bensinger WI, Buckner CD, Clift RA, et al. Plasma exchange for platelet alloimmunization. Transplantation 1986;41:602-5.

158. Shirey R, Ness P, Kickler T, et al. The association of anti-P and early abortion. Transfusion 1987;27:189-91.

159. Vicari AM, Folli F, Pozza G, et al. Plasmapheresis in the treatment of stiff-man syndrome (letter). N Engl J Med 1989;320:1499.

160. Wright RD, Larison PJ, Cook LO. Plasma exchange in the management of delayed hemolytic transfusion reaction. Transfus Sci 1990;11:91-6.

161. Graus F, Abos J, Roquer J, et al. Effect of plasmapheresis on serum and CSF autoantibody levels in CNS paraneoplastic syndromes. Neurology 1990;40:1621-3.

162. Humphreys D, Galacki D, Kent P, et al. Intensive plasma exchange in a patient with Wilson's disease (abstract). J Clin Apher 1992;7:31-2.

163. Beardall FV, Varma M, Martinez J. Normalization of plasma Factor X levels in amyloidosis after plasma exchange. Am J Hematol 1997;54:68-71.

164. Smith SV, Liles DK, White GC, Brecher ME. Successful treatment of transient acquired Factor X deficiency by plasmapheresis with concomitant intravenous immunoglobulin and steroid therapy. Am J Hematol 1998;57:245-52.

165. Schwab PJ, Fahey JL. Treatment of Waldenström's macroglobulinemia by plasmapheresis. N Engl J Med 1960;263:574-9.

166. Salmon SE. "Paraneoplastic" syndrome associated with monoclonal lymphocyte and plasma cell proliferation. Ann N Y Acad Sci 1974;230:228-39.

167. Kitano Y, Thompson GR. Role of LDL apheresis in the management of hypercholesterolaemia. Transfus Sci 1993;14:269-80.

168. Lian EC, Harkness DR, Byrnes JJ, et al. Presence of a platelet aggregating factor in the plasma of patients with thrombotic thrombocytopenic purpura (TTP) and its inhibition by normal plasma. Blood 1979;53:333-8.

169. Scott EA, Puca KE, Pietz BC, et al. Comparison and stability of ADAMTS13 activity in therapeutic plasma products. Transfusion 2007;47:120-5.

170. Nguyen L, Li X, Duvall D, et al. Twice-daily plasma exchange for patients with refractory thrombotic thrombocytopenic purpura: The experience of the Oklahoma Registry, 1989 through 2006. Transfusion 2008;48:349-57.

171. Knobl P, Jilma B, Gilbert JC, et al. Anti-von Willebrand factor aptamer ARC1779 for refractory thrombotic thrombocytopenic purpura. Transfusion 2009;49:2181-5.

172. Guillain-Barré Study Group. Plasmapheresis and acute Guillain-Barré syndrome. Neurology 1985;35:1096-1104.

173. vanderMeche FGA, Dutch Guillain-Barré Study Group. A randomized trial comparing intravenous immune globulin and plasma exchange in Guillain-Barré syndrome. N Engl J Med 1992;326:1123-9.

174. McLeod BC, Sassetti R. Plasmapheresis with return of cryoglobulin-depleted autologous plasma (cryoglobulinpheresis) in cryoglobulinemia. Blood 1980;55:866-70.

175. Perlmutter SJ, Leitman SF, Garvey MA, et al. Therapeutic plasma exchange and intravenous immunoglobulin for obsessive-compulsive disorder and tic disorders in childhood. Lancet 1999;354:1153-8.

In: McLeod BC, Szczepiorkowski ZM, Weinstein R, Winters JL, eds.
Apheresis: Principles and Practice, 3rd edition
Bethesda, MD: AABB Press, 2010

3

Physiology of Apheresis

Kendall P. Crookston, MD, PhD, and Deborah J. Novak, MD

THE USE OF APHERESIS IN BOTH the blood donor and therapeutic patient settings involves important physiologic considerations. Requirements for anticoagulation have a profound effect on several physiologic variables. The procedure itself leads to both hemodynamic and dilutional changes in donors and patients, and the physiologic impact of the procedure may result in adverse consequences. An understanding of the physiology of apheresis is necessary in order to minimize donor and patient reactions.

Anticoagulation

Apheresis procedures require anticoagulation, which serves to minimize activation of circulating cellular and plasma components (eg, plate-

lets and clotting factors), thereby insuring that extracorporeal blood remains in a fluid state. Citrate has become the anticoagulant of choice for apheresis; it chelates positively charged calcium ions, effectively blocking calcium-dependent clotting factor reactions.[1-2]

Citrate Anticoagulation

Citric acid (molecular weight 192) is a ubiquitous compound found in all human cells. It is also found in plant cells, with particularly high concentrations in citrus fruits. It contains three ionizable carboxyl groups, two of which may bind to divalent cations (eg, calcium and magnesium) while the last ionized carboxyl group maintains high solubility in physiologic solutions.[3] When citric acid binds to a positively charged ion, it becomes "citrate" (eg, sodium citrate). (See Fig 3-1.) Several citrate anticoagu-

Kendall P. Crookston, MD, PhD, Associate Professor, Departments of Pathology and Medicine, University of New Mexico School of Medicine; Medical Director, United Blood Services of New Mexico; and Associate Medical Director, TriCore Reference Laboratories, Albuquerque, New Mexico; and Deborah J. Novak, MD, Medical Director, University Hospital Blood and Tissue Banks, Department of Pathology, University of New Mexico School of Medicine, and Associate Medical Director, United Blood Services of New Mexico, Albuquerque, New Mexico

The authors have disclosed no conflicts of interest.

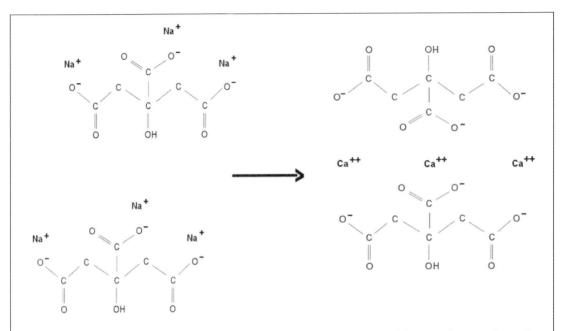

Figure 3-1. The chelation of calcium by citrate. Citrate, a molecule ubiquitous in living organisms, carries up to three negative charges at physiologic blood pH. Sodium citrate used for apheresis anticoagulation binds circulating calcium ions in the blood. In the simplest form, two molecules of trisodium citrate give up six single-charged sodium atoms and preferentially associate with three double-charged calcium ions. Fewer free calcium ions are left in circulation to participate in the clotting cascade, resulting in anticoagulation of the patient. If too many calcium ions are bound by citrate, the patient will experience side effects from ionized hypocalcemia.

lants have been used in apheresis, including acid-citrate-dextrose solution A (ACD-A), ACD-B, and 2% sodium citrate (see Table 3-1).[1,3] The challenge is in establishing a balance between adequate anticoagulation and potential toxicity. This requires an understanding of calcium metabolism and the effects of citrate infusion on calcium homeostasis.

Table 3-1. Common Citrate Formulations

Solution (Undiluted)	Citrate Ion Concentration	
	mmol/L	mg/mL
ACD-A	113	21.3
ACD-B	68	12.8
Trisodium Citrate (4%)	136	25.6

Overview of Calcium Homeostasis

Of the total body calcium, 99% is found in bone, where it exists in complex crystals with phosphate ion (eg, hydroxyapatite). A small proportion of skeletal calcium is in a noncrystalline form that can be rapidly mobilized to correct an extraosseous deficiency. Virtually all of the 1000 mg of nonosseous calcium is extracellular, with the normal plasma concentration being about 10 mg/dL (2.5 mmol/L). Roughly 40% of plasma calcium is bound to plasma proteins, primarily albumin, and 13% complexes with small anions such as citrate, phosphate, and lactate. Studies have shown that this anion-bound fraction is markedly increased when exogenous anions are introduced (eg, citrate).[4] The remaining 47% of plasma calcium is unbound (1.2 to 1.3 mmol/L). The unbound (ionized) calcium fraction, which participates in coagulation reactions, is chelated by added citrate. Thus, citrate infusion results in decreased ionized calcium, which underlies both the anti-clotting effect and the adverse symptoms associated with citrate anticoagulants.[1]

An adequate level of ionized calcium is essential for proper function of the calcium channels that mediate many cellular responses. Additionally, ionized calcium mediates bone mineralization. Its concentration in the blood is tightly regulated; when the ionized calcium level falls, hormonal homeostatic mechanisms lead to increased parathormone secretion by the parathyroid glands. This stimulates mobilization of calcium from the noncrystalline pool in bone and increased resorption of crystalline bone material. Parathormone also increases intestinal absorption and renal tubular reabsorption of calcium, thereby increasing new calcium uptake and decreasing excretion, respectively.[1]

Calcium Homeostasis During Apheresis

At physiologic pH, citrate ions have only moderate affinity for binding calcium. Data on platelet donors indicate that ionized calcium decreases by 0.1 mmol/L for each 0.5 to 0.6 mmol/L rise in plasma citrate.[5] Infusion rates used in many early apheresis procedures of about 80 mg/kg per hour of citrate solution delivered close to 11 grams of citrate ion to the subject during a procedure.[6] Assuming that all citrate remained in the blood stream, this could increase the plasma citrate concentration to as high as 76 mg/dL.[5] Fortunately, actual plasma citrate levels during apheresis are considerably lower than would be predicted by such a model, and therefore ionized calcium levels remain higher.

Dilution, redistribution, metabolism, and excretion of infused citrate are important factors protecting against profound hypocalcemia. Observed citrate levels have been reported to range from 17 mg/dL[5] to over 30 mg/dL.[7] During a plateletpheresis procedure, this typically leads to a 23% to 33% reduction in ionized calcium.[2,7] Renal excretion of the acute citrate load leads to an obligate increase in excretion of cations in the urine (eg, calcium, magnesium, sodium, potassium).[7] Serum and

urine citrate levels ordinarily return to baseline within 4 hours after infusion ceases.[2]

Some effect is also seen from calcium mobilization secondary to increased parathormone secretion during apheresis.[8] Studies have shown that parathormone rises rapidly within 5 to 15 minutes after citrate infusion has begun.[9] A study of seven plateletpheresis donors receiving fixed citrate infusion rates of 66, 84, and 96 mg/kg per hour showed that intact parathormone rises quickly, then levels off or slightly decreases during the remainder of the procedure.[7] Figure 3-2 illustrates the relationship between citrate levels, ionized calcium, and parathormone levels during plateletpheresis.

The net effect of exogenous citrate and endogenous parathormone levels on plasma calcium has been examined in several studies. In general, total calcium decreases most rapidly in the first 15 minutes of a procedure, attaining a 25% decrease by 90 minutes. In one study of platelet donors, however, total calcium declined during the first 15 minutes but increased slightly during the remainder and by 90 minutes was decreased only 6%.[9] Another study,[6] which reported 15 procedures on the Haemonetics Model 10 or Model 30 (Haemonetics Corp, Braintree, MA) using full-strength ACD, found that ionized calcium decreased by 32.4% during plateletpheresis. The average citrate concentration was 26.7 mg/dL in the post-apheresis samples. In 12 procedures using half-strength ACD, the ionized calcium decreased by only 16%, and the citrate concentration increased to only 12.5 mg/dL at the end of the procedure. Another study showed that a citrate infusion rate of 83 mg/kg per hour led to a 23% (±7.6%) fall in the ionized calcium level.[10] Olson et al[6] concluded from similar data that citrate infusion to donors at 65 to 95 mg/kg per hour was safe, although donor symptoms increased when the rate approached 100 mg/kg per hour. Hypomagnesemia contributed occasionally to donor symptoms.

When granulocyte donors received 2% sodium citrate at 3.8 to 5.4 mL/minute for 110 to 200 minutes, ionized calcium reductions and symptoms increased with procedure time. This suggested that, in addition to body weight,

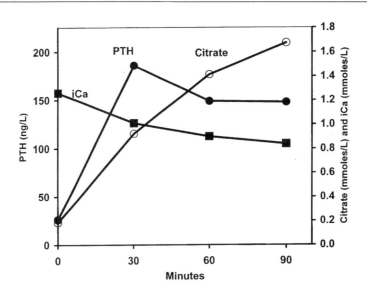

Figure 3-2. Changes in serum concentrations of citrate, calcium, and parathormone during plateletpheresis. Plateletpheresis at 1.4 mg citrate infusion per kg per minute was monitored in donors over 90 minutes. The ionized calcium (iCa) fell continuously over the procedures as the circulating citrate levels continuously increased. Serum levels of intact parathormone (PTH) rose quickly at 30 minutes and then declined, despite progressive decreases in calcium. (Adapted from Bolan et al.[14])

blood volume, and hematocrit, the *duration* of infusion may affect the presence of toxicity.[10] On the basis of this data, in 1993 a panel of experts recommended that citrate infusion be limited to 90 to 110 minutes for platelet collection and to 100 to 200 minutes for granulocyte collection.[10] Newer procedures, such as large-volume progenitor cell collections, sometimes avoid this limitation by supplementing the bag of citrate anticoagulant with heparin, which allows a dramatic reduction in the amount of citrate infused.[11]

Calcium homeostasis has also been studied in therapeutic plasma exchange (TPE). When the replacement is citrate-containing product, such as Fresh Frozen Plasma (FFP) or thawed plasma, TPE involves somewhat higher rates of citrate infusion than plateletpheresis, but the resultant effects on calcium homeostasis are similar. When a calcium-free, citrate-free replacement such as 5% albumin solution is used, the situation becomes more complex. Processed albumin itself can bind ionized calcium

and may account for early "citrate toxicity" during a typical exchange.[2,12] In TPE, much of the infused citrate is discarded with the separated plasma; nonetheless, an exchange still produces a net loss of calcium. In 21 such procedures using either the IBM/COBE 2997 (Caridian-BCT, Lakewood, CO) or the Haemonetics Model 30 on 10 patients with neurologic disease,[8] parathormone levels more than doubled during the procedures; cyclic adenosine monophosphate levels rose as well. Some centers depend on this increase in parathormone to obviate the need for routine supplementary calcium during TPE procedures. However, a number of centers routinely use conservative replacement with calcium gluconate in order to decrease citrate reactions.[11,13,14] Calcium gluconate may be added directly to the 5% albumin used in the procedures. A solution of calcium gluconate and saline may also be run separately with an intravenous pump, although care must be taken when infusing calcium with solutions such as thawed plasma or ceftriaxone, as these may precipitate from solution with severe consequences.[15]

Physiologic Effects of Citrate Infusion in Apheresis

Figure 3-3 illustrates the effects of citrate infusion on levels of serum analytes at the completion of plateletpheresis. The transient hypocalcemia associated with apheresis is usually well tolerated; nevertheless, certain physiologic consequences may be encountered. Decreases in ionized calcium can increase the excitability of nerve cell membranes, reducing the threshold for neural impulse triggering and resulting in spontaneous depolarization. This usually manifests as mild perioral and/or peripheral

paresthesias (ie, tingling sensations). Early investigators of donor plateletpheresis using ACD anticoagulation with the Haemonetics Model 30 reported reactions in the majority of donors (58% to 100%).[5,6,16] Other studies with the Model 30 and less concentrated citrate solutions such as ACD-B, or with continuous flow instruments, noted citrate toxicity in less than one-fourth of donors.[9] A smaller proportion may experience dysgeusia (unusual taste), nausea, and/or lightheadedness. Shivering, twitching, and tremors are rare but have been reported.[5,6]

Patients undergoing therapeutic cytapheresis have similar citrate exposure and presumably have a risk of toxicity comparable to platelet

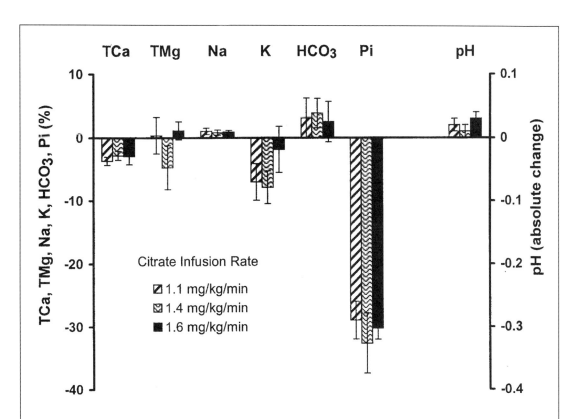

Figure 3-3. The effect of the infusion of citrate anticoagulant and preservative solution on serum analyte levels at the completion of plateletpheresis compared with the levels before plateletpheresis. Changes for total calcium (TCa), total magnesium (TMg), sodium (Na), potassium (K), bicarbonate (HCO₃), and phosphorus (Pi) are expressed as the percentage of change on the left axis. Changes in pH are shown as the absolute change (serum pH at completion minus serum pH before plateletpheresis) on the right axis. Error bars are the standard error of the mean. (Reprinted with permission from Bolan et al.[14])

donors. Conversely, patients receiving FFP replacement in TPE may be exposed to somewhat higher citrate concentrations. Despite their expected net calcium loss, patients receiving 5% albumin replacement have a considerably lower risk of symptomatic hypocalcemia. For example, in 17 patients reported by Rodnitzky and Goeken,[17] only 7.8% of 154 exchanges were associated with symptoms (152 intermittent flow, most with ACD-A), and no "significant" citrate toxicity was seen in the 21 procedures on 10 patients studied by Silberstein et al.[8] Some patients nevertheless may have unusual disease-specific citrate effects, such as intraprocedural worsening of myasthenic weakness.[18]

The threshold for developing symptoms of hypocalcemia depends on the rate of decrease as well as the absolute amount of ionized calcium present. Plasma pH, the presence of sedatives, and concomitant decreases in magnesium, potassium, and/or sodium may also affect the threshold. Severe hypocalcemia may cause continuous muscle contractions, initially as an involuntary carpopedal spasm (adduction of thumbs; extension of interphalangeal joints; and flexion of metacarpophalangeal, wrist, and elbow joints). If ionized hypocalcemia is not corrected, the symptoms can progress to frank tetany with spasms in other muscle groups, including life-threatening laryngospasm. In addition, grand mal seizures have also been reported. Appropriate physical examination may reveal evidence of neuromuscular irritability, such as Chvostek's sign (marked facial twitching when the facial nerve is tapped) and Trousseau's sign (carpal spasm seen with less than 3 minutes of cuff-induced arm ischemia) before the onset of spontaneous muscle spasms. The clinician should be aware that these symptoms and signs can also be seen with alkalosis, especially respiratory alkalosis caused by hyperventilation.[19]

Reductions of ionized calcium seen in apheresis can also lengthen the plateau phase of myocardial depolarization, which leads to QT interval prolongation on electrocardiogram (EKG). Several studies of plateletpheresis donors have documented QT interval prolon-gations averaging 0.07 to 0.08 seconds, or 103% to 113% of baseline, depending on the EKG lead and method of measurement.[5,6,16] Prolongation was generally less in donors who received ACD-B or half-strength ACD-A,[6] but it correlated only moderately well with symptoms and measured decreases in ionized calcium in individual donors.[16] No adverse cardiac consequences from QT interval prolongation were noted in any of these studies. Higher citrate levels can, in other settings, lead to lower ionized calcium levels, resulting in depressed myocardial contractility. In one such study,[20] the citrate infusion rates (between 222 and 444 mg/kg per hour) were several times those in most apheresis procedures, and increases in serum citrate ranged from 2.4 to 4.1 mmol/L (46 to 77 mg/dL). Total calcium was unchanged, but ionized calcium decreased to only 50% of normal, with definitive QT interval prolongation. Pulse rates rose, but stroke volumes and left ventricular work decreased. Mean arterial pressure decreased 16% to 38%, whereas pulse pressure fell 37% to 50%. Cardiac output, measured in five patients, was decreased in three, unchanged in one, and increased in one. Only the patient with the slowest infusion rate (222 mg/kg per hour) showed no change. Such changes have not been reported with apheresis; however, arrhythmias have been associated with deaths during therapeutic apheresis.[1]

Descriptions of citrate concentrations and anticoagulant ratios in the literature can seem confusing or even contradictory. The molar concentration of citrate ion would seem to be the most relevant quantity when discussing potential calcium binding; however, published concentrations may be based on the amount of sodium citrate added to the blood. Most sodium citrate powder comes as a dihydrate, with two water molecules attached. If the water of hydration is not accounted for in calculations based on weight, the results will be inaccurate. Further complicating the matter, ACD formulations contain not only sodium citrate but also citric acid. For example, ACD-A contains 2.2 g of trisodium citrate and 730 mg of citric acid per 100 mL[21]; both species contribute to the concentration of citrate ion, which is approximately 113 mmol/L (see Table 3-1). If one knows what species of citrate molecule is being considered, conversions between mmol/L and mg/dL can be made based on the approximate molecular weights in Daltons. For example, if citrate ion = 189, trisodium citrate = 258, and trisodium citrate dihydrate = 294, conversion from mmol/L to mg/dL can be accomplished by multiplying by 18.9, 25.8, or 29.4, respectively. In this example, ACD-A contains 2136 (113 × 18.9) mg/dL of citrate ion.

Adding to the confusion, the meaning of the phrase "anticoagulant ratio" depends on the investigator and the instrumentation used. For instance, from a mathematical point of view, a 1:13 ratio would describe the addition of one part anticoagulant to 13 parts of blood; the anticoagulant would actually be diluted to 1/14th of its original concentration. The anticoagulant panel on the COBE Spectra Apheresis System (CaridianBCT, Lakewood, CO), however, displays the reciprocal of the dilution and would call this an anticoagulant ratio of 14 (see Tables 3-2 and 3-3). Depending on the author, a "1:13" ratio could be interpreted as 1/13th or

Table 3-2. Example of Anticoagulant (AC) Ratio Determination by the Cobe Spectra Apheresis Machine*

Whole Blood:AC	Dilution Factor	Cobe Spectra "AC Ratio"
7:1	1/8th	8
12:1	1/13th	13
17:1	1/18th	18

*CaridianBCT, Lakewood, CO.

1/14th dilution, which could make a difference when comparing data from two papers using different conventions, especially when trying to extrapolate published ratios for local use.

Farrokhi and colleagues examined 1053 blood samples from 48 donors for the effect of gradual reduction of citrate on platelet clumping and activation of the coagulation cascade as measured by thrombin/antithrombin complex formation.[22] Some platelet clumping was

Table 3-3. Examples of Citrate Concentration and ACD-A Dilution by the Cobe Spectra Apheresis Machine During Apheresis*

| | AC Ratio | Citrate Ion Concentration | |
		mmol/L	mg/mL
Citrate concentration in whole blood	8	14.1	2.7
	13	8.7	1.6
	18	6.3	1.2
Citrate concentration in plasma[†]	8	21.2	4.0
	13	13.4	2.5
	18	9.8	1.9

*Adapted from a presentation by Larry J. Dumont at the American Society for Apheresis 23rd annual meeting, Orlando, FL, May 30, 2002. Used with permission.
[†]Assumes hematocrit = 38%.

observed at an ACD-A ratio of 1:18, and it increased at lower concentrations. There was also an increase in the mean value for thrombin/antithrombin complexes formed at a 1:18 ratio, though with significant variation among individual donors. They concluded that an ACD-A ratio of 1:14 was safe for their study population.

Most published descriptions concerning the incidence and manifestations of citrate toxicity appeared early in the development of apheresis technology and reported experience with ACD-A anticoagulation at a 1:8 ratio and intermittent flow instruments. Symptoms of citrate toxicity typically appeared or worsened during the reinfusion phase, when plasma only slightly diluted with red cells was often reinfused quite rapidly by gravity, producing transiently higher citrate dose rates.[6]

With current instruments, less citrate is added per unit volume of blood, and citrated plasma is returned at a more constant rate, even in intermittent flow procedures. Some instruments limit both dose rate and total citrate infused based on an estimate of subject blood volume calculated from sex, height, and weight. For instance, for the COBE Spectra Apheresis System, the default ACD-A infusion rate for a TPE is 0.8 mL ACD-A per minute per liter of the patient's blood volume (0.8 mL/min/L). The operator can change the inlet pump flow rate or the inlet:anticoagulant ratio to modify the procedure, but the instrument will not allow the citrate infusion rate to exceed a predetermined maximum and may force compensatory changes in the anticoagulant pump rate and/or the total length of the procedure. Because of features like these, modern instruments produce peak citrate and trough ionized calcium levels that are less extreme, with a lower incidence of citrate toxicity. However, significant citrate reactions can still be experienced during donor apheresis if the donor is on the verge of being hypocalcemic before the procedure begins.[23]

Studies of platelet donations on the COBE Spectra showed that total calcium was slightly reduced from 8.85 to 8.27 mg/dL, and ionized calcium was reduced from 4.53 to 3.73 mg/dL.[24] The continuous flow Spectra has also been compared to the older Haemonetics V50 and Model 30 intermittent flow instruments in a study with 49 patients undergoing therapeutic plateletpheresis or leukocyte reduction.[25] Adverse reaction rates were lower with the continuous flow instrument for plateletpheresis (8% vs 10%) and leukapheresis (14% vs 21%). In a study of the Fenwal CS3000 (Fenwal Inc, Lake Zurich, IL) paresthesias were seen in only 14%, a relatively low rate.[26] In a comparison of the Spectra and the CS3000, one study showed that calcium decreased 23% in platelet donors with both instruments, although the Spectra required more ACD-A. Symptoms were slightly less with the CS3000, but no procedures had to be stopped with either instrument.[27]

Comprehensive analyses of citrate effects by Bolan et al[7,14] showed that donor ionized calcium and magnesium levels decreased by means of 33% and 39%, respectively, in plateletpheresis and by means of 35% and 56%, respectively, in leukapheresis. They also confirmed that as citrate infusion rates increase, donor symptoms become more severe. An increase in urinary calcium and magnesium excretion was shown to accompany the renal excretion of a large citrate load.

Management of Citrate-Induced Hypocalcemia

Management of citrate overload during apheresis is straightforward in most cases. Communicative subjects should be asked to report if tingling or numbness is noted anywhere, particularly around the lips. They should also be questioned about paresthesias periodically during the procedure. In a noncommunicative patient, an EKG pattern may be monitored. QT interval prolongation is difficult to quantify and interpret on a monitor screen, but new arrhythmias and QRS interval widening are detectable entities that may be signs of clinically significant reductions in ionized calcium.[3] Where available, STAT ionized calcium levels may be drawn before and during procedures on patients who experience significant symptoms of hypocalcemia. This will help the clinician correlate patient signs and symptoms with the calcium level, monitor response to calcium infusion, and tailor future treatment to the specific patient.

If paresthesias are bothersome, either the total blood flow rate or the rate at which anticoagulant is added to whole blood in the instrument should be reduced. If tingling becomes severe or is associated with nausea, the procedure should be interrupted until symptoms subside and then resumed with a lower citrate flow rate. If unbearable paresthesias, carpopedal spasm, tetany, or EKG changes develop, parenteral calcium supplementation should be considered. Intravenous infusion of up to 10 mL of 10% calcium chloride over 10 to 15 minutes provides up to 273 mg (6.8 mmol = 13.6 mEq) of calcium and will usually correct the deficiency of ionized calcium. An alternative is 10% calcium gluconate, which is only one-third as potent with respect to calcium ions but has less potential for serious adverse events during routine administration.[2] Oral calcium supplementation, either before or during apheresis, may be useful in preventing mild reactions.[28]

In some centers, calcium gluconate is routinely added to 5% albumin infused during TPE. Magnesium and potassium supplementation have also been reported.[29] As early as 1976, it was suggested that supplemental calcium administration would be of benefit.[30] However, some experts believe that calcium should not be administered unless there are significant signs of hypocalcemia that cannot be treated in other ways (such as slowing down the procedure or changing the citrate ratio).[8]

A study of 636 TPEs using albumin replacement (predominantly in patients with neurologic disease) concluded that supplementation of the return fluid with calcium gluconate is an effective, convenient, and well-tolerated method for the prevention of citrate toxicity during therapeutic plasma exchange procedures using albumin-based return fluid.[31] Patients were assigned to one of three groups. The first group did not receive any intravenous calcium, and the second group received only small, periodic calcium boluses by intravenous drip in response to, or to prevent, reactions. These two groups experienced reactions 41% of the time, but this number fell to 24% in the third group, which received constant calcium infusion (10 mL of 10% calcium gluconate per liter of return fluid). The numbers of adverse events attributed to hypocalcemia were 32%, 25%, and 9%, respectively, in the three groups. The highest proportion of adverse events was seen in younger women (under age 50). These results must be interpreted with caution, however, as the study was not randomized or blinded, and the reaction rates in all categories were significantly higher than those reported elsewhere.

Bolan et al reported a 96% reduction in clinically significant paresthesias during peripheral blood stem cell donation by using calcium infusions (1 mmol Ca/10 mmol citrate; ie, 0.5 mg of calcium ion for every mL of ACD-A used).[14] Another study reported a 9-fold decrease in symptoms of hypocalcemia during TPE with calcium prophylaxis.[32] The prophylactic administration of calcium during therapeutic procedures is becoming more common, although a rigorous study is still needed to prove that it is beneficial in TPE.

In summary, hypocalcemia is the most common adverse event associated with anticoagulation use during TPE. This results mainly from 1) infusion of citrate anticoagulant, 2) infusion of calcium-avid albumin solutions, and/or 3) infusion of citrate-rich FFP.[12] The symptoms of hypocalcemia increase with the concentration of citrate used, the rate of infusion, and the duration of the procedure.

Hypomagnesemia

Citrate can chelate magnesium as well as calcium. In a study evaluating intravenous magnesium supplementation during large-volume progenitor cell collections, mean ionized magnesium levels fell 39% below baseline in the nonsupplemented group and 7.4% in the supplemented group.[33] Baseline ionized magnesium levels were lower with each successive procedure. Magnesium supplementation reduced the fall in ionized magnesium levels, but the clinical significance of this is not clear. Magnesium supplementation during large-volume collections is associated with a more pronounced parathyroid hormone response to lowered calcium levels[31]; however, it has not been shown to decrease mild citrate-related symptoms. Prophylactic magnesium supplementation is not recommended for plateletpheresis donations. Magnesium infusions may be considered in pediatric patients, in patients who have hypomagnesemia before a procedure, and possibly when repetitive large-volume procedures are anticipated in adults.[29,33]

Alkalosis

Metabolism of citrate consumes hydrogen ions. In patients with renal disease whose maximal bicarbonate excretion rate is reduced, infusion of citrate often leads to metabolic alkalosis.[34] This is observed with TPE, usually when the replacement fluid is FFP.[3,35] In addition to requiring increased respiratory work to maintain pH, alkalosis might make patients *more susceptible* to symptoms of hypocalcemia and could slow citrate metabolism.[3] Signs and symptoms might also include rapid breathing, headache, fatigue, nausea, vomiting, and diarrhea. Alkalosis induced by a citrate load from an apheresis procedure will resolve with time or dialysis. Once recognized, alkalosis may be minimized in subsequent procedures by adding less citrate for anticoagulation and, where clinically feasible, choosing noncitrated replacement fluids.[35]

Heparin Anticoagulation

Heparin anticoagulation can also be used during an apheresis procedure. Adequate anticoagulation requires a plasma heparin concentration of 0.5 to 2.0 IU/mL, which is roughly the same range (though extending somewhat higher) required for therapeutic heparinization in hospitalized patients (eg, for deep venous thrombosis). Heparin prevents clotting by potentiating the activity of plasma antithrombin at least 1000-fold. Antithrombin is a serine proteinase inhibitor (serpin) that inactivates Factors II, IX,

and X, which are important in the coagulation cascade. Heparin generally has low toxicity when given temporarily, as in an apheresis procedure. It has long been used in open-heart surgery during cardiac bypass and also in intensive care units to prevent coagulation in vascular access devices. Furthermore, if given in excess, it can be reversed by protamine.

Although heparin can be used with apheresis, it is not typically used in the United States, Canada, and northern Europe unless the separation method requires it (eg, Kaneka Liposober LDL-apheresis system, Kaneka America, New York, NY). Heparin's anticoagulant properties are neutralized by normal plasma, so that if blood were collected in heparin, it would need to be transfused within a short period. Therefore, it is a poor choice for anticoagulation of blood components derived from apheresis. Heparin enjoyed some use in the early days of therapeutic apheresis, but it has generally fallen out of favor because of the systemic anticoagulant impact on the patient and recently recognized side effects such as heparin-induced thrombocytopenia.[36] It has been suggested that the use of heparin flushes for maintaining central venous catheter patency might be avoided by the use of saline with or without specialized line caps or flushing techniques.[37] The addition of heparin into the bag containing citrate anticoagulant during an apheresis procedure allows the amount of citrate used in the procedure to be greatly reduced, thus providing more options for patients that experience severe reactions with citrate or those needing large-volume treatments (eg, certain progenitor cell collection protocols).

Fluid Shifts

The second major category of physiologic responses to apheresis is fluid shifts. These occur when whole blood is removed, one or another component is retained, and remaining components are returned, with or without a replacement product. Resultant changes in intravascular volume can induce hemodynamic alterations. Dilutional effects on plasma constituent levels may also be seen, especially in therapeutic procedures (see Chapter 14).

Hemodynamic Changes

Fluid overload may be a problem for patients with cardiac or renal impairment. In other situations, such as patients suffering malaise from a gastrointestinal or respiratory infection, hypovolemia may be a concern. There is a general sense that hemodynamic changes are more common with intermittent flow centrifugation than with continuous flow procedures. This probably relates to the greater extracorporeal volume associated with earlier models of intermittent flow machines. Newer machines attempt a "gentler" fluctuation in extravascular and intravascular volumes. A volume of blood in excess of 500 mL may be removed from the subject at the beginning of an apheresis procedure to prime the tubing, fill the centrifugal element, and fill any columns. The actual volume removed depends on the instrument, the procedure, and possibly even the hematocrit (in discontinuous machines using the Latham bowl). Examples of approximate extracorporeal volumes for various machines are as follows: 340 to 490 mL for the Fenwal CS3000, 169 mL for the Fresenius AS 104 (Fresenius AG, Bad Homburg, Germany), 170 mL for the Cobe Spectra, and 245 mL for the Haemonetics MCS+.[38]

Different procedures may produce differing hemodynamic effects. In simple plateletpheresis, a relatively small net volume deficit (approximately 300 mL plasma) develops gradually over 60 to 100 minutes. In leukapheresis, a somewhat larger volume of plasma may be removed along with the leukocytes, although infusion of a sedimenting agent with volume-expanding properties tends to offset this. Similarly, hematopoietic progenitor cell apheresis may remove a substantial amount of plasma. In plasmapheresis for source plasma (for manufacture of derivatives) or for apheresis donation of both platelets and plasma, 500 to 800 mL of plasma may be retained. The total volume removed in the latter procedures exceeds that removed during a whole blood donation; symp-

toms of hypovolemia may occur in these donors unless replacement fluid is given.

Nomograms based on height, weight, and hematocrit are used to predict the consequences of volume removal. Techniques vary as to whether saline replacement is given routinely, but if needed, it can be given more readily during an apheresis donation than during a whole blood donation. These matters are discussed further in Chapters 6 and 13.

Dilutional Effects

It is in TPE, where plasma is removed and replaced with substitution fluids, that the greatest potential exists for volume shifts and dilutional effects. These topics are considered in greater detail in Chapter 15; however, a summary of important concepts is presented here.

The equation that describes the removal of a substance of interest in TPE is

$$\frac{y}{y_0} = e^{-x}$$

where
y = final concentration,
y_0 = the initial concentration,
e = base of natural logarithm, and
x = number of times the patient's total plasma volume is exchanged.

The equation assumes that no reequilibration of the substance with extravascular stores occurs and that there is no additional synthesis. Further, it predicts that 37% (roughly one-third) of the initial quantity will remain at the end of a one-volume exchange, with 22% and 14% remaining at 1.5 and 2 volumes exchanged, respectively. Reequilibration does occur for some substances, reducing the apparent efficiency of removal.

A replacement fluid that can exert oncotic pressure—usually containing protein and/or complex carbohydrate (eg, pentastarch or hetastarch)—must be infused to replace the plasma that was removed. Four- to five-percent albumin solution in saline has become a popular replacement solution; it provides protein and, thereby, oncotic activity, and it is processed to prevent transmission of infection.[39] Five-percent albumin exerts an oncotic pressure that draws a small amount of extra fluid into vascular space by conclusion of the procedure. The French Apheresis Registry reports that a combination of pentastarch and albumin replacement gave the best results in a retrospective study analyzing 46,000 TPE procedures.[40] It has been suggested that pentastarch is preferable to hetastarch for use as a nonprotein oncotically-active replacement fluid during apheresis.[41] One study has suggested that pentastarch may be suitable for partial colloid replacement during the first half of TPE.[42] However, there are proponents of routinely using 3% hetastarch during the first part of the procedure, with albumin used in the latter part.[43,44] Replacement with FFP should be avoided unless it is 1) specifically indicated to treat a disease such as thrombotic thrombocytopenic purpura (TTP), 2) required to correct a plasma factor deficiency, or 3) required to prevent dilutional coagulopathy in a patient who is actively bleeding (eg, pulmonary renal syndrome).

When patient plasma is replaced during TPE with a solution other than plasma, four patterns of constituent removal have been reported in a study that sampled participants immediately before and after TPE with 5% albumin. The patterns vary based on how changes in measured concentration compare with predictions by the above equation.[45] In the first pattern, seen with fibrinogen, concentration decreases slightly more than predicted. A different pattern is seen with IgG and IgM, for which concentration changes essentially as predicted. In the third pattern, seen with the enzymes serum alanine aminotransferase, lactate dehydrogenase, and creatine phosphokinase, concentration decreases somewhat less than predicted, suggesting some reequilibration. A fourth pattern is seen with small inorganic solutes; their concentrations decrease much less than predicted because of rapid reequilibration with extravascular and/or intracellular fluids. This information can be useful for understanding adverse effects, as discussed

in Chapter 15. For example, patients rarely become hypokalemic during TPE, even when replacement solutions contain no potassium.

Most nonimmunoglobulin proteins recover to nearly 100% of baseline within 48 to 72 hours after TPE. The recovery of fibrinogen depends greatly on production, which may vary considerably, as it is an acute-phase protein. If TPE is performed at intervals greater than 72 hours, FFP replacement is almost never required. In contrast, FFP may be required if treatments are performed on more than 2 or 3 consecutive days because fibrinogen may be depleted. An overshoot phenomenon, in which the concentration of a particular analyte increases after plasma exchange because of increased synthesis, is uncommon.[46] However, during treatment of hyperglobulinemic patients, reequilibration after exchange often leads to rapid recovery of serum immunoglobulin levels.

Management of volume replacement has several subtle pitfalls. For example, up to two-thirds of the anticoagulant volume may be retained in removed plasma; therefore, a corresponding portion of the measured "volume removed" is not really plasma and need not be replaced. Clinicians familiar with dialysis procedures may request that fluid be "taken off" by TPE, but hypovolemic exchanges should be performed with great caution. Because plasma exchange modulates only intravascular volume, it has very different effects in reducing volume than has hemoperfusion or hemodialysis. Severe hypotension can occur with hypovolemic exchanges, even in patients who initially have volume overload.

Drug Interactions and Clearance

Because plasma exchange involves removal of plasma, pharmaceutical agents in the plasma may be removed in significant amounts.[47] Two situations in which this might be clinically relevant are 1) the potential use of plasma exchange in the setting of overdose and 2) the potential of plasma exchange to adversely affect therapeutic levels of medications.

The removal of pharmacologic agents by TPE has been documented for aspirin, tobramycin, phenytoin, propranolol, vancomycin, and many others.[48,49] The amount removed depends on the volume of distribution of the drug (intravascular vs other), the half-life of the drug in the circulation, and whether the agent is administered immediately before or during apheresis. For example, only about 1% of prednisone is removed by apheresis,[50] whereas therapeutic agents that remain in the circulation, such as intravenous immunoglobulin, will be removed in proportion to the amount of plasma processed and the efficiency of the procedure.

Ibrahim and colleagues examined the National Library of Medicine's PubMed/Medline database of the literature on the effects of plasma exchange on pharmaceutical agents over a 10-year period.[49] They suggest that many of the pharmacologic parameters typically used to describe drug clearance do not easily lend themselves to determination of the amount of drug removed. The most reliable method would be to quantify the drug in the removed plasma, but this is difficult and is not often done. They suggest that when there is no reliable data on the drug in question, as is often the case, the volume of distribution of the drug along with the amount of protein binding and the temporal association of drug administration with the apheresis treatment may be used to help predict the degree to which the drug may be eliminated. However, estimated removal of a circulating drug does not always correlate with measurements of drug concentration in the blood after plasma exchange. Other variables include drug elimination by the body, the duration of plasma exchange, the volume of plasma removed, and the frequency of plasma exchange.[49,51]

Kintzel et al recommend that antimicrobial agents be administered after plasma exchange, as this is when it can be reasonably assumed that intravascular drug concentration is at its lowest because extravascular tissue distribution from the previous dose has already occurred.[51] If the drug exerts its desired effect quickly, then removal by TPE may not be as clinically important. One example of this is rituximab, which clears CD20-positive B-lymphocytes from the circulation shortly after a single dose, even though this humanized antibody remains detectable in the circulation for days. Certainly, waiting as long as possible after administration of this type of drug before performing TPE would be advised. Physicians should be very cautious using apheresis on patients who are actively undergoing a course of cancer chemotherapy because no data exist on whether the course would be compromised by plasma exchange.

Cellular Loss

As large volumes of donor or patient blood circulate through an apheresis device, blood cells are intentionally or incidentally removed. The effects of single apheresis procedures have been studied extensively, especially in the setting of platelet donation, the most frequently performed cytapheresis procedure.

Plateletpheresis

In a 1981 study of 352 donors where the Haemonetics Model 30 was used, the postapheresis platelet count was below $100,000/\mu L$ in 2.7% of donors. If a preprocedure count above $150,000/\mu L$ was required, 3.7% of donors were deferred, but platelet counts dropped below $100,000/\mu L$ in only 1.3% of those drawn. Return to baseline was seen in 4 days, and a rebound increase above the baseline was seen 8 to 11 days after the procedure.[52] It has subsequently become clear that the rapid removal of platelets by apheresis leads to replenishment of the circulating pool from the spleen.[53]

Studies of plateletpheresis on healthy donors with the COBE Spectra at the time of its introduction[24] showed that mean pre- and postdonation platelet counts were $288,000/\mu L$ and $217,000/\mu L$, respectively, whereas mean white blood cell (WBC) counts dropped from $7000/\mu L$ to $6120/\mu L$. Mean hematocrit decreased from 44.9% to 43.6%, whereas mean hemoglobin increased slightly from 14.06 g/dL to

14.79 g/dL, and the mean red cell count was unchanged.

The Fenwal CS3000 was studied in 63 donors undergoing platelet collection. Comparison of pre- and postprocedure values showed mean platelet counts of 234,000 and 182,000/µL and mean hematocrits of 42% and 40%, respectively; there were no changes in WBCs.[26] Another study of 107 procedures on the CS3000 indicated that the platelet count was reduced by a mean of 19%.[54]

Another group has shown that extended collection procedures[55] (120 minutes in men and 140 minutes in women) for donors with low normal platelet counts decreased those counts by means of 34% in men and 45% in women. When the mean postprocedure count was 119,000/µL (±18,000), counts fell below 100,000/µL in 10 of 89 procedures, with the lowest postprocedure count being 69,000/µL. With a higher mean preprocedure count of 180,000/µL, the percentage of decrease was 37% to a mean postprocedure count of 124,000/µL (±14,000). The absolute lymphocyte count fell below 1000/µL in only 1 of 99 donations. The authors noted that historical counts and actual counts may not correlate. The safety of doing these extended procedures appeared to be demonstrated.

The thrust of all these studies is that individual apheresis donation procedures produce only modest decreases in circulating blood cell counts, which are not associated with any immediate toxicity. Although there is a theoretical risk for donors that leave with platelet counts less than 100,000/µL (for example, excess bleeding if involved in a motor vehicle accident), in healthy blood donors that have already been screened for bleeding diatheses and antiplatelet medications, this is likely very small.

There has been concern regarding the effect of regular, long-term plateletpheresis donations on the donor. These concerns include decreased lymphocyte counts with the possibility of inducing an immunodeficient state.[56] Studies of plateletpheresis donors have suggested that the impact of frequent long-term donation is minimal in terms of well-being. One large study[56] looked at samples drawn 3 weeks after the lat-

est procedure from 50 apheresis donors who had donated at least 25 times (range = 25 to 102) over a 3- to 9-year period, with a maximum of 12 procedures in any 1 year. There were 1743 plateletpheresis procedures and 206 granulocyte procedures on the Model 30, the V50 (without surge), and the CS3000. No significant changes were found in hemoglobin, platelet count, or WBC count with serial donation. Absolute lymphocyte counts were lower in apheresis donors compared with frequent whole blood donors, and there were more lymphocytopenic donors in the apheresis group. There was also a decrease in CD4+ cells. There was no difference in suppressor cells (CD8+), but the T4:T8 ratio was diminished. Responses to mitogens and alloantigens were not different, except that cytapheresis donors had lesser responses to phytohemagglutinin (PHA). Iron deficiency was less frequent in cytapheresis donors than in whole blood donors.

In another study, 25 volunteer donors who had undergone plateletpheresis 72 times on the Model 30 in periods of up to 8 years were compared with 25 age-matched controls. T cells, particularly those bearing the T4, T8, and Leu-7 antigens, were decreased, as was the T4:T8 ratio. T4-, T8-, and T11-positive cells appeared to be removed preferentially, and the T4- and T8-cell decreases were proportional to the number of donations. PHA and concanavalin A responsiveness was decreased but still within normal limits.[57]

In yet another study, 58 veteran donors were followed over 2 to 4 years in 1023 consecutive platelet donations that used the Fenwal CS3000 and Haemonetics V50.[58] The study examined donors who started with low lymphocyte counts. Lymphocyte counts below 1200/µL were found in 4.9% of donors, as predicted for a normal population (5%). No evidence of immune dysfunction was seen. In a different study, however, donors with 10 weekly platelet donations on the Model 30 showed a 20% decrease in lymphocytes, with a significant decrease in B cells in half the cases.

Twenty long-term platelet donors who had donated on the CS3000, V50, Spectra, and IBM 2997 dual-stage channel were compared with 29 whole blood donors and 27 nondonor controls. No significant differences were found among the groups in WBC counts, in percentages or absolute numbers of lymphocytes, or in percentages or absolute numbers of cells in lymphocyte subsets. There was also no difference when platelet donors with fewer than 45 lifetime donations were compared with those with more than 45. It was concluded that there are no significant immunologic changes associated with long-term plateletpheresis at the currently allowed donation frequency in the United States.[59]

Richa and colleagues examined the effect on platelet and WBC counts of double- and triple-apheresis donation of platelets.[60] A small but statistically significant *increase* in platelet count was seen (rather than a decrease) as the total number of apheresis platelet products collected per donor increased. A small decrease in lymphocyte count was seen, but the median lymphocyte count for each donor was within the normal range. The study authors concluded that limitations on the number of plateletpheresis products donated within 12 months do not seem warranted because of platelet or lymphocyte count changes.[60]

Thus, studies of cell depletion in platelet donors have generally shown no detrimental effects, and lymphocyte counts in most donors remain normal or near normal even with frequent donation.[59] In studies with older equipment, some of the donors showed lymphocyte counts lower than those of control subjects, but most were still in the normal range, and there was no clinical evidence of immune dysfunction. Current cell separators remove far fewer leukocytes so that yearly loss of lymphocytes with maximal donation is equivalent to loss with whole blood donations.[59]

In one report, a platelet donor donated for her sister 101 times over a 33-month period on the Haemonetics Model 30.[61] She had two machine-related complications, including the loss of one red cell unit and 150 mL of plasma. Her platelet count was reduced but still normal, and she developed mild anemia with iron deficiency. Her hepatic enzymes had increased but returned to normal during continued apheresis,

and no significant protein or immunoglobulin changes were seen. Six months after the donations, the donor was healthy and well. This reinforces the evidence that repeated plateletpheresis procedures are safe, with minimal chance of long-term effects. One study even suggested that selective recruitment of borderline anemic donors for plateletpheresis can be done safely, offering an alternative donation opportunity to otherwise excluded volunteer blood donors.[62]

Collection of Hematopoietic Progenitor Cells by Apheresis

Like plateletpheresis, large-volume leukapheresis for progenitor cell ("stem cell") collections in patients, discussed further in Chapter 24, has also been shown to be well tolerated.[14,63] Declines in hematocrit and platelet count may be seen, however. In a study involving daily collections, the platelet count decreased by 61% from baseline on day 1, by 75% on day 2, and by 81% on day 3.[63] In another study,[64] total WBC and lymphocyte counts were maintained, but there was a transient fall in platelet count at the end of 5 days on intensive schedules. A more recent study[65] of progenitor cell collection in healthy donors mobilized with granulocyte colony-stimulating factor (G-CSF) showed that platelet, neutrophil, and red cell counts decreased. Thrombocytopenia continued for 7 days, but platelet counts had recovered by 2 to 3 weeks after collection. Physiologic effects of G-CSF likely also contributed to the decrease in platelet counts. Although none of these decreases was clinically significant, platelet counts should probably continue to be monitored in this setting.[65]

Plasma Protein Interactions

Plasma contains enzymes and enzyme systems that can theoretically be activated during apheresis by contact with foreign surfaces. Activation of the clotting cascade is prevented by the anticoagulant, but other systems have also been of concern.

Filtration leukapheresis, in which heparinized donor blood flows over nylon fiber filters, has resulted in substantial activation of complement.[66] This was eventually linked to troublesome adverse effects such as priapism and peroneal pain, and it led to abandonment of the technique. Similar effects on complement were discovered with some plasma separator membranes.[67,68] These were more prominent with heparin anticoagulation and could be partially suppressed by the addition of citrate. Other studies have confirmed a lack of complement activation during centrifugation leukapheresis with hydroxyethyl starch.[69] Screening for complement activation has since become an integral part of the licensing evaluation for materials in apheresis instrument blood paths.

More recently, activation of enzymes in the kinin system has been discovered in association with the protein A immunoadsorption column and selective depletion columns for low-density lipoprotein removal, as well as during TPE, possibly, using some earlier albumin and/or plasma protein fraction lots.[70] Angiotensin-converting enzyme (ACE) inhibitors are relatively contraindicated in therapeutic procedures, as patients who take these medications may have decreased ability to inactivate bradykinin, which can lead to flushing, hypotension, and/or respiratory distress. In a record review of 299 consecutive patients undergoing TPE over a 13-year period, 14 patients were receiving ACE inhibitors at the time of apheresis. All 14 experienced atypical reactions, but only 20 of the remaining 285 patients experienced atypical reactions.[70] Preliminary data suggest that in certain patients experiencing hypotension, a metabolic anomaly of bradykinin metabolism may be involved.[71] This is a relative contraindication because the benefit of receiving a lifesaving apheresis treatment may outweigh the risks incurred when a patient experiences an atypical reaction.

Adverse Effects

Physiologic trends expected with apheresis can sometimes become severe enough to qualify as adverse effects. Those associated with citrate infusion and fluid shifts have been already discussed. Other adverse effects involve more radical departures from normal homeostasis, sometimes because of errors or avoidable risks. The remainder of this chapter discusses potential adverse effects of apheresis, principally from an etiologic standpoint. A more detailed discussion of the management of adverse effects can be found in Chapters 5, 12, and 14.

Vasovagal Reactions

Vasovagal reactions, the most common reactions seen with whole blood donation, are also observed during and after apheresis.[72] They generally manifest as pallor and diaphoresis, with associated hypotension and bradycardia. A full-blown attack appears to result from a combination of several interacting peripheral and central alterations, including imbalances in autonomic tone.[73] The following progression is often observed: 1) pallor and sweating begin, with the skin turning cold; 2) the pulse slows strikingly, sometimes to as low as 30 beats per minute; and 3) the blood pressure falls. More severe vasovagal reactions may progress to nausea, vomiting, and syncope, with involuntary defecation and/or convulsions. Vasovagal effects are more commonly seen in first-time donors and are thought to be less frequent with apheresis than with whole blood donation.[72] The slow pulse rate is the most useful sign in differentiating vasovagal effects from hypovolemia. Attacks are best treated by maintaining the donor or patient in a supine position with the head lower than the legs (Trendelenberg position). Further removal of blood should be postponed until the reaction is reversed.

Vascular Access

Adverse effects related to vascular access are a frequent concern. Hematoma, venous sclerosis, and thrombosis can complicate percutaneous needle puncture and may be more frequent with apheresis than with whole blood donation because of the longer indwelling time of the needle. Venipuncture is nonetheless the preferred means of access for all apheresis procedures and the only allowable method for most voluntary donations.

If venipuncture is not possible, insertion of an artificial access device may be indicated for patient procedures. As the catheter represents the single greatest risk factor for adverse events,[74] it should be avoided whenever possible. In one large series of studies,[75] unsatisfactory arm veins were seen in only 4.4% of patients, and only 5.4% of procedures were terminated because of access problems, although 20.7% required an additional venipuncture. The investigators concluded that arm veins should be used in most cases unless there is a clear need for access by artificial means. Subclavian vein catheterization has been found in one series[74] to carry a 0.98% risk of pneumothorax and a 0.02% risk of subcutaneous emphysema. The internal jugular and femoral veins may also be used. Sepsis and thrombosis are the complications of most concern in indwelling catheters, although experimental use of antibiotics in the line has reduced catheter-related infection.[76] Central lines are more likely to be needed in patients requiring frequent procedures over extended periods of time (eg, with TTP or pulmonary-renal syndrome) or with decreased muscle tone and/or autonomic instability (eg, myasthenic crisis, acute Guillain-Barré syndrome).[77,78] A more detailed discussion of vascular access catheters is found in Chapter 13.

Comparison of Therapeutic Apheresis, Donor Apheresis, and Whole Blood Donation

As might be expected, the overall rate of adverse effects is higher in therapeutic apheresis than in donor apheresis. This has been confirmed by several studies and surveys. One report surveyed 2418 procedures in 570 subjects using the Haemonetics PCS and V50, the Dideco instrument (Dideco, Mirandola Modena, Italy), the CS3000, and the Aminco Celltrifuge (Aminco, Silver Spring, MD). Therapeutic plasmapheresis was performed in 926 procedures on 181 patients, whereas therapeutic cytapheresis was performed in 305 procedures on 89 patients. Apheresis donations accounted for 1187 procedures. Only 11.6% of donors had reactions in 4.2% of procedures, although there were 225 complications in 107 patients for an overall incidence of 15.9% of procedures and 39.6% of patients. Hemodynamic effects, mostly vasovagal, accounted for 38% of the reactions in TPE, whereas 27% were attributed to citrate effects, 20% involved a technical problem, 9% were allergic reactions, and 6% were considered as miscellaneous. In therapeutic cytapheresis, 44% of reactions were citrate related, 25% were technical, 14% circulatory, 11% allergic, and 6% miscellaneous. In platelet donors, circulatory effects, mostly vasovagal, accounted for 51% of all reactions, whereas 36% were technical problems and 13% had other causes.[79]

In a survey study conducted by the Hemapheresis Committee of the AABB in 1995, data were received on immediate adverse events of 19,611 apheresis donation procedures. Ignoring expected minor citrate reactions, nonvenipuncture adverse-effect rates for donations of platelets, granulocytes, and plasma were 1.05%, 0.67%, and 0.37%, respectively.[72] In reports from United Blood Services (Blood Systems, Inc) comparing donor apheresis with whole blood donation, adverse event data were collected on over 1,000,000 whole blood and 380,000 donor apheresis procedures.[80] The authors concluded that automated collections are as safe as, or safer than, manual whole blood collections, with few concerns when procedures are performed according to manufacturers' instructions.[80,81]

Complications of Therapeutic Plasma Exchange

Immediate Complications

Several studies have focused on the adverse effects of TPE, because this is the most commonly performed therapeutic procedure. One study comprised 381 procedures in 63 patients who had 1.5 plasma volume exchanges for neurologic diseases, using the Fenwal CS3000,

COBE Spectra, Haemonetics PCS, or Fenwal Autopheresis C. It showed complications in 17% of procedures and in 49% of patients treated. Most adverse effects were either mild (55.4%) or moderate (35.4%) and did not prevent completion of the procedure. Citrate reactions and autonomic instability were the most frequent, as might be expected in patients with neurologic disease. Reactions were severe in 6.4% of procedures, with two fatalities: one was caused by catheter placement and the other by a cerebral hemorrhage that was probably disease related. Most of the severe events were related to catheter placement. Hypofibrinogenemia occurred in 11 patients, but bleeding was seen in only one patient, after the third exchange. Reversible hypotension was seen in four patients, and two had vasovagal syncope. Citrate effects led to nausea in seven instances and vomiting in two. No intravenous calcium was used in this group. There was one incident of urticaria, and one case each of staphylococcal bacteremia and hemopneumothorax.[82]

Adverse effects were studied in 17 patients with neurologic diseases who underwent 154 TPEs (152 on the Model 30 and 2 on the IBM 2997). Citrate reactions were seen in 7.8%, hypotension in 2.6%, and scotomata suggesting embolism in 1.3%. There was one case each of cardiac arrhythmia, fatal myocardial infarction, and hemolysis caused by a tubing problem. Fibrinogen was reduced to 58% at the end of procedures, and platelets dropped by 18%, but there were no serious infections.[17]

In the Canadian experience of 5235 procedures, there were adverse effects in 612 procedures (12%), with 40% of patients treated having at least one adverse event. Fever, chills, urticaria, muscle cramps, and paresthesias accounted for the majority. Hypotension was seen more often with the Haemonetics Model 30 (73 out of 1903) than with the COBE Spectra (31 out of 1931). Twenty-eight of the reactions were severe, including one cardiac arrest and two respiratory arrests. Five late deaths were recorded but deemed not to be procedure related.[83] An update of the Canadian data based on more than 80,000 TPE procedures

shows the rate of severe reactions fell from 0.8% to 0.3%.[84]

A 1996 review[85] of adverse reactions to TPE in Guillain-Barré syndrome identified a reduction from 12% in 1986 to 7% in 1992. Allergic reactions and hypotension were most common. Autonomic dysfunction caused by disease may be exacerbated by the apheresis, and mortality arising from this is estimated at 1 to 2 per 10,000 sessions in international registries. Bradycardia with cardiac consequences is of concern. However, similar autonomic dysfunction can occur independently of TPE and may be reduced if exchange therapy ameliorates the underlying disease.[78]

Seventy-one consecutive patients treated for TTP-HUS were followed prospectively for complications.[77] Thirty percent had major complications, including two deaths (from hemorrhage after line insertion and systemic infection). Minor complications occurred in 31% of patients, and 39% had no complications. The 27 major complications reported included hemorrhage after line insertion (2), pneumothorax (1), systemic infection (12), catheter thrombosis (7), venous thrombosis (2), hypoxemia and hypotension (2), and serum sickness (1).

The Swedish therapeutic apheresis registry reported data on 14,000 procedures performed between 1996 and 1999.[86] No fatalities occurred. Adverse events occurred in approximately 4% of procedures: 22% were paresthesias; 21%, hypotensive events; 14%, urticaria; 7%, nausea; and 7%, shivering.

One of the largest registry databases, the French Registry for Plasma Exchange, reported information on 126,770 therapeutic procedures on 14,183 patients.[40] The total number of early complications decreased from 11.9% in 1985 to 4.6% in 1998. This was attributed to improvement of the technical quality of TPE and use of albumin plus a nonalbumin colloid combination for replacement. The most common complication was symptomatic hypocalcemia; for instance, in 8135 procedures during 1998, there were 109 cases, with an overall reaction rate of 1.3%. A subset of cases replaced with albumin alone had a hypocalcemia rate of 1.7%. Other early complications (from most to least frequent) included allergic reactions, hypotension, hematoma at the access site, fever and chills, hemolysis, and nausea/vomiting.

A survey conducted by AABB looked at the frequency of immediate adverse effects associated with 3429 therapeutic procedures.[87] A total of 242 adverse events were reported in 163 procedures, for a rate of 4.75% overall (6.87% of first-time procedures and 4.28 % of repeat procedures). The incidence of transfusion reaction was 1.6%—nearly all in patients receiving plasma. Other documented events include citrate-related nausea/vomiting (1.2%), hypotension (1.0%), vasovagal nausea/vomiting (0.5%), pallor and/or diaphoresis (0.5%), tachycardia (0.4%), respiratory distress (0.3%), tetany or seizure (0.2%), and chills or rigors (0.2%). Rates for other events were 0.1% or less. Procedure-specific immediate adverse event rates were 10.3% for red cell exchange, 7.8% for TPE with plasma replacement, 3.4% for TPE without plasma, 5.7% for leukapheresis, and 1.7% for autologous stem cell collection. No adverse events were reported in 18 therapeutic plateletpheresis procedures.

Delayed Complications

Delayed complications can also be seen in TPE.[88] These include hemorrhage and thrombosis, viral infection related to FFP infusion, bacterial infections related to the catheter, anemia, and hypoproteinemia.

Mortality and Morbidity

Huestis reported a retrospective literature review including a total of 50 deaths reported associated with therapeutic apheresis. Sixty percent of deaths were classified as cardiac (16) or respiratory (14—all having received FFP). Other associated causes of death included anaphylactic reactions (3—1 TPE with albumin replacement and 2 with FFP), sepsis (2), pulmonary embolism (3), vascular perforations (3), and hemorrhagic disseminated intravascular coagulation (2). There were two late deaths from hepatitis in

exchanged patients who received donor plasma, and five deaths with incomplete data.[89] It was striking that FFP replacement increased the risks of mortality as well as of morbidity. Thus, restoration of immunoglobulins, coagulation factors, and other plasma proteins may not compensate for the adverse effects associated with plasma replacement. Nonfatal pyrogen reactions to albumin have been reported,[90] so although albumin replacement significantly reduces problems caused by replacement fluids, it does not totally eliminate them. With stricter adherence to established indications, and the realization that therapeutic apheresis is not a totally benign procedure, it was suggested that the actual fatality rate may be lower than the 3/10,000 reported in 1983.[89] The French registry calculated an overall mortality between 1/10,000 and 2/10,000.[40,91] The Swedish registry reported no fatalities in over 14,000 procedures.[86] Morbidity and mortality related to therapeutic procedures is greater in acutely ill patients treated in a hospital setting than in "routine" patients treated in an outpatient setting. This can often be directly attributed to the underlying disease.

Coagulopathy

When plasma is exchanged for a nonplasma replacement solution, coagulopathy caused by dilution of coagulation factors is a potential problem. Regardless of the replacement fluid used, coagulation testing in the hours after apheresis should be avoided, as the tests may be artifactually prolonged by the procedure. Waiting until the next morning to draw coagulation studies may give a better picture of the actual state of coagulation and prevent unnecessary angst for house staff or surgeons. A fibrinogen level is always useful in evaluating prolonged clotting tests in an apheresis patient. Though the removal of fibrinogen can be accurately predicted, the production of this acute-phase protein varies greatly among patients. When fibrinogen drops much below 100 mg/dL, clotting times may be prolonged in the absence of any other factor deficiency. In a patient with an extremely prolonged activated partial thromboplastin time (aPTT), it is not infrequently discovered that the specimen was drawn through a heparinized catheter. Potential coagulopathy is discussed in greater detail in Chapter 15 and in other specific contexts; however, the results of three studies are presented here.

In a group of 10 patients, the prothrombin time (PT) and aPTT increased after TPE and returned to baseline within 24 to 72 hours. After 24 hours, fibrinogen was still 52% below baseline, and it remained 32% below baseline at 72 hours. Platelet counts were also below normal after an exchange, but they were below baseline by only 11.4% at 24 hours and by 13.4% at 72 hours. No clinical bleeding was seen in the study, although it had been prompted by postprocedure bleeding in two previous patients.[92]

Hemostatic effects were also studied in 40 TPEs on 26 patients with immunologic disease. Protein C, antithrombin III, and prothrombin levels were all reduced to the extent expected for the volume exchanged. They returned to normal within 24 hours, and clinical evidence of hemostatic imbalance was not seen.[93]

A third study of the coagulation effects of TPE showed that PT often became prolonged after procedures, whereas aPTT was prolonged after the first procedure but had normalized by the next one. Thrombin time, however, was not prolonged. Factor II levels decreased to 57% of normal, and Factor V levels fell to 90%, although Factors VII, VIII, and IX were typically not decreased. Factor XI decreased to 50%, and fibrinogen decreased to 55% of normal levels. Sporadic hemorrhagic complications were seen. Antithrombin was normal in three patients. Thus, patients without disease-associated coagulopathy who are treated no more often than every 48 hours seldom need plasma replacement. Conversely, patients with pretreatment bleeding or diseases likely to be associated with consumption coagulopathy may require up to half of their replacement volume as plasma. Also, as mentioned above, patients treated daily for more than a few treatments may require plasma to correct hypofibrinogenemia. Fibrinogen measurements can guide such therapeutic decisions and help clinicians to determine how fast an individual patient is able to produce fibrinogen.[94]

Plasma Donation

Long-term plasma donation by plasmapheresis can be carried out by manual methods or on any of several machines, such as the Fenwal Autopheresis C, an instrument in the Haemonetics PCS series, and others. In the United States, a source plasma donor could theoretically donate 104 times per year (65 to 83 liters of plasma, depending on donor weight).[95] One study of 12 donors[96] showed that a majority expressed P-selectin within 48 hours after apheresis. Similar expressions were seen for glycoproteins, suggesting that the procedure caused platelet activation. Another study also suggested that regular plasmapheresis leads to platelet activation.[97] A comprehensive study of source plasma donors[98] showed that regular plasmapheresis (up to twice weekly) results in decreased serum protein, globulin, and IgG, with an increase in B cells and a decrease in suppressor and natural killer cells. It has been argued that this is a physiologic effect that has no associated clinical dysfunction.[95]

Leukapheresis

A large number of studies[41,99,100] have been concerned with the effects of hydroxyethyl starch (HES) used as a sedimenting agency in leukapheresis or as a fluid replacement alternative to albumin in TPE. HES has been implicated in weight gain and anemia and also has the potential to cause coagulation problems, given that it prolongs aPTT and lowers Factor VIII levels. However, it is unlikely that the modest abnormalities produced by these uses would lead to significant clinical bleeding.[41] Pentastarch has been found to have less pronounced effects on coagulation times, and lower-molecular-weight HES starch also seems to reduce the effect.[41]

Statistical analyses show lowered lymphocyte counts and T4:T8 ratios after leukapheresis for granulocyte donation, but the decreases do not appear to be clinically significant. An emerging concern with granulocyte collection procedures is the impact of G-CSF administration on donor safety; this is discussed in Chapter 11.

Miscellaneous Reactions

The administration of any blood component or product carries a small risk of various reactions and infections that are not addressed here. Miscellaneous apheresis reactions not specifically caused by a blood component include allergic reactions linked to ethylene oxide used in sterilization of the apheresis kit and also to HES. Prednisone used to stimulate WBC donors can cause headaches, insomnia, and irritability, and G-CSF (filgrastim) stimulation may lead to significant bone pain in some donors. Potential mechanical problems include hemolysis, clotting, and air embolism. Another potential problem is the temporary depletion of cholinesterase by TPE, which could increase the anesthesia risk if urgent surgery is required.

Summary

Apheresis procedures cause major physiologic changes in donors and patients, including hypocalcemia caused by citrate infusion, hemodynamic changes associated with fluid shifts, and depletion of cellular and plasma constituents. A knowledge of the physiology of apheresis may help the practitioner to avoid some of the adverse reactions described. As greater understanding of the physiology of apheresis has guided continued improvements in technology, the potential for untoward effects has been minimized so that most procedures are performed without adverse events. This is especially true of donation procedures, which have justifiably become very routine and are considered as safe or safer than whole blood donation.[80,81] Registry data show that overall rates of adverse reactions to therapeutic procedures have decreased significantly. Caution is in order if cell or plasma removal from donors exceeds current guidelines, or if patients have underlying instabilities that predispose them to untoward events.

References

1. Strauss RG, McLeod BC. Complications of therapeutic apheresis. In: Popovsky MA, ed. Transfusion reactions. 3rd ed. Bethesda, MD: AABB Press, 2007:405-33.
2. Hester JP, Ayyar R. Anticoagulation and electrolytes. J Clin Apher 1984;2:41-51.
3. Dzik WH, Kirkley SA. Citrate toxicity during massive blood transfusion. Transfus Med Rev 1988;2:76-94.
4. Roberts WH, Domen RE, Walters MI. Changes in calcium distribution during therapeutic plasmapheresis. Arch Pathol Lab Med 1984;108:881-3.
5. Szymanski IO. Ionized calcium during plateletpheresis. Transfusion 1978;18:701-8.
6. Olson PR, Cox C, McCullough J. Laboratory and clinical effects of the infusion of ACD solution during plateletpheresis. Vox Sang 1977;33:79-87.
7. Bolan CD, Greer SE, Cecco SA, et al. Comprehensive analysis of citrate effects during plateletpheresis in normal donors. Transfusion 2001;41:1165-71.
8. Silberstein LE, Naryshkin S, Haddad JJ, Strauss JF. Calcium homeostasis during therapeutic plasma exchange. Transfusion 1986;26:151-5.
9. Toffaletti J, Nissenson R, Endres D, et al. Influence of continuous infusion of citrate on responses of immunoreactive parathyroid hormone, calcium and magnesium components, and other electrolytes in normal adults during plateletapheresis. J Clin Endocrinol Metab 1985;60:874-9.
10. Hester JP, McCullough J, Mishler JM, Szymanski IO. Dosage regimens for citrate anticoagulants. J Clin Apher 1983;1:149-57.
11. Fontana S, Groebli R, Leibundgut K, et al. Progenitor cell recruitment during individualized high-flow, very-large-volume apheresis for autologous transplantation improves collection efficiency. Transfusion 2006;46:1408-16.
12. Weinstein R. Hypocalcemic toxicity and atypical reactions in therapeutic plasma exchange. J Clin Apher 2001;16:210-11.
13. Korach JM, Berger P, Giraud C, et al. Role of replacement fluids in the immediate complica-

tions of plasma exchange. Intensive Care Med 1998;24:452-8.

14. Bolan CD, Cecco SA, Wesley RA, et al. Controlled study of citrate effects and response to IV calcium administration during allogeneic peripheral blood progenitor cell donation. Transfusion 2002;42:935-46.

15. Bradley JS, Wassel RT, Lee L, Nambiar S. Intravenous ceftriaxone and calcium in the neonate: Assessing the risk for cardiopulmonary adverse events. Pediatrics 2009;123:e609-13.

16. Ladenson JH, Miller WV, Sherman LA. Relationship of physical symptoms, ECG, free calcium, and other blood chemistries in reinfusion with citrated blood. Transfusion 1978;18:670-9.

17. Rodnitzky RL, Goeken JA. Complications of plasma exchange in neurological patients. Arch Neurol 1982;39:350-4.

18. Wirguin I, Brenner T, Shinar E, Argov Z. Citrate-induced impairment of neuromuscular transmission in human and experimental autoimmune myasthenia gravis. Ann Neurol 1990;27:328-30.

19. Bruder JM, Guise TA, Mundy GR. Mineral metabolism. In: Felig P, Frohman LA, eds. Endocrinology and metabolism. 4th ed. New York: McGraw-Hill, 2001:1079-177.

20. Bunker JP, Bendixen HH, Murphy AJ. Hemodynamic effects of intravenously administered sodium citrate. N Engl J Med 1962;266:372-7.

21. Rock G, Tittley P, Fuller V. Effect of citrate anticoagulants on Factor VIII levels in plasma. Transfusion 1988;28:248-52.

22. Farrokhi P, Marion S, Samama M, et al. [Safety of donors, quality of products, how much to reduce the quantity of citrate]. Rev Fr Transfus Hemobiol 1991;34:233-42.

23. Bell AM, Nolen JD, Knudson CM, Raife TJ. Severe citrate toxicity complicating volunteer apheresis platelet donation. J Clin Apher 2007; 22:15-6.

24. Simon TL, Sierra ER, Ferdinando B, Moore R. Collection of platelets with a new cell separator and their storage in a citrate-plasticized container. Transfusion 1991;31:335-9.

25. Burgstaler EA, Pineda AA. Therapeutic cytapheresis: Continuous flow versus intermittent flow apheresis systems. J Clin Apher 1994;9: 205-9.

26. Katz AJ, Genco PV, Blumberg N, et al. Platelet collection and transfusion using the Fenwal CS-3000 cell separator. Transfusion 1981;21: 560-3.

27. Bertholf MF, Mintz PD. Comparison of plateletpheresis using two cell separators and identical donors. Transfusion 1989;29:521-3.

28. Kishimoto M, Ohto H, Shikama Y, et al. Treatment for the decline of ionized calcium levels during peripheral blood progenitor cell harvesting. Transfusion 2002;42:1340-7.

29. Krishnan RG, Coulthard MG. Minimising changes in plasma calcium and magnesium concentrations during plasmapheresis. Pediatr Nephrol 2007;22:1763-6.

30. Buskard NA, Varghese Z, Wills MR. Correction of hypocalcaemic symptoms during plasma exchange. Lancet 1976;2:344-5.

31. Weinstein R. Prevention of citrate reactions during therapeutic plasma exchange by constant infusion of calcium gluconate with the return fluid. J Clin Apher 1996;11:204-10.

32. Mokrzycki MH, Kaplan AA. Therapeutic plasma exchange: Complications and management. Am J Kidney Dis 1994;23:817-27.

33. Haddad S, Leitman SF, Wesley RA, et al. Placebo-controlled study of intravenous magnesium supplementation during large-volume leukapheresis in healthy allogeneic donors. Transfusion 2005;45:934-44.

34. Kelleher SP, Schulman G. Severe metabolic alkalosis complicating regional citrate hemodialysis. Am J Kidney Dis 1987;9:235-6.

35. Pearl RG, Rosenthal MH. Metabolic alkalosis due to plasmapheresis. Am J Med 1985;79: 391-3.

36. Warkentin TE, Sheppard JA, Horsewood P, et al. Impact of the patient population on the risk for heparin-induced thrombocytopenia. Blood 2000;96:1703-8.

37. Stephens LC, Haire WD, Tarantolo S, et al. Normal saline versus heparin flush for maintaining central venous catheter patency during apheresis collection of peripheral blood stem cells (PBSC). Transfus Sci 1997;18:187-93.

38. Winters JL, ed. Therapeutic apheresis: A physician's handbook. 2nd ed. Bethesda, MD: AABB, 2008.

39. Gilcher RO, Smith JW. Apheresis: Principles and technology of hemapheresis. In: Simon TL, Snyder EL, Solheim BG, et al, eds. Rossi's principles of transfusion medicine. 4th ed. Bethesda, MD: AABB Press, 2009:617-28.

40. Korach JM, Guillevin L, Petitpas D, et al. Apheresis registry in France: Indications, techniques, and complications. Ther Apher 2000; 4:207-10.

41. Strauss RG, Pennell BJ, Stump DC. A randomized, blinded trial comparing the hemostatic effects of pentastarch versus hetastarch. Transfusion 2002;42:27-36.

42. Goss GA, Weinstein R. Pentastarch as partial replacement fluid for therapeutic plasma exchange: Effect on plasma proteins, adverse events during treatment, and serum ionized calcium. J Clin Apher 1999;14:114-21.

43. Owen HG, Brecher ME. Partial colloid starch replacement for therapeutic plasma exchange. J Clin Apher 1997;12:87-92.

44. Brecher ME, Owen HG, Bandarenko N. Alternatives to albumin: Starch replacement for plasma exchange. J Clin Apher 1997;12:146-53.

45. Orlin JB, Berkman EM. Partial plasma exchange using albumin replacement: Removal and recovery of normal plasma constituents. Blood 1980;56:1055-9.

46. Derksen RH, Schuurman HJ, Gmelig Meyling FH, et al. Rebound and overshoot after plasma exchange in humans. J Lab Clin Med 1984;104:35-43.

47. Sketris IS, Parker WA, Jones JV. Effect of plasma exchange on drug removal. In: Valbonesi M, Pineda A, Briggs JC, eds. Therapeutic hemapheresis. Milan, Italy: Wichtig-Idito, 1986:15-20.

48. Foral PA, Heineman SM. Vancomycin removal during a plasma exchange transfusion. Ann Pharmacother 2001;35:1400-2.

49. Ibrahim RB, Liu C, Cronin SM, et al. Drug removal by plasmapheresis: An evidence-based review. Pharmacotherapy 2007;27:1529-49.

50. Stigelman WH Jr, Henry DH, Talbert RL, Townsend RJ. Removal of prednisone and prednisolone by plasma exchange. Clin Pharm 1984;3:402-7.

51. Kintzel PE, Eastlund T, Calis KA. Extracorporeal removal of antimicrobials during plasmapheresis. J Clin Apher 2003;18:194-205.

52. Lasky LC, Lin A, Kahn RA, McCullough J. Donor platelet response and product quality assurance in plateletpheresis. Transfusion 1981; 21:247-60.

53. Lee EJ, Schiffer CA. Evidence for rapid mobilization of platelets from the spleen during intensive plateletpheresis. Am J Hematol 1985; 19:161-5.

54. Buchholz DH, Porten JH, Menitove JE, et al. Description and use of the CS-3000 blood cell separator for single-donor platelet collection. Transfusion 1983;23:190-6.

55. Rogers RL, Johnson H, Ludwig G, et al. Efficacy and safety of plateletpheresis by donors with low-normal platelet counts. J Clin Apher 1995;10:194-7.

56. Prior CR, Coghlan PJ, Hall JM, Jacobs P. In itro study of immunologic changes in long-term cytapheresis donors. J Clin Apher 1991;6:69-76.

57. Matsui Y, Martin-Alosco S, Doenges E, et al. Effects of frequent and sustained plateletapheresis on peripheral blood mononuclear cell populations and lymphocyte functions of normal volunteer donors. Transfusion 1986;26:446-52.

58. Silva VA. Are frequent platelet apheresis donors with borderline lymphopenia at risk of worsening lymphopenia and of decreasing immunoglobulins? Transfus Sci 1994;15:67-72.

59. Lewis SL, Kutvirt SG, Bonner PN, Simon TL. Effect of long-term platelet donation on lymphocyte subsets and plasma protein concentrations. Transfus Sci 1997;18:205-13.

60. Richa E, Krueger P, Burgstaler EA, et al. The effect of double- and triple-apheresis platelet product donation on apheresis donor platelet and white blood cell counts. Transfusion 2008;48:1325-32.

61. Bongiovanni MB, Katz RS, Wurzel HA. Long-term plateletpheresis of a donor. Transfusion 1980;20:465-6.

62. Mendez A, Wagli F, Schmid I, Frey BM. Frequent platelet apheresis donations in volunteer donors with hemoglobin <125 g/L are safe and efficient. Transfus Apher Sci 2007;36:47-53.

63. Malachowski ME, Comenzo RL, Hillyer CD, et al. Large-volume leukapheresis for peripheral blood stem cell collection in patients with hematologic malignancies. Transfusion 1992; 32:732-5.

64. Jacobs P, Wood L. Lack of short-term effects on the donor during continuous-flow selective mononuclear cell collection. J Clin Apher 1987;3:151-3.

65. Stroncek DF, Clay ME, Smith J, et al. Changes in blood counts after the administration of granulocyte-colony-stimulating factor and the collection of peripheral blood stem cells from healthy donors. Transfusion 1996;36:596-600.

66. Nusbacher J, Rosenfeld SI, MacPherson JL, et al. Nylon fiber leukapheresis: Associated com-

plement component changes and granulocytopenia. Blood 1978;51:359-65.

67. McLeod BC, Viernes A, Sassetti RJ. Complement activation by plasma separator membranes. Transfusion 1983;23:143-7.

68. Nose Y. Blood purification procedures and their related short- and long-term effect on patients. Ther Apher 2002;6:333-47.

69. McLeod BC, Sassetti RJ. Effects of centrifugation leukapheresis with hydroxyethyl starch on the complement system of granulocyte donors. Transfusion 1981;21:405-11.

70. Owen HG, Brecher ME. Atypical reactions associated with use of angiotensin-converting enzyme inhibitors and apheresis. Transfusion 1994;34:891-4.

71. Cyr M, Hume HA, Champagne M, et al. Anomaly of the des-Arg9-bradykinin metabolism associated with severe hypotensive reactions during blood transfusions: A preliminary study. Transfusion 1999;39:1084-8.

72. McLeod BC, Sniecinski I, Ciavarella D, et al. Frequency of immediate adverse effects associated with apheresis donation. Transfusion 1998;38:938-43.

73. Sheldon R, Morillo C, Krahn A. Management of vasovagal syncope: 2004. Expert review of cardiovascular therapy 2004;2:915-23.

74. Spindler JS. Subclavian vein catheterization for apheresis access. J Clin Apher 1983;1:202-5.

75. Noseworthy JH, Shumak KH, Vandervoort MK. Long-term use of antecubital veins for plasma exchange. Transfusion 1989;29:610-3.

76. Dogra GK, Herson H, Hutchison B, et al. Prevention of tunneled hemodialysis catheter-related infections using catheter-restricted filling with gentamicin and citrate: A randomized controlled study. J Am Soc Nephrol 2002;13:2133-9.

77. Rizvi MA, Vesely SK, George JN, et al. Complications of plasma exchange in 71 consecutive patients treated for clinically suspected thrombotic thrombocytopenic purpura-hemolytic-uremic syndrome. Transfusion 2000;40:896-901.

78. Annane D, Baudrie V, Blanc AS, et al. Short-term variability of blood pressure and heart rate in Guillain-Barré syndrome without respiratory failure. Clin Sci (Lond) 1999;96:613-21.

79. Rossi PL, Cecchini L, Menichella G, et al. Comparison of the side effects of therapeutic cytapheresis and those of other types of hemapheresis. Haematologica 1991;76(Suppl 1):75-80.

80. Wiltbank TB, Giordano GF. The safety profile of automated collections: An analysis of more than 1 million collections. Transfusion 2007;47:1002-5.

81. Kamel H, Tomasulo P, Bravo M, et al. Delayed adverse reactions to blood donation. Transfusion 2010 (in press).

82. Couriel D, Weinstein R. Complications of therapeutic plasma exchange: A recent assessment. J Clin Apher 1994;9:1-5.

83. Sutton DM, Nair RC, Rock G. Complications of plasma exchange. Transfusion 1989;29:124-7.

84. Rock G, Buskard NA. Therapeutic plasmapheresis. Curr Opin Hematol 1996;3:504-10.

85. Raphael JC, Chevret S, Gajdos P. Plasma exchange in neurological diseases. Transfus Sci 1996;17:267-82.

86. Norda R, Berséus O, Stegmayr B. Adverse events and problems in therapeutic hemapheresis. A report from the Swedish registry. Transfus Apher Sci 2001;25:33-41.

87. McLeod BC, Sniecinski I, Ciavarella D, et al. Frequency of immediate adverse effects associated with therapeutic apheresis. Transfusion 1999;39:282-8.

88. Huestis DW. Complications of therapeutic apheresis. In: Valbonesi M, Pineda A, Briggs JC, eds. Therapeutic hemapheresis. Milan, Italy: Wichtig-Idito, 1986:179-86.

89. Huestis DW. Risks and safety practices in hemapheresis procedures. Arch Pathol Lab Med 1989;113:273-8.

90. Pool M, McLeod BC. Pyrogen reactions to human serum albumin during plasma exchange. J Clin Apher 1995;10:81-4.

91. Korach JM, Petitpas D, Poiron L, et al. 14 years of therapeutic plasma exchange in France. Transfus Apher Sci 2001;25:73-7.

92. Domen RE, Kennedy MS, Jones LL, Senhauser DA. Hemostatic imbalances produced by plasma exchange. Transfusion 1984;24:336-9.

93. Mannucci PM, D'Angelo A, Vigano S, et al. Decrease and rapid recovery of protein C after plasma exchange. Transfusion 1986;26:156-8.

94. Simon TL. Coagulation disorders with plasma exchange. Plasma Ther Transfus Technol 1982;3:147-52.

95. Crookston KP, Schreiber GB, Simon TL. Recruitment and screening of donors and the collection, processing, and testing of blood. In: Simon TL, Snyder EL, Solheim BG, et al, eds. Rossi's principles of transfusion medicine. 4th ed. Bethesda, MD: AABB Press, 2009:975-92.

96. Wun T, Paglieroni T, Holland P. Prolonged circulation of activated platelets following plasmapheresis. J Clin Apher 1994;9:10-6.

97. Wun T, Paglieroni T, Sazama K, Holland P. Detection of plasmapheresis-induced platelet activation using monoclonal antibodies. Transfusion 1992;32:534-40.

98. Lewis SL, Kutvirt SG, Bonner PN, Simon TL. Plasma proteins and lymphocyte phenotypes in long-term plasma donors. Transfusion 1994; 34:578-85.

99. Lawrence DA, Schell RF. Influence of hydroxyethyl starch on humoral and cell-mediated immune responses in mice. Transfusion 1985; 25:223-9.

100. Strauss RG, Stansfield C, Henriksen RA, Villhauer PJ. Pentastarch may cause fewer effects on coagulation than hetastarch. Transfusion 1988;28:257-60.

In: McLeod BC, Szczepiorkowski ZM, Weinstein R, Winters JL, eds.
Apheresis: Principles and Practice, 3rd edition
Bethesda, MD: AABB Press, 2010

4

Current Instrumentation for Apheresis

Edwin A. Burgstaler, MT, HP(ASCP)

 THIS CHAPTER GIVES AN OVER-view of methods and instruments used for donor collection or therapeutic applications to collect and/ or separate blood components by apheresis. It includes the most current and commonly used instruments in the United States and Canada. The chapter is divided into three sections: 1) a general review of the principles of cell separation, 2) a description of the instruments and of how they work, and 3) a comparison of instrument features. Further discussion of the operation and performance of specific instruments in other applications can be found in Chapter 12 (therapeutic apheresis), Chapter 21 (pediatric apheresis), Chapter 23 (collection of hematopoietic progenitor cells from apheresis), and Chapter 24 (ex-vivo cell processing).

Principles of Operation

The basic steps in apheresis are 1) the separation of blood components and 2) the removal of the desired component(s) using an online automated system. The ability of various techniques and equipment to carry out these basic steps determines collection efficiency and product purity.

Separation can be accomplished by filtration, centrifugation, or a combination of both. Filtration takes advantage of differences in particle size to separate blood plasma from the cellular elements. Centrifugation uses differences in specific gravity to separate and isolate blood components. Figure 4-1 lists components of blood and their specific gravity. There are small differences between platelets and lymphocytes and between lymphocytes and granulocytes,

Edwin A. Burgstaler, MT, HP(ASCP), Apheresis Research and Development Coordinator, Division of Transfusion Medicine, Mayo Clinic, Rochester, Minnesota
The author has disclosed no conflicts of interest.

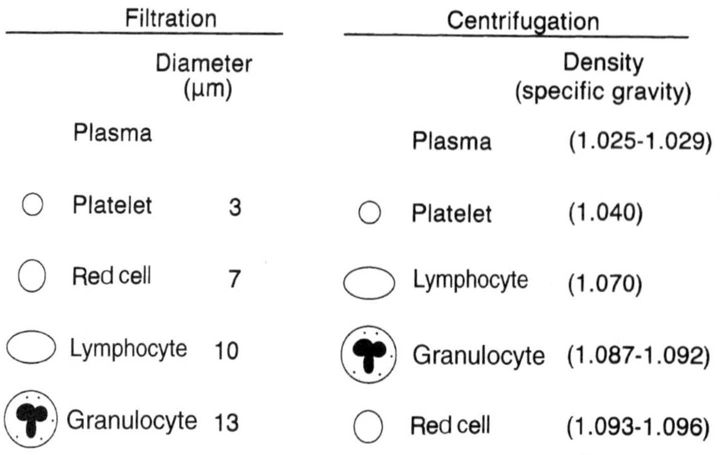

Filtration			Centrifugation		
Diameter (μm)			Density (specific gravity)		
	Plasma			Plasma	(1.025-1.029)
○	Platelet	3	○	Platelet	(1.040)
○	Red cell	7	⬭	Lymphocyte	(1.070)
⬭	Lymphocyte	10	🟤	Granulocyte	(1.087-1.092)
🟤	Granulocyte	13	○	Red cell	(1.093-1.096)

Figure 4-1. Distribution of blood components by size and weight. (Used with permission from Mayo Foundation for Medical Education and Research.)

but larger differences between platelets and granulocytes and between plasma and red cells.

Centrifugation

In a tube of blood that has reached equilibrium after the application of centrifugal force, mature red cells (the most dense component) would be located at the bottom, and plasma (the least dense component) would have risen to the top. In between, in order of decreasing density, would be neocytes (young red cells), granulocytes, mononuclear cells, and platelets. The granulocyte fraction contains neutrophils, basophils, and eosinophils. The mononuclear cell fraction contains lymphocytes, monocytes, peripheral blood progenitor cells, and, in some leukemic patients, blast cells. Unfortunately, a perfectly clean separation of these components is not usually achieved in apheresis instruments. Instead, there is some mixing; for example, small amounts of platelets and red cells may be mixed in with the white blood cells (WBCs).

In the apheresis field, centrifugal separators are classified as intermittent flow or continuous flow. In intermittent flow devices (also called discontinuous or semicontinuous flow), blood is processed in discrete batches. Separation can occur until the separation container is filled with the most dense component; then the container must be emptied before the next batch is processed. This is in contrast to continuous flow devices, in which low-, high-, and intermediate-density fractions can all be removed in an ongoing manner so that the separation container need not be emptied until the end of the procedure.

Filtration

Filtration or the use of membrane separators isolates blood components on the basis of differences in particle size. Usually, plasma is separated from the cellular elements. For example, the effective filter pore size may be 0.6 micron, whereas the diameter of the platelet, the smallest cellular element, is 2 to 3 microns. As whole blood flows by the membrane surface under pressure, plasma passes through the pores and is collected while the cellular elements are retained for return to the donor or patient.

Most membrane separators used in apheresis today are composed of a bundle of parallel, single, hollow fiber filters confined in a plastic cylinder. Each fiber resembles a straw with many holes in its walls. Whole blood under pressure enters at one end; as it flows through the hollow fibers, plasma is squeezed out the walls and a more concentrated cell suspension exits at the other end. In the most common layout, blood enters through a bottom port, cells exit from a top port, and plasma is withdrawn from a side port. An additional side port is usually provided to monitor pressure.

Centrifuge-Filter Combination

Filtration and centrifugal separation can be combined in a rotating filter. Whole blood enters an upper side port of a stationary cylindrical container. Rotation of a centrally located cylindrical filter imparts rotation to the blood, which fosters separation of cells and plasma. This pushes cellular components away from the filter surface and its pores, making the filter less likely to become clogged by cells and, therefore, more efficient for plasma removal. Plasma passes radially inward through the filter membrane and is collected while concentrated cellular elements are pumped off and returned to the donor. The combination of separation modalities permits the use of a lower *g* force and a smaller filter surface area than would be required if the modalities were used separately.

Instruments for Leukapheresis, Plateletpheresis, and/or Plasma Collection

Haemonetics Systems

The instruments built by the Haemonetics Corporation in Braintree, MA, collect plasma, platelets, WBCs, or red cells by intermittent flow centrifugation. Two differently shaped centrifugation bowls are offered; the choice between them depends on the component to be collected.

Latham Bowl

The conical Latham bowl (Fig 4-2) was used in the Haemonetics Model 10, Model 30, and Model V50 instruments discussed in Chapters 1 and 2 and is still found in the instruments designated MCS and MCS Plus (MCS+). Its stationary stem is joined to the bowl by a rotating seal. Friction in the seal is minimized by a graphite-based coating, which prevents heat buildup. Blood entering the stationary tube goes to the bottom of the rotating bowl where it is forced to the periphery and rises between two concentric conical surfaces. Centrifugal force causes vertical layers to form with red cells on the outside, plasma on the inside, and buffy coat (platelets and white cells) in between. As more whole blood is pumped into the bowl, accumulation of red cells pushes lighter components upward and inward. Lighter components eventually exit the bowl through an effluent tube in order of increasing density and are directed into appropriate containers. When the bowl becomes filled with red cells, the process must be stopped temporarily. The blood pump is reversed to empty the bowl, and another cycle is started.

The autosurge technique was developed to collect purer platelet and mononuclear cell components with Haemonetics instruments.

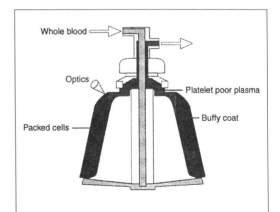

Figure 4-2. Latham bowl used with the Haemonetics systems. (Used with permission from Haemonetics Corporation.)

With this technique, whole blood enters the bowl until the buffy coat is detected by optical monitors mounted over the top of the bowl (Fig 4-2). Whole blood inflow is then stopped, and plasma from the plasma air bag is pumped rapidly (>200 mL/minute) into the rotating bowl. The recirculating plasma percolates through the cellular layers in the bowl, and as it exits the bowl, the lighter components—first platelets, then lymphocytes—are floated off. Eventually, granulocytes and red cells would come off too, but a sensor monitors the optical density of the bowl effluent and stops the surge cycle before this can happen.

The surge process is not used for granulocyte collection; instead, the entire or partial buffy coat (with considerable red cell content) is skimmed off into the product bag. Two bags are used, and red cells are sedimented out to be returned to the donor.

Plasmapheresis Bowl

The grenade-shaped plasmapheresis or blow mold bowl (Fig 4-3) is suitable only for plasma and red cell collection. It has the same basic parts as the Latham bowl, but its walls are cylindrical rather than conical. Whole blood

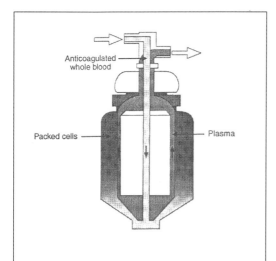

Figure 4-3. Plasmapheresis (blow mold) bowl used with the Haemonetics systems. (Used with permission from Haemonetics Corporation.)

entering the bowl through the stationary tube forms vertical layers of plasma and packed cells. As the bowl fills, packed cells accumulating on the outer wall displace the plasma inward, pushing it out the effluent tube. When the bowl has filled with packed cells, it must be stopped and emptied before the process can be repeated. This bowl is easier to fabricate; hence, plasmapheresis disposable sets are less expensive.

Model MCS

MCS stands for "Mobile Collection System," and portability is this instrument's major asset. This small apheresis instrument can be placed on a stand or tabletop, making it well suited for off-site or mobile collections.

The MCS (Fig 4-4) has an anticoagulant pump, a reversible blood pump, and air detectors on the anticoagulant and blood lines as well as two on the donor line. There are four electric valves, two pressure sensors, and a line sensor. The instrument is microprocessor controlled with minimal manual control. The controls and a light-emitting diode (LED) screen are built into the instrument's cover.

Extracorporeal volume (ECV) for this system is highly variable and depends on patient/donor hematocrit, time in the cycle, and time in the procedure, as well as on the size of the bowl used. ECV and monitors on the instrument are indicated in Table 4-1. Centrifuge pressure is monitored during plateletpheresis only. There is no built-in blood warmer. Single-vein access is used for plateletpheresis; either single- or double-vein access can be used for granulocyte collection.

MCS Plus LN9000

The LN9000 (Fig 4-5) is a modified version of the MCS. It has an additional plasma pump (see Fig 4-4) to promote better separation in the bowl and shorten the blood return cycle. During the withdrawal phase, plasma (when available) is pumped from the plasma air bag and mixed with whole blood to maintain blood flow into the bowl at a predetermined rate (critical

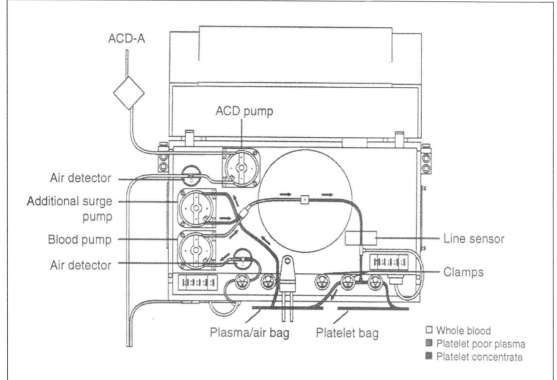

Figure 4-4. Flow diagram of plateletpheresis with the Haemonetics MCS Plus. (Used with permission from Haemonetics Corporation.)

flow). The plasma pump rate is controlled by the microprocessor and is dependent on hematocrit, draw rate, and anticoagulant ratio. It automatically compensates for decreases in whole blood outflow. The continual plasma recirculation enhances platelet separation from lymphocytes and facilitates collection of a leukocyte-reduced platelet product. This pump also operates during the autosurge phase of product collection. During reinfusion, the blood pump returns packed cells while the plasma pump returns plasma. Their actions are simultaneous rather than sequential, thus shortening the reinfusion cycle.

Advantages of the MCS and MCS+ include portability and quiet operation. Their platelet products contain fewer leukocytes than those of the V50 (the MCS+ with pre-attached filters is consistently capable of $<5\times10^6$ leukocytes per product).[1] The MCS+ is improved over the MCS for platelet collection, having lower leuko-

cyte content, higher blood-processing rates (42 mL/minute vs 37 mL/minute),[2] faster alarm recovery procedures, and a built-in platelet yield predictor. The LN9000 version of the MCS+ offers a larger viewing screen, online help screens, updated procedure statistics, and computer interface capabilities that allow several instruments to be monitored from one screen. Disadvantages include a large ECV, limited manual control, and longer procedure times than some continuous flow instruments. As of January 1, 2010, Haemonetics will support only platelet and plasma donation and therapeutic plasma exchange (TPE) on the LN9000.

Model PCS-2

The Haemonetics PCS-2 is a modified version of the MCS designed for plasma collection. It uses a simpler, less expensive disposable kit

Table 4-1. Apheresis Instrumentation Overview

	Haemonetics		Fenwal		CaridianBCT	Fresenius	
	MCS/MCS Plus	PCS-2	AMICUS	Autopheresis C	COBE Spectra	AS 104	COM.TEC
Type of system	IFC	IFC	CFC	IFCF	CFC	CFC	CFC
Weight (lb)	56	56	345	105	389	319	286
Height × width × depth (inches)	26 × 21.5 × 21.5	26.5 × 21.5 × 21.5	60 × 20.5 × 32	59 × 17 × 10	59.5 × 27.6 × 27.9	75.6 × 24 × 27.8	55 × 24 × 26
ECV (approx): Total/RBCs (mL)	<u>Variable</u> 225 bowl 480 (38% Hct)- 359 (52% Hct)/180	<u>Variable</u> 225 bowl 480 (38% Hct)- 359 (52% Hct)/ 182-187	<u>Double needle</u> 210/60	200	<u>Double needle</u> (with LRS) 272/52	<u>Double needle</u> 175	<u>Double needle</u> 175
	<u>Single needle</u> 329 mL (max) 64 + Max cycle volume × Hct				<u>Single needle</u> 361/93	<u>Single needle</u> 285	<u>Single needle</u> 285
					<u>Granulocyte</u> 285/114	<u>Granulocyte</u> 120	<u>Granulocyte</u> 120
Monitors:							
Draw pressure	Yes	Yes	Yes	Yes	Yes	Yes	Yes
Return pressure	Yes	Yes	Yes	Yes	Yes	Yes	Yes
Air present	Yes	Yes	Yes	Yes	Yes	Yes	Yes
AC delivery	Yes	Yes	Yes	No	Yes	Yes	Yes
Centrifuge pressure	Yes	Yes	Yes	Yes	Yes	No	No
Leak detector	No	No	Yes	No	Yes	Yes	Yes
Blood warmer	No	No	No	No	No	No (centrifuge 36 C)	No (centrifuge 36 C)
Donor applications	Plasma, platelets	Plasma	Platelets (plasma by-product)(red cells by-product)	Plasma	Platelets, granulocytes (plasma by-product)	Platelets, granulocytes (plasma by-product)	Platelets, granulocytes (plasma by-product)

*Not in the United States as of September 2009.

IFC = intermittent flow centrifugation; CFC = continuous flow centrifugation; IFCF = intermittent flow centrifugation and filtration; ECV = extracorporeal volume; RBCs = red blood cells; WB = whole blood; Hct = hematocrit; LRS = leukocyte reduction system; Max = Maximum; AC = anticoagulant.

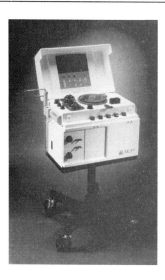

Figure 4-5. Haemonetics MCS Plus LN9000 blood cell separator. (Used with permission from Haemonetics Corporation.)

incorporating the plasmapheresis bowl (Fig 4-3), and it offers both portability and an automated procedure. The relatively high ECV can be offset with the use of an optional normal saline return. It is limited to single-needle procedures and has limited manual control.

Fenwal Systems

This section discusses two instruments from Fenwal, Inc (Lake Zurich, IL): 1) the AMICUS for plateletpheresis and 2) the Autopheresis C for plasma donation.

AMICUS

The Fenwal AMICUS (Fig 4-6) was approved by the Food and Drug Administration (FDA) for donor plateletpheresis in 1996. It is smaller, lighter, and more portable than its predecessor, making it potentially more suitable for bedside or off-site use. For AMICUS operation, the entire disposable tray is placed on the top panel and remains there during the procedure. The tray aligns six pumps and three cassettes, each

with 10 valves and four sensors. Solutions are hung from electric scales, and lines are placed in four clamps and an optical sensor.

The centrifuge is sealless with a multilumen harness that enters the instrument from above and loops around in a "J" configuration so that blood enters and exits the separation module from below. There is a unique centrifuge drive mechanism that contacts the tubing harness via a disposable bearing only in the outer portion of the loop. The harness is made of a fairly rigid plastic, and as it is turned around the separation module at an angular velocity ϖ by the drive mechanism, its inherent untwisting tendency causes rotation of the separator module about its bearing at an angular velocity of 2ϖ. Thus, there is no need for another drive mechanism for the separation module. The single direct drive enhances reliability while decreasing vibration and noise.

The rotating module contains separation and collection containers, which are configured like a belt wrapped around a spool. The controls and displays have been combined into a touch TV screen control monitor, which can be

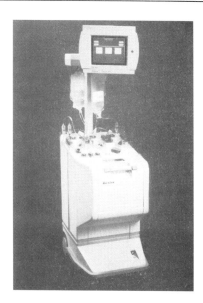

Figure 4-6. AMICUS blood cell separator. (Used with permission from Fenwal, Inc.)

moved and repositioned for operator or donor convenience. The instrument is microprocessor-driven and highly automated with limited manual control. There is a dedicated anticoagulant pump, which delivers anticoagulant at either a constant ratio or a specific weight-based infusion rate (mg of citrate per kg per minute).

As can be seen in the flow diagram in Fig 4-7, the AMICUS has unique separation steps. First, some of the platelet-rich plasma (PRP) coming from the separation chamber is recirculated back to the incoming whole blood to reduce its hematocrit before the blood enters the separation chamber. Second, as blood thus diluted enters the separation chamber (Fig 4-8), plasma separates and exits quickly, causing a countercurrent elutriation effect that pushes platelets up a ramp to exit the separation chamber at the same end where the whole blood entered. This elutriation will move large platelets that are missed during conventional separation. Third, as red cells flow through the separation chamber, they become more concentrated; the remaining platelets rise to the top and are drawn off with the PRP, while the granulocytes remain near the bottom of the chamber and exit with the red cells (Fig 4-8). Fourth, mononuclear cells float to the top as the hematocrit increases and begin to flow back with the PRP; when they encounter the more diluted red cell zone, however, they drop back down again. Hence, they tend to loop around the far end of the chamber, away from the PRP exit port (Fig 4-8). Fifth, the interface position is monitored and controlled throughout the procedure by an interface detector in the centrifuge itself. PRP that is not recirculated with whole blood is pumped into the collection chamber, where platelets are concentrated, and platelet-poor plasma (PPP) exits for collection or return (Fig 4-7).

With the double-needle system, anticoagulated whole blood is pumped continuously into the separation container while recombined packed cells and plasma flow back through a return line. With the single-needle system, the whole blood pump draws off more blood than the centrifuge can handle. The centrifuge pump takes what it needs, and the surplus is diverted into a draw reservoir attached to an electronic scale. As PPP leaves the collection container, it is pumped into a plasma transfer pack while the cellular elements leaving the separation chamber are diverted into a return reservoir. All reservoirs are monitored by electronic scales, and when specified maximum weights are reached, the instrument automatically switches from draw phase to return phase. The centrifuge pump continues to pump whole blood from the draw reservoir into the separation chamber. The whole blood pump reverses, returning PPP from the collection chamber, packed cells from the separation chamber, PPP from the plasma reservoir, and packed cells from the return reservoir through the needle. When specified minimum reservoir weights are reached, the instrument automatically switches back to the draw phase.

The monitors included on the AMICUS are listed in Table 4-1, as are the ECVs for single-needle and double-needle procedures. There is no integral blood warmer. With software Version 2.51, a PRP integrator was introduced to monitor platelets collected vs target yield. When enabled, the integrator will extend the procedure time as needed to reach the target yield. With software Version 3.1, the single needle procedure is enhanced, and details of each procedure can be printed out.

Advantages of the AMICUS include reliable anticoagulant delivery, shorter processing times, efficient platelet collection, a consistently low leukocyte cell content ($<1 \times 10^6$/product), a platelet yield predictor, PRP integrator, single- and double-needle procedure capability, low ECV, enhanced mobility, quiet operation, easy loading, and on-screen prompts.[3] Disadvantages include limited manual control, low-hanging saline containers that limit gravity flow rates for irrigation or saline bolus, and limited procedure capability (plateletpheresis with concurrent plasma and/or red cells and mononuclear cell collection).[3]

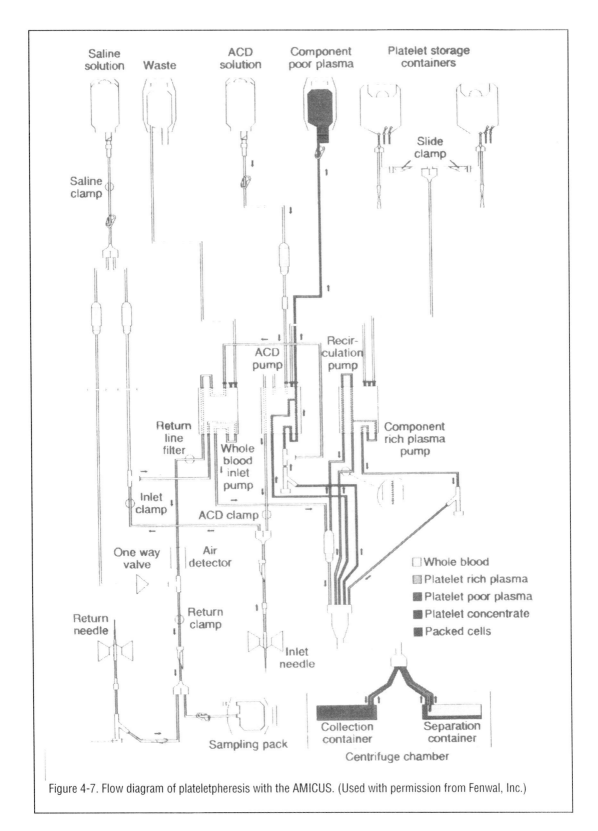

Figure 4-7. Flow diagram of plateletpheresis with the AMICUS. (Used with permission from Fenwal, Inc.)

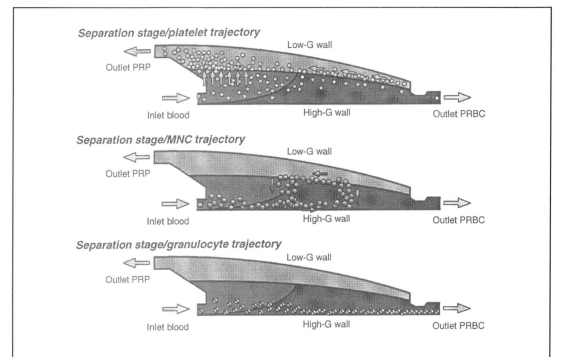

Figure 4-8. Platelet, mononuclear cell, and granulocyte flow in the AMICUS separation chamber. PRP = platelet-rich plasma; MNC = mononuclear cells; PRBC = packed red blood cells. (Used with permission from Fenwal, Inc.)

Autopheresis C

The Autopheresis C (Fig 4-9) is a single-access instrument that uses a rotating filter to separate and collect plasma. One pump delivers anticoagulant to the needle site (Fig 4-10), and anticoagulated whole blood is pumped into the separatory element (Fig 4-11). Metal parts on the filter module are induced to rotate by a rotating magnet; this causes the blood to rotate, much as a stirring bar imparts motion to a liquid. The sweeping action of the blood over the membrane and the radially outward packing of cells in rotating blood prevent cells from collecting on the centrally located membrane surface, where they could plug filter pores and reduce efficiency. Plasma passes inward through the filter and flows into a collection container, while packed cells are removed by another pump and delivered to a reservoir. When a detector determines that the reservoir is full, the machine automatically repositions

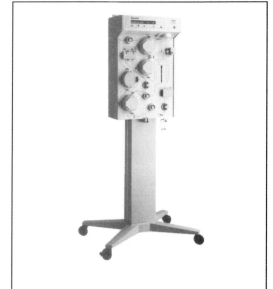

Figure 4-9. Fenwal Autopheresis C plasmapheresis system. (Used with permission from Fenwal, Inc.)

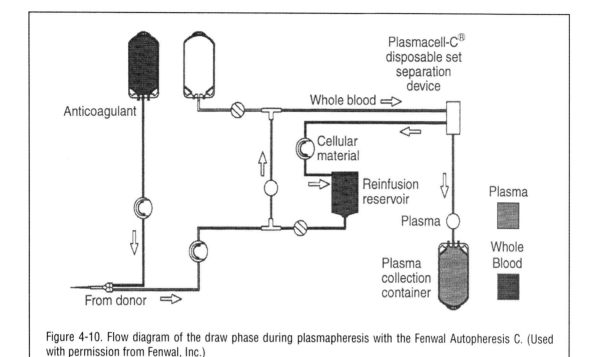

Figure 4-10. Flow diagram of the draw phase during plasmapheresis with the Fenwal Autopheresis C. (Used with permission from Fenwal, Inc.)

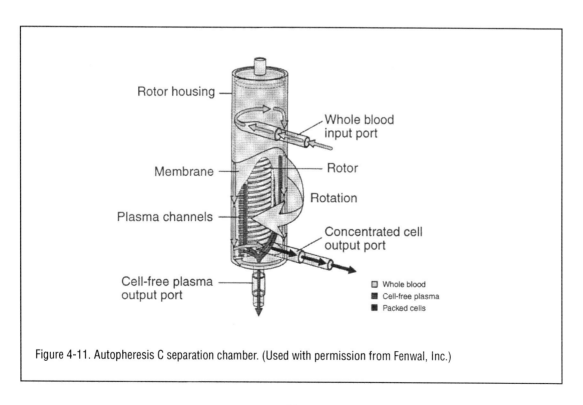

Figure 4-11. Autopheresis C separation chamber. (Used with permission from Fenwal, Inc.)

the valves and reverses the blood pump to empty the reservoir into the donor before another cycle starts. Collected plasma is weighed on an electronic scale. There are two pressure monitors as well as optical detectors on the blood line and plasma line.

The Autopheresis C is a microprocessor-controlled, combination centrifugation-filtration instrument that is limited to plasma collection. Its monitors are listed in Table 4-1. Anticoagulant is delivered by an adjustable dedicated pump. There is no integrated blood warmer.

Advantages include automated procedures, low ECV, single access, a low anticoagulant-to-blood ratio, moderate mobility, and easy loading. Disadvantages include limited manual control, moderate portability, and limitation to plasma collection.

CaridianBCT Instruments

Overview of the Spectra

The COBE Spectra (CaridianBCT, Lakewood, CO) (Fig 4-12) is also a highly automated, microprocessor-controlled instrument. It has preloaded programs for several procedures, but some manual control is also possible. The instrument uses hard plastic inserts to reinforce the shape of the soft plastic channels in which blood is separated. There are no rotating seals. A Leukoreduction System (LRS) was introduced for the Spectra to minimize the leukocyte content of platelet components. The LRS includes a modified dual-stage channel and modified computer software to regulate and monitor the pumps and sensors. Plateletpheresis can be performed with double- or single-needle disposables, with or without the LRS.

Anticoagulant is pumped to the needle site by a dedicated, adjustable pump (Fig 4-13). Anticoagulated whole blood is drawn through the access pressure sensor by the inlet pump and passes through a centrifuge pressure sensor and air detector/filter before entering the centrifuge. Plasma is withdrawn from the centrifuge by the plasma pump and is either collected into a transfer pack or returned to the subject, passing through a return pressure sen-

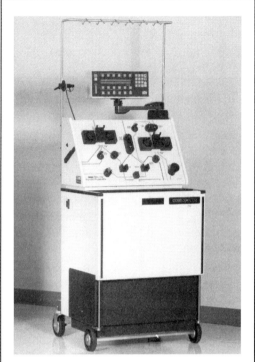

Figure 4-12. The COBE Spectra (CaridianBCT, Lakewood, CO) blood cell separator. (Used with permission from Mayo Foundation for Medical Education and Research.)

sor. Red cells exit the centrifuge under pressure arising from the difference between the inlet pump and plasma removal pump rates. They pass through a red cell detector (active only at the beginning of the procedure), then through an air detector/filter, through a return valve, and back to the subject. During collection procedures, the collection pump withdraws the component from the centrifuge and pumps it into collection bags.

For single-needle operation, the return line is attached to a small return bag placed in a spring-loaded monitor box. When a preset volume has accumulated in this bag, the instrument automatically stops drawing blood and returns the processed blood in the return bag. An improvement made in Version 4.0 and subsequent software versions provides for some of the processed blood to be recirculated through the centrifuge during return cycles. This pre-

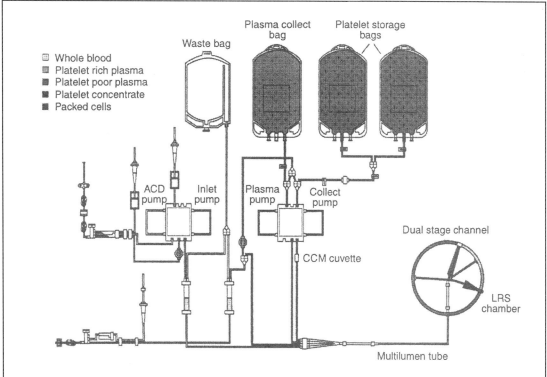

Figure 4-13. Flow diagram of plateletpheresis with the Spectra and Leukocyte Reduction System (LRS). CCM = collection concentration monitor. (Copyright, CaridianBCT, Inc, 2009. Used with permission.)

vents excessive packing of cells in the separation channel and facilitates interface maintenance and exclusion of leukocytes from platelet products.[4]

A unique feature of this instrument is the online collection concentration monitor (CCM). During plateletpheresis, this device monitors for leukocyte and red cell spillovers and estimates optically how many platelets have been collected. If a spillover occurs, the CCM repositions the collect valve to return the resulting contaminated product to the donor until the line has cleared, as determined by the operator. Before the LRS was introduced, the CCM triggered a spillover alarm at a 3% hematocrit. With the LRS system, the CCM is made more sensitive.

Dual-Stage Channel. The dual-stage channel is used for platelet collection only (Fig 4-14). Whole blood enters the first stage through the tube on the left in the diagram. Red cells

and leukocytes travel in a clockwise direction (viewed from above) until they encounter a "dam," where they change direction and go back toward the packed red cell exit, as discussed in Chapter 1. PRP spills over into the second stage, and platelets concentrated at the point of greatest radius are removed by the collection pump. PPP then continues around the chamber to a plasma exit, where most of the plasma is drawn off by the plasma pump. A small amount of plasma continues around to the small control tube. The remaining chamber contents, including leukocytes and red cells, exit at a fixed flow rate under positive pressure as described above. A competition to exit the separation chamber develops between red cells in the larger red cell tube and plasma in the smaller control tube; resolution of this competition occurs automatically and fixes the radial position of the red cell/plasma interface in the channel near the end of the control tube. If

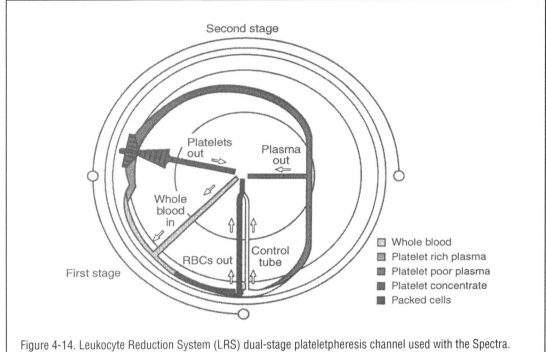

Figure 4-14. Leukocyte Reduction System (LRS) dual-stage plateletpheresis channel used with the Spectra. RBCs = red blood cells. (Copyright, CaridianBCT, Inc, 2009. Used with permission.)

there is excess plasma, it will travel through the control tube faster than red cells in the red cell tube because of its relatively lower viscosity, and red cells will accumulate, adjusting the interface radially inwards. Conversely, if red cells are in excess, a higher viscosity red cell/plasma mixture will enter the control tube, slowing flow there so that more red cells will flow out of the large tube, adjusting the interface radially outward. This system is capable of collecting platelets with $<5 \times 10^6$ leukocytes per unit; however, it does not do so consistently without the LRS system.[5]

Platelet collection was enhanced with software Version 7 (Turbo) by modifying the dual-stage channel and the computer programs to process blood faster during the establishment of the interface.[6] The second stage of the channel (Fig 4-14) was modified to include a sharp bend beyond the platelet collection port. This bend slows the flow of PRP through the second stage and reduces a swirling action of the platelets, allowing more platelets to be collected without altering white cell content.[6]

The conical LRS chamber (Fig 4-14) enhances separation of platelets from leukocytes with saturated, fluidized, particle bed filtration technology. The collection line contents enter the LRS chamber at a high speed, owing to the small tubing diameter, but slow down as they encounter the increased diameter of the chamber. Leukocytes tend to stay at the chamber entrance while platelets move radially inward. When the chamber has filled with platelets, they begin to exit. Two forces tend to keep leukocytes at the chamber entrance: 1) a higher g force in the outer portion of the chamber and 2) the mass of less dense platelets they would have to percolate through to exit the chamber. The system can consistently collect platelet components with $<1.0 \times 10^6$ leukocytes.[1,7-9] For optimal performance, the system requires constant g forces and pump rates. If the instrument detects changes in these parameters, or if the CCM detects a spillover, the operator is advised by a readout at the end of the procedure to measure the leukocyte content of the component.

Single-Stage Channels. A straightforward channel having an inlet line and exit lines for red cells and plasma is provided for blood exchange procedures. Another single-stage channel is used for leukocyte collections (Fig 4-15). Collection of different cell types can be emphasized by varying centrifugal force. Whole blood flows counterclockwise after entering the channel, and centrifugal force separates blood components on the basis of their densities. Plasma exits via the innermost port while most red cells exit via the outermost port; there is a buffy coat collection port at an intermediate radius just upstream from an interface barrier, as described in Chapter 1. Once again, a small diameter control tube joined to the red cell removal tube is used to help establish and maintain the interface. Leukocyte collections require some operator attention to monitor the collect-line color and some intervention to adjust the plasma pump speed. The system is susceptible to interface disruptions with changes in hematocrit, pump speeds, or resistance in the return access.

Spectra Summary. The operator communicates with the instrument through the control panel. Each procedure is customized on the basis of entered data such as height, weight, platelet count, and hematocrit. The instrument establishes optimal and maximal pump rates, with particular concern for anticoagulant delivery. It also calculates the amount of anticoagulant in the products. It has a platelet yield predictor, and the endpoint predictors are quite accurate.

The Spectra is a continuous flow instrument capable of double- or single-needle plateletpheresis and double-needle leukapheresis, as well as of therapeutic procedures such as TPE, mononuclear cell (MNC) collections [including hematopoietic progenitor cells (HPCs)], red cell exchange, therapeutic platelet and WBC depletions, and marrow processing. Plasma can be collected as a by-product during plateletpheresis, but the time requirements and the cost of disposables make the instrument impractical for 2-unit plasma donation alone.

Advantages of the Spectra include automated plateletpheresis, consistently leukocyte-

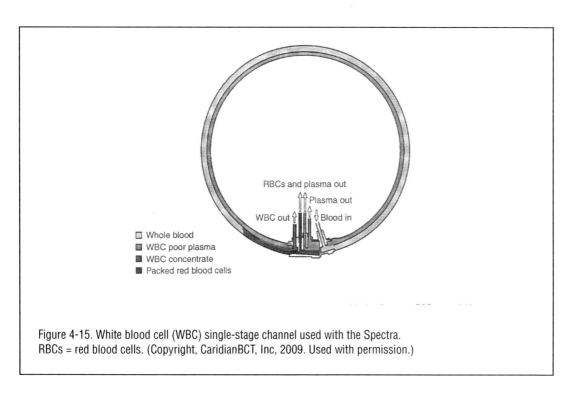

Figure 4-15. White blood cell (WBC) single-stage channel used with the Spectra. RBCs = red blood cells. (Copyright, CaridianBCT, Inc, 2009. Used with permission.)

reduced platelets without further processing, low ECV, moderate mobility, a reliable yield predictor (in the microprocessor), both single- and double-needle procedure capability, anticoagulant control, and availability of some manual control. Disadvantages include its relatively large size, an unstable interface during leukapheresis, and inconsistent CCM yield predictions with plateletpheresis.

Fresenius Instruments

Fresenius AS 104

The Fresenius AS 104 (Fresenius Kabi, Redmond, WA) (Fig 4-16) comes with several preprogrammed, automated procedures; customized programs can also be entered. It is no longer used for plateletpheresis; however, it can perform granulocyte collection, TPE, red cell exchange, MNC collection (including HPC collection), therapeutic platelet and WBC depletions, and marrow processing. It has four

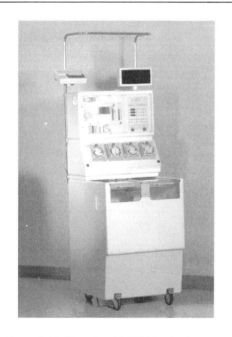

Figure 4-16. Fresenius AS 104 blood cell separator. (Used with permission from Mayo Foundation for Medical Education and Research.)

pumps (anticoagulant, whole blood, plasma, and collection), as well as access and return pressure sensors, and an air detector. The centrifugation system is sealless. Unique features include an anticoagulant drip monitor, a small printer that provides a hard copy of run data, a battery backup blood pump, and a "help" program in the microprocessor that contains the entire operator's manual.

A disposable single-stage channel is used for granulocyte collection (Fig 4-17). Operation is cyclical: buffy coat accumulates in the channel and then spills over; granulocytes are collected during spillovers, following which buffy coat is allowed to accumulate again; and so on.

The operator communicates with the instrument through a large LED screen and a series of displays and controls on the control panel. Continuous displays are provided that show inlet and return pressures as well as interface position. As can be seen in Table 4-1, this instrument has the lowest ECVs of the instruments reviewed herein.

Advantages include the low ECVs, an anticoagulant drip monitor, a printer as standard equipment, a battery backup blood pump, an extensive "help" program, some manual control, custom programmability, automated interface control without preprocedure counts, quick interface establishment with leukapheresis, and moderate mobility. Disadvantages include its large size and the inability to collect platelets.

Fresenius COM.TEC

The COM.TEC (Fresenius Kabi) is the latest microprocessor-driven apheresis instrument released from Fresenius (Fig 4-18). Though it uses the same disposables as the AS 104, it has several new features. The instrument is lighter (Table 4-1), quieter, and easier to move. Disposables are easier to load and the interface monitor is improved. The COM.TEC also has improved plateletpheresis capabilities over the AS 104. It is currently approved for platelet collection in Canada but not the United States.

A dual-stage spiral channel is provided for plateletpheresis (Figs 4-19 and 4-20). Anticoag-

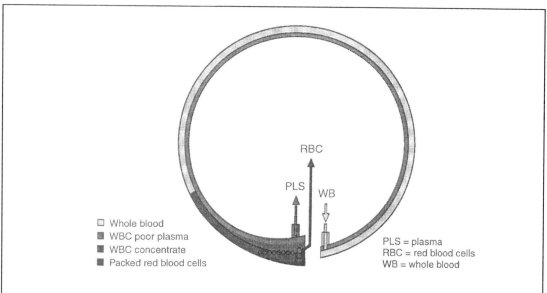

Figure 4-17. Granulocyte single-stage channel used with the Fresenius AS 104 and COM.TEC. WBCs are collected intermittently, during spillovers into the PLS line. (Used with permission from Fresenius Kabi.)

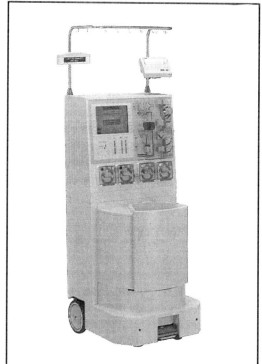

Figure 4-18. Fresenius COM.TEC. (Used with permission from Fresenius Kabi.)

ulated whole blood is pumped into the first stage and travels counterclockwise (viewed from above). A new feature is a recirculation pump that adds PPP to whole blood to obtain a hematocrit of 37% as the blood enters the centrifuge (Fig 4-19). Centrifugal force separates red cells and most of the leukocytes from PRP, which spills over into the second stage, where it also flows counterclockwise. Platelets are concentrated at a platelet exit port at the maximal radius and are removed by the cell pump (Fig 4-19). PPP continues counterclockwise around the second stage and is removed from a plasma exit port by the plasma pump. The position of the plasma/cell interface is monitored by an infrared camera and maintained automatically by the instrument. The PPP is either collected in a transfer pack or returned to the donor with cellular components separated in the first stage.

A single-stage channel is employed for granulocyte collection (Fig 4-17). Operation is identical to that in the AS 104.

The COM.TEC is capable of the same procedure applications as the AS 104; however, only TPE is approved in the United States at this time. Advantages of the COM.TEC include

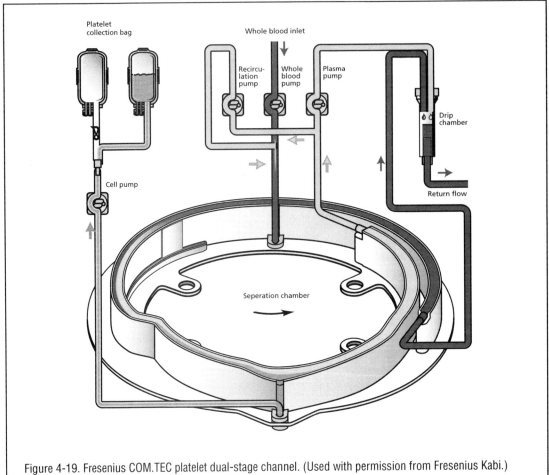

Figure 4-19. Fresenius COM.TEC platelet dual-stage channel. (Used with permission from Fresenius Kabi.)

adjustable centrifuge speed and cell/plasma interface monitoring.

Instruments for Red Cell and Other Component Collection

There are five systems capable of collecting red cells and other components. They offer standardized units of red cells and plasma because collection can proceed until a predetermined product volume is obtained, regardless of donor hematocrit. On-site component collection also obviates the need for further processing. In addition, automated component collection allows optimal utilization of available donors to meet inventory needs. For example, donors with higher blood volumes and hematocrits can donate double doses of red cells, whereas donors with lower blood volumes and hematocrits can donate a single unit of red cells and plasma and/or platelets, depending on blood type and current inventory needs.

CaridianBCT Trima Accel

CaridianBCT's Trima Accel (Version 5.1) is the latest in a series of modifications of computer software and disposables for the Trima instrument (Figs 4-21, 4-22, 4-23) for automated blood component collection. It is designed for donor procedures only. The fluid path is less

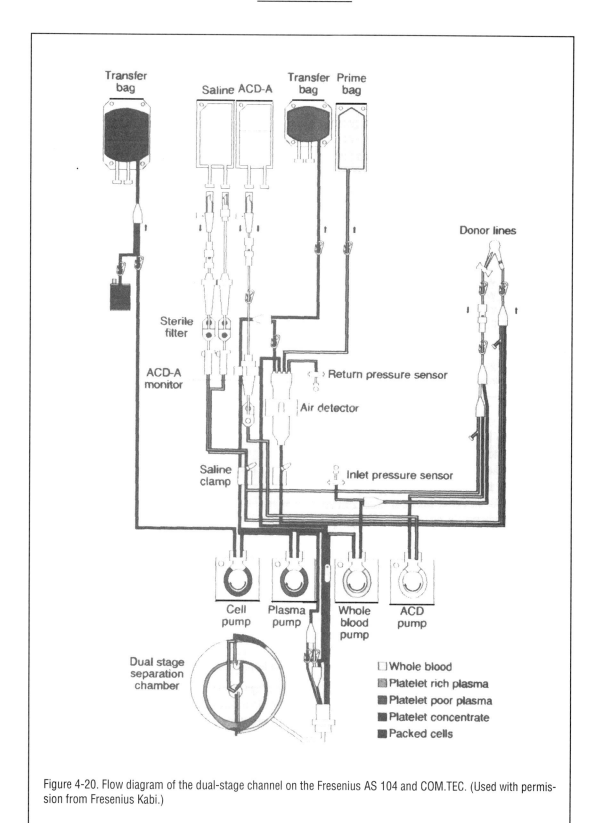

Figure 4-20. Flow diagram of the dual-stage channel on the Fresenius AS 104 and COM.TEC. (Used with permission from Fresenius Kabi.)

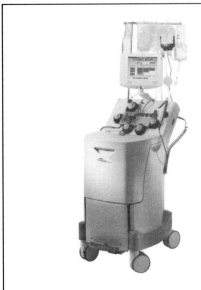

Figure 4-21. Trima Accel blood separator. (Copyright, CaridianBCT, Inc, 2009. Used with permission.)

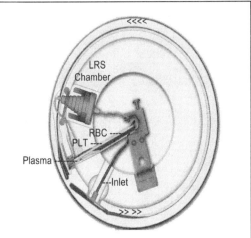

Figure 4-22. Trima Accel single-stage channel. (Copyright, CaridianBCT, Inc, 2009. Used with permission.)

complex and more compact than that of the Spectra. Most of the tubing is enclosed in a cassette with self-loading pump loops. The Trima

has five pumps: anticoagulant, inlet (draws blood), plasma (moves plasma to plasma collection bag or return reservoir), platelet (moves platelets to platelet collection bag or return reservoir; for red cell/plasma donation, it pumps saline to return reservoir), and return (returns blood). The Trima has three valves that direct

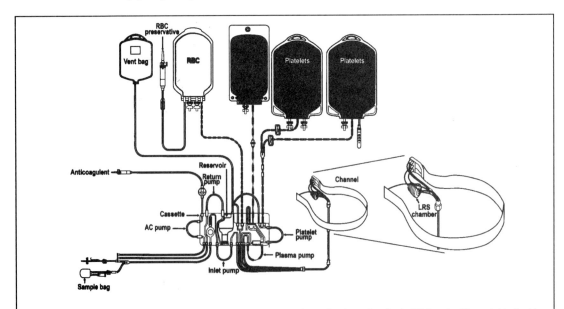

Figure 4-23. Blood flow diagram of the Trima Accel system for collection of a single RBC unit. (Copyright, CaridianBCT, Inc, 2009. Used with permission.)

the collection of platelets, plasma, or red cells. The operator communicates with the instrument via a touch screen. Commands are executed by touching icons on the screen. Graphs and icons display the status of the procedure.

The Trima Accel Version 5 incorporates modifications designed to increase platelet collection efficiency. Both channel and software were changed. The new channel is a single-stage channel that is less selective for platelets (vs WBCs) but more efficient in platelet collection. It has an oversized LRS chamber in the platelet collection line (Fig 4-22) that traps the excess WBCs and thus allows more efficient collection of a component that still qualifies as leukocyte reduced. A shelf was also added in the buffy coat area to help separate the platelets from the WBCs.

The Trima Accel uses single-needle venous access to provide intermittent flow to and from the donor but continuous flow to the centrifuge. Anticoagulated whole blood is pumped into the channel (Fig 4-22), from which platelets and plasma are drawn off by separate pumps to a collection bag and return reservoir, respectively. Packed red cells are pushed from the channel by the inlet pump and directed to either a collection bag or the return reservoir. When approximately 54 mL have accumulated in the return reservoir, the instrument automatically switches to the return cycle. The return pump delivers blood back to the donor until a low level is detected in the return reservoir. During this return phase, however, the inlet pump continues to run slowly, pumping some "return" blood back through the channel to maintain the plasma-cell interface. When the return cycle is complete, the instrument reverts to the draw cycle. Cycles continue until the programmed component volumes are collected. Collected red cells are then removed from the instrument, after which addition of preservative solution and leukocyte reduction by filtration (if desired) are carried out manually. Software Version 6.0, scheduled for release in 2010, will incorporate an online leukocyte reduction filter and addition of preservative solution by a pump. The platelet components are adequately leukocyte reduced.[10-13]

The Trima Accel is capable of collecting single or double Red Blood Cell (RBC) units; single, double, or triple plateletpheresis units; and/or plasma, with the choice depending on donor size, blood type, hematocrit, and platelet count as well as inventory needs. It has programmable settings for anticoagulant and blood flow rates that allow for shorter or longer procedure times.

Advantages of the instruments include simple set up and operation, multiple component collection, efficient platelet collection, consistent leukocyte reduction, low extracorporeal volume, and moderate mobility. Disadvantages include size (larger than the Haemonetics MCS+ or Fenwal ALYX described below) and manual red cell preservative addition and leukocyte reduction (which will be corrected with Version 6.0 software).

Haemonetics MCS+ LN8150

The Haemonetics MCS+ LN8150 (Fig 4-24) is similar to the LN9000, but less complex and capable of automated collection of both red cells and plasma. It uses intermittent flow via a

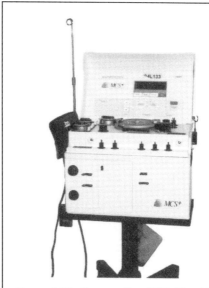

Figure 4-24. Haemonetics MCS Plus LN8150 blood separator. (Used with permission from Haemonetics Corporation.)

single needle. In the draw cycle, anticoagulated whole blood is pumped into a blow-molded bowl from which separated plasma emerges and is directed into a plasma/air bag (Fig 4-25). When the cell-plasma interface is detected by an optical sensor, the return cycle is initiated. The blood pump is reversed and red cells from the bowl are directed to a collection bag while an appropriate volume of saline replacement is pumped back to the donor by a separate pump. Draw/return cycles continue until the targeted volumes of plasma and red cells are collected, after which any residual plasma and red cells are returned to the donor. The solution pump is used to transfer preservative solution to the red cells. Three kits are available: kits for collecting 1) 2 RBC units; 2) a single RBC unit plus a jumbo plasma unit; and 3) 2 RBC units with an in-line leukocyte-reduction filter (leukocyte reduction is performed after collection by gravity flow through this filter).

Advantages of the MCS+ LN 8150 include a simple design, double RBC unit collection, and portability. Disadvantages include its large extracorporeal volume and inability to collect platelets.

Haemonetics Cymbal Automated Blood Collection System

The latest release from Haemonetics is a very small (about half the size of the MCS+ LN 8150), AC-plug-in or battery-powered, double-unit RBC collection instrument called the Cymbal Automated Blood Collection System (Fig 4-26). It is based on a new separation device called the Dynamic Disk (Fig 4-27), which consists of a hard plastic top over a flexible membrane (Fig 4-27). The disk can be filled or emptied by application of negative or positive pressure, respectively, in the space adjacent to the membrane. Anticoagulant is pumped to the whole blood line and the whole blood is pumped into the rotating disc (Fig 4-28). Red cells migrate to the radially outward wall while plasma goes radially inward and eventually flows out of a central exit port into a reinfusion bag (Figs 4-27 and 4-28). When the disk has

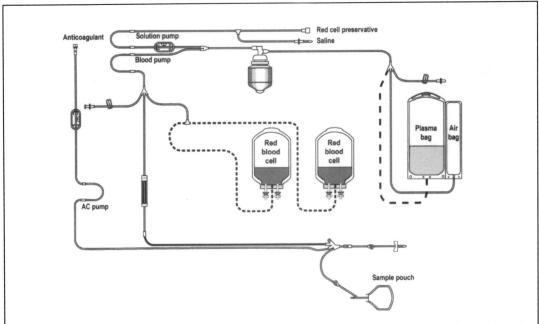

Figure 4-25. Blood flow diagram of the Haemonetics MCS Plus LN8150 system for collection of a double RBC unit. (Used with permission from Haemonetics Corporation.)

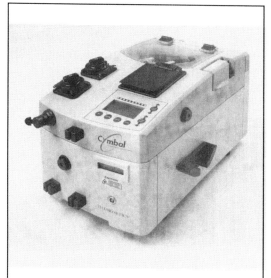

Figure 4-26. Haemonetics Cymbal System. (Used with permission from Haemonetics Corporation.)

filled with red cells, plasma plus saline are returned to the donor. The red cells are concentrated, and an additive solution (AS 3) is drawn into the disk and mixes with the red

cells. Positive pressure is then applied to the membrane; the red cell suspension exits the disk, passes through a leukocyte-reduction filter, and is delivered to the final collection bags (Fig 4-28). Blood withdrawal then resumes. The donation continues until four cycles have been completed and 2 units of leukocyte-reduced, AS-3 RBC units have been collected.

The Cymbal System has electric scales, two pumps, an air detector, pressure sensors, a sensor for red cells, and a bar-code reader. There are optional lithium ion rechargeable batteries to run the instrument, good for one day's collections. The size, weight, and ECV are presented in Table 4-2. At the time of this writing, the Cymbal can collect only a double red cell product, but additional capabilities are planned. Advantages of the Cymbal include the small size, bar-code reader, and low ECV.

Fenwal ALYX Component Collection System

In 2002, Baxter Fenwal introduced the ALYX (Fig 4-29) component collection system. The instrument is very portable and uses a pneu-

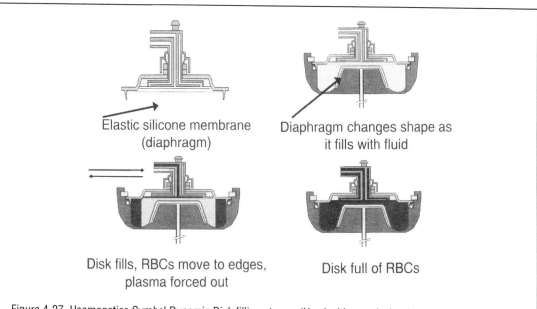

Elastic silicone membrane (diaphragm)

Diaphragm changes shape as it fills with fluid

Disk fills, RBCs move to edges, plasma forced out

Disk full of RBCs

Figure 4-27. Haemonetics Cymbal Dynamic Disk filling stages. (Used with permission from Haemonetics Corporation.)

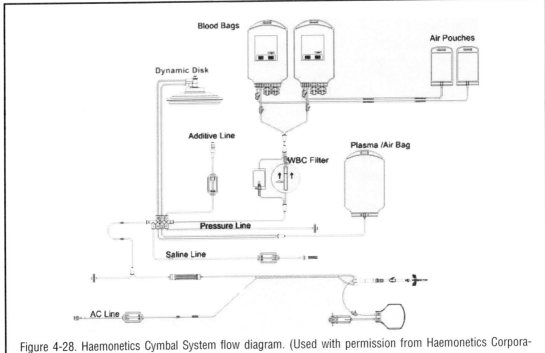

Figure 4-28. Haemonetics Cymbal System flow diagram. (Used with permission from Haemonetics Corporation.)

matic pressure pump system, rather than roller pumps, to move fluids. The pneumatic pumps have flexible chamber walls that are squeezed with air pressure and then allowed to fill again. The disposable separation chamber in the centrifuge is a preformed rigid plastic cylinder. The flow pattern is similar to that in the separation chamber of the AMICUS plateletpheresis set.

The ALYX also uses single-needle access and provides intermittent flow/return to the donor but continuous flow to the centrifuge. During the draw cycle, anticoagulated whole blood is withdrawn from the donor by a "donor pump" (Fig 4-30). Downstream, a separate "in-process" pump draws some blood from the inlet line and pumps it into the centrifuge. The donor pump runs faster than the in-process pump; excess blood accumulates in an "in-process" bag (Fig 4-30). Whole blood entering the centrifuge flows around the cylinder and is separated into red cells and plasma. Plasma is drawn off through a radially inward plasma port and pumped into a plasma bag. Packed

red cells are pushed through a radially outward port to a red cell bag. When a preset amount of blood has been withdrawn, the instrument switches to the return cycle, during which plasma from the plasma bag is returned to the donor by the donor pump along with saline replacement. Simultaneously, the in-process pump draws unprocessed blood from the in-process bag and delivers it to the centrifuge for separation. When the plasma bag has been emptied, the instrument advances to the next draw cycle. Draw/return cycles continue until the targeted volume of red cells has been collected, at which point the instrument returns any excess components to the donor. When collection is complete, the instrument adds preservative solution and pumps the red cell component through a single leukocyte-reduction filter and into two collection bags, mixing the two in-line.

The ALYX can collect 2 RBC units or a single RBC unit plus plasma. Advantages of the ALYX include simple design, portability, small

Table 4-2. Automated Component Collection Instrument Overview

| | CaridianBCT | Haemonetics | | | Fenwal | |
	Trima Accel	MCS+ LN 8150	Cymbal	ALYX	AMICUS	
Type of system	IFD, CFC	IFC	IFC	IFD, CFC	IFD, CFC	
Weight (lb)	185	56	29	51	345	
Height × width × depth (inches)	41.9 × 20.8 × 32	26.5 × 21.5 × 21.5	14 × 14 × 20	26 × 18 × 19	75.6 × 24 × 27.8	
ECV (approx):Without product Total	182-196	542 (38% Hct)-391 (54% Hct)	200 ml	110 + collect bags/(110 × Hct) + (IP/1.05 g/mL) + RBCs/1.08 g/mL	329 ml (max)	
Monitors:						
Draw pressure	Yes	Yes	Yes	Yes	Yes	
Return pressure	Yes	Yes	Yes	Yes	Yes	
Air present	Yes	Yes	Yes	Yes	Yes	
AC delivery	Yes	Yes	Yes	Yes	Yes	
Centrifuge pressure	Yes	Yes	Yes	Yes	Yes	
Leak detector	Yes	Yes	Yes	Yes	Yes	
Blood warmer	No	No	No	No	No	
Donor applications	Plts (1 or 2 units) Concurrent plasma RBCs (1 or 2 units)	Concurrent plasma RBCs (1 or 2 units)	RBCs (2 units)	RBCs (1 or 2 units) Concurrent plasma	Plts (1 or 2 units) Concurrent plasma Concurrent RBCs (1 unit)	

IFD = intermittent flow to donor; CFC = continuous flow to centrifuge; IFC = intermittent flow centrifugation; ECV = extracorporeal volume; Hct = hematocrit; max = maximum; IP = in-process bag; RBCs = Red Blood Cells; Plts = platelets.

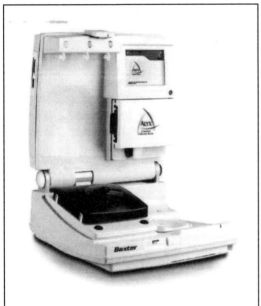

Figure 4-29. ALYX blood separator. (Used with permission from Fenwal, Inc.)

size, continuous whole blood processing, low extracorporeal volume, and automated preservative addition and leukocyte reduction. The major disadvantage of the ALYX at this time is its inability to collect platelets.

Fenwal AMICUS Red Cell Collection

As mentioned previously, the AMICUS can collect apheresis platelets using double- or single-needle kits. In 2002, Baxter Fenwal released Version 2.51 software that includes the option of collecting a single RBC unit in addition to single or double plateletpheresis units from eligible donors using the single-needle kit (Fig 4-31). The RBC unit is collected by not returning the red cells on the last cycle. After an RBC unit is removed from the instrument, addition of preservative and leukocyte reduction by filtration are carried out manually using an add-on kit. Disadvantages include size (larger than the MCS+ or ALYX) and the inability to collect 2 RBC units.

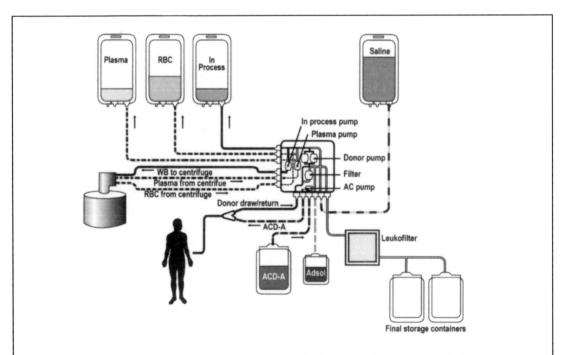

Figure 4-30. Blood flow diagram of the ALYX system during the draw cycle. (Used with permission from Fenwal, Inc.)

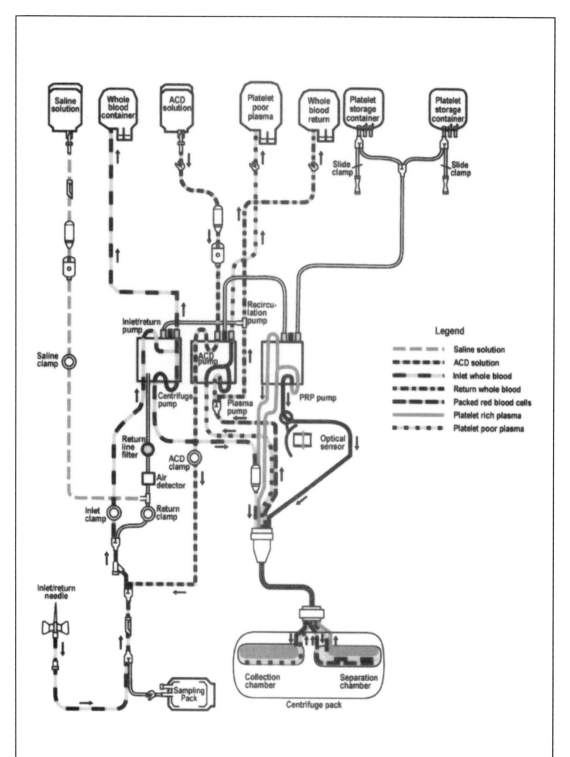

Figure 4-31. Blood flow diagram of the AMICUS single-needle system during the draw cycle. (Used with permission from Fenwal, Inc.)

Comparison of Donor Apheresis Systems

Features

Table 4-1 is a comparison of system types, dimensions, ECVs, monitors, and donor applications for platelet, granulocyte, and plasma collection. All systems listed have centrifugal separators except the Fenwal Autopheresis C, which combines centrifugation with filtration. All of the Haemonetics systems are intermittent flow, and the Autopheresis C is limited to intermittent processing by its single-needle configuration. CaridianBCT's COBE Spectra, Fresenius's AS 104 and COM.TEC, and Fenwal's AMICUS use continuous flow *processing*; however, when the available single-needle systems are used, blood *flow* can become intermittent.

When available space and portability are being considered, machine dimensions and weight are important issues. As can be seen in Table 4-1, the Haemonetics MCS models and PCS-2 are the smallest instruments at 56 pounds and 7 cubic feet, whereas Caridian-BCT's COBE Spectra is the largest at 389 pounds and 26.5 cubic feet.

ECV is another important consideration. The Fresenius AS 104 has the lowest ECV at 175 mL (dual needle), and the Haemonetics Latham bowl systems have the highest ECVs at 359 to 480 mL for donors. It should also be noted that with the AMICUS, some of the product is included in the ECV, whereas with the other systems, the product volume is in addition to the stated ECV. The ECVs quoted for CaridianBCT's COBE Spectra are tubing set volumes, as indicated in the operator's manual, to make them comparable to the other ECVs listed. CaridianBCT usually reports ECV in equivalent blood volume, which is calculated from the red cell volume in the set with a 40% hematocrit. Of the single-needle systems, the Autopheresis C has the lowest ECV at 200 mL.

Most instruments have several standard sensors, such as draw and return pressure sensors, air detectors, and centrifuge pressure detectors. An anticoagulant delivery detector is lacking only in the Autopheresis C. The MCS, MCS+, PCS-2, and COBE Spectra monitor for air in the anticoagulant tubing, the AS 104 has a drip counter to monitor anticoagulant delivery rate, and the AMICUS monitors bag weight. Centrifuge leak detectors are found in the COBE Spectra, AS 104, COM.TEC, and AMICUS.

The COBE Spectra and the two Fresenius instruments can collect platelets and granulocytes as well as plasma as a by-product. The Autopheresis C and PCS-2 can collect plasma only.

When considering automated component collection, several factors need to be addressed: versatility in types of products collected, portability, extracorporeal volume, simplicity of operation, and donor safety. Of the instruments reviewed, the Trima is the most versatile (Table 4-2). The Cymbal is the smallest and therefore the most readily portable machine available (Table 4-2). ECV is difficult to compare in these machines because they all operate with single access and have different ECVs depending on the access and the stage of the procedure (Table 4-2). It is assumed that donors can tolerate loss of at least one pint of blood and all of the instruments are within that ECV limit. All of the instruments reviewed are fairly simple to operate. Donor safety features are incorporated into all the instruments reviewed; however, citrate toxicity must still be monitored on the basis of individual donor tolerance.

Therapeutic Applications

HPC and MNC Collection

Fenwal AMICUS

Fenwal provides a separate MNC kit to collect HPCs and MNCs with the AMICUS (Fig 4-6), but it actually performs a plateletpheresis, in cycles, on the donor or patient. Collected platelets are continuously returned to the donor/patient as the MNC layer builds up (Fig 4-8). When sufficient MNCs have accumulated (usually from 1000-1400 mL whole blood processed), approximately 30 mL of packed red cells are collected and then slowly pumped into the separation chamber. As the cell/plasma interface rises, MNCs exit the PRP line, pass through an optical sensor, and flow into a collection bag outside the centrifuge. The optical sensor determines when to open and close the valve to the product bag and can be programmed for the optimal degree of cross-cellular content, favoring lymphocytes, monocytes, or a combination. The collection chamber in the channel is filled with normal saline for balance but is excluded from the blood flow path. The ECV is 163 mL. Software Version 3.1 includes additional anticoagulant ratios (up to 30:1), printable procedure reports, and more operator-controlled functions during the procedure.

Advantages include small ECV, good mobility, and platelet sparing technology. Disadvantages include limited therapeutic apheresis applications.

CaridianBCT COBE Spectra

All COBE Spectra (Fig 4-12) software versions except Version 6.0 Auto PBSC collect HPCs and MNCs, with the operator monitoring the collect line and making adjustments as needed (as in granulocyte collection). Anticoagulant ratios up to 30:1 are available. The ECV is 285 mL.

The Version 6.0 Auto PBSC program is a fully automated collection system that processes blood in a dual-stage channel (similar to Fig 4-14, but without the LRS chamber). MNCs accumulate and are transferred to a collection bag in discrete cycles. Flow rates are controlled by donor-specific data entered into the system; however, settings for harvesting MNCs are adjustable. The ECV is 282 mL.

Advantages include manual and automated formats and multiple therapeutic applications. Disadvantages include relatively high platelet loss, a requirement for current MNC counts with Auto PBSC, and only moderate mobility.

Frensenius AS 104 and COM.TEC

The AS 104 (Fig 4-16) and COM.TEC (Fig 4-18) can collect HPCs using three different dis-

posable kits. One kit has a single-stage channel (Fig 4-17) and collects in cycles, as for granulocyte collection. There are two versions of the dual-stage channel kit; both separate cell-rich plasma from packed red cells in the first stage; MNCs are concentrated in the second stage and then delivered to the collection bag. Packed red cells from the first stage and cell-poor plasma from the second stage are returned to the donor/patient. One of the dual-stage kits is capable of collecting a reduced-volume product. The cell/plasma interface is monitored automatically (with an infrared camera in the COM.TEC), and collection parameters can be adjusted. The ECV is 175 mL. The COM.TEC is not approved for HPC and MNC collection in the United States at this time.

Advantages include small ECV and multiple collection options. Disadvantages include moderate to poor mobility and unavailability of some applications in the United States.

Therapeutic Plasma Exchange and Absorption/Selective Removal

Several apheresis instruments can perform TPE. The continuous flow devices among these can also be adapted to provide a plasma stream for absorption/selective removal (ASR) of a plasma component, as described in Chapter 21.

CaridianBCT COBE Spectra

The COBE Spectra (Fig 4-12) can perform either TPE or ASR with a single-stage channel that has only plasma and cell exit ports (Fig 4-15). The cell/plasma interface is not monitored, but its position is dictated by algorithms derived from patient-specific data entered into the microprocessor. For TPE, the plasma is collected in a large waste bag. For ASR, plasma is usually perfused through the selective system and then into a reservoir bag for return to the patient by the replacement pump. The ECV for the double-needle disposable is 285 mL.

CaridianBCT Spectra Optia

CaridianBCT recently released the Spectra Optia (Fig 4-32) for TPE in the United States and Canada, with plans to add capability for all the therapeutic procedures and the granulocyte collection procedure that are possible with the COBE Spectra. The Spectra Optia is much smaller, quieter, and easier to move and operate than its predecessor. One major improvement is a cell/plasma interface-monitoring device called the Automated Interface Management (AIM) system. AIM includes a high-speed digital imaging system that monitors the cell/plasma interface in a single-stage channel. When buffy-coat components have accumulated to a maximum allowable thickness, a buffy-coat return phase begins. The plasma pump slows to 10% of the inlet rate; this increases passive outflow through the red cell line to accommodate the continuing inlet flow, which forces buffy-coat components out through the red cell line as plasma accumulates in the channel. When buffy-coat thickness has decreased, the plasma pump speeds up to re-establish the cell/plasma interface. The system intermittently repeats this process until the procedure is complete. Separated red cells and replacement fluids flow into a small reservoir, and a return pump controls the return to the patient from the reservoir.

The Spectra Optia has five pumps: anticoagulant, inlet, remove/plasma, replace/collect, and return (Fig 4-33). It has three pressure sensors: inlet, return, and centrifuge. It also has a tubing-set bar-code reader, a red cell detector, an anticoagulant fluid detector, a replacement fluid detector, and low- and high-level sensors for the reservoir. It has a touch screen operator interface that displays states of the procedure and suggests actions to address alarms. It also has the ability to print run data to an external printer or network file. Its dimensions are 41.9 inches (106.4 cm) high, 20.8 inches (52.7 cm) wide, and 32 inches (81.3 cm) deep; it weighs 202 pounds (91.8 kg). The ECV for TPE is 185 mL.

Advantages include a small ECV, the interface monitor, and the network or print run data option. A disadvantage is the limited number of applications (TPE and ASR only) in the United States.

Fresenius AS 104

For TPE and ASR, the AS 104 (Fig 4-16) is fitted with a single-stage channel similar to that in Fig 4-17. Advantages include a low ECV (175 mL), an automated interface detector, and a run data printer. Disadvantages include cumbersome loading of the channel insert and platelet loss at high flow rates.[14,15]

Fresenius COM.TEC

The COM.TEC (Fig 4-18) is approved for TPE and ASR in the United States and Canada with the same modified single-stage channel as the AS 104. The variable speed centrifuge in the COM.TEC has reduced the average platelet loss from the 19% seen with the AS 104 to 3%.[16]

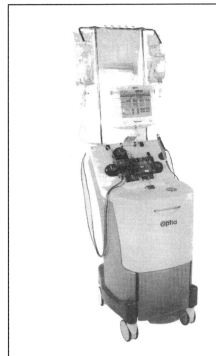

Figure 4-32. CaridianBCT Spectra Optia. (Copyright, CaridianBCT, Inc, 2009. Used with permission.)

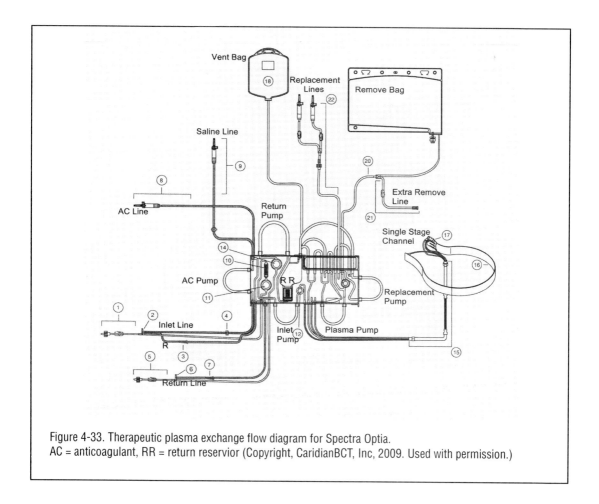

Figure 4-33. Therapeutic plasma exchange flow diagram for Spectra Optia.
AC = anticoagulant, RR = return reservoir (Copyright, CaridianBCT, Inc, 2009. Used with permission.)

Advantages include a more precise cell/plasma interface monitor (infrared camera), easier channel loading, low ECV (175 mL), a wireless download option, and low platelet loss. A disadvantage is the limited number of applications (TPE and ASR only) in the United States.

Haemonetics MCS LN9000

The Haemonetics MCS LN9000 (Fig 4-5) can perform TPE with either a 125-mL or 225-mL Latham bowl (Fig 4-2), depending on patient blood volume and hematocrit. The procedure is automated and can be performed with either single or double access. Maximum ECV for the LN9000 is 950 mL. The instrument notifies the operator when ECV has reached 15% of the patient's blood volume. Thereafter it limits

progression of the procedure in 100-mL increments until 950 mL is reached.

Advantages of the LN9000 include small size and mobility. Disadvantages include a large ECV and application that is limited to TPE.

Red Cell Exchange/Depletion

CaridianBCT COBE Spectra

The COBE Spectra (Fig 4-12) can perform red cell exchange with a single-stage channel (Fig 4-15) and a modified tubing set. The microprocessor determines the volume of red cells to remove and replace, based on patient-specific data entered for each procedure. The ECV in this application is 285 mL.

Fresenius AS 104 and COM.TEC

Both the AS 104 (Fig 4-16) and COM.TEC (Fig 4-18) can accomplish red cell exchange with a modified single-stage channel. The tubing set for red cell exchange is only slightly modified from the TPE set. The microprocessor calculates the volumes of red cells to be removed and replaced based on information entered for each procedure and patient. The COM.TEC is not approved for red cell exchange in the United States.

Therapeutic Cytapheresis (WBC or Platelet Depletion)

CaridianBCT COBE Spectra

A modification of the MNC procedure is used for therapeutic leukapheresis with the COBE Spectra. Differences include the hematocrit of the product as it is collected, a higher collection speed, and a higher product volume. Hydroxyethyl starch may be added to blood entering the centrifuge to enhance separation of WBCs from red cells. ECV in this application is 285 mL.

A modification of the dual-needle plateletpheresis procedure is used for therapeutic platelet depletion with the COBE Spectra. The channel lacks an LRS chamber. ECV in this application is 260 mL.

Fresenius AS 104 and COM.TEC

A dual-stage channel and plateletpheresis disposable serve for both platelet and leukocyte reduction on both the AS 104 and COM.TEC. Its ECV is 175 mL. The COM.TEC is not approved for depletion procedures in the United States.

Cholesterol Reduction

A more complete account of selective removal of cholesterol and lipoprotein can be found in Chapter 21. This section addresses only the equipment used.

Kaneka MA-03

The Kaneka MA-03 (Kaneka Corp, Osaka, Japan) is a recent replacement for the MA-01 used for selective removal of low-density lipoprotein (LDL), very-low-density lipoprotein (VLDL), and lipoprotein a (Lp^a) (Fig 4-34). Most of the high-density lipoprotein (HDL), which is considered desirable, is returned to the patient. A syringe pump delivers heparin anti-

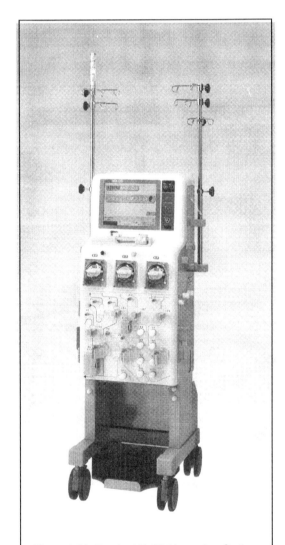

Figure 4-34. Kaneka MA-03 Liposorber System. (Used with permission from Kaneka Corporation.)

coagulant to the inlet line. A blood pump (Fig 4-35) delivers heparinized whole blood to a hollow fiber plasma separator, from which cell-free plasma is drawn off with a plasma pump while cells are returned to the patient. The plasma is routed to one of a pair of adsorption columns that contain dextran sulfate chemically bonded to cellulose beads. The negative charge of the dextran sulfate attracts the positive charges of LDL, VLDL, and Lp^a lipoproteins, but HDL passes through. Treated plasma passes through a filter and then a blood warmer before being recombined with packed cells for return to the patient. When 500 to 600 mL of plasma have passed through one column, the microprocessor automatically alters valve settings to direct plasma to the second column while "column one" is rinsed with buffer (lactated Ringer's solution). Plasma displaced from column one is returned to the patient, and priming solution displaced from "column two" is directed to waste. When plasma has been flushed from column one and column two has filled with plasma, the effluent

from column one is directed to waste and that from column two to the patient. Five-percent sodium chloride then enters column one to elute lipoproteins from the beads; the eluate is directed to waste. When elution is complete, column one is again filled with physiologic buffer. The sodium concentration in the waste line is monitored, and plasma cannot be routed to column one again until a physiologic salt concentration is reestablished. When approximately 500 mL plasma have been perfused through column two, the valves switch again, directing plasma to column one and buffer, followed by elution fluid, to column two. Plasma flow cycles back and forth between the two columns until the endpoint is reached.

The MA-03 has four pumps: heparin, blood, plasma, and regeneration. It also has seven pressure sensors, four air detectors, four fluid level sensors, a free hemoglobin detector, a blood warmer, a compact flash memory card, and an LCD touch screen/monitor. Its ECV is 400 mL: 230 mL plasma and 170 mL cells. The dimensions of the MA-03 are 54.8 inches

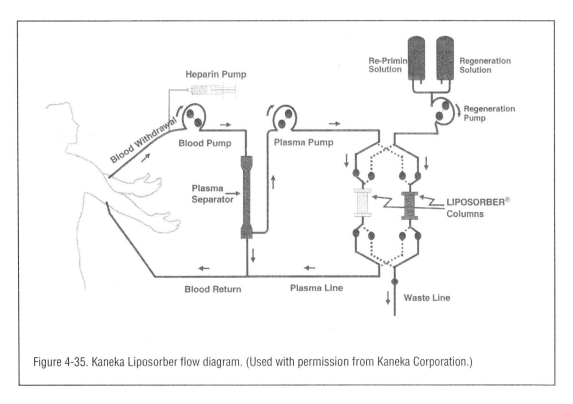

Figure 4-35. Kaneka Liposorber flow diagram. (Used with permission from Kaneka Corporation.)

(137 cm) high, 17.6 inches (44 cm) wide, and 13.8 inches (34.5 cm) deep; it weighs 169 pounds (77 kg).

Advantages of the MA-03 include good LDL reduction (66%-81%), an operator interface with a touch screen, and a memory card for each procedure.[17,18] Disadvantages include an expensive disposable set and long procedure times (a range of 2-4 hours for 1.5 plasma volumes).

B. Braun Heparin-Induced Extracorporeal LDL Precipitation (HELP) System

The HELP system (B. Braun Medical, Inc, Bethlehem, PA) is a multi-component system designed to remove LDL, VLDL, and Lp[a]. The system (Fig 4-36) includes a hollow fiber filter to separate plasma from heparinized whole blood. Plasma is diluted 1:1 with a heparin/sodium acetate solution, which lowers the pH. At pH 5.12, in the presence of (negatively charged) heparin, the positively charged lipo-proteins precipitate along with some fibrinogen. The precipitate is removed by a filter and the supernatant plasma is directed to a heparin adsorber to remove excess heparin. It then passes through a dialysis module that reduces volume and restores physiologic pH. The treated plasma is then combined with red cells and returned to the patient (Fig 4-37).

The HELP system has seven pumps: blood, heparin, plasma, buffer, recirculation, filtrate, and substitution. It also has one air detector, three level detectors, eight pressure sensors, and a monitor with operator interface. The ECV is 450 mL: 300 mL plasma and 150 mL blood. The dimensions of the HELP system are 62.4 inches (156 cm) high, 25 inches (62.5 cm) wide, and 22.4 inches (56 cm) deep; it weighs 219.3 pounds (99.7 kg).

Advantages of the HELP system include LDL reductions of 56% to 70% (better than TPE with similar procedure times).[19,20] Disadvantages include limited therapeutic applications.

Photopheresis

THERAKOS UVAR XTS Photopheresis System

The UVAR XTS Photopheresis System (THERAKOS, Raritan, NJ) is the second generation of the UVAR Photopheresis System (Fig 4-38). With several advancements in harvesting the cells, it uses a pneumatic pump (soft pillow chambers compressed by air), to move fluids, and a series of multiple valves and pressure sensors, all contained in the fluid logic module. It is a single-needle, intermittent flow instrument. A separate pump adds heparinized saline as anticoagulant to the blood line (Fig 4-39). Whole blood is withdrawn from the patient by a double-chambered pump and delivered to a Latham bowl (Fig 4-2). Sterile air and then plasma exit the bowl and flow to a plasma-air bag while red cell and buffy coat accumulate, as discussed above for Haemonetics systems. When the buffy coat reaches the shoulder of the bowl, an optical sensor is activated. Plasma from the plasma-air bag is pumped into the rotating bowl, dislodging WBCs from the buffy

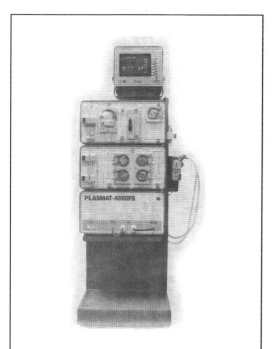

Figure 4-36. B. Braun HELP System. (Used with permission from B. Braun Medical, Inc.)

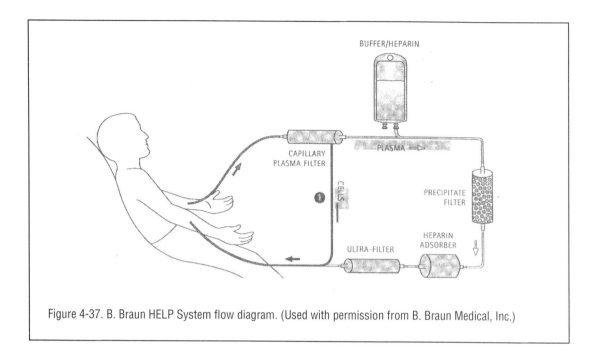

Figure 4-37. B. Braun HELP System flow diagram. (Used with permission from B. Braun Medical, Inc.)

coat layer (elutriation). Valves direct the buffy coat past a hematocrit sensor to the photoactivation chamber. When the elutriate hematocrit reaches the pre-set value, buffy coat collection ends. Plasma and red cells are returned to the patient, and another cycle begins.

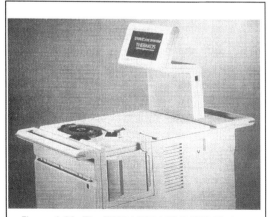

Figure 4-38. The THERAKOS UVAR XTS Photopheresis System. (Trademarks of THERAKOS, Inc; image copyright, THERAKOS, Inc, 2009.)

Depending on the patient's blood volume and hematocrit, a treatment consists of three cycles with a standard bowl (225 mL) or six cycles with a small bowl (125 mL). At the beginning of the last cycle, the photoactivation chamber is emptied and rinsed into the recirculation bag. Then the contents of the recirculation bag are emptied into the bowl and patient blood is used to complete the cycle. Instead of elutriation in the last cycle, 80 mL of additional plasma is collected into the photoactivation chamber.

Once the collection and the final return are completed, psoralen medication is added and the photoactivation mode begins. The ultraviolet A (UVA) lights turn on and the pump recirculates the buffy coat solution through the photoactivation chamber, the hematocrit sensor, and the recirculation bag. The photoactivation time is determined by the buffy coat volume and hematocrit as well as the intensity of the light source. When photoactivation is complete, the UVAR XTS System automatically returns the treated cells to the patient.

The UVAR XTS System has a fluid logic module, Latham bowl centrifuge, pressure sen-

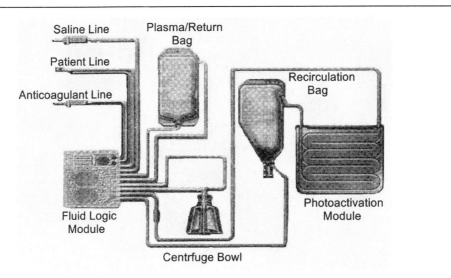

Figure 4-39. The THERAKOS UVAR XTS Photopheresis System flow diagram. (Trademarks of THERAKOS, Inc; image copyright, THERAKOS, Inc, 2009.)

sors, two air detectors, a hematocrit line sensor, ultraviolet light chamber, data key port to record each procedure, and a touch screen operator interface. ECV ranges from approximately 220 to 620 mL, depending on patient size, hematocrit, and stage of procedure. Its dimensions are 57 inches (144.1 cm) high, 18.6 inches (47.2 cm) wide, and 42.8 inches (108.7 cm) deep; it weighs 210 pounds (95 kg). The UVAR XTS System is capable of photopheresis only.

Advantages include an automated buffy coat harvest and customized photoactivation based on properties of the buffy coat collected. Disadvantages include difficulty in addressing low hematocrit in patients, large ECV, expensive disposables, and limited therapeutic applications.

THERAKOS CELLEX Photopheresis System.

The CELLEX Photopheresis System (THERAKOS) was approved by the FDA for photopheresis in the United States in early 2009. The CELLEX System (Fig 4-40) is a major change from the UVAR XTS System. It uses a single-harvest, continuous flow, sealless centrifuge bowl (Fig 4-41) that significantly reduces proce-dure time and ECV. It is also flexible in addressing high and low hematocrit, lipemic plasma, and dark plasma. It is capable of single- or double-needle access and can be switched from double-needle to single-needle during a procedure.

Whole blood is anticoagulated with heparin as it is drawn from the patient (Fig 4-42). It enters the spinning bowl in a tube near the axis of rotation that ends about halfway down into the vertical depth of the bowl (Fig 4-41). From there it migrates toward the outside wall of the bowl through a gap between upper and lower fixed plastic inserts. The geometry of the inserts confines plasma to the upper half, where it migrates toward the top center and is displaced out of the bowl by the addition of new whole blood and returned to the patient. Only packed red cells can reach the bottom of the bowl, where they are extracted by the red cell pump and returned to the patient. The buffy coat is sandwiched between the plasma and red cell layers and is retained in the bowl until 1500 mL of whole blood have been processed (Fig 4-41). The position of the buffy coat is monitored optically and managed by the speed of the red cell pump.

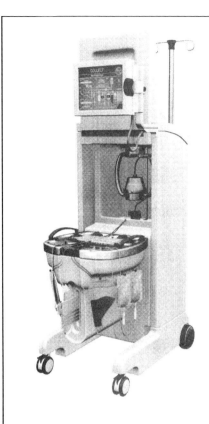

Figure 4-40. The THERAKOS CELLEX Photo-pheresis System. (Trademarks of THERAKOS, Inc; image copyright, THERAKOS, Inc, 2009.)

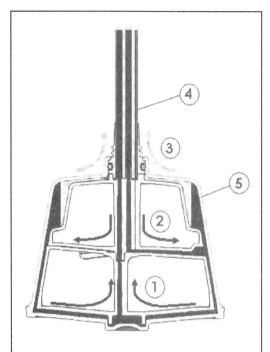

Figure 4-41. The THERAKOS CELLEX Photopher-esis System centrifuge bowl flow diagram. 1. Red cells out. 2. Whole blood in. 3. Plasma out. 4. Drive tube. 5. Continuous flow centrifuge bowl. (Trademarks of THERAKOS, Inc; image copyright, THERAKOS, Inc, 2009.)

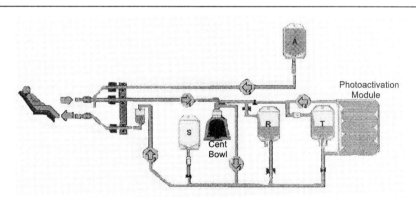

Figure 4-42. The THERAKOS CELLEX Photopheresis System flow diagram.
A = anticoagulant; S = saline; R = return bag; T = treatment bag. (Trademarks of THERAKOS, Inc; image copy-right, THERAKOS, Inc, 2009.)

Once the targeted amount of blood is processed, the red cells in additional whole blood are allowed to accumulate in the bowl and slowly float the buffy coat out of the upper, plasma exit, through a hematocrit sensor, and into the treatment bag (Fig 4-42). When the hematocrit reaches 24%, the buffy coat harvest is stopped. The bowl contents and a saline rinse are returned to the patient. The recirculation pump mixes the buffy coat with the prime solution (saline and anticoagulant), directing the flow through the hematocrit sensor. The instrument determines the photoactivation time from the product volume and hematocrit and the intensity of the UVA light source. Psoralen medication is added, and UVA photoactivation begins. When it is complete, the buffy coat is automatically reinfused to the patient, with a saline rinse at the end.

The usual procedure is one cycle and 1500 mL blood processed; however, the number of cycles and/or the volume processed per cycle can be adjusted for special circumstances. During single-needle operation, plasma and red cells are pumped into a return bag, the contents of which are intermittently returned to the patient, while the centrifuge continues to spin.

The CELLEX System has five pumps: anticoagulant, collect, red cell, return, and recirculation. It also has three pressure sensors, eight valves, five air detectors, one hematocrit sensor, and centrifuge and photoactivation chamber leak detectors. The operator interfaces with a touch screen that displays current fluid flow, states of the procedure, alarm codes, and procedure data. There is a smart card for each procedure that records data for diagnostic use. The ECV (procedural kit tubing volume) is 216 mL for a double-needle procedure or 266 mL for a single-needle procedure. The dimensions of the CELLEX System are 64 inches (163 cm) high, 23 inches (58.4 cm) wide, and 31 inches (79 cm) deep; it weighs 341 pounds (155 kg).

Advantages include low ECV, shortened procedure times, and flexible programming. Disadvantages include the high cost of disposables and limited therapeutic applications.

Summary

There are a number of apheresis systems available today. Each instrument has advantages and disadvantages; the "perfect" instrument has not yet appeared. Nevertheless, vigorous innovation by competing manufacturers continues to result in significant advances.

References

1. Burgstaler E, Pineda A, Wollan P. Plateletapheresis: Comparison of processing times, platelet yields, and white blood cell content with several systems. J Clin Apher 1997;12:170-8.
2. Burgstaler E, Pineda A, McCoy J. Plateletapheresis using the surge pump to increase blood processing rate and decrease white blood cell content (abstract). Transfusion 1994; 34(Suppl):2S.
3. Burgstaler E, Pineda A, Potter B, Brown R. Plateletapheresis with a next generation blood cell separator. J Clin Apher 1997;12:55-62.
4. Beeler S, Axelrod F. A comparison of platelet yields, processing time, and white blood cell content with COBE Spectra version 3.6 vs version 4 software single needle procedures (abstract). J Clin Apher 1995;10:30.
5. Burgstaler EA, Pineda AA, Brecher MA. Plateletapheresis: Comparison of platelet yields, processing time, and white blood cell content with two apheresis systems. Transfusion 1993;33:393-8.
6. Burgstaler EA, Pineda AA, Bryant SC. Prospective comparison of plateletapheresis using four apheresis systems on the same donors. J Clin Apher 1999;14:163-70.
7. Perseghin P, Mascaretti L, Riva M, et al. Comparison of plateletpheresis concentrates produced with Spectra LRS version 5.1 and LRS Turbo version 7.0 cell separators. Transfusion 2000;40:789-93.
8. Zingsem J, Glaser A, Weisbach V. Evaluation of a platelet apheresis technique for the preparation of leukocyte-reduced platelet concentrates. Vox Sang 1998;74:189-92.
9. Zingsem J, Zimmermann R, Reisbach V, et al. Comparison of COBE white cell-reduction and standard plateletpheresis protocols in the same donors. Transfusion 1997;37:1045-9.

10. Rugg N, Pitman C, Menitove JE, et al. A feasibility evaluation of an automated blood component collection system: Platelets and red cells. Transfusion 1999;39:460-4.

11. Elfath MD, Whitley P, Jacobson MS, et al. Evaluation of an automated system for the collection of packed RBCs, platelets, and plasma. Transfusion 2000;40:1214-22.

12. Valbonesi M, Florio G, Ruzzenenti MR, et al. Multicomponent collection (MCC) with the latest hemapheresis apparatuses. Int J Artif Organs 1999;22:511-15.

13. McAteer M, Kagen L, Graminske S, et al. Trima Accel improved platelet collection efficiency with the merging of single stage separation technology with leukoreduction performance of the LRS chamber (abstract). Transfusion 2002;42(Suppl):37S.

14. Burgstaler E, Pineda A. Therapeutic plasma exchange: A paired comparison of Fresenius AS104 vs. COBE Spectra. J Clin Apher 2001; 16:61-6.

15. Perdue J, Chandler L, Vesely S, et al. Unintentional platelet removal by plamapheresis. J Clin Apher 2001;16:55-60.

16. Sassi M, Bernuzzi G, Talarico E, Sauer GA. Reduced platelet loss in therapeutic plasma exchange using the blood cell separator Fresenius COM.TEC. Presented at the 36th Annual Meeting of the Deutsche Gesellschaft für Transfusionsmedizin und Immunhämatologie, Innsbruck, Austria, September 16-19, 2003.

17. Gordon B, Kelsey S, Dau P, et al. Long-term effects of low-density lipoprotein apheresis using an automated dextran sulfate cellulose absorption system. AM J Cardiol 1998;81:407-11.

18. Mabuchi H, Koizum J, Shimizu M. Long-term efficacy of low-density lipoprotein apheresis on coronary heart disease in familial hypercholesterolemia. Am J Cardiol 1998;82:1489-95.

19. Jaeger B. Evidence for maximal treatment of atherosclerosis: Drastic reduction of cholesterol and fibrinogen restores vascular homeostasis. Ther Apher 2001;5:207-11.

20. Seidel D. H.E.L.P. apheresis therapy in treatment of severe hypercholesterolemia: 10 years of clinical experience. Artif Organs 1996;20:303-10.

In: McLeod BC, Szczepiorkowski ZM, Weinstein R, Winters JL, eds.
Apheresis: Principles and Practice, 3rd edition
Bethesda, MD: AABB Press, 2010

5

Selection and Care of Apheresis Donors

Christina Anderson, RN, BSN, HP(ASCP)

 THE COLLECTION OF BLOOD components using automated apheresis technology began in the 1970s.[1] For over three decades, donors have been volunteering to undergo apheresis procedures, which involve prolonged venous access and infusion of anticoagulant and saline solutions, with relatively few serious consequences. In today's blood centers, more and more donations are obtained with automated apheresis devices instead of traditional whole blood collection. This change to the collection of red cells, platelets, and plasma through automated separation technology has allowed blood centers to better match available donors to the types of products needed.

The first part of this chapter will examine the selection of apheresis donors from a process perspective, covering donor and recipient safety issues pertaining to donor eligibility and suitability for the apheresis procedure. The second part will discuss care of the donor before, during, and after the apheresis procedure.

Selection of Apheresis Donors

Recruitment of Apheresis Donors

There are several potential sources of apheresis donors. In the hospital setting, patients' families, patients' friends, and hospital employees serve as the main source of apheresis donors. In the community blood center setting, the majority of donors come from the community, and resources are usually devoted to donor recruitment and retention. For many blood centers, whole blood donors serve as the foundation for identification of potential apheresis donors because they are already familiar with the donation process and have previously volun-

Christina Anderson, RN, BSN, HP(ASCP), Director, Clinical Apheresis, Carter BloodCare, Dallas, Texas
The author has disclosed no conflicts of interest.

teered to donate. Once donors have demonstrated successful completion of the whole blood donation process, including infectious disease testing, they may then be recruited to become apheresis donors. In some blood centers, whole blood donors are screened to identify those with high platelet counts. These individuals are then recruited in order to maximize yields when donating platelets by apheresis.

Scheduling apheresis donors to ensure an adequate supply of apheresis platelets is an integral part of a blood center's activities. This ensures the maximal use of available time slots and instruments and allows donors to commit to appointments ahead of time. Donors may be scheduled by blood center recruiters or they may schedule their own appointments using the blood center's Web site.

Eligibility Determination of Apheresis Donors

Determination of eligibility of potential apheresis donors focuses on two goals: 1) ensuring that the donation process is safe for the donor and 2) ensuring that the related transfusion will be safe for the recipient. In the United States, blood collection is regulated by the Food and Drug Administration (FDA).[2] Voluntary blood collection standards have been established by the AABB.[3] Additionally, other regulatory bodies and professional organizations have established standards and/or regulations that apply to blood collections, depending on the type and location of the blood collection center. These are covered in greater detail in Chapter 30.

All blood collection centers must have in place a set of written procedures and policies that define the blood donation process and specifically detail the measures taken to ensure safety for both the donor and the recipient. To facilitate understanding of how these two primary goals are achieved in donor apheresis programs, this chapter will approach donation from a process perspective, starting with a prospective donor and covering the steps leading up to acceptance or deferral.

Donation Record

Each prospective donor is directed to a special area to read the educational material provided and begin the screening process for eligibility determination. This must be done in a location that protects the donor's privacy and confidentiality. At that time, creation of the donation record, in the form of a written document or an electronic file, is begun. The donation record will document the entire donation process for each particular donor and specific donation. It covers the identification of the donor, the determination of eligibility, and the details of the component collected.

Donor Screening

Prospective donors must show adequate proof of identity to ensure that they are not attempting to donate under another name because of a previous deferral. Additionally, adequate identification confirms donors' addresses so that they can be contacted, if necessary, about positive test results, posttransfusion infectious disease investigations, or other matters. The age of the donor must also be verified. In most blood centers, donors must be of legal age, as defined by state law, to be acceptable. Some blood centers will permit minors to donate after their 16th birthday, with parental permission, if allowed by state law. The FDA does not specify an upper limit for donor age, but individual facilities may develop their own.

After identity and age are established, donors are asked questions about their health, travel, medications, and transfusion-transmitted disease risk factors. They are then given a "mini-physical examination" as described below.[4] Hematocrit is measured to identify anemic donors who are at risk for adverse effects of donation.

Medical History Interview

The purpose of the medical history interview is again twofold; it is used to obtain health information that could indicate either that the donation process would be unsafe for the donor or that the donated product would be unsafe for a recipient.

The interview consists of a series of questions that can be self-administered (ie, read and completed by the donor) or read to the donor by a trained, qualified employee. The questionnaire may be either a paper form or an electronic form in which the questions are presented on a computer screen for the donor to read and answer. The latter is known as computer-assisted screening.

To facilitate understanding by the donor, written educational material is usually provided. It customarily contains information about the donation process, explanations of the health history questions that will be asked, and information about medications that may disqualify individuals from donating blood. Donors should also be provided with educational materials concerning infectious diseases transmissible by blood transfusion, including a list of signs and symptoms of AIDS.[3(p15)]

The screening process should include an opportunity for the donor to ask questions and have those questions satisfactorily answered. This may involve contacting another donor center employee, such as a nurse or doctor, who is more knowledgeable about the screening and donation process.

Finally, some donor centers include a step that allows private and confidential self-deferral by donors who suspect that their blood is unsafe for transfusion to another person. This is called confidential unit exclusion.

Completion of the screening process should allow determination of a donor's eligibility. A donor who is deemed to be eligible may proceed to donation, whereas ineligible donors are deferred. The FDA requires that deferred donors be apprised of the reason for deferral, which will have a bearing on their future eligibility.

Regulations and standards focus on infectious disease risk and prescribe questions designed to protect the recipient. Questions that evaluate donor safety, such as those about cardiac conditions and certain medications, are left to the discretion of the blood center. As a result, donor acceptance criteria can vary between blood centers.

In October 2006, the FDA issued "Guidance for Industry: Implementation of Acceptable Full-Length Donor History Questionnaire and Accompanying Materials for Use in Screening Human Donors of Blood and Blood Components." This document recognized and accepted the donor history questionnaire (DHQ), version 1.1, prepared by the AABB Donor History Task Force, as an effective document for donor screening that met the FDA requirements outlined in the *Code of Federal Regulations* (21 CFR 640.3 and 21 CFR 640.63).[5] In February 2007, the AABB Donor History Task Force updated the DHQ to version 1.2, but as of this writing, that version had not yet been approved by the FDA.[6]

The DHQ is a standardized document that is available on the FDA[6] and AABB[7] Web sites. It is important to note that the DHQ contains questions related to issues not addressed by FDA requirements or guidance documents, such as cancer, pregnancy, and tissue grafts. Because the FDA does not require screening for these issues, blood centers can choose to exclude those questions and still be in compliance with FDA regulations. The Donor History Task Force also developed several ancillary documents to serve as tools for blood centers that implement the DHQ. These include a user brochure, a glossary, a list of references, a medication deferral list, and blood donor education materials.

History of Cardiac or Pulmonary Disease. Donors with a history of cardiac or pulmonary disease should be carefully evaluated. FDA regulations require that donors be free of acute respiratory disease.[8] Donor centers must define in their standard operating procedures how other cardiac and pulmonary conditions are handled. Donors should be assessed for the effect that the procedure may have on their condition, given the volume of blood in the apheresis circuit and the volume of products being collected.

Pregnancy. Pregnant women should not donate until 6 weeks following completion of the pregnancy.[3(p57)] Exceptions may be made in unusual circumstances, such as when a mother donates platelets for a fetus or newborn with neonatal alloimmune thrombocytopenia, if approved by the blood center medical director.

Medications. FDA regulations and AABB standards require that donors be questioned about a limited number of specific medications that could potentially harm a recipient, indicate an infectious disease risk in the donor, or adversely affect the function of the collected blood product. Both the FDA and AABB define medication deferral durations in relation to the last dose ingested. AABB standards also require that donors be asked if they are currently taking antibiotics or any other medications.[3(pp56,57)] Specific criteria for deferral are usually not mandated, and the donor center defines how donors taking such medications are handled. Medications for which specific requirements are mandated by FDA and/or AABB are described below:

- Finasteride (Proscar, Propecia) is given for prostatic hypertrophy or male pattern baldness; donors are deferred for 1 month after the last dose because of potential teratogenicity.
- Dutasteride (Avodart), also given for prostatic hypertrophy, requires a 6-month deferral.
- Isotretinoin (Accutane, Amnesteen, Claravis, and Sotret) is given for severe acne; it requires a 1-month deferral from the last dose because of potential teratogenicity.
- Acitretin (Soriatane) and etretinate (Tegison) are medications given for severe psoriasis that are also potential teratogens. Acitretin requires a 3-year deferral, and etretinate requires an indefinite deferral[3(p56)] because it is never completely excreted.

In addition, platelet donors should be evaluated for medications that could adversely affect platelet function and, thereby, the efficacy of the platelet product. Donors taking aspirin or medications containing aspirin should be deferred for 2 days after the last dose.[9] Platelet donors should also be screened for clopidogrel (Plavix) and ticlopidine (Ticlid) use as these medications, in addition to indicating potential underlying vascular disease, inhibit platelet function. Donors are deferred for 14 days after the last dose of either of these drugs.[9] Finally, AABB standards require that platelet donors be asked about piroxicam (Feldene) ingestion and deferred for 2 days following the last dose.[3(p57)]

Donors taking anticoagulants such as warfarin are deferred from plasma donation for 1 week following the last dose,[3(p57)] as their plasma would have reduced vitamin-K-dependent coagulation-factor activity. Some blood centers defer such donors from all donations because of concerns about bruising or bleeding at venipuncture sites.

Donors are also asked if they have received pituitary-gland-derived growth hormone or bovine/beef insulin. Growth hormone obtained from human pituitary glands can be contaminated with the agent that causes Creutzfeldt-Jakob disease (CJD). Bovine insulin imported from countries affected by bovine spongiform encephalopathy (BSE or mad cow disease) may have been contaminated and recipients may be at risk for variant CJD (vCJD). Receipt of either of these medications results in an indefinite deferral.[3(pp56,57)]

Finally, donors who have received hepatitis B immune globulin are deferred for 12 months from administration[7] because this medication is administered only when hepatitis B exposure has occurred. The 12-month deferral allows time for an infected donor to seroconvert and become detectable on donor testing.

Immunizations. Donors are asked about recent immunizations. Unlicensed immunizations require a 1-year deferral.[3(p58)] The length of deferral for other immunizations is variable. For live attenuated vaccines, deferrals range from 2 to 4 weeks.[3(p58)] An exception to this is deferral for smallpox vaccination, the length of which is determined by the date of vaccination, the date the scab fell off, and the presence or absence of complications.[10] For vaccines made from killed virus or bacteria components, no deferral is necessary.[3(p58)]

Receipt of Blood, Blood Components, or Other Human Tissues. Because of the possibility of disease transmission, donors are asked about blood transfusion in the preceding 12 months. A donor who has received an alloge-neic transfusion of red cells, platelets, plasma, or any other blood component is deferred for 12 months following the transfusion.[3(p57)] The indication for blood transfusion may also be a reason for deferral.

Individuals who have received any tissue or organ transplant should also be identified. Someone who has been exposed to allogeneic tissue through a transplant or graft should not serve as a blood donor for 12 months[3(p57)] fol-lowing exposure (receipt of the tissue or organ) because of the possibility of infectious disease transmission.

Tattoos and Other Percutaneous Expo-sures. Individuals who have received a tattoo or body piercing should be evaluated for possi-ble exposure to infectious diseases such as human immunodeficiency virus (HIV) and hep-atitis. Tattoos that have been applied with ster-ile needles and nonreusable ink at a state-regulated entity are acceptable. If a tattoo was performed in an unlicensed facility or in a state where such activities are not regulated, the donor is deferred for 12 months.[3(p59)]

Potential donors who have been exposed to another person's blood or body fluid via an open wound, nonintact skin, or a mucous membrane should be deferred for 12 months.[3(p59)] Individuals who have had a nee-dle-stick or other injury from any type of instru-ment that has been contaminated with blood from another person are also deferred for 12 months.[3(p59)]

Cancer. Deferral policies for donors with a history of cancer are not defined by either the FDA or the AABB.[11] Therefore, persons who have a history of cancer should be evaluated according to the donor center's standard oper-ating procedures. Most donor centers will per-manently defer a donor for hematologic malignancies such as leukemia.[12] Donors with other types of cancer may be allowed to donate provided they are cancer-free at the time of donation and have been free of disease for a period of time defined by the donor center. Minor types of localized skin cancers, such as basal cell or squamous cell carcinomas, are usually acceptable.[12]

Infectious Disease History and Risk: HIV and Hepatitis. There is a delay between the time of infection, the onset of symptoms, and seroconversion for most infectious diseases, including some that are transmitted by transfu-sion. A person who has been recently infected may not experience symptoms or have a posi-tive result in a screening test. Therefore, all blood donors are questioned about infectious disease risk factors, including travel and life-style activities.

The DHQ includes questions about sexual contact that are intended to identify risks for certain sexually transmitted diseases that can also be transmitted by blood transfusion. The questions emphasize sexual contact with others who are at risk for HIV infection.

Donors are asked if they have ever used needles to take drugs, steroids, or any other substance not prescribed by a physician and if they have had sexual contact with a person who has done so in the last 12 months. Individ-uals who have accepted drugs, money, or other forms of payment in return for sex are perma-nently deferred from donation because of an increased risk of HIV infection. Potential donors who have AIDS or have had a positive test for HIV are permanently deferred. Donors who have had sex with those who have accepted drugs, money, or any other form of payment in return for sex are deferred from blood donation for 12 months. Males who have had sexual contact with another male since 1977 are permanently deferred from donation. Females who have had sex with males who have had sex with another male are deferred for 12 months.[3(p59)] Individuals should not donate if they are experiencing symptoms asso-ciated with HIV such as unexplained weight loss, night sweats, blue or purple spots in the oral cavity or on the skin, swollen lymph nodes for more than one month, white spots or unusual sores in the mouth, persistent cough, persistent shortness of breath, diarrhea, or fever of more than 100.5 F for more than 10 days.[7]

Donors who were born in or have lived in certain central African countries since 1977, donors who received blood transfusion or other related treatment that involved blood in these countries, and donors who have had sexual contact with people from these selected areas are deferred because of possible exposure to a subgroup of HIV that is not consistently detected by all currently available tests. This subgroup, HIV-1 group O, is detected by some FDA-licensed donor screening tests; if one of these tests is used by the collection center, these questions need not be asked.[13]

As with HIV, the risk of hepatitis is also assessed through a series of questions. Individuals who have or had hepatitis, live with a person who has hepatitis, or have had sexual contact with a person who has hepatitis must be evaluated further. Generally, a history of viral hepatitis results in a permanent deferral. An exception is made if a donor has a history of viral hepatitis before the age of 11 because hepatitis A, a virus without a chronic carrier state, is the most common cause. Donors with a history of nonviral hepatitis, such as that resulting from medications, may be accepted. Donors who have been exposed to hepatitis are deferred for 12 months from the time of exposure. An exception is sexual contact with an individual with asymptomatic hepatitis C; such donors are eligible to donate.[3(p59)]

Other Sexually Transmitted Diseases. Classic venereal diseases are associated with a higher risk for HIV infection. Donors are therefore questioned concerning a history of syphilis or gonorrhea. A prospective donor who has had or has been treated for either is deferred for 12 months from diagnosis (but must have completed treatment by the time of donation).[3(p59)]

Travel History. Donors are questioned concerning travel that may have exposed them to infectious agents that could be transmitted by transfusion. For many of these agents, FDA-licensed donor testing is not available, and questioning donors is the only means to prevent disease transmission. Donors are asked about travel outside of the United States and Canada in order to identify travel to areas where malaria is endemic and to determine if European travel has increased their risk for vCJD. Donors who have traveled to malaria-

endemic areas are deferred for 12 months after returning. Those who have emigrated from such areas are deferred for 3 years.[3(p60)] Donors who spent 3 or more months in the United Kingdom between 1980 and 1996, were stationed at US military bases in Europe for 6 or more months between 1980 and 1996, or who have spent 5 or more years in Europe since 1980 are permanently deferred because of an increased risk of vCJD.[3,14] Potential donors who have traveled to Iraq are at risk for Leishmaniasis, a cutaneous disease caused by protozoa of the genus *Leishmania*, which are transmitted by the bite of a sandfly.[15] Donors are deferred for 12 months after departure from the country.[7]

Parasitic Infectious Diseases. Individuals who have had malaria are deferred for 3 years after becoming asymptomatic.[3(p60)] Donors are questioned concerning a history of infection with other parasites, including *Trypanosoma cruzi*, the causative agent of Chagas disease, and *Babesia spp*, the causative agents of babesiosis.[15] Donors with a history of infection with these agents are indefinitely deferred.[3(p59)]

Prion Diseases. Prions are proteins which, when their structure is altered through mutation or conversion by other abnormal prions, can behave like traditional infectious agents.[15] These proteins, which cause dementing neurologic diseases, may be transmitted by transfusion. As a result, potential donors are questioned concerning risk factors for these illnesses. The DHQ asks about CJD and vCJD. As described above in the section on travel questions, donors are queried about travel and residency risk factors for vCJD. In addition, donors are asked if they received a blood transfusion in the United Kingdom or France since 1980. Donors who have been exposed to blood components in these countries are permanently deferred. Questions are asked about dura mater transplants and family histories of CJD; both are risk factors for CJD that lead to indefinite deferral.[3(p57)]

Physical and Laboratory Assessment

General Appearance. In general, the donor should be in good health. The donor's overall appearance is usually assessed for evidence of illness, alcohol or drug intoxication, and cognitive impairment.

Arm Inspection. The donor's arms are evaluated for skin lesions, bruises, and scars, as described in the CFR.[16] If scarring or needle marks are present, the donor should be questioned about the cause. A donor with needle marks suggestive of drug abuse should be deferred. However, frequent blood donors may have multiple needle marks and scarring in the antecubital area of one or both arms from previous donations; this is not cause for deferral.

Weight. FDA regulations require that a blood donor weigh at least 110 pounds.[9] Depending on the type and number of products being collected, additional qualifications for weight and height may apply. The volume of blood that will be withdrawn by the apheresis machine will vary with the type of donation. If the amount of blood in the extracorporeal circuit is too large in comparison with a donor's total blood volume (which is proportional to weight), then the donor may be at increased risk for adverse consequences during the procedure. Apheresis devices used in the donor setting should not remove more than 15% of the donor's total blood volume, and most remove less than 10%.

Temperature, Heart Rate, and Blood Pressure. Body temperature, heart rate, and blood pressure are checked to ensure that a donor is in good health. The temperature should not exceed 99.5 F (37.5 C) as this could indicate an infection.[3(p56),16] Systolic and diastolic blood pressures must be normal.[17] Although the FDA and the AABB do not define normal ranges for blood pressure and heart rate, acceptable limits should be established by each facility. A heart rate between 50 and 100 beats per minute is usually considered normal. An athlete who has a high tolerance for exercise may be accepted with a lower heart rate, according to blood center procedure. Abnormal findings require approval from the medical director of the blood center and/or the donor's personal physician, depending on the circumstances. If abnormal values are observed, it is important that facilities define how often the parameters may be rechecked before accepting the value.

Hemoglobin/Hematocrit Determination. Allogeneic donors must have a hemoglobin level of at least 12.5 g/dL (or a hematocrit level of 38%).[18] This requirement is meant to protect the donor in the event the blood in the circuit cannot be returned at the end of the procedure. The AABB further stipulates that blood samples obtained from earlobe punctures cannot be used for the hemoglobin/hematocrit determination.[3(p18)] If 2 units of red cells are being collected from a donor using an apheresis device, a higher hemoglobin threshold is required. This is determined by the blood center's written procedures in accordance with the requirements of the apheresis instrument manufacturer.

Platelet Count. Platelet donors should have a platelet count of at least 150,000/µL. It is preferable that a platelet count be performed before the first donation, but if this is not possible, the FDA permits donation provided that a predonation sample is obtained and the result evaluated after the collection. When predonation platelet counts cannot be obtained, the FDA allows either an average of a donor's previous platelet counts or a default platelet count specified by the apheresis device manufacturer to be used to set the target platelet yield. Triple platelet products cannot be collected from first-time donors unless the donor's platelet count can be measured before the start of the procedure.[9]

Donation Interval and Red Cell/Plasma Loss

Guidance issued by the FDA in December 2007, "Guidance for Industry and FDA Review Staff: Collection of Platelets by Automated Methods,"[9] limits platelet donors to 24 collections during a rolling 12-month period.[9] The interval between donations should be at least 2 days, with no more than two procedures in a 7-day period. If the collection results in a double or triple platelet product, the interval until the next donation must be 7 days. The guidance document requires that the apheresis device be configured so that the postdonation platelet count is at least 100,000/μL.

Although this document's title suggests that it applies only to platelet donations, it also addresses red cell and plasma losses from whole blood donations and apheresis donations. Donors who have given 2 units of red cells by apheresis are not allowed to donate any type of component for at least 16 weeks. A donor of a unit of whole blood or a single unit of red cells by apheresis in the preceding 8 weeks cannot donate platelets unless the extracorporeal red cell volume of the device being used is less than 100 mL.[9]

The total volume of plasma, not including anticoagulant, collected during the apheresis platelet donation cannot exceed 500 mL for donors weighing less than 175 lb or 600 mL for donors weighing 175 lb or more. If the apheresis device used for the collection has a different prescribed plasma volume limit, such limit must not be exceeded.[9]

Care of the Apheresis Donor

Once it has been determined that a donor meets all eligibility criteria and has been accepted for donation, the donation process can begin. Care of the apheresis donor during the donation includes preparation of the donor for the procedure, completion of the procedure, and postdonation care of the donor.

Preparation of the Apheresis Donor for the Procedure

Consent and Release of Medical Information

Before an apheresis donation, consent must be obtained from the donor.[3(p15)] This should be done after information has been provided to the donor, including a general explanation of the procedure, a description of possible risks and side effects, the expected duration of the procedure, and a disclosure that testing will be performed on the donation for diseases that can be transmitted by transfusion. The specific items to be covered are outlined in FDA guid-

ance documents[5,19] and AABB Standards.[3(p15)] The information should be given to donors in an understandable manner, appropriate for education and language, and there should be adequate opportunity for questions in a location that allows for confidentiality. Consent is usually obtained in writing.

The consent may include permission from the donor to release information to others such as other members of the health-care or blood center team. The "release" of private health information concerning *patients* is protected under law, in the provisions of the Health Insurance Portability and Accountability Act (HIPAA).[20] HIPAA ensures that private health information is protected and guarantees that certain identifying information is not publicly released. Blood donor centers are explicitly excluded from the HIPAA provisions, except when providing therapeutic services, but centers may choose to comply with respect to donor information because of uncertainty about HIPAA's applicability to their specific practices.

Vein Selection

Proper vein selection and phlebotomy technique minimize donor discomfort and risks, help to ensure an adequate blood flow, and reduce the possibility of an incomplete collection. The antecubital fossae are the most common venipuncture sites for apheresis procedures. One or two suitable veins are needed for single- or dual-arm procedures, respectively.

After a tourniquet or blood pressure cuff is placed above the elbow, fist-closing motions by the donor will engorge the veins to facilitate location of suitable venipuncture sites. Donors may indicate preferences based on comfort or successful use in previous donations. Once a venipuncture site has been identified, the preparation procedure is performed.

Arm Preparation

The skin at the site of the needle insertion must be aseptically prepared before phlebotomy.[21] This is a critical step in the collection process because proper preparation helps to minimize the risk of bacterial contamination of the product(s). Numerous methods can be used to disinfect the skin surrounding the phlebotomy site. Most of them combine mechanical cleaning of the site (swabbing and/or scrubbing) with application of a chemical disinfectant such as chlorhexidine or iodine. Before starting the scrub, it is important to check that the donor is not allergic to the chemical being used. The scrub is performed for a period of time defined by standard operating procedures and in a manner such that the skin surrounding the needle insertion site is also treated. The venipuncture site should not be touched after the arm scrub has been performed; if this occurs, the arm must be scrubbed again. The technique for arm preparation should be established in the form of a written procedure and all staff should be routinely assessed for competency and compliance with the procedure.

Phlebotomy

After the site has been properly prepared, venipuncture can be performed. Most apheresis kits contain a preattached 17-gauge needle. If vascular access is not obtained with the first venipuncture, additional attempts may or may not be possible, depending on the blood center's policy and the type of apheresis device being used.

Apheresis Procedure

Separation of Blood and Collection of Products

Once venous access has been established, the apheresis procedure can begin. Current apheresis instruments are highly automated and require minimal operator input and intervention. At the beginning of the procedure, the apheresis operator enters information, such as the donor's height, weight, hematocrit, and platelet count, required by the apheresis device to optimize the procedure for the donor and the product(s) being collected. The duration of the procedure varies from 20 to 120 minutes, depending on the products being collected as

well as cell counts, donor size, vascular access, and any limitations placed on procedure length by the collection center. During the procedure, donors are made as comfortable as possible and offered entertainment such as TV or music to divert their attention from the collection procedure. One key to a successful donation is the demeanor of the apheresis operator. Apheresis personnel who are confident, attentive, reassuring, and knowledgeable are more likely to give the donor a positive experience and provide reinforcement that will minimize adverse events.

Prevention and Management of Donor Reactions

Although most apheresis donations are completed without significant adverse events, inherent risks exist for each and every one. Donation centers should implement practices that minimize the occurrence of adverse events and train apheresis personnel in the recognition and proper treatment of such events. This chapter will not discuss every adverse event that has been associated with apheresis because many are rare with current apheresis devices and practices. A more detailed account of reactions to apheresis donations and their physiology and treatment can be found in Chapter 3.

Apheresis facilities should have processes with corresponding written procedures to assess, investigate, and monitor adverse events related to donations.[3(p77)] If an adverse event occurs during an apheresis procedure, most facilities will document relevant information such as the type and severity of the reaction, the treatment provided, and the status of the donor following any interventions. The extent of documentation will depend upon the seriousness of the reaction. In addition, most centers will contact the donor after more significant events to follow up and determine outcome. Not only does this step collect important data, but it provides good customer service. Aggregate data can be periodically reviewed to search for trends.

Adverse effects of apheresis procedures can be categorized by severity (eg, mild, moderate, or severe) or by the nature of the reaction (eg, vasovagal, citrate toxicity, hypotension, etc). Some centers use a combination of the two.

The overall rate of adverse events with apheresis donation is approximately 10 times less than that seen with whole blood donation, with mild events outnumbering the more severe ones, although the frequency of events requiring hospitalization may be higher than with whole blood donation.[22] Hospitalization is still extremely rare; it occurred in 0.01% of donations in one study.[23]

Early recognition and intervention are the keys to minimize discomfort and/or consequences from adverse events and to allow completion of the donation. It can be challenging to recognize and distinguish between different adverse effects because they can share common symptoms. These may include inappropriate laughter, excessive talking, restlessness, irregular breathing, abdominal discomfort, flushing, pallor, cold and clammy hands, hyperventilation, and tachycardia.[24]

Hypotensive Reactions. Hypotension during apheresis donation can result from a number of causes, including intravascular volume depletion, vasovagal reactions, citrate toxicity, severe allergic reactions, and air embolism. Of these, the most common are vasovagal reactions and citrate toxicity. Hypovolemia is uncommon as a result of limitations on extracorporeal volume (10.5 mL/kg).[3(p56)] Air embolism is extremely rare because of air detectors on all current apheresis instruments.[22] Severe allergic reactions are also very rare.

Symptoms and signs of a vasovagal reaction include lightheadedness, hot flashes, pallor, diaphoresis, nausea, vomiting, decreased heart rate, and decreased blood pressure. These symptoms arise from excessive parasympathetic activation in the donor, which is believed to be a compensatory response to sympathetic activation induced by mild hypovolemia.[22] Because sympathetic activation has a psychological component, preventive steps include helping the donor feel comfortable and confident throughout the procedure. This is especially important for first-time apheresis donors, as they are more likely to be anxious about the procedure.

Treatment of vasovagal reactions includes pausing the procedure, lowering the head and raising the feet of the donor (Trendelenburg position), applying cold compresses to the forehead and neck, and reassuring the donor. If moderate or severe symptoms are present, the apheresis procedure should be discontinued. Of note, these interventions are identical to those for hypotension caused by hypovolemia, where, in addition, infusion of intravenous fluids and return of the blood within the extracorporeal circuit would be considered.[22]

Citrate reactions. Citrate reactions are the most common adverse effects seen with apheresis procedures. They result from ionized hypocalcemia caused by the infusion of citrate anticoagulant during the procedure. The lowered ionized calcium levels allow spontaneous depolarization of neurons. The resulting symptoms may include numbness and/or tingling in the lips and nose and sneezing. Moderate symptoms can include nausea and/or vomiting; progression of paresthesias to the hands, feet, and/or chest; intense vibrating sensation throughout body; chills; abdominal cramping; and lightheadedness or hypotension. Severe symptoms include painful muscle cramps, tetany, blurred or double vision, loss of consciousness, cardiac arrhythmia, and seizure.[22,24] These symptoms are usually progressive in adult donors, so moderate and severe symptoms can usually be avoided through close monitoring and treatment of earlier symptoms.[22,24]

Interventions for mild symptoms include reducing the return rate of the instrument or pausing the procedure to allow the donor to metabolize some citrate and release bound calcium. Additional treatments include administration of oral calcium carbonate or, in severe cases, an intravenous calcium solution (see Chapter 3).[22,24] Preventive measures in donors who have experienced citrate reactions can include encouragement to increase dietary intake of calcium-rich foods.[24]

Hematoma and Infiltrations. Complications of venous access can occur at any time during an apheresis donation. Hematoma formation, infiltration, and thrombosis are among possible acute complications. Symptoms include pain and/or pressure and bruising and/or swelling at the needle site. If venous access fails during the procedure, the procedure may not be completed and the resulting physical discomfort may influence the donor's decision about donating in the future.

Treatment includes discontinuing the collection, removing the needles, and applying pressure to the site. It may not be possible to return blood in the apheresis instrument as this could cause the hematoma to enlarge. Cold compresses may be used and may provide relief to the donor. Because a major risk factor for these reactions is inexperienced phlebotomy staff, prevention strategies include maintaining apheresis personnel competency. Preventive strategies for donors include encouraging donors to be well hydrated before the donation and instructing them to keep the needle sites secure and stable during the donation.

Loss of Consciousness and Seizures. Loss of consciousness is uncommon and usually occurs as a result of a vasovagal reaction or severe citrate toxicity. It may be accompanied by tonic-clonic jerking; however, this does not represent true seizure activity. A true seizure is rare during blood donation but can occur as a component of severe citrate toxicity or from an underlying donor seizure disorder. Should a donor become unconscious or experience a seizure, the procedure should be discontinued immediately.

Postdonation Care

Discontinuation of the Apheresis Procedure

At the end of the collection, the blood remaining in the circuit is returned to the donor. Needles are then removed and pressure is applied to the venipuncture site until bleeding has stopped. A pressure dressing is then applied to the phlebotomy site.

Postdonation Instructions

Following discontinuation of the apheresis procedure, postdonation instructions are given to the donor verbally and/or in writing. These will vary depending on each facility's policies. Common elements include encouragement to leave the bandage in place for a specified interval, to avoid strenuous activity such as lifting or pulling with the arms for a specified interval, and to eat well and drink plenty of fluids over the next 24 hours. Some facilities also discourage smoking and alcohol consumption after donation as smoking may induce hypotension and donors may experience greater effects from alcohol. Instructions are given concerning actions to be taken if the venipuncture site begins to bleed. Contact information is also usually offered so that, in the event of any unusual or adverse consequences after leaving the blood donation area, a donor can notify the donor center. Information may also include educational material about bruising and healing of phlebotomy sites.

In addition, facilities may include a special contact number so that donors may call with instructions not to use their blood. Possible reasons for such calls include the onset of illness or fever shortly after donation or a belated admission that the blood may not be safe.

Release of Donors

If donors are feeling well, they are typically assisted from the donor chair and asked to stand by the chair for a few moments to ensure that they do not experience hypotension. They are then escorted to the canteen/donor lounge where they are encouraged to eat and drink. Donors should be observed following apheresis donations[3(p16)] for about 15 minutes to ensure that no delayed negative effects occur. Most adverse reactions will occur within this time frame. Donors who are feeling well and have not experienced any adverse effects are then allowed to leave.

Special Types of Donations

Autologous donors may require special attention. The screening process is substantially different because such donors need not fulfill all the donor safety criteria described earlier in the chapter.[3(pp17,18)] In addition, because these individuals are "patients" with an underlying disease process, they are at greater risk for adverse reactions.

There are additional specific standards and regulations that apply to hematopoietic stem cell donors. Allogeneic hematopoietic progenitor cells are considered by the FDA to represent a tissue; such donations are therefore regulated under 21 CFR 1271.[25] These regulations focus solely on minimizing the risk of infectious disease transmission from allogeneic donor to recipient. Additional standards applicable to both allogeneic and autologous hematopoietic stem cell collection include the AABB *Standards for Cellular Therapy Product Services*[26] and the *FACT-JACIE International Standards for Cellular Therapy Product Collection, Processing, and Administration.*[27] These contain detailed standards for qualifying tissue and cellular therapy donors and cover all aspects of the collection, modification, and transplantation processes.

Conclusion

In summary, blood collection using apheresis technology is an integral and important part of the total blood collection effort in the United States. When carried out by qualified, trained personnel following institutional procedures that comply with applicable regulations and standards, donor apheresis is safe and effective.

References

1. Smith JW, Burgstaler EA. Blood component collection by apheresis. In: Roback JD, Combs MR, Grossman BJ, Hillyer CD, eds. Technical manual. 16th ed. Bethesda, MD: AABB, 2008: 229-39.
2. Code of federal regulations. Title 21 CFR. Washington, DC: US Government Printing Office, 2010 (revised annually).
3. Price TH, ed. Standards for blood banks and transfusion services. 26th ed. Bethesda MD: AABB, 2009.
4. Code of federal regulations. Title 21 CFR Part 640.3(a). Washington, DC: US Government Printing Office, 2010 (revised annually).
5. Food and Drug Administration. Guidance for industry: Implementation of acceptable full-length donor history questionnaire and accompanying materials for use in screening human donors of blood and blood components. (October 2006) Rockville, MD: CBER Office of Communication, Outreach, and Development, 2006.
6. AABB donor history questionnaire documents. Version 1.1 (June 2005). Bethesda, MD: AABB, 2005. [Available at http://www.fda. gov/Bio logicsBloodVaccines/BloodBloodProducts/Ap provedProducts/LicensedProductsBLAs/ Blood DonorScreening/ucm164185.htm (ac cessed February 1, 2010).]
7. Blood donor history questionnaire. Version 1.1 and version 1.2. Bethesda, MD: AABB, 2005/ 2007. [Available at http://www.aabb.org/Con tent/Donate_Blood/Donor_History_Question naires/Blood_Donor_History_Questionnaire/ (accessed February 1, 2010).]
8. Code of federal regulations. Title 21 CFR Part 640.3(b)(4-6). Washington, DC: US Government Printing Office, 2010 (revised annually).
9. Food and Drug Administration. Guidance for industry and FDA review staff: Collection of platelets by automated methods. (December 17, 2007) Rockville, MD: CBER Office of Communication, Outreach, and Development, 2007.
10. Food and Drug Administration. Guidance for industry: Recommendations for deferral of donors and quarantine and retrieval of blood and blood products in recent recipients of smallpox vaccine (vaccinia virus) and certain contacts of smallpox vaccine recipients. (December, 2002) Rockville, MD: CBER Office of Communication, Training, and Manufacturers Assistance, 2002.
11. Strauss RG. Rationale for medical director acceptance or rejection of allogeneic plateletpheresis donors with underlying medical disorders. J Clin Apher 2002;17:111-17.
12. Eder AF. Allogeneic and autologous blood donor selection. In: Roback JD, Combs MR, Grossman BJ, Hillyer CD, eds. Technical manual. 16th ed. Bethesda, MD: AABB, 2008: 137-87.
13. Food and Drug Administration. Guidance for industry: Recommendations for management of donors at increased risk for human immuno-

deficiency virus type 1 (HIV-1) group O infection. (August 2009) Rockville, MD: CBER Office of Communication, Training, and Manufacturers Assistance, 2009.

14. Food and Drug Administration. Guidance for industry: Revised preventive measures to reduce the possible risk of transmission of Creutzfeldt-Jakob disease (CJD) and variant Creutzfeldt-Jakob disease (vCJD) by blood and blood products. (January 9, 2002) Rockville, MD: CBER Office of Communication, Outreach, and Development, 2002.

15. Fiebig EW, Busch MP. Infectious disease screening. In: Roback JD, Combs MR, Grossman BJ, Hillyer CD, eds. Technical manual. 16th ed. Bethesda, MD: AABB, 2008:241-82.

16. Code of federal regulations. Title 21 CFR Part 640.3(a)(5,7). Washington, DC: US Government Printing Office, 2010 (revised annually).

17. Code of federal regulations. Title 21 CFR Part 640.3(b)(1,2). Washington, DC: US Government Printing Office, 2010 (revised annually).

18. Code of federal regulations. Title 21 CFR Part 640.3(b)(3). Washington, DC: US Government Printing Office, 2010 (revised annually).

19. Food and Drug Administration. Guidance for industry: Recommendations for collecting red blood cells by automated apheresis methods—technical correction February 2001. (February 2001) Rockville, MD: CBER Office of Communication, Outreach, and Development, 2001.

20. Code of federal regulations. Title 45 CFR Parts 160 and 164. Health Insurance Portability and Accountability Act of 1996. Washington, DC: US Government Printing Office, 2010.

21. Code of federal regulations. Title 21 CFR Part 640.5(f). Washington, DC: US Government Printing Office, 2010 (revised annually).

22. Winters JL. Complications of donor apheresis. J Clin Apher 2006;21:132-41.

23. Despotis GJ, Goodnough L, Dynis M, et al. Adverse events in platelet apheresis donors: A multivariate analysis in a hospital-based program. Vox Sang 1999;77:24-32.

24. Golden PJ. Complications of apheresis. In: Andrzejewski C, Golden P, Kong B, et al, eds. Principles of apheresis technology. 3rd ed. Vancouver, BC, Canada: American Society for Apheresis, 2002:85-99.

25. Code of federal regulations. Title 21 CFR Parts 1270 and 1271. Washington, DC: US Government Printing Office, 2010 (revised annually).

26. Padley D, ed. Standards for cellular therapy product services. 4th ed. Bethesda, MD: AABB, 2009.

27. FACT-JACIE international standards for cellular therapy product collection, processing and administration. 4th ed. Omaha, NE: Foundation for the Accreditation of Cellular Therapy and Joint Accreditation Committee—ISCT and EBMT, 2008.

In: McLeod BC, Szczepiorkowski ZM, Weinstein R, Winters JL, eds.
Apheresis: Principles and Practice, 3rd edition
Bethesda, MD: AABB Press, 2010

6

Automated Donations: Plasma, Red Cells, and Multicomponent Donor Procedures

James W. Smith, MD, PhD

 AS DESCRIBED IN CHAPTER 1, the Cohn-ADL centrifuge was developed for on-line blood component donation. The further advances in blood cell removal and collection that are now known as apheresis were responses to perceived needs for both therapeutic white cell removal and methods to collect platelets and white cells for transfusion. As apheresis technology progressed, it became possible to collect platelets and various white cell products, including granulocytes, lymphocytes, and hematopoietic progenitor cells. Collection of these products depended on the isolation of the buffy coat from whole blood passing through the apheresis instrument. It then became apparent that the same instruments could be used to collect other products from a donor's bloodstream. This fostered the notion that plasma could be collected by apheresis and the realization that doing so might increase the yield of plasma proteins while decreasing donation time for donors. Later advances engendered techniques for collecting red cells by apheresis. Subsequently, apheresis systems have been further enhanced to permit the collection of multiple components per donation. The goals of this approach are to improve product quality and consistency, to decrease donor exposures, to improve blood product availability, and to improve efficiency in terms of products per donor.

Because platelet donations are covered in detail in subsequent chapters, this chapter will deal primarily with plasma and red cell dona-

James W. Smith, MD, PhD, Medical Director, Oklahoma Blood Institute, Oklahoma City, Oklahoma
The author has disclosed no conflicts of interest.

tion. Plasma donation is reviewed first, followed by a discussion of red cell donations. Multiple component donations are then discussed. Comments on regulatory issues, operational concerns, recruitment and utilization issues, and financial considerations complete the discussion. Instrument design and operation are covered in Chapter 4.

Plasma Donation by Apheresis

The original method for plasma donation involved manual removal of whole blood into a plastic bag containing anticoagulant, with off-line separation of red cells and plasma in a laboratory centrifuge followed by reinfusion of red cells and supplemental saline to the donor. This cycle would be repeated several times during each donation procedure. The collected plasma was typically referred to as source plasma (vs recovered or whole-blood-derived plasma). Apheresis equipment, by contrast, has made it possible to collect plasma by automated techniques.[1] Whole blood is separated on-line in a centrifuge while confined in a sterile, single-use tubing set that remains attached to the donor's bloodstream throughout the donation procedure; this ensures that another donor's red cells are not infused by mistake. Red cells are returned immediately to the donor, whereas plasma is collected for freezing and/or further processing.

Uses for Apheresis Plasma

Donor plasma can be used for several purposes. The major uses for Fresh Frozen Plasma (FFP) are direct therapeutic transfusion to patients, usually to correct a coagulopathy, and infusion as a replacement fluid in therapeutic plasma exchange. Source plasma, which is also fresh frozen, is used to manufacture the full range of fractionation-derived blood products. Liquid or recovered plasma (ie, not fresh frozen) can be fractionated into some transfusable derivatives such as albumin and can also be used for diagnostic and other noninjectable products.

As the use of apheresis-derived plasma and plasma fractionation products has grown, techniques for plateletpheresis have been adapted to permit concurrent collection of plasma for fractionation or transfusion. As explained below, apheresis donation yields an increased volume of plasma with higher concentrations of specific proteins. Patient safety may also be enhanced with transfusable products such as FFP if an increase in volume collected per donor permits fewer donor exposures.

Sources of Plasma for Fractionation

On the basis of fractionation capacity, current worldwide use of plasma is estimated to be approximately 35 million liters per year.[2] It is also estimated that 5 million liters of plasma are transfused each year throughout the world in the form of FFP, thawed plasma, and other nonfractionated products. The distribution of plasma sources is indicated in Table 6-1, which shows that between 1993 and 2002, the amount of source plasma collected by apheresis in both the nonprofit (volunteer donor) and commercial (paid donor) sectors increased substantially. This expansion has been driven by a number of factors, including the increased yields of plasma proteins that are obtained in this way. These increases are carried through the plasma fractionation process and translate into higher final yields of fractionated products such as Factor VIII.

Between 1993 and 2002, the nonprofit sector's percentage of fractionation capacity decreased, with a corresponding increase in commercial sector capacity (Tables 6-1 and 6-2). There has been further growth in the plasma obtained by the commercial sector in Asia. Despite the availability of recombinant Factor VIII, the amount of plasma collected for fractionation has not declined since 1993 (Table 6-1). The 2007 National Blood Collection and Utilization Survey Report reflects a continuing increase in US collection and therapeutic usage of plasma products.[3] Approximately 1.7 million liters of plasma were collected by blood centers and hospitals in 2006, with approximately 1.0 million liters

Table 6-1. Trends in Procurement of Plasma for Fractionation (in Thousands of Liters)

	1993		2002	
	Whole-Blood-Derived	Plasmapheresis	Whole-Blood-Derived	Plasmapheresis
Europe				
Nonprofit	3300	600	1780	930
Commercial	1560	3830	4070	5420
North America				
Nonprofit	390	130	100	100
Commercial	630	6350	950	7630
Asia				
Nonprofit	491	950	400	1310
Commercial	110	870	250	2590

Adapted from Robert.[2]

transfused therapeutically. At least some of the 700,000-liter difference would have gone to fractionation, compared to 200,000 liters fractionated from nonprofit sources in 2002.[3]

Collection of source plasma is addressed in the *Code of Federal Regulations* (CFR), Title 21, Part 640, which is applicable to donors who give large-volume plasmapheresis units at frequent intervals.[4] Donors may give no more than 1000 mL (1200 mL for donors weighing ≤175 lb) every 48 hours and no more than 2000 mL (2400 mL for donors weighing ≥175 lb) within a 7-day period. Annual examination by a physician, measurement of immunoglobulin levels every 4 months, and measurement of plasma protein levels at each donation are required to ensure that such donors remain healthy. The blood banking community, however, makes greater use of the Food and Drug Administration (FDA) guidelines for infrequent plasmapheresis, which were issued on March 10, 1995,[5] as a revision of the original plasmapheresis guidelines published on August 27, 1982.[6] Under the revised recommendations,

Table 6-2. Plasma Capacities and Sources

	Capacity	Collection Method		Sector	
	(Liters)	Whole Blood (%)	Apheresis (%)	Nonprofit (%)	Commercial (%)
Europe	$14,890 \times 10^3$	48	52	80	20
North America	$11,040 \times 10^3$	12	88	13	87
Asia	$9,270 \times 10^3$	14	86	50	50

Adapted from Robert.[2]

plasma can be collected at intervals of 4 weeks as long as the donor meets all other criteria for whole blood donation. Plasma collected in this way can be used either as source plasma for fractionation or as FFP for transfusion. The maximal allowable plasma volume donated each year, excluding anticoagulant, is 12 L (14.4 L for donors weighing >175 lb). These guidelines are consistent with analogous recommendations for plateletpheresis donors; they also specify that donors may not participate in competing donation strategies that would exceed these overall limits.

Instrumentation

Most of the instruments used to collect plasma by apheresis in the United States are centrifugal separators, with most of the procedures being performed with the Haemonetics Plasma Collection System (PCS),[7] the PCS-2 (Haemonetics Corporation, Braintree, MA), or the Fenwal Autopheresis C (Fenwal Inc, Lake Zurich, IL).[8] The Autopheresis C uses a combination of centrifugal force and filtration (through a rotating membrane) to collect plasma. In several other regions, including Asia and Europe, "pure" membrane separation systems are used for on-line collection of plasma.

As mentioned above, instruments designed for plateletpheresis can also be used for automated plasma donation. The cost of these instruments and their associated disposables makes this fiscally impractical if plasma is the only product collected; however, these instruments can be configured for collection of plasma concurrently with apheresis platelets. Instruments such as the Fenwal CS3000 and AMICUS (Fenwal), the Spectra and Trima (CaridianBCT, Inc, Lakewood, CO), the Haemonetics Mobile Collection System (MCS) series, and the Fresenius AS 104 (Fresenius Kabi, Redmond, WA) are capable of concurrent plasma collection.

Product Quality

The factors favoring collection of plasma by apheresis are similar to those favoring collection of other apheresis products: the desires for better quality and for decreased donor exposure. These reasons apply equally well to plasma for either fractionation or transfusion. One advantage of apheresis instruments designed specifically for plasma collection over both the production of plasma from whole blood and the concurrent collection of plasma during plateletpheresis is that such instruments yield a more concentrated plasma by adding a smaller volume of a more concentrated anticoagulant. The Haemonetics PCS uses 4% sodium citrate at a 1:16 ratio; this reduces dilution by anticoagulant and increases the protein concentration. This is an advantage in a transfusion product and is also a benefit for fractionators, who obtain higher yields in factor concentrates. In addition, cost differences between automated and manual plasmapheresis have narrowed as disposables have been made less costly and the volume of plasma harvested has been increased.

Automated plasma donation by volunteer donors also can serve as a source of "jumbo" FFP units that may contain the equivalent of up to 3 units of whole-blood-derived FFP. It has been proposed that 400 mL is the minimal volume of plasma that should be considered a therapeutic dose for an adult.[9] Apheresis plasma products containing 450 mL provide a full therapeutic dose from each donor. The effects of citrate concentration have been further optimized in "red cells plus plasma" (RBCP) collections, in which 3% citrate-phosphate-dextrose-dextrose (CP2D) anticoagulant is used. Citrate and absolute plasma concentrations in plasma from alternative sources are noted in Table 6-3, which indicates that apheresis-derived plasma has an increased absolute plasma concentration and a decreased citrate content relative to plasma derived from whole blood donation.

Other Plasma Derivatives

Additional products may be derived from apheresis plasma units. One of these is apheresis cryoprecipitate, a material that is manufactured in a fashion completely analogous to cryopre-

Table 6-3. Fresh Frozen Plasma Comparison

	Whole-Blood-Derived	Apheresis Fresh Frozen Plasma	Red Cells Plus Plasma
Volume (mL)	200-250	500-600	450-550
Plasma (%)	80	90	90
Anticoagulant ratio	1:8	1:16	1:16
Anticoagulant type	3% citrate	4% sodium citrate	3% CP2D
Citrate content (g/100 mL plasma)	0.60	0.40	0.30

Adapted from Gilcher.[10]

cipitate from whole-blood-derived plasma.[11] Because the process starts with a larger volume of plasma than that derived from whole blood (approximately 500 mL/unit), it yields an increased cryoprecipitate protein content and a cryoprecipitate volume of approximately 80 mL.[10] A by-product of this process is apheresis cryoprecipitate-reduced plasma. This material, with a volume of approximately 400 mL/unit, has been found to be a useful replacement fluid in the treatment of thrombotic thrombocytopenic purpura.[12] Unfortunately, these products are not recognized by the FDA because of CFR definitions, and routine production is no longer practiced.

Cryoprecipitate can also be collected through sequential plasma exchange donations, particularly among donors of Factor VIII. This process was described by McLeod et al,[13] who supported hemophilic children entirely with repeated donations by one dedicated donor per child. Cryoprecipitate was prepared from the apheresis plasma collected from donors in a plasma exchange procedure, and the residual autologous cryoprecipitate-reduced plasma was used as the replacement fluid for the next in a series of regularly scheduled plasma exchange donations. Donors could be stimulated by 1-deamino-8-D-arginine vasopressin (DDAVP) to boost the yield of Factor VIII and/or von Willebrand factor (vWF) and thereby enhance the utility of the procedure for these purposes. The procedure has also been used as a source of dedicated-donor vWF and fibrinogen.[14]

Red Cell and Multicomponent Donation by Apheresis

Apheresis instruments can also be used to collect red cells. This capability was initially employed in therapeutic red cell exchange (eg, for sickle cell disease), as discussed further in Chapter 19. It has since been adapted to allow an appropriate volume of red cells to be collected from a healthy donor. Collection of red cells by apheresis has several inherent advantages related to quality and consistency in the units obtained. For example, apheresis systems can enhance consistency by collecting a defined volume of Red Blood Cells (RBCs) at a defined hematocrit. Optimization of these systems to reduce the content of undesired elements such as plasma, platelets, and leukocytes is also possible. The apheresis approach can also increase the volume of red cells collected per donor, through double red cell collections, in the same way that other apheresis donations facilitate the collection of an increased amount of other components. This can translate into reduced donor exposure for a recipient who receives both units from such a collection. As in other apheresis donations, the unwanted components are returned to the donor so that only the component of interest is collected. This can be desirable in terms of minimizing reactions.

Theoretically, any apheresis instrument that separates blood components by centrifugation could be adapted for RBC collection. However, cost has been a major concern in the development of donor red cell apheresis. Apheresis red blood cell collection procedures pull donors from the whole blood donor pool. Because of this, the cost of production of an apheresis RBC unit must be comparable to that produced through whole blood donation. Of the companies active in the area of donor apheresis, the Haemonetics Corporation was the first to pursue development of devices that would collect red cells by apheresis in a cost-effective manner. This section begins with a brief review of developmental work sponsored by Haemonetics. A summary is then provided of instruments developed by CaridianBCT and Fenwal for apheresis red cell and multiple component collections. Leukocyte reduction of apheresis red cells is covered briefly, particularly in relation to leukocyte-reduction filters for double red cell units.

Development of Red Cell Collection by Apheresis

Haemonetics PCS and MCS+

The early clinical experience with red cell collection by apheresis was part of a broader effort by Haemonetics to promote apheresis collection of all components of whole blood. In a project undertaken in the mid-1980s, a modified plasma collection system was fitted with an additional pump to allow red cells to be collected and the other components returned to the donor. Studies of the modified system were carried out at the Puget Sound Blood Center and the Oklahoma Blood Institute by Sherrill Slichter and Ronald Gilcher, respectively.

Slichter's studies, published in 1993,[15] investigated whether healthy individuals could donate two RBC units per sitting at intervals such that the volume of cells donated annually would be equal to that permitted with standard whole blood donations. The study was performed with a specially modified PCS that allowed donors to give 450 mL of red cells. Donors who gave three times a year in this way were compared with a control group of whole blood donors who gave approximately 225 mL of red cells six times a year. The main purpose of the study was to determine whether donors who gave two RBC units by apheresis three times per year maintained iron balance as well as the frequent whole blood donors did. The major side effects observed in this study were citrate reactions, primarily numbness and tingling. There was a higher rate of reactions in the apheresis donors; this was attributed to their receiving citrate anticoagulant, which had been added in a 1:8 ratio, in reinfused materials. Overall, however, donors in both groups tolerated the procedures very well if iron supplementation was used. If there was no iron supplementation, both groups showed depletion of iron stores as evidenced by measurement of serum ferritin and the red cell protoporphyrin-to-heme ratio.

The subsequent years brought development of the MCS configuration for Haemonetics instruments. With its more sophisticated programming, the MCS+ allows the collection of red cells and/or plasma. The device is based on the original PCS application, but many improvements have been incorporated, including accommodations for smaller needles (18- or 19-gauge) and for saline infusion. Blood is withdrawn from an antecubital vein as 3% CP2D anticoagulant is added in a 1:16 ratio. As the blow-molded centrifuge bowl described in Chapter 4 is filled, plasma is separated into a transfer bag and red cells are left in the bowl. The centrifuge stops, and the red cells are transferred to a bag containing an additive solution, while the donor's plasma is returned along with saline that replaces the lost red cell volume. To collect a second RBC unit, the cycle is repeated. This process is called "2RBC" collection. Another modification is that apheresis plasma may be collected in addition to red cells in the previously mentioned procedure called RBCP, which is, incidentally, quite similar to the original purpose that Cohn envisioned for the Cohn-ADL centrifuge described in Chapter 1. In this procedure, a targeted amount of plasma is collected in one or two cycles, and red cells are collected at the end of the "last" cycle so that the total extracorporeal volume is never excessive. This procedure also includes saline infusion to replace the lost red cell volume.

Further improvements were incorporated with time, and product quality was verified on the basis of in-vitro and in-vivo study results.[13-18] Representative collection data from studies involving autologous donors are provided in Table 6-4.[19,20] The average collection volume for RBC products from either a 2RBC or RBCP

protocol was 312 mL (including 100 mL of additive solution) at a hematocrit of 58%. The average absolute red cell volume per unit was 180 mL, and for RBCP procedures the target red cell volume was 180 mL, with an average plasma volume of 375 mL.

The experience with autologous donation using either the 2RBC or the RBCP procedure has been that donors are receptive to the idea and that both procedures are well tolerated. As indicated in Table 6-5, the overall rate of donor reactions is approximately 1%, which compares favorably with the reaction rate reported in the literature for autologous whole blood donations.[21] Most reactions have been vasovagal and/or transient hypovolemic events during the

Table 6-4. Phase II Autologous Red Blood Cell Apheresis Study

Statistics		2RBC (n = 1271)	RBCP (n = 1185)
Donor			
Age (years)		58	58
Weight (lbs)		197	174
Gender (% M/F)		73/27	33/67
Procedure			
Time (minutes)		50 ±10	31 ±8
Saline (mL)		500	498
Hct (% pre/post)		44/34	39/34
Product			
RBC-1	Vol (mL)	312 ±7	310 ±9
	Hct (%)	58 ±3	58 ±3
	RBC (mL)	182 ±9	179 ±11
RBC-2	Vol (mL)	312 ±8	N/A
	Hct (%)	58 ±3	N/A
	RBC (mL)	182 ±9	N/A
Plasma	Vol (mL)	N/A	375 ±56

Adapted from Smith et al.[19,20]
2RBC = 2-unit Red Blood Cell; RBCP = red cells plus plasma; Hct = hematocrit; RBC-1 = Red Blood Cell unit 1; Vol = volume; N/A = not applicable.

procedure and are easily managed by saline infusion. As experience was gained with this technique and as instrument programming was improved to allow earlier reinfusion of saline and/or plasma during the procedure, the reaction rate has decreased even further. In addition, assessments of donor tolerance and exercise capacity have confirmed donors' ability to give double units.[22-24]

On the basis of this work, the FDA approved autologous RBCP and 2RBC procedures in October 1995 and approved the RBCP protocol for allogeneic products in March 1996. On the basis of data comparing 2RBC and RBCP procedures for donor tolerance, the FDA approved 2RBC procedures in the allogeneic setting in April 1997.

CaridianBCT Trima and Trima Accel

CaridianBCT developed the Trima system based on the dual-stage separation technology used in the Spectra Apheresis System. Although initially designed for apheresis platelet collection, the Trima was adapted for multicomponent collection and is capable of collecting platelets, plasma, and/or red cells by apheresis. Various combinations of products and volumes of products are possible, using acid-citrate-dextrose (formula A, or ACD-A) as the anticoagulant.

More recently, CaridianBCT has redeveloped its single-stage separation technology in the format of the Trima Accel system. In addition to collecting platelets more efficiently, this system provides for the collection of red cells and/or plasma and/or platelets in single-donor procedures. Trima Accel uses ACD-A as the system's anticoagulant, but additive solution formula 3 (AS-3) is added to RBC units to permit 42-day storage. Studies by Greenwalt et al[25] and Taylor et al[26] confirmed acceptable in-vitro storage parameters for apheresis RBC units collected by Trima Accel (Table 6-6). These storage data are representative of RBC units collected with other manufacturers' multicomponent collection instruments.

Fenwal ALYX

Baxter (Fenwal) developed the ALYX system specifically targeting red cell collections by apheresis. Based on AMICUS technology, this system provides for 2RBC or RBCP collection. It uses ACD-A as the primary anticoagulant, with Adsol as the additive solution to permit 42-day storage. Studies by Snyder et al[27] and Taylor et al[28] confirmed acceptable in-vitro storage characteristics for apheresis red cells collected by ALYX.

Leukocyte Reduction

All three manufacturers (Haemonetics, CaridianBCT, and Fenwal) now provide leukocyte-reduction filter sets that permit collection of

---

Table 6-5. Autologous Donor Reactions and Red Cell Apheresis*

Donor Reaction	2RBC (n = 1271)	RBCP (n = 1185)
Vasovagal	4	3
Hypovolemic	0	4
Combined vasovagal/hypovolemic	4	3
Other	1	0
Total	9 (0.80%)	10 (1.19%)

*Based on unpublished data from Oklahoma Blood Institute.
2RBC = 2-unit red cell (collection); RBCP = red cells plus plasma.

Table 6-6. In-Vitro Storage Data for RBCs Collected with Trima Accel*

	Day 0	Day 42
Hemolysis (%)	0.10	0.32
Sodium (mEq/L)	150.0	114.0
Potassium (mEq/L)	1.8	45.0
ATP (% recovery)	–	70.0

*CaridianBCT, Lakewood, CO.
RBCs = Red Blood Cells; ATP = adenosine triphosphate.
Adapted from Greenwalt et al[25] and Taylor et al.[26]

leukocyte-reduced RBC units. These filters have been available in configurations that permit sterile connection to the product and off-line leukocyte reduction; however, all manufacturers are moving toward an integral filter and toward a single filter suitable for a 2RBC unit. Snyder et al[29] reported illustrative data using automated filtration on the ALYX. 2RBC units were filtered in 5.8 ±0.5 minutes [mean ± standard deviation (SD)], yielding residual white cell counts of 4.4 ±7.2 × 10^4 cell/unit (mean ±SD) with 91.9 ±2.7% postfiltration recovery (mean ±SD).

Donor Acceptance, Regulatory Concerns, and Administrative Issues

The implementation of automated donations for plasma, red cells, and multiple components can be accomplished successfully with planning and periodic evaluation.

Donor Acceptance and Safety

Collection of red cells by apheresis has generally been well accepted by donors. Indeed, centers implementing apheresis red cell donations have found donors quite interested in these newer versions of apheresis technology. The underlying motivation for blood donation is altruism, but there are additional factors to consider, especially with apheresis donations. The sense that they can help multiple recipients by donating multiple products in a single donation appeals to many donors. The "high-tech" nature of apheresis is also appealing to many donors, especially younger donors. Some donors view the extra time required for apheresis donations as a desirable feature. It affords the time to watch a movie, read, or simply relax while receiving attention from center staff. The access needles used with most apheresis systems are slightly smaller than those used in whole blood collections, and, for some donors, that makes a difference. Many of the systems also provide intravenous fluid infusion, and this hydration minimizes reactions caused by volume depletion.

General experience has demonstrated that red cell donations are well tolerated. Several studies have documented that the rate of adverse events for apheresis donations is lower than for traditional whole blood donations. Wiltbank[30] reported that the rate of severe donor reactions was 1.2 per 10,000 automated red cell donations, 1.1 per 10,000 apheresis platelet donations, and 1.5 per 10,000 whole blood donations. There were greater differences in moderate reactions, with rates of 6.8 per 10,000 apheresis red cell donations, 6.2 per 10,000 apheresis platelet donations, and 14.5 per 10,000 whole blood donations. A number of factors should be considered when analyzing such data (eg, gender, body weight, and percentage of first-time donors); nonetheless, some centers have observed an overall reduction in adverse events with apheresis red cell donations vs whole blood donations.[31]

Although the rates of moderate and severe side effects appear lower with 2RBC donations than with whole blood donations, it should be noted that a transient but significant 9-point decrease in hematocrit after 2RBC donation has been documented by Smith et al[32] and Taylor et al.[33] The return of donor plasma plus supplemental saline probably accounts for the greater-than-expected reduction in hematocrit. While contributing to the hematocrit reduction, saline infusion to maintain relative isovolemia has also helped to minimize immediate side effects, even in autologous donors.

Regulatory Considerations for Apheresis Red Cell, Plasma, and Multicomponent Donations

With FDA approval in the late 1990s for autologous and allogeneic collection of RBCP and 2RBC products by apheresis, a set of guidelines was established concerning donor acceptance criteria, frequency of donation, and quality control (QC) protocols.[34] Donor acceptance/eligibility criteria summarized in Tables 6-7 and 6-8 for 2RBC and RBCP allogeneic donations are from the Haemonetics MCS+ Operations Manual.[35,36] They are a simplified version of the FDA-approved algorithm, which considers gender, height, weight, and hematocrit to determine maximum allowable donation volumes.[34] Allogeneic 2RBC donations are restricted to every 112 days, whereas RBCP donations (one 180- to 210-mL RBC unit plus one 450- to 550-mL plasma unit) could be given every 56 days according to these original guidelines (considering extracorporeal volume in the apheresis system). The tables present criteria for allogeneic donors, but tables are also available for autologous donations, with parameters modified to more closely follow autologous donation practices. Based on postmarket studies, the height criteria for female donors has since been modified to greater than 5′ 3″.

As the other apheresis instrument manufacturers developed systems capable of red cell collections, the FDA approved changes in dona-

Table 6-7. Simplified Allogeneic 2RBC Donation Volumes for Donors of Different Weights[35,36]

Donor Weight (lb)	Donor Height	Donor Hematocrit (%)	Absolute Red Cell Volume (mL)
Male			
130-149	≥5′ 1″	≥40	180 × 2
		≥42	190 × 2
150-174	≥5′ 1″	≥40	200 × 2
		≥42	210 × 2
175 and over	≥5′ 1″	≥40	210 × 2
		≥42	210 × 2
Female			
150-174	≥5′ 5″	≥40	180 × 2
		≥42	190 × 2
175 and over	≥5′ 5″	≥40	200 × 2
		≥42	210 × 2

Table 6-8. Simplified Allogeneic RBCP Donation Volumes for Donors of Different Weights[35,36]

Weight (lb)	Hematocrit (%)	Settings	
		Red Cells (mL)	Plasma (mL)
Males			
≥110 ≤129	≥38	185	450
	≥42	190	450
≥130 ≤149	≥38	195	500
	≥42	200	500
≥150 ≤174	≥38	210	
	≥42	210	550
			550
≥175	≥38	210	
	≥42	210	550
			550
Females			
≥110 ≤129	≥38	180	450
	≥42	185	450
≥130 ≤149	≥38	190	450
	≥42	195	450
≥150 ≤174	≥38	190	500
	≥42	195	550
≥175	≥38	200	550
	≥42	210	550

tion guidelines based on extracorporeal volumes of the apheresis systems. The January 30, 2001 FDA guidance recognizes multicomponent apheresis collection of a single RBCP unit, a single unit of RBCs plus platelets, a single unit of RBCs plus platelets plus plasma, or double units of RBCs only.[37] This guidance requires that donor selection criteria from the device manufacturer's operator's manual be followed and that donors otherwise meet FDA criteria for allogeneic whole blood donations. The January 2001 guidance did not recommend the routine weighing of donors but did require that a quantitative method be used to measure predonation hemoglobin or hematocrit.[37]

The guidance retained the 112-day interval between collection of 2RBC units. However, two modifications were introduced. Platelets or plasma can be donated within 8 weeks after a single red cell donation if the extracorporeal red cell volume in the apheresis system is <100 mL. The new guidance also covers incomplete procedures. After an incomplete apheresis procedure with an absolute red cell loss <200 mL, a donor may donate again within 8 weeks. If a second red cell loss <100 mL occurs within 8 weeks, the donor is deferred for a further 8 weeks. If the donor loses >300 mL red cells within an 8-week period, the donor is deferred for 16 weeks.

Regarding apheresis RBC QC, the guidance requires a two-phase process. Initially, 100 consecutive RBC units must be tested for parameters described in the device manufacturer's operator's manual. If 95% of the units meet established specifications, the facility may proceed to routine QC in which 50 units must be tested each month for red cell content, with at least 95% meeting product specifications. This applies to red cells from all collection protocols on all devices at all sites.

In addition to these criteria for red cell donations by apheresis, existing regulations regarding apheresis platelet donations and infrequent plasma donations must also be considered. The October 7, 1988 FDA guidelines for platelets recommends a maximum of 24 donations per year.[38] The maximal frequency is every 48 hours, not to exceed two procedures within 7 days. The maximal allowable volume of plasma removed annually is 12.0 L (donor weight ≤175 lb) or 14.4 L (donor weight >175 lb). The requirements for infrequent plasmapheresis donors (March 10, 1995 revision) covers donations at intervals of ≥4 weeks.[5] The maximum allowable volume of plasma removed annually is 12.0 L (donor weight ≤175 lb) or 14.4 L (donor weight >175 lb). Further guidelines for automated donations have been updated.[39]

Because different automated collection devices use different primary anticoagulants and preservatives, apparently similar products collected on different devices are not interchangeable from a regulatory point of view. Thus, a facility using more than one type of device would need to assign a unique product code and maintain separate collection procedures and QC for each product from each instrument.

Implementation of Automated Donations

Implementation of automated procedures should proceed in stages. The overall strategy must include determining what kinds of products are needed, what equipment is needed to produce those products, how the new processes will integrate with other operations of the cen-

ter, how the products will be accepted and used by transfusing facilities, how the staff will accept and learn a new process, and how donors can be recruited for a new type of donation.

Recruiting donors for apheresis donations requires good communication with, and education of, both donors and staff. Management, recruitment staff, and phlebotomy staff all influence donors' perceptions of new procedures. An enthusiastic, knowledgeable staff plays an integral part in recruitment for new donation procedures. As mentioned, some donors view apheresis donations as "high technology" and are intrigued by the notion of providing multiple products in single donations. There are many ways to recruit donors, but emphasizing that multiple products help multiple patients seems to be generally successful. Also, it is important to encourage interest in giving the products that are needed.

The benefits of multicomponent donations to the blood collection centers and transfusion facilities are readily identified. They improve the availability, consistency, and quality of products while reducing testing costs, recruiting efforts, and donor exposures for recipients. Also, the prevalence of positive test results for viral disease is significantly lower in apheresis donors than in whole blood donors; thus, the former tend to be regarded as safer donors.[40]

Strategically defining the types of apheresis components to draw will affect the approach to donors and how donors of different blood groups will be utilized. Table 6-9 is an example of procedure preferences based on donor blood group, with types of collection procedures listed in decreasing order of preference. Multiple models can be constructed, depending on the center's automated capabilities, transfusion needs, donor factors, etc. Targeting Rh-negative donors of groups O, A, and B for 2RBC donations is a common approach. The model in Table 6-9 is based on the Oklahoma Blood Institute's practice of supplying platelets and plasma as apheresis products. The goal is to collect multiple platelet units from each platelet donation, and RBCP collections are performed to supply a whole-blood-equivalent red cell

Table 6-9. Procedure Preference by Blood Group*

Blood Group	Rh Positive	Rh Negative
A	PLAP RBCP AFFP WB	2RBC RBCP WB PLAP
B	RBCP PLAP 2RBC WB	2RBC RBCP WB PLAP
AB	AFFP PLAP	AFFP PLAP RBCP
O	PLAP 2RBC RBCP WB	2RBC RBCP WB PLAP

*Procedure preferences are listed in decreasing order of priority. From Oklahoma Blood Institute.
WB = Whole Blood; AFFP = Apheresis Plasma; RBCP = Red Blood Cell + Plasma; 2RBC = 2-unit Red Blood Cell;
PLAP = Apheresis Platelet.

dose plus a 500-mL plasma product from one donation.

Operationally, once a center has committed itself to certain products and procedures, it must place automated devices in all fixed collection sites and eventually in mobile settings to allow all donors to have access to apheresis donation equipment. Most centers have mean donation rates of <2 donations/year/donor. Conversion of a fraction of once- or twice-a-year donors to multicomponent donors (eg, converting a group-O-negative whole blood donor to a 2RBC donor) could help alleviate blood shortages.

Financial Considerations

Multiple analyses can be performed on cost and revenue data for automated collections. The value of an analysis will depend on the accuracy of the underlying assumptions. Some

key factors that must be considered are outlined in Table 6-10. In such data analysis, it is important to look at potential revenue not only for a single procedure but also in relation to donation frequency and potential revenue over time. Other factors that have an impact are market demand and licensure status, so that product utilization can be ensured.

Using a set of basic assumptions, one can derive a margin (revenue minus expense) for a whole blood donation. Substituting revenue and expense items in various automated procedures allows one to calculate potential margins for various procedure/product combinations. A whole blood donation that yields RBCs, platelet concentrate, cryoprecipitate, and cryoprecipitate-reduced plasma produces a margin that is $25 to $50 lower than that for 2RBC donation. However, other automated components (eg, RBCP with plasma converted to apheresis cryoprecipitate-reduced plasma plus apheresis cryo-

Table 6-10. Elements of Financial Modeling for Multiple Component Donations

1. Revenue is variable by procedure type and number of products.

2. Some costs are equal for all collections (may distribute over multiple products):

   a. Donor screening

   b. Donor infectious disease testing

   c. Postdonation communication/support/data entry

3. Some costs are variable between procedures:

   a. Disposable supplies/apheresis kits

   b. Product quality control

   c. Equipment placement/maintenance

   d. Collections labor

4. Other costs are less clearly defined:

   a. Recruitment cost

   b. Overhead

   c. Fixed-site collection cost (capacity evaluation)

   d. Component manufacturing cost

precipitate) may increase the margin by another $100. Apheresis platelets generate the largest margin, especially when multiple apheresis doses are collected in a single procedure.

Use of margin calculations to compare various products is helpful but requires that the expense and revenue estimates for the variables included be realistic. It may be difficult to estimate some expenses before implementing a new apheresis procedure. Also, the transition to automated collections involves additional activities to comply with current good manufacturing practice regulations (cGMP). Additional monitoring may increase some expenses; however, this increases the quality of products and ultimately leads to improved cGMP compliance in multiple areas involved with apheresis products. Margin calculations are useful for tracking expenses and predicting a revenue stream. However, other methods, such as Oklahoma Blood Institute's analysis of transfusable prod-

uct needs in the system, can be used to determine the product mix.

Summary

Apheresis donation procedures can now collect the full range of components that can be separated by centrifugation. From platelets, plasma, or red cells to combinations of multiple components, a single donation may now yield several products with improved quality, volume, reproducibility, and efficiency. This not only improves the availability of blood components but also their safety, reducing overall donor exposure for recipients. Multiple product donations allow many fixed donation costs to be distributed over several products. Automated, multiple component donations could help provide solutions to several ongoing needs in the field of transfusion medicine.

References

1. Gilcher RO. Plasmapheresis technology. Vox Sang 1986;51(Suppl 1):35-9.
2. Robert P. International directory of plasma fractionators. Orange, CT: Marketing Research Bureau, 2002.
3. The 2007 national blood collection and utilization survey report. Washington, DC: Department of Health and Human Services, 2008. [Available at http://www.aabb.org/Content/Programs_and_Services/Data_Center/NBCUS/nbcus.htm (accessed January 28, 2010).]
4. Code of federal regulations. Title 21 CFR Part 640.65. Washington, DC: US Government Printing Office, 2010 (revised annually).
5. Food and Drug Administration. Memorandum: Requirements for infrequent plasmapheresis donors. (March 10, 1995) Rockville, MD: CBER Office of Communication, Training, and Manufacturers Assistance, 1995.
6. Food and Drug Administration. Memorandum: Requirements for infrequent plasmapheresis donors. (August 27, 1982) Rockville, MD: CBER Office of Communication, Training, and Manufacturers Assistance, 1982.
7. Smith JW. The Haemonetics Plasma Collection System (PCS) for the automated collection of plasma and platelets. Plasmapheresis 1987;1:40-2.
8. Vezon G, Piquet Y, Manier C, et al. Technical aspects of different donor plasmapheresis systems and biological results obtained in collected plasma. Vox Sang 1986;51(Suppl 1):40-4.
9. Practice parameters for the use of fresh-frozen plasma, cryoprecipitate and platelets. Fresh-Frozen Plasma, Cryoprecipitate, and Platelets Administration Practice Guidelines Development Task Force of the College of American Pathologists. JAMA 1994;8:777-81.
10. Gilcher RO. Novel hemapheresis donations. In: Capon SM, Jeffries L, McLeod BC, eds. Selected topics in hemapheresis. Bethesda, MD: AABB, 1996.
11. Method 6-11. Preparing cryoprecipitated AHF from whole blood. In: Roback JD, Combs MR, Grossman BJ, Hillyer CD, eds. Technical manual. 16th ed. Bethesda, MD: AABB, 2008:956-7.
12. Owens MR, Sweeney JD, Tahhan RH, Fortkolt P. Influence of type of exchange fluid on survival in therapeutic apheresis for thrombotic thrombocytopenic purpura. J Clin Apher 1995;10:178-82.
13. McLeod BC, Sassetti RJ, Cole ER, Scott JP. A high-potency, single-donor cryoprecipitate of known Factor VIII content dispensed in vials. Ann Intern Med 1987;106:35-40.
14. McLeod BC, McKenna R, Sassetti RJ. Treatment of von Willebrand's disease and hypofibrinogenemia with single donor cryoprecipitate from plasma exchange donation. Am J Hematol 1989;32:112-16.
15. Meyer D, Bolgiano DC, Sayers M, et al. Red cell collection by apheresis technology. Transfusion 1993;33:819-24.
16. Bandarenko N, Rose M, Kowalsky RJ, et al. In vivo and vitro characteristics of double units of RBCs collected by apheresis with a single in-line WBC-reduction filter. Transfusion 2001;41:1373-7.
17. Holme S, Elfath MD, Whiteley P. Evaluation of in vivo and in vitro quality of apheresis-collected RBCs stored for 42 days. Vox Sang 1998;75:212-17.
18. Matthes G, Tofote U, Krause KP, et al. Improved red cell quality after erythroplasmapheresis with MCS-3P. J Clin Apher 1994;9:183-8.
19. Smith JW, Axelrod FB, Ness PM, Gilcher RO. Improved red blood cell products: Collection by apheresis (abstract). Transfusion 1995;35(Suppl):66S.
20. Smith JW, Gilcher RO. Red blood cells, plasma, and other new apheresis-derived blood products: Improving product quality and donor utilization. Transfus Med Rev 1999;13:118-23.
21. Pinkerton PH. Two-years' experience with a Canadian hospital-based autologous blood donor program. Transfus Med 1994;4:231-6.
22. Quintana R, Smith KJ, James DS, McDonough W. Exercise performance in blood donors: A randomized, double blind comparison of sham, 1U, and 2U red cell donation (abstract). Transfusion 1995;35(Suppl):15S.
23. Axelrod FB, Catton P, Beeler SA. A comparison of post donation reactions in 2-unit automated red cell apheresis collection using the Haemonetics MCS+ with 1 unit manual whole blood collection in autologous donors (abstract). Transfusion 1995;35(Suppl):65S.
24. Smith KJ, James DS, Hunt WC, et al. A randomized double-blind comparison of donor tolerance of 400 mL, 200 mL, and sham red cell donation. Transfusion 1996;36:674-80.

25. Greenwalt TJ, Rugg N, Gormas JF, et al. In vitro study of red blood cells collected by the Trima Accel System and stored in AS-3 for 42 days (abstract). Transfusion 2002;42(Suppl): 34S.

26. Taylor H, Sawyer S, Whitely P, et al. Clinical verification of single stage collection procedures for red blood cells, platelets and plasma on the Trima system (abstract). Transfusion 2002;42(Suppl):36S.

27. Snyder E, Basil L, Dincecco D, et al. In vitro and in vivo quality of red cells collected on the ALYX red cell/plasma collection system and stored in ACD-A and Adsol for 42 days (abstract). J Clin Apher 2002;17:144.

28. Taylor H, Sawyer S, Whitley P, et al. In vivo and in vitro quality of 42 days stored double red cells collected on the ALYX automated component collection system (abstract). Transfusion 2002;42(Suppl):34S.

29. Snyder E, Basil L, Taylor H, et al. Evaluation of leukoreduced red cells collected and automatically filtered using a new portable component collection system (abstract). Transfusion 2002; 42(Suppl):33S.

30. Wiltbank TB. Donor reaction rates: A preliminary comparison of automated vs whole blood procedures (abstract). Transfusion 2002;42 (Suppl):67S.

31. Moog R, Franck V, Pierce JA, Muller N. Evaluation of a concurrent multicomponent collection system for the collection and storage of WBC-reduced RBC apheresis concentrates. Transfusion 2001;41:1159-64.

32. Smith JW, Gilcher RO, Ford KE. Transient hemodilution accompanying colloid and/or crystalloid infusions during apheresis red cell collections. Presented at the Annual Meeting of the South Central Association of Blood Banks, New Orleans, LA, April 7, 1997.

33. Taylor H, Sawyer S, Whitley P, et al. Donor safety and physiologic response to automated collections of a double red cell collection on ALYX. J Clin Apher 2002;17:143.

34. Food and Drug Administration. Guidance for industry: Recommendations for collecting Red Blood Cells by automated apheresis methods; technical correction. (February 13, 2001) Rockville, MD: CBER Office of Communication, Training, and Manufacturers Assistance, 2001.

35. Haemonetics MCS+ for RBC apheresis owner's operating and maintenance manual (Rev H). Braintree, MA: Haemonetics Corporation, 2002:5-11 to 5-15.

36. Haemonetics MCS+ for RBC apheresis owner's operating and maintenance manual (Rev H). Braintree, MA: Haemonetics Corporation, 2002:7-11 to 7-13.

37. Food and Drug Administration. Guidance for industry: Recommendations for collecting Red Blood Cells by automated apheresis methods. (January 30, 2001) Rockville, MD: CBER Office of Communication, Training, and Manufacturers Assistance, 2001.

38. Food and Drug Administration. Memorandum: Guidelines for the collection of Platelets, Pheresis. (October 7, 1988) Rockville, MD: CBER Office of Communication, Training, and Manufacturers Assistance, 1988.

39. Food and Drug Administration. Guidance for industry and FDA review staff: Collection of platelets by automated methods. (December 17, 2007) Rockville, MD: CBER Office of Communication, Training, and Manufacturers Assistance, 2007.

40. Glynn SA, Schreiber GB, Busch MP, et al. Demographic characteristics, unreported risk behaviors, and the prevalence and incidence of viral infections: A comparison of apheresis and whole blood donors. Transfusion 1998;38: 350-8.

In: McLeod BC, Szczepiorkowski ZM, Weinstein R, Winters JL, eds.
Apheresis: Principles and Practice, 3rd edition
Bethesda, MD: AABB Press, 2010

7

Apheresis Platelet Collection, Storage, Quality Assessment, and Clinical Use

Ralph R. Vassallo, Jr, MD, FACP, and Scott Murphy, MD*

 FOLLOWING A BRIEF MENTION of the function and kinetics of platelets, this chapter reviews current thinking about the appropriate dose of transfused platelets because dose dictates the number of platelets that should be present in an apheresis product and, therefore, the characteristics of the container in which the product should be stored. Important considerations will then be described for the collection and storage of apheresis platelets, followed by an examination of product quality assessment and component modification.

Platelet Physiology

Hemostatic Function of Platelets

There are two major and extensively studied functions of platelets: adhesion to exposed subendothelium with subsequent formation of aggregates at the site of vessel injury, and facilitation of thrombin and fibrin formation to strengthen these aggregates. These two functions, discussed in detail by Jurk and Kehrel,[1] are illustrated in Fig 7-1 and described briefly in its legend. Both functions are required to prevent excessive bleeding during surgery and

Ralph R. Vassallo, Jr, MD, FACP, Heritage Division Chief Medical Officer, and Scott Murphy, MD (*now deceased), former Atlantic Division Chief Medical Officer, American Red Cross Blood Services, Penn-Jersey Region, Philadelphia, Pennsylvania

R. Vassallo has disclosed financial relationships with Fenwal, Terumo Corporation, and Pall Corporation.

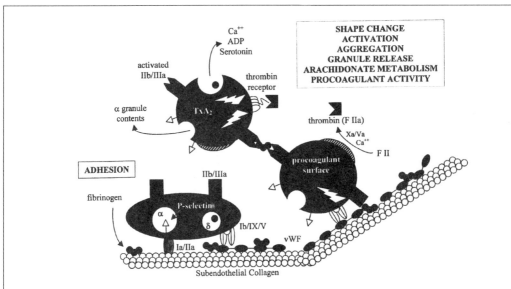

Figure 7-1. Vessel wall injury exposes the subendothelial collagen-containing matrix and results in adsorption of plasma proteins such as von Willebrand factor (vWF) and fibrinogen. These substances bind platelet surface glycoprotein (GP) receptors, causing platelet adhesion. This, in turn, triggers several events. The first, a discoid-to-spherical shape change, is accompanied by the appearance of a number of cytoplasmic markers of platelet activation. These result in the alteration of the GP IIb/IIIa receptor to an activated configuration, increasing affinity for fibrinogen, vWF, and other proteins, which results in aggregation (cross-linking of non-surface-adherent activated platelets). Platelet arachidonic acid is metabolized to thromboxane A_2 (TxA_2), a potent activator released into the microenvironment. Activated platelets also release the contents of their storage granules, particularly adenosine diphosphate (ADP), yet another potent activator. Finally, activated platelet membranes express previously sequestered phospholipids whose procoagulant activity facilitates the activation of plasma clotting factors. The conversion of prothrombin to thrombin generates yet another potent platelet agonist to activate and recruit liquid-phase platelets.

to stop bleeding from other areas of tissue injury, such as ulcerations of the gastrointestinal (GI) tract. It is the delay in aggregate formation that accounts for the prolonged bleeding time in thrombocytopenic patients, which begins when the platelet concentration is reduced to 80,000/μL or below.[2]

Apheresis platelets are transfused to treat bleeding in the setting of critically decreased circulating platelet concentrations or functionally abnormal platelets, and they are used prophylactically to prevent bleeding at prespecified low platelet concentrations. Although data from large, prospective studies would best aid physicians in the decision to transfuse individual patients, such information is lacking. As a result, expert advice based on clinical evidence and consensus statements often guide practice.

Guidelines published by the American Society of Anesthesiology succinctly state that prophylactic preoperative transfusion for hypoproliferative thrombocytopenia is rarely required for concentrations >100,000/μL, is usually required for concentrations <50,000/μL, and is guided by risk factors at intermediate concentrations.[3] Procedures with insignificant blood loss or vaginal deliveries can be performed at concentrations <50,000/μL without prophylactic transfusion.[3] Neurologic or ophthalmologic procedures require a platelet concentration of at least 100,000/μL.[4] Transfusion may be required with apparently adequate concentrations when known platelet dysfunction results in microvascular bleeding. Data regarding specific procedures are derived primarily from the oncology literature, but platelet concentrations of 50,000/μL are required for major invasive procedures, including central line placement, paracentesis, sinus aspiration, dental extraction, closed liver biopsy, lumbar puncture, and endoscopic GI and respiratory tract biopsies. Fiberoptic bronchoscopy (without biopsy) by an experienced operator may be safely performed at a platelet concentration $\geq$20,000/μL, and GI endoscopy without biopsy may be safely performed at platelet concentrations <20,000/μL.[5]

In the setting of a thrombocytopenic patient who is bleeding from an anatomic lesion such as a gastrointestinal ulcer, a goal of achieving a platelet concentration of 50,000 to 100,000/μL appears reasonable. There is, however, much less information regarding "spontaneous," nonsurgical bleeding in the patient with severe thrombocytopenia. Concern about disastrous, spontaneous hemorrhage, particularly into the central nervous system, drives most of the use of platelet transfusion worldwide. Two classic studies have addressed the question of what concentration of platelets is required to prevent endothelial weakening and spontaneous, disastrous hemorrhage.[6,7] Gaydos et al[6] described the relationship between platelet concentration and clinical hemorrhage in leukemia patients before platelet transfusions were available. Minor hemorrhage began when the platelet concentration fell below 50,000/μL (Fig 7-2). On the other hand, major hemorrhage began only when the platelet concentration was below 20,000/μL. The rate of major bleeding increased rapidly when the concentration fell below 5000/μL, reaching 33% of patient days when the platelet concentration was 0/μL. However, when the concentration was between 5000 and 20,000/μL, the incidence of major bleeding was only 3% of patient days. Using 20,000/μL as the transfusion trigger, Freireich et al[7] subsequently described how the repetitive transfusion of platelets affected a similar group of patients. The frequency of major hemorrhage was markedly reduced when the pretransfusion platelet concentration was less than 5000/μL, but it did not change substantially when the pretransfusion platelet concentration was between 5000 and 20,000/μL. Nonetheless, these data were widely interpreted to

establish the platelet transfusion trigger at 20,000/μL.

A number of randomized trials in patients with acute leukemia, hematopoietic stem cell transplants, and aplastic anemia have demonstrated the outcome equivalency of a prophylactic transfusion threshold of 10,000/μL instead of the 20,000/μL threshold derived empirically from older literature.[8-12] Patient-specific clinical data may alter the threshold at which prophylactic transfusion is desirable (eg, major vs minor bleeding, known anatomic lesions, coagulopathy, drug-induced platelet dysfunction, fever/sepsis, hyperleukocytosis, use of antithymocyte globulin, serious mucositis or cystitis, acute graft-vs-host disease (GVHD), sinusoidal obstructive syndrome/veno-occlu-

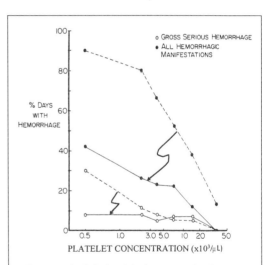

Figure 7-2. Relationship between platelet concentration and hemorrhage before and during the era of prophylactic platelet transfusion. The broken lines provide data on patients who were treated before platelet transfusion was available. The solid lines indicate results for patients who received prophylactic platelet transfusions if their platelet concentrations decreased below 20,000/μL. Serious hemorrhage was very rare when platelet concentration was greater than 20,000/μL. Prophylactic platelet transfusion had little impact on the risk in the range between 0 and 20,000/μL unless the platelet concentration was below 5000/μL. Redrawn from Freireich et al.[7]

sive disease, or a rapid decline in platelet concentration).

Patients with chronic, stable, severe thrombocytopenia seen in hypoproliferative states such as myelodysplasia and aplastic anemia tolerate a platelet count of ≥5000/μL without life-threatening hemorrhage in intercurrent periods between active treatment. Sagmeister et al[12] outlined just such a protocol, transfusing aplastic anemia patients routinely at concentrations ≤5000/μL, at 6000 to 10,000/μL with fever or minor hemorrhage, and at >10,000/μL when actively bleeding.

In solid tumor patients undergoing intensive chemotherapy regimens, the identification of a threshold platelet concentration for significant bleeding is more difficult. Major hemorrhage rates in excess of 10% in patients with platelet concentrations <10,000/μL suggest that most patients should be transfused at this level.[5] The greater risk of bleeding from bladder neoplasms and necrotic tumors may warrant transfusion at a platelet count of ≤20,000/μL. The serious impact of even minor bleeding in patients with limited physiologic reserve or with restricted access to platelet components also justifies transfusion at a platelet count of ≤20,000/μL.[5]

To summarize, spontaneous minor hemorrhage may occur when the platelet concentration decreases below 50,000/μL. Major hemorrhage is a substantial threat with concentrations ≤5,000/μL but is very unlikely with concentrations >20,000/μL. These considerations have implications concerning the indications for platelet transfusion. They also have implications for platelet dose because the dose chosen must be appropriate for the platelet concentration desired following a prophylactic transfusion.

Platelet Kinetics

Platelets are derived from the highly controlled disintegration of the cytoplasm of megakaryocytes, the giant platelet precursor cells in the marrow. Thrombopoietin (TPO), the major physiologic regulator of platelet production, is a glycoprotein produced constitutively in the liver that up-regulates platelet production by increasing the number and maturation of precursor megakaryocytes.[13] The body's platelet mass modulates the level of circulating TPO available to the marrow by binding and sequestering TPO through platelet c-Mpl receptors.

Detailed kinetic studies[14,15] indicate that in normal individuals, approximately 82% of platelets live out their normal potential life span of about 10.5 days; after that they leave the circulation because of a process of senescence, which is not completely understood. The other 18% leave the circulation prematurely in response to ongoing hemostatic needs; this percentage includes those platelets that prevent spontaneous hemorrhage. With increasing degrees of thrombocytopenia, irrespective of cause, there is a progressive shortening of mean platelet survival time (Fig 7-3), presumably because the fixed daily loss of approximately 7100 platelets/μL results in an increasing fraction of platelets leaving the circulation prematurely to provide ongoing hemostasis.[15] At some

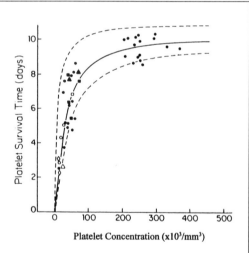

Figure 7-3. Mean platelet survival time compared with platelet concentration in the blood in patients with aplastic anemia. Survival time is shorter at lower platelet concentrations, presumably because an increasing fraction of the circulating platelets is consumed per unit time to meet ongoing hemostatic needs. Redrawn from Hanson and Slichter.[15]

level of extreme thrombocytopenia, all platelets are consumed in this ongoing function, and mean platelet life span is very short. Presumably, spontaneous hemorrhage occurs below this level.

These findings have major implications for platelet transfusion policies and platelet dose. Studies have confirmed what one would predict from the kinetic considerations just described.[16-19] For prophylactic transfusion in an adult, smaller doses (2 to 4 × 10^{11} platelets) are associated with a short survival of the transfused platelets, necessitating frequent transfusions (daily or every other day). It is presumed that most of the transfused platelets will be used in routine microvascular repairs. In contrast, very large doses (>8 × 10^{11} platelets) are associated with longer platelet survival and therefore less frequent transfusion (every 3-4 days). Fewer donor exposures, prolonged transfusion-free intervals, and lower costs related to infusion itself resulted from the higher-dose strategy in hematopoietic stem cell transplant patients using exclusively unsplit apheresis components (ie, units with greater numbers of platelets).[20] Further, the proportion of patients achieving posttransfusion platelet concentrations >20,000/μL was higher in those receiving high-dose platelet support. On the other hand, a mathematical model using whole-blood-derived (WBD) rather than apheresis platelets suggested the potential for lower overall platelet use and donor exposure by employing a low-dose strategy.[21] The platelet-sparing effect of lower-dose therapy was borne out in a large, prospective study demonstrating an 18% to 55% reduction in platelets transfused (and, potentially, in the acquisition cost for WBD platelets) with a low- vs medium- or high-dose strategy.[19] In this study, there was no difference in bleeding outcomes, but low-dose therapy did result in a 66% greater number of transfusion episodes, each of which incurs some additional cost for administration. The clinical equivalency of low, medium, and high doses lends credence to the conduct of studies comparing the outcome of therapeutic-only transfusion (ie, after visible, noncutaneous hemorrhage) to the current prophylactic administration strategy.[22]

Additional studies are necessary to guide optimal practice, as the results of available studies have been quite sensitive to changes in the cost of platelet components and the clinical setting (ie, inpatient vs outpatient, therapeutic vs prophylactic, targeted posttransfusion concentration vs empiric increment, etc).

Platelet Mass and Peripheral Concentration

At first glance, it would appear that total body platelet mass is not tightly regulated, as the normal range for platelet concentration in the blood (150,000-450,000/μL) is quite broad. However, two aspects must be considered in the relationship between peripheral platelet concentration and total body platelet mass. First, there is evidence[23,24] that the mean volume for individual platelets varies inversely with the platelet concentration. Second, not all of the body's platelets are in circulation. Roughly one-third are in a splenic pool, in exchangeable equilibrium with peripheral blood platelets.[25] The percentage of platelets residing in the splenic pool varies among normal individuals[24] so that those with a higher percentage have somewhat lower peripheral platelet concentrations. Splenic platelet sequestration is proportional to organ blood flow, demonstrates a relative affinity for larger platelets, and is affected by donor hematocrit, adrenergic state, and other, as yet undefined factors.[26-29] Platelet mass, therefore, may be more consistent from one individual to another than the variability in blood platelet concentration would suggest. However, it is the blood concentration that dictates the number of platelets available to the apheresis instrument, which is further dependent on individual variability in the immediate release of platelets from the splenic pool.

Figure 7-4(A) shows the wide distribution of platelet concentrations in the blood of apheresis donors at the Penn-Jersey Region of the American Red Cross Blood Services. With this variability, platelet yields in apheresis components are expected to be widely distributed when a fixed volume of blood is processed with a platelet separation device [Fig 7-4(B)]. Many

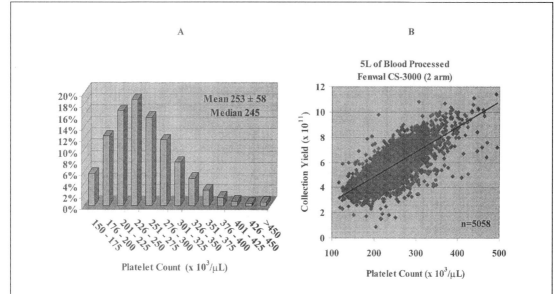

Figure 7-4. (A) Healthy individuals display a wide range of platelet concentrations when presenting for platelet-pheresis donations. (B) For a given volume of blood processed (or time spent on a given instrument) the yield of platelets will vary widely.

approaches can be taken in response to this donor heterogeneity. Some centers do not accept individuals with platelet concentrations below 200,000/μL. For donors with higher concentrations, centers may strive for very high yields (ie, 7 to 10×10^{11} platelets) so that two, or even three, patients can be treated with the components of one donation (by splitting the collection), or centers may collect a single unit of acceptable yield (3 to 4×10^{11} platelets) in less time.

Efforts to augment donor platelet yields by the administration of first-generation TPO analogues to increase a donor's platelet mass and circulating concentration have been abandoned in light of the occasional formation of TPO antibodies, which results in life-threatening thrombocytopenia.[30-32]

Platelet Transfusion Dose

The original principle behind the development of methods for producing platelet components by apheresis was that an entire therapeutic dose for an adult could be obtained from one donor at a single sitting. Thus, considerations of platelet dose should guide apheresis collection practice. Furthermore, storage conditions should enable the chosen dose to be stored optimally for 5 days or possibly longer; considerations of storage conditions are discussed later in this chapter.

Physiologic Considerations

As mentioned above, approximately one-third of infused platelets are pooled reversibly in a spleen of normal size. Therefore, the volume of distribution for transfused platelets is 50% greater than the recipient's blood volume. If the latter is taken to be 65 to 70 mL/kg body weight, then the "effective" volume of distribution is approximately 100 mL/kg. It is easy to calculate that the infusion of 1×10^{11} platelets into a 20-kg (44-lb) recipient should raise the platelet concentration by 50,000/μL. This concept is expressed graphically in Fig 7-5, which indicates the number of platelets (or the average number of WBD platelet units) required to

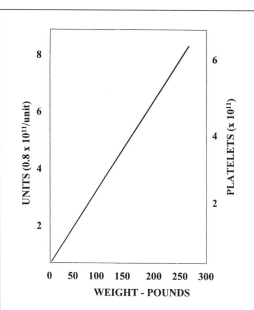

Figure 7-5. Theoretical platelet dose required to increase the platelet concentration by 50,000/µL. The dose is given both as units of whole-blood-derived platelet concentrates (left axis) and absolute platelet numbers (right axis). Because blood volume increases with body weight, so does the dose. The calculations, explained in the text, assume no complicating factors such as splenomegaly.

raise the platelet concentration by 50,000/µL at various patient body weights.

In practice, the average increment after transfusion may be half of that expected.[33] Many patients do not achieve the optimal, predicted response because of alloimmunization and/or clinical factors such as fever, infection, disseminated intravascular coagulation, bleeding, concomitant use of amphotericin B, GVHD, or other conditions.[34] Therefore, Fig 7-5 can be taken to indicate the dose of platelets required to raise the platelet concentration by at least 25,000/µL in the "average" ill, myelosuppressed patient transfused prophylactically for platelet concentrations below 10,000/µL. Thus, for the average 70-kg (155-lb) patient, a prophylactic dose of 3.5×10^{11} platelets will usually increase the platelet count by 30,000/µL. This represents a residual increment of 20,000/µL following an expected one-third

loss of platelets over the ensuing 24 hours.[35] Proportionately larger doses may be required in other situations, especially for surgical patients in whom a target platelet concentration is required (usually over 50,000/µL and occasionally as high as 125,000/µL).

Problems with a "Standard" Platelet Dose

On the basis of the above considerations, one can see that 3.5×10^{11} platelets is an acceptable dose for an average-sized patient transfused in the most common clinical setting (prophylaxis during marrow suppression) according to the most widely accepted transfusion trigger. But this is probably an inadequate dose for a large patient (eg, 90-100 kg), a patient whose enlarged spleen provides an expanded exchangeable platelet pool, a patient actively bleeding from an anatomic lesion, or a surgical patient in whom a higher increment is required. Also, physicians caring for outpatients often take advantage of the fact that larger doses extend the intervals between transfusions.[16-19] In these situations, a dose of 7 to 8 × 10^{11} is perfectly appropriate. It may seem inefficient to recombine components that have been previously divided (especially components from two different donors). On the other hand, it is probably wasteful to prepare high-yield components and then transfuse them indiscriminately to small patients who require only one or two platelet doses. Such a practice would also necessitate significantly more donations to meet national demand for transfusable doses and lead to wider swings in availability around holidays or with inclement weather, both of which proportionately reduce donor turnout.

The answer to this dilemma is not apparent, so individual blood center practice should probably be responsive to the therapeutic approaches of the clinicians and hospitals being served. Some have suggested that standardization of platelet content would allow clinicians to better predict patient response. However, unless one cares for patients with uniform body weights and blood volumes, patients will continue to either receive more platelets than necessary or require 2 units to achieve an acceptable increment, incurring an extra donor exposure. Considering the current safety of the blood supply,[36,37] the latter alternative is not as problematic as in the past. In practice, most blood centers ask donors to remain on the apheresis instrument as long as they are comfortable to achieve the highest product yield possible. Units are split into two or three transfusable doses when the yield is high enough to ensure a content of at least 3×10^{11} in 90% of components. This results in a slightly left-skewed distribution of yields in distributed components, with a mean content just below 4×10^{11}.[38]

When blood centers label their apheresis units with platelet contents, component assignment can be tailored to the needs of individual patients by the transfusion service if clinicians communicate their patients' required increments and values to estimate blood volume. This is a paradigm more often seen in Europe than the United States. It is more labor intensive, requiring re-education of clinicians about ordering, transfusion service calculations, and more complex hospital inventory practices. A new focus on unit content might also require changes in blood center reimbursement, with variable fees geared to content rather than a flat per-unit charge. Whether these changes are ultimately introduced will depend upon the perceived balance of cost and patient benefit.

As discussed below, because apheresis platelet storage containers have upper and lower content (and sometimes concentration) specifications, these values are determined for every component. In this process, blood centers identify nonstandard components with contents of 1.0 to 2.9×10^{11} platelets. Doses below 2×10^{11} are probably inadequate for most adult patients, and units with both lower concentration and content are probably inappropriate for children.

Liquid Storage of Platelets in Plasma

Most of what is known about platelet storage has been learned from studies of WBD platelet concentrates. As far as is known, the principles are the same for apheresis platelets. Fundamentals include 1) maintenance of appropriate temperature, 2) insurance of metabolic fuel availability, 3) storage in a plastic container allowing adequate delivery of oxygen to respiring platelets, and 4) continuous agitation. When stored for 5 days in accordance with these principles, apheresis platelets have had quite satisfactory in-vivo viability.[39-43]

Storage Temperature

In the 1960s, platelets were stored under refrigeration (1-6 C), but it was recognized that they survived for only a few hours after infusion, even after only 1 day of storage (Fig 7-6). Subsequently, it was determined that platelets survived normally, even after several days of storage, if they were kept at room temperature (20-24 C).[44] The superiority of storage at 20 to 24 C relative to 1 to 6 C has also been confirmed by studies in thrombocytopenic patients.[45,46] Measurable cryo-damage appears after 24 hours' storage at 18 C, 16 hours at 16 C, 10 hours at 12 C, and 6 hours at 4 C.[47] It is now recognized that storage of platelets at temperatures below 30 C results in membrane phase transitions that cluster phosphoinositide-rich lipid rafts.[48] This results in actin polymerization and dendritic shape change as well as creating clustered carbohydrate neoepitopes.[49,50] Cold-stored platelets appear to function normally despite these morphologic changes[51] but do not circulate long. An understanding of the mechanism underlying this rapid clearance is just emerging. At least two carbohydrate-dependent clearance mechanisms operate to remove cold-stored platelets from circulation.[50] Short-term refrigeration leads to clustering of platelet surface von Willebrand receptor GP1bα subunits, which are recognized by macrophage $\alpha_M\beta_2$ receptors and removed by hepatic Kupffer cells. Longer storage results in emergence of a different neoepitope recognized by hepatocyte asialoglycoprotein receptors, promoting platelet clearance by these cells. Ongoing studies seek to enzymatically alter these neoepitopes to prevent premature platelet clearance. Until such a solution is found, cold

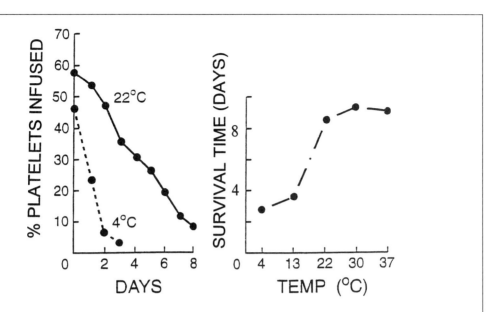

Figure 7-6. Autologous, radiolabeled, reinfusion studies of platelets stored overnight at various temperatures. The graph on the left shows that platelets stored at 22 C are essentially equivalent in survival to fresh platelets (approximately 8-10 days), whereas survival is very short after storage at 4 C. Recovery of only 50 to 60% of platelets immediately after infusion results from physiologic pooling[25] in the spleen and not from cell injury. The graph on the right shows that survival time is normal (8-10 days) when platelets are stored at 22 C or above but is reduced after storage at lower temperatures. Redrawn from Murphy and Gardner.[44]

storage, despite its potential to extend platelet shelf life, is simply not feasible.

Platelet storage below body temperature is known to confer salutary metabolic effects. Holme and Heaton have shown that platelet aging at a storage temperature of 22 C is 42% to 44% of that at 37 C.[52] Storage at temperatures above 24 C, however, appears to be inferior to that at 20 to 24 C,[44] principally because of increased platelet metabolism and the resultant accelerated accumulation of toxic metabolites in the storage container.

Platelet Metabolism and Oxygen Requirements during Storage

During storage in plasma at 20 to 24 C when there is an adequate oxygen supply, platelets use two major metabolic pathways: 1) glycolysis, which does not require oxygen, and 2) oxidative metabolism through the citric acid cycle[53] (Fig 7-7). In glycolysis, one molecule of glucose is converted into two molecules of lactic acid because little, if any, of the pyruvate intermediate derived from glucose enters the citric acid cycle. The production rate of lactic acid is approximately 0.1 to 0.15 mmoles/day/10^{11} platelets. At the same time, the cells consume oxygen at approximately the same rate using plasma-free fatty acids as the predominant substrate.[54]

The production of 1 lactate molecule fuels the regeneration of 1 adenosine triphosphate (ATP) molecule, and the consumption of 1 oxygen molecule regenerates up to 6 ATP molecules. Therefore, the cell derives 85% of its ATP regeneration from oxygen consumption through the citric acid cycle and 15% through glycolysis. If the demand for oxygen is not met, the cell will increase its glycolytic rate, the so-called Pasteur effect. In theory, a cell completely deprived of oxygen should increase its

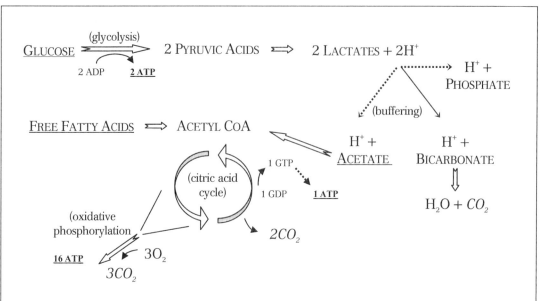

Figure 7-7. Metabolic pathways available to platelets when stored in plasma or platelet additive solution (PAS). Platelets use two plasma substrates, glucose and fatty acids, for energy production. Almost all glucose used is converted through pyruvate to lactate and a hydrogen ion. The hydrogen ion is buffered by bicarbonate (or, in PAS, acetate and phosphate). Acetyl CoA is produced and enters the citric acid cycle through metabolism of fatty acids and, in PAS, acetate. The cycle oxidizes acetyl CoA to carbon dioxide. Entry of oxygen and exit of carbon dioxide require a container with suitable gas permeability.
ADP = adenosine diphosphate; ATP = adenosine triphosphate; GDP = glucose diphosphate; GTP = glucose triphosphate.

glycolytic rate six- to sevenfold to regenerate the ATP not being regenerated by oxidative metabolism, and experiments have shown that this occurs.[55]

The end product of oxidative metabolism is carbon dioxide, a volatile acid that can leave the platelet suspension by passing through the walls of the plastic container. Lactic acid cannot do this; it must be buffered by the only significant plasma buffer, bicarbonate. As each molecule of lactic acid is buffered, bicarbonate is converted into water and carbon dioxide, which leaves through the wall of the container. There is enough bicarbonate in plasma to accommodate a rise in lactate concentration to approximately 20 mmoles. Beyond that concentration, the pH will fall to less than 6.8. As the pH falls from 6.8 to 6.2, there is progressive platelet swelling, disc-to-sphere transformation, aggluti-

nation, and lysis.[56] When radiolabeled and reinfused, these platelets demonstrate marked decreases in recovery and survival.[57]

Attempts to intervene in this downward cycle of hypoxic H^+ generation, decline in pH, and loss of platelet viability have driven improvements in storage container design to allow sufficient O_2 influx and CO_2 efflux.

Plastics do not have "pores" through which gases may pass; rather, the gases are soluble in the plastic and pass through when the plastic is saturated. Plastics vary in the ease with which gases penetrate. Adequacy of the oxygen supply has been linked to three major factors: 1) the number of platelets within the container (each cell needs one femtomole of oxygen per day), 2) the intrinsic permeability of the plastic, and 3) the surface area of the container. In practice, oxygen supply can be presumed adequate if there is an easily measurable oxygen tension (>40 mm Hg) throughout storage, and if the rise in the lactate concentration does not exceed 2 to 3 mmoles/day.

Of course, the situation is particularly complicated for apheresis platelets. An individual component may have as few as 2×10^{11} or as many as 10×10^{11} platelets. The component may be in one, two, or even three containers so that the surface area available for gas transport is variable. As discussed below, component volume is yet another variable that affects gas exchange. Manufacturers generally recommend an appropriate range of plasma volumes for a single container. Finally, each manufacturer of apheresis devices has a container constructed from a unique plastic, and some manufacturers market more than one plastic type. Observations concerning these complex interactions are presented in a subsequent section of this chapter.

Agitation during Storage

Platelet concentrates must be agitated during storage to obtain optimal results. AABB standards allow no more than 24 hours without agitation (eg, during shipping).[58(pp51-52)] When concentrates are left undisturbed, production of lactic acid accelerates and the pH decreases.[59,60] Furthermore, certain forms of agitation appear to be better than others. To summarize many studies, flatbed platform and "face-over-face" agitation have produced satisfactory results, whereas elliptical and Ferris-wheel forms have not.[61,62] In-vitro studies of WBD and apheresis platelet concentrates suggest that agitation may be discontinued for as long as 24 to 30 hours without ill effects.[60,63-65]

Although initially thought to promote oxygen diffusion throughout the container, agitation appears to exert a more complex effect on platelet metabolism. Oxygen tension (pO_2) is maintained in unagitated platelets, and in at least two studies, mixing even once daily has prevented deleterious pH drops in components with relatively low platelet contents.[66,67] Thus, agitation may either facilitate oxygen use by the platelets or prevent settling and contact-

mediated up-regulation of glycolytic metabolism.[60]

Platelet Containers

Platelets from apheresis collections are commonly stored in large containers to maximize the surface area for gas exchange. Within 24 hours of collection, assessment of platelet concentration and content determines whether storage throughout the remainder of platelet shelf life must be in one, two, or three containers. Each manufacturer determines limits for concentration and content that permit the maintenance of pH throughout storage based on the unique composition and surface-to-volume ratio of its containers. One can measure the rate of gas exchange, which varies considerably for the various containers.[68] There is an inverse relationship between the pO_2 within the container and its platelet content. In the steady state, pO_2 reflects the balance between inflow through the plastic walls of the container and platelet oxygen consumption. As platelet content rises, the pO_2 falls until it plateaus at the detection limit of the oxygen electrode. The point at which the plateau begins is the point at which just enough oxygen is available to meet the platelets' needs. Beyond this point, the platelets become hypoxic and up-regulate glycolysis. This results in accelerated lactate production and a progressive fall in pH.

Figure 7-8(A) shows data on day 3 of storage in a PL-732 container at two storage volumes, 100 and 200 mL. One can see that the pO_2 begins to plateau at approximately 3.5×10^{11} platelets for a 200-mL volume and between 2.5 and 3×10^{11} when the volume is 100 mL. This suggests that the gas exchange is somewhat better when the volume of the platelet suspension is larger. The results are similar for platelets stored in the PL-3014 container [Fig 7-8(B)]. In addition, because the PL-3014 container is more permeable to oxygen than PL-732 (Fig 7-9), the pO_2 is higher at any given platelet content.

The very first containers, made of polyvinylchloride (PVC) plasticized with di-(2-ethylhexyl) phthalate (DEHP) were originally intended for

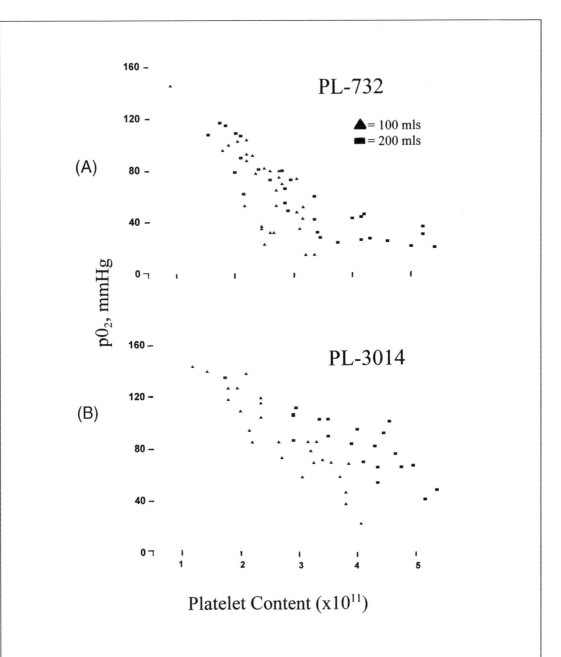

Figure 7-8. Relationship between oxygen tension (pO$_2$) and platelet content in one container on day 3 of storage. Figure 7-8(A) shows data for Baxter's PL-732 container with either 100- or 200-mL volumes per container. In a 200-mL volume, pO$_2$ reaches a minimum when the platelet content is 3.5 $\times$ 10^{11}. Above that value, there is inadequate oxygen transport to meet the demands of the platelets within the container. With a 100-mL volume, pO$_2$ is somewhat less for a given platelet content relative to 200 mL. Figure 7-8(B) shows similar data for storage in one PL-3014 container. Again, the difference between a 100-mL and 200-mL volume is evident. Further, from a comparison of (A) and (B), it is clear that, for a given platelet content, pO$_2$ is higher in the more oxygen-permeable PL-3014.

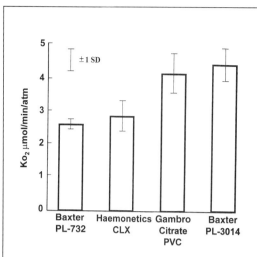

Figure 7-9. Oxygen transport capacity (KO_2) of containers for storage of apheresis platelets. Measurements were made[68] for two Baxter containers (PL-732 and PL-3014), the CLX container from the Haemonetics MCS, and the citrate-plasticized polyvinylchloride (PVC) container used with the Gambro Spectra. KO_2 is substantially higher for the PL-3014 and the Gambro container relative to the PL-732 and the CLX container.

Platelet Storage Duration

In 1986, following increasingly frequent reports of posttransfusion sepsis, platelet storage duration was reduced to 5 days from the 7-day period approved in 1984.[69] With the approval of bacterial culture techniques licensed for quality control testing, the FDA reauthorized the extension of shelf-life in 2005 to 7 days for apheresis platelets collected on specific automated platforms using a specified microbial testing schema. Following 32 months of mandated postmarketing surveillance, the sponsors terminated the study and, thus, the availability of extended shelf-life platelets that it had afforded. Interim analysis had raised statistical concerns that tested 7-day products may not be able to demonstrate a lower rate of contamination than untested 5-day products.[70] Thus, platelet shelf-life is critically affected by the multiplication of small numbers of bacteria present in as many as 1 in 2000 to 1 in 3000 apheresis collections.[71]

The American Red Cross's reported rate of septic transfusion reactions from 5-day apheresis platelets tested using the BacT/ALERT culture system (bioMérieux, Marcy l'Etoile, France) was approximately 1 per 75,000 transfused components.[71] This was as low as 1 per 193,000 units collected with apheresis technology, diverting the initial portion of blood into the sampling pouch rather than channeling it into the instrument. More septic transfusion reactions were reported from 5-day-stored platelets than the preceding 3 days combined, underscoring the potential for ongoing exponential growth to produce harmful levels of bacteria throughout progressively longer storage periods.

Viability of platelets stored in plasma is only minimally reduced after the additional 2 days of storage between days 5 and 7,[41,72,73] but acceptable recoveries and survival times in additive-solution-stored platelets containing second-messenger inhibitors have been reported for as long as 7 to 14 days after collection.[74,75] As a result, the storage duration of platelet concentrates is determined primarily by the relatively high risk of bacterial growth at room

freezing plasma. Not designed to maximize oxygen transport, these containers permitted the storage of WBD platelets for only 3 days before a significant percentage of units experienced deleterious drops in pH. So-called second-generation containers permit much longer periods of storage, up to 14 days in some cases, without deleterious falls in product pH. These containers are constructed from polyolefin, thinner PVC, or PVC plasticized with different compounds such as triethyl-hexyl trimellitate and butyryl-tri-hexyl citrate. These have nearly twice the oxygen permeability of DEHP-plasticized PVC containers.

When storing platelets, one should be cognizant of the importance of gas exchange. Containers should not substantially overlap or be covered with labels or other materials that impede oxygen diffusion.

temperature. Efforts to reduce the risk of bacterial contamination are reviewed elsewhere and in Chapter 10 of this text.[76-78] Suffice it to say that the relatively low detection rate of culture technologies, which appear to detect fewer than half of contaminated units, remains a significant barrier to the extension of platelet shelf life back to 7 days.[79] Point-of-issue detection technologies may be able to reduce the residual rate of septic transfusion reactions if they are sufficiently sensitive to detect harmful levels of bacterial contamination. Pathogen-reduction technologies face an uphill battle to demonstrate safety and efficacy against bacterial pathogens while maintaining platelet viability. Continued efforts are important, both to reduce patient morbidity and to extend platelet shelf-life. Prolonged platelet storage has been shown to provide logistical benefits for blood centers by reducing the number of platelet components that expire in inventory and by enhancing the reliability of the platelet supply.[80] Such an extension may also partially or fully offset the increased cost associated with mass implementation of new bacteria detection or pathogen-reduction technologies.

Liquid Storage of Platelets in Platelet Additive Solution

Synthetic media as platelet additive solutions (PAS) have been in routine use in Europe, where pooled buffy-coat-derived platelet concentrates are produced. They are also CE-marked either as stand-alone solutions for apheresis platelet storage or as solutions for apheresis platelets photochemically treated to inactivate pathogens and white cells by cross-linking nucleic acids.[81,82] Some of these media will likely be approved for use in the United States because of the increasingly appreciated benefits of reducing the amount of plasma in apheresis platelet components.[83]

The use of PAS allows 1) enhanced concurrent collection of apheresis plasma for transfusion, 2) diminution of allergic reactions and, possibly, other plasma-mediated reactions (eg, transfusion-related acute lung injury), 3) efficient employment of photochemical pathogen-reduction technologies, and 4) potential improvements in platelet storage through solutions engineered to enhance buffering capacity or improve maintenance of adenine nucleotide levels.

The composition of selected solutions is listed in Table 7-1. PAS consists of saline-based crystalloids with citrate anticoagulant and supplemental acetate to substitute for the plasma fatty acids that serve as fuel for aerobic platelet metabolism. Acetate enters the citric acid cycle while using a proton from the medium and providing an alkalinizing effect that ameliorates the decline in pH (Fig 7-7). Gluconate, phosphate, or bicarbonate are added to supplement the bicarbonate buffering capacity of the small fraction of remaining plasma.[84] Phosphate, a component of the base anticoagulant for WBD platelets, but not apheresis platelets collected in acid-citrate-dextrose, also appears to maintain adenine nucleotide levels.[81]

It has been recognized that even in the presence of alternate fuels, storage medium glucose exhaustion leads to adenine nucleotide depletion and loss of platelet viability.[84] Some percentage (20%-40%) of plasma carryover has therefore been required to provide adequate reserves of glucose and bicarbonate buffers. Glucose has been technically difficult to add to PAS because of caramelization during heat storage at neutral or slightly basic pH, so most solutions require higher fractions of plasma carryover to make up for this deficit. The addition of second-messenger inhibitors such as prostaglandin E$_1$, xanthines, forskolin, amiloride, sodium nitroprusside, quinacrine, dipyridamole, ticlopidine, and/or protease inhibitors has also been attempted with varying degrees of success to decrease activation-mediated platelet loss during storage.[85-87] Safety concerns in the setting of routine transfusion in varied patient populations significantly hinder their use and commercial applicability, however.

Table 7-1. Composition of Selected Platelet Additive Solutions

	T-Sol*	InterSol*	Composol†	SSP+‡	PAS-G§
NaCl	115.5	77.3	90	69.3	110
KCl	–	–	5	5	5
MgCl	–	–	1.5	1.5	3
Citric acid	–	–	–	–	7.5
Na citrate	10	10.8	11	10.8	–
Na acetate	30	32.5	27	32.5	15
Na bicarbonate	–	–	–	–	26.4
Na gluconate	–	–	23	–	–
Na phosphate	–	28.2	–	28.2	4
Glucose	–	–	–	–	30

*Fenwal, Inc, Lake Zurich, IL.
†Fresenius AG, Bad Homburg, Germany.
‡Macopharma, Tourcoing, France.
§Pall Corp, East Hills, NY.

Assessing Platelet Quality

Platelet Counting

In the discussion of how many platelets should be present in an apheresis platelet component to provide an adequate dose for a patient, it is assumed that the number can be accurately counted. To be sure that the number of platelets in a component does not exceed the gas transport capacity of the storage container, it is customarily assumed that what is counted is identical to what the manufacturer would count when developing guidelines to define the maximal number of platelets that the container can handle. In fact, this is clearly not the case.

In several studies,[88,89] it has been shown that different hematology analyzers yield different platelet concentrations for a standardized platelet suspension. In the most recent study, which used glutaraldehyde/formaldehyde-fixed human platelets at concentrations relevant for blood centers (750,000-2,000,000/µL), analyzer results ranged from a 35% underestimate to a

16% overestimate of mean values derived from 89 instruments.[90] Most coefficients of variation within instrument types were <10%, demonstrating that differences in the instruments themselves is primarily responsible for observed differences in counts. When instruments count too low, the pH may decrease during storage of higher-than-expected-yield components. When they count too high, components with inappropriately low platelet contents may be divided ("split"), thus leaving patients underdosed. Counts obtained by flow cytometry employing labeled platelet-specific antibodies and fluorescent counting beads produce highly linear results with good precision—important features for any potential standard method.[91] Automated immunoplatelet techniques are coming into use, but without an established, independent, "gold-standard" assay, the relevance of counts obtained using different impedance or optical counters is problematic.[92] Standardized techniques employing suspensions of platelet-like particles in assays that are linear over the range of platelet concentrations present in apheresis platelet containers (up to 2,500,000/μL) are clearly a research priority.

Quality Assessment Requirements

Aside from its leukocyte-reduction standards, the US Food and Drug Administration (FDA) has set two requirements for assurance of platelet component quality. The first stipulation is that, with 95% confidence, more than 95% of components must maintain a pH ≥6.2 through the end of storage. Second, with 95% confidence, more than 75% of components must contain at least 3.0×10^{11} platelets [although AABB requires that 90% meet this content standard[58(pp28-29)]].[93] FDA review of components collected or stored using new technologies, however, is subject to a pyramidal schema of additional data (Fig 7-10).[94] Given minimal levels of concern about potential platelet damage associated with new processes, evaluation of in-vitro tests of platelet function is felt to be

sufficient. These results can be used to decide whether the benefits anticipated for components with moderate potential concerns outweigh possible shortcomings before determination of radiolabeled platelet recovery and survival is required in healthy research subjects. Some components may require further assessment in a hemostasis clinical trial, based on higher levels of concern and data from preceding in-vitro and in-vivo studies. Postmarket studies may also be required when concerns regarding rare adverse events arise.

In-Vivo Studies of Radiolabeled Platelets

As predicted by initial results with platelet transfusions,[95] it has been apparent that efficacy correlates with a measurable sustained increase in platelet concentration in the blood. Therefore, research into the preparation and storage of platelets for transfusion has always stressed the maintenance of platelet viability—

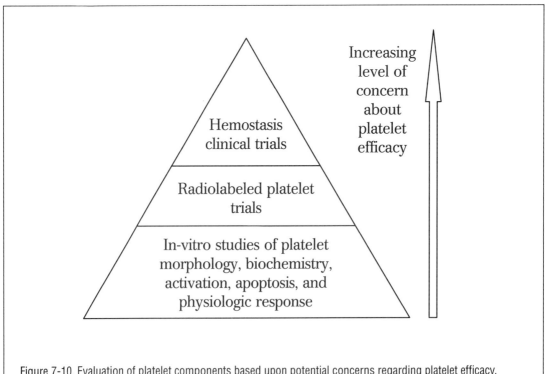

Figure 7-10. Evaluation of platelet components based upon potential concerns regarding platelet efficacy.

that is, the capacity of platelets to circulate without being removed by the recipient's phagocytic system because of cellular damage.

The ultimate test of this capacity has always been the measurement of increments in platelet concentration in thrombocytopenic patients. Unfortunately, clinical factors such as alloimmunization and nonimmune platelet consumption lead to variable patient responses, so that small differences in viability between two components may be obscured, or inordinately large numbers of trial participants are required to detect clinically significant differences. Therefore, the transfusion community has relied on autologous, radiolabeled reinfusion studies in normal, healthy volunteers using chromium-51 or indium-111.[96-98] In such studies, platelets are obtained and stored by the method being investigated; they are then radiolabeled and reinfused into the original donor along with an aliquot of freshly obtained WBD platelets collected on the day of infusion and radiolabeled with a different nuclide from the one used to label the test component. Samples are taken in the first few hours after infusion and for approximately 1 week thereafter. The data are generally reduced to two numbers: 1) the percentage of infused platelets recovered immediately after infusion and 2) the mean cell life (survival) over the subsequent week. The goal for any method of platelet preparation and storage is to achieve results similar to those of fresh platelets—that is, approximately 60% to 70% recovery and a mean cell life of approximately 8 to 9 days. The FDA has thus far informally defined standards based on the proposal of Murphy[96] that, with 95% confidence, test platelets retain at least 66% of control (fresh platelet) recovery and 58% of control survival by noninferiority analysis.

In-Vitro Assessment of Platelet Quality

In-vivo studies are difficult and expensive, and relatively few laboratories are equipped to perform them. It would therefore be preferable to have a simple in-vitro assay or group of assays that would predict in-vivo recovery, survival, and function. A review of the literature[99] concluded that three assays have consistently correlated with in-vivo recovery and survival: 1) the osmotic reversal reaction; 2) the morphology score by oil, phase microscopy; and 3) the extent of shape change. A multi-institutional study confirmed that these measurements can be made in a consistent, quantitative fashion.[100]

It is beyond the scope of this chapter to describe these or other methods in detail. Suffice it to say that the osmotic reversal reaction, also called the hypotonic shock response, exposes platelets to a hypotonic environment. Only metabolically active platelets are able to extrude water, and an estimate of the ability to restore normal cell volume can be obtained by light transmittance. Both the morphology score and the extent of shape change reflect retention of the cell's discoid shape. Normal, fresh, resting platelets have the appearance of thin discs with few or no projections. Platelets with this morphology usually circulate well after infusion, whereas disc-to-sphere transformation often predicts in-vivo failure. Platelet discoid shape is also reflected by the swirling or shimmering appearance of well-preserved concentrates during gross visual inspection. Another multi-institutional study indicated that this assessment could be performed in a reproducible fashion by a trained observer.[101] This method has potential as a quick, cost-effective quality control measure.

Other in-vitro studies of platelet activation during storage have been less useful in predicting recovery and survival—eg, agonist-induced aggregation or serotonin release, supernatant concentration of α-granule proteins (β-thromboglobulin, platelet factor 4, etc), surface activation markers (P-selectin, CD63, functional glycoprotein IIb/IIIa changes), and assessment of platelet procoagulant activity (phosphatidylserine expression) or cell lysis (lactate dehydrogenase). The results of these in-vitro studies become abnormal during storage of platelet concentrates that have been shown to be effective in vivo. Apparently, many of these activation-dependent changes are reversible and do not preclude platelet functional recovery following infusion.[102,103]

Problems with Current Methods

These methods present at least two problems that need to be stressed. First, although they predict the capacity of cells to circulate in normal volunteers and most clinically stable thrombocytopenic patients, there is no insurance that circulation is equivalent to hemostasis. Bleeding times after platelet transfusion have been measured in thrombocytopenic patients,[45,104-106] and, in general, a shortened bleeding time has been observed when stored platelets have retained their capacity to circulate. However, such studies are rarely performed now. Suitable patients generally have low granulocyte levels and decreased resistance to infection, so there is concern about infection of the bleeding-time incision. More recent trials have incorporated a standardized, reproducible daily bleeding score (World Health Organization) in an effort to quantitatively compare clinically relevant bleeding events during evaluation of the in-vivo efficacy of different platelet products.[19,107]

The other problem is less well defined. As mentioned above, many patients have poor in-vivo increments after platelet transfusions, attributable to a host of conditions leading to platelet consumption.[33] It has been proposed that some of these patients may respond to fresh platelets but not to stored ones, even if the latter pass all the in-vivo and in-vitro tests described above.[108] Thus, there may be clinically significant defects in some stored platelet preparations that go undetected by all current testing. There is, therefore, a pressing need to develop better in-vitro methods for predicting in-vivo platelet function after transfusion and to better define the reasons for the poor clinical responses of some thrombocytopenic patients.

Component Modification

Leukocyte Reduction

Demand for leukocyte-reduced apheresis platelets has been driven by a number of documented and purported benefits inherent in the transfusion of cellular products with reduced white cell (WBC) content.[109] The proven benefits of leukocyte reduction include reductions in cytomegalovirus (CMV) transmission,[110] HLA alloimmunization and platelet refractoriness,[111] and febrile nonhemolytic transfusion reactions.[109] Purported benefits include decreases in posttransfusion immunomodulation (resulting in lower rates of postoperative infection and tumor recurrence), avoidance of myocardial reperfusion injury, and reductions in bacterial contamination rates.[109]

Guidelines developed by the FDA[93] and the AABB[58(p29)] have established a standard of <5 × 10^6 WBCs per leukocyte-reduced unit. The Council of Europe has defined acceptable leukocyte reduction at a more stringent level of <1 × 10^6 WBCs.[112] Many newer apheresis devices incorporate leukocyte-reduction hardware or software, allowing the collection of components consistently containing <5 × 10^6 WBCs without secondary filtration. These technologies include fixed-particle-bed WBC separation (Spectra Turbo and Trima ACCEL, CaridianBCT, Lakewood, CO), and sophisticated software interface controls (AMICUS, Fenwal, Lake Zurich, IL). These low WBC levels challenge the accuracy and precision of current leukocyte-counting assays, leading to significant difficulties in process validation and the demonstration of process control. FDA guidelines recommend the testing of enough units to ensure, with 95% confidence, that 95% of units meet the 5 × 10^6 standard (in each container of a split product).[93] The principles of leukocyte counting and process control demonstration are discussed in detail by Dzik.[113] Of the more commonly used assays, automated techniques such as quantitative flow cytometry and volumetric capillary microfluorometry (IMAGN 2000, Biometric Imaging, a BD company, Mountain View, CA) outperform manual light microscopic enumeration using the Nageotte hemacytometer in accuracy and precision.[114]

Much has been published on sampling strategies to ensure consistent detection of intermittent process failures that occur as the result of leukocyte "spillover" from high donor WBC counts and operator or machine error.[115,116] Significant progress still remains to be made in the design of automated technologies invariably capable of producing highly leukocyte-reduced components. Because leukocyte-reduction failure rates can be up to 0.4%, some clinicians prefer CMV-negative, leukocyte-reduced components for their patients at risk for CMV to reduce the already low risk of CMV transmission from a leukocyte-reduced component.

Irradiation

Components containing viable lymphocytes (representing ~97% of WBCs in a leukocyte-reduced apheresis platelet unit) must be irradiated before transfusion to patients susceptible to GVHD.[117] Leukocyte reduction alone does not decrease the WBC content below the number necessary to cause GVHD. Unlike red cells, platelets tolerate irradiation at doses of approximately 25 Gy (15-50 Gy) administered as early as the day after collection; no significant effect on common platelet in-vitro parameters is detectable even after 7 days of storage.[118]

Volume Reduction and Platelet Washing

Apheresis platelets are concentrated approximately 6 times relative to the mean population value of 250,000/µL; consequently, further concentration is usually not necessary unless recipients are exquisitely volume sensitive (eg, critically ill neonates or for intrauterine platelet transfusions). Because relatively low volumes of platelets are required for these small recipients, WBD platelets may be preferred unless an institution can aliquot using a sterile connection device to avoid the 4-hour outdate of apheresis units entered by spiking. The AABB *Technical Manual* describes a procedure for volume reduction that, under certain conditions, has been reported to result in <15% loss of platelets and relatively preserved circulatory capacity.[119]

When recipients require removal of substances in the plasma (ie, proteins to which they are immunized or donor antibodies toward recipient antigens), platelet washing is preferred to volume reduction (maternal antibodies), or it is required (anti-IgA). Some institutions also wash platelets to remove ABO-incompatible plasma.[120] Washing, however, results not only in losses of 8% to 29% of a unit's platelet content but also in impaired circulation of the remaining platelets and possible impaired function of those that do circulate.[121-123] Apheresis platelets from appropriately matched donors [eg, IgA-deficient or human platelet antigen (HPA)-negative donors without HPA-specific antibodies] may thus be preferred to avoid the loss of content and potency and the resultant 4-hour outdate when washing is accomplished using an open system.

Red Cell Content

Although not a "modification" per se, the red cell content of apheresis platelet units may nevertheless be of clinical significance. Unlike WBD platelets, which may contain up to 0.5 mL of red cells per unit, apheresis platelets, by the nature of their collection, contain far fewer red cells. The few studies reporting mean red cell content of apheresis platelet units place it around 0.0002 to 0.005 mL per unit.[124-126] This is significantly below reported immunizing single doses of 0.03 mL and cumulative doses of 0.05 mL.[126] There are also reports that few Rh(D)-negative hematology/oncology patients transfused with Rh(D)-positive components form anti-D, even when transfused with WBD platelets. When Rh(D)-negative individuals must receive Rh(D)-positive platelets, anti-D immunoprophylaxis may be considered for children and women of child-bearing potential but foregone in others receiving apheresis platelets, especially immune-impaired patients. For immunocompetent patients, confirmatory measurements of low red cell content (ie, <0.03 mL) may justify not providing anti-D immunoprophylaxis in adult males or women without childbearing potential.

Conclusions

This chapter has reviewed many of the advances made in the preparation and storage of apheresis platelets over the past 50 years. This knowledge and technology are now widely available and have demonstrated clinical benefits. Ground rules for platelet storage are well developed, and guidelines concerning indications for transfusion and dose are emerging.

Much work remains to be done, however. A better understanding is needed of the pathophysiology of severe thrombocytopenia and the poor clinical responses of some patients to components that have been optimally prepared and stored. Many technical advances would also be welcome, including methods for assessing the functional capacity of components, simpler methods for storage, methods for reducing the risk of bacterial contamination, and standardization of platelet and residual leukocyte counting.

References

1. Jurk K, Kehrel BE. Platelets: Physiology and biochemistry. Semin Thromb Hemost 2005; 31:381-92.
2. Harker LA, Slichter SJ. The bleeding time as a screening test for evaluation of platelet function. N Engl J Med 1972;287:155-9.
3. Practice guidelines for perioperative blood transfusion and adjuvant therapies: An updated report by the American Society of Anesthesiologists Task Force on Perioperative Blood Transfusion and Adjuvant Therapies. Anesthesiology 2006;105:198-208.
4. British Committee for Standards in Haematology, Blood Transfusion Task Force. Guidelines for the use of platelet transfusions. Br J Haematol 2003;122:10-23.
5. Schiffer CA, Anderson KC, Bennett CL, et al. Platelet transfusion for patients with cancer: Clinical practice guidelines of the American Society of Clinical Oncology. J Clin Oncol 2001;19:1519-38.
6. Gaydos LA, Freireich EJ, Mantel N. The quantitative relation between platelet count and hemorrhage in patients with acute leukemia. N Engl J Med 1962;266:905-9.
7. Freireich EJ, Kliman A, Lawrence AG, et al. Response to repeated platelet transfusion from the same donor. Ann Intern Med 1963;59: 277-87.
8. Wandt H, Frank M, Ehninger G, et al. Safety and cost effectiveness of a $10 \times 10^9/L$ trigger for prophylactic platelet transfusions compared with the traditional $20 \times 10^9/L$ trigger: A prospective comparative trial in 195 patients with acute myeloid leukemia. Blood 1998;91: 3601-6.
9. Rebulla P, Finazzi G, Marangoni F, et al. The threshold for prophylactic platelet transfusions in adults with acute myeloid leukemia. N Engl J Med 1997;337:870-5.
10. Gil-Fernandez JJ, Alegre A, Fernandez-Villalta MJ, et al. Clinical results of a stringent policy on prophylactic platelet transfusion: Non-randomized comparative analysis in 190 bone marrow transplant patients from a single institution. Bone Marrow Transplant 1996;18:931-5.
11. Zumberg MS, del Rosario ML, Nejame CF, et al. A prospective randomized trial of prophylactic platelet transfusion and bleeding incidence in hematopoietic stem cell transplant recipients: 10,000/μL versus 20,000/μL trigger. Biol Blood Marrow Transplant 2002;8: 569-76.
12. Sagmeister M, Oec L, Gmür J. A restrictive platelet transfusion policy allowing long-term support of outpatients with severe aplastic anemia. Blood 1999;93:3124-6.
13. Kaushansky K. The molecular mechanisms that control thrombopoiesis. J Clin Invest 2005;115:3339-47.
14. Slichter SJ. Controversies in platelet transfusion therapy. Annu Rev Med 1980;31:509-40.
15. Hanson SR, Slichter SJ. Platelet kinetics in patients with bone marrow hypoplasia: Evidence for a fixed platelet requirement. Blood 1985;66:1105-9.
16. Benson K, Martinez S, Tolzmann L, Leparc G. Split vs whole apheresis platelets: Clinical response in thrombocytopenic patients (abstract). Transfusion 1996;36(Suppl):4S.
17. Norol F, Bierling P, Roudot-Thoraval F, et al. Platelet transfusion: A dose-response study. Blood 1998;92:1448-53.
18. Klumpp TR, Herman JH, Gaughan JP, et al. Clinical consequences of alterations in platelet transfusion dose: A prospective, randomized, double-blind trial. Transfusion 1999;39:674-81.

19. Slichter SJ, Kaufman RM, Assmann SF, et al. Effects of prophylactic platelet (Plt) dose on transfusion (Tx) outcomes (PLADO Trial) (abstract). Blood 2008;112:285.
20. Ackerman SJ, Klumpp TR, Guzman GI, et al. Economic consequences of alterations in platelet transfusion dose: Analysis of a prospective, randomized, double-blind trial. Transfusion 2000;40:1457-62.
21. Hersh JK, Hom EG, Brecher ME. Mathematical modeling of platelet survival with implications for optimal transfusion practice in the chronically platelet-transfusion-dependent patient. Transfusion 1998;38:637-44.
22. Blajchman MA, Slichter SJ, Heddle NM, Murphy MF. New strategies for the optimal use of platelet transfusions. Hematology Am Soc Hematol Educ Program 2008;198-204.
23. Bessman JD, Levin J. The inverse relation between platelet volume and platelet number. J Lab Clin Med 1983;101:295-307.
24. Thompson CB, Jakubowski JA. The pathophysiology and clinical relevance of platelet heterogeneity. Blood 1988;72:1-8.
25. Jandl JH, Aster RH. Increased splenic pooling and the pathogenesis of hypersplenism. Am J Med Sci 1967;253:383-97.
26. Wadenvik H, Kutti J. The spleen and pooling of blood cells. Eur J Hematol 1988;41:1-5.
27. Wadenvik H, Denfors I, Kutti J. Splenic blood flow and intrasplenic platelet kinetics in relation to spleen volume. Br J Haematol 1987;67:181-5.
28. Chamberlain KG, Tong M, Penington DG. Properties of the exchangeable splenic platelets released into the circulation during exercise-induced thrombocytosis. Am J Hematol 1990;34:161-8.
29. Peters AM, Lavender JP. Factors controlling the intrasplenic transit of platelets. Eur J Clin Invest 1982;12:191-5.
30. Kuter DJ, Goodnough LT, Romo J, et al. Thrombopoietin therapy increases platelet yields in healthy platelet donors. Blood 2001;98:1339-45.
31. Goodnough LT, Kuter DJ, McCullough J, et al. Prophylactic platelet transfusions from healthy apheresis platelet donors undergoing treatment with thrombopoietin. Blood 2001;98:1346-51.
32. Li J, Yang C, Xia Y, et al. Thrombocytopenia caused by the development of antibodies to thrombopoietin. Blood 2001;98:3241-8.

33. Bishop JF, McGrath K, Wolf MM, et al. Clinical factors influencing the efficacy of pooled platelet transfusions. Blood 1988;71:383-7.
34. Klumpp TR, Herman JH, Innis S, et al. Factors associated with response to platelet transfusion following hematopoietic stem cell transplantation. Bone Marrow Transplant 1996;17:1035-41.
35. Daly PA, Schiffer CA, Aisner J, Wiernik PH. Platelet transfusion therapy. One hour post-transfusion increments are valuable in predicting the need for HLA-matched preparations. JAMA 1980;243:435-8.
36. Dodd RY. Current risk for transfusion transmitted infections. Curr Opin Hematol 2007;14:671-6.
37. Stramer SL. Current risks of transfusion-transmitted agents: A review. Arch Pathol Lab Med 2007;131:702-7.
38. Vassallo RR Jr, Wahab F, Giordano K, Murphy S. Improving technology for collecting platelets by apheresis: Five-year experience in one blood center. Transfus Med Rev 2004;18:257-66.
39. Arnold DM, Heddle NM, Kulczycki M, et al. In vivo recovery and survival of apheresis and whole blood-derived platelets: A paired comparison in healthy volunteers. Transfusion 2006;46:257-64.
40. Cardigan R, Williamson LM. The quality of platelets after storage for 7 days. Transfus Med 2003;13:173-87.
41. Dumont LJ, AuBuchon JP, Whitley P, et al. Seven-day storage of single-donor platelets: Recovery and survival in an autologous transfusion study. Transfusion 2002;42:847-54.
42. Shanwell A, Larsson S, Aschan J, et al. A randomized trial comparing the use of fresh and stored platelets in the treatment of bone marrow transplant recipients. Eur J Haematol 1992;49:77-81.
43. Sweeney JD, Holme S, Moroff G. Storage of apheresis platelets after gamma radiation. Transfusion 1994;34:779-83.
44. Murphy S, Gardner FH. Platelet preservation. Effect of storage temperature on maintenance of platelet viability—deleterious effect of refrigerated storage. N Engl J Med 1969;280:1094-8.
45. Filip DJ, Aster RH. Relative hemostatic effectiveness of human platelets stored at 4 C and 22 C. J Lab Clin Med 1978;91:618-24.
46. Slichter SJ, Harker LA. Preparation and storage of platelet concentrates, II: Storage variables

influencing platelet viability and function. Br J Haematol 1976;34:403-19.

47. Holme S, Sawyer S, Heaton A, Sweeney JD. Studies on platelets exposed to or stored at temperatures below 20 C or above 24 C. Transfusion 1997;37:5-11.

48. Lopez JA, DelConde I, Shrimpton CN. Receptors, rafts and microvesicles in thrombosis and inflammation. J Thromb Haemost 2005;3:1737-44.

49. Hoffmeister KM, Falet H, Toker A, et al. Mechanisms of cold-induced platelet actin assembly. J Biol Chem 2001;276:24751-9.

50. Rumjantseva V, Hoffmeister KM. Novel and unexpected clearance mechanisms for cold platelets. Transfus Apher Sci 2009;42:63-70.

51. Kaufman RM. Uncommon cold: Could 4 C storage improve platelet function? Transfusion 2005;45:1407-12.

52. Holme S, Heaton A. In vitro platelet aging at 22 C is reduced compared to in vivo aging at 37 C. Br J Haematol 1995;91:212-18.

53. Kilkson H, Holme S, Murphy S. Platelet metabolism during storage of platelet concentrates at 22 C. Blood 1984;64:406-14.

54. Cesar J, DeMinno G, Alam I, et al. Plasma free fatty acid metabolism during storage of platelet concentrates for transfusion. Transfusion 1987;27:434-7.

55. Murphy S, Gardner FH. Platelet storage at 22 C; metabolic, morphologic, and functional studies. J Clin Invest 1971;50:370-7.

56. Holme S, Murphy S. Quantitative measurements of platelet shape by light transmission studies: Application to storage of platelets for transfusion. J Lab Clin Med 1978;92:53-64.

57. Murphy S. Platelet storage for transfusion. Semin Hematol 1985;22:165-77.

58. Price TH, ed. Standards for blood banks and transfusion services. 26th ed. Bethesda, MD: AABB, 2009.

59. Murphy S, Gardner FH. Platelet storage at 22 C: Role of gas transport across plastic containers in maintenance of viability. Blood 1975;46:209-18.

60. Hunter S, Nixon J, Murphy S. The effect of interruption of agitation on platelet quality during storage for transportation. Transfusion 2001;41:809-14.

61. Holme S, Vaidja K, Murphy S. Platelet storage at 22 C: Effect of type of agitation on morphology, viability, and function in vitro. Blood 1978;52:425-35.

62. Snyder EL, Pope C, Ferri PM, et al. The effect of mode of agitation and type of plastic bag on storage characteristics and in vivo kinetics of platelet concentrates. Transfusion 1986;26:125-30.

63. Moroff G, George VM. The maintenance of platelet properties upon limited discontinuation of agitation during storage. Transfusion 1990;30:427-30.

64. Wagner SJ, Vassallo R, Skripchenko A, et al. Comparison of the in vitro properties of apheresis platelets during 7-day storage after interrupting agitation for one or three periods. Transfusion 2008;48:2492-500.

65. Wagner SJ, Vassallo R, Skripchenko A, et al. The influence of simulated shipping conditions (24- or 30-hour interruption of agitation) on the in vitro properties of apheresis platelets during 7-day storage. Transfusion 2008;48:1072-80.

66. Wallvik J, Stenke L, Akerblom O. The effect of different agitation modes on platelet metabolism, thromboxane formation, and alpha-granular release during platelet storage. Transfusion 1990;30:639-43.

67. Mitchell SG, Hawker RJ, Turner VS, et al. Effect of agitation on the quality of platelet concentrates. Vox Sang 1994;67:160-5.

68. Murphy S. pH failure, filter clogging, and lack of clinical efficacy in apheresis platelets (AP). Role of inadequate oxygen supply and accelerated lactic acid production in AP with high platelet content. Vox Sang 1996;70(Suppl 2):145.

69. Food and Drug Administration. Memorandum to all registered blood establishments: Reduction of the maximum platelet storage period to 5 days in an approved container. (June 2, 1986) Rockville, MD: Office of Biologics Research and Review, 1986.

70. Kleinman S, Dumont LJ, Tomasulo P, et al. The impact of discontinuation of 7-day storage of apheresis platelets (PASSPORT) on recipient safety: An illustration of the need for proper risk assessments. Transfusion 2009;49:903-12.

71. Eder AF, Kennedy JM, Dy BA, et al. Bacterial screening of apheresis platelets and the residual risk of septic transfusion reactions: The American Red Cross experience (2004-2006). Transfusion 2007;47:1134-42.

72. AuBuchon JP, Taylor H, Holme S, Nelson E. In vitro and in vivo evaluation of leukoreduced

platelets stored for 7 days in CLX containers. Transfusion 2005;45:356-61.

73. Simon TL, Nelson EJ, Murphy S. Extension of platelet concentrate storage to 7 days in second-generation bags. Transfusion 1987;27:6-9.

74. Holme S, Heaton WAL, Whitley P. Platelet storage lesions in second-generation containers: Correlation with in vivo behavior with storage up to 14 days. Vox Sang 1990;59:12-18.

75. Holme S, Bode A, Heaton WAL, Sawyer S. Improved maintenance of platelet in vivo viability during storage when using a synthetic medium with inhibitors. J Lab Clin Med 1992; 119:144-50.

76. Goodrich RP, Gilmour D, Hovenga N, Keil SD. A laboratory comparison of pathogen reduction technology treatment and culture of platelet products for addressing bacterial contamination concerns. Transfusion 2009;49:1205-16.

77. Pietersz RN, Englefriet CP, Reesink HW, et al. Detection of bacterial contamination of platelet concentrates. Vox Sang 2007;93:260-77.

78. McCullough J. Pathogen inactivation: A new paradigm for blood safety. Transfusion 2007; 47:2180-4.

79. Benjamin RJ, Wagner SJ. The residual risk of sepsis: Modeling the effect of concentration on bacterial detection in two-bottle culture systems and an estimation of false-negative culture rates. Transfusion 2007;47:1381-9.

80. Hay SN, Immel CC, McClannan LS, Brecher ME. The introduction of 7-day platelets: A university hospital experience. J Clin Apher 2007; 22:283-6.

81. Ringwald J, Zimmermann R, Eckstein R. The new generation of platelet additive solution for storage at 22 degrees C: Development and current experience. Transfus Med Rev 2006; 20:158-64.

82. Gulliksen H. Platelet additive solutions: Current status. Immunohematology 2007;23:14-19.

83. Sweeney J. Additive solutions for platelets: Is it time for North America to go with the flow? Transfusion 2009;49:199-201.

84. Gulliksen H. Defining the optimal storage conditions for the long-term storage of platelets. Transfus Med Rev 2003;17:209-15.

85. Holme S, Bode A, Heaton WA, et al. Improved maintenance of platelet in vivo viability during storage when using a synthetic medium with inhibitors. J Lab Clin Med 1992;119:144-50.

86. Lozano ML, Rivera J, Bermejo E, et al. In vitro analysis of platelet concentrates stored in the presence of modulators of 3′,5′ adenosine monophosphate, and organic anions. Transfus Sci 2000;22:3-11.

87. Rivera J, Lozano ML, Corral J, et al. Quality assessment of platelet concentrates supplemented with second-messenger effectors. Transfusion 1999;39:135-43.

88. Dijkstra-Tiekstra MJ, Kuipers W, Setroikromo AC, de Wildt-Eggen J. Platelet counting in platelet concentrates with various automated hematology analysers. Transfusion 2007;47:1651-7.

89. Moroff G, Sowemimo-Coker SO, Finch S, et al. The influence of various hematology analyzers on component platelet counts. Transfus Med Rev 2005;19:155-66.

90. Van der Meer PF, Dijkstra-Tiekstra MJ, Mahon A, de Wildt-Eggen J. Counting platelets in platelet concentrates on hematology analyzers: A multicenter comparative study. Transfusion 2009;49:81-90.

91. Dickerhoff R, von Ruecker A. Enumeration of platelets by multiparameter flow cytometry using platelet-specific antibodies and fluorescent reference particles. Clin Lab Haematol 1995;17:163-72.

92. Johannesson B, Haugen T, Scott CS. Standardisation of platelet counting accuracy in blood banks by reference to an automated immunoplatelet procedure: Comparative evaluation of Cell-Dyn CD4000 impedance and optical platelet counts. Transfus Apher Sci 2001;25:93-106.

93. Food and Drug Administration. Guidance for industry and FDA review staff: Collection of platelets by automated methods. (December 17, 2007) Rockville, MD: CBER Office of Communication, Training, and Manufacturers Assistance, 2007.

94. Vostal JG. Efficacy evaluation of current and future platelet transfusion products. J Trauma 2006;60:S78-S82.

95. Hirsch EO, Gardner FH. The transfusion of human blood platelets. With a note on the transfusion of granulocytes. J Lab Clin Med 1952;39:556-69.

96. Murphy S. The case for a new approach for documenting platelet viability. Transfusion 2006;46:49S-52S.

97. Taylor HL, Whitley P, Heaton A. A historical perspective on platelet radiolabeling technique. Transfusion 2006;46:53S-58S.

98. Biomedical Excellence for Safer Transfusion (BEST) Working Party of the International Society of Blood Transfusion (ISBT). Platelet radiolabeling procedure. Transfusion 2006; 46:59S-66S.

99. Murphy S, Rebulla P, Bertolini F, et al. In vitro assessment of the quality of stored platelet concentrates. Transfus Med Rev 1994;8:29-36.

100. Holme S, Moroff G, Murphy S. A multi-laboratory evaluation of in vitro platelet assays: The tests for extent of shape change and response to hypotonic shock. Biomedical Excellence for Safer Transfusion Working Party of the International Society of Blood Transfusion. Transfusion 1998;38:31-40.

101. Bertolini F, Murphy S. A multicenter evaluation of reproducibility of swirling in platelet concentrates. Transfusion 1994;34:796-801.

102. Owens M, Holme S, Heaton A, et al. Post-transfusion recovery of function of 5-day stored platelet concentrates. Br J Haematol 1992;80:539-44.

103. Rinder HM, Ault KA. Platelet activation and its detection during the preparation of platelets for transfusion. Transfus Med Rev 1998;12: 271-87.

104. Murphy S, Kahn RA, Holmes S, et al. Improved storage of platelets for transfusion in a new container. Blood 1982;60:194-200.

105. Simon TL, Nelson EJ, Carmen R, Murphy S. Extension of platelet concentrate storage. Transfusion 1983;23:207-12.

106. Bertolini F, Rebulla P, Riccardi M. Evaluation of platelet concentrates prepared from buffy coats and stored in glucose-free crystalloid medium. Transfusion 1989;29:605-9.

107. McCullough J, Vesole DH, Benjamin RJ, et al. Therapeutic efficacy and safety of platelets treated with a photochemical process for pathogen inactivation: The SPRINT trial. Blood 2004;104:1534-41.

108. Norol F, Kuentz M, Cordonnier C, et al. Influence of clinical status on the efficiency of stored platelet transfusion. Br J Haematol 1994;86:125-9.

109. Vamvakas EC, Blajchman MA. Universal WBC reduction: The case for and against. Transfusion 2001;41:691-712.

110. Bowden RA, Slichter SJ, Sayers M, et al. A comparison of filtered leukocyte-reduced and cytomegalovirus (CMV) seronegative blood products for the prevention of transfusion-associated CMV infection after marrow transplant. Blood 1995;86:3598-603.

111. The Trial to Reduce Alloimmunization to Platelets Study Group. Leukocyte reduction and ultraviolet B irradiation of platelets to prevent alloimmunization and refractoriness to platelet transfusions. N Engl J Med 1997;337: 1861-9.

112. Council of Europe. Guide to the preparation, use and quality assurance of blood components. 14th ed. Strasbourg, France: Council of Europe Press, 2008.

113. Dzik WH. Leukocyte counting during process control of leukoreduced blood components. Vox Sang 2000;78(Suppl 2):223-6.

114. Dzik S, Moroff G, Dumont LJ. A multicenter study evaluating three methods for counting residual WBCs in WBC-reduced blood components: Nageotte hemocytometry, flow cytometry, and microfluorometry. Transfusion 2000; 40:513-20.

115. Dumont LJ, Dzik WH, Rebulla P, Brandwein H. Practical guidelines for process validation and process control of white cell-reduced blood components: Report of the Biomedical Excellence for Safer Transfusion (BEST) Working Party of the International Society of Blood Transfusion (ISBT). Transfusion 1996;36:11-20.

116. Adams MR, Fisher DM, Dumont LJ, et al. Detecting failed WBC-reduction processes: Computer simulations of intermittent and continuous process failure. Transfusion 2000;40: 1427-33.

117. Garritsen HS, Sibrowski W. Flow cytometric determination of leukocytes and lymphocyte subsets in thrombocytapheresis products. Beitr Infusionsther Transfusionsmed 1994;32:401-4.

118. Van der Meer PF, Pietersz RNI. Gamma irradiation does not affect 7-day storage of platelet concentrates. Vox Sang 2005;89:97-9.

119. Method 6-14. Removing plasma from platelets (volume reduction). In: Roback JD, Combs MR, Grossman BJ, Hillyer CD, eds. Technical manual. 16th ed. Bethesda, MD: AABB, 2008: 960-1.

120. Heal JM, Blumberg N. Optimizing platelet transfusion therapy. Blood Rev 2004;18:149-65.

121. Kalmin ND, Brown DJ. Platelet washing with a blood cell processor. Transfusion 1982;22: 125-7.

122. Vo TD, Cowles J, Heal JM, Blumberg N. Platelet washing to prevent recurrent febrile reactions to leukocyte-reduced transfusions. Transfus Med 2001;11:45-7.

123. Pineda AA, Zylstra VW, Clare DE, et al. Viability and functional integrity of washed platelets. Transfusion 1989;29:524-7.

124. Heim MU, Bock M, Kolb HJ, et al. Intravenous anti-D gammaglobulin for the prevention of Rhesus isoimmunization caused by platelet transfusion in patients with malignant diseases. Vox Sang 1992;62:165-8.

125. Atoyebi W, Mundy N, Croxton T, et al. Is it necessary to administer anti-D to prevent RhD immunization after the transfusion of RhD-positive platelet concentrates? Br J Haematol 2000; 111:980-3.

126. Lozano M, Cid J. The clinical implications of platelet transfusions associated with ABO or Rh(D) incompatibility. Transfus Med Rev 2003; 17:57-68.

In: McLeod BC, Szczepiorkowski ZM, Weinstein R, Winters JL, eds.
Apheresis: Principles and Practice, 3rd edition
Bethesda, MD: AABB Press, 2010

8

Provision of Apheresis Platelet Transfusions: Patient and Producer Perspectives

Thomas H. Price, MD

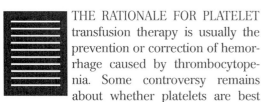 THE RATIONALE FOR PLATELET transfusion therapy is usually the prevention or correction of hemorrhage caused by thrombocytopenia. Some controversy remains about whether platelets are best given prophylactically[1] or therapeutically[2]; nevertheless, the overall efficacy of platelet transfusion is well established and universally accepted. The optimal "transfusion trigger" platelet counts for various clinical conditions are considered in Chapter 7. Most other aspects of the day-to-day management of thrombocytopenic patients are outside the scope of this volume, although excellent discussions of that topic have recently been published elsewhere.[3-5] This chapter considers apheresis platelets, focusing on their distinctive features as seen from the perspectives of both producers and recipients of platelet transfusions.

Usage Trends

The use of platelet transfusion in the United States has grown substantially over the last 20 years as medical therapy has become more complex. Increases in hematopoietic progenitor cell transplantation, intensive chemotherapy for malignancy, complicated cardiovascular surgical procedures, and aggressive care of trauma victims have all contributed to this growth. As shown in Table 8-1, red cell demand between 1987 and 2006, the last year for which figures

Thomas H. Price, MD, Executive Vice-President and Medical Director, Puget Sound Blood Center, and Professor of Medicine, University of Washington, Seattle, Washington

The author has disclosed no conflicts of interest.

Table 8-1. Units Transfused in the United States (Thousands)*

	1987	1989	1992	1994	1997	1999	2001	2004	2006
Allogeneic whole blood/red cells	11,612	11,703	10,704	10,625	11,099	12,022	13,539	14,830	15,840
Whole-blood-derived platelets	4,855	5,146	4,688	3,582	3,397	3,036	2,614	1,537	1,296
Apheresis platelets[†]	1,572	2,112	3,642	4,284	5,640	6,018	7,582	8,338	9,092
Total platelets[†]	6,427	7,258	8,330	7,866	9,037	9,054	10,196	9,875	10,388
Apheresis platelets (% of total)	24	29	44	54	62	66	74	84	88

*Data from Wallace et al,[6-8] Sullivan et al,[9-11] and the Department of Health and Human Services et al.[12]
†Whole-blood-derived platelet equivalents, considering 1 apheresis platelet unit as equivalent to 6 whole-blood-derived platelet units, divided units included.

are available, was relatively constant for 10 to 12 years, then increased more sharply, for an overall increase of about 36%.[6-12] Overall platelet use increased approximately 62% between 1987 and 2006. During this same period, the fraction of platelets obtained by apheresis increased from 24% to 88%. The platelet equivalent values in Table 8-1 should be considered only as an approximation because they are based on the assumption that a unit of apheresis platelets contains the same number of platelets as 6 units of whole-blood-derived (WBD) platelets. Whether or not this is true depends on what values are used to represent a standard WBD platelet concentrate, the details of the apheresis collection procedure, and the fraction of divided units produced. Figure 8-1 shows component production data for the Puget Sound Blood Center in Seattle, WA. The total number of platelets produced increased dramatically in the early years but has remained relatively constant for the last 15 years. The number of apheresis platelet units collected increased from 1988 to 1992 as platelet demand increased, then decreased over the next few years as overall demand decreased and as efforts at cost containment shifted the mix toward WBD platelets. Since

1996, there has been a constant increase in both the number of apheresis platelet units provided as well as the proportion of platelets collected by this method. Over the 20-year time span, the fraction of platelets collected as apheresis platelets has increased from approximately 30% to 65%.

There are several reasons for the increasing preferential use of apheresis platelets over the last 10 to 15 years. In many locations, platelet inventory needs cannot be met by increasing the production of WBD platelets, requiring an increased reliance on apheresis techniques. This was the case in Seattle before 1999. In addition, the demand for apheresis platelets has increased in many areas as clinicians have concluded that these products might offer medical advantages to their patients. These perceived advantages, discussed in more detail below, include reduced donor exposures and possible beneficial effects on rates of adverse transfusion reactions. Finally, whether driven by demand or not, many collection facilities have increased production of apheresis platelets— some provide only apheresis platelets—because of the same perceived advantages as well as for reasons of productivity and efficiency.

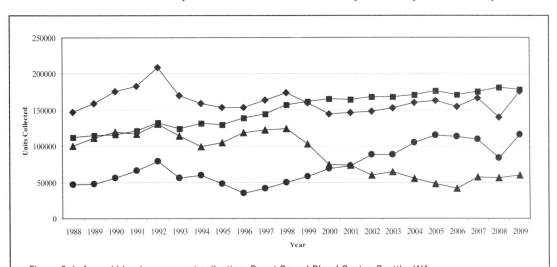

Figure 8-1. Annual blood component collection, Puget Sound Blood Center, Seattle, WA.
■ = whole blood; ◆ = total platelets; ▲ = whole-blood-derived platelets; ● = apheresis platelets. Total platelets and apheresis platelets are expressed as whole-blood-derived platelet equivalents, considering 1 apheresis platelet unit as equivalent to 6 whole-blood-derived platelet units.

Characteristics of Apheresis and Pooled Platelets

Donors

Platelet donors and whole blood donors together make up the majority of volunteer community blood donors. In most institutions, these two groups of donors are not mutually exclusive; that is, on different occasions, individuals may donate either whole blood or platelets. However, platelet donors are much less likely to be first-time donors, and they tend to give more often than the average whole blood donor.

Units of whole blood are not usually selected for platelet preparation because of any particular characteristic of the donor. For example, there is no attempt to select blood from frequent donors or donors with high platelet counts. By contrast, these sorts of selections are often made with plateletpheresis donors—sometimes actively and sometimes because the donors available for apheresis are already frequent donors. The donor's platelet count before donation is determined for all plateletpheresis procedures, although the results are often not available until after the collection. Even if acceptable in terms of regulatory limits, facilities may elect to discourage donors with lower platelet counts, who would likely donate a low-yield product, and recruit those with higher counts for more frequent donation. Donors with higher counts are particularly valuable in that one is more likely to collect a concentrate that can be divided into more than one platelet transfusion dose. Thus, it is possible to build quality-enhancing mechanisms into plateletpheresis donation programs that are not feasible when platelet concentrates are prepared from whole blood.

Both plateletpheresis and whole blood donors must pass the same basic screening criteria as determined by the US Food and Drug Administration (FDA)[13] and the AABB.[14] Plateletpheresis donors must refrain from ingesting irreversible inhibitors of platelet function (eg, aspirin or aspirin-containing com-

pounds) for suitable periods of time before donation (48 hours for aspirin).

Matched-platelet donors are those whose platelets lack HLA or platelet-specific antigens to which the intended recipient has or may become alloimmunized. They may be community donors or members of the patient's family. Although basic screening criteria for matched donors are the same as those for unmatched donors, situations may arise in which it is medically justified to collect and transfuse platelets from matched donors who do not meet all the usual criteria. Such donations may be accepted only if written justification and approval are provided by a physician and if no suitable alternative donors are available at the time to meet the patient's medical needs. If the criterion in question is one intended for the protection of the donor (eg, the donor has a hematocrit of 36% instead of $\geq 38\%$), the justification and approval must be provided by the apheresis physician. If the criterion in question is intended to protect the patient (eg, the donor has recently travelled to a malaria risk area), the justification and approval must be provided by the patient's physician.

Dedicated plateletpheresis donors are those who give platelets repeatedly for the same recipient. They may also be matched donors. For these donors, the FDA requires that infectious disease testing be performed only every 30 days once the first transfusion has been administered.[13]

Whole-Blood-Derived Platelets

In the United States, platelet concentrates are separated from whole blood by first preparing platelet-rich plasma (PRP) and then concentrating the platelets with a second centrifugation. In Europe, the buffy coat technique is most prevalent; the buffy coat is isolated from whole blood by a hard spin and resuspended, after which platelets are separated by a second, softer centrifugation. Mean platelet yields from the two techniques are approximately the same, and there are no differences in the quality of these products.[15] The yield in an individual platelet concentrate depends on the platelet count of the donor, a value that has quite a wide normal distribution. It is also highly dependent on proper technique. However, variations tend to even out when the transfusion product is a pool of 4 to 8 platelet concentrates. In the United States, FDA requirements are that the platelet content be at least 0.55×10^{11} per unit in 75% of the units tested.[16] It is important to keep in mind that this value has no particular significance in terms of the clinical goals for platelet transfusions; it is merely useful to indicate whether the preparation techniques are adequate. At the Puget Sound Blood Center, the mean number of platelets contained in a unit of WBD platelets is currently 0.86×10^{11}.

Apheresis Platelets

There is also wide variation in the number of platelets obtained from plateletpheresis donations. Variability may stem from differences in apheresis instruments used, in donor platelet counts, and/or in collection parameters us discussed in Chapters 4 and 7. Because the traditional transfusion dose for an adult patient was 6 units of pooled platelets, many institutions originally adopted plateletpheresis collection parameters that, on average, yielded the equivalent number of platelets—namely, 4.5 to 5.0 $\times$ 10^{11}. In the past, when there was no way to directly predict the final platelet yield, procedure endpoints were specified in terms of the collection time, the volume of blood processed, or the number of batches processed; the parameters chosen were those likely to result in the desired yields. More modern apheresis instruments display a predicted yield based on the donor's size, platelet count, and hematocrit. This information allows the operator or the facility to customize run parameters so that the desired yield is more likely to be achieved for each donor.

The most recent FDA guidelines require that apheresis platelet concentrates contain at least 3×10^{11} platelets.[13] AABB standards require that 90% of concentrates meet the same quantitative standard.[14] This value of 3×10^{11} platelets was established many years

ago as a process control indicator and was never meant to imply a medical determination that 3×10^{11} platelets represented a standard or minimum transfusion dose. Nevertheless, over the years, the value of 3×10^{11} has become more and more often interpreted as the minimum acceptable transfusion dose, even though this concept has no biologic basis. As discussed in Chapter 7, the appropriate dose of platelets depends on a number of clinical factors, including the patient's underlying condition, the patient's size and platelet count, whether the patient is bleeding, and the patient's expected response to a given transfusion dose. A knowledgeable ordering physician will take these factors into account in determining the optimal platelet product for a patient. The recently completed randomized controlled trial on platelet dosing in patients being transfused prophylactically demonstrated that doses as low as $1.1 \times 10^{11}/m^2$ (approximately 2×10^{11} platelets in an average-size adult) were just as effective hemostatically as doses of $4.4 \times 10^{11}/m^2$.[17]

By extending collection times and/or selecting donors with high platelet counts, collection facilities can use the predictive yield features of modern apheresis instruments to achieve yields large enough to divide the collected component into two or three transfusion doses, each containing enough platelets to meet the 3×10^{11} standard. The fraction of platelet collections that can be divided in this manner can be as high as 60% to 80%, depending on the particular strategies used as well as on the platelet yields that are considered acceptable for clinical use. From the producer's point of view, there are two advantages to this approach. First, more platelet concentrates can be obtained from a given number of apheresis donors, making more efficient use of the donors and making additional transfusion doses available for the community. Second, the cost of production per transfusion dose is reduced because two or more units can be prepared for little more than the cost usually associated with one.

The practice of dividing collected platelets, which is usually based on considerations of inventory management and revenue for producers, is not so obviously advantageous to patients or to physicians ordering platelets. Patients receiving the split units are, on average, being given fewer platelets for the same price. If there is a mix of units that have and have not been split, uncertainty about the dose delivered rises substantially. The difference between the lower- and higher-dose apheresis platelet units is generally obscured because both are marketed as apheresis platelet units with little emphasis on the actual platelet content. Therefore, clinicians may not be aware of the variation in platelet content and may assume incorrectly that one apheresis platelet unit is equivalent to any other. In addition, in most collection facilities, the fees for "split" platelet concentrates are identical to those charged for components that have not been split.

Platelet Dose from a Quality Perspective

One measure of quality in a product, whether it be a blood component, an aspirin tablet, or a chocolate bar, is the predictability and consistency of the content. From this perspective, the variability commonly seen in apheresis platelet content (3.0 to 6.0 × 10^{11} cells) is disappointing. As indicated above, dose is an important aspect of appropriate platelet transfusion therapy. This is reflected in the ordering of pooled platelets when clinicians specify the number of units of platelets to be pooled. Although tailoring apheresis platelet collection to individual recipient dose needs would be ideal and might even be possible in certain settings, it is not practical for the most part. Another approach would be for collection facilities to generate different apheresis platelet products with different specified dose ranges or, alternatively, to label the platelet concentrates with the actual platelet content. The charge for these components would ideally be proportional to the actual platelet content. Clinicians could then assess the patient's needs and specifically order the appropriate number of platelet units for transfusion. Although it may be preferable from a quality point of view, such a system would be more complicated to manage for the collection

facility, it would require clinicians to be familiar with the actual number of platelets needed by their patients, and it would require the FDA to recognize that the appropriate dose for many patients is less than 3.0 × 10^{11} platelets. A system of two different doses of apheresis platelets as described above was in place for several years at the Puget Sound Blood Center but ultimately failed because of these issues.

Leukocyte Content

As outlined in Chapter 4, the leukocyte content of apheresis platelet units depends on the apheresis instrument used. Modern instruments are capable of reliably producing apheresis platelet units containing <10^6 leukocytes, either directly off the machine or after subsequent in-line filtration, easily meeting current regulatory requirements for leukocyte reduction (<5 × 10^6).[18] The leukocyte content of platelet units made from whole blood also depends on the method used. Platelet concentrates made from PRP commonly contain 1.0 to 1.5 × 10^8 leukocytes.[15] Thus, for a dose of platelets equivalent to that obtained in an apheresis component (4 to 6 units), the patient would receive approximately 4 to 9 × 10^8 leukocytes. Single-unit leukocyte content is on the order of 10^7 cells in platelet concentrates prepared with the use of the buffy coat technique common in Europe.[15] Filtration of any of these components with third-generation leukocyte-reduction filters results in a component containing fewer than 5 × 10^6 leukocytes.

Advantages and Disadvantages of Apheresis Platelets

There is little evidence to suggest any substantive difference between apheresis platelets and WBD platelets in terms of transfusion efficacy. Direct comparisons have shown posttransfusion platelet corrected-count increments or postinfusion recovery and survival to be equivalent or modestly (20%-30%) better with apheresis platelets.[19-21] The magnitude of the storage defect through 5 days has been shown to be the same with both types of platelet components.[19,20] There are other considerations or clinical conditions, however, for which there may be an advantage of one type over the other,[22,23] some of which are discussed below.

Provision of Components from Selected Donors

Apheresis techniques are required when one must obtain adequate doses of platelets from selected donors. The most common reason to do this is to provide HLA-selected platelets to alloimmunized patients, as discussed in Chapter 9. Additional reasons include the collection of maternal platelets for newborns with neonatal alloimmune thrombocytopenia or the use of IgA-deficient donors for patients with anti-IgA.

Disease Transmission

In spite of rigorous donor screening criteria and the battery of infectious disease tests currently performed on each whole blood or plateletpheresis donor, transfusion is still associated with a small residual risk of infectious disease transmission. This risk is attributable to false-negative results in the screening procedures, window-period donations, and the prevalence of infectious diseases for which no screening is performed. Studies of Glynn et al have suggested that the prevalence of viral infection is 50% higher in whole blood donors than in apheresis donors,[24] implying that apheresis donors are intrinsically safer. Apart from this possibility, apheresis platelet units pose less risk to recipients than do pooled platelets because fewer donors are involved. Although the risk of exposure to infectious agents is not strictly linearly proportional to the number of donor exposures, it is nearly so when the risk per donor is extremely low (eg, <1%).[25] Thus, for most infections of concern (eg, hepatitis, human immunodeficiency virus), the risk of transmission with 1 apheresis platelet unit is one-sixth of that with 6 units of pooled platelets. This relationship is true no matter how much the safety of the blood supply improves. For example, in 2009 the risk of hepatitis C virus transmission with 6 units of WBD platelets was estimated to be approximately 1:300,000, whereas the risk for the same number of platelets given as 1 apheresis platelet unit was estimated to be 1:1,800,000.[26]

As discussed in Chapter 10, with modern viral marker technology, the highest risk of infection transmission by platelets is from bacterial contamination. Most studies have shown that this risk is five to six times higher with pooled platelet concentrates than it is with apheresis units,[27,28] presumably because of the multiple donors, venipunctures, and laboratory manipulations associated with the production of pooled platelet components. Over the last several years, these differences in risk were magnified as collection facilities instituted bacterial culturing methods to detect contaminating bacteria in apheresis platelets. More recently, the bacterial contamination risk for both components has been reduced approximately 50% with the use of diversion techniques to discard the first 30 to 50 mL of blood drawn from the donor. In addition, systems for bacteria detection in pooled WBD platelets have become available. Current estimates for the risk of bacterial contamination if diversion techniques and culture-based detection systems are used is 1:60,000 for apheresis platelets and 1:12000 for pooled WBD platelets.[29]

Alloimmunization

Platelet alloimmunization occurs in 30% to 70% of patients receiving chronic transfusion support[30] and may cause substantial difficulty in providing patients with platelet components that are clinically efficacious. Because there is some evidence that the likelihood of alloimmunization depends on the number of transfusions received, one of the strategies advocated for the prevention of alloimmunization has been to limit the number of donors to which the patient is exposed. Such a goal can be accomplished by transfusing less often or, alternatively, by providing apheresis platelets as the platelet component of choice. Although there are older studies to suggest that this strategy might be effective,[31-33] it was clearly shown by the Trial to Reduce Alloimmunization to Platelets (TRAP) that if all products are leukocyte reduced, the provision of apheresis platelets provides no advantage in terms of alloimmunization.[34]

Leukocyte Content

Leukocyte reduction of blood components is effective in the prevention of 1) febrile hemolytic transfusion reactions, 2) transmission of cytomegalovirus infection, and 3) platelet alloimmunization.[35-37] Whether the provision of leukocyte-reduced components is important to avoid the purported effects of transfusion-mediated immunomodulation, such as increased rates of postoperative infection and tumor recurrence, is highly controversial.[36,37] In the largest trial to date (2780 patients), there was no advantage in terms of mortality, length of stay, or total cost of hospitalization for patients randomly assigned to receive leukocyte-reduced blood components.[38] Neither PRP nor buffy coat platelet concentrates can be considered leukocyte reduced by the current standard ($<5 \times 10^6$ cells per container) as they are initially prepared. They must be filtered to qualify as leukocyte reduced, a process that may result in the loss of up to 15% of the platelets. Apheresis platelets collected using the modern apheresis techniques almost invariably contain fewer than 10^6 leukocytes and require no further manipulation to be labeled as leukocyte reduced, an advantage in terms of both platelet loss and, compared to platelets that must be leukocyte reduced at issue by the transfusion service, the speed with which the component can be issued to the patient.

Transfusion Reactions

Febrile nonhemolytic transfusion reactions have classically been attributed to the reaction of leukocyte antibodies in the recipient with donor leukocytes in the transfused platelets. Reactions caused by this mechanism generally occur only if the transfused component contains at least 5×10^8 leukocytes, and they can

essentially be eliminated by leukocyte reduction. Febrile transfusion reactions are still fairly common with the use of leukocyte-reduced platelet components, however, and recent studies have demonstrated that a large fraction of these are attributable to cytokines released by leukocytes during the period of room temperature storage.[39] These latter reactions can largely (but not totally) be prevented by prestorage leukocyte reduction, but the problem is not prevented by leukocyte reduction immediately before transfusion because the inflammatory cytokines are already present. Prestorage leukocyte reduction is almost always achieved with apheresis platelets collected using modern apheresis instruments. It is also achieved with prestorage pooling of whole blood platelets using collection and pooling systems recently approved by the FDA.

It is not clear that either type of platelet component is superior in the prevention of allergic transfusion reactions (usually caused by recipient antibody directed toward a donor plasma protein). The development of transfusion-related acute lung injury (TRALI), often attributable to antibodies in the donor plasma directed toward recipient leukocyte antigens, is usually associated with the transfusion of components containing relatively large amounts of plasma and might be expected to be more likely in apheresis platelets. On the other hand, the likelihood of encountering an incompatible donor will be several times higher in WBD platelets. The limited data available to date does not suggest a difference in TRALI risk between apheresis platelets and pooled WBD platelets.[29] In the future, the risk will likely be reduced for apheresis platelets to the extent that these components are collected from male donors or from female donors at reduced risk for the presence of HLA antibodies.

Inventory Management

Optimal management of platelet inventory can be complicated for a number of reasons. First, platelet demand may change dramatically from day to day, and the maximum storage period is only 5 days, not long enough to dampen the effect of these daily fluctuations on the overall inventory. The situation is further complicated if efforts are made to supply platelets that are ABO compatible with the patient. Therefore, it makes sense for a producer to have the capability to make rapid changes in platelet production. There is added flexibility in this regard if platelets are obtained both from whole blood and by apheresis. One can envision a system in which a certain fraction of the needed platelets is routinely supplied as WBD platelets, and the remainder (probably the majority) is produced by a steady, reliable flow of apheresis donors. When there are sudden changes in platelet demand, there can be correspondingly rapid changes in the fraction of whole blood units processed into platelets. If the baseline fraction of whole blood processed for platelets is not too high, substantial leeway will be available to increase platelet production. Similarly, a sudden decrease in demand can be accommodated easily by reducing the fraction of whole blood units processed into platelets, a maneuver that can be accomplished without contacting donors and changing apheresis collection schedules.

If individual whole blood platelet units are pooled at issue for a specific patient as a transfusion dose, they incur a 4-hour expiration time because the pooling processing involves entering each unit. If the transfusion is delayed or the patient no longer needs the platelets, the component is usually wasted. However, assuming that no additional secondary processing is required, a 4-hour expiration time need not apply to apheresis platelet units or to prestorage pooled WBD platelets assigned to a particular patient; such units would retain their original 5-day shelf life. In regard to the effect of shipping, a number of studies have shown that interruption of continuous agitation for as long as 24 hours does not adversely affect platelet function.[40-42]

A final issue is that occasionally platelets are needed quickly. There may be a clinically important difference between delivering platelets in 15 minutes and delivering them in 30 minutes. As noted above, one advantage of apheresis platelet units or prestorage pooled WBD platelets is that the time necessary for pooling is eliminated. In addition, both of these components are usually already leukocyte reduced and tested for bacteria contamination, saving crucial time for emergent orders.

Cost

By conventional calculation, it is more expensive to prepare 1 apheresis platelet unit than it is to prepare a pool of 4 to 6 units of WBD platelets.[43] Capital expenditures are required for instruments, and the cost of disposable kits, nurse/technician time, and supplies per unit equivalent are higher than the costs of separating platelets from whole blood units. In addition, revenue generated from the sale of WBD platelets reduces the net cost of red cell production; this revenue is lost if platelets are produced only by plateletpheresis.

However, there are a number of offsetting factors to be considered. The cost per unit of production is subject to economies of scale and will decrease as the number of apheresis procedures increases. Depending on the needs of the particular institution, it may be advantageous from the standpoint of donor recruiting costs to increase the proportion of apheresis platelets. If the driving force is a need for red cells, whole blood donors must be recruited anyway, and recruiting plateletpheresis donors is an added expense. On the other hand, if red cell collections are adequate and the need is for additional platelet components, recruiting dollars can probably be spent more wisely by increasing the number of platelet donors, apheresis representing a more efficient use of any one donor in terms of the numbers of platelets obtained, particularly if one is able to produce two or three transfusion doses of platelets from one donor.

With apheresis platelet production, it is necessary to perform testing (ABO, antibody screen, infectious disease markers) only once for the equivalent of 6 to 10 units of WBD platelets. Because pooling is not necessary, there is also a savings in the time, materials, and personnel costs of component preparation and secondary processing. Leukocyte reduction of apheresis products is relatively inexpensive if performed as part of the production procedure, and it may substantially reduce the incremental costs associated with providing this component. For example, at the Puget Sound Blood Center, the charge for 6 units of leukocyte-reduced WBD platelets in 2009 was $544; a leukocyte-reduced apheresis platelet unit was $580.

Whether the use of apheresis platelets is worth additional cost has been a matter of debate.[43,44] Lopez-Plaza et al, using a decision analysis model and sensitivity analysis, concluded that the use of apheresis platelets was not likely to be cost effective (<$50,000 per quality adjusted life years gained) until the cost differential was reduced to $40.[45] In the current competitive environment, producers must also consider the cost of not providing apheresis platelet units. From a customer service point of view, there are advantages to having a component that can be produced as leukocyte reduced, carries a lower risk of disease transmission, can be issued much more quickly than a pooled component, and has a shelf-life in the transfusion service of up to 4 days rather than 4 hours. The last two of these advantages will, of course, not apply if the comparison is to prestorage pooled WBD platelet components.

Summary

Despite a somewhat higher cost, clinical use of apheresis platelet units has grown steadily since their introduction in the 1960s. These platelets can offer definite advantages to recipients, including increased consistency of dose, decreased donor exposure, speed of availability, and the possibility for matched platelet transfusions. To producers, they offer the advantages of increased flexibility in processing and inventory management and an optimal use of the available donor pool.

References

1. Baer MR, Bloomfield CD. Controversies in transfusion medicine; prophylactic platelet transfusion: Pro. Transfusion 1992;32:377-80.
2. Patton E. Controversies in transfusion medicine; prophylactic platelet transfusion revisited after 25 years: Con. Transfusion 1992;32:381-5.
3. Slichter S. Platelet transfusion therapy. Hematol Oncol Clin N Am. 2007;21:697-729.
4. McCullough J. Current issues with platelet transfusion in patients with cancer. Semin Hematol 2000;37:3-10.
5. Murphy S. Preservation and clinical use of platelets. In: Beutler E, Lichtman MA, Coller BS, et al, eds. Williams' hematology. 6th ed. New York: McGraw-Hill, 2001:1905-16.
6. Wallace EL, Surgenor DM, Hao HS, et al. Collection and transfusion of blood and blood components in the United States, 1989. Transfusion 1993;33:139-44.
7. Wallace EL, Churchill WH, Surgenor DM, et al. Collection and transfusion of blood and blood components in the United States, 1992. Transfusion 1995;35:802-12.
8. Wallace EL, Churchill WH, Surgenor DM, et al. Collection and transfusion of blood and blood components in the United States, 1994. Transfusion 1998;38:625-36.
9. Sullivan MT, McCullough J, Schreiber GB, Wallace EL. Blood collection and transfusion in the United States in 1997. Transfusion 2002;42:1253-60.
10. Sullivan MT, Wallace EL. Blood collection and transfusion in the United States in 1999. Transfusion 2005;45:141-8.
11. Sullivan MT, Cotton R, Read EJ, Wallace EL. Blood collection and transfusion in the United States in 2001. Transfusion 2007;47:385-94.
12. The 2007 national blood collection and utilization survey report. Washington, DC: Department of Health and Human Services, 2008.
13. Food and Drug Administration. Guidance for industry and FDA review staff: Collection of platelets by automated methods. (December 2007) Rockville, MD: CBER Office of Communication, Training, and Manufacturers Assistance, 2007. [Available at http://www.fda.gov/BiologicsBloodVaccines/GuidanceCompliance RegulatoryInformation/Guidances/Blood/ucm073382.htm (accessed December 8, 2009).]
14. Price TH, ed. Standards for blood banks and transfusion services. 26th ed. Bethesda, MD: AABB, 2009.
15. Murphy S, Heaton WA, Rebulla P. Platelet production in the old world—and the new. Transfusion 1996;36:751-4.

16. Code of federal regulations. Title 21 CFR Part 640.24(c). Washington, DC: US Government Printing Office, 2009 (revised annually).
17. Slichter SJ, Kaufman RM, Assmann SF, et al. Effects of prophylactic platelet (plt) dose on transfusion (tx) outcomes (PLADO trial) (abstract). Blood 2008;112:111.
18. Food and Drug Administration. Memorandum to registered blood establishments: Recommendations and licensure requirements for leukocyte-reduced blood products. (May 29, 1996) Rockville, MD: CBER Office of Communication, Training, and Manufacturers Assistance, 1996.
19. Kelley DL, Fegan RL, Ng AT, et al. High-yield platelet concentrates attainable by continuous quality improvement reduce platelet transfusion cost and donor exposure. Transfusion 1997;37:482-6.
20. Slichter SJ, Grabowski M, Townsend-McCall D, et al. Prospective randomized transfusion trial to directly compare fresh and stored apheresis platelets (AP) and pooled random donor platelet concentrates (PC) in thrombocytopenic patients (abstract). Blood 1998;92(Suppl):672a.
21. Arnold DM, Heddle NM, Kulczycky M, et al. In vivo recovery and survival of apheresis and whole blood-derived platelets: A paired comparison in healthy volunteers. Transfusion 2006; 46:257-64.
22. Ness P, Cambell-Lee SA. Single donor versus pooled random donor platelet concentrates. Opin Hematol 2001;8:392-6.
23. Chambers LA, Herman JH. Considerations in the selection of a platelet component: Apheresis versus whole blood-derived. Transfus Med Rev 1999;13:311-22.
24. Glynn SA, Schreiber GB, Busch MP, et al. Demographic characteristics, unreported risk behaviors, and the prevalence and incidence of viral infections: A comparison of apheresis and whole-blood donors. Transfusion 1998;38:350-8.
25. Lynch TL, Weinstein MJ, Tankersley DL, et al. Considerations of pool size in the manufacture of plasma derivatives. Transfusion 1996;36:770-5.
26. Dodd, RY. Current risk for transfusion transmitted infections. Curr Opin Hematol 2007;14:671-6.
27. Ness P, Braine H, King K, et al. Single-donor platelets reduce the risk of septic platelet transfusion reactions. Transfusion 2001;41:857-61.
28. Yomtovian R, Lazarus HM, Goodnough LT, et al. A prospective microbiologic surveillance program to detect and prevent the transfusion of bacterially contaminated platelets. Transfusion 1993;33:902-9.
29. Vamvakas, EC. Relative safety of pooled whole blood-derived versus single-donor (apheresis) platelets in the United States: A systematic review of disparate risks. Transfusion 2009; 49:1874-83.
30. Slichter SJ. Prevention of platelet alloimmunization. Prog Clin Biol Res 1986;211:83-116.
31. Sintnicolaas K, Vriesendorp HM, Sizoo W, et al. Delayed alloimmunisation by random single donor platelet transfusions. Lancet 1981;1:750-4.
32. Gmür J, von Felten A, Osterwalder B, et al. Delayed alloimmunization using random single donor platelet transfusions: A prospective study in thrombocytopenic patients with acute leukemia. Blood 1983;62:473-9.
33. Slichter SJ, O'Donnell MR, Weiden PL, et al. Canine platelet alloimmunization: The role of donor selection. Br J Haematol 1986;63.713-27.
34. TRAP Trial Study Group. A randomized trial evaluating leukocyte-reduction and UV-B irradiation of platelets to prevent alloimmune platelet refractoriness. N Engl J Med 1997;337:1861-9.
35. Dzik WH, AuBuchon J, Jeffries L, et al. Leukocyte reduction of blood components: Public policy and new technology. Transfus Med Rev 2000;14:34-52.
36. Vamvakas EC, Blajchman MA. Universal WBC reduction: The case for and against. Transfusion 2001;41:691-712.
37. Ratko TA, Cummings JP, Oberman HA, et al. Evidence-based recommendations for the use of WBC-reduced cellular blood components. Transfusion 2001;41:1310-19.
38. Dzik WH, Anderson JK, O'Neill EM, et al. A prospective, randomized clinical trial of universal WBC reduction. Transfusion 2002;42:1114-22.
39. Heddle NM, Klama L, Singer J, et al. The role of the plasma from platelet concentrates in transfusion reactions. N Engl J Med 1994;331:625-8.
40. Simon TL, Sierra ER. Lack of adverse effect of transportation on room temperature stored platelet concentrates. Transfusion 1982;22:496-7.

41. Hunter S, Nixon J, Murphy S. The effect of the interruption of agitation on platelet quality during storage for transfusion. Transfusion. 2001;41:809-14.

42. Dumont L, Gulliksson H, van der Meer P, et al. Interruption of agitation of platelet concentrates: A multicenter in vitro study by the BEST Collaborative on the effects of shipping platelets. Transfusion 2007;47:1666-2172.

43. Sweeney JD, Petrucci J, Yankee R. Pooled platelet concentrates: Maybe not fancy, but fiscally sound and effective. Transfus Sci 1997;18: 575-83.

44. Zeger G, Williams CT, Shulman IA. Single donor platelets: Can we afford to use them? Can we afford not to use them? Transfus Sci 1997;18:585-8.

45. Lopez-Plaza I, Weissfeld J, Triulzi DJ. The cost-effectiveness of reducing donor exposures with single-donor versus pooled random-donor platelets. Transfusion 1999;39:925-32.

In: McLeod BC, Szczepiorkowski ZM, Weinstein R, Winters JL, eds.
Apheresis: Principles and Practice, 3rd edition
Bethesda, MD: AABB Press, 2010

9

Matched Apheresis Platelets

Janice G. McFarland, MD

 THE TERMS *ALLOIMMUNIZA-tion* and *refractoriness* are often used interchangeably in discussions of platelet transfusion responses. The former refers to the immune system's response to foreign antigens, usually the production of antibodies, whereas the latter describes a clinical state in which the anticipated rise in platelet count from a platelet transfusion is not achieved. Although the detection of alloimmunization is fairly straightforward—demonstration of antibodies reactive with HLA or other blood cell antigens in the patient's serum—the designation of refractoriness is somewhat arbitrary. This chapter discusses both alloimmunization and refractoriness and considers the selection of apheresis platelets based on avoidance of the patient's immune response in the management of alloimmunized patients.

Although the two conditions can be closely related, refractoriness does not necessarily imply alloimmunization. Only about 30% of HLA-alloimmunized patients develop clinical refractoriness to platelet transfusions,[1,2] and most cases are caused not by alloimmunization but rather by nonimmune factors that result in decreased platelet recovery and survival.[3-5] A number of clinical factors have been reported to negatively influence the outcome of platelet transfusion, including fever, splenomegaly, sepsis, antibiotics, antifungal medications, disseminated intravascular coagulation, and marrow transplantation.

Other factors may be more or less important, depending on the population of patients studied and the platelet components received.[4-11] A storage lesion in platelet components may also result in poorer responses to transfusions in some patient groups. In a study of 39

Janice G. McFarland, MD, Medical Director, Platelet and Neutrophil Immunology Laboratory, BloodCenter of Wisconsin, Inc, Milwaukee, Wisconsin
The author has disclosed no conflicts of interest.

patients receiving platelet transfusions, stable patients responded as well to stored platelets as to those transfused within 24 hours of collection. In contrast, patients with sepsis, fever, or active bleeding responded better to fresh platelets.[12]

HLA Alloimmunization and Platelet Transfusions

HLA antibodies are the most important cause of alloimmune platelet transfusion refractoriness. Exposure during pregnancy and/or blood transfusion leads to the development of HLA antibodies. Such antibodies do not appear to be "naturally occurring." Before the widespread use of leukocyte-reduced red cell and platelet transfusions, up to 70% of multitransfused patients developed HLA antibodies.[13] More recent studies have found that rates of HLA alloimmunization among patients receiving non-leukocyte-reduced transfusions are somewhat lower at 45% and 19%.[2,14]

With rare exceptions,[15] Class II HLA molecules are not present on the platelet membrane, and until recently, it was thought that of the Class I molecules, only the A- and B-locus antigens were significantly represented. A recent report from Japan, however, suggests that anti-HLA-C antibodies might mediate between 5% and 10% of alloimmune refractoriness. In this study, patients refractory to HLA-A- and -B-matched and -C-mismatched platelets but responsive to platelets that were matched for all three Class I antigens were shown, using careful absorption and elution techniques, to have antibodies reactive with HLA-C antigens on the -C-mismatched platelets.[16] The failure to detect HLA-C antigens on platelets in earlier studies was probably the result of limitations of serologic typing reagents and techniques used in the past.[17] Like HLA-A and -B antigens, HLA-C markers can be determined using DNA-based methods, and increasingly, recommendations are made to include HLA-C typing of both alloimmune refractory platelet recipients and donors to allow matching for these specificities.[17,18]

The contaminating white cells (WBCs) in blood components appear to be most responsible for primary HLA alloimmunization occurring with transfusion. A number of studies in animals and humans demonstrate that when platelets devoid of WBCs are transfused, primary HLA immunization is very much delayed or does not occur at all, whereas unmodified platelet concentrates are associated with high rates of HLA immunization.[2,19] These observations implicate leukocytes in both platelet and red cell transfusions as the source of primary alloimmunization. However, studies in mice reveal that platelets in the absence of WBCs can stimulate a primary immune response including transformation of T lymphocytes and subsequent programming of B lymphocytes to produce antibody to the major histocompatibility complex.[20] Additional studies[21,22] suggest that neither intact platelets nor intact WBCs are essential to the process of primary alloimmunization to platelet HLA antigens, because cell-free supernatant plasma from platelet concentrates stored without prior leukocyte reduction contains immunizing fragments thought to have been derived from WBCs. There may then be at least two possible pathways for the primary immune response to HLA antigens on platelets to develop: one dependent on WBCs and another, less efficient mechanism, independent of leukocytes.[20,23]

There is consensus that primary alloimmunization to HLA is unlikely to occur before 3 to 4 weeks after the first transfusion in patients receiving multiple transfusions. HLA antibodies detected sooner than this most likely represent secondary immune responses in patients with remote histories of pregnancy or transfusion. In one early study when non-leukocyte-reduced blood components were used, the patients' responses to random-donor platelet transfusions could be correlated with the time of appearance of the lymphocytotoxic antibodies.[24] Patients alloimmunized at the beginning of the study had the poorest responses to transfusions of random-donor platelets, those who did not develop lymphocytotoxic antibodies had the best responses, and those whose antibodies developed during the period of observation had intermediate responses.

Although the risk of HLA alloimmunization may be reduced by removing or inactivating contaminating WBCs, it has not been eliminated, particularly in those patients who have been sensitized through pregnancy. Remote exposure to HLA antigens appears to increase the risk of sensitization when multiple transfusions are given, even if the serologic evidence of sensitization is lacking at the outset of the transfusion course.[2,25] This appears to be the case in the Trial to Reduce Alloimmunization to Platelets (TRAP) trial,[2] a randomized, controlled trial of platelet transfusion components, the aim of which was to reduce alloimmune refractoriness. In this study, previously pregnant patients experienced a rate of HLA antibody formation twice that of women who had never been pregnant (62% vs 33%). Moreover, although patients in this study who had been pregnant previously and were receiving components modified to reduce or inactivate contaminating WBCs had lower rates of alloimmunization compared to previously pregnant patients who received unmodified platelets, they had rates that were three to five times that of patients who had not been previously sensitized and who received treated products (33% vs 7-15%). These trends were confirmed in a later retrospective study of the impact of prestorage leukocyte reduction on rates of alloimmunization in platelet transfusion recipients.[14]

The underlying disease for which transfusions are required also influences the likelihood of HLA alloimmunization. Patients with aplastic anemia were found to have a significantly higher frequency of HLA sensitization compared with those with hematologic malignancies.[26] In a 1987 study, patients undergoing intensive induction chemotherapy for acute myelogenous leukemia (AML) were significantly more likely to become alloimmunized to HLA antigens than were patients being treated with similarly intensive therapy for acute lymphoblastic leukemia (ALL) (44% vs 18%).[27] The lower sensitization rate in the ALL patients may be the result of a decreased immune responsiveness attributable to the underlying disease, or of the immunosuppressive effects of high-dose corticosteroids given to these patients and not to the AML group. Other studies note that alloimmunization also appears to occur sooner in AML patients than in ALL patients.[28]

A dose-response relationship between donor exposures in platelet transfusion and the rate of HLA alloimmunization is not always evident. One group failed to detect such a relationship in AML patients receiving induction therapy,[29] but others have demonstrated a dose-response relationship in animal studies.[30] More recently, a large-scale study of patients receiving multiple platelet transfusions found that exposure to 13 or more apheresis platelet transfusions was among the few factors significantly associated with higher rates of HLA alloimmunization, the others being prior pregnancy or transfusion and receipt of non-leukocyte-reduced components.[14]

As important as they appear to be in determining responses to platelet transfusions, lymphocytotoxic antibodies are often a transient finding, disappearing in more than half the patients who develop them. Lymphocytotoxic antibodies can be lost despite a patient's continued exposure to random-donor platelet transfusions.[31] One group reported that in two-thirds of patients demonstrating decreased anti-HLA reactivity despite continued transfusion exposure, anti-idiotypic antibodies had developed that were reactive with the variable region of HLA antibodies.[32] In 36% of these, sera collected after anti-HLA reactivity had been lost actually blocked binding of the patients' own HLA antibodies (in older samples) to appropriate lymphocyte targets. A history of pregnancy did not affect a patient's ability to produce anti-idiotypic antibodies. In patients with persistently detectable HLA antibodies, anti-idiotypic antibodies did not develop. HLA antibodies detected before the onset of transfusion therapy (ie, those that developed as a result of remote transfusion or pregnancy) tend to persist, whereas those that develop de novo during a transfusion support episode are more likely to be transient, decreasing in strength or disappearing altogether despite continued exposure to allogeneic blood and platelets.[31]

A number of factors have changed in the last decade that may have reduced the risk of alloimmunization in the average patient receiving multiple platelet transfusions. More blood components are being leukocyte reduced, and there is a trend to supply apheresis platelets for transfusion rather than pools of concentrates.[33] In addition, most institutions have lowered the platelet-count level at which prophylactic platelet transfusions are given.[34,35] These trends—leukocyte reduction, increased use of apheresis platelets, and lowering of the platelet transfusion trigger—have resulted in fewer donor HLA exposures being necessary to support patients receiving multiple platelet transfusions. These changes are largely responsible for lower rates of alloimmunization, particularly in patients without prior exposure to HLA antigens through pregnancy.[2,14]

ABH Antigens and Platelet Transfusion

The ABH blood group system is also an important antigen system represented on platelets. The amount of ABH substance on platelets varies not only from person to person but also among platelets in the same individual. Dunstan and Simpson demonstrated the variable distribution of group A substance on platelets using flow cytometry.[36] This distribution of ABH could explain why, in some platelet transfusions, there is a rapid destruction of a subset of ABO-incompatible cells followed by near-normal survival of the remaining cells, as described first by Aster.[37] Greater recovery was seen for group B platelets than for group A platelets—attributable, perhaps, to the lower levels of B antigens on donor platelets (about half that of A sites)[38] and the lower levels of B-specific isoagglutinins in recipient plasma.[37] The number of A antigens per platelet is highly variable and donor dependent. It is important for the purpose of platelet donor selection for recipients with high anti-A or anti-A,B titers to note that individuals of the subgroup A_2 have no detectable A antigens on their plate-

lets,[38-41] and A_2 platelets can be substituted successfully for group O.[39,42]

Ogasawara et al[43] reported highly variable ABH expression on the surface of platelets from a group of Japanese blood donors, with "high" A or B antigen expressers accounting for about 7% of non-group-O individuals. The high or low expression of A and B substances was independent of secretor phenotype and correlated with high levels of glycosyltransferase measured in donor serum.[43] More recently, Curtis et al confirmed these findings in studies of 200 blood donors of European ethnicity and further defined two subgroups of high expressers of platelet A_1 antigens, termed Type I and Type II.[38] Type I high expressers had elevated platelet A_1 antigen levels (about three times the normal expression), elevated serum A^1-glycosyltransferase activity, and a heterogeneous distribution of A_1 antigens on individual platelets. Type II high expressers were characterized as having platelet A_1 antigen levels that averaged seven times the normal expression, higher A^1-glycosyltransferase activity than even Type I individuals, and homogeneous distribution of platelet A_1 antigens on platelets, the majority of which were associated with platelet glycoproteins GPIIb and the platelet endothelial cell adhesion molecule (PECAM).[38] This inherited pattern of high and low ABH expression may offer an explanation for the variable refractory responses some patients develop to ABO-incompatible platelet transfusions.

Heal et al reexamined the importance of ABO blood groups in platelet transfusion therapy.[44] Forty patients with hematologic diseases receiving platelet transfusions were randomized to receive either ABO-identical or ABO-unmatched platelets. The responses in the group of patients receiving ABO-unmatched transfusions (ie, when either the recipient would be expected to have isoagglutinins to the ABH antigens on the transfused platelets or the donor had such antibodies directed at the recipient's blood type) were significantly worse than those observed in patients receiving ABO-identical platelet transfusions [mean corrected count increment (CCI) = 6600 vs 5200; p <0.01]. Analyzing the first 25 transfusions in each group, the authors noted this effect was most important in the first 10 transfusion episodes and tended to predict subsequent alloimmunization and refractoriness to platelet transfusions. This finding seemed to be in conflict with earlier reports in which a minor, clinically insignificant impact of ABO mismatching was observed. The newer data were then reanalyzed using the earlier definitions of ABO "compatibility" (the patient lacks isoagglutinins to donor ABH antigens) and "incompatibility" (the patient has isoagglutinins reactive with donor ABH antigens). In the reanalysis, no benefits of ABO compatibility were detected,[45] suggesting that there is a significant negative impact of *both major and minor* ABO incompatibility in platelet transfusions.

A later publication by Heal et al reported that ABO-incompatible transfusions were correlated with inferior outcomes in leukemia treatment independent of transfusion responses.[46] An increased frequency of refractoriness in patients receiving ABO-unmatched platelet transfusions was also observed by Carr et al in a study of 26 patients (69% vs 58%; p = 0.001).[47] Since then, large studies of factors affecting platelet transfusion have likewise identified ABO mismatching as detrimental to platelet transfusion responses.[2,14,48]

The mechanism for platelet destruction in platelet ABO-incompatible transfusions (the patient has isoagglutinins reactive with donor ABH antigens) is not difficult to ascertain. Presumably, IgM and IgG anti-A or anti-B in the recipient interact with A and B substances on the transfused platelets, resulting in their premature exit from the circulation. The suboptimal response of the plasma-incompatible transfusions (the donor has isoagglutinins to patient ABH antigens) is more difficult to explain. Heal et al postulate that immune complexes involving soluble recipient ABH substance and donor anti-A or -B antibodies form.[49,50] These immune complexes interact secondarily with the transfused platelets via the FcγRIIα receptor, or the complement receptors cC1q-R and gC1q-R, and mediate platelet destruction. Some experimental evidence supports this theory, in that anti-A has been detected in an immune-complex fraction of group A recipient plasma after transfusion with group O platelets,[50] and that these immune complexes bind to IgG FcγRIIα and the cC1q-R and gC1q-R receptors on group O platelets.[49]

Platelet-Specific Antigens and Platelet Transfusions

To date, 24 platelet-specific alloantigens have been described, including localization to platelet surface glycoprotein structures, quantification of their density on the platelet surface, and determination of DNA polymorphisms in genes encoding for them (Table 9-1).[51,52] Several others have been described serologically, but genetic polymorphisms underlying these have not yet been determined. Many of the recognized platelet alloantigens have been implicated in cases of neonatal alloimmune thrombocytopenic purpura (NATP) and posttransfusion purpura (PTP), and a few have been determined to be relevant in platelet transfusion responses.

Evidence implicating platelet-specific antigens in the destruction of transfused platelets is that not all transfusions of HLA-matched platelets in patients refractory to random-donor platelets are successful.[9,54] When the HLA match between donor and recipient is very close, a transfusion failure caused by HLA antibodies would be unexpected. The failure of platelet transfusions despite HLA matching indicates that other antigens, perhaps platelet-specific, are involved. Additional evidence involves the demonstration of platelet-reactive antibodies in the absence of HLA antibodies. The conclusion drawn is that these antibodies are directed at platelet-specific antigens.[31]

Although there are a few well-documented cases of transfusion failures attributable to platelet-specific antibodies,[25,55-57] most platelet-specific reactivity in refractory recipients does not seem to influence transfusion responses.[2] This is perhaps because many of the platelet-specific antibodies detected in such patients are directed against platelet antigens present in a minority of the general population, and they are therefore unlikely to cause refrac-

Table 9-1. Human Platelet Alloantigens*[51,52]

Nucleotide Alloantigens	Other Names	Phenotypic Frequencies	Glycoprotein Location/Amino Acid Change	Nucleotide Substitution
HPA-1a (Pl^{A1})	Pl^A, Zw	72% a/a	GPIIIa/Leu→Pro$_{33}$	T:C196
HPA-1b (Pl^{A2})		26% a/b		
HPA-1c[53]		2% b/b	GPIIIa/Leu→Val$_{33}$	C:G175
		<1% a/c		
HPA-2a (Ko^b)	Ko, Sib	85% a/a	GPIb/Thr→Met$_{145}$	C:T524
HPA-2b (Ko^a)		14% a/b		
		1% b/b		
HPA-3a (Bak^a)	Bak, Lek	37% a/a	GPIIb/Ile→Ser$_{843}$	T:G622
HPA-3b (Bak^b)		48% a/b		
		15% b/b		
HPA-4a (Pen^a)	Pen, Yuk	>99.9% a/a	GPIIIa/Arg→Gln$_{143}$	G:A526
HPA-4b (Pen^b)		<0.1% a/b		
		<0.1% b/b		
HPA-5a (Br^b)	Br, Hc, Zav	80% a/a	GPIa/Glu→Lys$_{505}$	G:A648
HPA-5b (Br^a)		19% a/b		
		1% b/b		
HPA-6bw	Ca^a, Tu	<1%	GPIIIa/Arg→Gln$_{489}$	A:G1564
HPA-7bw	Mo^b	<1%	GPIIIa/Pro→Ala$_{407}$	G:C1317
HPA-8bw	Sr^a	<0.1%	GPIIIa/Arg→Cys$_{636}$	T:C2004
HPA-9bw	Max^a	<1%	GPIIb/Val→Met$_{837}$	A:G2603
HPA-10bw	La^a	1%	GPIIIa/Arg→Gln$_{62}$	A:G281
HPA-11bw	Gro^a	<0.5%	GPIIIa/Arg→His$_{633}$	A:G1996
HPA-12bw	Iy^a	1%	GPIb$_\beta$/Gly→Glu$_{15}$	A:G 141
HPA-13bw	Sit^a	<1%	GPIa/Met→Thr$_{799}$	T:C2531
HPA-14bw	Oe^a	1%	GPIIIa/Del Lys$_{611}$	AAG1929-31

Table 9-1. Human Platelet Alloantigens*[51,52] (Continued)

Nucleotide Alloantigens	Other Names	Phenotypic Frequencies	Glycoprotein Location/Amino Acid Change	Nucleotide Substitution
HPA-15a (Gov[b]) HPA-15b (Gov[a])	Gov	35% a/a 42% a/b 23% b/b	CD109/Tyr→Ser$_{703}$	A:C2108
HPA-16bw	Duv[a]	<1%	GPIIIa/Thr→Ile$_{140}$	C:T517
HPA-17bw	Va[a]	<1%	GPIIIa/Thr→Met$_{195}$	C:T622
NA[†]	Nak[a]	99.8% (European ethnicity) 97% (African ethnicity) 96% (Asian ethnicity)	CD36 (GPIV)	T:G1264 C:T478

*Phenotypic frequencies for the antigens shown are for people of European ethnicity only. Significant differences in gene frequencies may be found in populations of African and Asian ethnicities.
[†]Sensitization to CD36 (GPIV) is an example of isoimmunization. Anti-CD36 antibodies have been implicated in cases of neonatal alloimmune thrombocytopenic purpura and posttransfusion purpura and are therefore included in the list of platelet alloantigens that have also been associated with these disorders.
HPA = human platelet antigen; GP = glycoprotein.

tory responses to a majority of attempted platelet transfusions. In the TRAP study, approximately 8% of study patients developed platelet-specific antibodies during the trial, regardless of assigned treatment arm; and similar to earlier studies, there did not appear to be any significant contribution of these antibodies to refractory responses.[2] Alloimmunization to high-frequency, platelet-specific antigens presents a major challenge in finding compatible platelets to support a patient requiring multiple platelet transfusions. Fortunately, these cases are rare.[25,58,59] An exception to this experience is isoimmunization to glycoprotein IV (GPIV, or CD36). There are now several reports of platelet transfusion refractoriness caused by such antibodies in patients who are GPIV defi-

cient.[60,61] These patients are difficult to support because virtually all platelet components available for transfusion would be incompatible.

Diagnosis of Alloimmune Refractoriness

Clinical Diagnosis of Refractoriness

The diagnosis of alloimmune refractoriness rests first on demonstrating that platelet transfusions from randomly selected donors are not successful. Ordinarily, platelet transfusion recipients receive single-donor apheresis platelet concentrates or pooled whole-blood-derived (WBD) platelet concentrates for their initial platelet support. In adults of average size, the expected increment in platelet count after a platelet transfusion is roughly 5000 to 10,000/µL per single concentrate (or per 0.75×10^{11} platelets) transfused. Therefore, after a six-donor pool of WBD platelet concentrates is transfused, the expected platelet count increment at 1 hour after transfusion is approximately 30,000 to 60,000/µL. In patients with leukemia or other hematologic malignancies requiring platelet support, the platelet count increment per unit transfused is often not optimal because of coincidental clinical factors (see earlier this chapter).

The corrected count increment (CCI), which normalizes transfusion responses for patient blood volume and platelet dose, is calculated using the following formula:

$$CCI = \frac{[\text{Posttransfusion} - \text{pretransfusion platelet count (/µL)}] \times \text{body surface area (m}^2)}{\text{Number of platelets transfused } (\times 10^{11})}$$

Most would agree that a 1-hour posttransfusion platelet count increment expressed in terms of a CCI of less than 5000 to $7500/\text{m}^2/10^{11}$ platelets transfused on two consecutive occasions adequately defines the refractory state. Although a 1-hour posttransfusion platelet count is often recommended for determination of the CCI, one study found that a posttransfusion count taken as early as 10 minutes after the transfusion was as reliable.[62] However, a second report casts doubt on the reliability of posttransfusion platelet counts taken sooner than 60 minutes after the transfusion in detecting refractoriness.[63] These investigators, using indium-111-labeled platelets in both healthy and thrombocytopenic volunteers, demonstrated that transfused platelets do not reach intravascular equilibrium before 1 hour after transfusion.

Although measurements of platelet transfusion response such as the CCI or the posttransfusion platelet recovery (PPR), which both take into account the patient's blood volume and the dose of platelets administered, are commonly used to assess the success of platelet transfusions, these calculations may be misleading, particularly when smaller doses of platelets are administered. In a reevaluation of TRAP study data, the authors argue that absolute posttransfusion platelet count increments are more useful in assessing the impact of different manipulations of platelet components, such as leukocyte reduction by filtration, particularly if the manipulations result in lower doses of platelets in the final component transfused. In the setting of large transfusion studies, where sufficient numbers of patients and transfusions can be analyzed, the posttransfusion platelet count increment together with multiple immune and nonimmune factors, blood volume, and platelet dose can be analyzed by multiple regression analysis to better assess the impact of different manipulations of the platelet components on transfusion response.[64]

Diagnosis of HLA Alloimmunization

When refractory responses to randomly selected platelet components are evident, particularly in the absence on nonimmune clinical factors that may affect transfusion success, testing the patient for the presence of HLA antibodies can confirm the diagnosis of alloimmune refractoriness. Typically, multiple specificity or broadly reactive HLA antibodies affect the 1-hour posttransfusion platelet response.[65] However, early in the course of alloimmunization, the interval between transfusions begins to deteriorate before the 1-hour posttransfusion platelet count is affected.[64] If 24-hour posttransfusion increments are consistently poor in the absence of nonimmune clinical factors that might explain shortened platelet survival, the possibility of HLA alloimmunization should be considered.

Because many clinical factors can influence platelet transfusion success, a laboratory test to help diagnose alloimmune platelet refractoriness is useful. Many centers use periodic (eg, weekly) HLA antibody screening to predict when patients might be developing a need for HLA-selected platelet transfusions. In the past, the standard assay to evaluate platelet transfusion recipients for alloimmunization was lymphocyte cytotoxicity or antihuman-globulin-enhanced, complement-dependent cytotoxicity

(AHG-CDC). A standard lymphocyte panel consists of frozen aliquots of cells from 30 to 60 individuals representing common HLA antigens in the population. The cells are plated into microtiter tray wells, each well containing cells from a single individual. The panel-reactive antibody score (PRA) is calculated by dividing the number of wells containing significant numbers of lysed cells, as demonstrated by the uptake of dye into the cell, by the total number of wells in the assay × 100. Alloimmunization can be stringently defined as at least *one* well with >60% of cells lysed, or at least two wells with >40% of cells lysed.[2] Alternatively, in detecting a degree of HLA sensitization that is more closely associated with refractoriness, many centers use a PRA of 20% as a threshold for defining HLA alloimmunization.[66]

In recent years, more sensitive HLA antibody assays have been developed, primarily for use in screening potential renal transplant recipients. One such method is the flow cytometric PRA, in which patient serum is incubated with microparticles coated with purified Class I or Class II antigens derived from 30 separate Epstein-Barr virus transformed cell lines representing the majority of serologically defined HLA antigens.[67,68] The sensitized microparticles are incubated with FITC-conjugated antihuman IgG and assessed by flow cytometry. When more than 5% of Class I or Class II beads exhibit fluorescence above a negative control, the result is considered positive. Flow cytometric PRA appears to be more sensitive and specific in detecting Class I and II antibodies than the AHG-CDC, and it is now recommended as a screening procedure for prospective recipients of renal allografts in order to identify which patients will require pretransplant crossmatch testing with prospective donor lymphocytes.[67,68] Another test for determining whether patients are HLA alloimmunized is an enzyme-linked immunosorbent assay (ELISA) in which pooled, purified Class I HLA isolated from the platelets of a large number of donors serves as the target substance. Using this test, HLA antibodies can be detected in patient serum in approximately 4 hours.[67]

Diagnosis of Platelet-Specific Alloimmunization

When patients fail HLA-matched, ABO-compatible platelet transfusions and clinical factors are insufficient to explain the poor response, a platelet-specific antibody should be suspected. Certain specialty laboratories offer platelet antibody detection and identification services. Alternatively, some hospital laboratories offer screening with a commercially available solid-phase red cell adherence method.[69] This intact platelet antibody screen cannot distinguish between HLA- and platelet-specific antibodies when untreated target platelets are used, but prior treatment of target platelets with chloroquine may alter HLA structures sufficiently to allow detection of a platelet-specific reaction.[70,71] Newer, commercially available glycoprotein-based platelet antibody detection kits are also now available for detecting platelet-specific antibodies in such patients.[72]

Matched Platelets in the Management of the Alloimmunized Patient

The refractory state in which patients fail to benefit from random-donor platelet transfusions has been found in various series in 19% to 100% of patients receiving multiple transfusions.[73] Refractoriness, if related to HLA alloimmunization, can be transient or persistent. Several approaches to selecting more compatible platelets for transfusions are possible.

HLA-Selected Platelet Transfusions

A standard approach to supporting a patient who is refractory to random-donor platelet transfusions is to supply HLA-matched apheresis platelet concentrates.[74] Because the primary cause of alloimmune refractoriness is sensitization to Class I HLA antigens, it follows that avoidance of incompatible HLA antigens in platelet components should result in more successful responses. In practice, 65% to 90% of refractory patients benefit from these components.[1,9] Moreover, even though HLA-matched apheresis platelets are generally more expensive to provide than either pools of WBD platelet concentrates or random-donor apheresis platelets, provision of well-matched HLA-selected platelets can be more cost-effective in supporting alloimmunized refractory patients than the use of those alternative components.[75]

The HLA antibodies formed by multitransfused refractory patients are typically broadly reactive when tested against panels of randomly chosen lymphocytes. These antibodies often react with only one or a few "public" determinants shared by HLA antigens in the same cross-reactive group (CREG).[76,77] Indeed, these shared determinants are the basis of the cross-reactivity. Public epitopes differ from the "private" determinants that account for the extreme polymorphism of the HLA system.[76]

Duquesnoy[74] took advantage of the fact that certain "private" HLA antigens can be segregated into these CREGs, defined by antisera that react with several different but structurally related Class I specificities. It was proposed that selection of platelet donors having antigens from the same CREGs as those of the patient's antigens might result in the patient's immune system being relatively unable to recognize these donor antigens. Application of the cross-reactive associations of HLA antigens greatly increases the number of potentially successful platelet donors in a given pool (Table 9-2), decreasing the donor pool size necessary to ensure a reasonable chance of finding matched donors for most patients—from 10,000 random donors for sufficient numbers of rigorously HLA-compatible matches to only 500 donors for HLA-matched and selectively mismatched transfusions (Table 9-3). Others have confirmed the success of selectively mismatched platelet transfusions based on this system.[79,80] Recent studies confirm that the need for high degrees of HLA matching in HLA-selected platelet components is probably confined to those patients with broad, multispecific HLA antibodies and PRAs greater than 60% to 70%. Other, less broadly alloimmunized patients may be adequately supported by selectively mismatched platelets[81] or random-donor platelets.[25]

Because the expression of some Class I antigens on platelets is highly variable, platelet transfusions from donors with very low expression of mismatched HLA antigens can be successful. The B12 Class I antigens (B44 and B45) are most notable in this regard; individuals may differ by 35-fold in the expression of these antigens.[82] Schiffer et al[83] selectively mismatched for the B12 antigen using B12-positive

Table 9-2. Donor/Recipient HLA Match Grades (HLA-A and -B Antigens)

Grade	Interpretation
A	All four donor antigens identical to those in recipient.
B1U	All donor antigens identical to those in recipient; only three antigens detected in donor (probable homozygous antigen).
B2U	All donor antigens identical to those in recipient; only two antigens detected in donor (probable homozygous haplotype).
B1X	Three donor antigens identical to those in recipient; the fourth is cross-reactive with a recipient antigen.
B2UX	Two donor antigens identical to those in recipient; a third is cross-reactive; only three antigens detected in donor (probable homozygous antigen).
B2X	Two donor antigens identical to those in recipient; two are cross-reactive.
C	One donor antigen is mismatched (not cross-reactive) with antigens in the recipient.

Table 9-3. Projected (and Observed) Yields of Well-Matched Platelet Donors from HLA-Typed Donor Pools of Various Sizes

Donor Pool Size	Yield of Matched Donors				Reference
	A	A,B1U,B2U	A,B1U,B2U, B1X,B2X, B2UX	A,B1U,B2U, B1X,B2X, B2UX,B3,B4	
440				3.4	79
500	0.20	2.4	27		74
750	0.25	3.8	43		74
1000	0.30	5.2	59		74
1157				58	78
1157				127*	78
1500	0.40	9	89		74
2000	0.54	12	120		74
3000	0.88	18	183		74
3405				92†	78
3405				215*	78
4000	1.10	24	243		74
4562				150†	78
4562				342*	78
5000	1.50	31	306		74
20,000‡	19.00	155	816		

*Projected well-matched donor yields for patients of European ethnicity using an HLA platelet donor pool predominantly of European ethnicity.

†Projected well-matched donor yields for patients of African ethnicity using an HLA platelet donor pool predominantly of European ethnicity.

‡Data from BloodCenter of Wisconsin's matched platelet program, based on donor lists generated for 50 consecutive local patients.

donors for platelet-refractory patients lacking this antigen. In a study of 162 transfusions given to 31 patients, they found that 69% were successful, some despite positive lymphocytotoxic crossmatches between recipient sera and donor lymphocytes and despite specific B12 antibody detected in recipient plasma. They postulated that the variable expression of B12 on platelets might account for the discrepancy between the serologic data and the platelet transfusion responses.

Recently, Petz et al extended the use of HLA-typed platelets by using the patient's HLA antibody specificity as the basis for selecting a platelet component. They recognized that A and B match grade platelets are frequently unavailable for some patients and that crossmatching of platelet transfusions has limitations. Using antibody specificity prediction

(ASP),[84] they selected platelet components from donors who lacked HLA antigens to which the patient had raised an antibody, as detected in the AHG-CDC assay. These platelet components were often frank mismatches for some or all of the Class I antigens. For comparison, they selected platelets by standard HLA-matching criteria and by platelet crossmatching using a solid-phase red cell adherence assay (SPRCA). The PPR was determined in 1621 platelet transfusions in 114 patients. HLA-matched, crossmatched and ASP-selected platelet transfusions were found to have similar platelet recoveries, whereas randomly selected control platelets had significantly lower PPR. Interestingly, they found that for 29 alloimmunized patients, the mean number of potential donors found in a file of 7247 donors was only six when grade A HLA matches were required, and 39 when BU matches were added. However, 1426 potential donors (20% of the total) were identified by the ASP method. They recommended that careful identification of HLA antibody specificity could greatly enhance the number of potential donors by identifying nonmatched components that lack those HLA antigens. Zimmerman et al, also using a computerized analysis of the lymphocytotoxic assay for private and public HLA Class I epitopes in platelet recipients confirmed that there is value in carefully identifying HLA antibody specificities, allowing selection of many more donors by simply avoiding the HLA antigens against which the antibodies are directed.[85]

A variation of the ASP method involves analysis of patient antibody specificities detected in sensitive assays [either flow-cytometry[67] or luminex–based (Luminex Corp, Austin, TX)[86,87] platforms] where single HLA antigens are represented on discrete and identifiable populations of beads. Reactivity of the patient's serum with the specific bead populations yields both the specificity and the relative strength of antibody binding to specific HLA antigens represented on the beads. Bead populations that lack reactivity with patient serum identify HLA antigens that could be used in donor selection even though they may not be matched to the patient's HLA type using more

classic criteria for HLA matching. The identification of so-called "permissive" HLA antigens is modeled on a strategy used for identifying potentially compatible, deceased-donor kidney grafts for HLA-sensitized, renal graft recipients.[68,88] This is yet another way to expand the donor pool to provide platelets that would be compatible with the patient's HLA antibodies.

In a recent innovation in the use of HLA typing to find suitable platelet donors for highly alloimmunized refractory patients, Duquesnoy employs a computerized algorithm—HLA Matchmaker—for evaluation of the molecular similarities and differences between HLA Class I epitopes.[89] The strategy is based on the concept that immunogenic epitopes are represented by amino acid triplets on exposed parts of protein sequences of the Class I alloantigens that are accessible to alloantibodies. An updated version of the strategy uses an expanded definition of these HLA Class I alloimmunogenic epitopes to include longer sequences of amino acids and discontinuous residues that, in the tertiary structure of the molecule, form discrete sites for antibody binding, or *eplets*.[17] Using this scheme, Class I HLA antigens that are classified as mismatches to a patient's HLA type have no incompatible exposed eplets and therefore would not be expected to elicit an antibody response. The pool of potentially compatible HLA-selected donors is thereby greatly expanded. The clinical usefulness of HLA Matchmaker in refining and expanding platelet donor selection for refractory patients has been demonstrated.[90]

HLA-compatible platelets may be beneficial when used with other strategies to improve platelet responses in refractory patients. In a study of intravenous immunoglobulin (IVIG) therapy for platelet refractory patients, Zeigler et al[91] found that very-high-dose (median dose = 6 g/kg) of IVIG could reverse the refractory response in patients who had failed to respond to HLA-selected, lymphocytotoxic crossmatch-compatible platelet transfusions. Thirteen of 19 patients in their study responded to IVIG with improvement of 1-hour PPR of HLA-matched platelets. Responsiveness was not restored for incompatible platelets, indicating the possible involvement in such patients of several mechanisms of platelet destruction, only some of which are amenable to IVIG modulation. Interestingly, the most highly alloimmunized patients—those with more than 85% PRA—responded less well to IVIG (2 of 8), and those with less than 85% PRA responded best (11 of 11).

Platelets Matched for Platelet-Specific Antigens

In those infrequent instances in which a platelet-specific antibody reaction is contributing to poor platelet transfusion responses, it is possible to select platelet donors using platelet antigen typing. Antibodies to platelet-specific antigens, even low-incidence antigens, may be a problem with regard to consistent transfusion support in patients who also have broad specificity HLA alloimmunization.[92] In these instances, it may be necessary to screen HLA-matched donors for the platelet antigen in question to be more certain of a successful transfusion response. In a single report, GPIV negative platelets were obtained by large-scale screening of donor populations with a higher frequency of GPIV deficiency (donors of African ethnicity), and transfusion of those platelets resulted in positive platelet increments for the patients.[61]

Platelet Crossmatching

HLA-matched and selectively mismatched platelet components provide satisfactory support for the majority of patients with alloimmune refractoriness. However, as many as 20% to 25% of all refractory patients fail to respond adequately to HLA-matched platelets,[73] even in the absence of the nonimmune clinical factors that can decrease transfused platelet survival. These failures might be explained by ABO incompatibility, undetected HLA incompatibility (eg, antibodies to HLA-C antigens), platelet-specific antibodies, or, as recently proposed, antibodies to epitopes that appear on stored platelets.[93]

Platelet transfusion failures caused by immunization can often be predicted with pretransfusion platelet crossmatching assays that test reactions of patient serum with donor platelets. Although virtually any platelet or lymphocyte antibody detection method can be used as a platelet compatibility test, the method that has gained greatest acceptance for this purpose is the commercially available SPRCA assay.[94] First described by Shibata et al[95] and later by Rachel et al,[69,96] the test is rapid and sensitive, particularly for detecting HLA antibodies.

Although crossmatching of single-donor apheresis platelets is most often recommended as a strategy to identify an adequate dose of compatible platelets for an individual alloimmunized patient, two studies explored the utility of crossmatching WBD platelet concentrates. In moderately alloimmunized patients, Freedman et al[97] showed that nearly 70% of WBD pooled platelet transfusions judged to be compatible by a radiolabeled antiglobulin technique were successful. By contrast, in a highly alloimmunized, refractory population of leukemic patients, O'Connell and Schiffer[98] found that only 41% of transfusions judged compatible by either a micro-ELISA or a SPRCA test produced satisfactory increments. Moreover, because only 15% to 24% of the platelet concentrates were negative in these tests, large numbers of platelet concentrates had to be screened to provide each "compatible" transfusion. Indeed, for 43% of their patients, only one or two compatible concentrates could be identified. Crossmatching of WBD platelet concentrates may be helpful in patients with limited alloimmunization; however, for severely refractory patients it might not be worthwhile.

O'Connell et al[99] suggest contacting donors of WBD platelet concentrates found to be compatible in crossmatching tests and arranging single-donor apheresis platelet collections to support refractory patients. Such a strategy allowed good support of eight patients reported; however, two additional patients receiving apheresis platelets selected with SPRCA testing had poor responses because of newly developed HLA antibodies. A potential risk of using crossmatch-compatible, HLA-incompatible platelets in partially immunized patients is that the HLA antibodies can broaden in specificity, eventually limiting compatible donors to those who are very closely HLA matched.

Another study compared available platelet crossmatching techniques with HLA-based platelet donor selection in supporting platelet-refractory patients.[100] This multicenter study used three different platelet antibody tests, depending on the site. At least one set of 2 apheresis platelet units was transfused to each patient: 1 was selected by prospective HLA matching and the other by prospective crossmatching. When 1-hour PPRs were compared, the HLA-selected transfusions were successful slightly more often than the crossmatch-selected transfusions, but the difference was not statistically significant. However, the HLA-selected transfusions were significantly more likely to produce a satisfactory 24-hour recovery, particularly when only A and BU matches were considered. The authors concluded that if HLA-typed donors are available, an A or BU HLA match is preferable to a random component selected by any of the crossmatch methods used. Nevertheless, platelet crossmatching remains an option for hospitals that lack access to adequate numbers of HLA-typed donors.

The transfusion success rate in such studies is highly dependent on the quality of the HLA match. In one recent study in which HLA-matched platelets did not seem superior to crossmatch-selected platelets, the matched platelets were seldom of A or BU match grade with the recipients.[101] Another recent trial in which SPRCA crossmatching appeared to be a superior predictor of transfusion outcome was likewise confounded by inclusion of "HLA-ordered" apheresis platelets that were not well matched.[102]

Several studies demonstrate that combining HLA-based donor selection with crossmatching can improve transfusion results. Using relatively well-matched donor-recipient pairs, Sintnicolaas and Lowenberg[103] showed that a flow cytometric crossmatch could accurately predict the success of HLA-matched platelets in 81% of transfusions. The predictive value of the test decreased, however, in ABO-incompatible transfusions and in the presence of nonimmune clinical factors.

Elements of a Matched Donor Program

HLA-Typed Donor Pool

Given a pool of HLA-typed donors, the number of suitable donors that will be available for a patient depends on the answers to several questions:

- First, is the patient's HLA type common or uncommon? Common patient HLA types generate larger numbers of compatible prospective donors.
- Second, is the patient broadly alloimmunized or is alloimmunization limited to one or a few private HLA specificities? The breadth of alloimmunization and the presence of antibodies against public epitopes determine the success of using selectively HLA-mismatched donors. Initially, patients may have limited alloimmunization and respond well to platelets from donors with cross-reactive HLA antigens, but eventually they may become more broadly alloimmunized, requiring progressively better-matched products.
- Third, does the patient have evidence of ABO or platelet-specific antigen immunization affecting HLA-matched component response? Restriction of HLA-matched donor lists to ABO-identical donors, or to those lacking a particular platelet-specific antigen, will further reduce the number of donors available for the patient.
- Fourth, how many HLA-typed donors are in the pool? The larger the pool, the better the chance of finding compatible donors.

Several investigators have calculated the average number of suitable donors per patient based on the size of the HLA-typed pool (Table 9-3). In general, the smaller the pool, the more likely that cross-reactive associations will have to be used to generate a reasonable number of matched donors for a given patient. Relatively small pools may be adequate for patients with common HLA types but insufficient for patients with unusual types. In a 1996 publication,[78] ethnicity was examined as a factor in determining the number of well-matched donors available for refractory patients. On average, patients of European ethnicity had twice as many well-matched (A or BU) donors as patients of African ethnicity when the same, predominantly European-ethnicity donor pool was used (Table 9-3).

One successful strategy for establishing an HLA-typed donor pool is to recruit donors from files of existing whole blood donors. Donors known to be willing to come in repeatedly to donate whole blood are more likely to become reliable apheresis platelet donors, and their familiarity with the regional center and the process of blood donation facilitates the education process about apheresis donation. At the author's center, such donors are first recruited to give a random (non-HLA-typed) platelet donation. This allows them to become familiar with the apheresis process and the time commitment involved. Only donors who express a willingness to return for repeated platelet donations are HLA typed. The retention of such individuals in a pool of HLA-typed donors is likely to be superior to that of first-time donors. The expense of typing each new donor dictates that there be a high likelihood of the donor's remaining in the program, accessible for repeated platelet donation for several years at least.

Once a pool of HLA-typed donors is established, resources must be dedicated to ongoing recruitment and HLA typing of new donors to ensure maintenance of an adequate pool size. Estimates are that 10% to 20% of donors in such files are lost to attrition each year. Reasons for attrition include donor relocation, development of medical conditions that preclude further donation, and changes in donors' schedules that make them less accessible for a lengthy collection procedure required on short notice. Expanding a pool requires even larger investments for recruitment and HLA typing of new donors. Maintenance of an HLA-typed platelet donor pool can be supported by a "matching surcharge" on HLA-matched platelet components. This generates enough revenue to cover the expenses of updating HLA types and recruiting new donors.

HLA-Matching Computer Programs

A number of different computer programs have been developed to assist in identifying matched platelet donors. All use the cross-reactive associations between Class I HLA antigens to allow more donors to be identified as compatible for each patient. One example of a straightforward computer algorithm for HLA matching was described by Jorgensen et al.[79] In this system, about 500 HLA-typed donors were entered into the file. Information added included a unique donor identifier, ABO group, Rh type, HLA-A and -B antigens, and donor contact information. To generate a list of matched donors for a specific patient, the computer compared each donor antigen with those of the patient and, using an algorithm to assign categories of exact match, split, and cross-reactivity, assigned an antigen match grade for each donor antigen. The combination of antigen match grades then gave rise to a donor-recipient match grade (Table 9-2). Donors were ranked and displayed in order of match grade with the patient—that is, A, B1U, B2U, B1X, B2UX, B2X, B3UX, or B3X. Most matching programs allow users to specify that donors with certain HLA antigens or ABO types be excluded from the list of potential donors. This allows the use of information about antibody specificities obtained from previous transfusion responses and lymphocytotoxic studies.

Newer computer algorithms to assist in finding compatible donors among an HLA-typed file function based on individual patients' HLA antibody specificities[84] or, alternatively, use information about the Class I antigen secondary structure and amino acid sequences of exposed regions to find compatible platelet donors among those formerly classified as frank HLA mismatches by more traditional criteria.[89] These two strategies result in the generation of larger lists of potential donors for a given patient from existing HLA-typed donor files. Because the latter strategy attempts to avoid using donors whose HLA peptide sequences are discordant with those of the recipient at antibody-accessible sites in the molecules' secondary structure, molecular rather than serologic HLA typing of both donor and recipient is recommended.[90]

References

1. Murphy MF, Waters AH. Clinical aspects of platelet transfusions. Blood Coagul Fibrinolysis 1991;2:389-96.
2. Trial to Reduce Alloimmunization to Platelets Study Group. Leukocyte reduction and ultraviolet B irradiation of platelets to prevent alloimmunization and refractoriness to platelet transfusions. N Engl J Med 1997;337:1861-9.
3. Hod E, Schwartz J. Platelet transfusion refractoriness. Br J Haematol 2008;142:348-60.
4. Alcorta I, Pereira A, Ordinas A. Clinical and laboratory factors associated with platelet transfusion refractoriness: A case-control study. Br J Haematol 1996;93:220-4.
5. Doughty HA, Murphy MF, Metcalfe P, et al. Relative importance of immune and non-immune causes of platelet refractoriness. Vox Sang 1994;66:200-5.
6. McFarland JG, Anderson AJ, Slichter SJ. Factors influencing the transfusion response to HLA-selected apheresis donor platelets in patients refractory to random platelet concentrates. Br J Haematol 1989;73:380-6.
7. Bock M, Muggenthaler KH, Schmidt U, Heim MU. Influence of antibiotics on posttransfusion platelet increment. Transfusion 1996;36:952-4.
8. Legler TJ, Fischer I, Dittmann J, et al. Frequency and causes of refractoriness in multiply transfused patients. Ann Hematol 1997;74:185-9.
9. Klingemann HG, Self S, Banaji M, et al. Refractoriness to random donor platelet transfusions in patients with aplastic anaemia: A multivariate analysis of data from 264 cases. Br J Haematol 1987;66:115-21.
10. Bishop JF, Matthews JP, McGrath K, et al. Factors influencing 20-hour increments after platelet transfusion. Transfusion 1991;31:392-6.
11. Bishop JF, McGrath K, Wolf MM, et al. Clinical factors influencing the efficacy of pooled platelet transfusions. Blood 1988;71:383-7.
12. Norol F, Kuentz M, Cordonnier C, et al. Influence of clinical status on the efficiency of stored platelet transfusion. Br J Haematol 1994;86:125-9.
13. Triulzi DJ, Dzik WH. Leukocyte-reduced blood components: Laboratory and clinical aspects. In: Simon TL, Snyder EL, Solheim BG, et al, eds. Rossi's principles of transfusion medicine. 4th ed. Bethesda, MD: AABB Press, 2009: 228-46.
14. Seftel MD, Growe GH, Petraszko T, et al. Universal prestorage leukoreduction in Canada decreases platelet alloimmunization and refractoriness. Blood 2004;103:333-9.
15. Boshkov LK, Kelton JG, Halloran PF. HLA-DR expression by platelets in acute idiopathic thrombocytopenic purpura. Br J Haematol 1992;81:552-7.
16. Saito S, Ota S, Seshimo H, et al. Platelet transfusion refractoriness caused by a mismatch in HLA-C antigens. Transfusion 2002;42:302-8.
17. Duquesnoy RJ. Structural epitope matching for HLA-alloimmunized thrombocytopenic patients: A new strategy to provide more effective platelet transfusion support? Transfusion 2008;48:221-7.
18. Vassallo RR. Changing paradigms in matched platelet support. Transfusion 2008;48:204-6.
19. Eernisse JG, Brand A. Prevention of platelet refractoriness due to HLA antibodies by administration of leukocyte-poor blood components. Exp Hematol 1981;9:77-83.
20. Semple JW, Freedman J. Recipient antigen-processing pathways of allogeneic platelet antigens: Essential mediators of immunity. Transfusion 2002;42:958-61.
21. Blajchman MA, Bardossy L, Carmen RA, et al. An animal model of allogeneic donor platelet refractoriness: The effect of the time of leukodepletion. Blood 1992;79:1371-5.
22. Bordin JO, Bardossy L, Blajchman MA. Experimental animal model of refractoriness to donor platelets: The effect of plasma removal and the extent of white cell reduction on allogeneic alloimmunization. Transfusion 1993;33:798-801.
23. Semple JW, Speck ER, Milev YP, et al. Indirect allorecognition of platelets by T helper cells during platelet transfusions correlates with anti-major histocompatibility complex antibody and cytotoxic T lymphocyte formation. Blood 1995;86:805-12.
24. Howard JE, Perkins HA. The natural history of alloimmunization to platelets. Transfusion 1978;18:496-503.
25. Novotny VM, van Doorn R, Witvliet MD, et al. Occurrence of allogeneic HLA and non-HLA

antibodies after transfusion of prestorage filtered platelets and red blood cells: A prospective study. Blood 1995;85:1736-41.

26. Holohan TV, Terasaki PI, Deisseroth AB. Suppression of transfusion-related alloimmunization in intensively treated cancer patients. Blood 1981;58:122-8.

27. Lee EJ, Schiffer CA. Serial measurement of lymphocytotoxic antibody and response to nonmatched platelet transfusions in alloimmunized patients. Blood 1987;70:1727-9.

28. Pamphilon DH, Farrell DH, Donaldson C, et al. Development of lymphocytotoxic and platelet reactive antibodies: A prospective study in patients with acute leukaemia. Vox Sang 1989; 57:177-81.

29. Dutcher JP, Schiffer CA, Aisner J, Wiernik PH. Alloimmunization following platelet transfusion: The absence of a dose-response relationship. Blood 1981;57:395-8.

30. Slichter SJ, O'Donnell MR, Weiden PL, et al. Canine platelet alloimmunization: The role of donor selection. Br J Haematol 1986;63:713-27.

31. Murphy MF, Metcalfe P, Ord J, et al. Disappearance of HLA and platelet-specific antibodies in acute leukaemia patients alloimmunized by multiple transfusions. Br J Haematol 1987; 67:255-60.

32. Atlas E, Freedman J, Blanchette V, et al. Downregulation of the anti-HLA alloimmune response by variable region-reactive (anti-idiotypic) antibodies in leukemic patients transfused with platelet concentrates. Blood 1993; 81:538-42.

33. Sullivan MT, Cotten R, Read EJ, Wallace EL. Blood collection and transfusion in the United States in 2001. Transfusion 2007;47:385-94.

34. Rebulla P, Finazzi G, Marangoni F, et al. The threshold for prophylactic platelet transfusions in adults with acute myeloid leukemia. Gruppo Italiano Malattie Ematologiche Maligne dell'Adulto. N Engl J Med 1997;337:1870-5.

35. Beutler E. Platelet transfusions: The 20,000/μL trigger. Blood 1993;81:1411-13.

36. Dunstan RA, Simpson MB. Heterogeneous distribution of antigens on human platelets demonstrated by fluorescence flow cytometry. Br J Haematol 1985;61:603-9.

37. Aster RH. Effect of anticoagulant and ABO incompatibility on recovery of transfused human platelets. Blood 1965;26:732-43.

38. Curtis BR, Edwards JT, Hessner MJ, et al. Blood group A and B antigens are strongly

expressed on platelets of some individuals. Blood 2000;96:1574-81.

39. Skogen B, Rossebo Hansen B, Husebekk A, et al. Minimal expression of blood group A antigen on thrombocytes from A2 individuals. Transfusion 1988;28:456-9.

40. Santoso S, Kiefel V, Mueller-Eckhardt C. Blood group A and B determinants are expressed on platelet glycoproteins IIa, IIIa, and Ib. Thromb Haemost 1991;65:196-201.

41. Hou M, Stockelberg D, Rydberg L, et al. Blood group A antigen expression in platelets is prominently associated with glycoprotein Ib and IIb. Evidence for an A1/A2 difference. Transfus Med 1996;6:51-9.

42. Cooling LL, Kelly K, Barton J, et al. Determinants of ABH expression on human blood platelets. Blood 2005;105:3356-64.

43. Ogasawara K, Ueki J, Takenaka M, Furihata K. Study on the expression of ABH antigens on platelets. Blood 1993;82:993-9.

44. Heal JM, Rowe JM, McMican A, et al. The role of ABO matching in platelet transfusion. Eur J Haematol 1993;50:110-17.

45. Heal JM, Rowe JM, Blumberg N. ABO and platelet transfusion revisited. Ann Hematol 1993;66:309-14.

46. Heal JM, Kenmotsu N, Rowe JM, Blumberg N. A possible survival advantage in adults with acute leukemia receiving ABO-identical platelet transfusions. Am J Hematol 1994;45:189-90.

47. Carr R, Hutton JL, Jenkins JA, et al. Transfusion of ABO-mismatched platelets leads to early platelet refractoriness. Br J Haematol 1990; 75:408-13.

48. Heim D, Passweg J, Gregor M, et al. Patient and product factors affecting platelet transfusion results. Transfusion 2008;48:681-7.

49. Heal JM, Masel D, Blumberg N. Interaction of platelet fc and complement receptors with circulating immune complexes involving the ABO system. Vox Sang 1996;71:205-11.

50. Heal JM, Masel D, Rowe JM, Blumberg N. Circulating immune complexes involving the ABO system after platelet transfusion. Br J Haematol 1993;85:566-72.

51. Santoso S. Human platelet alloantigens. Transfus Apher Sci 2003;28:227-36.

52. Blumberg N, McFarland J. Human leukocyte and platelet antigens. In: Kaushansky K, Lichtman M, Beutler E, et al, eds. Williams hematology. New York: McGraw Hill Professional, 2010 (in press).

53. Santoso S, Kroll H, Andrei-Selmer CL, et al. A naturally occurring LeuVal mutation in beta3-integrin impairs the HPA-1a epitope: The third allele of HPA-1. Transfusion 2006;46:790-9.

54. Peters AM, Porter JB, Saverymuttu SH, et al. The kinetics of unmatched and HLA-matched ^{111}In-labelled homologous platelets in recipients with chronic marrow hypoplasia and anti-platelet immunity. Br J Haematol 1985;60:117-27.

55. Taaning E, Jacobsen N, Morling N. Graft-derived anti-HPA-2b production after allogeneic bone-marrow transplantation. Br J Haematol 1994;86:651-3.

56. Murata M, Furihata K, Ishida F, et al. Genetic and structural characterization of an amino acid dimorphism in glycoprotein Ib alpha involved in platelet transfusion refractoriness. Blood 1992;79:3086-90.

57. Saji H, Maruya E, Fujii H, et al. New platelet antigen, Siba, involved in platelet transfusion refractoriness in a Japanese man. Vox Sang 1989;56:283-7.

58. Uhrynowska M, Zupanska B. Platelet-specific antibodies in transfused patients. Eur J Haematol 1996;56:248-51.

59. Langenscheidt F, Kiefel V, Santoso S, Mueller-Eckhardt C. Platelet transfusion refractoriness associated with two rare platelet-specific alloantibodies (anti-Baka and anti-PlA2) and multiple HLA antibodies. Transfusion 1988;28:597-600.

60. Curtis BR, Aster RH. Incidence of the Nak(a)-negative platelet phenotype in African Americans is similar to that of Asians. Transfusion 1996;36:331-4.

61. Lee K, Godeau B, Fromont P, et al. CD36 deficiency is frequent and can cause platelet immunization in Africans. Transfusion 1999;39:873-9.

62. O'Connell B, Lee EJ, Schiffer CA. The value of 10-minute posttransfusion platelet counts. Transfusion 1988;28:66-7.

63. Brubaker DB, Marcus C, Holmes E. Intravascular and total body platelet equilibrium in healthy volunteers and in thrombocytopenic patients transfused with single donor platelets. Am J Hematol 1998;58:165-76.

64. Slichter SJ, Davis K, Enright H, et al. Factors affecting posttransfusion platelet increments, platelet refractoriness, and platelet transfusion intervals in thrombocytopenic patients. Blood 2005;105:4106-14.

65. Contreras M. Consensus conference on platelet transfusion. Final statement. Blood Rev 1998;12:239-40.

66. Hogge DE, Dutcher JP, Aisner J, Schiffer CA. Lymphocytotoxic antibody is a predictor of response to random donor platelet transfusion. Am J Hematol 1983;14:363-9.

67. Gebel HM, Bray RA. Sensitization and sensitivity: Defining the unsensitized patient. Transplantation 2000;69:1370-4.

68. Bray RA, Nolen JD, Larsen C, et al. Transplanting the highly sensitized patient: The Emory algorithm. Am J Transplant 2006;6:2307-15.

69. Rachel JM, Sinor LT, Tawfik OW, et al. A solid-phase red cell adherence test for platelet cross-matching. Med Lab Sci 1985;42:194-5.

70. Lown JA, Ivey JG. Evaluation of a solid phase red cell adherence technique for platelet antibody screening. Transfus Med 1991;1:163-7.

71. Neumuller J, Tohidast-Akrad M, Fischer M, Mayr WR. Influence of chloroquine or acid treatment of human platelets on the antigenicity of HLA and the 'thrombocyte-specific' glycoproteins Ia/IIa, IIb, and IIb/IIIa. Vox Sang 1993;65:223-31.

72. Ziman A, Klapper E, Pepkowitz S, et al. A second case of post-transfusion purpura caused by HPA-5a antibodies: Successful treatment with intravenous immunoglobulin. Vox Sang 2002;83:165-6.

73. Curtis BR, McFarland JG. Platelet immunology and alloimmunization. In: Simon TL, Snyder EL, Solheim BG, et al, eds. Rossi's principles of transfusion medicine. 4th ed. Bethesda, MD: AABB Press, 2009:168-86.

74. Duquesnoy RJ. Donor selection in platelet transfusion therapy of alloimmunized thrombocytopenic patients. In: Greenwalt TJ, Jamieson GA, eds. The blood platelet in transfuion therapy. New York: Alan R. Liss, 1978:229-43.

75. McFarland JG, Larson EB, Hillman RS, Slichter SJ. Cost-benefit analysis of a plateletapheresis program. Transfusion 1986;26:91-7.

76. Schwartz BD, Luehrman LK, Lee J, Rodey GE. A public antigenic determinant in the HLA-B5 cross-reacting group—a basis for cross-reactivity and a possible link with Behcet's disease. Hum Immunol 1980;1:37-54.

77. Schwartz BD, Luehrman LK, Rodey GE. Public antigenic determinant on a family of HLA-B molecules. J Clin Invest 1979;64:938-47.

78. King KE, Ness PM, Braine HG, Armstrong KS. Racial differences in the availability of human

leukocyte antigen-matched platelets. J Clin Apher 1996;11:71-7.

79. Jorgensen DW, McFarland JG, Hillman RS, Slichter SJ. Plateletapheresis program. II. Computer selection of HLA compatible donors. Transfusion 1984;24:292-8.

80. Dahlke MB, Weiss KL. Platelet transfusion from donors mismatched for crossreactive HLA antigens. Transfusion 1984;24:299-302.

81. Hussein MA, Lee EJ, Fletcher R, Schiffer CA. The effect of lymphocytotoxic antibody reactivity on the results of single antigen mismatched platelet transfusions to alloimmunized patients. Blood 1996;87:3959-62.

82. Szatkowski NS, Aster RH. HLA antigens of platelets. IV. Influence of "private" HLA-B locus specificities on the expression of Bw4 and Bw6 on human platelets. Tissue Antigens 1980;15:361-8.

83. Schiffer CA, O'Connell B, Lee EJ. Platelet transfusion therapy for alloimmunized patients: Selective mismatching for HLA B12, an antigen with variable expression on platelets. Blood 1989;74:1172-6.

84. Petz LD, Garratty G, Calhoun L, et al. Selecting donors of platelets for refractory patients on the basis of HLA antibody specificity. Transfusion 2000;40:1446-56.

85. Zimmermann R, Wittmann G, Zingsem J, et al. Antibodies to private and public HLA Class I epitopes in platelet recipients. Transfusion 1999;39:772-80.

86. Tait BD. Solid phase assays for HLA antibody detection in clinical transplantation. Curr Opin Immunol 2009;21:573-7.

87. Tait BD, Hudson F, Cantwell L, et al. Review article: Luminex technology for HLA antibody detection in organ transplantation. Nephrology (Carlton) 2009;14:247-54.

88. Tambur AR, Ramon DS, Kaufman DB, et al. Perception versus reality?: Virtual crossmatch—how to overcome some of the technical and logistic limitations. Am J Transplant 2009;9:1886-93.

89. Duquesnoy RJ. HLA Matchmaker: A molecularly based algorithm for histocompatibility determination. I. Description of the algorithm. Hum Immunol 2002;63:339-52.

90. Nambiar A, Duquesnoy RJ, Adams S, et al. HLAMatchmaker-driven analysis of responses to HLA-typed platelet transfusions in alloimmunized thrombocytopenic patients. Blood 2006;107:1680-7.

91. Zeigler ZR, Shadduck RK, Rosenfeld CS, et al. Intravenous gamma globulin decreases platelet-associated IgG and improves transfusion responses in platelet refractory states. Am J Hematol 1991;38:15-23.

92. Schnaidt M, Northoff H, Wernet D. Frequency and specificity of platelet-specific alloantibodies in HLA-immunized haematologic-oncologic patients. Transfus Med 1996;6:111-14.

93. Skodlar J, Bolgiano D, Teramura G, Slichter SJ. Distinguishing between mechanisms of platelet refractoriness: Abnormal post-storage platelet viability vs immune destruction (abstract). Blood 1992;90(Suppl 1):1030a.

94. Bock M, Heim MU, Schleich I, et al. Platelet crossmatching with Capture P: Clinical relevance. Infusionstherapie 1989;16:183-5.

95. Shibata Y, Juji T, Nishizawa Y, et al. Detection of platelet antibodies by a newly developed mixed agglutination with platelets. Vox Sang 1981;41:25-31.

96. Rachel JM, Summers TC, Sinor LT, Plapp FV. Use of a solid phase red blood cell adherence method for pretransfusion platelet compatibility testing Am J Clin Pathol 1988;90:63-8.

97. Freedman J, Hooi C, Garvey MB. Prospective platelet crossmatching for selection of compatible random donors. Br J Haematol 1984;56:9-18.

98. O'Connell BA, Schiffer CA. Donor selection for alloimmunized patients by platelet crossmatching of random-donor platelet concentrates. Transfusion 1990;30:314-17.

99. O'Connell BA, Lee EJ, Rothko K, et al. Selection of histocompatible apheresis platelet donors by cross-matching random donor platelet concentrates. Blood 1992;79:527-31.

100. Moroff G, Garratty G, Heal JM, et al. Selection of platelets for refractory patients by HLA matching and prospective crossmatching. Transfusion 1992;32:633-40.

101. Friedberg RC, Donnelly SF, Mintz PD. Independent roles for platelet crossmatching and HLA in the selection of platelets for alloimmunized patients. Transfusion 1994;34:215-20.

102. Friedberg RC, Donnelly SF, Boyd JC, et al. Clinical and blood bank factors in the management of platelet refractoriness and alloimmunization. Blood 1993;81:3428-34.

103. Sintnicolaas K, Lowenberg B. A flow cytometric platelet immunofluorescence crossmatch for predicting successful HLA matched platelet transfusions. Br J Haematol 1996;92:1005-10.

In: McLeod BC, Szczepiorkowski ZM, Weinstein R, Winters JL, eds.
Apheresis: Principles and Practice, 3rd edition
Bethesda, MD: AABB Press, 2010

10

Bacterial Contamination of Platelet Products

Sara C. Koenig, MD; Mark E. Brecher, MD; and Yara A. Park, MD

 OVER THE PAST THREE DEcades, significant improvements have been made in reducing the risk of viral transmission by transfusion.[1-3] For several reasons, much less attention has been paid to the issue of bacterial contamination of blood components until the last decade. First, transfusion-related sepsis, while a significant cause of morbidity and mortality, received less public attention than did human immunodeficiency virus and hepatitis C virus. Unlike those agents, bacteria do not cause a chronic disease; in general, either recovery or death rapidly follows acute bacterial infection. In the absence of a large cohort of patients with chronic disease clamoring for resolution of their problem and the resulting media coverage, this risk never gained significant public recognition.

Although the overall bacterial contamination rate of red cell components is similar to that of platelet components,[1(p257)] differences in how the two components are stored account for a large discrepancy between rates of transfusion-related infection in recipients of these components. Red cells are refrigerated products, stored at 1 to 6 C; significant bacterial growth at these temperatures is uncommon and is principally limited to a few gram-negative organisms. Bacteria cannot proliferate in frozen plasma and cryoprecipitate (although there are rare reports of contamination of these components by waterborne organisms in the water baths used for thawing[4,5]). In contrast, platelets

Sara C. Koenig, MD, Fellow, University of North Carolina, Chapel Hill, North Carolina; Mark E. Brecher, MD, Chief Medical Officer, Laboratory Corporation of America, Burlington, North Carolina, and Adjunct Professor, University of North Carolina, Chapel Hill, North Carolina; and Yara A. Park, MD, Assistant Professor, University of North Carolina, Chapel Hill, North Carolina

S. Koenig and Y. Park have disclosed no conflicts of interest. M. Brecher has disclosed financial relationships with bioMérieux, Pall, Fenwal, Verax, and Cerus.

must be stored at 20 to 24 C, which is a favorable temperature for bacteria proliferation.

Multiple studies using aerobic culture systems have shown that 1 in 1000 to 1 in 3000 platelet units are contaminated with bacteria.[6-9] Based on data estimating that a severe episode of transfusion-associated bacterial sepsis occurs with one-sixth of contaminated units[10] and that one-fifth to one-third of the clinically significant septic infections result in death,[11-13] the risk of death from sepsis is estimated between 1 in 18,000 and 1 in 100,000 per platelet unit transfused. This estimate is consistent with a 2001 publication from The Johns Hopkins Hospital reporting a fatality rate of 1 in 17,000 with pooled, whole-blood-derived (WBD) platelets, and 1 in 61,000 with apheresis platelets.[14] In 2000, University Hospitals of Cleveland reported a fatality rate of 1 in 48,000 per WBD platelet unit.[15] From October 1, 1995 to September 30, 2004, 85 deaths from transfusion-transmitted bacterial infections were reported to the US Food and Drug Administration (FDA),[16] with an average of 11.7 deaths per year between 2001 and 2003.[3] From 1986 to 1991, 29 fatalities from bacterial contamination were reported to the FDA,[17] and from 1976 to 1985, 26 such fatalities were reported.[18] Reported cases may represent only a fraction of the total, however, as the relationship to transfusion may not be recognized clinically in all cases.

By the early part of this century, a vocal cohort of concerned members of the blood banking community brought the issue of transfusion-related sepsis to the forefront of the debate on infectious disease testing in blood banking and transfusion medicine through an open letter to the transfusion medicine community. As a result, in 2002, the College of American Pathologists (CAP) added a phase 1 item to its laboratory accreditation checklist, requiring laboratories to have a "system to detect the presence of bacteria in platelet components."[19] Similarly, in 2003, the AABB added a new standard to its *Standards for Blood Banks and Transfusion Services,* requiring accredited facilities to have a process to limit and detect bacterial contamination in all platelet components.[20]

This standard was later changed to address the emerging interest in pathogen-inactivation technologies, as discussed later.

By mandating procedures to limit and detect bacterial contamination in platelet components, AABB and CAP were a force for addressing concerns of component safety. From a practical perspective, a culture-based system was feasible with apheresis platelet units because of their larger volume, but such an approach was not appropriate for WBD platelets in countries where prepooling of WBD platelets was not allowed. As a result, in such countries, two testing models have emerged. Apheresis platelets are tested with a liquid culture-based system; those with a positive culture are immediately withdrawn from available inventory, and confirmatory testing is performed on the component. Alternative, less sensitive methods of bacteria detection have been used for WBD platelets, most commonly pH and/or glucose measurements performed just before platelet pooling.[21] However, the AABB requires the use of FDA-approved methods or those validated to have equivalent sensitivity.[22]

The full effect of the AABB and CAP requirements addressing the risk of bacterial contamination of platelet components may not become clear for a number of years; however, preliminary studies comparing the rates of clinical bacterial infection before and after these measures were put in place are encouraging. According to FDA data, mortality from bacterially contaminated apheresis platelet components declined precipitously from an average of 9.4 cases per year between 1995 and 2004[16] to 1 fatality per year between 2006 and 2008.[23] A review of a total of 49,625 platelet transfusions at The Johns Hopkins Hospital after implementation of bacteria testing of apheresis platelets showed a 67% decrease in septic transfusion reactions—from 6.6 to 2.0 per 100,000 platelet transfusions (Fig 10-1).[24] The American Red Cross estimated the residual risk of a septic transfusion reaction from its apheresis platelet components at 1 in 74,807 after implementation of screening for bacterial contamination, with a fatality rate of 1 in 498,711 per transfused unit.[25] The estimate represents a

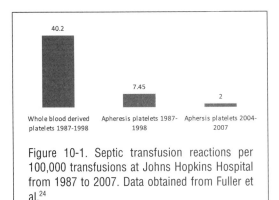

Figure 10-1. Septic transfusion reactions per 100,000 transfusions at Johns Hopkins Hospital from 1987 to 2007. Data obtained from Fuller et al.[24]

decrease of approximately 50% in reaction and fatality rates from those observed before implementation of bacterial detection. It should be noted that reaction and fatality rates from WBD platelets tested for pH and/or glucose levels were not examined.

Clinical Presentation of Septic Transfusion Reactions

There are several challenges in the accurate and timely diagnosis of transfusion-related bacterial sepsis. The clinical presentation of sepsis related to platelet transfusions is more varied and often less severe than that of sepsis related to contaminated red cell components.[26] The patients who are most likely to receive platelet transfusions are those with compromised immune systems, primarily hematology/oncology and transplant patients, many of whom are on chemotherapy or other immunosuppressant regimens (Fig 10-2).[2,24,27] These patients may not exhibit the typical signs and symptoms of infection, such as fever. Additionally, fever in these patients may be attributed to other causes, and shock and death may be ascribed to underlying illness. Milder reactions may not be easily distinguished from febrile non-hemolytic transfusion reactions. A delay in onset of clinical manifestations of infection can also contribute to missed diagnoses. For example, an outbreak of *Salmonella cholerasuis* sepsis affecting seven patients at the National Institutes of Health Clinical Care Center was traced to a repeat platelet donor subsequently found to have an occult chronic osteomyelitis. The onset of illness in these recipients ranged from 5 to 12 days (mean = 8.6) after transfusion of the implicated units.[28] In another case, the death of a WBD platelet recipient caused by *Serratia liquefaciens* sepsis was not recognized to be related to the platelet transfusion until investigation connected the platelets to a whole blood donation from which the red cells had been implicated in a case of sepsis.[29]

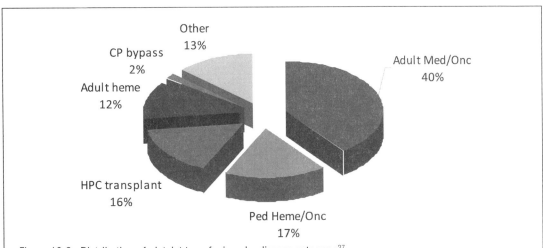

Figure 10-2. Distribution of platelet transfusions by disease category.[27]
Med/Onc = medical oncology; Heme/Onc = hematology/oncology; HPC = hematopoietic progenitor cell; heme = hematology; CP = cardiopulmonary.

Organisms and Sources

Although skin commensal bacteria such as *Staphylococcal* and *Streptococcal* species are the most commonly reported contaminating organisms in platelet concentrates (Fig 10-3), gram-negative bacteria (mostly *Enterobacteriaceae*) account for the majority of fatalities.[21,30] Combined data from the Bacterial Contamination (BaCon), Serious Hazards of Transfusion (SHOT), and BACTHEM (part of the French hemovigilance system) studies show an overall fatality risk of 10% in transfusion-related infection with gram-positive organisms and 45% in cases of sepsis with gram-negative organisms.[21] In transfusion-related fatalities involving platelet components reported to the FDA from 1976 to 1998, *Staphylococcus aureus*, *S. epidermidis*, and *Streptococcus* and *Bacillus* species were the most frequently reported gram-positive organisms.[31] Gram-negative organisms—in particular, *Escherichia coli* and *Klebsiella* and *Serratia* species—are implicated in the majority of deaths caused by transfusion-associated sepsis.[23,31]

In some cases, the source of the bacterial contamination is not readily identified. Donor bacteremia may be asymptomatic and donors may not be aware of risk factors without explicit questioning. An example is a report of *Salmonella enteric* sepsis in two patients who were recipients of apheresis platelet components from the same donor. Upon follow-up questioning, it was found that the donor owned a pet boa constrictor and was treated with antibiotics for bloody diarrhea before his donation.[32] Another unusual case involved a platelet pool that resulted in a fatal septic transfusion reaction in a leukemic patient. The contaminating organism, *Clostridium perfringens*, was subsequently cultured from the antecubital skin of one of the donors, who had two young children and frequently changed their diapers.[33] Other cases have been associated with scarring or dimpling of skin at the venipuncture sites as a result of repeated donations. Such areas may contain recessed pits that are difficult to disinfect adequately during the arm scrub. In one report, three episodes of platelet contamination, resulting in four cases of gram-positive sepsis in recipients, were traced to a single donor with a "dimpled" venipuncture site.[34]

Methods to Reduce the Risk of Transfusion-Acquired Sepsis

Broadly speaking, three approaches are being used to avoid bacterial transfusion-related sep-

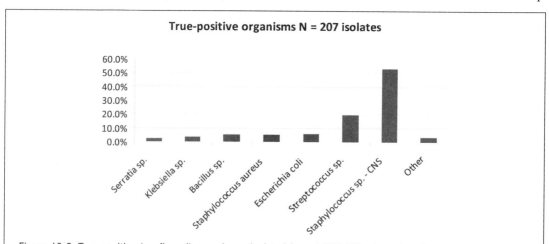

Figure 10-3. True-positive (confirmed) organisms, isolated from 1,237,177 apheresis cultures tested with 4 mL in an aerobic BacT/ALERT bottle. Examples of organisms isolated only once or twice were grouped in the "other" category. These included examples of *Micrococcus* sp., *Diptheroids/Corynebacterium*, *Enterococcus avium* (n = 2), *Granulicatella adiacens*, *Citrobacter* sp., *Lactobacillus* sp., and *Enterobacter aerogenes*. (Adapted from Pietersz et al.[30])

sis from platelet components, although variability exists in their implementation among blood collection centers and transfusion services within the United States, and further differences exist between protocols used in the United States and those used in Canada and several European countries. The first and perhaps most obvious tactic is to prevent bacterial contamination of the components. The second is to detect contaminated units before issue in order to prevent infection of a recipient. The third approach is to inhibit, inactivate, or destroy pathogens that may be present in the component, a tactic that has seen partial adoption in Europe.

Avoidance of Bacterial Contamination

Donor Screening

To some extent, reduction of bacterial contamination is achieved through the process of donor screening. The presence of fever (body temperature >37.5 C or 99.5 F) requires deferral.[35(p162)] The donor history questionnaire contains several questions designed to exclude donors with possible bacteremia, including those addressing the donor's subjective state of health, current antibiotic use, and any other current medications.[35(p165)] Individual blood centers may set additional limitations on donor eligibility, such as those pertaining to breastfeeding, recent dental work, or the presence of an atrophic or paralytic neurologic disease that may predispose the donor to urinary tract infection.[36-37] A downside to such short term deferrals is a significant negative impact on the likelihood of subsequent donations.[38] Unfortunately, signs and symptoms of bacteremia may be absent, as in the case of the patient with occult chronic osteomyelitis mentioned earlier.[28] In particular, questioning donors about gastrointestinal (GI) symptoms has been shown to lack specificity and sensitivity. In one study, 13% of donors reported GI symptoms in the 30 days before donation.[39] Conversely, when questioned retrospectively, only half of donors implicated in *Yersinia enterocolitica* red cell

transfusion-related sepsis described GI symptoms in the 30 days before donation.[40-42]

Blood Collection Practices

Skin Preparation. Contamination at the time of blood collection is the most frequent cause of bacterial contamination of platelet components.[43] Skin disinfection, although of proven benefit in reducing skin bacterial load, does not sterilize the phlebotomy site. The adequacy of disinfection, technique employed, timing of disinfection, and training of the phlebotomists all contribute to reducing the risk of contamination.[44] Even with the most meticulous preparation, however, a sterile venipuncture site cannot be guaranteed because microorganisms exist in sebaceous glands and hair follicles that may be inaccessible to the disinfectant. This fact is reflected in the relatively high rate of false-positive blood cultures caused by skin contamination in clinical practice. Several studies have demonstrated that 1% to 3% of blood cultures are contaminated with skin flora, even when the samples are collected by highly trained personnel.[45] In the donation scenario, such organisms may be present in skin fragments drawn into the component bag at the time of venipuncture. They proliferate during storage and can become a significant inoculum for the recipient.[46-47] Areas of pitting and scarring provide a particular challenge to disinfection because bacteria can be present in areas inaccessible to the topical disinfectant.[34]

Typically, a tincture of iodine, providone iodine, or chlorhexidine is used for skin preparation before donation.[2,48] The use of a protocol using a cetrimide/chlorhexidine disinfectant solution followed by isopropyl alcohol has also been studied but showed no benefit over the use of providone-iodine followed by isopropyl alcohol.[48] The skin of donors who are allergic to iodine is often cleansed with a chlorhexidine solution or by a method in which the venipuncture site is scrubbed twice with isopropyl alcohol.[2] The use of green soap has been explicitly prohibited by AABB standards[49(p21)] because of unacceptable levels of contamination. In one study, 13 of 30 subjects grew more bacterial colonies after skin decontamination with green soap and isopropyl alcohol than before disinfection.[50]

Even with appropriate disinfectant selection, reagent contamination may remain a threat. Skin disinfection materials, including swab sticks impregnated with iodine or alcohol, have been reported to be contaminated with various bacterial species,[43] although no instances of blood component contamination from such sources have been reported.

Diversion of Initial Blood Draw. Several studies have demonstrated a reduction in the rate of bacterial contamination during whole blood collection by diverting the first 10 to 15 mL of donor blood drawn. In one study, a French group cultured the first and second 15 mL aliquots from 3385 donations. Although contamination was found in 76 (2.2%) of the first 15 mL samples, only 21 of the second 15 mL aliquots were culture positive, suggesting that diversion of the first 15 mL may have prevented the contamination of 55 of the 76 primary product bags.[51] Several other studies have reported 40% to 90% reductions in bacterial load introduced into blood components through the removal of the initial 10 to 40 mL of blood following venipuncture.[51-55] As would be expected, diversion is most effective in decreasing the rate of contamination with skin flora.[51,54] This limits its effectiveness against fatal septic transfusion reactions because the majority of such reactions are caused by gram-negative organisms, which are more likely to be present with asymptomatic donor bacteremia and therefore not intercepted by diversion.

Apheresis Collection vs Pooling. Because bacterial contamination results from donor-specific factors, it might be expected that pooled platelet components should have a higher risk of contamination than apheresis platelets. This supposition is supported by studies from The Johns Hopkins Hospitals and University Hospitals of Cleveland. From 1986 to 1998, the incidence of septic events related to platelet transfusions at Johns Hopkins decreased from 1 in 4818 to 1 in 15,098 transfusions as the hospital transitioned from administering 48.3% random platelet pools to 99.4% apheresis

platelet components.[14] The overall clinical sepsis rates were approximately 1 in 2500 for WBD components and 1 in 13,400 for apheresis components, whereas contamination-related mortality rates were approximately 1 in 17,000 and 1 in 61,000, respectively.[14] University Hospitals of Cleveland cultured all apheresis and WBD platelets at issue and reported a culture positivity rate of 1 in 2184 for apheresis platelets and 1 in 1821 for WBD platelet components.[56] Transfusion of the latter in pools of 6 units would be predicted to result in a culture-positivity rate of about 1 in 310 transfusions. It should also be noted that a septic reaction to a 6-unit pool implicates five donors whose blood may not be contaminated. Nevertheless, related components from these donors must be pulled from inventory and discarded at a significant financial loss.

Bacteria Detection

Bacteria detection techniques vary in complexity and sensitivity but follow a general rule: the more rapid an assay, the lower its sensitivity. Because of this, many of the older, less sophisticated techniques of screening for contamination have been replaced with newer culture-based assays. Approaches to testing vary according to the type of platelet component, as discussed earlier. Apheresis platelets are typically tested with a culture-based system in which sampling occurs at least 24 hours after collection to allow time for a small inoculum to grow, if present, increasing the likelihood that bacteria will be present in the small sample taken for culture. Culture-based methods are effective only when the culture becomes positive while the platelet component is still in inventory. Platelets from whole blood are generally evaluated for bacterial contamination at the time of issue, but available methods are significantly less sensitive than the culture-based methods. Two major technologies, the Verax Platelet Pan Genera Detection (PGD) Test (Verax Biomedical, Inc, Worcester, MA) and the Acrodose PL system (Pall Medical, East Hills, NY), described in the sections that follow, have recently emerged to address the challenge of detecting bacterial contamination in WBD platelets since the promulgation of AABB and CAP requirements.

Acrodose PL System

In 2005, the FDA licensed the Pall Acrodose PL system for the production of prestorage, prepooled, leukocyte-reduced, WBD platelets. In this system, bacterial culture testing of WBD platelets is performed at the manufacturing blood center using either the enhanced Bacterial Detection System (eBDS, Pall Medical), a second-generation assay that replaced the original Pall BDS, or the BacT/ALERT 3D (bioMérieux, Durham, NC) culture system. After collection and processing, 4 to 5 ABO-identical WBD platelet concentrates are pooled using sterile connections into a single 1.5-L storage bag. The volume of the platelets after pooling is large enough that an adequate sample can be removed for bacterial culture without reducing the overall platelet content to an unacceptable level. This allows the significantly more sensitive culture-based methods to be applied to WBD platelets, avoiding the less sensitive surrogate markers that are currently used at the point of issue for this component. In one study by the American Red Cross, the rate of bacteria detection using the Acrodose system for 5 pooled units of platelets was 5.8 times the rate of detection for apheresis platelets.[57] This likely reflects the effect of an increased number of donors, with the corresponding increased number of venipunctures needed to create these pools.

Bacteria Growth Characteristics and the Timing of Detection

Initial bacterial concentrations in blood components at the time of collection may be less than 1 colony-forming unit (CFU) per mL.[58] In contrast to viral testing, where much of the methodology depends on the measurement of antibodies to viral antigens, bacterial culture depends on detecting a minimum threshold population of organisms. During storage at 22 C, bacteria proliferate readily, resulting in a much higher bacterial load at the time of transfusion (often on day 4 or 5) than at the time of collection. Thus, it is crucial to consider the kinetics of bacterial growth, the relative sensitivities of different detection methods, and the timing of component sampling when establishing guidelines for bacterial culture detection for platelets. This must be reconciled with an understanding of the direct relationship between 1) the virulence of the particular bacterial species and the bacterial load and 2) the clinical severity of a septic transfusion reaction.

In a study from University Hospitals at Case Medical Center in Cleveland, Ohio, using a combination of passive and active surveillance over a 15-year period, the clinical severity of each transfusion reaction was graded and correlated with the bacterial load in a culture at the time of transfusion and the species detected in the contaminated units. Reaction severity was defined on a 5-point scale, from no reaction to fatal septic reaction. Grade 3 represented a severe reaction, defined as a change in vital signs requiring intervention, and grade 2 was defined as a change in vital signs resolving in 24 hours and requiring minimal or no intervention. In the analysis of 44 culture-positive units transfused, all severe reactions (grade 3 or above) were associated with bacterial loads of $\geq 10^5$ CFU/mL and/or more virulent bacteria species (*Pseudomonas aeruginosa*, *Serratia marcescens*, *Staphylococcus aureus*, *Bacillus cereus* and *Streptococcus bovis*).[59] An ideal system would be capable of detecting extremely low levels of highly virulent species, such as endotoxin-producing gram-negative bacteria, and be capable of detecting clinically significant levels of other pathogens.

In a study of bacterial growth characteristics, 165 platelet units were inoculated on the day of collection with 1 to 1000 CFU/mL of one of the following: *B. cereus*, *P. aeruginosa*, *Klebsiella pneumoniae*, *S. marcescens*, *S. aureus*, or *S. epidermidis*.[60] All examples of *B. cereus*, *P. aeruginosa*, *K. pneumoniae*, *S. marcescens*, and *S. aureus* had concentrations $\geq 10^2$ CFU/mL by day 3 following inoculation. By day 4, all units with these organisms contained $\geq 10^5$ CFU/mL. Units contaminated with *S. epidermidis* showed slower and more varied growth.[60] This study suggests that an assay capable of detecting 100 CFU/mL on day 3 of storage would detect the vast majority of contaminated platelets. It also demonstrated that with a variety of organisms, plateau growth is typically achieved by day 3 or 4 of storage. Such studies suggest that detection would be optimized if sufficient time is allowed for bacteria proliferation before sampling.

Bacterial Culture

BioMerieux BacT/ALERT. The BacT/ALERT is an automated liquid culture system that is widely used in clinical microbiology laboratories. Typically, 4 to 8 mL of platelet component is added to an aerobic culture bottle (and possibly an anaerobic culture bottle as well) and incubated for 5 to 7 days. A closed system is maintained during sampling so that component outdate is not altered. A colorimetric sensor at the bottom of the culture bottles changes color in the presence of carbon dioxide produced by bacteria. The readout from the sensor is monitored at approximately 10-minute intervals by an automated system, and computer software evaluates both the absolute degree and the rate of change. Two studies have validated this instrument with 15 bacterial species inoculated into day-2 apheresis platelets at concentrations of 10 and 100 CFU/mL. The mean time to detection in replicate 10-CFU/mL cultures was less than 25.6 hours for all bacterial species tested except *Propionibacterium acnes*, which is of questionable clinical significance.[61,62] Culture bottles used in this system have since been upgraded to eliminate venting of the aerobic bottle and to replace a sensor disk with an emulsion-based colorimetric sensor. These bottles have been shown to be equivalent for bacterial detection in apheresis platelets.[63]

The question of whether to use a single aerobic bottle or both an aerobic and anaerobic bottle for culture has been explored in a number of studies. Although most bacteria implicated in septic transfusion reactions are aerobic organisms, certain aerobic bacteria grow faster in the anaerobic bottle, mostly likely because of differences in the nutrient broth. This difference in time may be most significant at very low levels of inoculum. Considering that most centers use a 4-mL inoculum per bottle, use of an anaerobic bottle in addition to the standard aerobic bottle could reduce the time to detection of bacteria and thus prevent the transfusion of contaminated units. Alternatively, some proponents of the one-bottle system argue that increasing the size of the inoculum in the aerobic bottle, instead of splitting the tested volume of platelets between two bottles, would achieve a similar reduction in time to detection. One study comparing the one- and two-bottle culture systems for bacterial detection in apheresis platelets did not show a statistically significant increase in the yield of true-positive cases with the use of the two-bottle system.[64] This study also confirmed the decreased time to positive results for selected organisms in the anaerobic bottle when compared to the aerobic bottle, although for those culture results deemed to be true positives (ie, showing growth in both the culture bottle and the platelet component and/or blood culture from the transfused patient), both bottles turned positive before the units were released (after 24 hours), resulting in no change in clinical outcome.[64]

Pall eBDS. In a second culture system that is used for monitoring platelet contamination, the Pall eBDS samples are again obtained from the platelet component in a way that maintains a closed system. Approximately 2 to 3 mL of leukocyte-reduced platelet concentrate passes into a culture bag fitted with a one-way valve.[65] The culture bag contains trypticase soy broth (TSB) and sodium polyanethol sulfonate (SPS).[65] The TSB provides an excellent culture medium for bacterial growth, and the SPS neutralizes naturally occurring bacterial inhibitors in blood. The SPS also induces aggregation of platelets, reducing any platelet oxygen metabolism that could confound the test results. After incubation, the oxygen content in the space above the sample (head space) is read on the gas analyzer included with the Pall eBDS system.[65] Oxygen content of 9.4% or less is considered positive for bacterial growth.[65]

The Pall eBDS differs from the original Pall BDS in that it lacks a filter, which had been shown to reduce the sensitivity of the culture, and that incubation temperature is constant at 35 C, rather than 35 C for the first 24 hours and 22 C thereafter.[65] A study comparing the Pall eBDS with the BacT/ALERT system showed similar sensitivities between the systems, both on the order of 1 CFU/mL for the most common clinically significant contaminants.[65] One notable drawback of the Pall eBDS is that because it measures oxygen consumption, it is not designed to detect anaerobic organisms.

Molecular-Based Bacteria Detection

The high sensitivity and specificity of molecular techniques make them appealing for detection of bacteria in blood components. However, a number of factors limit the direct application of broad-range bacteria nucleic acid amplification to components. Among the most important of these are 1) contamination of laboratory materials and polymerase chain reaction (PCR) reagents (particularly the bacteria-derived enzymes) by bacteria DNA and 2) the presence of blood-associated bacteria DNA sequences.

Flow Cytometry

Several groups have developed methods based on flow cytometry to detect bacterial contamination in platelets.[66] Advantages of this approach include the ability to distinguish viable bacteria from nonviable bacteria by using cellular enzymes to cleave fluorochromes, causing fluorescence of viable bacteria.[66] Evolving technology in this field represents a potentially useful method for point-of-issue testing, requiring little sample volume and providing relatively quick results.

Verax Platelet PGD Test

The Verax Platelet PGD system is a rapid, qualitative immunoassay for the detection of aerobic and anaerobic gram-positive and gram-negative bacteria in leukocyte-reduced apheresis platelets.[67] It is currently approved by the FDA as an adjunct quality control measure to licensed culture-based testing methods.[2] The PGD system is a single-use, lateral-flow device. After mixing with a reagent, a drop of resuspended platelet pellet is placed into a central sample well. Capillary action simultaneously pulls the sample into two oppositely positioned immunoassay columns impregnated with dye, which test for the presence of the conserved antigens lipoteichoic acid (LTA) or lipopolysaccharide (LPS) found on gram-positive and gram-negative bacteria, respectively. A precipitation line in either test result window indicates a positive result. This test suffers from drawbacks common to other immunoassay platforms. False positives may occur in the presence of heterophile antibodies, hypergammaglobulinemia, or autoantibodies, most notably rheumatoid factor.[67] Unlike nucleic-acid-based testing platforms, the PGD system does not require extensive purification of the sample or dedicated clean working space. The level of sensitivity is 10^4 to 10^5 CFU/mL.

Other Methods of Bacteria Detection

Microscopic Examination. Microscopic examination of gram-stained samples is an inexpensive method that is relatively insensitive, particularly when components are tested early in their shelf-life. One study found 80% sensitivity and 99.96% specificity in platelets aged 1 to 5 days.[10] In 4- to 5-day-old platelets, the sensitivity improved to 100%, with a specificity of 99.93%. The reported bacteria surveillance program using culture and Gram's stain evolved over time. It was first limited to components implicated in reactions. It was then extended to all pooled platelet concentrates and eventually to all platelets stored for 4 and 5 days (in addition to reaction-associated concentrates).[10] Less promising results were obtained in a study of 5334 platelet units in which only two of eight positive Gram's stains were confirmed by a positive culture.[68]

Multireagent Strips. Another approach to rapid detection of bacteria in platelet components is the use of multireagent strips that measure glucose and pH. Overall sensitivity is approximately 10^7 CFU/mL.[69,70] In a large prospective surveillance study of 3093 platelet units screened with reagent strips, 30 units had a glucose or pH reading outside the reference range; however, only two of these units were culture-positive.[71] This resulted in 9.7 platelet units per 1000 being discarded.[71] None of the units with negative test results by multireagent strip resulted in clinical sepsis after transfusion, although many of the transfused patients were already being treated with antibiotics or were immunocompromised, which may have masked signs of infection.[71]

Visual Inspection for Platelet Swirling. The morphology of platelets is predictive of their viability. Discoid platelets, which have better viability, will reflect light to produce a "swirling" or "streaming" phenomenon. Nondiscoid (spherical) platelets do not show this effect. Swirling is diminished at a lower pH, which can be a consequence of bacteria metabolism. Platelets have been noted to lose their "swirl" at bacteria levels of 10^7 to 10^8 CFU/mL.[70] However, up to 18% of 5-day-old platelets have been reported not to "swirl," so the specificity of this approach to detection of bacteria is quite low.[72] The swirling technique is not recommended by CAP as a sole method for detection of bacterial contamination because of its very low sensitivity.[73]

Growth Inhibition

Cold Storage

Cold storage of red cells, plasma and cryoprecipitate prevents growth of most bacteria and thereby decreases the risk of transfusion-associated sepsis. Refrigerated platelets have been shown to have better in-vitro function than those maintained at room temperature, but once transfused they are rapidly cleared from the blood and provide little in-vivo efficacy.[74] There have been attempts to circumvent the adverse effects of cold storage on platelet function. In one study, second-messenger stimulators were added to platelets stored at 4 C, mimicking the endogenous inhibition of plate-

let activation.[75] Platelets stored for 9 days under these conditions retained partial function and displayed no decrease in cell number.[75] Another option may be to modify platelet binding sites to decrease the clearance of cold-stored platelets by hepatic macrophages after transfusion.[74] Further research is needed in this field, but the development of a safe and effective method for cold storage of platelets could not only decrease the risk of bacterial contamination but also enhance inventory control by extending platelet shelf-life.

Elimination of Contaminating Organisms— Platelet Pathogen-Reduction Technologies

While stringent donor selection policies, optimized collection techniques, and improvements in pathogen detection have reduced the overall risk of infection from transfused components, continued efforts to create a "zero-risk" blood supply have fueled the development of technologies designed to inactivate microbial pathogens. Although there are currently no FDA-approved platelet pathogen inactivation systems available in the United States, AABB revised Standard 5.1.5.1 (effective November 2009) to require blood banks or transfusion services to "have methods to limit and to detect *or inactivate* bacteria in all platelet components" (emphasis added).[49(p11)] This statement reflects increasing support among transfusion medicine practitioners for pathogen inactivation strategies such as those currently in use in Europe and acknowledges that methods to eliminate microbial contamination of platelet components, although valuable, may never reach 100% efficacy. One advantage of pathogen inactivation is its potential to inactivate emerging blood-borne pathogens for which no reliable, cost-effective testing methods are available.

The current approach to emerging infectious diseases in blood components is set in motion once a disease is identified as a public safety threat, whereupon the pathogen causing disease is identified, epidemiologic risk factors are analyzed to expand donor deferrals, and an assay is developed and implemented to test for the presence of the infectious agent (or an antibody to it) in collected components.[76] In contrast, the institution of pathogen inactivation systems represents a proactive rather than reactive approach to emerging infectious disease risks. Not only could pathogen inactivation presumably prevent or mitigate the majority of novel infectious disease agents, but it might also enhance the blood supply by reducing further donor deferral requirements, each of which reduces the pool of eligible donors, and possibly allow for the removal of some current restrictions.

An ancillary benefit of most pathogen-reduction strategies is the reduction or elimination of graft-vs-host disease (GVHD). The DNA damage that occurs during pathogen inactivation prevents replication not only of microbial agents, but also of donor lymphocytes.[77,78] Thus, these technologies should effectively eliminate the need for irradiation of components. This expectation is supported by the lack of an increase in GVHD in several European medical centers after discontinuation of irradiation of pathogen-inactivated platelets.[78,79]

Currently, there are three main technologies for pathogen inactivation in platelets, discussed below, none of which are licensed for clinical use in the United States or Canada.

INTERCEPT Blood System. The INTERCEPT platelet system (Cerus Corp, Concord, CA) is currently in clinical use in several European countries. In this system, platelet components are treated with amotosalen, a psoralen compound which intercalates between DNA strands. The component is then subjected to ultraviolet (UV) light (320-400 nm), which results in irreversible cross-linking of complementary strands and inhibition of DNA and RNA replication.[76,80,81] Following UV light exposure, the platelets are held for 4 to 16 hours in a separate container containing a compound adsorption device (CAD), which removes unreacted amotosalen and photoproducts.[76]

There is conflicting data on the survival of psoralen/UV-light-treated platelets compared to conventional, untreated platelets. One European study of 166 thrombocytopenic patients showed no difference in platelet-count increments in patients transfused with psoralen/UV-light-treated platelets compared to patients given untreated platelets.[82] A larger US study with 635 patients demonstrated lower 1-hour posttransfusion increments and a corresponding increase in the number of platelet transfusions required by patients receiving treated platelets.[81] Extensive toxicology, mutagenicity, and carcinogenicity studies have established the safety of platelet components subjected to this method of pathogen inactivation.[83,84] To date, the FDA has permitted only investigational use of the INTERCEPT system.

Mirasol PRT. The Mirasol Pathogen Reduction Technology (PRT) system for platelets (CaridianBCT Biotechnologies, Lakewood, CO) adds riboflavin (vitamin B_2) to platelet components, followed by exposure to UV light (265-370 nm).[76] The riboflavin acts as a photosensitizing agent. It intercalates between DNA strands and, upon UV light exposure, oxidizes guanine residues, generating reactive-oxygen species. Platelets so treated may be transfused without further processing,[76] because riboflavin and its photoproducts are naturally occurring substances found in a wide range of foods, and their catabolites are detectable in normal blood.[85] The safety of riboflavin is supported by extensive clinical experience in the treatment of neonatal jaundice. Although one study has shown the in-vitro cell quality parameters of riboflavin-treated platelets to be inferior to conventional platelets, recovery and survival results of treated platelets in human subjects are clinically acceptable.[86] One randomized controlled study using radiolabeled platelets showed a recovery of 65% in untreated platelets vs a 50% recovery in treated platelets at day 5 of storage.[86]

Theraflex UV for Platelets. In the Theraflex UV system for platelets (MacoPharma, Tourcoing, France), platelets are suspended in a storage solution containing magnesium and potassium. They are then placed into bags, which form a thin layer of platelets (approximately 4-5 mm). The platelets are then subjected to monochromatic UV light (254 nm) with intense agitation for approximately 1 minute.[87,88] Nucleic-acid damage is caused, presumably by cyclobutyl ring formation within the component.[76] No photoactive compound is added and, similar to the Mirasol PRT system, no further processing is required. In contrast to the INTERCEPT and Mirasol technologies, fewer studies are available examining the efficacy and safety of this approach. In-vitro platelet parameters do not seem to be significantly affected by this process.[87] Initial results suggest that although short-wave UV light with agitation is effective in eliminating bacteria and viruses in a dose-dependent manner, the effect on spore-forming bacteria, such as *B. cerus*, is much weaker.[87]

Conclusion

Bacterial contamination of platelets continues to be a serious threat to transfusion safety despite encouraging data on the effect of mandatory bacterial testing. The variety of clinical manifestations of transfusion-associated sepsis presents a challenge to the clinician and may often delay or prevent diagnosis and appropriate treatment. Strict donor criteria and improved collection practices have had a measurable effect on the rates of bacterial contamination but have not been able to eliminate the risk entirely. Similarly, bacteria detection methods appear to be successful in reducing the rate of transfusion-associated sepsis. The rates of efficacy may differ, however, for different platelet components, detection methods, and testing times. Pathogen-inactivation technologies show promise and may be an appropriate solution for both recognized and emerging pathogens. Implementation of more comprehensive methods of bacteria testing or inactivation may not only improve the overall safety of transfusion practices, but also enhance blood bank inventories by allowing a longer shelf-life for platelet components.

References

1. Fiebig EW, Busch MP. Infectious disease screening. In: Roback JD, Combs MR, Grossman BJ, Hillyer CD, eds. Technical manual. 16th ed. Bethesda, MD: AABB, 2008:241-82.
2. Park YA, Brecher ME. Bacterial contamination of blood products. In: Simon TL, Snyder EL, Solheim BG, et al, eds. Rossi's principles of transfusion medicine. 4th ed. Bethesda, MD: AABB, 2009:773-90.
3. Blajchman MA, Vamvakas EC. The continuing risk of transfusion-transmitted infections. N Engl J Med 2006;355:1303-5.
4. Casewell MW, Slater NG, Cooper JE. Operating theatre water-baths as a cause of *Pseudomonas septicaemia*. J Hosp Infect 1981;2:237-47.
5. Rhame FS, McCullough JJ, Cameron S. *Pseudomonas cepacia* infections caused by thawing cryoprecipitate in a contaminated water bath (abstract). Transfusion 1979;19:653.
6. Claeys H, Verhaegle B. Bacterial screening of platelets (abstract). Vox Sang 2000;78(Suppl 1):374.
7. Schelstaete B, Bijnens B, Wuyts G. Prevalence of bacteria in leukodepleted pooled platelet concentrated and apheresis platelets: A 3-year experience (abstract). Vox Sang 2000;78 (Suppl 1):373.
8. Leiby D, Ferr K, Campos J, et al. A retrospective analysis of microbial contaminants in outdated random-donor platelets from multiple sites. Transfusion 1997;37:259-63.
9. Dykstra A, Jacobs M, Yomtovian R. Prospective microbiologic surveilance (PMS) of random donor (RDP) and single donor apheresis (SDP) platelets (abstract). Transfusion 1998;38(Suppl):104S.
10. Yomtovian R, Lazarus HM, Goodnough LT, et al. A prospective microbiologic surveillance program to detect and prevent the transfusion of bacterially contaminated platelets. Transfusion 1993;33:902-9.
11. Perez P, Salmi LR, Follea G, et al. Determinants of transfusion-associated bacterial contamination: Results of the French BACTHEM case-control study. Transfusion 2001;41:862-72.
12. Serious hazards of transfusion. SHOT summary/report 2001/2002. Manchester, UK: SHOT, 2002. [Available at http://www.shotuk.org/SHOT%20reports%20&%20Summaries%202001-02.htm (accessed December 16, 2009).]
13. Kuehnert MJ, Roth VR, Haley NR, et al. Transfusion-transmitted bacterial infection in the United States, 1998 through 2000. Transfusion 2001;41:1493-9.
14. Ness P, Braine H, King K, et al. Single-donor platelets reduce the risk of septic platelet transfusion reactions. Transfusion 2001;41:857-61.

15. Engelfriet CP, Reesink HW, Blajchman MA, et al. Bacterial contamination of blood components. Vox Sang 2000;78:59-67.

16. Niu MT, Knippen M, Simmons L, Holness LG. Transfusion-transmitted Klebsiella pneumoniae fatalities, 1995 to 2004. Transfus Med Rev 2006;20:149-57.

17. Hoppe PA. Interim measures for detection of bacterially contaminated red cell components. Transfusion 1992;32:199-201.

18. Sazama K. Reports of 355 transfusion-associated deaths: 1976 through 1985. Transfusion 1990;30:583-90.

19. Shulman IA. College of American Pathologists laboratory accreditation checklist item TRM.44955. Phase I requirement on bacterial detection in platelets. Arch Pathol Lab Med 2004;128:958-63.

20. Fridey J, ed. Standards for blood banks and transfusion services. 22nd ed. Bethesda, MD: AABB, 2003:13.

21. Brecher ME, Hay SN. Bacterial contamination of blood components. Clin Microbiol Rev 2005;18:195-204.

22. Interim Standard 5.1.5.1.1. Association bulletin #10-02. Bethesda, MD: AABB, 2010.

23. Food and Drug Administration. Fatalities reported to FDA following blood collection and transfusion: Annual summary for fiscal year 2008 (Fig 5). Rockville, MD: CBER Office of Communication, Outreach, and Development, 2009. [Available at http://www.fda.gov/BiologicsBloodVaccines/SafetyAvailability/ReportaProblem/TransfusionDonationFatalities/ucm 113649.htm.]

24. Fuller AK, Uglik KM, Savage WJ, et al. Bacterial culture reduces but does not eliminate the risk of septic transfusion reactions to single-donor platelets. Transfusion 2009;49:2588-93.

25. Eder AF, Kennedy JM, Dy BA, et al. Bacterial screening of apheresis platelets and the residual risk of septic transfusion reactions: The American Red Cross experience (2004-2006). Transfusion 2007;47:1134-42.

26. Morrow JF, Braine HG, Kickler TS, et al. Septic reactions to platelet transfusions: A persistent problem. JAMA 1991;266:555-8.

27. Cummings JP. Technology assessment: Platelet transfusion guidelines. Oak Brook, IL: University HealthSystem Consortium, 1998.

28. Rhame FS, Root RK, MacLowry JD, et al. Salmonella septicemia from platelet transfusions. Study of an outbreak traced to a hematogenous carrier of Salmonella cholerae-suis. Ann Intern Med 1973;78:633-41.

29. Roth VR, Arduino MJ, Nobiletti J, et al. Transfusion-related sepsis due to Serratia liquefaciens in the United States. Transfusion 2000;40:931-5.

30. Pietersz RN, Engelfriet CP, Reesink HW, et al. Detection of bacterial contamination of platelet concentrates. Vox Sang 2007;93:260-77.

31. Lee JH. FDA surveillance for bacterial safety of blood. Presented at the FDA/CBER bacterial contamination of platelets workshop, Bethesda, MD, September 24, 1999. [Available at http://www.fda.gov/downloads/BiologicsBloodVaccines/NewsEvents/WorkshopsMeetingsConferences/TranscriptsMinutes/UCM055446.pdf.]

32. Jafari M, Forsberg J, Gilcher RO, et al. Salmonella sepsis caused by a platelet transfusion from a donor with a pet snake. N Engl J Med 2002;347:1075-8.

33. McDonald CP, Hartley S, Orchard K, et al. Fatal Clostridium perfringens sepsis from a pooled platelet transfusion. Transfus Med 1998;8:19-22.

34. Anderson KC, Lew MA, Gorgone BC, et al. Transfusion-related sepsis after prolonged platelet storage. Am J Med 1986;81:405-11.

35. Eder AF. Allogeneic and autologous blood donor selection. In: Roback JD, Combs MR, Grossman BJ, Hillyer CD, eds. Technical manual. 16th ed. Bethesda, MD: AABB, 2008:137-87.

36. Newman B. Blood donor suitability and allogeneic whole blood donation. Transfus Med Rev 2001;15:234-44.

37. Sellors JW, Hayward R, Swanson G, et al. Comparison of deferral rates using a computerized versus written blood donor questionnaire: A randomized, cross-over study [ISRCTN 84429599]. BMC Public Health 2002;2:14.

38. Halperin D, Baetens J, Newman B. The effect of short-term, temporary deferral on future blood donation. Transfusion 1998;38:181-3.

39. Grossman BJ, Kollins P, Lau PM, et al. Screening blood donors for gastrointestinal illness: A strategy to eliminate carriers of Yersinia enterocolitica. Transfusion 1991;31:500-1.

40. Tipple MA, Bland LA, Murphy JJ, et al. Sepsis associated with transfusion of red cells contaminated with Yersinia enterocolitica. Transfusion 1990;30:207-13.

41. Centers for Disease Control and Prevention. Red blood cell transfusions contaminated with Yersinia enterocolitica—United States, 1991-1996,

and initiation of a national study to detect bacteria-associated transfusion reactions. MMWR Morb Mortal Wkly Rep 1997;46:553-5.

42. Centers for Disease Control and Prevention. Update: *Yersinia enterocolitica* bacteremia and endotoxin shock associated with red blood cell transfusion, United States, 1991. MMWR Morb Mortal Wkly Rep 1991;40:176-8.

43. Hillyer CD, Josephson CD, Blajchman MA, et al. Bacterial contamination of blood components: Risks, strategies, and regulation. Joint ASH and AABB educational session in transfusion medicine. Hematology Am Soc Hematol Educ Program 2003:575-89.

44. Yomtovian R. Bacterial contamination: An overview of key issues. Presented at FDA/CBER workshop, Safety and efficacy of methods for reducing pathogens in cellular blood products used in Transfusion, August 7-8, 2002, Bethesda, MD.

45. Weinstein MP. Blood culture contamination: Persisting problems and partial progress. J Clin Microbiol 2003;41:2275-8.

46. Lilly HA, Lowbury EJ, Wilkins MD. Limits to progressive reduction of resident skin bacteria by disinfection. J Clin Pathol 1979;32:382-5.

47. Gibson T, Norris W. Skin fragments removed by injection needles. Lancet 1958;2:983-5.

48. Lee CK, Ho PL, Chan NK, et al. Impact of donor arm skin disinfection on the bacterial contamination rate of platelet concentrates. Vox Sang 2002;83:204-8.

49. Price TH, ed. Standards for blood banks and transfusion services. 26th ed. Bethesda, MD: AABB, 2009.

50. Reading FC, Brecher ME. Transfusion-related bacterial sepsis. Curr Opin Hematol 2001;8:380-6.

51. Bruneau C, Perez P, Chassaigne M, et al. Efficacy of a new collection procedure for preventing bacterial contamination of whole-blood donations. Transfusion 2001;41:74-81.

52. de Korte D, Curvers J, de Kort WL, et al. Effects of skin disinfection method, deviation bag, and bacterial screening on clinical safety of platelet transfusions in the Netherlands. Transfusion 2006;46:476-85.

53. McDonald CP, Roy A, Mahajan P, et al. Relative values of the interventions of diversion and improved donor-arm disinfection to reduce the bacterial risk from blood transfusion. Vox Sang 2004;86:178-82.

54. de Korte D, Marcelis JH, Verhoeven AJ, Soeterboek AM. Diversion of first blood volume results in a reduction of bacterial contamination for whole-blood collections. Vox Sang 2002;83:13-16.

55. Wagner SJ, Robinette D, Friedman LI, Miripol J. Diversion of initial blood flow to prevent whole-blood contamination by skin surface bacteria: An in vitro model. Transfusion 2000;40:335-8.

56. Leiby DA, Kerr KL, Campos JM, Dodd RY. A retrospective analysis of microbial contaminants in outdated random-donor platelets from multiple sites. Transfusion 1997;37:259-63.

57. Benjamin RJ, Kline L, Dy BA, et al. Bacterial contamination of whole-blood-derived platelets: The introduction of sample diversion and prestorage pooling with culture testing in the American Red Cross. Transfusion 2008;48:2348-55.

58. Murphy WG, Foley M, Doherty C, et al. Screening platelet concentrates for bacterial contamination: Low numbers of bacteria and slow growth in contaminated units mandate an alternative approach to product safety. Vox Sang 2008;95:13-19.

59. Jacobs MR, Good CE, Lazarus HM, Yomtovian RA. Relationship between bacterial load, species virulence, and transfusion reaction with transfusion of bacterially contaminated platelets. Clin Infect Dis 2008;46:1214-20.

60. Brecher ME, Holland PV, Pineda AA, et al. Growth of bacteria in inoculated platelets: Implications for bacteria detection and the extension of platelet storage. Transfusion 2000;40:1308-12.

61. McDonald CP, Rogers A, Cox M, et al. Evaluation of the 3D BacT/ALERT automated culture system for the detection of microbial contamination of platelet concentrates. Transfus Med 2002;12:303-9.

62. Brecher ME, Means N, Jere CS, et al. Evaluation of an automated culture system for detecting bacterial contamination of platelets: An analysis with 15 contaminating organisms. Transfusion 2001;41:477-82.

63. Brecher ME, Heath DG, Hay SN, et al. Evaluation of a new generation of culture bottle using an automated bacterial culture system for detecting nine common contaminating organisms found in platelet components. Transfusion 2002;42:774-9.

64. Su LL, Kamel H, Custer B, et al. Bacterial detection in apheresis platelets: Blood systems experience with a two-bottle and one-bottle

culture system. Transfusion 2008;48:1842-52.

65. McDonald CP, Pearce S, Wilkins K, et al. Pall eBDS: An enhanced bacterial detection system for screening platelet concentrates. Transfus Med 2005;15:259-68.

66. Dreier J, Vollmer T, Kleesiek K. Novel flow cytometry-based screening for bacterial contamination of donor platelet preparations compared with other rapid screening methods. Clin Chem 2009;55:1492-502.

67. Platelet PGD test package insert. Worcester, MA: Verax Biomedical, Inc, 2009.

68. Barrett BB, Andersen JW, Anderson KC. Strategies for the avoidance of bacterial contamination of blood components. Transfusion 1993; 33:228-33.

69. Burstain JM, Brecher ME, Workman K, et al. Rapid identification of bacterially contaminated platelets using reagent strips: Glucose and pH analysis as markers of bacterial metabolism. Transfusion 1997;37:255-8.

70. Wagner SJ, Robinette D. Evaluation of swirling, pH, and glucose tests for the detection of bacterial contamination in platelet concentrates. Transfusion 1996;36:989-93.

71. Werch JB, Mhawech P, Stager CE, et al. Detecting bacteria in platelet concentrates by use of reagent strips. Transfusion 2002;42:1027-31.

72. Bertolini F, Murphy S. A multicenter evaluation of reproducibility of swirling in platelet concentrates. Biomedical Excellence for Safer Transfusion (BEST) Working Party of the International Society of Blood Transfusion. Transfusion 1994;34:796-801.

73. College of American Pathologists. Transfusion medicine checklist. TRM.449552009. Northfield, IL: CAP, 2009.

74. Snyder EL, Rinder HM. Platelet storage—time to come in from the cold? N Engl J Med 2003; 348:2032-3.

75. Connor J, Currie LM, Allan H, Livesey SA. Recovery of in vitro functional activity of platelet concentrates stored at 4 degrees C and treated with second-messenger effectors. Transfusion 1996;36:691-8.

76. Stramer SL, Hollinger FB, Katz LM, et al. Emerging infectious disease agents and their potential threat to transfusion safety. Transfusion 2009;49(Suppl 2):1S-29S.

77. Fast LD, Dileone G, Li J, Goodrich R. Functional inactivation of white blood cells by Mirasol treatment. Transfusion 2006;46:642-8.

78. Corash L, Lin L. Novel processes for inactivation of leukocytes to prevent transfusion-associated graft-versus-host disease. Bone Marrow Transplant 2004;33:1-7.

79. Osselaer JC, Doyen C, Sonet A, et al. Routine use of platelet components prepared with photochemical treatment (INTERCEPT platelets): Impact on clinical outcomes and costs (abstract). Blood 2004;104:3629.

80. Pineda A, McCullough J, Benjamin RJ, et al. Pathogen inactivation of platelets with a photochemical treatment with amotosalen HCl and ultraviolet light: Process used in the SPRINT trial. Transfusion 2006;46:562-71.

81. McCullough J, Vesole DH, Benjamin RJ, et al. Therapeutic efficacy and safety of platelets treated with a photochemical process for pathogen inactivation: The SPRINT Trial. Blood 2004;104:1534-41.

82. Van Rhenen D, Gulliksson H, Cazenave JP, et al. Transfusion of pooled buffy coat platelet components prepared with photochemical pathogen inactivation treatment: The euro-SPRITE trial. Blood 2003;101:2426-33.

83. Ciaravino V. Preclinical safety of a nucleic acid-targeted Helinx compound: A clinical perspective. Semin Hematol 2001;38(Suppl 11):12-19.

84. Ciaravi V, McCullough T, Dayan AD. Pharmacokinetic and toxicology assessment of INTERCEPT (S-59 and UVA treated) platelets. Hum Exp Toxicol 2001;20:533-50.

85. Solheim BG, Seghatchian J. Pathogen inactivation. In: Simon TL, Snyder E, Solheim BG, et al, eds. Rossi's principles of transfusion medicine. 4th ed. Bethesda, MD: AABB Press, 2009:801-10.

86. AuBuchon JP, Herschel L, Roger J, et al. Efficacy of apheresis platelets treated with riboflavin and ultraviolet light for pathogen reduction. Transfusion 2005;45:1335-41.

87. Mohr H, Gravemann U, Bayer A, Müller TH. Sterilization of platelet concentrates at production scale by irradiation with short-wave ultraviolet light. Transfusion 2009;49:1956-63.

88. Mohr H, Steil L, Gravemann U, et al. A novel approach to pathogen reduction in platelet concentrates using short-wave ultraviolet light. Transfusion 2009;49:2612-24.

In: McLeod BC, Szczepiorkowski ZM, Weinstein R, Winters JL, eds.
Apheresis: Principles and Practice, 3rd edition
Bethesda, MD: AABB Press, 2010

11

Granulocyte (Neutrophil) Transfusion

Ronald G. Strauss, MD

THE PRIMARY ROLE OF BLOOD neutrophils (PMNs) is to kill or inactivate pathogenic microorganisms, particularly pyogenic bacteria, yeast, and fungi. Generally, this is accomplished by phagocytosis of organisms, followed by the delivery of various microbicidal factors—including oxidants, enzymes, and cationic proteins—to the phagocytic vesicles. As an alternative to phagocytosis, PMNs will adhere to large organisms or infected cells and inflict damage by secreting microbicidal factors onto the surface of these targets. While PMNs, eosinophils, and basophils all fit the definition of blood granulocytes, PMNs are the most plentiful of the three cell types and are most phagocytically active. As described in the following section, PMNs perform a number of coordinated functions to provide an optimal antimicrobial defense. Because granulocyte transfusions are given to neutropenic patients primarily to provide adequate numbers of functional PMNs, the number and quality of PMNs transfused are critical in determining the efficacy of granulocyte transfusions.

Life-threatening bacterial, yeast, and fungal infections continue to be a consequence of either severe neutropenia ($<0.5\times10^9$/L PMN blood leukocytes) or disorders of PMN function. The usual clinical setting is neutropenic infection either during hematopoietic progenitor cell transplantation or intense chemotherapy for hematologic malignancies. Such infections cause considerable morbidity, occasionally are fatal, and add considerable cost to the treatment of these patients.

Many studies have shown granulocyte transfusions to be beneficial as treatment for infections in certain clinical settings, both in animals and in humans.[1] However, the use of therapeutic granulocyte transfusions has diminished strikingly over the past several years. Although this can be explained by the development of more effective antimicrobial agents to treat

Ronald G. Strauss, MD, Professor Emeritus, Pathology and Pediatrics, University of Iowa College of Medicine, Iowa City, Iowa

The author has disclosed no conflicts of interest.

infections, by the use of transfusions of hemato-poietic progenitor cells from apheresis (HPC-A) to hasten marrow recovery and, possibly, by the treatment of neutropenic patients with recombinant hematopoietic growth factors, many physicians hold strong negative opinions about the value of granulocyte transfusions—believing them to have little, if any, role in the management of infected neutropenic patients.[2] These negative opinions have been reinforced by knowledge that PMN concentrates collected for transfusion—particularly in past years—have contained woefully inadequate numbers of PMNs[1] and by the occasional occurrence of life-threatening pulmonary toxicity and other complications following granulocyte transfu-sions.[3] However, because it is now possible to collect very large numbers of PMNs from cytokine-stimulated donors,[4-6] a critical reas-sessment of the role of granulocyte transfusions is prudent.

Neutrophil (PMN) Physiology

All hematopoietic cells arise from a self-renew-ing pool of pluripotent stem cells that, under the influence of growth-promoting cytokines called colony-stimulating factors, become com-mitted to a major cell line (granulocyte-mono-cyte, erythrocyte, or megakaryocyte). The major lineage-specific growth factor for PMNs is granulocyte colony-stimulating factor (G-CSF). Once committed to the PMN cell line, the precursors progress in an orderly manner through stages of proliferation (myeloblast, pro-myelocyte, and myelocyte) and maturation (metamyelocyte and segmented PMNs). Mature PMNs can be stored in the marrow until their release into the peripheral blood, where they are equally divided into marginated and circu-lating pools. Then, after a circulating half-life of approximately 7 hours, they leave the blood in random fashion and do not return to the blood from tissues.

To participate in an inflammatory reaction in tissue, PMNs first roll along the walls of capil-laries and venules. Eventually, each PMN adheres to vascular endothelium and emigrates

from the bloodstream to enter tissues by pene-trating a narrow gap between endothelial cells. This process requires calcium and magnesium, depends on energy (adenosine triphosphate) production from glucose, and is enhanced by the presence of adhesion molecules and chemotactic factors.

A number of profound and complex cellular events are triggered by the binding of chemot-actic factors to the PMN plasma membrane. Within seconds of chemotactic factor binding, the PMN becomes more fluid, the concentra-tion of cyclic adenosine monophosphate dou-bles, the electrical charge of the cell changes, and calcium is mobilized from the PMN memb-rane into the cytosol. Other findings that have been described within the first few minutes of chemotactic factor binding include secretion of granular contents, movements of ions (potas-sium, sodium, and calcium), activation of enzymes, cellular swelling, and an increase in microtubule assembly. Many humoral and cel-lular factors promote optimal chemotaxis. Simi-larly, several processes suppress PMN locomotion, halting further migration to con-centrate these cells at the inflammatory site. In addition, these suppressive mechanisms may protect normal tissues by limiting the inflamma-tory response.

Phagocytosis, the internalization of parti-cles, is the first step in the bactericidal process. Plasma proteins are necessary for the efficient phagocytosis of most pathogenic microorgan-isms because they promote the interaction of microbial antigens with receptors on the PMN plasma membrane. Heat-stable opsonins are antibodies with specificity against microbial surface antigens. Often, the opsonic activities of specific antibodies are enhanced via recruit-ment of heat-labile opsonins of the complement system. To ingest a microorganism attached to the PMN surface, pseudopodia extend out and around the particle in cup-like fashion until they fuse. This movement requires energy, cal-cium, and a functioning cytoskeleton. Before ingestion is complete, cytoplasmic granules approach the phagocytic vesicle, fuse with it, and discharge their contents into it (degranu-late) to form a phagolysosome. Many aspects of the molecular biology of degranulation, granule secretion (exocytosis), and chemotaxis are similar. PMNs consume glucose and oxygen during phagocytosis. Glucose is metabolized via anaerobic glycolysis to provide adenosine triphosphate as energy for ingestion.

A burst of oxidative metabolism accompanies phagocytosis. Oxygen is consumed, initially reduced to form superoxide anion, and then reduced further to hydrogen peroxide. Also, human PMNs produce a variety of reactive molecules such as hydroxyl radical (OH•) and singlet oxygen ($^1O_2$). A number of other biochemical reactions are associated with the postphagocytic oxidative burst, including the generation of chemiluminescence, reduction of tetrazolium dyes, oxidation and depletion of glutathione, iodination of proteins, cellular binding of estradiol, and generation of lipoxygenase and cyclooxygenase products from arachidonic acid.

Microorganisms within phagolysosomes are killed by various oxygen-dependent mechanisms, the most important of which is the myeloperoxidase-hydrogen peroxide-halide system. Myeloperoxidase is present in the primary granules and is delivered to the phagolysosomes by degranulation. Hydrogen peroxide is generated during the postphagocytic oxidative burst. Chloride ions are present within the cytosol and serve as the halide. Although PMNs are capable of killing microorganisms by non-oxidative means, the oxidative mechanisms seem to have greatest importance. This is evidenced by the life-threatening infections manifested by patients with chronic granulomatous disease, a syndrome marked by diminished ability to reduce oxygen to its oxidant forms.

Clinical Experience and Limitations of Granulocyte Transfusions

Historical Experience with Therapeutic Granulocyte Transfusions in Neutropenic Patients

In the earlier editions of this book, an extensive discussion was presented of reports published in the 1970s and 1980s, in which PMNs were collected from donors who were stimulated either with corticosteroids alone or with nothing. The discussion in this edition will be shortened, and to obtain an historical perspective regarding the efficacy of therapeutic granulocyte transfusion (ie, granulocytes collected without donor G-CSF stimulation), only the seven controlled studies will be analyzed briefly.[7-13] In these seven studies, the response of infected neutropenic patients to treatment with granulocyte transfusion plus antibiotics (study group) was compared with that of comparable patients given antibiotics alone (control group) and evaluated concurrently. The design, size, and results of these seven studies are presented in Table 11-1. Three of the seven studies reported a significant overall benefit for granulocyte transfusion.[10-12] In two additional studies,[7,9] overall success was not demonstrated for granulocyte transfusion, but certain subgroups of patients were found to benefit significantly. Thus, some measure of success for granulocyte transfusion was evident in five of the seven historical controlled studies. However, this success was counterbalanced by four studies that reported negative results in some respect—two with negative overall results[8,13] and two with negative results for some types of patients.[7,9]

An explanation for these inconsistent results is evident on critical analysis of the adequacy of granulocyte transfusion support (Table 11-1). Patients in the three successful trials received relatively high doses of PMNs (generally $\geq 1.7 \times 10^{10}$/day), and donors were selected to be both erythrocyte and leukocyte compatible.[10,12] By contrast, the four controlled studies reporting overall or partial negative results can legitimately be criticized. Two of the four studies with negative findings used PMNs collected by filtration leukapheresis for some patients.[7,9] It is now established that such PMNs are defective and this method is no longer used for collection of granulocytes. In the negative studies using PMNs collected by centrifugation leukapheresis,[7,9,13] the dose was extremely low (0.41 to 0.56×10^{10} per granulocyte transfusion). As another factor, investigators in two of the four

Table 11-1. Seven Historical Controlled Studies of Granulocyte Transfusions in Neutropenic Patients

Reference	Transfusion Group				Control Group		
	Patients	Survival (%)	Dose × 10^10	HLA-WBC*	Patients	Survival (%)	Success
Alavi et al[7]	12	82	5.9 (F)	No-No	19	62	Partial
Fortuny et al[8]	17	78	0.4 (C)	No-Yes	22	80	No
Graw et al[9]	39	46	2.0 (F) 0.6 (C)	No-Yes	37	30	Partial
Herzig et al[10]	13	75	1.7 (C) 0.4 (C)	No-Yes	14	36	Yes
Higby et al[11]	17	76	2.2 (F)	No-Yes	19	26	Yes
Vogler et al[12]	17	59	2.7 (C)	Yes-Yes	13	15	Yes
Winston et al[13]	48	63	0.5 (C)	No-No	47	72	No

*Donor-recipient compatibility was enhanced by HLA match or white cell crossmatch.
F = filtration leukapheresis; C = centrifugation leukapheresis.

negative studies[7,13] made no provision for the possibility of leukocyte alloimmunization, as donors were selected solely on the basis of erythrocyte compatibility. Finally, control subjects responded particularly well to antibiotics alone in three of the four negative studies,[7,8,13] suggesting that these patients fared relatively well with conventional treatment alone, and it was not possible to document additional benefit by adding granulocyte transfusion.

The results of the historical seven controlled granulocyte transfusion trials have been analyzed by formal meta-analysis,[14] and conclusions were that the low doses of PMNs transfused and the relatively high survival rate of the nontransfused control subjects were primarily responsible for the differing rates of success of these historical studies. In clinical settings in which the survival rate of nontransfused control subjects was low,[9-12] study subjects benefited from receiving adequate doses of granulocytes—prompting the authors to suggest that severely neutropenic patients with life-threatening infections should be considered for granulocytes given in high doses.[14]

In a somewhat similar meta-analysis of historical reports, prophylactic granulocyte transfusions were of marginal value.[15] The findings confirmed that variability in the dose of PMNs transfused, inconsistent attempts to provide leukocyte-compatible granulocyte transfusions and the varying duration of severe neutropenia in different patient groups were primarily responsible for the differing success rates in the reported controlled trials. It was recommended that high doses of compatible PMNs be transfused if future trials of prophylactic granulocyte transfusion are to be conducted.[15] The remainder of this chapter will focus only on therapeutic granulocyte transfusion.

Modern Experience with Therapeutic Granulocyte Transfusions in Neutropenic Patients

A modern therapeutic granulocyte transfusion is defined as a transfusion in which PMNs are obtained from donors stimulated with G-CSF with or without corticosteroids (optimally with both), with collection by centrifugation leukapheresis using an erythrocyte-sedimenting agent during the processing of relatively large volumes of donor blood. Specifically, the requirements of an ideal PMN collection include 1) at least 400 µg G-CSF given subcutaneously plus 8 mg dexamethasone given orally to the donor approximately 12 hours before leukapheresis is begun, 2) hetastarch infused throughout the leukapheresis procedure at a ratio of 1 part starch to 12 to 14 parts donor blood, and 3) processing of 8 to 10 L of donor blood. The goal should be to transfuse 6 to 8×10^{10} neutrophils per granulocyte transfusion, with a lower limit of 4×10^{10}.

At this time, no randomized clinical trials of modern therapeutic transfusion of granulocytes collected after G-CSF and dexamethasone donor stimulation have been reported to establish either the efficacy or the potential toxicity of modern granulocyte transfusion. However, many case reports suggest success. For example, Clark et al[16] and Catalano et al[17] each reported single patients with aplastic anemia, undergoing progenitor cell transplantation, with fungal infections that responded favorably. Ozsahin et al[18] and Bielorai et al[19] each reported single patients with chronic granulomatous disease and fungal infections that responded favorably to granulocyte transfusion during the transplantation period. Bielorai et al[20] reported a single patient with acute leukemia and sepsis with vancomycin-resistant *Enterococcus* that cleared slowly with granulocyte transfusion. Similarly, Lin et al[21] reported a single patient with multidrug-resistant *Pseudomonas* sepsis who underwent a successful HPC-A transplant supported by granulocyte transfusion. It is impossible, in these single reports of very complicated patients, to firmly ascribe the positive outcome to the granulocyte transfusion. Moreover, the techniques of PMN collection and granulocyte transfusion were quite varied.

Studies of larger numbers of infected, neutropenic patients given granulocyte transfusion from G-CSF-stimulated donors are listed in Table 11-2.[6,22-26] Even with investigation of

larger numbers of patients, the benefits of granulocyte transfusion are unclear because of the lack of concurrent control patients treated with antibiotics alone. Hester et al[6] transfused 15 patients with hematologic malignancies and infections. PMNs were collected from donors stimulated only with G-CSF and selected without regard for leukocyte compatibility. Although granulocyte transfusions were successful in most patients, it was not possible to distinguish responses of fungal vs yeast infections. Grigg et al[22] transfused 11 patients. Eight patients had hematologic malignancies and progressive infections—five of the eight undergoing progenitor cell transplantation and three receiving chemotherapy. Three additional patients who were undergoing progenitor cell transplantation had stable fungal infections. PMNs were collected from donors stimulated only with G-CSF and selected without regard for leukocyte compatibility. Success was excellent for bacterial and stable fungal infections, but was quite poor for progressive fungal infections with organ dysfunction, a troubling pattern reported later by others.[23,24] Peters et al[25] transfused 30 patients with hematologic disorders—18 undergoing progenitor cell transplantation. PMNs were collected from donors stimulated with G-CSF or prednisolone and selected without regard for leukocyte compatibility. The exact PMN dose transfused is uncertain, but values from 0.9×10^{10} to 14.4×10^{10} were estimated from data reported. It was impossible to distinguish the success of granulocyte transfusion from G-CSF-stimulated vs prednisolone-stimulated donors. However, the outcome of bacterial infections overall appeared to be superior to that of fungal infections.

Price et al[24] transfused 19 patients (Table 11-2) with hematologic malignancies, 16 of whom had received progenitor cell transplants and three of whom had not. PMNs were collected from donors stimulated with G-CSF and dexamethasone. Although donors were selected without regard for leukocyte compatibility, recipients were documented not to exhibit evidence of leukocyte alloimmunization at study entry. Bacterial infections responded well and yeast infections responded modestly. Despite

Table 11-2. Modern Studies of Therapeutic Granulocyte Transfusions Using PMNs Collected from G-CSF-Stimulated Donors in Neutropenic Patients

Reference	PMNs ×10^10/ Transfusion	Stimulation	Leukapheresis	Outcomes
Hester et al[6]	4.1	G-CSF 5 µg/kg	Pentastarch 7 L processed	60% (9 of 15) success with fungus (11 patients) and yeast (4 patients)
Grigg et al[22]	5.9*	G-CSF 10 µg/kg	Dextran 10 L processed	100% (3 of 3) success with bacterial infection; 0% (0 of 5) success with progressive fungus; 67% (2 of 3) success with stable fungus
Peters et al[25]	3.5*	G-CSF 5 µg/kg or Prednisolone	Hetastarch 6.4 L processed	82% (14 of 17) success with bacterial infection; 54% (7 of 13) success with fungal infection
Price et al[24]	8.2	G-CSF 600 µg/kg plus Dexamethasone 8 mg	Hetastarch 10 L processed	100% (4 of 4) success with bacterial infection; 0% (0 of 8) success with invasive fungus; 57% (4 of 7) success with yeast infection.
Hubel et al[23]	4.6-8.1	G-CSF 600 mg/kg with or without Dexamethasone 8 mg	Hetastarch or Pentastarch 10 L processed	55% (unrelated donor) success bacterial infection; 75% (family donor) success bacterial infection; 70% (unrelated donor) success yeast infection; 40% (family donor) success yeast infection; 15% (unrelated donor) success fungal infection; 25% (family donor) success fungal infection
Lee et al[26]	5.1-10.6	G-CSF 5 µg/kg and/or Dexamethasone 3 mg/m^2	Pentastarch 6-10 L processed	40% (10 of 25) success with multiple-organism infections

*Assumptions made as PMN dose expressed ×10^10 unclear in these reports. Dose calculated that would be given to a 70 kg recipient for Clarke et al,[24] Bielorai et al,[27] and Peters et al[25]; PMN dose calculated using values for range of leukocytes collected, percentage of collected cells being myeloid, and volume of units collected (Grigg et al[22]).

very high PMN doses, success for invasive fungal infections was dismal. Hübel et al[23] expanded the study of Price et al[24] to a total of 74 patients experiencing progenitor cell transplants. Comparisons were made to historical control patients (n = 74) who did not receive granulocyte transfusion. PMNs were collected either from unrelated donors given G-CSF alone or in combination with dexamethasone or from family members given G-CSF only. Hetastarch was used for single leukapheresis procedures, and pentastarch was used when donors experienced repeated leukapheresis procedures. Comparative success in nontransfused historical control patients was approximately 90% for bacterial infections, 40% for yeast infections, and 30% for fungal/mold infections—values similar to those achieved by granulocyte transfusion recipients. Nontransfused controls had better success than PMN recipients for bacterial infections (p = 0.04). As a potential adverse effect, allogeneic transplant recipients transfused with granulocytes from unrelated donors experienced significantly more (p = 0.04) Grade IV graft-vs host disease than controls who were not given granulocyte transfusion. However, relatively few patients were assessed for this endpoint, and firm conclusions are not warranted.

Lee et al[26] transfused 25 patients with hematologic malignancies, many of whom were infected with multiple organisms. Thus, the outcome of infections with specific types of individual organisms could not be determined. PMNs were collected from donors stimulated with G-CSF alone (66% of donors), G-CSF plus dexamethasone (25% of donors), or dexamethasone alone (8% of donors). Of patients with sepsis, 50% (two of four) responded favorably, and 38% (8 of 21) of patients with progressive localized infections responded favorably.

Two studies reported results in ways that did not lend themselves to tabulation. Illerhaus et al[27] transfused 42 neutropenic patients with granulocytes collected from donors stimulated with 5µg/kg G-CSF. Eighteen of the patients had severe infections with a variety of organisms and each received a median of three granulocyte transfusions, each containing a median

of 2.6×10^{10} leukocytes. Of these 18 patients, eight (44%) improved, four (22%) stabilized and six (33%) deteriorated—with four of these last six dying of pulmonary aspergillosis. Rutella et al[28] transfused 20 patients with hematologic malignancies and neutropenic infections. Donors were HLA-identical siblings, and each received 5 µg/kg G-CSF. Favorable responses were seen in 54% of patients with bacterial infections and 57% with fungal infections. Underlying cancer status (ie, complete or partial remission achieved) and recovery of blood PMN counts to •0.5×10^9/L were significantly correlated with a favorable response to granulocyte transfusion.

No firm conclusions can be drawn from these larger, but still somewhat anecdotal, reports of modern therapeutic granulocyte transfusion for several reasons: 1) no concurrent control subjects were included (ie, randomly assigned to receive antimicrobial drugs but no granulocyte transfusion); 2) the number of patients reported, generally, was quite small; and 3) PMN collection methods were variable, with a broad range of PMN doses transfused. Based on these preliminary findings, bacterial infections appeared to respond quite well to modern granulocyte transfusion, and relatively mild fungal and yeast infections responded modestly well. However, serious fungal infections with tissue invasion often resisted even the large doses of PMNs transfused with modern granulocyte transfusion.[22-27] The precise role of modern therapeutic granulocyte transfusions, where granulocytes are collected from donors stimulated with G-CSF plus corticosteroids, in the management of infected, neutropenic, oncology/transplant patients awaits definition by randomized clinical trials. One such trial that is currently enrolling patients is being conducted by the Transfusion Medicine/Hemostasis Clinical Trials Group of the National Heart, Lung, and Blood Institute.[29]

Experience with Therapeutic Granulocyte Transfusions in Neonates and Children

Neonates and children are susceptible to severe bacterial and viral infections. Bacterial infections occur at an overall rate of 1 to 4 per 1000 births, with nearly 6% of premature neonates being infected when born more than 18 hours after premature rupture of the membranes. PMNs isolated from the blood of neonates exhibit both quantitative and qualitative abnormalities that may contribute to the increased incidence, morbidity, and mortality of bacterial infections. Abnormalities of neonatal PMNs include neutropenia, diminished chemotaxis, abnormal adhesion and aggregation, defective cellular orientation and receptor capping, decreased deformability, inability to alter membrane potential during stimulation or to mobilize intracellular receptors to the surface, imbalances of oxidative metabolism, and a diminished ability to withstand oxidant stress. Thus, a rationale exists for combining granulocyte transfusions with antibiotics to treat septic neonates—subjects in whom both neutropenia and PMN dysfunction have been demonstrated.

Six controlled trials[30-35] (Table 11-3) have assessed the role of granulocyte transfusions in treating neonatal infections. Although four of the six[30-33] found a significant benefit for transfusion, the controlled studies, when assessed by meta-analysis, were insufficiently homogeneous to permit clear recommendations regarding the efficacy of granulocyte transfusions.[14] The dose of PMNs transfused was identified as the primary reason for disagreements between studies. When leukapheresis PMN concentrates were transfused, the transfusions were beneficial. When buffy coats were transfused, the transfusions were not beneficial.[14] Thus, the role of therapeutic granulocyte transfusions for neonatal infections is unclear at present and, because they are transfused only rarely at this time, they will not be discussed further in this chapter.

Therapeutic granulocyte transfusions are prescribed for children with marrow failure and severe neutropenic infections using the same criteria as for adults. In a study by Sachs et al,[36] 27 children with hematologic/oncologic disorders and neutropenic infections received granulocyte transfusions every other day. PMNs were collected from crossmatch-compatible donors

Table 11-3. Six Controlled Trials of Granulocyte Transfusions for Neonatal Infections

| Reference | Randomized | Transfused Neonates | | Control Neonates | |
		Transfused	Survival (%)	Untrans-fused	Survival (%)
Laurenti et al[30]	No	20	90*	18	28
Christensen et al[31]	Yes	7	100*	9	11
	No†	—	—	10	100
Cairo et al[32]	Yes	13	100*	10	60
Cairo et al[33]	Yes‡	21	95*	14	64
Baley et al[34]	Yes	12	58	13	69
Wheeler et al[35]	Yes	4	50	5	40
	No†	—	—	11	91

*Survival was significantly better among the transfused than among the nontransfused.
†Additional control patients were not randomly selected because all had adequate marrow storage pools.
‡The expanded and modified version of a study reported in 1984.

stimulated with G-CSF only. The average dose of PMNs per each granulocyte transfusion was 8×10^8 kg recipient body weight. This corresponds to 5.6×10^{10} PMNs for a 70-kg adult. granulocyte transfusions were very successful, with 93% of patients able to clear infections—including all those with invasive pulmonary aspergillosis infections—and with an 82% survival 1 month later.

Most patients with congenital disorders of PMN dysfunction have adequate numbers of blood PMNs, but they are susceptible to serious infections because their PMNs fail to kill pathogenic microorganisms. Patients with severe forms of PMN dysfunction are relatively rare, and no randomized clinical trials have been reported to establish the efficacy of therapeutic granulocyte transfusion in their management. Firm recommendations about the use of granulocyte transfusion to treat patients cannot be made. However, several patients with chronic granulomatous disease, complicated by progressive life-threatening fungal infections, have been reported to benefit.[37-45] Because of the possibility of alloimmunization to leukocyte and RBC antigens, particularly to the Kell blood group, plus the risk of transfusion-transmitted infections, therapeutic granulocyte transfusions are recommended only for progressive infections that cannot be controlled with antimicrobial drugs. Because of lifetime problems with infections, prophylactic granulocyte transfusions are impractical.

Technology of Granulocyte Collection and Transfusion

A major limitation of granulocyte transfusion has been the inability to consistently transfuse adequate numbers of perfectly functioning PMNs. In any attempt to transfuse satisfactory granulocyte concentrates, PMNs must be collected by automated leukapheresis with the use of an erythrocyte-sedimenting agent such as hydroxyethyl starch (HES).[46,47] In addition, donors must be stimulated with a drug such as adrenal corticosteroid (eg, dexamethasone) and G-CSF a few hours before collection to

increase the donor blood PMN count. Granulocyte concentrates should be transfused as soon as possible after collection—preferably within 6 hours—because PMN functions begin to deteriorate rapidly. Some delay between collection and transfusion is inevitable; thus, granulocyte concentrates are usually stored briefly at 22 C with little or no agitation. Because aberrations of nearly all functions become evident within 24 to 72 hours and PMNs are collected using an "open" system, granulocyte concentrates stored for more than 24 hours should not be transfused. However, G-CSF diminishes PMN apoptosis and, eventually, the length of storage for granulocyte concentrates might be lengthened.

Preleukapheresis Donor Stimulation

Under the stress of a severe bacterial infection, marrow in an otherwise healthy adult will produce between 10^{11} and 10^{12} PMNs in 24 hours. Granulocyte concentrates collected from healthy donors who are not stimulated with corticosteroids or G-CSF will contain between 10^9 and 10^{10} PMNs, about 1% of healthy marrow output. Obviously, donor stimulation is mandatory to achieve even a hope of a reasonable PMN dose for each granulocyte transfusion. Donor stimulation with properly timed corticosteroids (≥ 4 hours before leukapheresis) will permit collection of 1 to 2.5×10^{10} PMNs.[47] Stimulation with G-CSF alone or in combination with corticosteroids will produce granulocyte concentrates with quite variable PMN yields, depending on the G-CSF dose and schedule of administration. Yields of 4 to 8×10^{10} PMNs are achieved regularly, with some investigators reporting yields as great as 14.4×10^{10}, 10.3×10^{10}, and 11.6×10^{10} PMNs.[4,5,48]

Donor stimulation with G-CSF and corticosteroids is extremely promising as a means to achieve reasonable doses of PMNs for transfusion. However, experience with G-CSF in normal donors is still somewhat limited. Donors have received varying doses of G-CSF by a variety of routes and schedules of administration. When given as a single dose of 300 µg or as 5 µg/kg, G-CSF seems to have acceptable acute toxicity—usually minor musculoskeletal pain that can be relieved by acetaminophen or ibuprofen.[24] Although the long-term effects of recombinant cytokines in humans can be established only after years of observations, it is widely believed that G-CSF will exert no long-term adverse effects when administered briefly to healthy individuals.[49] In contrast, many real and theoretical adverse effects of repeated doses of G-CSF to stem cell donors and to patients have been reported, and written consent should be obtained.[49]

Currently, optimal donor stimulation is achieved by giving 8 mg of dexamethasone orally and 400 µg of G-CSF subcutaneously approximately 12 hours before beginning leukapheresis.[48] Because flexibility of timing often is of importance for scheduling PMN donation, a "window" of 8 to 16 hours between dexamethasone and G-CSF administration and leukapheresis will permit adequate PMN collection. Of note, a recent report suggested that adrenal corticosteroids might cause posterior subcapsular cataracts in PMN donors.[50] Although this report was not confirmed by study of larger numbers of PMN donors, it seems logical to include this cautionary information in donor consent forms until a definitive answer is available.[51,52]

Leukapheresis Techniques

Optimal granulocyte transfusion therapy depends on the consistent preparation of satisfactory granulocyte concentrates that contain large numbers of functional PMNs. Each transfusion must deliver at least an acceptable modern dose for treating adults of $\geq 4 \times 10^{10}$ PMNs per transfusion.

Each center must perform quality assessments to ensure the manufacture of adequate granulocyte concentrates. There is general agreement that donors must be stimulated with corticosteroids and G-CSF, that an erythrocyte-sedimenting agent must be used throughout the leukapheresis procedure, and that large volumes of donor blood (eg, 10 L) should be processed using a continuous flow cell separator.

Erythrocyte-Sedimenting Agents

It has been known for decades that an erythrocyte-sedimenting agent such as HES, dextran, or modified fluid gelatin is required during centrifugation leukapheresis for optimal granulocyte collection.[53] Many cytapheresis centers prefer HES over the other agents because it has proven to be relatively safe. However, concern has been raised over the long persistence of hetastarch in the bloodstream after leukapheresis.[54] Thus, efforts have been made to replace hetastarch with pentastarch, an HES solution that has been reported to enhance PMN yields during leukapheresis yet is promptly eliminated from the bloodstream and has fewer effects on coagulation.[46,55] However, the efficacy of pentastarch has been questioned, and it has fallen into disuse.[56]

HES is a complex polysaccharide consisting of glucose units connected primarily by $\alpha(1-4)$ glycosidic linkages, with $\alpha(1-6)$ linkages serving as branch points. Hydroxyethyl groups are attached by ether linkages to carbon atoms C2, C3, and/or C6. Solutions of HES contain mixtures of HES molecules that vary in size rather than being of uniform size and weight. The weight average molecular weight (the average molecular weight of all molecules present in the solution) of hetastarch commonly used in the United States (Hespan, DuPont Pharmaceuticals, Wilmington, DE) is estimated to be 450,000 Da, with a number average molecular weight (the molecular weight of the fraction of molecules present in the greatest quantity) of 69,000 Da. The molar substitution of hydroxyethyl groups is 0.7 (ie, 70 molecules of hydroxyethyl moiety are present for every 100 glucose units contained in the HES; some glucose units contain more than one hydroxyethyl moiety). The average PMN yield obtained by processing 10 L of donor blood following only corticosteroid stimulation and using hetastarch at a 1:13 starch:donor blood ratio should be between 1.5 and 2.5×10^{10}; after corticosteroid plus G-CSF stimulation, the PMN yield should be consistently between 4.0 and 8.0×10^{10}.

Future of Granulocyte (Neutrophil) Transfusions

Because a major criticism of granulocyte transfusions has been the relatively small doses of PMNs available in granulocyte concentrates, the feasibility of stimulating normal donors with G-CSF to obtain markedly increased numbers of PMNs for transfusion has renewed interest in this therapy as a treatment for infections in neutropenic patients. However, other medical advances—including treatment of patients directly with G-CSF and other recombinant growth factors, the availability of more effective antimicrobial agents, and the use of HPC transfusions—have lessened the likelihood of progressive and unresponsive infections in severely neutropenic patients. Thus, it is ironic that now, when more effective doses of PMNs could be transfused, they seem to be needed only occasionally.

Each institution must assess local needs. If, despite optimal antimicrobial and other supportive therapy, neutropenic patients suffer significant morbidity or mortality from infections, granulocyte transfusions should be considered. Once therapeutic transfusions have been prescribed, they must be given effectively: $\geq 2 \times 10^{10}$ PMNs per dose with corticosteroid stimulation, $\geq 4\text{-}8 \times 10^{10}$ PMNs per dose with corticosteroid plus G-CSF, and never less than 1×10^{10} PMNs per dose. Transfusions are continued daily until the infection has resolved or until blood PMN levels rise above 0.5×10^9/L.

On the basis of studies of the circulation and migration of indium-111-labeled PMNs,[57,58] it seems logical that patients with evidence of alloimmunization (platelet refractoriness, leukocyte antibodies, repeated febrile transfusion reactions, or posttransfusion pulmonary infiltrates) should receive granulocyte transfusions from donors selected to be leukocyte compatible by HLA matching and/or leukocyte crossmatching. Dutcher et al[57] found that transfused, labeled PMNs failed to reach sites of infection in 78% of alloimmunized patients, whereas localization of PMNs was normal in nonalloimmunized patients. McCullough et al[58] reported similar findings and also documented reduced recovery and circulating half-life in some alloimmunized patients. However, it has not been clearly shown that attempts to improve leukocyte antigen compatibility increase the success of granulocyte transfusions in alloimmunized patients.

References

1. Strauss RG. Therapeutic granulocyte transfusion in 1993. Blood 1993;81:1675-8.
2. Strauss RG. Granulocyte transfusions: Uses, abuses and indications. In: Kolins J, McCarthy LJ, eds. Contemporary transfusion practice. Arlington, VA: AABB, 1987:65-83.
3. Wright DG, Robichaud KJ, Pizzo PA, et al. Lethal pulmonary reactions associated with the combined use of amphotericin B and leukocyte transfusions. N Engl J Med 1981;304:1185-9.
4. Bensinger WI, Price TH, Dale DC, et al. The effects of daily recombinant human granulocyte colony stimulating factor administration on normal granulocyte donors undergoing leukapheresis. Blood 1993;81:1883-7.
5. Caspar CB, Reinhard AS, Burger J, et al. Effective stimulation of donors for granulocyte transfusions with recombinant methionyl granulocyte colony-stimulating factor. Blood 1993; 81:2866-9.
6. Hester JP, Dignani MC, Anaissie EJ, et al. Collection and transfusion of granulocyte concentrates from donors primed with granulocyte stimulating factor and response of myelosuppressed patients with established infection. J Clin Apher 1995;10:188-93.
7. Alavi JB Root RK, Djerassi I, et al. A randomized clinical trial of granulocyte transfusions for infection in acute leukemia. N Engl J Med 1977;296:706-11.
8. Fortuny IE, Bloomfield CD, Hadlock DC, et al. Granulocyte transfusion: A controlled study in patients with acute non-lymphocytic leukemia. Transfusion 1975;15:548-58.
9. Graw RG Jr, Herzig G, Perry S, et al. Normal granulocyte transfusion therapy. N Engl J Med 1972;287:367-71.
10. Herzig RH, Herzig GP, Graw RG, et al. Successful granulocyte transfusion therapy for gram-negative septicemia. A prospectively randomized controlled study. N Engl J Med 1977; 296:701-5.

11. Higby DJ, Yates JW, Henderson ES, et al. Filtration leukapheresis for granulocytic transfusion therapy. N Engl J Med 1975;292:761-6.
12. Vogler WR, Winton EF. A controlled study of the efficacy of granulocyte transfusions in patients with neutropenia. Am J Med 1977;63:548-55.
13. Winston DJ, Ho WG, Gale RP. Therapeutic granulocyte transfusions for documented infections: A controlled trial in 95 infectious granulocytopenic episodes. Ann Intern Med 1982;97:509-15.
14. Vamvakas EC, Pineda AA. Meta-analysis of clinical studies of the efficacy of granulocyte transfusions in the treatment of bacterial sepsis. J Clin Apher 1996;11:1-9.
15. Vamvakas EC, Pineda AA. Determinants of the efficacy of prophylactic granulocyte transfusions: A meta-analysis. J Clin Apher 1997;12:74-81.
16. Clarke K, Szer J, Shelton M, et al. Multiple granulocyte transfusions facilitating unrelated bone marrow transplantation in a patient with very severe aplastic anemia complicated by suspected fungal infection. Bone Marrow Transplant 1995;16:723-6.
17. Catalano L, Fontana R, Scarpato N, et al. Combined treatment with amphotericin-B and granulocyte transfusion from G-CSF-stimulated donors in an aplastic patient with invasive aspergillosis undergoing bone marrow transplantation. Haematologica 1997;82:71-2.
18. Ozsahin H, von Planta M, Müller I, et al. Successful treatment of invasive aspergillosis in chronic granulomatous disease by invasive aspergillosis in chronic granulomatous disease by bone marrow transplantation, granulocyte colony-stimulating factor-mobilized granulocytes, and liposomal amphotericin-B. Blood 1998;92:2719-24.
19. Bielorai B, Toren A, Wolach B, et al. Successful treatment of invasive aspergillosis in chronic granulomatous disease by granulocyte transfusions followed by peripheral blood stem cell transplantation. Bone Marrow Transplant 2000;26:1025-8.
20. Bielorai B, Neumann Y, Avigad I, et al. Successful treatment of vancomycin-resistant Enterococcus sepsis in a neutropenic patient with G-CSF-mobilized granulocyte transfusions. Med Pediatr Oncol 2000;34:221-3.
21. Lin YW, Adachi S, Watanabe K, et al. Serial granulocyte transfusions as a treatment for sepsis due to multidrug-resistant Pseudomonas aeruginosa in a neutropenic patient. J Clin Microbiol 2003;41:4892-3.
22. Grigg A, Vecchi L, Bardy P, et al. G-CSF stimulated donor granulocyte collections for prophylaxis and therapy of neutropenic sepsis. Aust N Z J Med 1996;26:813-18.
23. Hübel K, Carter RA, Liles et al. Granulocyte transfusion therapy for infections in candidates and recipients of HPC transplantation: A comparative analysis of feasibility and outcome for community donors versus related donors. Transfusion 2002;42:1414-21.
24. Price TH, Bowden RA, Boeckh M, et al. Phase I/II trial of neutrophil transfusions from donors stimulated with G-CSF and dexamethasone for treatment of patients with infections in hematopoietic stem cell transplantation. Blood 2000;95:3302-9.
25. Peters C, Minkov M, Matthes-Martin S, et al. Leucocyte transfusions from rhG-CSF or prednisolone stimulated donors for treatment of severe infections in immunocompromised neutropenic patients. Br J Haematol 1999;106:689-96.
26. Lee JJ, Chung IJ, Park MR, et al. Clinical efficacy of granulocyte transfusion therapy in patients with neutropenia-related infections. Leukemia 2001;15:203-7.
27. Illerhaus G, Wirth K, Dwenger A, et al. Treatment and prophylaxis of severe infections in neutropenic patients by granulocyte transfusions. Ann Hematol 2002;81:273-81.
28. Rutella S, Pierelli L, Sica S, et al. Efficacy of granulocyte transfusions for neutropenia-related infections: Retrospective analysis of predictive factors. Cytotherapy 2003;5:19-30.
29. Price TH. Granulocyte transfusion therapy. J Clin Apher 2006;21:65-71.
30. Laurenti F, Ferro R, Isacchi G, et al. Polymorphonuclear leukocyte transfusion for the treatment of sepsis in the newborn infant. J Pediatr 1981;98:118-23.
31. Christensen RD, Rothstein G, Anstall HB, et al. Granulocyte transfusions in neonates with bacterial infection, neutropenia, and depletion of mature marrow neutrophils. Pediatrics 1982;70:1-6.
32. Cairo MS, Rucker R, Bennets GA, et al. Improved survival of newborns receiving leukocyte transfusions for sepsis. Pediatrics 1984;74:887-92.
33. Cairo MS, Worcester C, Rucker R, et al. Role of circulating complement and polymorphonuclear leukocyte transfusion in treatment and

outcome in critically ill neonates with sepsis. J Pediatr 1987;110:935-41.

34. Baley JE, Stork EK, Warkentin PI, et al. Buffy coat transfusions in neutropenic neonates with presumed sepsis: A prospective, randomized trial. Pediatrics 1987;80:712-20.

35. Wheeler JG, Chauvenet AR, Johnson CA, et al. Buffy coat transfusions in neonates with sepsis and neutrophil storage pool depletion. Pediatrics 1987;79:422-5.

36. Sachs UJH, Reiter A, Walter T, et al. Safety and efficacy of therapeutic early onset granulocyte transfusions in pediatric patients with neutropenia and severe infections. Transfusion 2006;46:1909-14.

37. Maybee DA, Millan AP, Ruymann FB. Granulocyte transfusion therapy in children. South Med J 1977;70:320-4.

38. Yomtovian R, Abramson J, Quie P, et al. Granulocyte transfusion therapy in chronic granulomatous disease: Report of a patient and review of the literature. Transfusion 1981;21:739-43.

39. Raubitschek AA, Levin AS, Stites DP, et al. Normal granulocyte infusion therapy for aspergillosis in chronic granulomatous disease. Pediatrics 1973;51:230-3.

40. Chusid MJ, Tomasulo PA. Survival of transfused normal granulocytes in a patient with chronic granulomatous disease. Pediatrics 1978;61:556-9.

41. Pedersen FK, Johansen KS, Rosenkvist J, et al. Refractory Pneumocystis carinii infection in chronic granulomatous disease: Successful treatment with granulocytes. Pediatrics 1979;64:935-8.

42. Buescher ES, Gallin JI. Leukocyte transfusion in chronic granulomatous disease: Persistence of transfused leukocytes in sputum. N Engl J Med 1982;307:800-3.

43. Brzica SM, Rhodes KH, Pineda AA, et al. Chronic granulomatous disease and the McLeod phenotype: Successful treatment of infection with granulocyte transfusion resulting in subsequent hemolytic transfusion reaction. Mayo Clin Proc 1977;52:153-6.

44. Bujak JS, Kwon-Chung KJ, Chusid MJ. Osteomyelitis and pneumonia in a boy with chronic granulomatous disease of childhood caused by a mutant strain of Aspergillus nidulans. Am J Clin Pathol 1974;61:361-7.

45. Haddad HL, Beatty DW, Dowdle EB. Chronic granulomatous disease of childhood. S Afr Med J 1976;50:2068-72.

46. Strauss RG, Rohret PA, Randels MJ, et al. Granulocyte collection. J Clin Apher 1991;6:241-3.

47. Strauss RG, Hester JP, Vogler WR, et al. A multicenter trial to document the efficacy and safety of a rapidly excreted analog of hydroxyethyl starch for leukapheresis with a note on steroid stimulation of granulocyte donors. Transfusion 1986;26:258-64.

48. Liles WC, Rodger E, Dale DC. Combined administration of G-CSF and dexamethasone for the mobilization of granulocytes in normal donors: Optimization of dosing. Transfusion 2000;40:642-4.

49. McCullough J, Kahn J. Hematopoietic growth factors—use in normal blood and stem cell donors: Clinical and ethical issues (summary of a conference). Transfusion 2008;48:2008-25.

50. Ghodsi Z, Strauss RG. Cataracts in neutrophil donors stimulated with adrenal corticosteroids. Transfusion 2001;41:1464-8.

51. Burch JW, Mair DC, Meny GM, et al. The risk of posterior subcapsular cataracts in granulocyte donors. Transfusion 2005;45:1701-8.

52. Strauss RG, Lipton KS. Glucocorticoid stimulation of neutrophil donors: A medical, scientific, and ethical dilemma. Transfusion 2005;45:1697-9.

53. Mishler JM, Hadlock DC, Fortuny IE, et al. Increased efficiency of leukocyte collection by the addition of hydroxyethyl starch to the continuous flow centrifuge. Blood 1974;44:571-81.

54. Maguire LC, Strauss RG, Koepe JA, et al. The elimination of hydroxyethyl starch from the blood of donors experiencing single or multiple intermittent-flow centrifugation leukapheresis. Transfusion 1981;21:347-53.

55. Treib J, Baron J-F, Grauer MT, Strauss RG. An international view of hydroxyethyl starches. Intensive Care Med 1999;25:258-68.

56. Lee JH, Leitman SF, Klein HG. A controlled comparison of the efficacy of hetastarch and pentastarch in granulocyte collections by centrifugal leukapheresis. Blood 1995;86:4662-6.

57. Dutcher JP, Schiffer CA, Johnston GS, et al. Alloimmunization prevents the migration of transfused indium-111-labeled granulocytes to sites of infection. Blood 1983;62:354-8.

58. McCullough J, Weiblen BJ, Clay ME, et al. Effect of leukocyte antibodies on the fate in vivo of indium-111-labeled granulocytes. Blood 1981;58:164-9.

In: McLeod BC, Szczepiorkowski ZM, Weinstein R, Winters JL, eds.
Apheresis: Principles and Practice, 3rd edition
Bethesda, MD: AABB Press, 2010

12

Management of the Therapeutic Apheresis Patient

Vishesh Chhibber, MD, and Karen E. King, MD

THE CLINICAL ROLE OF THERapeutic apheresis (TA) continues to expand as new disease entities are defined and as pathogenetic mechanisms of both newly described and familiar disorders are elucidated, revealing rationales for TA. Because of the variety of diseases treatable by TA, apheresis physicians and staff must evaluate and care for a diverse group of patients, ranging from neonates to the elderly, who are referred by physicians from a wide range of medical and surgical specialties. The acuity of referred patients may vary from stable outpatients to inpatients in an intensive care setting. The apheresis service must have expertise in performing all TA modalities and addressing problems that may arise during treatment. Consequently, apheresis physicians and staff members must be familiar with the current literature related not only to TA but also to the diseases and patient populations requiring treatment. This chapter focuses on the management of adult patients; pediatric apheresis is covered in detail in Chapter 21.

The Therapeutic Apheresis Service

A TA service is ideally organized as a clinical consultative service, typically consisting of a physician who has the role of medical director, potentially additional physicians, several nurses and/or other personnel trained to perform apheresis, and possibly additional ancillary staff to aid with supportive tasks. The physicians pro-

Vishesh Chhibber, MD, Associate Medical Director, Transfusion Medicine, UMass Memorial Medical Center, and Assistant Professor of Medicine and Pathology, University of Massachusetts Medical School, Worcester, Massachusetts, and Karen E. King, MD, Medical Director, Hemapheresis and Transfusion Support; Associate Director, Transfusion Medicine; and Associate Professor of Pathology and Oncology, Johns Hopkins Medical Institutions, Baltimore, Maryland

The authors have disclosed no conflicts of interest.

vide medical oversight and consequently must have formal training or have accumulated sufficient experience in TA.[1] The formal training of apheresis physicians varies; many have been trained in clinical pathology or hematology with subsequent subspecialty training or experience in transfusion medicine. Some have not completed a formal transfusion medicine fellowship program but have been trained in other medical specialties, such as internal medicine, nephrology, or anesthesia, and have acquired extensive experience in TA.

Professionals performing TA should maintain documentation to support their qualification by training and/or experience. As of December 31, 2008, the American Society for Clinical Pathology's Board of Registry no longer offers hemapheresis practitioner or apheresis technician certification; consequently, a record of both training and experience is the only way to document competence. Although staff other than nurses may perform apheresis, the majority of apheresis services employ at least some nurses because of their skills in evaluating patients and managing clinical issues that may arise during procedures.[2] In addition, nurses are able to administer medications that may be needed during a procedure.

In many institutions, the TA service is associated with a blood donor center, in part because the same or similar equipment can be used to perform both TA and apheresis donor collections. Additionally, the training required to perform these procedures may overlap, and the physicians providing oversight for TA are often trained in handling donor issues as well.

The Therapeutic Apheresis Consultation

An encounter with a patient for possible TA ideally begins with a request for consultation that may come from a variety of subspecialties. The services most frequently requesting consultation at the time of writing are hematology/oncology, neurology, nephrology, transplant surgery, and rheumatology. When consulted to perform TA, the apheresis physician must eval-

uate two crucial points. The first is whether TA is appropriate for the patient's diagnosis. The second is whether a clinical evaluation reveals risk factors that may influence the patient's ability to tolerate TA. Once these steps are completed, the apheresis physician must decide on a course of therapy, discuss the risks and benefits of this therapy with the requesting physician and the patient, obtain informed consent, and, finally, write orders for the procedures to be performed.

Some consultations are more challenging than others. The service requesting consultation may be confident of the patient's diagnosis and know that TA is appropriate for management. Conversely, the consulting service may not be sure of the diagnosis or of the role of TA in the patient's care. In the latter cases the consultant may be able to aid in diagnosis as well as assess whether TA should be considered for the patient. Although the expertise of the clinical service requesting consultation should be respected, the apheresis physician should make an independent evaluation. After a diagnosis is agreed on, the decision to perform TA should be based on the published evidence for efficacy of TA in that condition.

A widely accepted synopsis of available literature and categorization of TA indications is published periodically by the American Society for Apheresis (ASFA) as a special issue of the *Journal of Clinical Apheresis*. The most recent issue, published in 2010,[3] contains summaries of the evidential basis for TA in covered disease entities and assigns them to indication categories based on the strength of the evidence and the quality of the literature. Diseases are assigned to one of four categories:

1. TA is accepted as first-line therapy, either as a primary stand-alone treatment or in conjunction with other modes of treatment.
2. TA is accepted as second-line therapy, either as a stand-alone treatment or in conjunction with other modes of treatment.
3. The optimal role of TA is not established, and decision making should be individualized.
4. There is no evidence of benefit.

A grade of recommendation and the quality of evidence available are also listed for each disease entity. Although this is an excellent tool and a good starting point, a review of the primary literature may still be of value, particularly if the patient has a rare disease, if circumstances are unusual, or if important new data have been published. It is also important to understand available alternative therapies, including their risks and efficacy.

In addition to the strength of the indication, the risk/benefit assessment for TA must take account of the patient's ability to tolerate the procedure. As described in Table 12-1, critical elements of the medical evaluation include hemodynamic stability, the presence of anemia or coagulopathy, and any history of cardiac, renal, or hepatic dysfunction. Vascular access, allergies, and current medications must also be reviewed. Once the decision to perform TA has been made, the magnitude of the procedure must be determined, and appropriate replacement fluids chosen, if applicable. The planned course of therapy and the risk/benefit assessment should be discussed with both the patient and the clinical team.

Informed consent is required before treatment. When obtaining consent, the apheresis physician should provide the patient with a detailed explanation of the procedure, the indication to perform TA, and any alternative therapy. Potential complications and adverse events, including the associated signs and symptoms, should be presented to the patient (see "Management of Adverse Events"), along with a risk/benefit estimate. In some circum-

stances this information should be shared with a family member or health-care advocate who will provide consent, though when consent is obtained from a proxy, an attempt should still be made to explain the procedure to the patient. The patient should have an opportunity to ask questions and express concerns. Many patients have never heard of TA and may be anxious about it; such patients can be reassured that TA procedures are performed often and are generally safe and well tolerated. Written documentation of consent must be retained in the medical record.

The apheresis physician should write the orders for TA. These should include the specifications for the procedure, any premedications needed, laboratory tests to be drawn before and/or after the procedure, and if applicable, instructions for flushing the vascular access catheter. Some physicians choose to stipulate the total number and timing of procedures in advance and provide standing orders for the management of the most common potential complications, should they arise. Regardless, the patient should be reassessed before each procedure to ensure that TA is still needed and safe. Orders may be adjusted if needed based on the preprocedure assessment, as discussed below.

Extracorporeal Volume Evaluation and Management

In planning TA, several quantities related to blood volume must be calculated, including the

---

Table 12-1. Components of the Medical Evaluation for Therapeutic Apheresis Patients

Type of Evaluation	Components
General physical	Vital signs
	Height and weight
	Current vascular access

(Continued)

Table 12-1. Components of the Medical Evaluation for Therapeutic Apheresis Patients (Continued)

Type of Evaluation	Components
Hematologic	Hemoglobin and hematocrit (concern for anemia)
	Platelet count (exclude thrombocytopenia)
	Coagulation status and anticoagulation therapy (exclude coagulopathy, assess risk of bleeding)
	History of thrombosis or hypercoagulable state
Cardiopulmonary	Adequate oxygenation
	Adequate cardiac function (blood pressure, ejection fraction if known)
	History of or current cardiac disease, arrhythmias, or coronary artery disease
	Hemodynamic stability
	Sepsis/systemic inflammatory response syndrome
Renal/metabolic	Volume status and fluid balance
	Electrolyte abnormalities (Ca, K, Mg)
	History of renal or hepatic dysfunction
Neurologic	Mental status, including ability to participate in informed consent process and ability to report symptoms during procedure
	History of seizures or cerebrovascular accidents
	Autonomic dysfunction or neuropathy that may impact peripheral access
Medication	Allergies
	Protein-bound drugs
	Angiotensin-converting enzyme inhibitors
	Other blood pressure medications
	Anti-seizure drugs
	Immunoglobulin preparations
	Anticoagulants (heparin, coumadin, plavix, ASA)
	Vasopressors
	Consideration of timing of drug dosing
Disease-specific testing (some examples)	ADAMTS13, LDH, and reticulocytes for TTP
	Anti-GBM for Goodpasture syndrome
	Acetylcholine receptor antibodies for myasthenia gravis
	ABO and/or HLA antibody titers for incompatible kidney transplant recipients
	Percent hemoglobin S for patients with complications of sickle cell disease

ASA = aspirin; ADAMTS13 = von-Willebrand-factor-cleaving enzyme; LDH = lactate dehydrogenase; TTP = thrombotic thrombocytopenic purpura; GBM = glomerular basement membrane.

total blood volume (TBV), plasma volume (PV), and red cell volume (RCV) of the patient. These values are used to determine details of the TA order, such as the size of an exchange (the "apheresis dose") and hence the amount of replacement fluid that will be required. In therapeutic plasma exchange (TPE), the size of a procedure is customarily conceived in terms of patient PV, typically 1.0 to 1.5 PV. In peripheral blood progenitor cell harvests, the size of the procedure is often conceived in terms of the number of TBVs processed, which may be between 2 and 6 per procedure. For red cell exchange in the setting of severe malaria or babesiosis, the exchange volume may be 1 to 2.5 times the patient's RCV. These general goals must be converted to the requisite number of liters or units in a procedure order. An alternative approach may be used for situations in which a particular endpoint is desired. This approach can be used for red cell exchange in patients with complications of sickle cell disease when a specific final hematocrit and final percent hemoglobin S are specified, and for therapeutic leukapheresis in leukemic patients with leukostasis when a final white cell count is targeted.

Several methods are available to estimate TBV; the two most common approaches are included in Table 12-2 (A). The simplest formula, known as Gilcher's Rule of Fives, is derived from body weight.[4] Although it is easy to use and fairly accurate in average-sized adults, this method may overestimate TBV in obese patients, as adipose tissue is significantly less vascular than other tissues. A more accurate approach that can be used for adults is Nadler's formula, which derives TBV from both height and weight.[5] This method is used in the software of some apheresis instruments that calculate TBV. For obese patients, it is also reasonable to perform TBV calculations using lean body weight plus 20% as the patient's total weight. RCV is usually taken as TBV × hematocrit, and PV, as TBV × (1 − hematocrit).

Once TBV, PV, and RCV are determined and the "apheresis dose" has been decided, the apheresis physician must assess the extracorporeal volume (ECV) and extracorporeal red cell volume (ERCV) for the procedure as percentages of TBV and RCV, respectively. Most patients without significant cardiovascular or pulmonary disease will tolerate an ECV and an ERCV of up to 15%.[6] If the ECV or ERCV of a standard procedure will exceed 15%, or if the patient has significant cardiovascular disease, measures such as priming the circuit with a colloid or red cells should be considered.

Another approach used to assess how well a patient may tolerate red cell loss is to estimate the intraprocedure hematocrit using the formula in Table 12-2 (F). This formula assumes that an isovolemic state is being maintained during the procedure. Most patients will tolerate an intraprocedure hematocrit of 24% without any adverse events, and many will tolerate a lower level.

Different replacement fluids are recommended for different types of TA and clinical indications. Specific recommendations are described in detail in subsequent chapters. Table 12-3 presents an overview of the advantages and disadvantages of various replacement fluids.

Vascular Access

Vascular access capable of supporting an appropriate blood flow rate is needed for TA. In an adult, the optimal withdrawal rate is usually between 60 and 150 mL/minute, allowing most procedures to be performed in less than 3 hours. The most important factors limiting flow rate are the length and diameter of the needle or catheter used. The maximum usable flow rate may also be affected by physiologic factors such as blood viscosity or the patient's tolerance of citrate. Peripheral veins are often adequate, but placement of a double-lumen central venous catheter (CVC) is sometimes required. Less commonly, one can use a CVC as a draw line and a peripheral venous access as the return; this approach may be planned, or it may be employed when a double-lumen apheresis catheter has one port that is not functioning well.

Table 12-2. Calculations for Therapeutic Apheresis, Including Total Blood Volume, Plasma Volume, and Red Cell Volume

A. Two Methods of Calculating Total Blood Volume (TBV)

Gilcher's Rule of Fives

	Blood Volume (mL/kg of Body Weight)			
Patient	Fat	Thin	Normal	Muscular
Male	60	65	70	75
Female	55	60	65	70

Nadler's Formula

Patient	Total Blood Volume (mL)
Male	$(0.006012 \times H^3)/(14.6 \times W) + 604$
Female	$(0.005835 \times H^3)/(15 \times W) + 183$

H = height in inches; W = weight in pounds.

B. Plasma Volume (PV)
$(1 - \text{Hematocrit}) \times \text{TBV} = \text{PV}$
(Hematocrit should be written as a decimal.)

C. Red Cell Volume (RCV)
$\text{Hematocrit} \times \text{TBV} = \text{RCV}$
(Hematocrit should be written as a decimal.)

D. Extracorporeal Volume (ECV) as a Percentage of Total Blood Volume
$(\text{ECV/TBV}) \times 100 = \%\ \text{ECV}$
(ECV is provided by the instrument manufacturer for each specific tubing set.)

E. Extracorporeal Red Cell Volume (ERCV) as a Percentage of Total Red Cell Volume
$(\text{ERCV/RCV}) \times 100 = \%\ \text{ERCV}$
(ERCV is provided by the instrument manufacturer for each specific tubing set.)

F. Intraprocedure Hematocrit
$(\text{Initial RCV} - \text{ERCV/TBV}) \times 100 = \text{Intraprocedure hematocrit (\%)}$

Peripheral Access

Peripheral venous access is preferable, when possible, because it spares the patient the risks of CVC placement. Peripheral access usually includes at least one 17-gauge-or-larger steel needle for the draw line. The antecubital veins (median cubital, cephalic, and basilic veins) are most commonly chosen for withdrawal because they are large, superficial, and not close to major nerve trunks. The return line is often an 18-gauge-or-larger catheter that can typically allow a flow rate >80 mL/minute. The maximal flow rate for smaller catheters will usually be lower, generally <70 mL/minute. The return line can be placed in a forearm or hand vein or, rarely, at other sites such as the foot or the ankle; placement in a nonantecubital vein, if possible, allows the patient to move one arm freely and saves the antecubital vein for a draw

Table 12-3. Replacement Fluids: Advantages, Disadvantages, and Special Issues

Replacement Fluid	Advantages	Disadvantages	Special Issues
Normal Saline (crystalloid)	Inexpensive; no risk of allergic reactions; no risk of disease transmission	Hypo-oncotic; lacks coagulation factors and immunoglobulins	
Albumin (colloid)	Iso-oncotic; low risk of reactions and disease transmission	More expensive; lacks coagulation factors and immunoglobulins	
Plasma	Contains coagulation factors and immunoglobulins	Risk of transfusion reactions, especially allergic reactions; increased citrate content	Special transfusion requirements (ie, appropriate plasma type for ABO-incompatible transplant recipients)
Red Blood Cells		Risk of transfusion reactions	History of red cell alloimmunization

line in subsequent procedures. The draw and the return lines should not be placed in the same extremity, but if this is unavoidable, the draw line should be placed upstream from (ie, distal to) the return line to prevent recirculation of returned blood.

To evaluate and access antecubital veins, a tourniquet or a blood pressure cuff inflated to the patient's diastolic blood pressure is applied about 3 inches above the elbow. The antecubital veins are then visually assessed and palpated; they should feel compressible and spongy. Once a vein is chosen, the skin over it should be prepared in the same manner as for a donor, to avoid infections: an approximately 3-inch area of skin around the venipuncture site is swabbed with povidone-iodine followed by either isopropyl alcohol or chlorhexidine gluconate.[7,8] Topical EMLA cream (eutectic mixture of local anesthetic; lidocaine 2.5% and prilocaine 2.5%; AstraZeneca, Wilmington, DE) or injected lidocaine 1% can provide local anesthesia before venipuncture. They are useful in patients who are particularly anxious about needle sticks. In patients who do not have good peripheral veins, techniques such as arm exercises and warm compresses may be helpful. During a procedure, intermittently opening and closing the fist to squeeze a compressible object will increase venous blood flow; this is usually helpful and often required.

Variable success rates have been reported for gaining peripheral access. One study found that only 4.4% of subjects with multiple sclerosis had inadequate antecubital access for TPE. Furthermore, 89 of the 93 patients who had initially adequate antecubital access were able to complete the course of TPE with it.[9] Other studies have reported successful peripheral access in 30% to 50% of neurology patients undergoing TA.[10,11] Patients who may not be candidates for peripheral access include those with poor vascular or muscle tone, those who are unable to contract muscles to increase blood flow in the upper extremity, and those who are uncooperative or have altered mental status, weakness, or fatigue.[12]

Central Venous Access

CVC placement carries significant risks and should not be undertaken without good reason. If peripheral access cannot be obtained, the decision is straightforward. Factors that may favor central access in marginal cases include very long TA procedures, a long course of TA with many procedures planned, a need for venous access for other reasons, and the availability of adequate catheter care if the patient is to be discharged.

A CVC must be able to support adequate blood flow rates. Catheters that can support hemodialysis will be adequate for TA. However, many catheters intended for infusion of medications or for withdrawing blood for tests—such as standard double- or triple-lumen catheters, peripherally inserted central catheters, or ports—cannot provide adequate outflow rates. Catheters for TA must be sufficiently rigid that they do not collapse when negative pressure is applied during blood withdrawal at high flow rates. The flexibility of percutaneous polyurethane catheters exhibits temperature sensitivity. They are more rigid during placement at room temperature, then soften at body temperature for increased comfort after placement; however, they remain sufficiently rigid to support high draw rates.[13] Shorter catheters offer less resistance to flow and allow anticoagulant to be mixed with blood sooner. Double-lumen catheters generally have lumens coded as red and blue. The former is shorter and occasionally thicker and is intended as the access or draw line. The latter is intended as the return line; its more downstream tip minimizes recirculation during TA.

A CVC can be placed in an internal jugular, subclavian, or femoral vein. Femoral catheters do not entail risks of pneumothorax or hemothorax, require less specialized skill than jugular or subclavian catheter placement, and can be placed at the bedside. Consequently, femoral catheters are sometimes chosen for emergent TA. Disadvantages of femoral catheters include higher risks of infection, thrombosis, and kinking, as well as restrictions on patient positioning and mobility.[14]

Internal jugular or subclavian catheters should ideally be placed under imaging guidance. Catheter position should be confirmed with a radiograph to ensure proper placement without kinks or bends. The right internal jugular vein is preferred, as it allows almost straight line access to the superior vena cava and right atrium and avoids accidental lodging of the catheter tip within the azygous root. A left-sided approach requires bending the catheter to reach optimal position. The ideal tip location for these catheters is somewhat controversial. Some prefer that it be 1 to 2 cm above the junction of the right atrium and superior vena cava, believing that infusion of cold and/or citrate-containing fluids directly into the right atrium can cause arrhythmias. Others prefer the tip to be in the right atrium, believing that arrhythmias are uncommon and may be partially prevented with use of a blood warmer, while intra-atrial placement carries a lower risk of thrombosis and vascular erosion and allows higher flow rates with less recirculation.[13,15]

Central lines can be tunneled or nontunneled. Tunneled catheters are often soft silicone based and may have antimicrobial cuffs; they have a lower risk of infection with prolonged use.[16-18] A tunneled catheter is preferable if it will be needed for a prolonged period of time, and it may be advantageous if TA is performed in an outpatient setting.

Less common access alternatives include arteriovenous fistulas or grafts, and ports. Fistulas and grafts may be found in patients who also require vascular access for dialysis, including patients with sickle cell disease who require both dialysis and chronic red cell exchange, and incompatible kidney transplant patients who require dialysis and are also undergoing TPE for rejection or in preparation for incompatible transplantation. Indwelling (implanted) high-flow ports, sometimes called vortex ports, are being used more frequently for TA in patients with sickle cell disease who need chronic red cell exchange.[19,20] Patients may have two single ports, one single port plus one peripheral access, or even a double port. If a high-flow port is used for TA, care must be taken to use an appropriate, noncoring needle to avoid damaging the diaphragm.[19-21] Additionally, achievable flow rates may be lower, compared to CVCs, and high-flow ports may require instillation of fibrinolytics before use.

Catheter Care

Central catheters require care and maintenance, including regular dressing changes and inspection of the insertion site for redness, swelling, or drainage. If there is evidence of infection, the catheter should be removed before the patient develops catheter-related sepsis. Catheters must also be flushed with saline and filled with a heparin solution after each use and at regular intervals if unused, to prevent thrombosis. The concentration of heparin may vary from 100 units/mL to 5000 units/mL, depending on the expected interval between flushes. If the concentration exceeds 1000 units/mL, the solution should be aspirated before use of the catheter, because flushing the catheter without removing the heparin could systemically anticoagulate the patient.

Recirculation

Recirculation occurs when red cells and fluid returning from the instrument are withdrawn again through the access line, thus compromising the efficiency of the procedure. A small amount of recirculation, usually less than 10%, may occur with CVC access, even when procedures are uneventful[22-24]; however, several circumstances may increase recirculation, such as a thrombus on the catheter that affects blood flow, a fibrin sheath at the tip of the catheter, or a thrombus within the central vein where the catheter is placed. Recirculation is influenced by the relationship between blood flow rates in the central vein and the catheter. Ordinarily the rate of blood flow past the more distal access port is sufficient to keep recirculation to a minimum. However, if the ports on the catheter are reversed so that the blue port is being used for withdrawal and the red port for return, recirculation may amount to as much as 20% of total blood flow through the instrument.[25-27] If this configuration is necessary, an increase in the total amount of blood processed may be appropriate.

Technical Difficulties and Catheter-Related Complications

Technical problems that may be encountered during TA include defects in the manufacturing of the disposable kits, malfunctions of the apheresis instrument, difficulty maintaining adequate blood flow through the catheter, and air in the system. The instrument should receive regular maintenance and quality control checks to ensure proper functioning. One difficulty that may be encountered is air entering the circuit. Most instruments have sensors that will detect the air, activate an alarm, and stop the pumps. Air is then diverted into the waste bag; once it has cleared from the circuit the procedure can resume. At the current time, air embolism remains a risk associated with CVC placement but is seldom related to TA. Leaks within the tubing may uncommonly be seen; if this occurs, the procedure should be stopped, the disposable kit replaced, and the procedure restarted with a new tubing set. Depending on the patient's baseline hemoglobin and hematocrit, a red cell transfusion may be necessary to replace blood lost in the defective tubing.

Probably the most common technical difficulty encountered during TA is inadequate access flow. This may be caused by kinking, malpositioning, or thrombosis of a catheter, but the exact cause may not be known. Commonly, a limb of the catheter can be flushed easily but does not provide adequate blood outflow. If the catheter appears to be positioned properly, instillation of a fibrinolytic agent such as alteplase or t-PA (tissue plasminogen activator; 1-2 mg/mL) may be tried. Suitable caution should be exercised to prevent its entry into the systemic circulation. Only the actual volume of the catheter lumen should be instilled. If one lumen seems clotted, it may be wise to treat the other lumen as well. It is occasionally preferable to use the blue port as the draw line, for better flow, recognizing the likelihood of increased recirculation. If there is a hole between the two ports of the catheter, shunting between the draw and return lines may occur. This should be suspected if the fluid in the draw line appears clear or dilute (because of the priming solution entering the draw line) or if the instrument is unable to establish an interface.

A number of severe complications are associated with CVCs. These include pneumothorax, hemothorax, arterial puncture, air embolism, infection, sepsis, life-threatening hemorrhage, cardiac arrhythmias, thrombosis, and stenosis of a central vein.[11] Studies have suggested that the most common and severe complications of TA are related to use of a CVC.[10] Central vein thrombosis and arteriovenous fistula formation can limit vascular access in the future. Vascular erosion from a CVC, although rare, can cause acute hemothorax or hemopericardium that may be fatal.[28]

Intraprocedural Care and Monitoring

Following a thorough initial evaluation for TA, patients often have multiple procedures; for example, 5 to 10 TPEs over several weeks or a monthly red cell exchange for years. Patients should have a brief medical evaluation before each TA procedure that includes an interval history and a review of pertinent vital signs, laboratory data, and any changes in medications. A brief physical examination may sometimes be indicated. A decision to withhold or delay a medication before a procedure may be required, especially for inpatients who may be on intravenous medications or fluids; such adjustments should be discussed with the primary team. Additional vascular access may be needed if medications or fluids must be infused during apheresis. Information acquired during reevaluation may warrant adjustment or postponement of the procedure; for example, a patient whose hemoglobin has decreased may require a red cell transfusion before TA.

Several steps are required to prepare an apheresis instrument for use. All preventive maintenance and routine quality control must be up to date. The disposable kit must be properly installed and primed, and patient-specific information must be entered. Internal software will perform many of the required calculations and will monitor the instrument during the procedure. Most instruments also maintain fluid balance according to instructions entered by the operator.

Although modern apheresis instruments are highly automated, a trained and alert operator is still needed to visually check for kinks or leaks in the tubing and for the appropriate color in the solutions and to visually monitor the flow of blood and solutions in the instrument as well as the material that is being removed, to confirm proper functioning of pumps. The operator must also monitor the volume of anticoagulant and replacement fluids consumed to confirm that they are correct. Although most instruments have detectors and alarms for air in the tubing, the operator must also be vigilant and check for this because as little as 50 to 100 mL of air can be fatal. This volume of air can be aspirated through an 18-gauge catheter in 1 second if the pressure difference is 4 cm H_2O.[29]

The operator must also monitor the patient for adverse events. During the informed consent process, the patient should have been counseled to report symptoms related to possible adverse effects (Table 12-4). Vital signs should be measured at regular intervals during the procedure (usually every 15-30 minutes). Occasionally a critically ill patient or a patient with a cardiac arrhythmia will require cardiac monitoring. Such patients are frequently in an intensive care or other monitored setting where the primary team can continue to monitor the patient during therapy. If such a patient becomes unstable during TA, the procedure should be halted while the primary team evaluates and resuscitates the patient; TA can be reinitiated, if appropriate, once the patient has been stabilized.

Table 12-4. Complications of Therapeutic Apheresis and Suggested Management

Type of Complication	Signs and Symptoms	Suggested Management
Procedure Related		
Anxiety with hyperventilation	Tachycardia, hypertension or hypotension, tingling of fingers and/or toes, diaphoresis	Have patient breathe into a paper bag. Offer supportive, calm reassurance. For hypotensive patients, place in Trendelenburg and administer normal saline bolus. Consider anxiolytics for subsequent procedures.
Vasovagal reaction	Bradycardia, hypotension, diaphoresis, pallor and nausea	Place patient in Trendelenburg, give normal saline bolus. Place cool moist towels on forehead. Stimulate patient. Consider ammonia spirits.
Hypocalcemia	Paresthesias, initially circumoral but may progress to involve other parts of body; vibration in jaw; nausea, vomiting, and diarrhea; chest tightness; hypotension; prolonged QT interval on EKG; tetany	Pause procedure. Slow citrate infusion by decreasing whole blood flow rate or increasing WB:ACD ratio. Administer calcium, either oral or IV. Add calcium to colloid or crystalloid replacement fluid for continuous replacement procedures (do not add calcium to plasma).
Hypovolemia or antihypertensive therapy	Hypotension, diaphoresis, tachycardia (the latter may not occur in patients on beta blockers)	Place patient in Trendelenburg, and give normal saline bolus. For subsequent procedures, increase colloid replacement, decreasing crystalloid replacement when applicable; consider holding antihypertensive dose until after apheresis, when applicable.
ACE inhibitor use	Flushing, hypotension	Hold apheresis for 24 to 48 hours after last ACE inhibitor dose.
Reaction to ethylene oxide	Burning eyes, periorbital edema, other allergic symptoms	Stop procedure; if feasible, perform double prime for subsequent procedures.

(Continued)

Table 12-4. Complications of Therapeutic Apheresis and Suggested Management (Continued)

Type of Complication	Signs and Symptoms	Suggested Management
Replacement Fluid Related		
Allergic	Itching, urticaria, facial edema, change in voice, difficulty swallowing, wheezing, shortness of breath, hypotension	Administer IV diphenhydramine, IV methylprednisolone, and/or subcutaneous epinephrine.
Transfusion reaction (including nonhemolytic febrile, allergic, acute hemolytic, TRALI, etc)	Signs and symptoms will vary based on type of transfusion reaction but include fever (nonhemolytic febrile), itching, hives and wheezing (allergic), respiratory compromise	Stop infusion of blood product and follow transfusion reaction protocol.
Vascular Access Related		
Sepsis	Hypotension, positive blood cultures	Treat patient with appropriate antimicrobials, hold apheresis until new catheter is placed, and use peripheral access if feasible.
Thrombosis	Catheter cannot be flushed, high-pressure alarms indicate suboptimal flow	Radiograph to assess placement if appropriate; instill thrombolytic agent.

WB = whole blood; ACD = acid-citrate-dextrose; IV = intravenous; EKG = electrocardiogram; ACE = angiotensin-converting enzyme; TRALI = transfusion-related acute lung injury.

Management of Special Patient Populations

Some complications of TA are related to the patient's underlying medical condition. It is important to identify these conditions in the initial evaluation so that the TA procedure can be adjusted to prevent or at least minimize such complications.

Patients with an Increased Risk of Bleeding

Adverse events related to bleeding, though not common, are possible, especially in patients undergoing TPE. Patients who do not have a predisposition to hemorrhage typically receive a 5% albumin replacement solution that does not contain coagulation factors.[30,31] As described in Chapter 15, this will cause a drop in coagulation factor activity of 40% to 70% after the procedure, which is evident in a mild prolongation of the prothrombin time and activated partial thromboplastin time.[30,32] These values, though increased from baseline, may still be in the normal range and will return to baseline in 1 to 2 days.[32] Fibrinogen is also affected by TPE and may take 2 to 3 days to return to normal levels.[31]

Plasma should be avoided whenever possible because of the risks of disease transmission and allergic or hypocalcemic reactions.[33] However, for patients with an increased risk for bleeding, such as those who have recently undergone invasive procedures, those with liver disease or other coagulopathies, and those undergoing intensive daily TPE, repletion of fibrinogen and other coagulation factors with plasma replacement should be considered.

Although citrate is the anticoagulant of choice for TA, heparin can also be used.[34] With a half-life of approximately 90 minutes, heparin is not metabolized as rapidly as citrate; consequently its use during TA results in systemic anticoagulation of the patient. When plasma is not being removed, as in patients undergoing peripheral blood progenitor cell collection or leukocyte reduction, a combination of acid-citrate-dextrose and heparin is sometimes chosen; this allows a lower amount of each anticoagulant to be used, resulting in decreased hypocalcemia and minimal systemic anticoagulation despite high flow rates.[35]

Patients with Anemia

The ERCV will constitute a greater percentage of RCV for an anemic patient. Such patients are therefore less likely to tolerate the temporary shift of that portion of their red cells into the extracorporeal circuit. As described above, if the patient's intraprocedure hematocrit is too low or ERCV exceeds 15% of RCV, the patient may become symptomatic during TA.[6] Acutely anemic patients are more likely to be symptomatic than those with chronic anemia at the same hematocrit level. Patients at risk from anemia should be transfused before or during TA, or the circuit should be primed with red cells. Anemic patients with preexisting cardiovascular disease, especially those with signs or symptoms possibly related to anemia such as chest pain, shortness of breath, tachycardia, headache, dizziness, or confusion, should be transfused before TA. For patients with an unstable hemoglobin, including those with active blood loss, thrombotic thrombocytopenic purpura, hemolytic uremic syndrome, acute leukemia, or sickle cell disease, a timely hematocrit measurement should guide decisions. Anemic patients with hyperviscosity caused by paraproteinemia or hyperleukocytosis should not have red cell transfusions until their blood viscosity has been decreased by either TPE or leukapheresis, respectively.[36] In severely anemic patients with hyperleukocytosis, the authors have transfused red cells slowly through a separate peripheral IV line after leukapheresis has been initiated.

Patients with Heart Disease or Hemodynamic Instability

Some patients who would benefit from TA are hemodynamically unstable from cardiovascular disease or other causes. These patients are less likely to tolerate the blood volume changes related to TA. In such situations the apheresis physician, in consultation with the patient's primary care team, must decide if TA is needed urgently or if it can be withheld until the patient's clinical situation improves. These patients may benefit from cardiac monitoring if they are not already in a monitored setting. Patients receiving vasopressors for blood pressure support may need dose adjustments during TA. Removal of pressors during apheresis is generally not a significant problem, because of their short half-life.[37,38] Critically ill patients may deteriorate for reasons unrelated to TA. In these situations, TA is generally halted while the patient is resuscitated, after which TA can resume if appropriate. In the authors' experience, TA can be performed safely in patients on cardiopulmonary support devices, including pulmonary oscillators, intra-aortic balloon pumps, ventricular assist devices, and extracorporeal membrane oxygenators.

Patients with Fluid-Volume Abnormalities

Some patients requiring TA may have preexisting fluid-volume abnormalities. The apheresis team may be asked to leave a volume-overloaded patient in negative fluid balance after TPE; however, this is not necessarily the best management option. Patients with renal failure often have low albumin and serum protein levels; such patients left in negative fluid balance after TPE are at risk for symptomatic hypotension from a decrease in plasma oncotic pressure. Also, these patients typically have a large proportion of the excess fluid in the extravascular space, which is not immediately accessible by TA. Diuresis and/or dialysis are more appropriate and effective methods to remove excess volume. If volume reduction is desired with TPE, it should be limited to no more than 5% to 10% of plasma volume.

Managing TA patients with decreased intravascular volumes resulting from hemorrhage or dehydration can also be a challenge. Patients with significant blood loss and anemia should be transfused. Dehydrated patients should be resuscitated with crystalloid before or during TA, because they may not tolerate volume loss into the extracorporeal circuit. In patients undergoing TPE, the fluid balance can be adjusted so that replacement exceeds removal by 10% to 25% (110-125% replacement), and a portion of the replacement can be crystalloid. Patients who have just completed hemodialysis may be marginally hypovolemic and thus may not tolerate TA well; if a patient requires both procedures on the same day, TA should generally be performed first. Alternatively, the two procedures can be performed in tandem using a four-way stopcock attached to the draw line to connect the TPE circuit in parallel with the low-pressure side of the hemodialysis circuit.[39]

Patients with Serum Protein Abnormalities

Patients with elevated serum protein levels, such as those with Waldenström macroglobulinemia or multiple myeloma, may need TPE for the treatment of hyperviscosity or other problems, as discussed in Chapter 16. These patients usually have an expanded plasma volume and may have symptoms related to volume overload. Clinicians may request a negative fluid balance in these patients; however, this should be limited to 10% or less, as it could dehydrate the patient and increase serum viscosity. In patients with nephrosis and hypoproteinemia, some recommend a positive fluid balance to prevent hypotension, but it is not

clear that this helps, and many practitioners will simply maintain euvolemia for these patients. Some authors have noted that removal of immunoglobulins from patients with paraproteins appears less efficient than in other patients; this may be related to underestimation of the patient's plasma volume by standard formulas.[40,41] However, because viscosity decreases logarithmically as a function of protein concentration, even small exchanges will have a salutary effect on symptoms of hyperviscosity.[42]

Patients with Abnormalities of Citrate Metabolism

Most patients can metabolize the citrate infused during TA and will not develop significant symptoms related to hypocalcemic toxicity. However, patients who have renal or liver disease are at a higher risk of developing symptoms. Patients with severe liver disease may have severe hypocalcemic toxicity because of an inability to metabolize citrate. This problem is further exacerbated because they typically require plasma as the replacement fluid, exposing them to even higher amounts of citrate. Such patients will need monitoring of ionized calcium levels at regular intervals (every 15-30 minutes) and may require intravenous calcium infusions during the procedure.

Patients with Cryoglobulinemia or Cold Agglutinin Syndrome

Patients with cryoglobulinemia or cold agglutinin syndrome may have exacerbation of symptoms from cooling of blood in the extracorporeal circuit. Cooling can be minimized if TPE is performed with a continuous-flow device at a relatively rapid flow rate. Nevertheless, the solutions and replacement fluids can be prewarmed, and a blood warmer should also be used. Raising the temperature of the patient's room and using warming blankets may be of additional benefit; however, one must be careful to avoid hypotension related to dehydration or vasodilatation. Additionally, the instrument should be closely monitored to be sure there is no malfunction related to overheating. A reliable vascular access is especially important in such patients because agglutination or precipitation may occur in blood in the instrument if a procedure must be halted because of loss of access.

Pregnant Patients

TA can be performed safely on pregnant women if appropriate adjustments are made. During pregnancy, TBV increases by approximately 40%, PV by 45% to 55%, and RCV by 20% to 30%.[43,44] The volumes calculated and programmed into the apheresis instrument should be adjusted appropriately. Positioning the patient during TA is also important; if a patient is not positioned appropriately on her left side, the gravid uterus may compress the inferior vena cava, causing diminished venous return, decreased efficiency of the procedure, and possibly hypotension.

Patients with Drug Interactions

Some drugs can predispose to adverse events. Beta blockers, calcium channel blockers, nitrates, and other antihypertensive medications may prevent or inhibit physiologic compensatory cardiovascular responses. For example, beta blockers may make a patient more susceptible to hypotension because of a blunted adrenergic response leading to an inability to achieve a needed increase in heart rate. Calcium channel blockers and nitrates may prevent vasoconstriction needed to maintain a normal blood pressure. One group has attributed hypotension during TPE in patients taking angiotensin-converting enzyme inhibitors (ACEi) to a mechanism other than the antihypertensive effect of the drug.[45] It is postulated that these reactions are caused by small amounts of prekallikrein-activating factor (PAF) in albumin replacement solutions. PAF could lead to generation of bradykinin, inactivation of which might be blocked by ACEi through inhibition of the enzyme kininase II. Reactions of this type have complicated procedures in which foreign surfaces activate PAF, including hemodialysis, protein A immunoadsorption, and red cell transfusion with bedside leukocyte-reduction filters.[46,47] However, a relationship of hypotension during TPE to PAF or any other contaminant in albumin has never been confirmed by actual measurement. Some physicians prefer to delay TPE until ACEi have been held for 24 to 48 hours, depending on the duration of action of the patient's ACEi. Others have observed many uneventful TPEs in patients on ACEi and reason that even if the PAF contaminant hypothesis is correct, reactions to albumin are likely to be lot specific. They therefore proceed with TPE and hold ACEi only if a hypotensive reaction occurs. Other proposed options (of unproven worth) include performing TPE with an alternative replacement fluid such as FFP or hydroxyethyl starch, with or without partial crystalloid replacement.

Certain drugs can be partially removed by TPE. Removal of agents such as antiseizure medications and antiarrhythmics can cause adverse events from loss of therapeutic effect. Drugs are more likely to be affected if they have a small volume of distribution and/or if a significant portion of the drug is bound to plasma proteins. Therapeutic immunoglobulin preparations such as antithymocyte globulin, intravenous immune globulin, and monoclonal antibodies such as rituximab may be removed by TPE. Ideally they should be given after a course of TPE is completed.

Theoretically, dosing of drugs immediately before TPE should be avoided,[48] especially if the drug is given infrequently (once daily or less); however, there is no evidence to prove that this approach is superior. TPE may be performed without regard to the dosing schedule for drugs given multiple times during the day. There are little objective data, but what there are suggests that dosing need not be adjusted with prednisone, digoxin, cyclosporine, ceftriaxone, ceftazidime, valproic acid, and phenobarbital.[48-50]

Another mechanism of interaction between TPE and medications is illustrated by the case of succinylcholine, which is inactivated by a plasma enzyme. Replacing plasma with albumin or crystalloid in TPE lowers the level of the enzyme enough to delay metabolism of succinylcholine and prolong its effects.

Management of Adverse Events

Complications of TA can be related to vascular access, to replacement fluids, or to the procedure itself (Table 12-4). A common complaint during TA is the sensation of being cold or even developing chills; this is likely related to infusion of replacement fluids that are colder than body temperature. A blood warmer in the return line and/or an electric heating pad placed under the patient may be helpful in preventing or ameliorating this feeling. Some patients prefer several blankets, including one around their head. Other common adverse events are hypocalcemia, allergic reactions to blood products, hypotension related to hypovolemia or antihypertensive medications, and vasovagal reactions. The first response to any adverse reaction is to pause the machine; further treatment is specific to the type of reaction observed (Table 12-4).

Hypocalcemic Toxicity

The signs and symptoms of hypocalcemia begin with circumoral paresthesias that may spread to other areas of the body. Symptoms may progress to include tremors, muscle cramps, nausea, vomiting, diarrhea, anxiety, lightheadedness, chest tightness, hypotension, prolonged QT interval on EKG, and ultimately tetany and/or grand mal seizures. During TA, the apheresis operator should ask the patient about such symptoms. For patients unable to report symptoms because of intubation or mental status issues, it may be prudent to monitor the ionized calcium level at intervals.

Calcium metabolism is controlled by several interrelated mechanisms, as described in detail in Chapter 3. Approximately half of the calcium in blood is bound to albumin, while most of the remaining half exists as an ion within the plasma. It is a low level of ionized calcium that causes the signs and symptoms of hypocalcemia. Mild metabolic alkalosis caused by citrate metabolism may be seen in patients undergoing TA; this can result in hypokalemia in addition to exacerbating the hypocalcemia.

The most common cause of ionized hypocalcemia related to TA is infusion of citrate anticoagulant, especially when it is infused rapidly and/or for a prolonged period of time. As already mentioned, patients with hepatic or renal disease are at increased risk because of decreased ability to metabolize citrate. Patients with pre-existing hypocalcemia are also at increased risk.

Another mechanism that may contribute to hypocalcemia during TPE relates to the infusion of fractionated albumin that has empty calcium binding sites (so-called stripped albumin). After infusion, such albumin can bind ionized calcium in plasma and contribute to ionized hypocalcemia.

There are several approaches to treating citrate-induced hypocalcemia. For very mild signs or symptoms, the whole blood flow rate can be decreased, thereby reducing the rate of citrate infusion. If this is not possible or effective, the whole-blood-to-anticoagulant ratio can be altered to reduce the flow of citrate. If symptoms persist, calcium supplementation should be used. Oral supplementation with calcium-containing antacids may be tried for patients with minor symptoms but may be of limited efficacy.[51] For persistent or severe symptoms, intravenous calcium should be given, using either calcium gluconate or calcium chloride infused via a drip or slow push.[51-54] Ten-percent calcium chloride has approximately three times as much calcium per unit of volume as 10% calcium gluconate (Table 12-5),[52,55,56] and studies have suggested that it ionizes faster than calcium gluconate when given intravenously to massively transfused patients.[55] Intravenous calcium supplementation with frequent monitoring of ionized calcium is recommended for patients with severe liver failure. One observational study showed that the percentage of TPE procedures in which patients had symptoms related to hypocalcemia was reduced from 35.6% to 8.6% when a continuous infusion of calcium gluconate was provided.[51]

Patients undergoing leukapheresis, whether for leukostasis or for peripheral blood progenitor cell collection, are at increased risk of citrate-induced hypocalcemia from high flow rates

Table 12-5. Comparison of Calcium Gluconate and Calcium Chloride

	Calcium Gluconate	Calcium Chloride
Molecular weight	430 kD	111 kD
Elemental calcium per gram	93 mg	272 mg
Milliequivalents per gram	4.65 mEq	13.6 mEq
Formulations available commercially	100 mg/mL in 10-, 50-, or 100-mL vials	100 mg/mL in 10-mL vial
Cardiac monitoring	Not required	Often required
Administration (IV)	Central or peripheral	Central only
Amount used per liter of albumin during therapeutic plasma exchange (published)	4.65 mEq,[51] 2 mEq[54]	4.07 mEq (2 mmol)[53]

and prolonged procedures. Several strategies have been employed to reduce complications related to citrate. As mentioned above, the amount of citrate infused can be reduced by anticoagulating with a mixture of citrate and heparin that anticoagulates adequately with less citrate.[57] Alternatively, calcium can be given via a slow intravenous infusion throughout the procedure; eg, 1 gram of calcium chloride or 2 to 3 grams of calcium gluconate in 100 to 250 mL of saline infused over several hours. The infusion should be given via a separate peripheral intravenous line, if possible.

To combat hypocalcemia from calcium binding by manufactured albumin, some apheresis facilities add calcium to the albumin solution.[51,53,54] The exact amount of calcium added varies by institution (see Table 12-5), but in uncontrolled trials the strategy has seemed effective in reducing symptoms.[51,53,54] This should not be done if intermittent flow instruments are being used, because of the possibility of clotting of extracorporeal blood during the procedure.[51]

Allergic Reactions

Allergic reactions may present as itching, hives, cutaneous erythema, facial swelling, or a burning sensation in the eyes. More severe reactions include wheezing, dyspnea, hypotension, and tachycardia. Allergic reactions during TA are most often caused by plasma or red cells, but hydroxyethyl starch and even albumin are occasionally implicated.

Mild allergic reactions can be treated with 25 to 50 mg of diphenhydramine intravenously. If symptoms do not improve, a corticosteroid such as methylprednisolone, 100 mg intravenously, can be administered. If the reaction is severe, epinephrine 1:1000, 0.3 mL to 0.5 mL, can be administered subcutaneously, and that dose can be repeated after 10 to 15 minutes if no improvement is noted. Such patients should be closely monitored.

In patients with a history of allergic reactions, some advocate premedication regimens that may include an H_1 receptor antagonist such as diphenhydramine or hydroxyzine, an H_2 receptor antagonist such as ranitidine or famotidine, and even corticosteroids. The efficacy of these regimens has not been established. In the setting of allergic transfusion reactions, premedication regimens have not been proven to be effective, but better studies are needed.[58] In patients with persistent moderate-to-severe allergic reactions despite premedication, a continuous infusion of 50 to 100 mg of diphenhydramine in 100 to 250 mL of saline during TA might be considered. Such patients may be premedicated with diphenhydramine and/or a corticosteroid approximately 30 minutes before

TA; the infusion is started approximately 15 to 30 minutes after the TA begins and continues to the end of the procedure.

A rare patient may have an allergic reaction to ethylene oxide, a gas used to sterilize disposable apheresis tubing sets. Such patients typically complain of a burning sensation involving their eyes, followed by the development of periorbital edema and tearing soon after initiation of the TA procedure.[59,60] Upon recognition of such a reaction, the procedure should be stopped and the patient treated with antihistamines and possibly steroids, depending on severity. If additional procedures are required, repeated priming of the tubing may help to wash out ethylene oxide to prevent subsequent reactions. (The feasibility of repriming may be limited for some instruments.)

Hypovolemia

Hypovolemia is a relatively common adverse effect of TA. The signs and symptoms include dizziness, lightheadedness, nausea, diaphoresis, tachycardia, and hypotension. A drop in blood pressure without symptoms may also be seen. The most likely cause of hypotension is the fluid shifts that occur during TA. Treatment usually involves halting the procedure, placing the patient in the Trendelenburg position, and giving a bolus of saline or colloid. The majority of patients will respond to this treatment, and the procedure can then resume. Adjustments in subsequent apheresis procedures, such as increasing the fluid balance or increasing the ratio of colloid to crystalloid in the replacement fluid, may prevent repeat episodes of hypovolemia.

Patients on antihypertensive medications may have hypotensive reactions that mimic hypovolemic reactions. As mentioned above, beta blockers and calcium channel blockers interfere with normal physiologic responses that help to maintain blood pressure during volume shifts. To prevent hypotension, it may be advisable to withhold such medications until after TA, if feasible. It should be noted that patients with chronic hypertension may experience symptoms of hypotension at blood pressures that, while normal, are lower than their usual readings. Such symptoms will usually respond to the standard treatments described above.

Orders

As mentioned above, orders must be written by the apheresis physician for all TA procedures. Although not required, it may be helpful to have preprinted order forms for TA, especially in institutions where the volume of procedures is high. Forms that cover a course of therapy increase efficiency and make it less likely that an order will be omitted accidentally. In addition, preprinted order forms provide more consistent communication between physicians and apheresis operators. When multiple physicians cover the apheresis service, preprinted orders help to maintain consistency in orders.

It is advisable to have PRN orders to manage the more common adverse effects, because prompt treatment will often minimize morbidity. The physician should still be notified promptly of such reactions, because additional diagnostic or therapeutic actions may be warranted, and adjustments to the procedure may be necessary.

Records

Meticulous records should be maintained for all patients undergoing TA. The medical record is indispensable as a means to document the apheresis procedure and as a method to communicate important information to other physicians, nurses, or teams treating the patient. If well documented and easily available, the record can be referenced by the apheresis team as needed, enabling review of prior adverse reactions or facilitating response to a recall of kits or reagents. The record should include the patient's vital signs, all run parameters, and the identity of staff who performed the procedure. All records generated must be signed by the physician or nurse performing the documentation. Many apheresis services maintain a chart in the apheresis center for each patient. An original procedure note is placed in the hospital chart and a copy is kept in the apheresis chart if the patient is admitted to the hospital. In the case of outpatients, one copy of the procedure note should be sent to the hospital medical records department and another copy should be placed in the apheresis chart. It is especially important that procedure notes in the hospital chart document adverse effects, unexpected findings, and medications given during TA; this information may be useful in treating patients after apheresis, in adjusting subsequent procedures, and in managing future adverse events.

Most institutions are developing policies for outpatient visit records that allow wide access to the documents, as there may be information in them that could affect management of the patient by other consultants. This can be accomplished by placing a note in a patient's electronic record that can be easily accessed by all services associated with the institution.

Conclusion

In order to appropriately manage the TA patient, well-qualified physicians, nurses, and technicians are required. Although most apheresis procedures are well tolerated, adverse effects may occur and must be recognized and properly managed to prevent minor adverse effects from becoming major complications. The apheresis staff must be well versed in the principles of apheresis and the indications for TA, as well as the issues and problems that may be encountered during apheresis procedures. An understanding of the patient's underlying disease is also necessary. A thorough evaluation of each patient before treatment will provide information that is crucial in making adjustments during a procedure. If patients are managed appropriately, serious adverse effects are less likely to be encountered.

References

1. Guidelines for therapeutic apheresis clinical privileges. J Clin Apher 2007;22:181-2.

2. Howell C. The challenging role of the therapeutic apheresis nurse. Transfus Apher Sci 2008;38:213-15.

3. Szczepiorkowski ZM, Winters JL, Bandarenko N, et al. Guidelines on the use of therapeutic apheresis in clinical practice—evidence-based approach from the Apheresis Applications Committee of the American Society for Apheresis. The fifth special issue. J Clin Apher 2010; 25:83-177.

4. Gilcher RO, Smith JW. Apheresis: Principles and technology of hemapheresis. In: Simon TL, Snyder EL, Solheim BG, et al, eds. Rossi's principles of transfusion medicine. 4th ed. Bethesda, MD: AABB Press, 2009:617-28.

5. Klein HG, Anstee DJ, eds. Mollison's blood transfusion in clinical medicine. 11th ed. Oxford, UK: Blackwell Publishing Ltd, 2005: 849-50.

6. Huestis DW. Risks and safety practices in hemapheresis procedures. Arch Pathol Lab Med 1989;113:273-8.

7. Methods Section 6: Blood collection, component preparation, and storage. In: Roback JD, Combs MR, Grossman BJ, Hillyer CD, eds. Technical manual. 16th ed. Bethesda, MD: AABB, 2008:941-61.

8. Goldman M, Roy G, Frechette N, et al. Evaluation of donor skin disinfection methods. Transfusion 1997;37:309-12.

9. Noseworthy JH, Shumak KH, Vandervoort MK. Long-term use of antecubital veins for plasma exchange. The Canadian Cooperative Multiple Sclerosis Study Group. Transfusion 1989;29: 610-13.

10. Couriel D, Weinstein R. Complications of therapeutic plasma exchange: A recent assessment. J Clin Apher 1994;9:1-5.

11. Grishaber JE, Cunningham MC, Rohret PA, Strauss RG. Analysis of venous access for therapeutic plasma exchange in patients with neurological disease. J Clin Apher 1992;7:119-23.

12. Hodgson WJB, Mercan S. Hemapheresis listening post: Optimal venous access. Transfusion Sci 1991;12:274.

13. Schwab SJ, Beathard G. The hemodialysis catheter conundrum: Hate living with them but can't live without them. Kidney Int 1999;56:1-17.

14. Bambauer R, Latza R. Complications in large-bore catheters for extracorporeal detoxification methods. Artif Organs 2004;28:629-33.

15. Athirakul K, Schwab SJ, Conlon P. Adequacy of hemodialysis with cuffed central vein catheters. Nephrol Dial Transplant 1998;13:745-9.

16. Broadwater JR, Henderson MA, Bell J, et al. Outpatient percutaneous central venous access in cancer patients. Am J Surg 1990;160:676-80.

17. Wagman LD, Kirkemo A, Johnston MR. Venous access: A prospective, randomized study of the Hickman catheter. Surgery 1984; 95:303-8.

18. Maki DG, Cobb L, Garman JK, et al. An attachable silver-impregnated cuff for prevention of infection with central venous catheters: A prospective randomized multicenter trial. Am J Med 1988;85:307-14.

19. Jones R. Use of vortex MP ports in therapeutic red cell exchanges (abstract). J Clin Apher 2006; 21:43.

20. Van Kirk R, Koncsol J, Gutin H, et al. A single-center experience with double and single lumen vortex ports for chronic erythrocytopheresis in pediatric patients with sickle cell anemia (abstract). J Clin Apher 2006; 21:42.

21. Powers ML, Lublin D, Eby C, et al. Safety concerns related to use of unapproved needles for accessing implantable venous access devices. Transfusion 2009;49:2008-9.

22. Leblanc M, Bosc JY, Vaussenat F, et al. Effective blood flow and recirculation rates in internal jugular vein twin catheters: Measurement by ultrasound velocity dilution. Am J Kidney Dis 1998;31:87-92.

23. Sencal L, Saint-Sauveur E, Leblanc M. Blood flow and recirculation rates in tunneled hemodialysis catheters. ASAIO J 2004;50:94-7.

24. Depner TA. Catheter performance. Semin Dial 2001;14:425-31.

25. Graber DA, Dinerstein C. The Quinton Mahurkar dual lumen subclavian catheter—preliminary clinical evaluation. Dial Transplant 1983;12:847-50.

26. Vanholder R, Ringoir S. Vascular access for hemodialysis. Artif Organs 1994;18:263-5.

27. Uldall PR, Dyck RF, Woods F, et al. A subclavian cannula for temporary vascular access for hemodialysis or plasmapheresis. Dial Transplant 1979;8:963-6.

28. Duntley P, Siever J, Korwes ML, et al. Vascular erosion by central venous catheters: Clinical features and outcome. Chest 1992;101:1633-8.

29. Polderman KH, Girbes AJ. Central venous catheter use. Part 1: Mechanical complications. Intensive Care Med 2002;28:1-17.

30. Chirnside A, Urbaniak SJ, Prowse CV, Keller AJ. Coagulation abnormalities following intensive plasma exchange on the cell separator. II. Effects on factors I, II, V, VII, VIII, IX, X and antithrombin III. Br J Haematol 1981;48:627-34.

31. Keller AJ, Chirnside A, Urbaniak SJ. Coagulation abnormalities produced by plasma exchange on the cell separator with special reference to fibrinogen and platelet levels. Br J Haematol 1979;42:593-603.

32. Flaum MA, Cuneo RA, Appelbaum FR, et al. The hemostatic imbalance of plasma-exchange transfusion. Blood 1979;54:694-702.

33. McLeod BC, Sniecinski I, Ciavarella D, et al. Frequency of immediate adverse effects associated with therapeutic apheresis. Transfusion 1999;39:282-8.

34. Davenport RD. Therapeutic apheresis. In: Roback JD, Combs MR, Grossman BJ, Hillyer CD, eds. Technical manual. 16th ed. Bethesda, MD: AABB, 2008:697-713.

35. Murea S, Goldschmidt H, Hahn U, et al. Successful collection and transplantation of peripheral blood stem cells in cancer patients using large-volume leukaphereses. J Clin Apher 1996; 11:185-94.

36. Miller K, Pihan G. Clinical manifestations of acute myeloid leukemia. In: Hoffman R, Benz E, Shattil S, et al, eds. Hematology: Basic principles and practice. 5th ed. Philadelphia: Churchill Livingstone, 2009:933-63.

37. Product information: Norepinephrine bitartrate injection. Irvine, CA: Sicor Pharmaceuticals, 2005.

38. Product information: Epinephrine IV injection, intracardiac, endotracheal. Lake Forest, IL: Hospira, 2005.

39. Mahmood A, Sodano D, Dash A, Weinstein R. Therapeutic plasma exchange performed in tandem with hemodialysis for patients with M-protein disorders. J Clin Apher 2006;21:100-4.

40. Chopek M, McCullough J. Protein and biochemical changes during plasma exchange. In: Berkman EM, Umlas J, eds. Therapeutic hemapheresis. Washington, DC: AABB, 1980:13-52.

41. Berkman EM, Orlin JB. Use of plasmapheresis and partial plasma exchange in the manage-

ment of patients with cryoglobulinemia. Transfusion 1980;20:171-8.

42. Beck JR, Quinn BM, Meier FA, Rawnsley HM. Hyperviscosity syndrome in paraproteinemia. Managed by plasma exchange; monitored by serum tests. Transfusion 1982;22:51-3.

43. Longo LD. Maternal blood volume and cardiac output during pregnancy: A hypothesis of endocrinologic control. Am J Physiol Regulatory Integrative Comp Physiol 1983;245:720-9.

44. Pritchard JA. Changes in the blood volume during pregnancy and delivery. Anesthesiology 1965;26:393-9.

45. Owen HG, Brecher ME. Atypical reactions associated with ACE inhibitors and apheresis. Transfusion 1994;34:891-4.

46. Kammerl MC, Schaefer RM, Schweda F, et al. Extracorporal therapy with AN69 membranes in combination with ACE inhibition causing severe anaphylactoid reactions: Still a current problem? Clin Nephrol 2000;53:486-8.

47. Cyr M, Eastlund T, Blais C, et al. Bradykinin metabolism and hypotensive transfusion reactions. Transfusion 2001;41:136-50.

48. Ibrahim RB, Liu C, Cronin SM, et al. Drug removal by plasmapheresis: An evidence-based review. Pharmacotherapy 2007;27:1529-49.

49. Pramodini BK, Woo MW. A review of the effects of plasmapheresis on drug clearance. Pharmacotherapy 1997;17:684-95.

50. Stigelman WH, Henry DH, Talbert RL, Townsend RJ. Removal of prednisone and prednisolone by plasma exchange. Clin Pharm 1984;3:402-7.

51. Weinstein R. Prevention of citrate reactions during TPE by constant infusion of calcium gluconate with the return fluid. J Clin Apher 1996;11:204-10.

52. Bolan CD, Cecco SA, Wesley RA, et al. Controlled study of citrate effects and response to i.v. calcium administration during allogeneic peripheral blood progenitor cell donation. Transfusion 2002;42:935-46.

53. Krishnan RG, Coulthard MG. Minimizing changes in plasma calcium and magnesium concentrations during plasmapheresis. Pediatr Nephrol 2007;22:1763-6.

54. Kankirawatana S, Huang ST, Marques MB. Continuous infusion of calcium gluconate in 5% albumin is safe and prevents most hypocalcemic reactions during therapeutic plasma exchange. J Clin Apher 2007;22:265-9.

55. White RD, Goldsmith RS, Rodriguez R, et al. Plasma ionic calcium levels following injection of chloride, gluconate and glucipate salts of calcium. J Thorac Cardiovasc Surg 1976;71:609-13.

56. Trissel L. Handbook on injectable drugs. 15th ed. Bethesda, MD: American Society of Health-System Pharmacists, 2009.

57. Malachowski ME, Comenzo RL, Hillyer CD, et al. Large volume leukapheresis for peripheral blood stem cell collection in patients with hematologic malignancies. Transfusion 1992; 32:732-5.

58. Tobian AA, King KE, Ness PM. Transfusion premedications: A growing practice not based on evidence. Transfusion 2007;47:1089-96.

59. Leitman SF, Boltansky H, Alter HJ, et al. Allergic reactions in healthy plateletpheresis donors caused by sensitization to ethylene oxide gas. N Engl J Med 1986;315:1192-6.

60. Purello D'Ambrosio F, Savica V, Gangemi S, et al. Ethylene oxide allergy in dialysis patients. Nephrol Dial Transplant 1997;12:1461-3.

In: McLeod BC, Szczepiorkowski ZM, Weinstein R, Winters JL, eds.
Apheresis: Principles and Practice, 3rd edition
Bethesda, MD: AABB Press, 2010

13

Therapeutic Leukocyte and Platelet Depletion

Nicholas Bandarenko, MD, and Evelyn Lockhart, MD

EXCESSIVE LEUKOCYTE OR platelet counts may be associated with significant morbidity and mortality in a variety of acute or chronic disorders. In some, leukocytes or platelets that have been activated by immune and autoimmune inflammatory triggers may result in organ damage and poor patient outcomes. Apheresis technology has been applied in these settings to remove pathologic leukocytes or platelets from the circulation using leukapheresis, plateletpheresis, or selective apheresis systems that incorporate special columns or filters. Therapeutic apheresis has been recommended in a number of clinical settings and even prescribed as primary treatment in some. However, its effect on long-term patient outcome in many of them is still uncertain, and it is more typically employed as an adjunct or bridge to the effects of more definitive therapy.

Hyperleukocytosis and Leukostasis

Whereas leukocytosis may occur in response to infection, inflammation, or certain pharmaceutical interventions, *hyper*leukocytosis (HL) refers to extreme increases in white cells (WBCs) seen in myeloproliferative disorders and leukemias. In and of itself, HL may not result in leukostasis, which is the pathologic accumulation of leukocytes occluding the microcirculation that may lead to endothelial injury, thrombosis, and/or hemorrhage.[1] The development of leukostasis depends on a number of factors, including the absolute WBC count, the abundance of circulating leukoblasts,

Nicholas Bandarenko, MD, Associate Professor of Pathology, and Evelyn Lockhart, MD, Assistant Professor of Pathology, Duke University Medical Center, Durham, North Carolina

The authors have disclosed no conflicts of interest.

potential interactions with both cytokines and adhesion molecules, and endothelial damage.

Description of Disease

Freireich et al[1] were among the first to report an increased incidence of fatal cerebrovascular hemorrhage in acute leukemia patients with HL. At autopsy, the brains of these patients were characterized histologically by distinctive, symmetrical, sharply circumscribed nodules of leukemic leukocytes surrounded by hemorrhage. Another observed microscopic lesion was called "leukostasis," which referred to dilated, thin-walled, intracerebral vessels that were filled with an almost pure population of leukemic cells.

HL, which is usually defined as a circulating WBC count exceeding 50,000 to 100,000/μL, may occur in acute or chronic leukemias of either myeloid or lymphocytic lineage. Most ominous are the blast crises of acute adult and pediatric myelogenous leukemias, which portend a high risk of early mortality.[2-4] In acute myelogenous leukemia (AML), the threshold WBC count for symptomatic hyperleukocytosis is typically >100,000/μL, while for monoblastic or monocytic subtypes, symptoms may appear at WBC counts <50,000/μL. In lymphoblastic leukemias, symptoms seldom appear unless the WBC count exceeds 400,000/μL. Caution is advised because patients may be asymptomatic initially but then deteriorate rapidly. It is also important to recognize that significant symptoms have been described at lower WBC counts.[4]

Clinical Features

Clinical signs and symptoms of leukostasis are variable but most often involve the brain and/or the lungs. Cerebral leukostasis is clinically defined as a constellation of signs and symptoms of cerebrovascular insufficiency in the presence of HL. Symptoms can include headache, visual impairment, confusion, somnolence, delirium, coma, and focal neurologic deficits.[5] Clinical evidence of pulmonary leukostasis includes dyspnea, tachypnea, hypoxemia without hypercapnea, and radiographic findings of interstitial or alveolar infiltrates without laboratory or clinical evidence of pneumonia. Fever is another characteristic feature.

Risks and Complications

The risks of leukostasis appear to be greatest in AML, acute myelomonocytic leukemia, acute monocytic leukemia, and the accelerated phase or blast crisis of chronic myelogenous leukemia (CML). HL is associated with a higher incidence of fatal hemorrhage in the first 8 days of therapy and a shorter duration of complete remission (CR) in AML.[6] Early deaths are frequently caused by central nervous system (CNS) hemorrhage.[3] Although the overall remission rate was found in one study to not differ between patients with or without HL, it was significantly lower for those presenting with signs of leukostasis. Of the patients who failed to achieve CR, nearly half died during induction therapy from complications of pulmonary leukostasis, particularly elderly patients with HL.[7]

Patients with HL in the chronic or accelerated phase of CML or chronic myelomonocytic leukemia (CMML) may have an increased proportion of circulating immature myeloid cells and are therefore at risk for leukostasis. A higher incidence of HL and leukostasis in childhood vs adult CML has been reported.[8] Autopsy data from 206 patients with CML or AML demonstrated that 40% had leukemic thromboaggregates that were widely distributed in the vascular system, most commonly in the lungs and CNS.[9] All patients with a WBC count of at least 200,000/μL showed either thrombi or aggregates, and 46% of myeloid leukemia patients with a WBC count of 50,000 to 200,000/μL showed thromboaggregates. Patients with chronic lymphocytic leukemia (CLL) usually had a WBC count of at least 300,000/μL before thrombi were seen.

Pathophysiologic and Laboratory Correlates of Leukostasis

The fact that not all patients with HL have leukostasis symptoms indicates that factors other than the WBC count may contribute to the sequelae of HL.[4] The leukocrit (the percentage of whole blood volume represented by leukocytes) is related to the size as well as the number of leukocytes in the circulation. The mean corpuscular volume of leukoblasts is higher in AML than in acute lymphoblastic leukemia (ALL), which could underlie the higher incidence of leukostasis in AML. Blood viscosity will increase at progressively higher leukocrits, although definitive in-vivo correlation of leukostasis with hyperviscosity is challenging to ascertain because the extreme WBC count elevations required to cause hyperviscosity are uncommon in clinical practice.[10] Furthermore, the increase in viscosity from HL is countered in part by a lower hematocrit–ie, anemia. Postmortem studies demonstrate that leukemic aggregates are more prevalent in pulmonary, CNS, and cardiac tissue. It appears that leukostasis has a propensity for certain organs, and therefore its development may be related to organ-specific characteristics of the vasculature.[11]

The fact that leukostasis is occasionally reported in patients with relatively low blast counts also suggests that factors other than sheer cell numbers may be involved, such as chemo-attractant events and complement mediated injury.[4] An extensive literature has been published on the role that cell adhesion plays in the proliferation, differentiation, and function of cells. Hematopoietic cells are particularly rich in adhesion molecules that include integrins, selectins, immunoglobulins, and proteoglycans. As described by McEver[12]:

Cells routinely make transitions between nonadherent and adherent phenotypes during differentiation and in response to stimuli in the circulation or extravascular tissue. During inflammation, neutrophils and monocytes adhere to endothelium and emigrate into tissue where they phagocytose invading pathogens; lymphocytes adhere to antigen-presenting macrophages, and during hemorrhage, activated platelets stick to endothelium.

Leukocytes also adhere to activated platelets, a mechanism linking hemostasis and inflammatory responses. Liesveld reported that adhesion receptors expressed on AML blasts represent all the main classes of such receptors but found no correlation between the adhesion receptor phenotype and the morphologic or clinical features of AML.[13] Studies by Stucki et al tested the hypothesis that adhesion receptors and cytokines secreted by blast cells, tumor necrosis factor alpha (TNFα), and interleukin (IL)-1β in particular might play a major role in leukostasis. Their study elucidated the heterogeneity of expression of L-selectin, CD11b, CD18, CD49d, CD49e, CD49f, and other molecules based on the FAB class of AML (M0 to M7).[14] Porcu et al[4] suggested that the "leukemic cell's ability to respond to cytokines and its expression of specific adhesion molecules are probably more important in determining whether leukostasis will develop than is the number of circulating blasts." This could explain why leukostasis does not develop in all patients with HL. It might also explain why some patients with WBC counts well below 100,000/μL manifest signs and symptoms of leukostasis.

Role of Leukapheresis in Hyperleukocytosis

In the past decade several single-institution studies have reported that preinduction therapy, including cytoreductive leukapheresis, is associated with reduction in early mortality in patients presenting with HL.[15-18] Leukapheresis has reduced the risk of mortality in AML patients with HL during the first 4 weeks of induction chemotherapy.[19] Statistical analysis of 482 AML patients [excluding acute promyelocytic leukemia (APL)] indicated that the CR and cumulative death rates at 4 weeks for patients who underwent leukapheresis for WBC counts >100,000/μL were 63% and 26%, respectively, compared with 36% and 64% for patients who had not undergone leukapheresis (p = 0.03). In a separate publication, the outcome of 146 AML patients with HL, 49% of whom underwent leukapheresis, were reported in terms of CR rates, early mortality, and overall survival of those who received leukapheresis vs those who did not.[15] Taking into account the risk factors of age, Zubrod performance status, and cytogenetics as well as infection status and renal and hepatic function, statistical analysis demonstrated evidence (p = 0.006) that leukapheresis reduced the 2-week mortality rate, suggesting (p = 0.06) that this resulted in a higher CR rate. However, there was no evidence it lengthened overall survival time.[15]

In an analysis of 806 newly diagnosed AML patients, treatment complications and deaths in the first 4 weeks of induction therapy were reviewed.[20] In this study, the leading causes of death in the first 2 weeks were infection (71%) and hemorrhage (43%) that occurred primarily in pulmonary tissue. A twofold increase in mortality rate was demonstrated in patients with WBC counts >50,000/μL. In addition to the known risk factors of age, performance status, and cytogenetics, hyperuricemia and plasma levels of TNFα also appeared to be associated with mortality within 4 weeks of starting induction therapy. Although 4-week mortality was lower in those receiving leukapheresis (specifically 36 % vs 48%), overall survival was worse in the leukapheresis group. The author suggested a possible selection bias for treating with leukapheresis and recommended a prospective randomized trial. Other investigators have reported no impact of leukapheresis in reducing early mortality[11,21,22] and suggested that the interaction between leukoblasts and the vasculature may exert a more significant effect in determining the clinical outcome than reduction in absolute WBC counts. A clinical leukostasis grading score has been found to be a reliable indicator of HL patients at risk for early mortality.[2]

Rationale for Therapeutic Leukapheresis

There is consensus in the literature that high WBC counts have a negative effect on early survival and CR rates and that leukapheresis may be beneficial for some, but not all, AML patients with HL. The role of leukapheresis is to reduce the leukocyte concentration in the peripheral blood. For AML patients with HL, if up-regulated expression of adhesion molecules is the mechanism for leukostasis whether the up-regulation is inherent in the malignant clone or is a response to inflammatory cytokines, then leukapheresis offers the potential to decrease morbidity and mortality by removing large quantities of these activated cells. The most opportune time for leukapheresis is presumed to be in the interval between diagnosis and the onset of chemotherapy-induced leukemic cell lysis. Leukapheresis may also have an adjunctive role in chronic disorders characterized by leukocytosis such as CML, CMML, and CLL when symptoms related to leukocytosis appear, as well as in treatment of patients resistant to therapy or for whom therapy is contraindicated. One example is the use of leukapheresis to avoid the teratogenic effects of chemotherapy in early pregnancy when complicated by myeloproliferative disorders.[23]

One one hand, both the American Society for Apheresis (ASFA) and the AABB consider clinical leukostasis to be a Category I (Grade 1b) indication for leukapheresis (the category for which therapeutic apheresis is standard and acceptable as a first-line therapy or as a valuable adjunct to other initial therapies).[5,24] On the other hand, it is less clear if performing leukapheresis prophylatically in asymptomatic patients can meaningfully reduce the renal and metabolic complications associated with rapid lysis of chemo-sensitive leukemic cells (tumor lysis syndrome). One potential consideration is the relatively small proportion of malignant cells in the circulation available to the leukapheresis procedure for removal compared to the total body tumor burden of leukemic cells.[25] Therefore, use of leukapheresis for this purpose is controversial.[26] Prophylaxis of asymptomatic HL and prevention of tumor lysis syndrome are rated as Category III (2c) indications for leukapheresis by ASFA (evidence is conflicting or insufficient to establish efficacy).[5] APL is associated with a severe coagulopathy that could be worsened by leukapheresis.[27]

Leukapheresis Procedural Considerations

Processing 8 to 10 liters of blood (1.5 to 2 blood volumes) is a typical goal for therapeutic leukapheresis. ASFA and AABB guidelines[5,24] indicate that success has been most consistent in procedures of this magnitude; however, the guidelines do not address what level of cytoreduction (postprocedure absolute WBC count and/or percent reduction) must be achieved to reverse signs and symptoms of leukostasis.

The yield (number of leukocytes removed) is related to the total circulating quantity of leukocytes available to be collected and the blood volume processed. Additional factors that influence leukocyte yield and patient response include the following: 1) the use of an erythrocyte-sedimenting agent such as hydroxyethyl starch (HES) to enhance separation of immature and mature myeloid cells from red cells, 2) the volume of cells to be removed, and 3) mobilization of cells from marrow and extramedullary sites into the intravascular space during the procedure.

In the past, studies using a continuous flow apheresis device illustrated that with the standard anticoagulant, acid-citrate-dextrose-A (ACD-A), 70% to 90% of circulating normal donor mononuclear cells and about 20% of mature myeloid cells are separated from whole blood during passage through the centrifugal field. The fraction of leukocytes cleared from whole blood rises to about 60% when 6% HES is added to the anticoagulated blood entering the centrifuge.[28] Experience with therapeutic leukapheresis for acute and chronic leukemia has shown similar patterns of separation. The leukocytes to be removed are usually a heterogeneous mixture of cells of different lineages (myeloid, lymphoid, monocytic, erythroid, megakaryocytic) and may therefore differ in size and density, but HES appears to improve the collection efficiency for all leukocyte lineages. The use of HES is obligatory if the predominant cell type to be removed is the mature myeloid cell. Lymphoid and monocytic cells may be removed efficiently with ACD-A alone. Decisions to use HES, with its associated plasma volume-expanding properties and reliance on renal function for excretion, may thus relate both to the lineage of cells to be removed and the patient's cardiovascular and renal function. All these factors make therapeutic leukapheresis procedures significantly more complex than normal donor platelet or granulocyte collections because they introduce the need for a medical assessment of organ function and medical management of fluid and electrolyte changes induced by the procedure.

Because leukocytes are 20 to 70 times larger than platelets, a much larger volume of cell concentrate must be removed in treating leukocytosis than in treating thrombocytosis. The volume of cells collected relates to the total blood processed and the rate of removal, and it correlates inversely with the capacity of individual apheresis devices to concentrate WBCs. Assuming that devices can concentrate WBCs to levels of 500,000 to 750,000/μL, removing one circulating leukemic cell mass in an adult patient would require removing 0.5 to 1.0 liter of cells per 100,000/μL of preprocedure WBC count. Some of this volume loss is compensated by HES solution if this is used; however, for patients with WBC counts of 200,000/μL or higher, the volume removed will exceed 1.0 L and additional replacement fluids may be required.

Observations suggest that leukemic cells may be mobilized from extramedullary sites into the intravascular space during leukapheresis. A decrease in hepatosplenomegaly has been reported in CML patients following repeated leukapheresis procedures.[29] Pre- and postleukapheresis cell cycle analysis has demonstrated recruitment of leukemic cells in S phase from the marrow into the circulation.[16] Finally, the reduction in the postprocedure WBC count is often less than that expected from the quantity of WBCs removed during the procedure. Mobilization of leukocytes during leukapheresis is not predictable at the present time and thus cannot be integrated into calculation of procedure parameters. Clearly the total body tumor burden of leukemia is only fractionally represented in the circulation within reach of the apheresis procedure. This imparts special importance to prompt initiation of cytotoxic therapy, as leukapheresis will only transiently influence the pathologic effects of leukemia.

Given the variability in the threshold WBC count for leukostasis symptoms, defining a specific postprocedure WBC count for reversal of leukostasis is problematic. Early morbidity and mortality may still occur after reduction of circulating WBC counts to "safe" levels (<100,000/μL).[4] In a study of one blood volume processed, WBC count reduction ranged from 15% to 46%.[30] A 50% to 86% reduction was noted in another study when two patient blood volumes were processed.[31] Current experience suggests that removing an average of 85% of the pretreatment circulating cell mass will provide an average of 50% reduction in the peripheral blood WBC count. That a greater reduction is not observed may be attributable to cell mobilization during the procedure. For a patient whose pretreatment WBC count was 100,000/μL, a 50% reduction might be satisfactory. For patients with WBC counts of 200,000/μL or greater, a 50% reduction might be inadequate to reverse leukostasis. For such patients, options would include processing additional blood and removing additional cells or performing a second procedure if a 24-hour WBC count remained above 100,000/μL.

The observation that adequate cytoreduction correlates with CR suggests that developing procedure parameters to achieve predictable cytoreduction could be valuable for medical and technical personnel responsible for these procedures.[7,18] However, given existing uncertainties in WBC removal efficiency, it is prudent to monitor the WBC count at intervals during therapeutic leukapheresis to ensure that a reasonable reduction has been achieved before the procedure is discontinued. Additional procedures may be performed to sustain a desirable level of circulating WBCs (<50,000/μL for AML and <300,000/μL for ALL, for example).

Additional Procedural Considerations

Medical oversight and apheresis experience are desirable to ensure patient safety and optimal removal of leukocytes. Replacement of removed blood volume (ie, the volume of leukocyte waste product) with crystalloid, 5% albumin, and/or plasma is recommended with large-volume leukapheresis. Because of the risk of anemia, which typically accompanies emergent presentations for leukapheresis, assessment of the intraprocedural hematocrit and the patient's tolerance of a further decrease in red cell oxygen-carrying capacity are necessary. Transfusion of red cells in asymptomatic patients with HL has been associated with rapid development of leukostasis.[4] Addition of red cells into the circulation of a symptomatic patient requires deliberate planning. Options to ensure an adequate intraprocedure hematocrit include priming the apheresis device with red cells or slow infusion of red cells via a peripheral line over the course of the procedure. Conducting the procedure in a monitored clinical setting may be warranted. Placement of a large-bore central venous catheter is typically required to maintain adequate apheresis flow rates in the setting of leukostasis. Repeated daily leukapheresis may be required to maintain adequate leukocyte reduction and resolution of symptoms of leukostasis.

Selective Leukocyte Apheresis

Automated apheresis devices rely on centrifugal separation to isolate leukocytes and can target the removal of mononuclear cells or granulocytes with relative efficiency. An attractive concept would be to target the removal of more specific pathologic subsets of leukocytes that may be relevant to the pathogenesis of clinical disease, with the goal of modulating or suppressing the disease process. Selective leukocyte apheresis applies this concept using specialized columns or filters to remove leukocytes from whole blood. It has been shown to remove 4 times more WBCs than centrifugation[32] and has been applied to several inflammatory diseases, such as inflammatory bowel disease (IBD), systemic lupus erythematosus, and rheumatoid arthritis.[33] Removal or modification of activated leukocytes and their associated proinflammatory cytokines implicated in the mechanism of disease has shown promise as an alternative or adjunct to pharmacologic treatment.[34]

Two selective leukocyte apheresis devices are currently available in some countries and have been evaluated for therapeutic benefit in several diseases: the leukocyte adsorptive apheresis system (LCAP, marketed as Cellsorba by Asahi Kasei Medical Co, Tokyo, Japan) and the granulocyte/monocyte adsorptive apheresis system (GMA, marketed as Adacolumn by JIMRO, Takasaki, Japan). For both, vascular access is obtained by antecubital venipuncture. The patient's whole blood is drawn from one arm and anticoagulated, passed through a column where removal of certain cell populations occurs, and then returned to the patient's opposite arm. Treatments with either device are typically carried out at weekly intervals, with blood being processed at 30 to 50 mL/min for 60 to 90 minutes.

Cellsorba consists of a 2-stage filter composed of nonwoven polyester fabric that removes leukocytes through filtration and adhesion. The efficiency of removal is related to the small diameter (0.8 to 2.8 microns) of the inner filter fibers. The complete system uses a Plasauto LC pump and monitor unit along with the filter column and circuit lines.[35] LCAP has been shown to remove about 99% of granulocytes and monocytes and 40% to 60% of lymphocytes from processed blood.[35,36] The device has been approved by the Japan Ministry of Health for the treatment of patients with active ulcerative colitis and rheumatoid arthritis and is also available in Europe.

The Adacolumn filter component consists of a column (335-mL capacity) filled with 220 g of cellulose acetate beads (2 mm in diameter) and immersed in 130 mL of isotonic saline.[37] Adacolumn selectively adsorbs approximately 65% of granulocytes and 55% of monocytes without significantly adsorbing lymphocytes.[38] It is approved for use in Europe for the treatment of Crohn disease, ulcerative colitis (UC), rheumatoid arthritis, systemic lupus erythematosus, and ocular Behçet disease, and in Japan for ulcerative colitis.

Proposed Mechanisms of Action

Both GMA and LCAP remove cells from the patient's circulating whole blood by taking advantage of varying degrees of attachment of leukocytes and lymphocytes to artificial surfaces. The cells targeted for removal are presumed to be disease promoting and to be either increased in number or activated. However, the precise mechanism by which the columns might produce a therapeutic effect remains unclear. Although selective leukocyte apheresis effectively filters and removes high proportions of circulating WBCs, the number of leukocytes in peripheral blood does not fall below the normal range.[34,38] Furthermore, calculations related to leukocyte removal and normal production kinetics suggest that mere leukocyte depletion is unlikely to account for any benefits that may be conferred by these devices.[25] Normal daily neutrophil (polymorphonuclear cell, or PMN) production is reported as 0.85 to 1.6 × 10^9/kg,[39] which equates to 6 to 11 × 10^{10} PMNs/day for a 70-kg person. GMA retains 65% of the granulocytes that enter it.[34,40] If the starting PMN count is estimated to be 10,000/μL, processing the recommended 1800 mL whole blood (30 mL/minute × 60 min) could deplete 1.2 × 10^{10} PMNs [(0.65 × 10^4 PMNs/μL) × (1800 mL × 10^3 μL/mL)], which is 11% to 20% of normal daily PMN production and only 1.6% to 2.9% of normal weekly production. The removal rate could be increased by intensifying frequency or duration of treatments; however, the percentage removal would be less at lower PMN counts or at the substantially higher PMN production rates expected in chronic inflammatory disease states.[25]

Activated proinflammatory leukocytes removed from the circulation appear to be replaced by less inflammatory (or more naive) leukocytes from the marginal pool into the bloodstream.[41] A decrease in inflammatory response might result from naive leukocytes being less responsive to proinflammatory mediators.

Other mechanisms of action that have been postulated for selective leukocyte apheresis include modulation of cytokine production and alteration of cell-surface moieties for trafficking and transmigration. GMA and LCAP appear to modulate cytokine responses. GMA has been shown to significantly diminish the release of soluble TNF receptors I and II in patients with active UC.[37,42,43] Suppression of production of the proinflammatory cytokines TNFα, IL-1β, IL-6, and IL-8; suppression of leukocyte adhesion molecule (L-selectin), IL-8 chemotaxis, and granulocyte adhesion to IL-1β-activated endothelial cells; and an increase in the number of CD10-negative premature granulocytes (from marrow) have been observed.[44] Down-regulation of L-selectin reduces the number of granulocytes that migrate into mucosal tissue.[38,45] After selective apheresis, the granulocytes remaining in the circulation tend to have a shortened life span because apoptosis is accelerated.[45] In a small clinical trial of LCAP, blood levels of the proinflammatory cytokine IL-6 were decreased following treatment in 6 of 19 patients with active UC.[46] In addition, increased secretion of IL-10, an anti-inflammatory cytokine, and a decrease in the percentage of reactive oxygen-producing leukocytes were observed.[46]

It should be noted that data cited above that have been interpreted to suggest clinical benefit and potential mechanisms of action for GMA or LCAP are preliminary and are not derived from adequately controlled studies. Well-controlled studies comparing therapies (including placebo/sham apheresis) are crucial to determine whether reported changes in peripheral immunologic markers are related to disease activity itself or are specific sequelae of selective leukocyte apheresis.

Clinical Experience in Inflammatory Bowel Disease

Most data on selective leukocyte apheresis to date are from prospective open-label studies or case series of patients with IBD.[45,47-58] Contrary to the favorable results that had accumulated in these studies, a large pivotal randomized sham-controlled clinical trial in North America involving GMA did not demonstrate effectiveness in the induction of remission or clinical response in patients with moderate-to-severe UC. Post-hoc analysis indicated a potential difference in both clinical remission and overall response rates in a subgroup of severely affected patients,[59] suggesting the possibility that a more selective study design might have disclosed clinical benefits that were anticipated based on previous smaller studies. A recent meta-analysis of seven randomized controlled trials in IBD (only one of which was fully blinded) suggested that clinical remission was obtained in a higher proportion of patients treated with GMA than in those treated by conventional therapy, with a relative likelihood of response or remission at 6 or 12 weeks of 1.42 or 1.41, respectively.[60] Other benefits reported include avoidance of or reduction in corticosteroid or other pharmacotherapy to manage clinical symptoms.[47,61-63] A postmarket surveillance study in Japan involving 656 patients treated with GMA demonstrated favorable safety and efficacy data for GMA in patients with UC.[63] Selective leukocyte apheresis has been applied anecdotally to other diseases, including human immunodeficiency virus, hepatitis C virus, pyoderma gangrenosum, and psoriasis; however, available data are limited.[37,64] Currently, IBD is regarded by ASFA as a Category II (2B) indication for selective leukocyte apheresis.[5]

Safety in Patients with Inflammatory Bowel Disease

Treatment-related adverse events reported in studies of LCAP and GMA have mostly been of mild-to-moderate severity. These have included headache, fever, hypotension, nausea, dizziness, diarrhea, venous access or flow rate problems, posttreatment hematoma, or difficulty in returning blood. Clotting and sagittal vein thrombosis have been reported in patients undergoing apheresis with LCAP and GMA, but neither of these was seen in the North American GMA trial or the postmarket surveillance study in Japan.[59,63,65,66]

Thrombocytosis

Thrombocytosis, generally defined as a platelet count exceeding 450,000 to 500,000/μL, may be caused by a reactive process (secondary thrombocytosis) or by an underlying clonal marrow disorder (primary thrombocytosis).[67] Thrombocytosis is often an incidental finding during routine hematology testing. Secondary thrombocytosis is far more common than primary thrombocytosis, accounting for 80% to 90% of all patients with an elevated platelet count. Causes of secondary thrombocytosis include iron-deficiency anemia, tissue damage from major surgery, infection, cancer, and chronic inflammation. Distinguishing between primary and secondary thrombocytosis can be challenging. However, this distinction is of significant clinical importance because primary thrombocytosis can be accompanied by potentially life-threatening hemostatic derangements and may require therapeutic interventions, including plateletpheresis.[5] Secondary thrombocytosis, while sometimes presenting with an alarmingly high platelet count, virtually never shows such derangements and resolves with treatment of the underlying condition.[67] It is worth noting that although secondary thrombocytosis may rarely cause direct complications, the underlying condition (such as occult malignancy) may have significant potential for morbidity and mortality. Therefore, unexpectedly high platelet counts found on peripheral blood analysis warrant a thorough investigation for the root cause. The literature on therapeutic plateletpheresis for secondary causes of thrombocytosis is limited to a small number of case reports and series and provides little evidence of clinical benefit.[5] Better evidence exists to support treatment of thrombotic or hemorrhagic complications of primary thrombocytosis with plateletpheresis and is reviewed below.

Primary Thrombocytosis: Description and Pathophysiology

Myeloproliferative neoplasms (MPNs) are disorders defined by the clonal proliferation of one or more myeloid cell lineages.[68] Because these disorders are clonal, all cell lines that derive from the affected hematopoetic stem cell share the same molecular lesion. Primary thrombocytosis is most often associated with essential thrombocythemia (ET); however, other MPNs such as polycythemia vera (PV), CML, and myelofibrosis with myeloid metaplasia may also present with thrombocytosis.[67] All of these disorders can display atypical megakaryocytic hyperplasia and megakaryocyte clusters, with some overlap in morphologic marrow findings.[68]

A variety of genetic lesions have been implicated in the pathogenesis of MPNs. Thrombopoietin (TPO), a glycoprotein hormone produced by the liver and kidney, is a regulator of megakaryocyte development and platelet production. Mutated *TPO* alleles have been reported in cases of familial thrombocytosis.[69] The TPO receptor, c-Mpl, has likewise been implicated both in cases of familial thrombocytosis as well as sporadic mutations associated with cases of ET.[69] Most importantly, recent investigations elucidated the single amino acid change V617F in the JAK2 kinase as a molecular lesion common to the MPNs.[70,71] This mutation has been reported in over 95% of PV cases and 50% of ET cases.[72] The multilineage cellular proliferation seen in these disorders becomes more understandable when one considers that the erythropoietin receptor, the TPO receptor, and the granulocyte colony-stimulating factor receptor all signal by association with JAK2 kinase.[69]

Epidemiology and Clinical Findings

PV and ET are rare disorders. Review of the literature shows a prevalence for PV ranging from 0.02 to 2.8 cases per 100,000 and for ET ranging from 0.1 to 2.4 per 100,000.[73] The median age at diagnosis of PV is 60 years, with 1.2:1 male preponderance.[72] ET affects primarily middle-aged persons, with a female preponderance of around 1.8:1.[74] In one study, 100 ET patients were first diagnosed by abnormal blood counts and were queried about hemostatic abnormalities. Of the 24 who had symptoms, 89% reported thrombotic symptoms, while 11% reported bleeding symptoms.[75] Thrombotic and hemorrhagic complication rates at the time of diagnosis of ET from 21 retrospective cohort studies were reviewed by Barbui et al. The frequency of thrombotic events ranged from 9% to 84%, while that of hemorrhage ranged from 3.9% to 63%.[76]

Both bleeding and thrombosis are well-recognized causes of morbidity and mortality in MPNs, particularly ET and PV.[67] Mucocutaneous hemorrhages, such as bruising, epistaxis, gum bleeding, and mucosal bleeding from the gastrointestinal or genitourinary tracts, are the most common bleeding manifestations; deep tissue bleeds and hemarthroses are rare. Significant thrombotic complications include stroke, transient ischemic attack, myocardial infarction, angina pectoris, peripheral arterial thrombosis, retinal artery occlusion, deep venous thrombosis, and pulmonary embolism.[76] Microcirculatory manifestations include vascular headaches, dizziness, visual disturbances, acrocyanosis, paresthesias, and erythromelalgia, a characteristic burning pain in the palms of the hands and soles of the feet. The thrombophilia seen in older patients with ET and PV is most likely multifactorial, as MPNs often affect individuals who already have other risk factors such as atherosclerosis, familial thrombophilia, or acquired hypercoagulable states related to smoking or malignancy.[76]

Because ET affects more women than men and a subset of affected patients are of childbearing age, it is possible for patients to present with both pregnancy and ET concurrently. Thrombotic or hemorrhagic complications in such patients increase the risks of fetal loss; cytoreductive therapy for the mother is also potentially harmful to the fetus.[77] Although there appears to be a spontaneous decline in platelet count through the course of pregnancy, reaching a nadir of 40% of the peak platelet count seen early on,[78] these pregnancies are threatened by complications such as placental infarction, placental abruption, spontaneous abortion, preterm birth, and postpartum thrombosis.[79] The first trimester appears to be a particularly vulnerable period, as several studies have shown an increased first-trimester miscar-

riage rate in ET patients.[77] The largest of these studies, by Passamonti et al,[80] followed 96 non-terminated pregnancies in 58 women with ET to determine pregnancy complications. The rate of live births was 64%, with 51% of all pregnancies experiencing no maternal complications. However, the risk of fetal loss was 3.4-fold higher than that in the general population, with 91% of all fetal loss resulting from abortion. The authors concluded that while many instances of pregnancy in ET may be uneventful, the risk of fetal loss is significant, and that the JAK2 mutation may be associated with higher risks of pregnancy complications.

Laboratory Correlates of Thrombotic or Hemorrhagic Risk

Patients with ET and PV have shortened platelet survival and increased circulating markers of platelet activation such as platelet factor 4, beta-thromboglobulin, and thrombomodulin.[81] It has been proposed that these changes, which are aspirin sensitive, may represent platelet hypersensitivity and a greater tendency of the abnormal platelet clone to activate in the high shear stress of the microcirculation. This may explain why a proportion of circulating platelets in patients with MPNs appear hypogranular; ie, they may have released granule contents during in-vivo activation. It is important to emphasize that although several features of platelet dysfunction have been identified in MPNs, no single defect has consistently been associated with a higher risk for either bleeding or thrombosis. The diagnostic utility of platelet function testing in MPNs as a predictor of hemostatic risk is not established. However, an associated consequence of markedly elevated platelet counts (>1,500,000/µL) is an acquired von Willebrand disease with a pathologic reduction in the plasma concentration of large von Willebrand factor (vWF) multimers.[82] The loss of these multimers may result from several contributing factors, including increased binding of vWF to the circulating abnormal platelets, elevated shear stress exposing platelet glycoprotein binding sites on vWF, and increased proteolysis of vWF (as is reflected by the increased circulating vWF fragments found in patients with MPN). Functional assays to measure the amount of vWF activity and antigen will show reduction, and vWF multimer analysis will show the loss of the large and ultralarge vWF multimers in plasma. Prolongation of both the bleeding time and the closure time measured with a PFA-100 platelet function analyzer also reflect defective platelet-vessel wall interaction attributable to the deficiency of large vWF multimers.

The increased hematocrit in PV contributes to the thrombotic risk seen in these patients. The most important factor contributing to whole blood viscosity is the red cell mass, and blood viscosity increases dramatically as hematocrit rises above 55%. There is a positive correlation between the hematocrit and the incidence of thrombotic events in PV.[67] This may be due in part to the altered mechanical stresses on platelets generated by the expanded red cell mass, the most significant being shear stress. Shear stress is generated within a vessel by the frictional interaction between cellular elements flowing at different rates.[83,84] Blood flow within the vessel will concentrate red cells toward the luminal center, where they flow faster (as they deform and align within the axial

zone of blood flow) but with less shear stress than that experienced by platelets in the plasma-rich mural zone (Fig 13-1). A high hematocrit enlarges the axial red cell zone; the concomitant contraction of the mural plasmatic zone increases the shear forces to which platelets are subjected, as well as increasing platelet/vessel wall interaction. The increased thrombotic risk in PV patients with very high hematocrits may in part be caused by these aberrations.[85]

Tests for the JAK2 V617F and c-Mpl mutations are now standard measures in the evaluation of potential MPNs. The JAK2 gain-of-function mutation also shows enticing potential as a diagnostic marker for thrombotic and/or hemorrhagic risk. Carobbio et al recently compared the JAK2 V617F allele status of 415 PV patients and 867 ET patients.[86] They found that patients with wild-type ET, ET with the V617F mutation, and PV patients (all with the V617F mutation) showed thrombotic rates of 1.4%, 2.1%, and 2.7%, respectively. However, use of JAK2 mutational analysis for estimating thrombotic risk in this setting is still under investigation and not used routinely.

Another parameter under investigation as a marker for thrombotic risk is the WBC count.

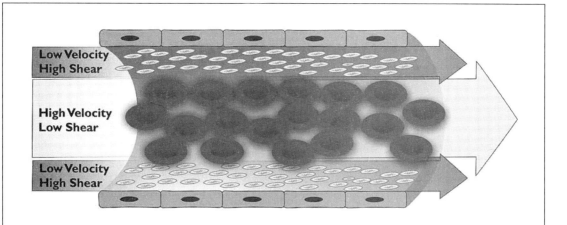

Figure 13-1. Blood rheology in erythrocytosis. Blood flow in vessels separates into an axial stream containing the red cell mass and a mural plasmatic zone containing platelets within the plasma. As the hematocrit rises, the concentration of the platelets in the plasmatic zone increases, subjecting platelets to greater activating shear stress and platelet/vessel wall interactions and increasing thrombotic risk.

In earlier studies, de Gaetano et al demonstrated that activated granulocytes can activate platelets.[87] P-selectin-mediated adhesion of activated platelets to granulocytes facilitates the transcellular metabolism of arachidonic acid, resulting in production of both thromboxane B2 and leukotriene C4. Kaplar et al[88] report a significant increase of monocyte-platelet aggregates in MPN patients with high platelet counts and suggest that adhesion involves a greater activation of platelets manifested by increased production of platelet-derived growth factor as well as enhanced tissue factor. More recent epidemiologic studies suggest that a baseline WBC count above 10,000/μL is an independent predictor of major thrombosis, particularly coronary syndromes, in both ET and PV.[89] The clinical significance of leukocytosis in this population is debatable, however, as most patients who are at high risk of thrombosis will be managed with cytoreductive agents that will lower both platelet and leukocyte counts.[90]

Management

The mainstay of therapy for patients with ET is a combination of an anti-platelet agent such as aspirin and a cytoreductive agent such as hydroxyurea, anagrelide, or interferon alpha (IFNα), with a target platelet count of 400,000/μL; currently recommended regimens stratify the treatment based on risk factors.[76] Pregnant women who present with ET are often managed with low-dose aspirin and either IFNα or hydroxyurea, with concerns regarding the teratogenicity of hydroxyurea favoring the use of IFNα.

Rationale for Therapeutic Plateletpheresis

Therapeutic plateletpheresis of MPN patients can rapidly reduce an elevated platelet count to help mitigate either thrombotic or hemorrhagic complications. Such short-term reduction can provide symptomatic relief and a therapeutic bridge to the delayed effects of cytoreductive therapy. While the primary aberration in PV is an increased red cell mass, the increased concentration of platelets subjected to increased

activating shear force within the mural plasmatic zone is a significant contributor to thrombotic risk in these patients, and they can potentially benefit from rapid, short-term reduction of the platelet count. Although long-term use of plateletpheresis has been described in both pregnancy and patients intolerant of chemotherapy,[91] this does not represent the norm, as often the reduction in platelet count is short-lived. Plateletpheresis has also been employed in MPN patients with rebound thrombocytosis after splenectomy, although a target platelet count has not been well defined in these patients.[5] In 1975, Greenberg and Watson-Williams reported six procedures in one patient.[92] Between 3.8 and 8.8×10^{12} platelets were removed per procedure, and patient platelet counts were reduced by 33% to 66%. Taft et al performed plateletpheresis on five patients, processing 3 to 11 L of blood.[93] The mean platelet count of 1,529,000 ±994,000/μL before treatment was reduced to 708,000 ±643,000/μL after procedure. Most patients required two or three procedures for an effective reduction. Burgstaler and Pineda demonstrated a 43% ±17% reduction in platelet count in 34 patients after a single procedure using the COBE Spectra (Caridian BCT, Lakewood, CO) and a 53% ±19% reduction in 32 patients after a single procedure using the Haemonetics (Braintree, MA) V50 and M30 instruments.[94]

Just as there is currently no absolute platelet count that correlates with the onset of symptoms, so too there is neither an absolute level to which the platelet count must be reduced with plateletpheresis nor a standardized procedure by which such a targeted goal could be achieved. Review of the evidence supporting the use of therapeutic plateletpheresis by the ASFA Clinical Applications Subcommittee in 2010 led to a Category II rating for its use in symptomatic thrombocytosis and a Category III rating for prophylaxis.[5] Demonstration of the procedure's efficacy is based on clinical observations of regression of symptoms. Rapid reduction of an elevated platelet count can help replenish large and ultralarge vWF multimers in patients with ET and acquired von Willebrand syndrome, ameliorating bleeding symptoms.

Plateletpheresis Procedural Considerations

The goal of therapeutic plateletpheresis in patients with acute thrombotic or hemorrhagic disorders is reduction of the platelet count to a normal or near-normal level (typically ≤400,000/μL); such a procedure can be expected to reduce the platelet count by 30% to 60%.[95] The current ASFA guidelines[5] recommend processing anywhere from 1.5 to 2 total blood volumes (TBV), with the anticoagulant-to-blood ratio ranging from 1:8 to 1:12. Heparin should be avoided as an anticoagulant because of its tendency to cause platelet clumping within the apheresis circuit. The frequency of procedures can be tailored to the patient's response and can usually be reduced as cytoreductive therapy takes effect. Daily plateletpheresis may be necessary to achieve the desired short-term effect, with periodic procedures repeated as needed for short-term maintenance.

All currently available centrifugal apheresis instruments have the capacity to perform therapeutic cytoreductions; however, procedural recommendations in operator manuals for such cytoreductions are limited and nonspecific. Knowledge gained in platelet collection from normal donors in the IBM 2997 and the Spectra devices resulted in predictable platelet yields from normal donors and helps to highlight principles that may be applied to therapeutic plateletpheresis.[96] Those principles are 1) that the platelet yield is some fraction of the total circulating cellular quantity (platelet concentration times the estimated blood volume) and 2) that the fraction of available cells collected (the yield) is related to the fraction of the patient's blood volume that is processed. Normal donor collections process about 1.0 blood volume and remove about 250 to 500 mL of platelets and plasma. The resulting fractional reduction in donor platelet count averages 25% or less. Because the circulating platelet mass in MPN patients can be 3 to 12 times that in healthy donors, it seems intuitive that a greater volume of the patient's blood must be processed and a larger volume of cells removed if a reduction in platelet count greater than 25% is to be achieved. With the Spectra, the volume removed is a function of 1) the maximum platelet concentration achievable in the collection line, 2) the collection rate, and 3) the procedure time. In the CS3000 (Fenwal, Lake Zurich, IL), the volume removed relates to the number of times the 200-mL collection bag is emptied, while in Haemonetics devices, the volume removed relates to the number of cycles performed and the volume removed per cycle.

The physiologic changes of pregnancy are accompanied by significant hematologic changes. The average expansion of blood volume can be up to 50% (with considerable individual variability), with women carrying multiple fetuses having a greater blood volume expansion than those carrying one. The red cell mass also increases during pregnancy, but disproportionate expansion of the plasma volume creates the "physiologic anemia of pregnancy."[97] The increased blood and plasma volumes may be underestimated by typical methods of volume calculation; thus caution should be used when approaching these patients, with careful attention to signs and symptoms of hypovolemia. Positioning the patient on her left side will help prevent uterine compression of the inferior vena cava, which could lead to hypotension during the procedure.[23]

Conclusion

Clinical signs and symptoms arising from HL or thrombocytosis are variable and unpredictable. Without specific laboratory assays to identify patients at risk for complications, guidelines for therapeutic apheresis procedures to lower peripheral blood concentrations of platelets and leukocytes may have to continue to rely on diagnosis, clinical findings, and peripheral blood counts alone. Multivariate statistical analyses of risk factors influencing early mortality, CR rates, and survival of patients who receive leukapheresis as part of their disease management will have to include quantitative data on cell quantities removed and percent reduction in cell counts achieved, or the relationship between cytoreduction and clinical outcome will remain difficult to demonstrate.

Selective leukapheresis has been applied in a variety of inflammatory diseases, most notably IBD. Clinical improvements similar to those obtained with pharmacologic therapies have been reported. Results from open-label trials in Japan and Europe suggested that GMA and LCAP might be useful as an adjunctive or alternative therapy in patients who fail to respond adequately or who are refractory to or unable to tolerate systemic therapies. However, a large, randomized, double-blind, sham-controlled, pivotal trial in North America failed to demonstrate improvement in remission rate or clinical response with GMA. Future investigations are necessary.

References

1. Freireich E, Thomas L, Rei E, et al. A distinctive type of intracerebral hemorrhage associated with "blastic crisis" in patients with leukemia. Cancer 1960;13:146-54.
2. Piccirillo N, Laurenti L, Chiusolo P, et al. Reliability of leukostasis grading score to identify patients with high-risk hyperleukocytosis (letter). Am J Hematol 2009;84:381-2.
3. Dutcher J, Schiffer C, Wiernik P. Hyperleukocytosis in adult acute nonlymphocytic leukemia: Impact on remission rate and duration and survival. J Clin Oncol 1987;5:1364-72.
4. Porcu P, Cripe LD, Ng EW, et al. Hyperleukocytic leukemias and leukostasis: A review of pathophysiology, clinical presentation and management. Leuk Lymphoma 2000;39:1-18.
5. Szczepiorkowski ZM, Winters JL, Bandarenko N, et al. Guidelines on the use of therapeutic apheresis in clinical practice—evidence-based approach from the Apheresis Applications Committee of the American Society for Apheresis. The Fifth Special Issue. J Clin Apher 2010; 25:83-177.
6. Hug V, Keating M, McCredie K, et al. Clinical course and response to treatment of patients with acute myelogenous leukemia presenting with a high leukocyte count. Cancer 1983;52: 773-9.
7. Ventura G, Hester J, Smith T, et al. Acute myeloblastic leukemia with hyperleukocytosis: Risk factors for early mortality in induction. Am J Hematol 1988;27:34-7.
8. Rowe J, Lichtman M. Hyperleukocytosis and leukostasis: Common features of childhood chronic myelogenous leukemia. Blood 1984; 63:1230-4.
9. McKee C, Collins R. Intravascular leukocyte thrombi and aggregates as a cause of morbidity and mortality in leukemia. Medicine 1974; 53:463-78.
10. Lichtmann MA. Rheology of leukocytes, leukocyte suspensions, and blood in leukemia. J Clin Invest 1973;52:350-8.
11. Tan D, Hwang W, Goh YT. Therapeutic leukapheresis in hyperleukocytic leukaemias—the experience of a tertiary institution in Singapore. Ann Acad Med 2005;34:229-34.
12. McEver RP. Cell adhesion. In: Hoffman R, Benz EJ Jr, Shattil SJ, et al, eds. Hematology: Basic principles and practice. 3rd ed. New York: Churchill Livingstone, 2000:49-56.
13. Liesveld JL. Expression and function of adhesion receptors in acute myelogenous leukemia: Parallels with normal erythroid and myeloid progenitors. Acta Haematol 1997;97:53-62.
14. Stucki A, Rivier AS, Gikic M, et al. Endothelial cell activation by myeloblasts: Molecular mechanisms of leukostasis and leukemic cell dissemination. Blood 2001;97:2121-9.
15. Giles FJ, Shen Y, Kantarjian HM, et al. Leukapheresis reduces early mortality in patients with acute myeloid leukemia with high white cell counts but does not improve long term survival. Leuk Lymphoma 2001;42:67-73.
16. Thiebaut A, Thomas X, Belhabri A, et al. Impact of pre-induction therapy leukapheresis on treatment outcome in adult acute myelogenous leukemia presenting with hyperleukocytosis. Ann Hematol 2000;79:501-6.
17. Bug G, Anargyrou K, Tonn T, et al. Impact of leukapheresis on early death rate in adult acute myeloid leukemia presenting with hyperleukocytosis. Transfusion 2007;47:1843-50.
18. Cuttner J, Holland JF, Norton L, et al. Therapeutic leukapheresis for hyperleukocytosis in acute myelocytic leukemia. Med Pediatr Oncol 1983;11:76-8.
19. Giles FJ, Kantarjian H, O'Brien SM, et al. Leukapheresis reduces early risk of mortality in AML patients with high white cell counts receiving first induction therapy (abstract). Blood 1998;92(Suppl):237a.
20. Estey E. Reducing mortality associated with immediate treatment complications of adult

leukemias. Semin Hematol 2001;38(Suppl 10): 32-7.

21. Chang MC, Chen TY, Tang JL, et al. Leukapheresis and cranial irradiation in patients with hyperleukocytic acute myeloid leukemia: No impact on early mortality and intracranial hemorrhage. Am J Hematol 2007;82:976-80.

22. Porcu P, Danielson C, Orazi A, et al. Therapeutic leukapheresis in hyperleucocytic leukaemias: Lack of correlation between degree of cytoreduction and early mortality rate. Br J Haematol 1997;98:433-6.

23. Owen HG, Brecher ME. Therapeutic apheresis of the pregnant patient. In: Sacher RA, Brecher ME, eds. Obstetric transfusion practice. Bethesda, MD: AABB, 1993:95-110.

24. Smith JW, Weinstein R, Lankford K. Therapeutic apheresis—a summary of current indication categories endorsed by AABB and ASFA. Transfusion 2003;43:820-2.

25. McLeod B, Gottschall J, eds. Therapeutic apheresis: A physician's handbook. 2nd ed. Bethesda, MD: AABB, 2008.

26. Marbello L, Ricci F, Nosari AM, et al. Outcome of hyperleukocytic adult acute myeloid leukaemia: A single-center retrospective study and review of literature. Leuk Res 2008;32: 1221-7.

27. Blum W, Porcu P. Therapeutic apheresis in hyperleukocytosis and hyperviscosity syndrome. Semin Thromb Hemost 2007;33:350-4.

28. Hester JP, Kellogg RM, Freireich EJ. Mononuclear cell collection by continuous-flow centrifugation. J Clin Apher 1983;1:197-201.

29. Vallejos CS, McCredie KB, Brittin GM, et al. Biological effects of repeated leukapheresis of patients with chronic myelogenous leukemia. Blood 1973;42:925-33.

30. Huestis D, Price J, White R, et al. Leukapheresis of patients with chronic granulocytic leukemia using the Haemonetics blood processor. Transfusion 1976;16:255-9.

31. Sleeper T, Smith J, McCullough J. Therapeutic cytapheresis using the Fenwal CS3000 blood cell separator. Vox Sang 1985;48:193-200.

32. Daibutsu M, Takagi T, Ogawa H, et al. Treatment of chronic rheumatoid arthritis by lymphocytapheresis. Ther Plasmapheresis 1987;7: 257-60.

33. Bosch T. Therapeutic apheresis—state of the art in the year 2005. Ther Apher Dial 2005;9: 459-68.

34. Pineda AA. Developments in the apheresis procedure for the treatment of inflammatory bowel disease. Inflamm Bowel Dis 2006;12 (Suppl 1):S10-14.

35. Sawada K. Leukocytapheresis as an adjunct to conventional medication for inflammatory bowel disease. Dis Colon Rectum 2003;46 (Suppl 10):S66-77.

36. Shibata H, Kuriyama T, Yamawaki N. Cellsorba. Ther Apher Dial 2003;7:44-7.

37. Saniabadi AR, Hanai H, Takeuchi K, et al. Adacolumn, an adsorptive carrier based granulocyte and monocyte apheresis device for the treatment of inflammatory and refractory diseases associated with leukocytes. Ther Apher Dial 2003;7:48-59.

38. Saniabadi AR, Hanai H, Suzuki Y, et al. Adacolumn for selective leukocytapheresis as a non-pharmacological treatment for patients with disorders of the immune system: An adjunct or an alternative to drug therapy? J Clin Apher 2005;20:171-84.

39. Smith CW. Production, distribution and fate of neutrophils. In: Lichtman MA, Beutler E, Kipps TJ, et al, eds. Williams hematology. 7th ed. New York: McGraw-Hill, 2006:855-61.

40. Yamamoto T, Saniabadi AR, Maruyama Y, et al. Factors affecting clinical and endoscopic efficacies of selective leucocytapheresis for ulcerative colitis. Dig Liver Dis 2007;39:626-33.

41. Fukuda Y, Matsui T, Suzuki Y, et al. Adsorptive granulocyte and monocyte apheresis for refractory Crohn's disease: An open multicenter prospective study. J Gastroenterol 2004;39:1158-64.

42. Hanai H, Watanabe F, Yamada M, et al. Correlation of serum soluble TNF-alpha receptors I and II levels with disease activity in patients with ulcerative colitis. Am J Gastroenterol 2004;99:1532-8.

43. Hanai H, Watanabe F, Yamada M, et al. Adsorptive granulocyte and monocyte apheresis versus prednisolone in patients with corticosteroid-dependent moderately severe ulcerative colitis. Digestion 2004;70:36-44.

44. Kashiwagi N, Sugimura K, Koiwai H, et al. Immunomodulatory effects of granulocyte and monocyte adsorption apheresis as a treatment for patients with ulcerative colitis. Dig Dis Sci 2002;47:1334-41.

45. Shimoyama T, Sawada K, Hiwatashi N, et al. Safety and efficacy of granulocyte and monocyte adsorption apheresis in patients with

active ulcerative colitis: A multicenter study. J Clin Apher 2001;16:1-9.

46. Hanai H, et al. Decrease of reactive-oxygen-producing granulocytes and release of IL-10 into the peripheral blood following leukocytapheresis in patients with active ulcerative colitis. World J Gastroenterol 2005;11:3085-90.

47. Amano K, Amano K. Filter leukapheresis for patients with ulcerative colitis: Clinical results and the possible mechanism. Ther Apher 1998;2:97-100.

48. Sawada K, et al. Multicenter randomized controlled trial for the treatment of ulcerative colitis with a leukocytapheresis column. Curr Pharm Des 2003;9:307-21.

49. Nishioka C, Aoyama N, Maekawa S, et al. Leukocytapheresis therapy for steroid-naive patients with active ulcerative colitis: Its clinical efficacy and adverse effects compared with those of conventional steroid therapy. J Gastroenterol Hepatol 2005;20:1567-71.

50. Hanai H, Watanabe F, Takeuchi K, et al. Leukocyte adsorptive apheresis for the treatment of active ulcerative colitis: A prospective, uncontrolled, pilot study. Clin Gastroenterol Hepatol 2003;1:28-35.

51. Naganuma M, Funakoshi S, Sakuraba A, et al. Granulocytapheresis is useful as an alternative therapy in patients with steroid-refractory or dependent ulcerative colitis. Inflamm Bowel Dis 2004;10:251-7.

52. Tanaka T, Okanobu H, Saniabadi R, et al. Efficacy of Adacolumn selective leukocytapheresis in patients with steroid naive and steroid dependent with moderate to severe ulcerative colitis. Presented at Digestive Disease Week, Los Angeles, CA, May 20-25, 2006.

53. Sawada K, Ohnishi K, Kosaka T, et al. Leukocytapheresis therapy with leukocyte removal filter for inflammatory bowel disease. J Gastroenterol 1995;30(Suppl 8):124-7.

54. Kusaka T, Sawada K, Ohnishi K, et al. Effect of leukocytapheresis therapy using a leukocyte removal filter in Crohn's disease. Intern Med 1999;38:102-11.

55. Matsui T, Nishimura T, Matake H, et al. Granulocytapheresis for Crohn's disease: A report on seven refractory patients. Am J Gastroenterol 2003;98:511-12.

56. Kusaka T, Fukunaga K, Ohnishi K, et al. Adsorptive monocyte-granulocytapheresis (M-GCAP) for refractory Crohn's disease. J Clin Apher 2004;19:168-73.

57. Domenech E, Hinojosa J, Esteve-Comas M, et al for the Spanish Group for the Study of Crohn's Disease and Ulcerative Colitis (GETECCU). Granulocytapheresis in steroid-dependent inflammatory bowel disease: A prospective, open, pilot study. Aliment Pharmacol Ther 2004;20:1347-52.

58. Sands BE. Pilot feasibility studies of leukocytapheresis with the Adacolumn apheresis system in patients with active ulcerative colitis or Crohn disease. J Clin Gastroenterol 2006;40:482-9.

59. Sands BE, Sandborn WJ, Feagan B, et al. A randomized, double-blind, sham-controlled study of granulocyte/monocyte apheresis for active ulcerative colitis. Gastroenterology 2008;135:400-9.

60. Habermalz B, Sauerland S. Clinical effectiveness of selective granulocyte, monocyte adsorptive apheresis with the Adacolumn device in ulcerative colitis. Dig Dis Sci 2010;55:1421-8.

61. Hanai H. Leucocytapheresis for inflammatory bowel disease in the era of biologic therapy. Eur J Gastroenterol Hepatol 2008;20:596-600.

62. Martin de Carpi J, Vilar P, Prieto G, et al. Safety and efficacy of granulocyte and monocyte adsorption apheresis in paediatric inflammatory bowel disease: A prospective pilot study. J Pediatr Gastroenterol Nutr 2008;46:386-91.

63. Hibi T, Sameshima Y, Sekiguchi Y, et al. Treating ulcerative colitis by Adacolumn therapeutic leucocytapheresis: Clinical efficacy and safety based on surveillance of 656 patients in 53 centres in Japan. Dig Liver Dis 2009;41:570-7.

64. Novelli G, Rossi M, Ferretti G, et al. Adacolumn treatment in kidney transplant patients with hepatitis C virus. Transplant Proc 2009;41:1195-200.

65. Nagase K, Sawada K, Ohnishi K, et al. Complications of leukocytapheresis. Ther Apher 1998;2:120-4.

66. Kruis W, Dignass A, Steinhagen-Thiessen E, et al. Open label trial of granulocyte apheresis suggests therapeutic efficacy in chronically active steroid refractory ulcerative colitis. World J Gastroenterol 2005;11:7001-6.

67. Schafer A. Thrombocytosis. N Engl J Med 2004;350:1211-19.

68. Thiele J, Kvasnicka HM. The 2008 WHO diagnostic criteria for polycythemia vera, essential thrombocythemia, and primary

myelofibrosis. Curr Hematol Malig Reports 2009;4:33-40.

69. Skoda RC. Thrombocytosis. Hematol Am Soc Hematol Educ Program 2009:159-67.

70. Kralovics R, Passamonti F, Buser AS, et al. A gain-of-function mutation of JAK2 in myeloproliferative disorders. N Engl J Med 2005;352:1779-90.

71. Levine RL, Wadleigh M, Cools J, et al. Activating mutation in the tyrosine kinase JAK2 in polycythemia vera, essential thrombocythemia, and myeloid metaplasia with myelofibrosis. Cancer Cell 2005;7:387-97.

72. Tefferi A. Polycythemia vera: A comprehensive review and clinical recommendations Mayo Clin Proc 2003;78:174-94.

73. Kutti J, Ridell B. Epidemiology of the myeloproliferative disorders: Essential thrombocythaemia, polycythaemia vera and idiopathic myelofibrosis. Pathol Biol 2001;49:164-6.

74. Mesa RA, Silverstein MN, Jacobsen SJ, et al. Population-based incidence and survival figures in essential thrombocythemia and agnogenic myeloid metaplasia: An Olmstead County study. Am J Hematol 1999;61:10-15.

75. Cortelazzo S, Viero P, Finazzi G. Incidence and risk factors for thrombotic complications in a historical cohort of 100 patients with essential thrombocythemia. J Clin Oncol 1990;8:556-62.

76. Barbui T, Barosi G, Grossi A, et al. Practice guidelines for the therapy of essential thrombocythemia: A statement from the Italian Society of Hematology, the Italian Society of Experimental Hematology and the Italian Group for Bone Marrow Transplantation. Haematologica 2004;89:215.

77. Tefferi A, Passamonti F. Essential thrombocythemia and pregnancy: Observations from recent studies and management recommendations. Am J Hematol 2009;84:629-30.

78. Wright CA, Tefferi A. A single institutional experience with 43 pregnancies in essential thrombocythemia. Eur J Haematol 2001;66:152-9.

79. McColl MD, Ramsay JE, Tait RC, et al. Risk factors for pregnancy associated venous thromboembolism. Thromb Haemost 1997;78:1183-8.

80. Passamonti F, Randi ML, Rumi E, et al. Increased risk of pregnancy complications in patients with essential thrombocythemia carrying the JAK2 (617V>F) mutation. Blood 2007;110:485-9.

81. Michiels JJ, Berneman Z, Schroyens W, et al. The paradox of platelet activation and impaired function: Platelet-von Willebrand factor interactions, and the etiology of thrombotic and hemorrhagic manifestations in essential thrombocythemia and polycythemia vera. Semin Thromb Hemost 2006;32:589-604.

82. Mohri, H. Acquired von Willebrand syndrome: Features and management. Am J Hematol 2006;81:616-23.

83. Kroll MH, Hellums JD, McIntire LV, et al. Platelets and shear stress. Blood 1996;88:1525-41.

84. Nesbitt W, Magnin P, Salem H, et al. The impact of blood rheology on the molecular and cellular events underlying arterial thrombosis. J Mol Med 2006;84:989-95.

85. Pearson TC. Hemorheology in the erythrocytoses. Mt Sinai J Med 2001;68:182-91.

86. Carobbio A, Finazzi G, Antonioli E, et al. JAK2V617F allele burden and thrombosis: A direct comparison in essential thrombocythemia and polycythemia vera. Exp Hematol 2009;37:1016-21.

87. de Gaetano G, Cerletti C, Evangelista V, et al. Recent advances in platelet polymorphonuclear leukocyte interaction. Hemostasis 1999;74:1225-30.

88. Kaplar M, Kappelmayer J, Kiss A, et al. Increased leukocyte-platelet adhesion in chronic myeloproliferative disorders with high platelet counts. Platelets 2000;11:183-4.

89. Barbui T, Carobio A, Rambaldi A, et al. Perspectives on thrombosis in essential thrombocythemia and polycythemia vera: Is leukocytosis a causative factor? Blood 2009;114:759-63.

90. Tefferi A. Leukocytosis as a risk factor for thrombosis in myeloproliferative neoplasms—biologically plausible but clinically uncertain. Am J Hematol 2010;85:93-4.

91. Greist A. The role of blood component removal in essential and reactive thrombocytosis. Ther Apher 2002;6:36-44.

92. Greenberg B, Watson-Williams E. Successful control of life-threatening thrombocytosis with a blood processor. Transfusion 1975;15:620-2.

93. Taft EG, Babcock RB, Scharfman WB, et al. Plateletpheresis in the management of thrombocytosis. Blood 1977;50:927-33.

94. Burgstaler E, Pineda A. Therapeutic cytapheresis: Continuous flow versus intermittent flow apheresis systems. J Clin Apher 1994;9:205-9.

95. Grima K, Therapeutic apheresis in hematological and oncological diseases. J Clin Apher 2000; 15:28-52.

96. Hester J, Ventura G. Boucher T. Platelet concentrate collection in a dual-stage channel using computer-generated algorithms for collection and prediction of yield. Plasma Ther Transfus Technol 1987;8:377-85.

97. Gordon MC. Maternal physiology. In: Gabbe SG, Niebyl JR, Simpson JL, eds. Obstetrics: Normal and problem pregnancies. 5th ed. New York: Churchill Livingstone, 2007:56-80.

In: McLeod BC, Szczepiorkowski ZM, Weinstein R, Winters JL, eds.
Apheresis: Principles and Practice, 3rd edition
Bethesda, MD: AABB Press, 2010

14

Basic Principles of Therapeutic Blood Exchange

Robert Weinstein, MD

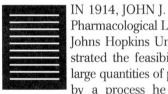

IN 1914, JOHN J. ABEL, OF THE Pharmacological Laboratory of The Johns Hopkins University, demonstrated the feasibility of removing large quantities of plasma from dogs by a process he called "plasmapheresis" (apheresis from the Greek *apairesos* or Roman *aphairesis*, meaning "to take away by force").[1] Subsequent use of plasmapheresis as a therapeutic modality was predicated upon assumptions that a disease state is causally related to a substance found in the plasma, and that the pathogenic substance can be removed via the plasma efficiently enough to permit resolution of the illness.[2] The earliest application of this principle to clinical medicine was the treatment of hyperviscosity syndrome in Waldenström's macroglobulinemia during the 1950s.[3-5] The offending immunoglobulin in this disease, IgM, is known to be predominantly intravascular and therefore can be readily removed from the plasma, even by manual plasmapheresis, as described in Chapter 3.

Subsequent development of the automated blood processor broadened the potential applicability of therapeutic apheresis to other disease states that fit the fundamental assumptions stated above as well as to other procedures, including therapeutic removal of cellular elements from the blood.[2,6-9] In addition, it brought into focus the need to assess more clearly the dynamics of changes in blood composition brought about by these therapies. Most of this chapter focuses on changes in plasma protein distribution among various body compartments as they relate to therapeutic plasma exchange (TPE), but some of the most fundamental concepts are also applicable to whole blood and red cell exchanges.[10]

Robert Weinstein, MD, Professor of Medicine and Pathology, University of Massachusetts Medical School, and Chief, Division of Transfusion Medicine, UMass Memorial Medical Center, Worcester, Massachusetts

The author has disclosed no conflicts of interest.

Modeling the Effects of Plasma Exchange

The effectiveness of a TPE depends on the volume of plasma removed relative to the patient's total plasma volume, the distribution between the intravascular and extravascular compartments of the pathogenic substance to be removed with the plasma, and the rapidity with which that substance equilibrates between compartments.[11,12] Figure 14-1 depicts a simple model of these compartments and the movement of a soluble substance between them during TPE. The model assumes that a newly synthesized soluble substance, such as a plasma protein, preferentially enters the intravascular space. The model accommodates proteins that enter the lymphatic circuit upon synthesis, such as immunoglobulins, by assuming that the proteins rapidly enter equilibrium with the intravascular space.[13] In other words, synthesis of a plasma protein proceeds at what is called a synthetic rate (S), which is equal to the rate of the protein's degradation and/or excretion from the plasma (the fractional catabolic rate, or FCR). Because S and FCR preferentially affect the intravascular mass of the protein and are

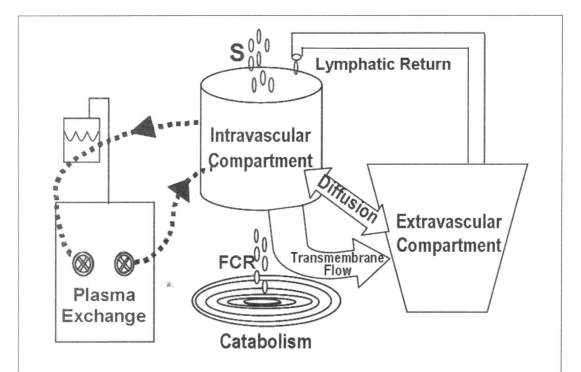

Figure 14-1. A model for the interaction between intravascular and extravascular compartments and the effects of plasma exchange. A soluble substance enters the body through the intravascular compartment at synthetic rate S and is catabolically removed from the body at its fractional catabolic rate (FCR). Movement from the intravascular compartment to the extravascular compartment takes place primarily by diffusion, whereas a smaller component of transmembrane flow occurs by other mechanisms. Soluble substances return from the extravascular compartment back to the intravascular compartment mainly through the lymphatic system, although a small component of back-diffusion takes place. Plasma exchange directly removes soluble substances only from the intravascular compartment. S, FCR, and intracompartment movement of solutes are balanced and in a steady state, and they proceed much more slowly than the removal of plasma from the intravascular compartment by plasma exchange. Therefore, for the purpose of therapeutic plasma exchange, the intravascular compartment is considered to be an isolated system that can be depleted of its soluble contents by the exchange of plasma for a replacement fluid.

balanced, the intravascular mass is in a steady state, in equilibrium with the proportion of the protein that resides in the extravascular compartment.[10,13,14]

The Isolated Intravascular Compartment: The "One-Compartment" Model

Mathematical models used to predict the outcome of TPE (see "Mathematical Models for Removal of Plasma Constituents by TPE" later this chapter) fundamentally assume that the intravascular plasma volume represents a closed compartment,[10-12,15-19] and thus that the intravascular mass of the substance to be removed is *isolated* from the extravascular compartment of the body (see Fig 14-1). In functional terms, this assumes that removal of a substance by TPE proceeds rapidly and efficiently so as not to be affected by the transfer of the substance between the intravascular and extravascular compartments. It also assumes that the steady state between endogenous synthesis and catabolism is not effectively altered during the TPE procedure.[10,11] In clinical practice, these assumptions apply fairly well to IgM and IgG (or immune complexes),[10,11,15,17,18] removal of which is the object of a large proportion of TPE procedures,[2] and to other large intravascular molecules, such as low-density lipoprotein (LDL).[14]

The extent to which TPE depletes a substance from the whole body is a function not only of the substance's intravascular mass but also of its distribution between intravascular and extravascular compartments.[10,16,17,20] Table 14-1 lists the metabolic characteristics of certain plasma proteins, some of which are particularly relevant to TPE.[10] From these data it can be seen that, in the course of a single TPE procedure, removal from the body of proteins such as IgM, fibrinogen, and α_2-macroglobulin, which are located predominantly in the *intra*vascular compartment, would be more complete than removal of proteins such as albumin or IgG, which are predominantly *extra*vascular in distribution.

Protein Transfer between Intravascular and Extravascular Compartments

Transfer of the protein from the intravascular compartment to the extravascular compartment proceeds mainly by diffusion down a concentration gradient, although a component of convective transport across biologic membranes also takes place (Fig 14-1).[13,21,22] The predominant transfer of extravascular protein back to the intravascular compartment proceeds via the lymphatic system.[21,22] The major barrier to the movement of large molecules from the intravascular to the extravascular compartment is the vascular capillary wall, with the permeability of large molecules being a function of both molecular weight and the Stokes-Einstein radius.[23,24] Small molecules and solutes are transferred in equilibrium between the two compartments largely via diffusion, with the other two mechanisms playing a lesser role.[13,23] A system of pores of 4-nm radius plus a few larger pores of approximately 80-nm radius or pinocytotic vesicles of approximately 25-nm radius may explain these transfer phenomena.[23,24] Although they are unable to pass across the capillary endothelium, larger molecules (>3 nm) approach their steady-state lymph concentrations faster than smaller ones because of "gel column" exclusion effects in the interstitial space.[25] Chopek and McCullough[10] refer to the combined rate of egress of a protein (or other soluble substance) from the intravascular space into the extravascular compartment as the transcapillary escape rate of that substance (Table 14-1).

The transfer of proteins such as IgG from the intravascular compartment to the extravascular compartment can be quantified as the fraction of the intravascular compartment transferred per unit of time, and this can be expressed as a clearance (the volume of plasma completely stripped of the substance of interest per unit time, quantified in mL/hour).[13] Such clearances, on the order of 5 to 20 mL per hour, are slow compared to plasma flow rates of 15 to 40 mL/minute typically achieved during TPE procedures.[13] Hence, the decrement in plasma IgG achieved by TPE can be predicted by the one-compartment model, which consid-

Table 14-1. Metabolic Characteristics of Some Plasma Proteins*

Protein	mg/mL[†]	Molecular Weight (kDa)	Percent Intravascular	FCR[‡] (%)	Change in FCR with ↓Concentration	TER[§] (%)
IgG	12.1	150	45	6.7	→	3
IgA	2.6	$(160)_n$	42	25	constant	
IgM	0.9	950	76	18	constant	1-2
IgD	0.02	175	75	37	←	
IgE	0.0001	190	41	94	←	
Albumin	42 ±3.5	66	40	10	→	5-6
Fibrinogen	2-4	340	80	25	constant	2-3
C_3	1.5	240	53	56	constant	
α_2-macroglobulin	2.6	820	100	8.2	constant	

* Adapted with permission from Chopek and McCullough.[10]
[†]Concentration in normal serum or plasma.
[‡]Fractional catabolic rate: as percentage of intravascular mass per day.
[§]Transcapillary escape rate: total transfer of protein from intravascular compartment to extravascular compartment as percentage of intravascular mass per hour.

ers only the physical removal of plasma and its solubilized immunoglobulins from the intravascular compartment during the TPE procedure.[10,11,14]

Patterns of Protein Catabolism

The plasma survival time, FCR, and response of FCR to changes in the concentration of serum proteins will all factor into the effectiveness with which a TPE will deplete the body of these soluble substances. Serum immunoglobulins are catabolized in a compartment that is in rapid equilibrium with the intravascular mass of the protein and at a rate that depends, in part, on the metabolic rate and thyroid function.[25]

The IgG Pattern of Catabolism

The catabolic rates of IgG and albumin are directly proportional to their serum concentrations.[26-29] IgG molecules have a longer survival and lower FCR than most other serum proteins.[26] The normal mean survival half-time of IgG is about 21 days (7.5-9 days for IgG_3[26]), and about 6.3% of the intravascular pool is catabolized daily. In patients with elevations of IgG from inflammation, liver disease, and multiple myeloma, the half-time of survival of IgG may decrease by almost half, and the FCR may increase almost three-fold.[26,28] Conversely, the FCR decreases in patients with primary IgG deficiency caused by chronic lymphocytic leukemia, hypogammaglobulinemia, or other lymphoproliferative disorders.[29] Patients with secondary IgG deficiency (eg, multiple myeloma with decreased normal IgG, renal homograft, nephrotic syndrome) may demonstrate an increased FCR and decreased serum half-life of their IgG.[26,29] These effects on IgG catabolism are related to the serum concentration of IgG and not to the concentrations of other proteins or immunoglobulins. For example, albumin infusion does not affect the catabolism of IgG.[30] This specificity of removal is determined by the Fc component of the gamma heavy chain.[26]

Waldmann and Strober[26] have presented a model explaining the relationship between plasma IgG concentration and the FCR, wherein a fixed fraction of the intravascular IgG pool is isolated for catabolism daily, with a saturable percentage of the isolated fraction somehow protected from catabolism and released back into the circulating pool. Brambell et al[31] hypothesized a protective receptor in tissues and on the vascular endothelium, a hypothesis that has been validated with the description of the FcRn receptor.[32-35] According to the model of Waldmann and Strober,[26] the fraction of the plasma pool isolated per day is 0.18 (the fraction of the intravascular pool catabolized per day at infinite IgG concentration), and the quantity of IgG protected per day at full saturation is approximately 5.5×10^{17} molecules of IgG/kg. A plot of FCR vs serum IgG concentration, using 41 measurements taken from patients with a variety of diseases affecting IgG concentration, closely correlated with a theoretical curve calculated according to the Waldmann/Strober model. It is not known whether the automated removal of IgG in exchange for albumin is analogous to primary gamma globulin deficiency, with a resulting decrease in FCR and increase in survival, or is simply a model for increased FCR by removal of a fixed proportion of the intravascular mass of IgG. However, experimental data predict that the FCR of IgG will decrease after the removal of immunoglobulin by TPE.[13]

The IgM Pattern of Catabolism

Predominantly intravascular in distribution, IgM demonstrates a catabolic pattern different from that of IgG and albumin, with the FCR *independent* of the serum concentration.[36,37] This pattern implies clearance of IgM from a constant volume of plasma per unit of time by a concentration-independent mechanism. This pattern may be explained by pinocytosis of plasma followed by intracellular catabolism, presumably in lysosomes. Other proteins, including fibrinogen, IgA, and ceruloplasmin, share this catabolic pattern. The FCR of IgM is two to three times that of IgG, its survival half-time is one-third to one-half that of IgG, and its synthetic rate in normal humans is one-fifth that of IgG.[10,26]

Saturable Catabolism

IgD, haptoglobin, and transferrin demonstrate an inverse relationship between serum concentration and FCR. This pattern suggests a saturable clearance mechanism wherein a fixed mass of protein is removed per unit of time. This would result in a reduction in the proportion of protein mass cleared as its concentration increased.[10,26]

Mathematical Models for Removal of Plasma Constituents by TPE

Plasma proteins with relatively high FCRs and a predominantly intravascular distribution, such as IgM and fibrinogen, are efficiently removed during TPE.[10,15,17] Given the apparent absence of a relationship between serum concentration and either FCR or synthetic rate, restoration of plasma levels of these proteins after TPE should be predictable. IgG, which is predominantly extravascular, demonstrates a fall in FCR with declining serum concentration.[26] However, as the intravascular mass of IgG is restored following TPE, the FCR should steadily adjust upward.[38] The synthetic rate of a specific autoantibody of the IgG class would depend on the status of the underlying autoimmune disease to be treated.[38] The extent to which clinical observations in patients treated with TPE reflect these theoretical predictions is discussed further below. Plasma protein catabolism is apparently regulated by the intravascular mass of protein,[26] and the rate of removal of plasma proteins by TPE exceeds the rate of reequilibration of proteins from the extravascular compartment to the intravascular compartment.[13] Hence it is reasonable to explore whether a one-compartment model of protein distribution, focusing on the intravascular compartment, is predictive of the outcome of TPE.

Continuous Flow Plasma Exchange

Clinical experience with exchange transfusion for liver failure provides a working model for the outcome of TPE.[39] The intravascular mass of a substance (eg, an immunoglobulin) can be determined from its concentration in the plasma (y) and the patient's plasma volume (V).[11,39] If the substance in vivo is predominantly located in the intravascular space (eg, IgM), its clearance from the plasma by TPE depends on the fraction of the plasma volume removed, at a rate of (b) milliliters per unit time, during the exchange. The fraction of the substance remaining in the intravascular space at any time (t) during the TPE is thus dependent on the *fractional rate* of exchange (r).[11] These relationships can be easily expressed as

Formula 1:

$$y_t = y_0 e^{-rt}$$

where y_0 represents the starting concentration of the compound in the patient's plasma, y_t is the concentration at time t, and e is the natural logarithm base (a constant valued at approximately 2.718281828459045). The fractional rate of exchange (r) is obtained by

Formula 2:

$$r = b/V$$

These formulas are simplest to use when t is expressed in hours and b is volume exchanged per hour. In common practice,[10] formula 1 is simplified as

Formula 3:

$$y_t = y_0 e^{-x}$$

where x refers to the number of plasma volumes exchanged at time (t) during the procedure.

According to formula 1, it is possible to generate a family of straight-line plots (on semilogarithmic axes) that predict the disappearance of an intravascular substance on the basis of the amount of plasma exchanged from a patient with a given plasma volume.[12] Chopek and McCullough[10] have used formula 3 to plot a curve predicting the disappearance of such a substance from the blood of any patient according to the number of plasma volumes removed during the exchange (Fig 14-2). Formulas 1 and

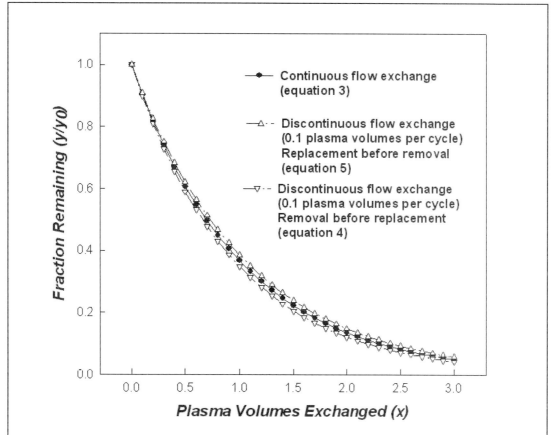

Figure 14-2. Theoretical depletion of soluble substances from the plasma by plasma exchange according to the one-compartment model. A fixed proportion of the remaining intravascular mass of a soluble substance is removed with each increment of plasma volume removed. (Adapted with permission from Chopek and McCullough.[10])

3 assume that the plasma is removed and replaced continuously by a fluid devoid of the substance whose disappearance is desired. In addition, these formulas assume complete mixing of the replacement fluid with the remaining intravascular plasma volume.[11] As described herein, these formulas ignore the formed elements of the blood, which are assumed to be returned to the patient. (Actual changes in cell counts resulting from TPE are discussed in detail later in this chapter) As a practical point, given the exclusively intravascular location of red cells, these formulas also accurately predict the decrement in the fraction of patient red cells remaining during a whole blood or red cell exchange by apheresis if whole blood or

red cell volume, respectively, is substituted for plasma volume in the calculations. The therapeutic application of apheresis to red cell exchange is described in detail in Chapter 19.

Kellogg and Hester[14] described the kinetics of TPE using a mathematical model that took into account the diffusion coefficient, transmembrane sieving coefficient, and lymphatic return flow rate for transfer of the substance of interest between intravascular and extravascular compartments. Their model also accounts for the volumes of the extravascular space and intravascular space, the constant rate of removal of the substance of interest from each compartment, the volume of the continuous flow blood processor, plasma and anticoagulant flow rates, and the anticoagulant dilution ratio. This complex model is predicated upon assumptions similar to those of the one-compartment model described above (ie, synthesis affects only the intravascular compartment, and mixing is instantaneous and complete). Applying their model to the removal of cholesterol from a patient with familial hypercholesterolemia, Kellogg and Hester[14] demonstrated that removal of the relatively nondiffusible marker cholesterol (bound to high-molecular-weight LDLs) is predictable with greater than 90% accuracy. Furthermore, postexchange reequilibration of cholesterol between the intravascular and extravascular compartments occurred over a 6- to 7-hour period, validating a primary assumption of the one-compartment model— namely, that the removal of a substance by TPE occurs much faster than intracompartment equilibration. Removal of paraproteins may deviate from prediction by as much as 50%, presumably because conventional formulas tend to substantially underestimate plasma volume in patients with paraproteinemic conditions.[10,15,16,40]

Kellogg and Hester[14] applied their model to the removal of bilirubin by TPE from a patient with metastatic colon carcinoma who was rendered acholic by partial hepatectomy. Their model predicted depletion of the relatively diffusible substance bilirubin to 55% of the starting serum concentration by an exchange of 1.5 plasma volumes, as compared with the depletion of cholesterol to approximately 30% of the starting serum concentration. Lower-molecular-weight compounds that are diffusible or subject to active homeostatic regulation in the plasma (such as calcium or potassium) are removed less efficiently by TPE, in effect behaving as though their intravascular and extravascular masses were being exchanged simultaneously.[10,17]

Discontinuous Flow Plasma Exchange

Berkman and Orlin[16] applied a method previously used for expressing the proportion of blood remaining after exchange transfusion to predict the efficiency with which cryoglobulins are removed by discontinuous TPE. The proportion of cryoglobulin remaining in the postapheresis intravascular pool (ie, y_t/y_0) is calculated as a function of the patient's plasma volume (V) and of the volume of plasma removed with each cycle (Δx) of the discontinuous exchange over n cycles.[10,16] Thus, for discontinuous TPE during which a volume of plasma (Δx) is removed before infusion of replacement fluid,

Formula 4:

$$y_t/y_0 = \left[\frac{V - \Delta x}{V}\right]^n$$

Formula 4 is similar to formula 1 in its dependence on the effective fractional exchange rate and the number of cycles of exchange (analogous to the number of plasma volumes removed). If the replacement fluid is infused before the plasma is removed, formula 4 is modified[10] so that

Formula 5:

$$y_t/y_0 = \left[\frac{V}{V + \Delta x}\right]^n$$

Chopek and McCullough[10] have demonstrated that when (Δx) does not exceed 0.1 plasma volume, the disappearance curves for discontinuous TPE closely follow the curve for continuous flow procedures (Fig 14-2).

Removal of nonparaprotein IgM or IgG by discontinuous TPE according to formula 4 results in the disappearance of immunoglobulin from the plasma within 2% of prediction,[17] again validating the assumption that equilibration of immunoglobulin between the intravascular space and extravascular pools does not occur rapidly enough during the exchange procedure to affect the result of the exchange. Paraproteins are removed less efficiently,[16] reflecting either a more rapid equilibration between compartments or, more likely, an expanded (and therefore underestimated) plasma volume. Formulas for modeling discontinuous TPE can be modified to accommodate equilibration between intravascular and extravascular compartments during the exchange.[16] For a fully equilibrating substance, the model predicts that approximately 55% of the total body pool of the substance of interest would remain after a 1.5-volume TPE, similar to what would be expected with the continuous flow model.[10,16]

Reduction of Blood Constituent Levels with Therapeutic Plasma Exchange

The models described above were originally used to predict the removal and residual mass of partially diffusible substances, such as bilirubin, during either exchange transfusion or cross-circulation for the treatment of liver failure.[39] The models were appreciated to take into account redistribution between compartments, catabolism, and synthesis by the healthy liver.[14] The one-compartment model has now gained wide acceptance as being predictive of the outcome of TPE, and it is taken as the basis for routine and automated methods for predicting outcome, in concert with knowledge of blood and plasma volume and anticoagulant flow rate.[10,11,15,18,41] Table 14-2 presents a broad summary of the anticipated alterations in certain blood constituents following a 1.0-volume TPE with albumin replacement fluid.

Plasma Proteins

Chopek and McCullough[10] have presented data on 14 patients treated with TPE. Among the 10 patients without paraproteins, removal of plasma proteins was related to the number of plasma volumes exchanged as predicted by the one-compartment model (formula 3). In other words, a fixed proportion of the remaining intravascular mass of the substance of interest was removed with each additional plasma volume removed. This applied to immunoglobulins, fibrinogen, Factor V, ferritin, transferrin, lactate dehydrogenase (LDH), serum glutamic-oxaloacetic transaminase (aspartate aminotransferase), and alkaline phosphatase.[10] Linear regression (Fig 14-3) showed a fit to formula 3 within 94% of prediction. The small deviation from prediction was attributed to errors in measurement of proteins, of the volume of plasma removed, or of patients' plasma volumes, and to reequilibration and/or metabolism during exchange. The four patients with multiple myeloma also demonstrated a linear relationship between the natural logarithm of protein remaining and the number of plasma volumes exchanged (Fig 14-3), but the slope of the curve distinguished this group from the patients without paraproteins.[10] Removal of proteins

---

Table 14-2. Alteration in Blood Constituents by a 1-Plasma-Volume Exchange*

Constituent	Percent Decrease from Baseline	Percent Recovery 48 Hours after Plasma Exchange
Clotting factors	25-50	80-100
Fibrinogen	63	65
Immunoglobulins	63	~45
Paraproteins	30-60	Variable
Liver enzymes	55-60	100
Bilirubin	45	100
C_3	63	60-100
Platelets	25-30	75-100

*Replacement fluid consisting of 4% to 5% albumin in 0.9% sodium chloride.

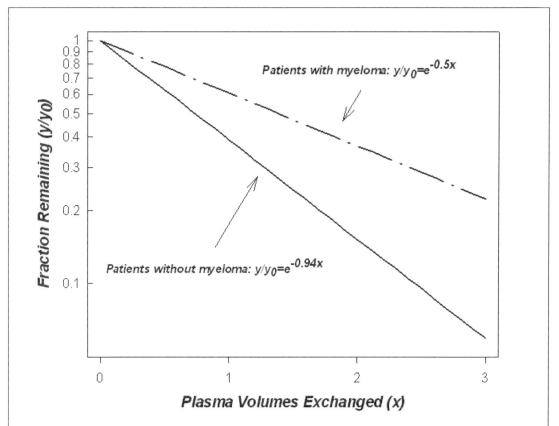

Figure 14-3. Linear regression plots depicting the observed removal of plasma proteins by therapeutic plasma exchange, using albumin replacement fluid, in patients without multiple myeloma (solid line) and with multiple myeloma (dashed line). Formulas depicted were derived from actual measurements that were applied to the one-compartment model by Chopek and McCullough.[10] Plasma protein removal from patients without myeloma approximated the ideal one-compartment model (formula 3) within 6%. Removal of proteins from patients with myeloma deviated from the one-compartment model by 50%. (Adapted with permission from Chopek and McCullough.[10])

from the group with multiple myeloma deviated from prediction by 50%, consistent with the tendency of the plasma volume to be increased in patients with paraproteinemias.[15,40]

Normal Immunoglobulins

Keller and Urbaniak[42] reported the lowering of IgG, IgA, and IgM to 34.6% ±2.6%, 39.1% ±5.2%, and 31.1% ±3.9%, respectively, of their starting concentrations by one continuous exchange of 4 or 5.2 L of plasma for immunoglobulin-free replacement fluid. They did not express the volumes exchanged as multiples of

the plasma volumes of their patients. In addition, six of 10 patients had IgG myeloma (although about 75% of the procedures were performed when the serum M component was less than 1.0 g/dL). Serum immunoglobulin levels did not reach (or slightly exceed) baseline until 3 days after TPE. Given the elements of uncertainty surrounding the amount of plasma exchanged relative to the patients' plasma volumes, the results suggest successful processing of about 1 plasma volume according to the one-compartment model, with the anticipated results. The relatively low serum M-component concentrations of their patients with multiple myeloma would not be expected to increase the patients' plasma volumes enough to affect the result.[40]

Orlin and Berkman[17] described eight patients with immune-mediated diseases (seven of whom were on immunosuppressive medication) and two healthy individuals who underwent discontinuous TPE with albumin replacement. Removal of IgG and IgM was within 1.6% of that predicted by the one-compartment model [ie, about 63% removal for a single volume of plasma exchanged (formula 4)]; recovery was approximately 44% by 48 hours after exchange. Recovery of IgG was 67% and 75% in the two healthy individuals at 2 weeks after exchange. These recovery rates likely reflect the balance of removal, reequilibration, catabolism, and synthesis after exchange. The authors contrasted their IgG and IgM recovery rates with those reported by Keller and Urbaniak[42] and concluded that the differences likely reflected the method used to calculate recovery. The method used by Keller and Urbaniak has been criticized by Chopek and McCullough.[10]

Volkin et al[43] performed discontinuous exchanges of 0.5 plasma volume on 17 patients with a variety of immune-mediated disorders. Many of their patients were concurrently treated with immunosuppressive medication. IgG, IgA, and IgM were decreased by 34% ±3%, 37% ±3%, and 34% ±3%, respectively, and remained at 19% ±9%, 13% ±8%, and 19% ±8%, respectively, below baseline by 48 hours after exchange. These findings closely approximate removal as predicted by the one-compartment model (formula 4). Recovery at 48 hours reflects reequilibration, catabolism, and synthesis and reasonably approximates the findings of Orlin and Berkman.[17] Nilsson et al[44] found similar degrees of removal of IgG, IgM, and IgA by small-volume TPE using discontinuous equipment and immunoglobulin-free replacement fluid.

Wood and Jacobs[45] performed continuous flow exchanges of 1.5 plasma volumes on patients with immune-mediated diseases or homozygous hyperlipidemia. They described a 37% recovery of IgG, IgA, and IgM from the nadir of a course of TPE in the first week after

stopping treatment. Thereafter, Ig levels increased 10% to 20% per week, reaching baseline or pretreatment levels by the fifth week after TPE.

The removal of immunoglobulins from patients whose plasma volumes can be reasonably estimated by standard measures is adequately predicted by the one-compartment model (formula 3 for continuous exchange or formula 4 for discontinuous exchange).[10,15,17] Recovery after apheresis is governed by a balance of reequilibration between compartments, catabolism (to include the effects of altered serum concentration on the FCR in the case of IgG), and synthesis. The administration of immunosuppressive drugs may affect the contribution of synthesis to the recovery of immunoglobulins after TPE.[10]

Paraproteins

Removal of immunoglobulins may seem less efficient from patients with multiple myeloma, Waldenström's macroglobulinemia, and other paraproteinemic states than from patients with nonparaproteinemic states.[10,16] Chopek and McCullough[10] observed that the removal of immunoglobulins by TPE from patients with multiple myeloma was about half of that predicted according to formula 3. They attributed the difference to the increase in plasma volume that may occur in patients with paraproteins. The measured plasma volume of one of their patients was 1.5-fold greater than expected. Berkman and Orlin[16] noted a similar decrease in the apparent efficiency with which monoclonal IgG cryoglobulin was removed in a patient with multiple myeloma. Beck et al[18] recorded a marked reduction of paraprotein level compared to prediction according to formula 3. They noted that the improvement in symptoms in three patients with hyperviscosity syndrome caused by multiple myeloma or Waldenström's macroglobulinemia correlated with the decrease in serum viscosity, which was a logarithmic function of plasma volume processed. Keller and Urbaniak[42] observed no significant difference in the removal of IgG between myeloma patients and patients without paraproteins. Orlin and Berkman[17] noted that paraprotein depletion from some patients with cryoglobulinemia could be predicted fairly closely by a one-compartment model according to formula 4.

These differences in reported experiences may be explained by two factors. First, the finding of an increased plasma volume in patients with paraproteins depends somewhat on the paraprotein concentration, being especially likely at an IgG concentration greater than 4 g/dL.[35] Sixty-seven percent of patients with macroglobulinemia may have an expanded plasma and red cell volume.[40] Second, some patients with multiple myeloma have been found to have a higher proportion of IgG in the intravascular space (56%-85%), perhaps accounting for unexpected efficiency in removing paraproteins despite an expanded plasma volume.[46] It is also likely that, as paraprotein is removed during TPE, plasma volume decreases progressively, thereby somewhat improving the efficiency of paraprotein removal during the procedure.[15] These latter two factors likely explain why the removal of paraproteins may sometimes be *greater* than the one-compartment model would predict.[11,15]

It is important to bear in mind that when TPE is performed for the treatment of hyperviscosity syndrome, the desired endpoint is a decrease in serum viscosity and an improvement of the patient's symptoms.[3-5,18,47,48] Although removal of 5 to 6 L of plasma will reliably deplete more than 80% of the M component from patients with Waldenström's macroglobulinemia,[47] symptomatic relief and reduction of serum viscosity may be achieved by removal of only 1 to 3 L in many patients.[18] Treatment can be individualized according to measurements of serum viscosity and patient response.[18]

Complement and Immune Complexes

The third component of complement (C3) is a high-molecular-weight protein, with a high FCR, that is almost equally distributed between the intravascular and extravascular compartments (see Table 14-1).[10] These features of the protein would predict efficient removal by TPE but rapid recovery of its intravascular mass afterwards. Keller and Urbaniak[42] reported on the removal of C3 and C4 by TPE in 10 patients. Removal of these components appeared to be as predicted by the one-compartment model; recovery to the original serum concentration was almost 90% at 24 hours after exchange and was complete by 48 hours after exchange. Orlin and Berkman[17] reported that removal of C3 by TPE was as predicted or slightly more than predicted by the one-compartment model in eight patients, with 63% recovery at 48 hours after exchange. Similar experience was reported by Volkin et al,[43] who performed small (0.5-plasma volume) exchanges on 17 patients. C3 and C4 were decreased by a mean of 40% $\pm$2.3% and 36% $\pm$2.7%, respectively, as predicted, but were almost at preexchange levels after 48 hours. Wood and Jacobs[45] found that the decrease in C3 was less than predicted, and the decrease in C4 was as predicted. In both cases, a significant return toward baseline had occurred after 24 hours. According to Calabrese et al,[11] removal of circulating immune complexes could be accurately predicted from formula 3 in five of eight patients treated with TPE for vasculitis or rheumatoid arthritis. Recovery was variable, taking up to several weeks. Most of their patients were also on immunosuppressive medication after TPE.

Coagulant Proteins

The predominantly intravascular distribution of fibrinogen (Table 14-1) would predict a significant fall in this important coagulant protein with TPE when the replacement fluid does not contain fibrinogen. No significant fall in plasma fibrinogen nor change in the activated partial thromboplastin time (aPTT) is observed when Fresh Frozen Plasma (FFP) is the replacement fluid.[10] But the aPTT rises rapidly and fibrinogen falls rapidly by the end of the procedure when an exchange of at least 1.3 plasma volumes is performed and less than 50% of the replacement fluid is FFP.[10]

Keller et al[49] reported the hemostatic alterations encountered in 179 continuous flow TPE procedures performed on 18 patients. All underwent exchange of 4.0 or 5.2 L of plasma, most with coagulation-factor-free replacement fluid. All patients received heparin anticoagulation during the procedures and protamine sulfate afterward to reverse the effect of heparin. Fibrinogen levels were lowered to 25% ±1.2% of preapheresis levels and recovered to baseline after 2 to 3 days. With consecutive daily TPE, fibrinogen remained below 10% of the starting preapheresis concentration but still recovered to normal in an average of 3 days after cessation of TPE. Thrombin times, reptilase times, and aPTT were prolonged after apheresis; platelet counts also fell with treatment but recovered within 24 hours. Minor hemorrhagic events, all associated with severe thrombocytopenia, occurred in three patients (2.2%). The authors concluded that the minimal hemorrhagic risk of TPE militated against the routine use of FFP to prevent bleeding.

In a follow-up study, the same group of investigators reported on alterations in specific coagulation factors with daily TPE.[50] Once again, fibrinogen fell significantly to 30% ±12% of baseline; prothrombin fell to a similar extent (33% ±10% of baseline). Factors VII, VIII, and IX were less affected by TPE, falling to 48% ±11%, 45% ±24%, and 62% ±11% of preapheresis levels, respectively. Factors V and X both fell to 38% ±11% of preapheresis levels. Antithrombin activity fell to 40% ±16% of the pretreatment level, but antithrombin antigen only fell to 68% ±24% of baseline, suggesting that enzyme-inhibitor complexes were formed between antithrombin and activated clotting factors generated during the procedures. Most clotting factors returned to 85% to 100% of normal within a day after TPE, and all but Factor X and fibrinogen were thus restored within 2 days. The authors concluded that a single TPE does not deplete coagulation factors below the levels nominally required for normal hemostasis.

Using continuous flow equipment and coagulation-factor-free replacement fluid, Sultan et al[51] performed 18 TPEs (1.6 plasma volumes per exchange) on seven patients with myasthenia gravis. Procedures occurred at 2- or 3-day intervals. Fibrinogen decreased by a mean of 78.3%. Factors V, VII, IX, X, XI, and XII fell 71%, 69%, 55%, 84%, 66%, and 66%, respectively. All had returned to baseline 48 to 96 hours later when remeasured just before a subsequent TPE. Factor VIII decreased variably after TPE, always remaining in the hemostatic range, and was found to have increased when remeasured before a subsequent TPE. Antithrombin antigen fell an average of 84% after TPE, recovering substantially, but not completely to baseline, when remeasured. There were no hemorrhagic complications, but two thrombotic events occurred, possibly related to inadequate anticoagulation.

Flaum et al[52] performed TPE of 1.2 plasma volumes using continuous flow equipment and coagulation-factor-free replacement fluids. They noted prolongation of prothrombin time (PT), aPTT, and thrombin time (TT) immediately after apheresis. The aPTT and TT returned to the normal range after 4 hours, and the PT was normal after 24 hours. Fibrinogen was approximately 30% of baseline after apheresis but had substantially recovered toward baseline after 24 hours. Factor V and VIII activity were decreased by approximately 50% after apheresis, but Factor VIII activity was back to baseline after 4 hours and Factor V was at baseline after 24 hours. Factor IX activity was decreased by only 26% by TPE, remaining within the normal hemostatic range, and was at baseline 4 hours after TPE. Factor X was about 67% depleted but was in the normal range 24 hours after TPE. Ristocetin cofactor activity was decreased by approximately 50% after the procedure but had recovered to baseline after 4 hours. Antithrombin antigen was decreased by 58% immediately after TPE (similar to the observation of Chirnside et al[50]) and remained 40% below normal 4 hours after completion of the procedure, rising toward baseline after about 24 hours. Despite these hemostatic alterations, no hemorrhagic complications were noted; however, the authors cautioned that similar changes in clotting parameters could be clinically significant if TPE were performed on an otherwise hemostatically compromised patient.

Simon[53] found no significant decrease in Factors V, VII, VIII, or IX resulting from TPE with albumin-containing replacement fluid in 10 patients. Modest prolongation of PT and aPTT were attributed to decreases in pro- thrombin (57%) and Factor XI (50%) to levels that do not compromise hemostasis. Fibrinogen fell to 50% of baseline after procedures but returned to baseline after 2 to 3 days. Five patients receiving FFP as replacement did not experience a fall in Factor XI, prothrombin, or fibrinogen. Two patients receiving albumin replacement fluid bled but were considered to be at high risk for hemorrhage. Simon concluded[53] that routine supplementation of clotting-factor-free replacement fluid with FFP is unnecessary but should be considered when there is a preexisting hemostatic risk, or when fibrinogen does not rebound to "clearly safe" levels within a "reasonably short period of time."

Chopek and McCullough[10] observed the exponential lowering of fibrinogen concentra- tion, as predicted by the one-compartment model, to a 75% decrease when 1.5 plasma volumes were exchanged for albumin-con- taining replacement fluid. At between 1.0 and 1.5 plasma volumes, the aPTT approached 180 seconds. The PT also increased above the nor- mal range when 1.0 plasma volume was exchanged, and it increased rapidly when more than 1.5 plasma volumes were exchanged. Fol- lowing exchange, plasma fibrinogen concentra- tion recovered with a half-time of about 26 hours and returned toward baseline between 48 and 72 hours after exchange, consistent with the prediction based on expected reequili- bration (which Chopek and McCullough assumed to be equivalent to the transcapillary escape rate) and synthesis (which they assumed to be equivalent to the FCR, as summarized in Table 14-1). The aPTT returned to the normal range for their laboratory between 24 and 48 hours after TPE.

Orlin and Berkman[17] performed TPE on 10 subjects using intermittent flow equipment. The replacement fluid was 5% albumin in normal

saline. They observed that the amount of fibrinogen removed was predictable according to a one-compartment model using formula 4. The actual removal was modestly higher than the formula predicted, suggesting that some fibrinogen was consumed during the proce- dures. Plasma fibrinogen recovered to 63% of preapheresis levels by 48 hours. In one normal subject, the plasma levels of coagulation Fac- tors VIII and IX were monitored during a 5-L TPE. Although both factors fluctuated during the procedure, they remained above 50% of the preapheresis activity level and were within normal limits by the end of the procedure. Fibrinogen, however, had decreased to about 25% of the preapheresis level. Orlin and Berk- man attributed the observed increase of aPTT and PT (to more than 3.2 and almost 2.0 times their respective control values) to the removal of fibrinogen. Commenting on the relative pau- city of reports of bleeding complications from TPE, and in light of their findings, the authors did not recommend supplementation of the albumin-containing replacement fluid with FFP or other sources of clotting factors for most routine applications of TPE.

Immediately following the exchange of 0.5 plasma volume for 5% albumin/saline solution, Volkin et al[43] noted a rise in the aPTT from 32.6 ±1.7 seconds to 37.2 ±2.1 seconds (nor- mal range = 26-34 seconds) and no significant increase in the PT. Fibrinogen fell by 52% but was only slightly below the lower limit of nor- mal; it remained 40% below baseline after 2 days. Factors V, VII, VIII, and IX decreased by 27%, 26%, 29%, and 23%, respectively, remaining within the normal range. Factors II (prothrombin), X, XI, and XII fell by 42%, 40%, 46%, and 55%, respectively, with only Factor XII dropping below the normal range. All factors had returned to baseline after 2 days except for Factors II, XI, and XII, which remained 25% to 40% below baseline. PT and aPTT were normal 2 days after TPE. In three patients who were treated with TPE every other day for three exchange procedures, fibrinogen remained 51% below baseline by 48 hours following the last exchange. All other factors were within the normal range except

Factor XII, which was modestly below normal and 30% below baseline. PT and aPTT were not prolonged, however.

Domen et al[54] prospectively studied the hemostatic imbalances produced in 10 patients treated with intensive TPE using 5% albumin in 0.9% saline as the return fluid. The PT was prolonged immediately after TPE, compared to the preapheresis measurement, in all 10 patients; however, only one measurement was outside the normal range. Similarly, all patients had a prolonged aPTT after apheresis, but in only one patient was the aPTT outside the normal range. In any case, all values returned to baseline within 24 to 72 hours (ie, by the next scheduled TPE). Plasma fibrinogen concentration fell significantly in each patient. Eight of the 10 had a plasma fibrinogen level below normal after their first exchange; five remained below normal at 24 to 72 hours after the first exchange; and seven remained below the lower limit of normal 24 to 72 hours after the fourth exchange. There were no clinically significant bleeding complications in any of the patients.

Wood and Jacobs[45] carried out 100 exchanges of 1.5 plasma volumes on seven patients at biweekly intervals using continuous flow equipment and replacement fluid containing 4% albumin in a balanced electrolyte solution. Median fibrinogen concentration fell by 76% and remained 40% below baseline 24 hours after apheresis; median Factor VIII fell by 82% and was still 38% below baseline 24 hours after apheresis; and median antithrombin fell by 70% and was still 18% below baseline after 24 hours. All three, however, had returned to baseline by 48 hours after apheresis. The median aPTT increased from 36 seconds (reference range = 32-40 seconds) before TPE to 59 seconds immediately after TPE and then dropped back down to 38 seconds by 24 hours after TPE. There were no hemorrhagic or thrombotic complications. The authors concluded that, in the absence of an underlying hemostatic defect or liver disease, it is unnecessary to supplement with FFP unless daily large-volume TPE is contemplated.

As a rule, FFP should be avoided as the replacement fluid for TPE, except when needed to treat thrombotic microangiopathies. Its use is associated with risks of hypersensitivity reactions, citrate toxicity, and infectious complications such as hepatitis; furthermore, it consumes a valuable blood product that should be kept available for repletion of coagulation factors in bleeding patients. The use of albumin solutions or other coagulation-factor-free replacement fluids is rarely associated with hemorrhage. In 381 TPE procedures performed on 63 patients, Couriel and Weinstein[55] observed a fibrinogen level below 150 mg/dL after only 14 procedures (3.7%) in 11 patients (17.5%). Bleeding occurred in only one of these patients, who was also vitamin K deficient. In certain inflammatory disorders, such as the acute Guillain-Barré syndrome, the plasma concentration of fibrinogen, an acute phase reactant, may remain normal or elevated, despite daily TPE, until the disorder begins to abate in response to treatment.[56] It seems desirable to be able to assess the hemorrhagic risk of patients about to undergo a course of TPE. Where the risk is clinically unacceptable, the replacement fluid can be supplemented with FFP or Cryoprecipitated AHF.

Other Plasma Proteins and Constituent Molecules

Orlin and Berkman[17] noted that removal of LDL cholesterol, alkaline phosphatase, and alanine aminotransferase (ALT) occurred within 1.6% of prediction by the one-compartment model. Aspartate aminotransferase (AST), LDH, amylase, and creatine phosphokinase (CPK) were removed an average of 17% less than predicted by the model. By 48 hours after TPE, mean recovery of ALT, AST, and amylase was complete (111%), whereas that of LDH, alkaline phosphatase, and CPK was 60%. LDL cholesterol had recovered 44% by 48 hours after TPE. Chopek and McCullough[10] described the removal characteristics of AST, LDH, transferrin, and ferritin as being similar to those of IgM (ie, within 6% of prediction by a one-compartment model). The difference between the observations by these two groups of investigators may be explained by differences in the characteristics of the patients treated in their studies. Production of nonhepatic AST, LDH, and CPK in the group treated by Orlin and Berkman[17] may have affected the apparent removal of these enzymes from their plasma.

Cornelissen et al[57] observed that reduction of α_2-macroglobulin, α_1-antitrypsin, α_1-acid glycoprotein, haptoglobin, and β_2-microglobulin differed from prediction according to the one-compartment model. β_2-microglobulin, molecular weight 12,000 Da, was removed substantially less than predicted, suggesting that diffusion and reequilibration were factors in its final plasma concentration. Kellogg and Hester[14] noted that, because of its diffusibility, bilirubin remained at 55% of its starting concentration after a 1.5-volume TPE. This result is highly dependent on the volume of the patient's extravascular compartment.

Electrolytes and Small Molecules

Because of diffusibility, removal of electrolytes and small molecules deviates from prediction according to the one-compartment model.

Potassium, Bicarbonate, Glucose, Uric Acid, Sodium, and Chloride

Orlin and Berkman[17] observed the reduction of serum uric acid and potassium to be 53% less than predicted according to the one-compartment model. The concentrations of bicarbonate ion and glucose, on the other hand, did not fluctuate during TPE procedures. Sodium ion and chloride ion also did not change during TPE, but the authors note that these ions were included with the replacement fluid.

Chopek and McCullough[10] observed a fall in potassium of approximately 0.25 mEq/L after 1.3 to 2.1 plasma volumes were exchanged with albumin replacement fluid, and a fall of up to 0.7 mEq/L after similar volumes were exchanged using FFP replacement. However, they felt that potassium supplementation was probably not necessary during exchange for most patients. They noted a fall in bicarbonate ion of 6 mEq/L and a rise in chloride ion of 4 mEq/L with albumin replacement, and a "mirror image" rise in bicarbonate ion of 3 mEq/L

and fall in chloride ion of 6 mEq/L with FFP replacement. The authors attributed these differences to the higher concentration of citrate anticoagulant in FFP compared to albumin solutions (17.4 mM/L vs 4.4 mM/L, respectively). They did not observe significant changes in serum sodium ion in their patients, regardless of replacement fluid. Indeed, all manufactured protein solutions for infusion must have a sodium ion concentration of 130 to 160 mEq/L.

Citrate and Calcium

Changes in citrate and calcium ions during apheresis are described in detail in Chapter 3; the following summarizes changes associated with TPE. Ionized calcium falls in the plasma of patients undergoing TPE as a result of citrate anticoagulant infusion, removal of calcium in the patient's plasma, and the intrinsic calcium-binding properties of albumin, which is infused as replacement fluid.[58-60] From their experience and review of the literature, Hester et al[59] observed that infusion of citrate between 1.0 and 1.8 mg/kg per minute, typical of donor and therapeutic apheresis procedures, results in a 25% to 35% reduction in blood levels of ionized calcium. This reduction may lead to mild hypocalcemic symptoms such as paresthesias. In some patients, the reduction in ionized calcium may be associated with prolongation of the QT interval. Hypocalcemic toxicity can be encountered in upwards of 10% of TPE procedures; however, it usually does not result in termination of the procedure,[55,61,62] and it can be prevented by adjusting the whole blood processing rate and/or the anticoagulant flow rate.[60,63] In addition, supplemental calcium replacement by the oral route or by intravenous boluses (eg, 5-10 mL of 10% calcium gluconate infused over 15 minutes as needed for symptoms) or constant infusion (eg, 10 mL of 10% calcium gluconate per liter of replacement fluid) may obviate symptoms without restoring ionized calcium to its baseline concentration.[45,55,58-60,62] Calcium should not be added directly to FFP.

Orlin and Berkman[17] found that removal of total calcium was approximately 60% less than predicted by the one-compartment model. Silberstein et al[63] found the reductions in total calcium, ionized calcium, phosphate ion, and magnesium to be less than predicted by 108%, 106%, 101%, and 134%, respectively. All were at preapheresis levels by 48 hours after TPE. The authors felt that in their patients, a rapid, compensatory increase in parathyroid hormone, associated with a rise in nephrogenous cyclic adenosine monophosphate, explained the relative maintenance of calcium homeostasis during TPE.

Chopek and McCullough[10] point out that the effects of TPE on calcium levels and the clinical response of patients to differing ionized calcium levels may be mostly a function of the rate (rather than the size) of the exchange and the sensitivity of individual patients to a given ionized calcium concentration. In their series, average citrate concentration increased more in patients exchanged with FFP than in those exchanged with albumin (1.1 mM/L vs 0.2 mM/L, respectively), in accord with the citrate content of the two fluids (17.4 mM/L vs 4.4 mM/L, respectively). The authors estimated that, given the citrate concentration in FFP, it would be safe to infuse FFP as replacement fluid at a rate of 1.0 mL/kg per minute, or 1.5 plasma volumes per hour, although this estimate does not take into account the citrate used to anticoagulate the patient's blood in the extracorporeal circuit, some of which does return to the patient. They noted a greater fall in total calcium with albumin as opposed to FFP replacement fluid, consistent with the higher concentration of total calcium in FFP. However, ionized calcium fell to a similar extent with both replacement fluids. Supplementation of the albumin with calcium prevented the fall in total, but not ionized, calcium. Hester and Ayyar[60] pointed out that the serum levels underestimate the extent to which ionized calcium is removed from the body during TPE. The deficit in plasma concentration is corrected within 2 to 4 hours after cessation of the procedure.

Formed Elements of the Blood

Despite the efficiency of modern equipment, the process of exchanging plasma for replacement fluid may result in a decrease in red cells, white cells, and platelets. Changes may relate to the physical removal of blood cells and hemodilution.

Red Cells

Chopek and McCullough[10] noted as much as a 12% drop in hemoglobin concentration immediately after exchanges of 1.3 plasma volumes for 5% albumin, with recovery of hemoglobin concentration within 24 hours. Hemoglobin did not change, however, when FFP was the sole replacement fluid. They attributed these observations to an expansion of the plasma volume when 5% albumin is used as the replacement fluid. In their patients, baseline albumin concentrations were between 3.0 and 4.0 g/dL. Isovolumetric replacement with 5% albumin, therefore, expanded the plasma volume, whereas FFP, with an albumin concentration of 3.4 g/dL, did not. They recommended that a combination of albumin and crystalloid be used to produce an albumin concentration of 3.5 to 4.0 g/dL for patients whose serum albumin concentration before isovolumetric TPE is normal or near normal. Wood and Jacobs[45] performed 100 therapeutic exchanges of 1.5 plasma volumes on seven patients, using a replacement fluid that contained 4% albumin in an electrolyte solution. Median hemoglobin concentration was 13.1 g/dL before TPE and fell to 11.5 g/dL immediately after TPE. After 24 hours, median hemoglobin had risen to 12.5 g/dL. These findings were also attributed to alterations in intravascular volume and appear to corroborate the findings of Chopek and McCullough.[10]

White Blood Cells

Chopek and McCullough[10] reported a transient increase in granulocyte count (2.2×10^9/L) after TPE. They attributed this observation to shifts in the marginated pool. For their part,

Wood and Jacobs[45] did not observe a change in the median white cell count after TPE in their patients.

Platelets

Flaum et al[52] noted a 33% decrease in mean platelet count (from 240,000/µL to 161,000/µL) after 1.2-volume TPEs performed on three patients using continuous flow equipment. There were no bleeding complications. Keller et al[44] analyzed 179 TPEs performed on 18 patients using continuous flow equipment. Platelet counts were lowered to 50.1% ±1.8% of preapheresis values. Patients undergoing daily TPE experienced continued reduction to 20.7% and 23.3% of the initial preapheresis platelet count after the fifth and the tenth exchange, respectively. Platelet counts recovered to 83% ±5% of the count preceding the previous apheresis after a rest of 24 hours, and they had completely recovered to the previous preapheresis value after 48 hours. Regardless of the platelet count after TPE, it took a maximum of 2 to 3 days for platelet counts to return to more than 100,000/µL. Sultan et al[51] noted a mean platelet reduction of 52.6% (range = 20%-78%) after 1.6-volume TPEs using continuous flow equipment in seven patients.

Chopek and McCullough[10] performed exchanges of 1.3 to 2.1 plasma volumes in 14 patients. Platelet counts fell an average of 30% in patients whose preapheresis platelet counts had been normal, or an average of 18% if the patients had been thrombocytopenic (50-150,000/µL) preceding TPE. Among those patients with normal platelet counts before TPE, the fall in platelet count with TPE averaged 22% with intermittent flow equipment and 32% with continuous flow equipment. The half-time for the platelet count to return to baseline after exchange was 30 hours.

A series of 10 patients treated by Domen et al,[54] with an average 2.0-L TPE, experienced a mean decrease in platelets of 14.2% immediately after the first exchange. Platelet counts were still 13.4% below their starting point by 24 to 72 hours after the first exchange, and

they were 30.6% below their initial value 24 to 72 hours after four TPEs. Wood and Jacobs[45] observed a 33% fall in median platelet count, from 396,000/µL before apheresis to 264,000/µL immediately after 1.5-volume TPE performed on seven patients. By 24 hours after TPE, the median platelet count was 278,000/µL (30% below baseline).

The Intensity of Therapeutic Plasma Exchange: Volume and Schedule

The recommended size and frequency of TPE relate primarily to the plasma volume of the patient, the distribution of the substance to be removed between intravascular and extravascular compartments, and the rate at which the substance is synthesized. If the one-compartment model is applied, it is evident from Fig 14-2 that the marginal benefit from removing additional plasma rapidly declines after the first 1.0 to 1.5 plasma volumes exchanged. Clinical data concerning the application of these considerations to the treatment of specific diseases are presented elsewhere in this book. Table 14-3 presents general recommendations.

Removal of Autoantibodies and Other Offending Substances

The therapeutic benefit of TPE in most clinical applications is likely the result of the removal of antibodies.[2,11,38] This may apply to monoclonal immunoglobulins, paraproteins, polyclonal autoantibodies, or antibodies in immune complexes. As indicated above, only 45% of IgG is in the intravascular compartment; therefore, exchange of 1.25 plasma volumes for replacement fluid removes only 32% of total body IgG. Reequilibration between intravascular and extravascular compartments may be complete after 24 hours. Thus, depletion of total body IgG by about 85%, as was found to be effective in severe myasthenia gravis,[64] requires five exchanges of 1.25 plasma volumes on an alternate-day treatment schedule.[38] IgM, being about 75% intravascular but with a faster rate of synthesis than IgG, is reduced a similar

Table 14-3. Targets and Goals for Therapeutic Plasma Exchange

Reason for Apheresis	Treatment Volume (mL/kg)	Treatment Interval (in hours)	Treatment Endpoint
Autoantibodies	40-60	24-48	Four to six treatments
Immune complexes	40-60	24-48	Treat for response
Paraproteins	40-60	24	Treat for response
Cryoproteins	40-60	24-48	Treat for response
Toxins	40-60	24-72	Treat for response
Thrombotic thrombocytopenic purpura/hemolytic uremic syndrome	40	24	Treat to establish remission
Immunologic rebound	40-60	24-48	Two to three treatments followed by immunosuppressive medication

amount after three to four such alternate-day exchanges (see Table 14-1).[38]

The North American Guillain-Barré Syndrome Study Group trial used a treatment schedule that would accomplish this degree of immunoglobulin reduction (200-250 mL/kg of plasma removed in 7-14 days) and demonstrated the effectiveness of TPE in treating the acute Guillain-Barré syndrome.[65] A single course of treatment is adequate if the underlying stimulus to autoantibody production has abated. Guillian-Barré is usually a monophasic illness, but early relapses may occur in approximately 10% of patients.[66] As demonstrated by Vriesendorp and coworkers, patients treated by TPE demonstrate a rapid fall in IgM autoantibodies directed against peripheral nerve myelin.[67] In some patients, however, clinical relapse is heralded by a rebound in antibody titer after 2 to 3 weeks. Additional treatment again results in antibody clearance and clinical improvement in responding patients.[68]

Diseases that are not self-limited may require repeat courses of TPE, depending on the kinetics of autoantibody resynthesis (eg, IgG with an approximate 21-day half-life vs IgM with a 5- to 6-day half-life) and the ability of pharmaceutical intervention to slow synthesis and/or control symptoms after the initial course of TPE.[11,12,15,16,38,41] Non-antibody-mediated illnesses (eg, Refsum's disease) are similarly treated on a schedule that lowers the initial plasma concentration (eg, of phytanic acid) and then responds to the reappearance of that substance in the plasma.[69]

Thrombotic thrombocytopenic purpura (TTP) is one condition for which FFP is the preferred replacement fluid for TPE.[70] It is now clear that the salutary effect of TPE is related to the infusion of a deficient von Willebrand factor-cleaving protease (ADAMTS13) in the replacement plasma[71] and the removal from the patient's plasma of an immunoglobulin inhibitor of the patient's endogenous ADAMTS13.[72] Before recognition of the role of ADAMTS13 inhibitors in TTP, the effect of TPE was attributed, in part, to the removal of ultralarge multimeric forms of von Willebrand factor that interact with platelets.[73] Although the approach to treatment is not standardized, the clinical urgency of this condition has led to a typical approach of intensive (40-60 mL/kg) daily TPE, followed by an empirical tapering schedule as the platelet count returns to normal and hemolysis abates.[70,74] The proper endpoint of treatment has not been established; however, stopping too early (ie, as soon as the platelet count returns to normal) may be associated with an excessive rate of relapse.[75]

Hyperviscosity Syndrome

The treatment of hyperviscosity syndrome in patients with malignant paraproteinemias is also based on the need to remove immunoglobulins from the plasma, but for different reasons than considered above. The concentration of paraprotein at which patients develop clinical hyperviscosity is highly variable, so programs of TPE for patients with this condition must be individualized.[16,18] IgM paraproteins can be removed from patients with Waldenström macroglobulinemia without stimulating the rapid resynthesis of the protein by the tumor cells,[47] and TPE can be used intermittently to control clinical hyperviscosity. Initial treatment should remove 70% to 80% of the paraprotein. Subsequently, less intense courses may be performed every few weeks to months, depending on symptoms, paraprotein concentration, and serum viscosity.[18,47]

Immunologic Rebound

The removal of immunoglobulins by TPE may be followed after treatment ceases by an increase in specific antibody titers to levels even higher than baseline.[17,33,76,77] Although not accepted by all investigators, this phenomenon has been the basis of clinical trials of combinations of TPE with immunosuppressive agents for the treatment of various immune-mediated diseases.[78-82] The assumption that the increase in plasma immunoglobulins results from a "rebound" phenomenon (eg, biofeedback stimulation of increased immunoglobulin synthesis) is not supported by experiments with FcRn-deficient "knock-out" mice, which are congenitally deficient in IgG but whose IgG synthetic rate is the same as that of normal mice.[83] Recent work by Goldammer et al demonstrates that immunoadsorption apheresis does not stimulate an increase in immunoglobulin synthesis in patients with autoimmune diseases.[84] Another approach to the phenomenon of immunologic rebound holds that, in principle, the accelerated proliferation[85] and synthetic activity[86] of B-lymphocyte clones in response to the removal of their relevant antibodies (and, perhaps, the coincident removal of "blocking factors" to the immune response) may render those clones more susceptible to the effects of immunosuppression.[87] Although some protocols use a full course of intensive TPE as described above,[86] others call for an abbreviated course of two to three exchanges (100-180 mL/kg) over 3 to 4 days.[79-81] Then, 24 hours after the last exchange, at a time when the increased lymphocyte activity can be detected experimentally,[85,86] the immunosuppressive drug is administered. An abbreviated course of TPE is deemed acceptable in this setting because the aim of therapy is to induce immunologic rebound and thereby maximize the effect of immunosuppression.[87] In addition, there is less removal of normal immunoglobulins at a time when the patient will be treated with potent immunosuppressive drugs.

Replacement Fluids for Plasma Exchange

Most indications for TPE call for human serum albumin as the replacement fluid.[2,88] As indicated above, the standard formulation of 5% albumin may be relatively hyperoncotic for patients, resulting in a mild to moderate dilutional anemia.[10] Standard practice in many centers is to use a 5% albumin solution for at least 60% of the replacement volume. Achieving 100% replacement with 5% albumin is unlikely because the extracorporeal circuit is primed with crystalloid fluid and because part of the crystalloid anticoagulant solution is returned to the patient with the reinfused red cells. Alterations in hemostatic system proteins, other plasma proteins, and formed elements of the blood associated with albumin replacement fluid are discussed above. Occasional hypotensive reactions in patients taking medications that contain angiotensin-converting enzyme inhibitors[89] have been reported, as have rare pyrogen reactions.[90]

FFP is usually chosen to treat TTP and related disorders.[70] Some patients refractory to TPE using FFP may respond to plasma from which the cryosupernatant fraction has been removed.[91,92] FFP may also be used as a supplement to albumin-containing return fluid to obviate the transient, dilutional coagulopathy of TPE.[10] FFP is less likely than albumin to cause dilutional anemia, but it does pose a higher risk of allergic reactions and transfusion-transmitted infections. Development of antibodies to plasma constituents may limit the long-term use of FFP as the replacement fluid for some patients with TTP.

Plasma protein fraction is now seldom used as a replacement fluid for TPE. Derived from human plasma, it is formulated as a 5% solution consisting of at least 83% albumin, and no more than 1% of the total protein can be gamma globulin.[93] Although it does not protect against the transient coagulopathy of TPE, plasma protein fraction does not result in dilutional anemia. However, it is associated with frequent hypotensive reactions, attributable to the presence of prekallikrein-activating factor,[94] and more frequent allergic reactions than albumin, thus negating its cost advantage over albumin.[10]

Hetastarch (3% or 6% solution) is sometimes used as a supplement to albumin for TPE.[95,96] Although it is less expensive than albumin, hetastarch is associated with more frequent urticarial and pruritic reactions than albumin, and it may result in a coagulopathy caused by interference with Factor VIII function if more than 20 mL/kg is infused in a 24-hour period.[97] Occasional atypical reactions, such as severe back and head pain, have been observed with hetastarch infusion during TPE.[95] Currently, there is no consensus supporting its use in TPE.[98] A low-molecular-weight hydroxyethyl starch, pentastarch, has also been demonstrated to be a safe alternative to albumin for therapeutic plasma exchange.[99,100] Pentastarch appears to convey a significantly lower risk of hypocalcemic toxicity than is associated with the use of 5% albumin, and it may obviate the need to give supplemental calcium to prevent such toxicity during plasma exchange.[100,101]

Pentastarch may also cause fewer hemostatic abnormalities than hetastarch, particularly when used in large volumes.[102-104]

Conclusions

TPE can remove pathogenic substances from the blood in a predictable manner that can be quantitatively expressed as a one-compartment model. Given the rapidity and reasonable efficiency of automated apheresis, removal of these substances from the body is generally limited to their removal from the intravascular compartment. In clinical circumstances where the outcome of TPE appears to deviate from prediction according to the one-compartment model (ie, removal of paraproteins), the deviation can be attributed to inaccuracies in estimation of parameters such as patients' plasma volumes or plasma immunoglobulin concentrations. The one-compartment model, with awareness of the metabolic characteristics of immunoglobulins and other proteins of interest, has led to a rational approach to the application of TPE to the treatment of diverse disease states that share two key characteristics.[87] First, something can be identified to have an actual (or believed) causal relationship to the presence of a pathogenic substance in the plasma. Second, enough of the pathogenic substance can be removed from the body through the removal of plasma to permit resolution or substantial improvement of the disease state. Choices concerning scheduling, replacement fluids, and anticoagulation for TPE can be made on the basis of a vast accumulation of clinical experience and an increasingly advanced understanding of the mechanisms of diseases treated by TPE and the mechanism of action of TPE in resolving these diseases.

References

1. Abel JJ, Rowntree LG, Turner BB. Plasma removal with return of corpuscles (plasmapheresis). J Pharmacol Exp Ther 1914;5:625-41.

2. Shumak KH, Rock GA. Therapeutic plasma exchange. N Engl J Med 1984;310:762-71.
3. Reynolds WA. Late report of the first case of plasmapheresis for Waldenström's macroglobulinemia. JAMA 1981;245:606-7.
4. Schwab PJ, Fahey JL. Treatment of Waldenström's macroglobulinemia by plasmapheresis. N Engl J Med 1960;263:574-9.
5. Solomon A, Fahey JL. Plasmapheresis therapy in macroglobulinemia. Ann Intern Med 1963;58:789-800.
6. Lockwood CM. Plasma-exchange: An overview. Plasma Ther 1979;1:1-12.
7. Wenz B, Barland P. Therapeutic intensive plasmapheresis. Semin Hematol 1981;18:147-62.
8. Kennedy MS, Domen RE. Therapeutic apheresis. Applications and future directions. Vox Sang 1983;45:261-77.
9. Balow JE. Plasmapheresis: Development and application in treatment of renal disorders. Artif Organs 1986;10:324-30.
10. Chopek M, McCullough J. Protein and biochemical changes during plasma exchange. In: Berkman EM, Umlas J, eds. Therapeutic hemapheresis. Washington, DC: AABB, 1980:13-52.
11. Calabrese LH, Clough JD, Krakauer RS, Hoeltge GA. Plasmapheresis therapy of immunologic disease. Cleve Clin Q 1980;47:53-72.
12. Jones JV, Clough JD, Klinenberg JR, Davis P. The role of therapeutic plasmapheresis in the rheumatic diseases. J Lab Clin Med 1981;97:589-98.
13. Charlton B, Schindhelm K, Smeby LC, Farrell PC. Analysis of immunoglobulin G kinetics in the non-steady state. J Lab Clin Med 1985;105:312-20.
14. Kellogg RM, Hester JP. Kinetics modeling of plasma exchange: Intra- and post-plasma exchange. J Clin Apher 1988;4:183-7.
15. Russell JA, Toy JL, Powles RL. Plasma exchange in malignant paraproteinemias. Exp Hematol 1977;5S:105-16.
16. Berkman EM, Orlin JB. Use of plasmapheresis and partial plasma exchange in the management of patients with cryoglobulinemia. Transfusion 1980;20:171-8.
17. Orlin JB, Berkman EM. Partial plasma exchange using albumin replacement: Removal and recovery of normal plasma constituents. Blood 1980;56:1055-9.
18. Beck JR, Quinn BM, Meier FA, Rawnsley HM. Hyperviscosity syndrome in paraproteinemia.
Managed by plasma exchange; monitored by serum tests. Transfusion 1982;22:51-3.
19. Randerson DH. Kinetics of continuous apheresis: A theoretic basis for the comparison of centrifugal and membrane systems. Plasma Ther Transfus Technol 1983;4:199-204.
20. Morgenthaler JJ, Nydegger UE. Synthesis, distribution and catabolism of human plasma proteins in plasma exchange. Int J Artif Organs 1984;7:27-34.
21. Drinker CK, Field ME. The protein content of mammalian lymph and the relation of lymph to tissue fluid. Am J Physiol 1931;97:32-9.
22. Field ME, Drinker CK. The permeability of the capillaries of the dog to protein. Am J Physiol 1931;97:50-1.
23. Garlick DG, Renkin EM. Transport of large molecules from plasma to interstitial fluid and lymph in dogs. Am J Physiol 1970;219:1595-605.
24. Carter RD, Joyner WL, Renkin EM. Effects of histamine and some other substances on molecular selectivity of the capillary wall to plasma proteins and dextran. Microvasc Res 1974;7:31-48.
25. Watson PD, Grodins FS. An analysis of the effects of the interstitial matrix on plasma-lymph transport. Microvasc Res 1978;16:19-41.
26. Waldmann TA, Strober W. Metabolism of immunoglobulins. Prog Allergy 1969;13:1-110.
27. Strober W, Wochner RD, Barlow MH, et al. Immunoglobulin metabolism in ataxia telangiectasia. J Clin Invest 1968;47:1905-15.
28. Wells JV, Fudenberg HH. Metabolism of radioiodinated IgG in patients with abnormal serum IgG levels, I: Hypergamma-globulinaemia. Clin Exp Immunol 1971;9:761-74.
29. Wells JV, Fudenberg HH. Metabolism of radioiodinated IgG in patients with abnormal serum IgG levels, II: Hypogamma-globulinaemia. Clin Exp Immunol 1971;9:775-83.
30. Fahey JL, Robinson AG. Factors controlling serum-globulin concentration. J Exp Med 1963;118:845-68.
31. Brambell FWR, Hemmings WA, Morris IG. A theoretical model of γ-globulin catabolism. Nature 1964;203:1352-5.
32. Simister NE, Mostov KE. An Fc receptor structurally related to MCH class I antigens. Nature 1989;337:184-7.
33. Junghans RP, Anderson CL. The protection receptor for IgG catabolism is the β2-microglo-

bulin-containing neonatal intestinal transport receptor. Proc Natl Acad Sci U S A 1996;93: 5512-16.

34. Leach JL, Sedmak DD, Osborne JM, et al. Isolation from human placenta of the IgG transporter, FcRn, and localization to the syncytiotrophoblast: Implications for maternal-fetal antibody transport. J Immunol 1996;157: 3317-22.

35. Ghetie V, Ward ES. FcRn: The MHC class I-related receptor that is more than an IgG transporter. Immunol Today 1997;18:592-8.

36. Barth WF, Asofsky R, Liddy TJ, et al. Metabolism of human gamma macroglobulins. J Clin Invest 1964;43:1036-48.

37. Cohen S, Freeman T. Metabolic heterogeneity of human γ-globulin. Biochem J 1960;76:475-87.

38. Dau PC. Immunologic rebound. J Clin Apher 1995;10:210-17.

39. Marsaglia G, Thomas ED. Mathematical considerations of cross circulation and exchange transfusion. Transfusion 1971;11:216-19.

40. Alexanian R. Blood volume in monoclonal gammopathy. Blood 1977;49:301-7.

41. Dau PC. The fundamental basis for therapeutic plasmapheresis in autoimmune diseases. Transfus Sci 1996;17:235-44.

42. Keller AJ, Urbaniak SJ. Intensive plasma exchange on the cell separator: Effects on serum immunoglobulins and complement components. Br J Haematol 1978;38:531-40.

43. Volkin RL, Starz TW, Winkelstein A, et al. Changes in coagulation factors, complement, immunoglobulins, and immune complex concentrations with plasma exchange. Transfusion 1982;22:54-8.

44. Nilsson T, Rudolphi O, Cedergren B. Effects of intensive plasmapheresis on the haemostatic system. Scand J Haematol 1983;30:201-6.

45. Wood L, Jacobs P. The effect of serial therapeutic plasmapheresis on platelet count, coagulation factors, plasma immunoglobulin, and complement levels. J Clin Apher 1986;3:124-8.

46. Gabuzda TG. The turnover and distribution of myeloma and macroglobulin proteins. J Lab Clin Med 1962;59:65-80.

47. Buskard NA, Galton DAG, Goldman JM, et al. Plasma exchange in the long-term management of Waldenström's macroglobulinemia. Can Med Assoc J 1977;117:135-7.

48. Avnstorp C, Nielsen H, Drachmann O, Hippe E. Plasmapheresis in hyperviscosity syndrome. Acta Med Scand 1985;217:133-7.

49. Keller AJ, Chirnside A, Urbaniak SJ. Coagulation abnormalities produced by plasma exchange on the cell separator with special reference to fibrinogen and platelet levels. Br J Haematol 1979;42:593-603.

50. Chirnside A, Urbaniak SJ, Prowse CV, Keller AJ. Coagulation abnormalities following intensive plasma exchange on the cell separator, II: Effects on Factors I, II, V, VII, VIII, IX, X and antithrombin III. Br J Haematol 1981;48:627-34.

51. Sultan Y, Bussel A, Maisonneuve P, et al. Potential danger of thrombosis after plasma exchange in the treatment of patients with immune disease. Transfusion 1979;19:588-93.

52. Flaum MA, Cuneo RA, Appelbaum FR, et al. The hemostatic imbalance of plasma-exchange transfusion. Blood 1979;54:694-702.

53. Simon TL. Coagulation disorders with plasma exchange. Plasma Ther Transfus Technol 1982; 3:147-52.

54. Domen RE, Kennedy MS, Jones LL, Senhauser DA. Hemostatic imbalances produced by plasma exchange. Transfusion 1984;24:336-9.

55. Couriel D, Weinstein R. Complications of therapeutic plasma exchange: A recent assessment. J Clin Apher 1994;9:1-5.

56. Sanjay R, Flanagan J, Sodano D, et al. The acute phase reactant, fibrinogen, as a guide to plasma exchange therapy for acute Guillain-Barré syndrome. J Clin Apher 2006;21:105-10.

57. Cornelissen JJ, Golterman AFL, Kerckhaert JAM, et al. Fixed IgM reduction in plasma exchange: A standardized method for calculating the volume to be removed per session. Plasma Ther Transfus Technol 1984;5:365-70.

58. Buskard NA, Varghese Z, Wills MR. Correction of hypocalcemic symptoms during plasma exchange. Lancet 1976;2:344-5.

59. Hester JP, McCullough J, Mishler JM, Szymanski IO. Panel IV: Dosage requirements for citrate anticoagulants. J Clin Apher 1983;1:149-57.

60. Hester JP, Ayyar R. Anticoagulation and electrolytes. J Clin Apher 1984;2:41-51.

61. Sutton DM, Nair RC, Rock G, et al. Complications of plasma exchange. Transfusion 1989; 29:124-7.

62. Mokrzycki MH, Kaplan AA. Therapeutic plasma exchange: Complications and management. Am J Kidney Dis 1994;23:817-27.

63. Silberstein LE, Naryshkin S, Haddad JJ, Strauss JF III. Calcium homeostasis during therapeutic plasma exchange. Transfusion 1986;26:151-5.

64. Dau PC. Plasmapheresis therapy in myasthenia gravis. Muscle Nerve 1980;3:468-82.

65. Guillain-Barré Syndrome Study Group. Plasmapheresis and acute Guillain-Barré syndrome. Neurology 1985;35:1096-104.

66. Ropper AH. The Guillain-Barré syndrome. N Engl J Med 1992;326:1130-6.

67. Vriesendorp FJ, Mayer RF, Koski CL. Kinetics of anti-peripheral nerve myelin antibody in patients with Guillain-Barré syndrome treated and not treated with plasmapheresis. Arch Neurol 1991;48:858-61.

68. Rudnicki S, Vriesendorp F, Koski CL, Mayer RF. Electrophysiologic studies in the Guillain-Barré syndrome: Effects of plasma exchange and antibody rebound. Muscle Nerve 1992; 15:57-62.

69. Gibberd FB. Plasma exchange for Refsum's disease. Transfus Sci 1993;14:23-6.

70. Rock GA, Shumak KH, Buskard NA, et al. Comparison of plasma exchange with plasma infusion in the treatment of thrombotic thrombocytopenic purpura. N Engl J Med 1991;325: 393-7.

71. Tsai HM. Von Willebrand factor, ADAMTS13, and thrombotic thrombocytopenic purpura. J Mol Med 2002;80:639-47.

72. Tsai HM, Lian EC. Antibodies to von Willebrand factor-cleaving protease in acute thrombotic thrombocytopenic purpura. N Engl J Med 1998;339:1585-94.

73. Moake JL. Thrombotic thrombocytopenic purpura. Thromb Haemost 1995;74:240-5.

74. Taft EG. Thrombotic thrombocytopenic purpura and dose of plasma exchange. Blood 1979;54:842-9.

75. Dawson RB, Brown JA, Mahalati K, et al. Durable remissions following prolonged plasma exchange in thrombotic thrombocytopenic purpura. J Clin Apher 1994;9:112-15.

76. Derksen RHWM, Schuurman HJ, Gmelig FHJ, et al. Rebound and overshoot after plasma exchange in humans. J Lab Clin Med 1984; 104:35-43.

77. Nasca TJ, Muder RR, Thoman DB, et al. Antibody response to pneumococcal polysaccharide vaccine in myasthenia gravis: Effect of therapeutic plasmapheresis. J Clin Apher 1990;5:133-9.

78. Khatri BO, McQuillen MP, Hoffmann RG, et al. Plasma exchange in chronic progressive multiple sclerosis: A long-term study. Neurology 1991;41:409-11.

79. Clark WF, Dau PC, Euler HH, et al. Plasmapheresis and subsequent pulse cyclophosphamide versus pulse cyclophosphamide alone in severe lupus: Design of the LPSG trial. J Clin Apher 1991;6:40-7.

80. Pestronk A, Lopate G, Kornberg AJ, et al. Distal lower motor neuron syndrome with high-titer serum IgM anti-GM1 antibodies: Improvement following immunotherapy with monthly plasma exchange and intravenous cyclophosphamide. Neurology 1994;44:2027-31.

81. Blume G, Pestronk A, Goodnough LT. Anti-MAG antibody-associated polyneuropathies: Improvement following immunotherapy with monthly plasma exchange and IV cyclophosphamide. Neurology 1995;45:1577-80.

82. Bernvil SS. Proposal for an international controlled randomized multicenter study of plasma exchange followed by pulsed cyclophosphamide versus pulsed cyclophosphamide in treatment of severe Behcet's disease. Transfus Sci 1994;15:149-54.

83. Junghans RP. IgG biosynthesis: No "immunoregulatory feedback." Blood 1997;90:3815-18.

84. Goldammer A, Derfler K, Herkner K, et al. Influence of plasma immunoglobulin level on antibody synthesis. Blood 2002;100:353-5.

85. Dau PC. Increased proliferation of blood mononuclear cells after plasmapheresis treatment of patients with demyelinating disease. J Neuroimmunol 1990;30:15-21.

86. Dau PC. Increased antibody production in peripheral blood mononuclear cells after plasma exchange therapy in multiple sclerosis. J Neuroimmunol 1995;62:197-200.

87. Euler HH, Schroeder JO. Antibody depletion and cytotoxic drug therapy in severe systemic lupus erythematosus. Transfus Sci 1992;13: 167-84.

88. Szczepiorkowski ZM, Bandarenko N, Kim HC, et al. Guidelines on the use of therapeutic apheresis in clinical practice: Evidence-based approach from the Apheresis Applications Committee of the American Society for Apheresis. J Clin Apher 2007;22:106-75.

89. Owen HG, Brecher ME. Atypical reactions associated with the use of angiotensin-convert-

ing enzyme inhibitors and apheresis. Transfusion 1994;34:891-4.

90. Pool M, McLeod B. Pyrogen reactions to human serum albumin during plasma exchange. J Clin Apher 1995;10:81-4.

91. Byrnes JJ, Moake JL, Klug P, Periman P. Effectiveness of the cryosupernatant fraction of plasma in the treatment of refractory thrombotic thrombocytopenic purpura. Am J Hematol 1990;34:169-74.

92. Obrador GT, Zeigler ZR, Shadduck RK, et al. Effectiveness of cryosupernatant therapy in refractory and chronic relapsing thrombotic thrombocytopenic purpura. Am J Hematol 1993;42:217-20.

93. Code of federal regulations. Title 21 CFR Part 640.91. Washington, DC: US Government Printing Office, 2009 (revised annually).

94. Alving BM, Hojima Y, Pisano JJ, et al. Hypotension associated with prekallikrein activator (Hageman-factor fragments) in plasma protein fraction. N Engl J Med 1978;299:66-70.

95. Owen HG, Brecher ME. Partial colloid replacement for therapeutic plasma exchange. J Clin Apher 1997;12:87-92.

96. Brecher ME, Owen HG, Bandarenko N. Alternatives to albumin: Starch replacement for plasma exchange. J Clin Apher 1997;12:146-53.

97. Kapiotis S, Quehenberger P, Eichler HG, et al. Effect of hydroxyethyl starch on the activity of blood coagulation and fibrinolysis in healthy volunteers. Crit Care Med 1994;22:606-12.

98. Vermeulen LC Jr, Ratko TA, Erstad BL, et al. A paradigm for consensus. The University Hospital Consortium guidelines for the use of albumin, nonprotein colloid, and crystalloid solutions. Arch Intern Med 1995;155:373-9.

99. Rock G, Sutton DMC, Freedman J, et al. Pentastarch instead of albumin as replacement fluid for therapeutic plasma exchange. J Clin Apher 1997;12:165-9.

100. Goss GA, Weinstein R. Pentastarch as partial replacement fluid for therapeutic plasma exchange: Effect on plasma proteins, adverse events during treatment, and serum ionized calcium. J Clin Apher 1999;14:114-21.

101. Weinstein R. Prevention of citrate reactions during therapeutic plasma exchange by constant infusion of calcium gluconate with the return fluid. J Clin Apher 1996;11:204-10.

102. Strauss RG, Stansfield C, Henriksen RA, Villhauer PJ. Pentastarch may cause fewer effects on coagulation than hetastarch. Transfusion 1988;28:257-60.

103. Stoll M, Treib J, Schenk JF, et al. No coagulation disorders under high-dose volume therapy with low-molecular-weight hydroxyethyl starch. Haemostasis 1997;27:251-8.

104. Strauss RG, Pennell BJ, Stump DC. A randomized, blinded trial comparing the hemostatic effects of pentastarch versus hetastarch. Transfusion 2002;42:27-36.

In: McLeod BC, Szczepiorkowski ZM, Weinstein R, Winters JL, eds.
Apheresis: Principles and Practice, 3rd edition
Bethesda, MD: AABB Press, 2010

15

Therapeutic Apheresis in Neurologic Disorders

Bruce C. McLeod, MD

 MYASTHENIA GRAVIS WAS ONE of the first diseases to be treated successfully with automated plasma exchange. The technique was tried subsequently with other neurologic disorders in which an immune etiology was known or suspected, and this category of disease soon evolved into an important group of indications for therapeutic plasma exchange (TPE). In the ensuing years, understanding of the etiology of these diseases has advanced. As previously known autoantibodies to structures in the nervous system have been better characterized, and more such antibodies have been identified, the value of TPE has become established in a number of neurologic diseases. The fifth special Clinical Applications issue (2010) of the *Journal of Clinical Apheresis*, prepared by the American Society for Apheresis (ASFA), reviews neurologic indications for apheresis therapy.[1] The format of the clinical applications assessment is described in detail in Chapter 12. The ASFA positions with respect to the use of TPE in neurologic disorders are summarized here in Table 15-1. The following pages describe the pathophysiology of, and treatment options for, neurologic diseases in which TPE has or has been thought to have therapeutic value. The discussion begins with diseases of the peripheral nervous system and moves to those affecting the central nervous system (CNS).

Guillain-Barré Syndrome

Clinical Features

The Guillain-Barré syndrome (GBS) is an acute progressive illness affecting the peripheral ner-

Bruce C. McLeod, MD, Professor of Medicine and Pathology, Rush Medical College, and Director, Blood Center, Rush University Medical Center, Chicago, Illinois

The author has disclosed no conflicts of interest.

Table 15-1. ASFA Indication Categories for Therapeutic Apheresis in Neurologic Disorders[1]

Disease	Procedure	Indication Category
Guillain-Barré syndrome	Plasma exchange	I
Chronic inflammatory demyelinating polyradiculoneuropathy	Plasma exchange	I
Polyneuropathy with IgG/IgA monoclonal protein	Plasma exchange	II
Polyneuropathy with IgM monoclonal protein	Plasma exchange	II
Myasthenia gravis	Plasma exchange	I
Lambert-Eaton myasthenic syndrome	Plasma exchange	II
Stiff-person syndrome	Plasma exchange	IV
Paraneoplastic neurologic syndromes	Plasma exchange	III
Multiple sclerosis	Plasma exchange	III
Neuromyelitis optica (Devic syndrome)	Plasma exchange	II
Refsum disease	Plasma exchange	II
Polymyositis or dermatomyositis	Plasma exchange	IV
	Leukapheresis	IV
Rasmussen encephalitis	Plasma exchange	II
Sydenham chorea	Plasma exchange	I
PANDAS	Plasma exchange	I
Schizophrenia	Plasma exchange	IV
Amyotrophic lateral sclerosis	Plasma exchange	IV

PANDAS = pediatric autoimmune neuropsychiatric disorders associated with streptococcal infections.

vous system. With an annual incidence of 1 to 2 cases per 100,000 population, it is the most common cause of acute areflexic paralysis in the United States and Europe. The typical case begins with symmetrical leg weakness and distal paresthesias. These symptoms worsen and spread as the arms and face become similarly involved. Respiratory and oropharyngeal weakness occur in more severe cases, and there may be dysautonomia with fluctuations in pulse and blood pressure. A minority of patients remain ambulatory, while about one-third need mechanical ventilation at some point. In the worst cases, patients have quadriplegia, ophthalmoplegia, and a marked sensory deficit and

may remain ventilator-dependent for months. Overall mortality is 4% to 15%, and although eventual recovery is the rule in survivors, 15% to 20% have residual disability at 1 year.[2]

It is now recognized that GBS patients are not a homogenous group. Most patients have motor and sensory deficits caused by loss of peripheral nerve myelin (acute inflammatory demyelinating polyradiculoneuropathy, or AIDP). However, in a minority of patients, similar clinical findings are associated with pathologic evidence of axonal damage or degeneration (acute motor sensory axonal neuropathy, or AMSAN). Others have axonal findings limited to motor nerves (acute motor axonal neuropathy, or AMAN). In the Miller Fisher syndrome, ophthalmoplegia and ataxia predominate, and peripheral findings may be limited to asymptomatic areflexia. Finally, in a few patients, signs of autonomic neuropathy such as postural hypotension predominate. These variants are summarized in Table 15-2. Progression is brisk in all types. Most patients are maximally weak by 2 weeks after onset of symptoms; a nadir is reached within 4 weeks in virtually all cases.[3]

While GBS remains largely a clinical diagnosis, certain tests may be helpful. The cerebrospinal fluid usually shows a moderate elevation in protein level without pleocytosis. Electrodiagnostic studies usually demonstrate conduction block caused by myelin loss; however, inexcitable motor nerves may be found in the "axonal" forms described above. The 4-week nadir helps to distinguish GBS from chronic inflammatory demyelinating polyneuropathy (CIDP), which may have similar electrodiagnostic findings.[3]

Pathophysiology

Demyelination, usually with some evidence of associated inflammation, is the pathologic hallmark of GBS. In a minority of cases, axonal change is prominent and may correlate with inexcitability in electrodiagnostic studies. An autoimmune process has long been suspected on the basis of the pathology and the similarity of clinical disease to animal models having an immune etiology. Although a cellular immune component has not been excluded, a growing body of evidence suggests that GBS is the consequence of a misdirected humoral immune response to a preceding infectious illness. As many as 75% of GBS patients give a history of an infectious illness in the weeks preceding the onset of weakness.[4] Links to *Campylobacter jejuni*, cytomegalovirus, Epstein-Barr virus, varicella-zoster virus, Lyme disease, mycoplasma, and human immunodeficiency virus (HIV) have been mentioned in developed countries,[5-7] and numerous other associations have been reported in other parts of the world. Some outbreaks have been linked to particular vaccines, such as that for the 1976 "swine flu."[8] The evidence implicating *C. jejuni* infection is particularly strong, with about 30% of patients having an indication of recent infection. An AMAN syndrome in rural Chinese children occurs in unmistakable epidemics, and more than 90% of those affected have evidence of recent infection with *C. jejuni*.[9] In Western countries, however, there is no apparent association between any specific infectious agent and any particular clinical variant.[10]

It is likely that implicated antibodies are directed against determinants found both on microorganisms and on gangliosides in the outer membrane of Schwann cells and/or axons. The specificity of some antibodies correlates with the clinical syndrome. For example, antibody to ganglioside GQ1b, which is enriched in ocular nerves, can block transmission across their neuromuscular junctions and is found in over 90% of patients with the Miller Fisher variant of GBS, which includes ophthalmoplegia, and in some patients with "classic" GBS that includes ophthalmoplegia. Antibodies to gangliosides GM1, GD1a, and GM1b are prevalent in the axonal forms of GBS.[3,6] An antibody associated with the more typical AIDP has yet to be identified. The antibodies most often associated with GBS and CIDP are listed in Table 15-3.

Other major points supporting an antibody-mediated etiology are the passive transfer of GBS-like disease to experimental animals with

---

Table 15-2. Variants of Guillain-Barré Syndrome

- Acute inflammatory demyelinating polyradiculoneuropathy
- Acute motor sensory axonal neuropathy
- Acute motor axonal neuropathy
- Acute sensory neuropathy
- Miller Fisher syndrome
- Acute panautonomic neuropathy

Table 15-3. Antibodies Associated with Demyelinating Neuropathies

Antigen	Disease
GM1	AMSAN, AMAN, CIDP, PNMP
GM1b	AMSAN, AMAN
GD1a	AMSAN, AMAN
GalNac-GD1a	AMAN
GD1b	ASN
GQ1b	MFS
GT1a	MFS
P0	CIDP
MAG	CIDP, PNMP

MAG = myelin-associated glycoprotein; AMSAN = acute motor sensory axonal neuropathy; AMAN = acute motor axonal neuropathy; CIDP = chronic inflammatory demyelinating polyneuropathy; PNMP = peripheral neuropathy with monoclonal protein; ASN = acute sensory neuropathy; MFS = Miller Fisher syndrome.

patient immunoglobulin preparations[11] and fluctuations in patient antibody levels that correlate with changes in clinical states, including the relationship between the more rapid lowering of titers and the faster pace of improvement in patients undergoing TPE.[8,12]

Therapy

The foregoing might predict a decline in antibody levels as the immune response to an inciting microbe subsides. For whatever reason, spontaneous recovery is the rule in GBS. Thus, a major challenge is to provide the supportive care, up to and including mechanical ventilation, that will allow patients to survive the paralytic phase of the illness. Modern intensive care techniques have surely contributed to improved survival. Rehabilitation techniques are also important for those with prolonged disability and/or permanent neurologic deficits.[3-7]

Corticosteroids were once used empirically, but a trial involving 124 treated patients has shown that pulse steroids as monotherapy are not helpful.[13] TPE was the first treatment modality shown to favorably alter the course of the disease. Open trials were undertaken when an autoimmune etiology was suspected, and when these suggested efficacy, several large randomized controlled trials documented the effectiveness of TPE in shortening recovery time and reducing disability.[14-16]

The North American Guillain-Barré Study Group trial enrolled 245 patients. At 4 weeks after entry, 59% of the treated (TPE) patients had improved by one clinical grade compared with 39% of the control patients; mean improvements at 4 weeks were 1.1 and 0.4 grades, respectively. Treated patients also reached important milestones of recovery significantly earlier. For example, the median times to improve one clinical grade were 19 and 40 days, respectively, and the respective times to reach clinical grade 2 (walk unassisted) were 53 and 85 days. For patients requiring mechanical ventilation, the median times to weaning were 24 days for treated patients and 48 days for control patients, while the times to reach clinical grade 2 were 97 and 169 days, respectively.[14]

The French Cooperative Group trial produced similar results. The median time to onset of recovery was 6 days for treated patients compared with 13 days for control patients, while the times to walk unassisted were 70 and 111 days, respectively. Only 21% of treated patients required mechanical ventilation compared with 43% of control patients, and in the ventilated subgroup, the median times to weaning were 18 and 31 days, respectively.[15] Follow-up at 1 year revealed full recovery of muscle strength in 71% of the TPE group compared with only 52% of the control group.[16] Advantages for patients receiving TPE were reported in other controlled trials in adults[17,18] and in more recent studies in pediatric patients.[19] Furthermore, TPE seems equally effective in sensory and motor GBS variants.[20] GBS was placed in indication Category I by ASFA.[1]

The North American and French trials have provided the models for clinical treatment protocols. In these studies, treated patients underwent TPE with 200 to 250 mL of plasma per kilogram of body weight (approximately 5-6 plasma volumes) over 7 to 14 days, beginning within 14 days after the onset of symptoms.[14,15] An "optimal" schedule has never been defined, but a French study showed that more exchanges (up to six) were better than fewer in patients with mild, moderate, and severe disease.[21]

A typical treatment schedule might be five or six exchanges of 1 to 1.5 plasma volumes carried out every other day over 10 to 12 days. The mounting evidence for an autoantibody could justify more frequent exchanges for more severely affected patients, who may have higher antibody titers, and a longer course of therapy when improvement or stabilization is delayed. Some patients relapse after a favorable response to an initial course of TPE,[22] perhaps because the immune response cross-reacting with peripheral nerve antigens has not yet run its course; such patients will usually respond favorably to another course of treatment. Albumin solutions are the preferred replacement fluid; Fresh Frozen Plasma causes more adverse effects in GBS patients[23] but offers no advantage in terms of therapeutic response.[16] Peripheral venipunctures are preferred over the use of central venous catheters when possible because of a lower incidence of vascular-access-related complications.[24] Treatment teams should be aware that autonomic neuropathy can make GBS patients especially prone to hemodynamic instability during TPE; these patients are more comfortably handled in an intensive care setting.[25] Despite this, however, TPE has been shown to reduce overall nursing care demands for GBS patients.[26]

The use of intravenous immunoglobulin (IVIG) to alter the course of GBS has also been studied. Dutch investigators compared IVIG with TPE in a randomized trial involving 150 patients.[27] The proportion of patients improving at least one grade in 4 weeks was 53% in the IVIG group and 34% in the TPE group, while the median times to improve one grade were

27 and 41 days, respectively, and the median times to walk unassisted were 55 and 69 days, respectively. It was perplexing that the TPE group in this trial did quite poorly compared to similarly treated patients in previous randomized trials. A second randomized comparison in 50 Canadian patients indicated equivalency between the two therapies, with more complications in the TPE group.[28] A subsequent multinational trial compared TPE alone, IVIG alone, and TPE followed by IVIG. With 121 to 130 patients per treatment group, some outcome measures favored sequential TPE/IVIG therapy, but none of the differences were statistically significant.[29] Many centers now regard IVIG as preferable because it is simpler to administer.[30] Cost analyses have differed on whether IVIG is more[31] or less[32] expensive than TPE.

Chronic Inflammatory Demyelinating Polyneuropathy

Clinical Features

CIDP is a persisting acquired neuropathy that may have either a continuously or an intermittently progressive course. Weakness usually predominates over sensory loss, and proximal as well as distal muscles are usually affected; reflexes are depressed. Proximal weakness is an important clinical discriminator from other chronic neuropathies, while progression for more than 2 months serves to differentiate CIDP from GBS.[33] A number of variants have been described in recent years.

Recognition of CIDP is important because it is a treatable condition that accounts for about one-third of initially undiagnosed neuropathies. Several laboratory studies can help to confirm the diagnosis. Electrodiagnostic studies reveal evidence of demyelination with slow conduction, conduction block, and prolonged distal latencies in more than one nerve.[34] In some cases conduction changes are confined to motor nerves (multifocal motor neuropathy, or MMN).[35] Cerebrospinal fluid protein usually exceeds 55 mg/dL, and the cell count is less than 10/μL. Superficial nerve biopsies most often reveal demyelination but may also show axonopathy, both, or neither. Patchy inflammatory cell infiltrates may be seen; these are also often demonstrated in nerve roots in autopsy studies. Suspected cases can be categorized as definite, probable, or possible on the basis of published criteria, but treatment is recommended for all three groups, and observed responses to treatment are similar.[34]

CIDP may occur in isolation or may coexist with one of several associated disorders. Some otherwise typical cases occur in patients with immune disorders such as chronic active hepatitis, inflammatory bowel disease, Hodgkin disease, connective tissue diseases, and HIV infection. Other patients develop a CIDP-like syndrome in the context of a monoclonal gammopathy.[33] The latter are considered separately in the next section.

Pathogenesis

The pathogenesis of CIDP remains uncertain. The pathology, the disease associations, and the similarity to GBS all suggest an immune etiology. Currently much attention is focused on a cellular immune response; however, the association with monoclonal gammopathy has suggested an antibody-mediated process, at least in some cases. Indeed, some monoclonal proteins (MPs) can be shown to react with peripheral nerve tissue. One report described antibodies specific for beta-tubulin, a myelin component, in a patient with CIDP and a monoclonal gammopathy of undetermined significance (MGUS) and in 57% of 70 other CIDP patients, but in only 2% of 483 control patients.[36] Later studies have reported lower prevalence rates.[37] Antibodies to GM1, myelin-associated glycoprotein (MAG), and P0, a peripheral nerve myelin protein, have also been described (Table 15-3).[37-40] A clear cause-and-effect relationship has yet to be documented for any of these antibodies, but the responsiveness of CIDP to TPE provides further suggestive evidence of an immune etiology.

Treatment

It has been known for decades that prednisone and other corticosteroids are effective in CIDP; almost 90% of patients improve within 3 months after initial treatment. Patients who fail to respond or who relapse when prednisone is tapered present more difficult management problems and may be treated with other immunosuppressive agents such as azathioprine, cyclophosphamide, or cyclosporine.[33,34] Children are especially likely to achieve complete and lasting remissions,[41] but MMN responds poorly to corticosteroids and may be exacerbated by their myopathic effects.[35]

Plasma Exchange

Dyck et al[42] reported a sham-controlled trial of TPE in 29 CIDP patients in 1986. After twice-weekly treatment for 3 weeks, the TPE group had significantly better motor function, motor amplitudes, and nerve conduction. Clinical improvement in treated patients far outpaced that in control patients, three of whom later improved markedly when true TPE was administered. Similar findings were reported in a later randomized sham-controlled trial that enrolled 18 patients.[43] TPE has been recommended as initial therapy for CIDP patients who cannot walk and as an alternative therapy for those who cannot be tapered from prednisone and/or do not respond to IVIG. A recommended treatment schedule is three 1-plasma-volume TPEs per week for 2 weeks, followed by two TPEs per week for 4 additional weeks. Five percent albumin with saline is the recommended replacement fluid.[44] ASFA has placed CIDP in indication Category I.[1]

Intravenous Immunoglobulin

Controlled trials have shown that IVIG also confers short-term benefit, approximately equivalent to that of TPE or prednisone, in CIDP.[45-47] Some neurologists consider IVIG simpler to administer[9,30] and would therefore reserve TPE for patients who do not respond to IVIG.[34]

Peripheral Neuropathy with Monoclonal Gammopathy

MPs are detected when single B-lymphocyte clones escape normal control of proliferation and secrete abnormal quantities of immunoglobulin molecules having, perforce, identical structures. This scenario may occur in amyloidosis, Type II cryoglobulinemia, and several well-defined B-cell malignancies such as myeloma and macroglobulinemia. MPs may mediate a variety of adverse effects, most of which are discussed in Chapter 16. In the nervous system they may cause peripheral nerve dysfunction in amyloidosis through infiltration and in cryoglobulinemia through inflammation; these conditions are not considered further in this chapter. In recent decades, increased attention has been paid to the association of peripheral neuropathy with MPs, particularly in patients who have no evidence of hematologic disease. Because some of these patients eventually develop a defined disease, they are said to have an MGUS.[48-50]

MPs are found in about 10% of patients with otherwise unexplained peripheral neuropathy, in 1% to 3% of adults over age 50, and in 3% to 5% of adults over age 70.[48,50,51] Conversely, clinically detectable neuropathy is found in more than 30% of patients with an IgM MP and in 5% to 10% of patients with an IgG or IgA MP.[50,52] Among IgM-MP patients, neuropathy correlates with moderate MP levels (<1.5 g/dL) and high titers of antibody activity against a MAG antigen.[53,54] In MGUS, the 17% of patients with IgM have 59% of the neuropathies, while the 60% of patients with IgG have only 27% of the neuropathies. Thus, IgM is overrepresented and IgG underrepresented in MGUS patients with neuropathy.[49,55] In osteosclerotic myeloma, however, the prevalence of neuropathy is quite high, sometimes as a component of the POEMS syndrome (*p*olyneuropathy, *o*rganomegaly, *e*ndocrinopathy, *m*onoclonal protein, *s*kin changes), even though all the patients have an IgG or IgA MP.[56]

Clinical and Pathologic Features

Peripheral neuropathies associated with MPs are clinically heterogeneous, having both sensory and motor components as well as demyelinating, axonal, or mixed patterns on electrodiagnostic testing. Initial symptoms of IgM-associated MP neuropathy are most often sensory (vs motor in CIDP), whereas progression is slower overall but at a more constant rate and with less likelihood of spontaneous improvement than in CIDP in which motor symptoms predominate at the onset of disease. Nerve biopsies usually show mixed pathology with fiber loss, demyelination, and axonal degeneration. Demyelination tends to predominate in IgM-associated cases, which may also demonstrate IgM and complement deposition in myelin sheaths and abnormally wide myelin spacing.[49,57]

Immunopathogenesis

Antibody activity directed against a number of peripheral nerve antigens has been identified in MPs of patients with neuropathy. About half of patients with IgM MGUS show reactivity with a carbohydrate epitope found on MAG. The same epitope also occurs on myelin glycoprotein P0 and on gangliosides in peripheral nerve cell membranes. Other patients demonstrate antibody to myelin sheath sulfatides and/or to chondroitin sulfate C moieties in neuronal and axonal membranes. A few MPs have antibody activity against GM-1, as mentioned above. These findings are summarized in Table 15-3. Thus, patients with MP and peripheral neuropathy demonstrate antibody activities that could account for either demyelination, axonal damage, or both.[51,54,58]

The prevalence of nerve antibody activities, the binding of IgM and complement to myelin in some cases, and the observation that anti-MAG IgM induces demyelination in animals when injected into nerves could all suggest a causal role for MP. However, anti-nerve activity is lacking in other cases, and MP deposition is not found in all cases where such activity is present. Causality is currently considered likely in IgM-associated cases that exhibit antibody to MAG or other relevant neural antigens or show immunoglobulin or complement deposition in nerve biopsies. In other cases a different immune mechanism may be operative.[57]

Treatment

Patients with B-cell malignances should be treated for these, although the neuropathy does not always improve. Patients with neuropathy and MGUS are often treated with immunosuppressive regimens similar to those used in CIDP.[49,57] In a sham-controlled trial with 39 patients, TPE was shown to be effective in MGUS neuropathy. Disability scores, weakness scores, and summed compound motor action potentials all improved in patients exchanged twice weekly for 3 weeks in the blinded portion of the trial, and these subsequently improved in sham-treated patients who received true TPE in an open continuation.[59] Another study suggested a higher rate of response to TPE in neuropathy associated with MGUS than in idiopathic CIDP (10 of 12 responding vs 11 of 27; $p = 0.02$).[60] Paradoxically, improvement in the sham-controlled studies was more apparent in patients with IgG or IgA MPs than in those with IgM.[59] It has been suggested that this trend, which has also been seen in other studies,[61,62] may be the result of slower mobilization of (larger) IgM molecules bound to nerve tissues, which in turn might necessitate a longer duration of TPE treatment in IgM cases.[63] Neuropathy with an IgG or IgA MP has been placed in indication Category II by ASFA, and neuropathy with an IgM MP has also been placed in Category II.[1] An exception is the POEMS syndrome, in which the neuropathy does not respond to TPE; this has been placed in Category IV.[2]

Myasthenia Gravis

Clinical Features

Myasthenia gravis is characterized clinically by muscular weakness and/or fatigue. Symptoms may be limited to ptosis and diplopia when only ocular muscles are involved; however, most patients have a more generalized disease that affects a variable combination of skeletal muscles. Several subtypes are recognized based on age at onset, antibody status (see below) and the presence or absence of thymoma. Bulbar involvement is the most ominous manifestation; swallowing difficulty can lead to aspiration or inadequate nutrition, and diaphragmatic weakness can lead to respiratory compromise. In the past, myasthenia was often fatal—hence, the adjectival "gravis." Fortunately, with modern therapy the outlook is much improved.[64,65]

Pathophysiology

Pathologic findings in myasthenia are localized to the motor end plate structures on the myocyte side of the neuromuscular junction. The most common morphologic finding is simplification of the normally convoluted junctional folds, which bear receptors for the junctional neurotransmitter, acetylcholine. Some biopsies also reveal inflammatory cell infiltrates surrounding these areas. Immunofluorescence microscopy demonstrates deposition of IgG and complement components.[66,67]

It is well established that damage to motor end plates in most myasthenic patients is mediated by IgG antibodies directed against a portion of the α-subunit of the acetylcholine receptor (AChR; Table 15-4).[68] High-affinity antibodies to this antigen can be demonstrated by various assays in the serum of 80% to 85% of patients with myasthenia. Absolute titers of anti-AChR do not always correlate with disease severity, but titer fluctuations in an individual patient often mirror changes in disease activity.[64,65,67,68] Pathogenic antibodies increase turnover of AChR in a manner that depends on crosslinking of adjacent receptors. They also mediate damage to junctional folds by both complement and inflammatory cell attacks. In addition, AChR antibodies may establish a competitive blockade that limits neurotransmitter access to intact receptors.[64,69] All of these antibody activities can inhibit electrical activation of affected muscle fibers in response to

Table 15-4. Antibodies Associated with Defective Neuromuscular Transmission

Antigen	Disease
Acetylcholine receptor	Myasthenia gravis
VGCC	LEMS
VGKC	Neuromyotonia
GQ1b (in ocular nerve endings)	Miller Fisher syndrome

VGCC = voltage-gated calcium channel; VGKC = voltage-gated potassium channel; LEMS = Lambert-Eaton myasthenic syndrome.

acetylcholine released from nerve endings; they can therefore account for weakness. Fatigability probably arises from exhaustion of the acetylcholine supply at the nerve ending.[64,65,67,69]

About half of patients lacking readily demonstrable AChR antibodies have antibody to an adjacent motor end plate structure, muscle-specific tyrosine kinase (MuSK), and anti-MuSK may well be pathogenic in these patients via an effect on AChR number and distribution.[70] A low-affinity anti-AChR has recently been detected in most of the remaining "seronegative" patients. In addition, some myasthenics, especially among more severely affected patients, exhibit antibodies, which may or may not be pathogenic, to certain proteins in skeletal muscle cytoplasm (titin, ryanodine receptor, rapsyn).[71]

Conventional Treatment

Drugs

Several classes of drugs are useful in myasthenia. Normally the duration of action of acetylcholine released from the nerve ending is limited by enzymatic degradation at the motor end plate. Inhibitors of cholinesterase enzymes will prolong and thereby amplify stimulation by released acetylcholine; oral or parenteral administration of drugs such as pyridostigmine and neostigmine can temporarily enhance patient strength by this mechanism. Immunosuppressive drugs, such as prednisone, azathioprine, cyclosporin, or mycophenolate mofetil, may decrease damage to motor end plates, either by anti-inflammatory effects or by reduction of autoantibody synthesis. Most patients with myasthenia will have a good response to one or a combination of these agents.[64,65,72]

Thymectomy

Malignant thymoma is strongly associated with myasthenia gravis; a gradual improvement in muscle strength is sometimes observed after thymectomy in these patients. This observation led to trials of thymic extirpation in patients without apparent tumor, who may also improve. Complete remission is possible after thymectomy, especially in younger patients, although it is by no means guaranteed.[65,72]

Plasma Exchange

TPE was reported to be beneficial in myasthenia in the 1970s, and the authors of many subsequent observational studies have concurred.[73-78] The lowering of plasma AChR antibody levels after repeated TPE correlates well, in the individual patient, with clinical improvement.[73] TPE can also be effective when assays for high-affinity anti-AChR are negative, suggesting that these assays may not detect all pathogenic antibodies. The efficacy of TPE in myasthenia is widely accepted even though it has never been subjected to a controlled trial, and ASFA has placed it in indication Category I.[1]

Despite this, TPE is not recommended for all patients with myasthenia. Rather, it is reserved for those having more severe disease. Thus, TPE might be a part of initial therapy for patients with impaired respiratory function, inability to swallow, or loss of locomotion. It can also be appropriate in established disease when there is precipitous deterioration (myasthenic crisis) or when response to drugs has stabilized at an unsatisfactory level. In many cases, an immunosuppressive drug such as azathioprine is given simultaneously to inhibit further antibody synthesis. Finally, a brief course of TPE before thymectomy or other surgery may help to optimize muscle function and lower the risk of myasthenic crisis.[64,65,72]

Various treatment schedules have been proposed, depending on the circumstances. For severely affected patients, daily treatments, which may produce faster improvement,[79] may be scheduled initially and then tapered gradually to a treatment schedule that would apply to more chronically affected patients. TPE is usually prescribed in isolated courses that address specific episodes of deterioration, but an occasional patient may benefit from indefinite "maintenance" therapy at 2- to 4-week intervals.[80] The standard treatment in myasthenia gravis is a 1- to 1.5-plasma-volume exchange with 5% albumin and saline replacement.[1] Fresh Frozen Plasma is seldom needed.

Intravenous Immunoglobulin

IVIG has seemed beneficial for myasthenia in some studies.[81] A randomized trial in 87 patients found that three TPEs and 1.2 g/kg IVIG were equally beneficial; paradoxically, both were superior to 2.0 g/kg IVIG.[82] A retrospective multicenter review of 54 treatment episodes compared five TPEs to 2.0 g/kg IVIG and found that TPE led to faster improvement.[83] TPE and IVIG were statistically equivalent in a retrospective comparison of preparatory therapy for thymectomy, although more TPE-treated patients improved (9/9 vs 5/9, respectively).[84] Thus, the relative roles of TPE and IVIG in myasthenia remain uncertain, and both treatments are in common use.

Lambert-Eaton Myasthenic Syndrome

Clinical Features

The Lambert-Eaton myasthenic syndrome (LEMS) is characterized by fatigue, weakness, and sometimes pain in both trunk and extremity musculature, along with signs of dysautonomia, such as dry eyes and dry mouth, and sometimes orthostatic hypotension. In contrast to myasthenia gravis, brain stem symptoms such as diplopia and dysarthria are uncommon. LEMS is a paraneoplastic syndrome in about half of cases, with small-cell carcinoma of the lung being by far the most frequently associated tumor. Most other cases are associated with an immune disorder.[85,86]

Pathophysiology

The symptoms of LEMS patients, like those of myasthenia patients, are caused by impaired signal transmission at the neuromuscular junction. In LEMS, however, the defect is in the nerve endings, where there is subnormal release of acetylcholine in response to arriving stimuli. LEMS is caused by circulating autoantibodies directed against P/Q- and/or N-type voltage-gated calcium channels (VGCCs; Table 15-4). The P/Q-type VGCC is involved in neuromuscular transmission; it is also found in the nerve endings of autonomic neurons. This fits well with the weakness and dysautonomia seen in LEMS. VGCCs are also abundant in small-cell lung cancer tissue.[85-87]

Treatment

Drug treatment is less satisfactory in LEMS than in myasthenia gravis; the efficacy of cholinesterase inhibitors is less impressive, while their side effects seem more frequent. Alternative agents such as 3,4-diaminopyridine have been reported as quite helpful. Prednisone and azathioprine are also used. In LEMS cases associated with malignancy, resection, radiation, or other effective antitumor therapy may lead to gradual remission. Antibody removal by TPE can also cause gradual temporary improvement in LEMS, regardless of the underlying disorder. IVIG has been reported to effect similar temporary improvement.[85-87] LEMS has been placed in indication Category II by ASFA.[1]

Stiff-Person Syndrome

Clinical Features

Stiff-person syndrome (SPS), originally known as stiff-man syndrome, is characterized by progressive rigidity and/or spasms of trunk and proximal limb muscles. Most patients have high titers of circulating antibody to glutamic acid decarboxylase (GAD), which is the rate-limiting enzyme in the synthesis of γ-aminobutyric acid (GABA), the neurotransmitter for the majority of inhibitory CNS synapses.[88,89]

Pathophysiology

SPS has interesting immunologic associations. Pancreatic β-cells are also rich in GAD, and low-titer anti-GAD can be found in some patients with diabetes mellitus. SPS may be found in association with diabetes and with several other autoimmune diseases as well. Because anti-GAD can be found in the cerebrospinal fluid of SPS patients and because their IgG inhibits GAD in animal brain extracts, it is believed to have a pathogenic role, even though neuronal GAD should be a cytoplasmic enzyme, not accessible to antibody. CNS histology is normal in SPS, suggesting that anti-GAD causes functional rather than structural changes.[88,89]

About 5% of SPS cases are associated with cancer, usually breast cancer. Anti-GAD is not found in these cases. Instead, most such patients have antibodies to amphiphysin, a 128-kD presynaptic vesicle protein. In one case associated with an undifferentiated carcinoma, antibody to a postsynaptic protein called gephyrin was identified. Gephyrin is associated with receptors for GABA and for glycine, another inhibitory neurotransmitter.[88,89] The antibodies associated with SPS are included in Table 15-5.

Treatment

Symptoms often respond to diazepam or other agents that increase CNS GABA levels. Immu-

Table 15-5. Antibodies Directed Against Central Nervous System Neurotransmitter/Receptor Complexes

Antigen	Disease
GAD	Stiff-person syndrome
Glu R3	Rasmussen encephalitis
Amphiphysine	Stiff-person syndrome
Gephyrin	Stiff-person syndrome

GAD = glutamic acid decarboxylase; Glu R3 = glutamate R3 receptor.

nomodulatory therapies such as TPE and IVIG have also seemed beneficial in individual cases, but no controlled trials have been performed. In paraneoplastic cases improvement may follow removal of the malignancy.[88,89] ASFA has nevertheless classified SPS as a Category IV indication for TPE.[1]

Other Paraneoplastic CNS Syndromes

Several syndromes involving the CNS may be associated with circulating autoantibodies to CNS structures in patients with underlying malignant disease. Antibody elicited by the tumor and synthesized within the CNS is believed to play a role in mediating the syndromes, which may be evident before the tumor is diagnosed.[90-94] Some antibodies associated with paraneoplastic CNS syndromes are listed in Table 15-6.

Paraneoplastic Encephalomyelitis

Patients with paraneoplastic encephalomyelitis may have symptoms and pathologic findings in

Table 15-6. Antibodies Associated with Central Nervous System Paraneoplastic Syndromes

Antigen	Disease
Amphiphysine	SPS
Gephyrin	SPS
Hu	PEM
ANNA-3	PEM, others
Ma1	PEM, PCD
Ma2	PEM
VGKC	PEM
CRMP5/CV2	PEM, PCD
PCA-2	PEM, PCD
Yo	PCD
Tr	PCD
Zic4	PCD
mGluR1	PCD
Ri	PCD, OMS
Recoverin	CAR
Bipolar retinal cells	MAR

VGKC = voltage-gated potassium channel; SPS = stiff-person syndrome; PEM = paraneoplastic encephalomyelitis; PCD = paraneoplastic cerebellar degeneration; OMS = opsoclonus-myoclonus syndrome; CAR = cancer-associated retinopathy; MAR = melanoma-associated retinopathy.

rian teratoma is associated with antibody to the NR1/NR2 heteromer of the N-methyl-D-aspartate receptor.[90-93]

Paraneoplastic Cerebellar Degeneration

Paraneoplastic cerebellar degeneration is found in association with ovarian and breast cancers as well as with small-cell lung tumors and Hodgkin disease. Clinically, it is characterized by purely cerebellar manifestations such as ataxia, nystagmus, and dysarthria. Many patients have a circulating antibody (anti-Yo) to 34- and 62-kD cytoplasmic antigens in Purkinje cells, but antibodies reacting with the CNS antigens Tr and Zi may also mediate the syndrome.[90-93]

Paraneoplastic Opsoclonus-Myoclonus Syndrome

This disorder is marked by dysrhythmic conjugate eye movements in both vertical and horizontal planes, along with myoclonus. Some cases occur in children with neuroblastoma or in adults with breast, lung, or other tumors. Patients with breast or fallopian tube cancer may have an autoantibody (anti-Ri) that reacts with neuronal nuclei.[90-93]

Cancer-Associated Retinal Degeneration

Antibody to a retinal antigen called recoverin is found in some patients with cancer-associated retinal degeneration. Melanoma-associated retinal degeneration, a similar but more rapidly progressive syndrome, is associated with a different antibody (See Table 15-6).[90-93]

Treatments

Antitumor therapy sometimes produces dramatic remissions, though these are not guaranteed. More often, responses of these syndromes to antineoplastic and/or immunosuppressive treatments are disappointing. Syndromes mediated by antibodies that interfere with neurotransmission, as do those in LEMS and SPS, are the most amenable to therapy. Case reports

one or several CNS regions (eg, limbic, cerebellar, brain stem) and may sometimes have subtle evidence of LEMS as well. The syndrome is most often seen in patients with small-cell lung cancer. It is associated in the majority of cases with an antibody (anti-Hu) directed against a 38- to 40-kD protein found in the nuclei of neurons and of small-cell lung cancer cells. Antibody to antigens, including amphiphysin, Ma2, or CV2/CRMP5, may be found in other cases. Limbic encephalitis in patients with ova-

describing improvement of CNS syndromes after TPE have been published for several paraneoplastic syndromes,[95-98] and trials of immunotherapies, including TPE, are still recommended[90-93]; however, in the compilation by Das et al[99] only 22% of 158 patients treated with TPE, many of whom presumably had LEMS, had any positive response. ASFA has placed these syndromes in indication Category III.[1]

Multiple Sclerosis and Neuromyelitis Optica

Clinical Features

Multiple sclerosis (MS) is a demyelinating disease that involves discrete zones in the central nervous system, resulting in localized neurologic dysfunction. Dysfunction may develop rather quickly, giving the typical clinical picture of an acute attack that resolves, either fully or partially, with time. Prevalence studies show that about 80% of patients have discrete attacks (relapsing-remitting MS), while in about 20% the disease seems gradually and continuously progressive from its onset (primary progressive MS). With time the frequency of attacks may decline and some patients whose illness begins with a relapsing-remitting pattern may transition to a continuously progressive course (secondary progressive MS).[100,101]

Neuromyelitis optica (NMO), also called Devic syndrome, is the diagnosis applied to a group of patients with attacks of CNS demyelination that affect the optic nerves and/or the spinal cord, often severely. Cord lesions are typically extensive in both diameter and length, with transverse myelitis involving three or more vertebral segments, in contrast to the shorter, more circumscribed lesions typical of myelitis in MS. The brain is usually spared in NMO patients, at least initially.[102]

Pathogenesis

Pathologically, MS is characterized by discrete areas or "plaques" of demyelination in white matter. New plaques have an inflammatory appearance with prominent infiltration of T lymphocytes and monocytes, whereas older ones are scarred and show evidence of axon loss. Plaques are well visualized by magnetic resonance imaging (MRI), and the degree of gadolinium enhancement gives an estimate of a lesion's age.[100,101,103]

The etiology of MS remains unknown, but most authorities believe it to be an immune disorder that occurs in genetically susceptible people.[100,101,104] Hypotheses about the pathogenesis of demyelination and neuron loss in MS emphasize cellular immune processes because active lesions are rich in T cells and their cytokines[101] and because experimental allergic encephalomyelitis, the most satisfactory animal model of MS, can be passively transferred with T cells but not with circulating antibody.[105] A possible role for locally secreted antibody is suggested by the finding of oligoclonal immunoglobulin in cerebrospinal fluid and antibodies to various myelin antigens (notably myelin oligodendrocyte glycoprotein) in the serum and/or cerebrospinal fluid of some MS patients.[106] More recent studies have detected immunoglobulin gene rearrangements characteristic of a specific immune response in B cells from MS patients[107] and evidence of immunoglobulin and complement deposition in plaques in some patients.[108] Whether these are primary or secondary changes is not known, however, and absent some prior (ie, primary) insult, it is not clear how circulating antibody could cross the blood-brain barrier. Thus, at present there is little evidence that any circulating antibody contributes to the pathogenesis of MS.[109]

The cause of NMO is also unknown, but it often occurs in the context of a more general autoimmune propensity. Autoantibodies to nuclear antigens, including ENA and SSA, are often detected in the blood of NMO patients, who may meet criteria for other diagnoses such as thyroiditis, systemic lupus erythematosus, or Sjogren syndrome.[110] The lesions of NMO are more intensely inflammatory, with eosinophils and neutrophils among the infiltrating leukocytes. Immunoglobulin, predominantly IgM, and complement are commonly found in a "vasculocentric" pattern that may not extend to areas of ongoing demyelination.[111,112] Recently a circulating IgG antibody to aquaporin-4 (AQP-4), a molecule involved in cell water homeostasis, has been demonstrated by several groups in about 70% of NMO patients. AQP-4 expression is enhanced in renal tubules, cerebellum, and the foot processes of CNS astrocytes. Anti-AQP-4 appears to be a useful diagnostic marker for NMO; in particular it may be useful in distinguishing NMO from MS with ocular and spinal involvement at presentation.[110] However, it has not yet been shown to be pathogenic. The predominance of IgM in NMO lesions and the inability to produce disease in animals with anti-AQP-4 argue against pathogenicity.[112,113]

Treatment

Studies of treatments for MS and NMO are made difficult by natural fluctuations in disease activity, especially the tendencies for acute attacks to subside spontaneously and for attack frequency to decrease with time. The latter can be particularly problematic in patients chosen for studies, whose pretreatment attack frequency is often higher than "average." The natural history of MS is one of progressive disability in most cases. Clinical measurement tools, such as the Disability Status Scale and the Expanded Disability Status Scale, have been devised in an effort to quantify both short- and long-term changes. Although undoubtedly useful, these tools are arithmetically arbitrary and subject to inter-observer inconsistency. MRI may prove to be a more accurate and objective indicator of disease activity and progress, though many lesions identified in this way are never associated with symptoms.[114,115]

Pharmacologic Agents

Corticosteroids and adrenocorticotropic hormone are believed to hasten the resolution of acute MS attacks and are usually prescribed when such an attack is diagnosed. Oral prednisone and intravenous methylprednisolone are the most common choices and are usually given for a total of 5 to 10 days. These agents probably lessen inflammation and edema around new plaques, allowing quicker return of function. It is not clear that these measures, as usually employed, alter the long-term course of the disease or the progressive disability it entails.[100,116]

Immunomodulatory agents are widely used to prevent MS relapses. Interferon beta has been studied in randomized trials involving multiple sites and many hundreds of patients. When given early in the course of disease, it can reduce the frequency of relapses and the extent of MRI changes in the ensuing 2 to 3 years. It is less clear that it prevents progression of long-term disability. Glatiramer acetate, a mixture of synthetic polypeptides rich in the amino acids prevalent in myelin basic protein, has also been extensively studied in randomized trials and can also reduce the relapse rate under these circumstances. Natalizumab, a monoclonal antibody to α-4 integrin, blocks an interaction of vascular endothelial cells with circulating lymphocytes and monocytes, thereby reducing transmigration of the latter into sites of inflammation. It has seemed quite effective in reducing MS disease activity, but its association with a rare and devastating CNS infection has limited its use. Cyclosporine and cytotoxic immunosuppressive drugs such as cyclophosphamide, azathioprine, methotrexate, cladribine, and mitoxantrone have also been tried in MS. Despite concern about their therapeutic:toxic ratios, they continue to be used by neurologists in difficult MS cases. Rituximab has also been tried. All of these measures are aimed at preventing or ameliorating acute attacks. Once the disease progresses to scarring and axonal loss, no therapy is effective.[101,115,116]

Controlled data for treatment of NMO are generally lacking. Attacks are usually treated with high-dose intravenous corticosteroids. The immunomodulatory agents that prevent relapses in MS have seemed ineffective in NMO, leaving immunosuppressive measures as the only approach to relapse prevention. Azathioprine plus oral prednisone is a popular regimen, and rituximab has been tried.[102]

Plasma Exchange

TPE was investigated in MS patients in the 1980s on the basis of the unconfirmed suspicion that circulating antibody or mediators might play a role in the disease. Several uncontrolled reports described encouraging results.[117-119] In controlled studies, however, it has been difficult to discover an important advantage, even with intensive TPE regimens.[120,121] For example, among 20 chronic progressive MS patients treated with azathioprine for 1 year, the 10 who also received TPE did no better than the controls.[121] A double-blind, randomized, sham-controlled study of 54 stable patients with chronic progressive MS was reported to show significant benefit for the group receiving TPE in addition to prednisone and cyclophosphamide.[122] This study has been questioned, however, because of statistical anomalies and because five of the 26 patients in the TPE group improved by three or more points on the Disability Status Scale rating, an extremely unusual occurrence in chronic progressive patients that has not been reproduced in other studies.[123,124] It is speculated that some of these may have been misclassified patients who were recovering from acute attacks.[125] No benefit was found for chronic progressive patients in two later sham-controlled studies.[126,127] In one of these, the authors commented on a trend toward faster recovery from acute attacks in the 39 (of 76) patients with relapsing-remitting disease who received TPE in addition to adrenocorticotropic hormone and cyclophosphamide.[126] However, this trend reached marginal significance (p = 0.04) only at the second of eight scheduled observations (at 1 month after treatment). Because adjustments for multiple outcomes measurement were not made in the statistical analysis, the clinical significance of this observation is questionable.[115,123,125,128] No such trend was seen in the other sham-controlled trial, which enrolled 168 patients.[127] No controlled trials of TPE in NMO have been published.

Given the expense and morbidity associated with TPE and the modest level of benefits seen in the most enthusiastic trials, TPE is not recommended for progressive MS,[115,129] although a meta-analysis published in 1995 suggested that it might yet be found useful in certain subgroups of MS patients.[130] ASFA has placed MS in indication Category III.[1]

Despite the generally negative experience with TPE in controlled trials, many authors of review articles now recommend TPE for unusually severe attacks of MS and NMO that do not improve with high-dose corticosteroid treatment in the expected timeframe.[100,102,106,107,109,110,115,129,131-135] All these authors base their recommendations on the conclusions of a single study published in 1999.[136] It is therefore worthwhile to consider this study in some detail. It was a sham-controlled crossover trial that enrolled only 22 patients with acute severe cases of "idiopathic inflammatory demyelinating disease" (IIDD) of the CNS. As proposed then by the authors, the concept of IIDD included MS as well as NMO and several other illnesses that were then, and are currently, distinguished from MS by most neurologists. Twelve patients in the trial had MS, four had NMO and six had other diagnoses. The primary analysis was a qualitative assessment (meaningful improvement or not, as judged by two blinded neurologists). This revealed a statistically significant advantage for TPE over sham (p = 0.011 and p = 0.032, respectively, for the two neurologists). Secondary analyses included three more quantitative assessments. One (power score) showed a significant advantage for TPE (p = 0.027); the other two did not (p = 0.066 for Expanded Disability Status Scale; p = 0.252 for gait). There is no separate analysis of the MS subgroup.

A major problem with this study, apart from the lack of a documented pathogenic antibody in any of the patients studied, was the inclusion of patients with multiple diagnoses, which risked meaningless comparisons of "apples and oranges". Having subsequently been instrumental in the discovery of anti-AQP-4 in NMO patients, some of the same investigators have recently been at pains to insist that NMO be "recognized as [a] … disease that is distinct from MS"[131] and that it is important to preserve "the validity of therapeutic trials for MS by not enrolling patients with NMO."[110] When the latter caveat is applied to the 1999 study, it is apparent that the inclusion of patients with multiple diagnoses in a single analysis of efficacy was not justifiable and that the study was underpowered to draw conclusions about MS, NMO, or any other illness separately. The need for confirmatory studies was acknowledged by the authors,[100,136] but these have not been forthcoming. Absent such confirmation, in the opinion of this author, conclusions of this flawed study, along with all therapeutic recommendations subsequently based on them, should be regarded as invalid. Nevertheless, largely on the basis of this report, ASFA has placed NMO in indication Category II.[1]

Other Neurologic Syndromes

Refsum Disease

Refsum disease results from a genetic deficiency of the enzyme phytanoyl-CoA hydroxylase that initiates metabolism of phytanic acid, a fatty acid acquired mainly through ingestion of ruminant fats.[137] Accumulation of phytanic acid can cause a number of neurologic manifestations. These can be partially reversed or prevented by a regimen of TPE and dietary restriction,[138] even in mature adults.[139] Cascade filtration has also been reported effective.[140] Refsum disease was placed in indication Category II by ASFA.[1]

Polymyositis and Dermatomyositis

These are inflammatory diseases involving skeletal muscle. An autoimmune etiology has been suspected, and steroids or other immunosuppressive drugs are often helpful, but an autoantibody to muscle has never been unequivocally implicated in pathogenesis.[141] Nevertheless, TPE was tried, and initial anecdotal reports were favorable.[142-144] In 1992, however, published results of a blinded, sham-controlled trial in 39 patients with chronic disease revealed that neither 12 TPEs nor 12 therapeutic leukapheresis procedures offered any advantage over sham

apheresis.[145] TPE for both polymyositis and dermatomyositis has been placed in indication Category IV for both TPE and therapeutic leukapheresis by ASFA.[1]

Rasmussen Encephalitis

Rasmussen encephalitis is a rare, acquired disorder beginning in childhood. Frequent seizures are a prominent feature, but in contrast to idiopathic epilepsy, these are accompanied by progressive neurologic deficits such as hemiparesis and dementia. Brain histopathology shows inflammation and atrophy.[146] One group reported that three of four patients tested had autoantibodies to the Glu R3 receptor for the CNS neurotransmitter glutamate (Table 15-5).[147] Another study suggested the antibody might arise as a response to a cross-reactive microbial antigen.[148] Both TPE[147,149] and IVIG[150] have been reported to reduce seizure frequency and improve neurologic function in some patients. In subsequent studies, however, antibodies to Glu R3 were found in some patients with other types of localized epilepsy and not found in many patients with Rasmussen encephalitis.[146,151] In addition, autoantibodies to other synaptic structures have been reported in Rasmussen patients.[152] Thus both the specificity and clinical significance of Glu R3 antibodies are uncertain at present. Immunotherapy, including TPE, is nevertheless still recommended for some patients who are not candidates for surgery.[146] ASFA has placed Rasmussen encephalitis in indication Category II.[1]

Sydenham Chorea and PANDAS

Sydenham chorea is a movement disorder that develops in some children after a group A streptococcal infection. Many children with chorea also have clinical manifestations of obsessive compulsive disorder (OCD). Other children with OCD, tics, and neurologic symptoms other than chorea also have evidence of recent group A streptococcal infection. The term *p*ediatric *a*utoimmune *n*europsychiatric *d*isorders *a*ssociated with *s*treptococcal infection (PANDAS) has been coined to describe such children. Some evidence suggests that a streptococcal antibody cross-reactive with neurons in the basal ganglia causes the symptoms in these patients.[153] Controlled trials have shown that both TPE and IVIG can be beneficial in these illnesses.[154,155] By contrast, TPE was of no benefit in OCD patients who lacked evidence of streptococcal infection.[156] ASFA has placed Sydenham chorea and PANDAS in indication Category I.[1]

Neuromyotonia, Morvan Syndrome, and Limbic Encephalitis

Neuromyotonia, also called Isaac syndrome, is a rare acquired disorder whose manifestations include myokymia, muscle cramps, weakness, and hyperhidrosis; a minority of cases are paraneoplastic.[157] Several recent reports indicate that it may be caused by antibody to the voltage-gated potassium channel (VGKC) in presynaptic nerve endings (Table 15-4) and that it responds to TPE.[72,158-160] Morvan syndrome, a related entity that also includes encephalopathy, and some cases of limbic encephalitis have also been associated with anti-VGKC and have also been reported to respond to TPE.[161-163] None of these illnesses has been assigned an indication category by ASFA.

Miscellaneous

Controlled trials have shown that TPE is ineffective in amyotrophic lateral sclerosis[164-166] and schizophrenia,[167] both of which were placed in indication Category IV by ASFA.[1]

Summary

Autoantibodies to a variety of structures in the nervous system have been characterized. Pathogenicity has not always been easily proven, but evidence that autoantibodies can cause disease is quite strong for some illnesses and is accumulating for others, though not for all. The evidence may include studies that show clinical benefit from TPE. Taken together, immunologic and clinical studies have estab-

lished a clear role for TPE in the management of many of the diseases discussed in this chapter. As a result, use of TPE for neurologic illnesses may constitute a major fraction of the procedures in a therapeutic apheresis facility. The patients' immobility and/or hemodynamic lability may pose special challenges in treatment; however, with due care and attention to proper procedure, patients can derive considerable benefit from TPE, without excessive risk.

References

1. Szczepiorkowski ZM, Winters JL, Bandarenko N, et al. Guidelines on the use of therapeutic apheresis in clinical practice—evidence-based approach from the Apheresis Applications Committee of the American Society for Apheresis. The Fifth Special Issue. J Clin Apher 2010 (in press).
2. Shaz BH, Linenberger ML, Banderenko N, et al. Category IV indications for therapeutic apheresis: ASFA fourth special issue. J Clin Apher 2007;22:176-80.
3. Hughes RAC, Cornblath DR. Guillain-Barré syndrome. Lancet 2005;366:1653-66.
4. Winer JB. Guillain-Barré syndrome. Mol Pathol 2001;54:381-5.
5. Ropper AH. The Guillain-Barré syndrome. N Engl J Med 1992;326:1130-6.
6. Kissel JT, Cornblath DR, Mendell JR. Guillain-Barré syndrome. In: Mendell JR, Kissel JT, Cornblath DR, eds. Diagnosis and management of peripheral nerve disorders. New York: Oxford University Press, 2001:145-72.
7. Pascuzzi RM, Fleck JD. Guillain-Barré syndrome and related disorders. Neurol Clin 1997;15:529-47.
8. Koski CL, Gratz E, Sutherland J, et al. Clinical correlation with anti-peripheral myelin antibodies in Guillain-Barré syndrome. Ann Neurol 1986;19:573-7.
9. McKhann GM, Cornblath DR, Griffen JW, et al. Acute motor axonal neuropathy: A frequent cause of flaccid paralysis in China. Ann Neurol 1993:33:333-42.
10. Hadden RDM, Karch H, Hartung H-P, et al. Preceding infections, immune factors, and outcome in Guillain-Barré syndrome. Neurology 2001;56:758-65.

11. McFarlin DE. Immunological parameters in Guillain-Barré syndrome. Ann Neurol 1990; 27(Suppl 1):525-9.

12. Vriesendorp FJ, Mayer RF, Koski CL. Kinetics of anti-peripheral nerve myelin antibody in patients with Guillain-Barré syndrome treated and not treated with plasmapheresis. Arch Neurol 1991;48:858-61.

13. Guillain-Barré Syndrome Steroid Trial Group. Double-blind trial of intravenous methylprednisone in Guillain-Barré syndrome. Lancet 1993;341:586-90.

14. Guillain-Barré Syndrome Study Group. Plasmapheresis and acute Guillain-Barré syndrome. Neurology 1985;35:1096-104.

15. French Cooperative Group on Plasma Exchange in Guillain-Barré Syndrome. Efficiency of plasma exchange in Guillain-Barré syndrome: Role of replacement fluids. Ann Neurol 1987;22:753-61.

16. French Cooperative Group on Plasma Exchange in Guillain-Barré Syndrome. Plasma exchange in Guillain-Barré syndrome: One-year follow-up. Ann Neurol 1992;32:94-7.

17. Osterman PG, Lundemo G, Pirskanen R, et al. Beneficial effects of plasma exchange in acute inflammatory polyradiculoneuropathy. Lancet 1984;2:1296-9.

18. Greenwood RJ, Newsom-Davis J, Hughes RA, et al. Controlled trial of plasma exchange in acute inflammatory polyradiculoneuropathy. Lancet 1984;1:877-9.

19. Jansen PW, Perkin RM, Ashwal S. The Guillain-Barré syndrome in childhood: Natural course and efficacy of plasmapheresis. Pediatr Neurol 1993;9:16-20.

20. Hadden RDM, Cornblath DR, Hughes RAC, et al. Electrophysiological classification of Guillain-Barré syndrome: Clinical associations and outcome. Ann Neurol 1998;44:780-8.

21. French Cooperative Group on Plasma Exchange in Guillain-Barré Syndrome. Appropriate number of plasma exchanges in Guillain-Barré syndrome. Ann Neurol 1997;41:298-306.

22. Rudnicki S, Vriesendorp F, Koski CL, Mayer RF. Electrophysiologic studies in the Guillain-Barré syndrome: Effects of plasma exchange and antibody rebound. Muscle Nerve 1992;15:57-62.

23. Bouget J, Chevret S, Chastang C, et al. Plasma exchange in Guillain-Barré syndrome: Results from the French prospective, double-blind, randomized, multicenter study. Crit Care Med 1993;21:651-8.

24. Grishaber JE, Cunningham MC, Rohret PA, Strauss RG. Analysis of venous access for therapeutic plasma exchange in patients with neurological disease. J Clin Apher 1992;7:119-23.

25. McLeod BC. The technique of therapeutic apheresis. J Crit Illn 1991;6:487-95.

26. Farkkila M, Penttila P. Plasma exchange therapy reduces the nursing care needed in Guillain-Barré syndrome. J Adv Nurs 1992;17:672-5.

27. van der Meché FGA, Schmitz PIM, and the Dutch Guillain-Barré Study Group. A randomized trial comparing intravenous immune globulin and plasma exchange in Guillain-Barré syndrome. N Engl J Med 1992;326:1123-9.

28. Bril V, Ilse WK, Pearce R, et al. Pilot trial of immunoglobulin versus plasma exchange in patients with Guillain-Barré syndrome. Neurology 1996;46:100-3.

29. Plasma Exchange/Sandoglobulin Guillain-Barré Syndrome Trial Group. Randomised trial of plasma exchange, intravenous immunoglobulin, and combined treatments in Guillain-Barré syndrome. Lancet 1997;349:225-30.

30. Hughes RAC. Systematic reviews of treatment for inflammatory demyelinating neuropathy. J Anat 2002;200:331-9.

31. Nagpal S, Benstead T, Shumak K, et al. Treatment of Guillain-Barré syndrome: A cost-effectiveness analysis. J Clin Apher 1999;14:107-13.

32. Tsai C-P, Wang K-C, Lin C-Y, et al. Pharmacoeconomics of therapy for Guillain-Barré syndrome: Plasma exchange and intravenous immunoglobulin. J Clin Neuroscience 2007; 14:635-9.

33. Köller H, Kieseier BC, Jander S, Hartung H-P. Chronic inflammatory demyelinating polyneuropathy. N Engl J Med 2005;352:1343-56.

34. Hughes RAC, Bouche P, Cornblath DR, et al. European Federation of Neurological Societies/Peripheral Nerve Society guidelines on management of chronic inflammatory demyelinating polyradiculoneuropathy: Report of a joint task force of the European Federation of Neurological Societies and the Peripheral Nerve Society. Eur J Neurol 2006;13:326-32.

35. Nobile-Orazio E. Multifocal motor neuropathy. J Neuroimmunol 2001;115:4-18.

36. Connolly AM, Pestronk A, Trotter JL, et al. High-titer selective anti-beta-tubulin antibod-

ies in chronic demyelinating polyneuropathy. Neurology 1993;43:557-62.

37. Hughes RAC, Allen D, Makowska A, Gregson N. Pathogenesis of chronic inflammatory demyelinating polyneuropathy. J Peripher Nerv Syst 2006;11:30-46.

38. Simone IL, Annunziata P, Maimone D, et al. Serum and CSF anti-GM1 antibodies in patients with Guillain-Barré syndrome and chronic inflammatory demyelinating polyneuropathy. J Neurol Sci 1993;114:49-55.

39. Khalili-Shirazi A, Atkinson P, Gregson N, Hughes RAC. Antibody response to P_0 and P_2 myelin proteins in Guillain-Barré syndrome and chronic inflammatory demyelinating polyradiculoneuropathy. J Neuroimmunol 1993;46: 245-52.

40. Allen D, Giannopoulos K, Gray I, et al. Antibodies to peripheral nerve myelin proteins in chronic inflammatory demyelinating polyradiculoneuropathy. J Peripher Nerv Syst 2005;10: 174-80.

41. Connolly AM. Chronic inflammatory demyelinating polyneuropathy in childhood. Ped Neurol 2001;24:177-82.

42. Dyck PJ, Daube J, O'Brien P, et al. Plasma exchange in chronic inflammatory demyelinating polyradiculoneuropathy. N Engl J Med 1986;314:461-5.

43. Hahn AF, Bolton CF, Pillay C, et al. Plasma-exchange therapy in chronic inflammatory demyelinating polyneuropathy. Brain 1996; 119:1055-66.

44. Mendell JR. Chronic inflammatory demyelinating polyradiculopathy. Annu Rev Med 1993;44:211-9.

45. Dyck PJ, Litchy WJ, Kratz KM, et al. A plasma exchange versus immune globulin infusion trial in chronic inflammatory demyelinating polyradiculoneuropathy. Ann Neurol 1994;36: 838-45.

46. Hahn AF, Bolton CF, Zochodne D, Feasby TE. Intravenous immunoglobulin treatment (IVIG) in chronic inflammatory demyelinating polyneuropathy (CIDP): A double-blind placebo-controlled cross-over study. Brain 1996;119: 1067-78.

47. Hughes RAC, Bensa S, Willison HJ, et al. Randomized controlled trial of intravenous immunoglobulin versus oral prednisolone in chronic inflammatory demyelinating polyradiculoneuropathy. Ann Neurol 2001;50:195-201.

48. Kyle RA. Monoclonal proteins in neuropathy. Neurol Clin 1992;10:713-34.

49. Bosch EP, Smith BE. Peripheral neuropathies associated with monoclonal proteins. Med Clin North Am 1993;77:125-39.

50. Kissel JT, Mendell JR. Neuropathies associated with monoclonal gammopathies. In: Mendell JR, Kissel JT, Cornblath DR, eds. Diagnosis and management of peripheral nerve disorders. New York: Oxford University Press, 2001:272-96.

51. Kyle RA, Rajkumar SV. Epidemiology of the plasma cell disorders. Best Pract Res Clin Haematol 2007;20:637-64.

52. Nobile-Orazio E, Barbieri S, Baldini L, et al. Peripheral neuropathy in monoclonal gammopathy of undetermined significance: Prevalence and immunopathogenetic studies. Acta Neurol Scand 1992;85:383-90.

53. Baldini L, Nobile-Orazio E, Guffanti A, et al. Peripheral neuropathy in IgM monoclonal gammopathy and Waldenström's macroglobulinemia: A frequent complication in elderly males with low MAG-reactive serum monoclonal component. Am J Hematol 1994; 45:25-31.

54. Nobile-Orazo E. IgM paraproteinemic neuropathies. Curr Opin Neurol 2004;17:599-605.

55. Latov N. Evaluation and treatment of patients with neuropathy and monoclonal gammopathy. Semin Neurol 1994;14:118-22.

56. Miralles GD, O'Fallon JR, Talley NJ. Plasma-cell dyscrasia with polyneuropathy: The spectrum of POEMS syndrome. N Engl J Med 1992; 327:1919-23.

57. Hadden RDM, Nobile-Orazo E, Sommer C, et al. European Federation of Neurological Societies/Peripheral Nerve Society guidelines on management of paraproteinemic demyelinating neuropathies: Report of a joint task force of the European Federation of Neurological Societies and the Peripheral Nerve Society. Eur J Neurol 2006;13:809-18.

58. Gabriel JM, Erne B, Miescher GC, et al. Expression patterns of human PNS myelin proteins in neuropathies associated with anti-myelin antibodies. Schweiz Arch Neurol Psychiatr 1994; 145:22-3.

59. Dyck PJ, Low PA, Windebank AJ, et al. Plasma exchange in polyneuropathy associated with monoclonal gammopathy of undetermined significance. N Engl J Med 1991;325:1482-6.

60. Gorson KC, Gregory A, Ropper AH. Chronic inflammatory demyelinating polyneuropathy: Clinical features and response to treatment in 67 consecutive patients with and without a

monoclonal gammopathy. Neurology 1997;48:
321-8.

61. Oksenhendler E, Chevret S, Leger JM, et al.
    Plasma exchange and chlorambucil in poly-
    neuropathy associated with monoclonal IgM
    gammopathy. J Neurol Neurosurg Psychiatry
    1995;59:243-7.

62. Bleasel AF, Hawke SH, Pollard JD, McLeod JG.
    IgG monoclonal paraproteinemia and periph-
    eral neuropathy. J Neurol Neurosurg Psychiatry
    1993;56:52-7.

63. Toyka KV, Hartung HP, Steck A. Plasma-
    pheresis in chronic demyelinating polyneurop-
    athy (letter). N Engl J Med 1992;326:1090-1.

64. Richman DP, Agius MA. Treatment of autoim-
    mune myasthenia gravis. Neurology 2003;61:
    1652-61.

65. Romi F, Gilhus NE, Aarli JA. Myasthenia
    gravis: Clinical, immunological and therapeutic
    advances. Acta Neurol Scand 2005;111:134-
    41.

66. Maselli RA, Pathophysiology of myasthenia
    gravis and Lambert-Eaton syndrome. Neurol
    Clin 1994;12:285-303.

67. Vincent A. Unravelling the pathogenesis of
    myasthenia gravis. Nat Rev Immunol 2002;2:
    797-804.

68. Lindstrom JM, Seybold ME, Lennon VA, et al.
    Antibody to acetylcholine receptor in myasthe-
    nia gravis. Neurology 1976;26:1054-9.

69. Richman DP, Wollman RL, Maselli RA, et al.
    Effector mechanisms of myasthenic antibodies.
    Ann N Y Acad Sci 1993;681:264-73.

70. Vincent A, Leite MI. Neuromuscular junction
    autoimmune disease: Muscle specific kinase
    antibodies and treatments for myasthenia
    gravis. Curr Opin Neurol 2005;18:519-25.

71. Lindstrom J. "Seronegative" myasthenia gravis
    is no longer seronegative. Brain 2008;131:
    1684-5.

72. Skeie GO, Apostolski S, Evoli A, et al. Guide-
    lines for the treatment of autoimmune neuro-
    muscular transmission disorders. Eur J Neurol
    2006;13:691-9.

73. Seybold ME. Plasmapheresis in myasthenia
    gravis. Ann N Y Acad Sci 1987;505:584-7.

74. Dau PC, Lindstrom JM, Cassel CK, et al. Plas-
    mapheresis and immunosuppressive drug ther-
    apy in myasthenia gravis. N Engl J Med 1977;
    297:1134-40.

75. Dau PC. Plasmapheresis therapy in myasthenia
    gravis. Muscle Nerve 1980;3:468-82.

76. Pollard JD, Basten A, Hassall JE, et al. Current
    trends in the management of myasthenia

gravis: Plasmapheresis and immunosuppressive
therapy. Aust N Z J Med 1989;10:212-17.

77. d'Empaire G, Hoaglin DC, Perlo VP, Pontoppi-
    dan H. Effect of pre-thymectomy plasma
    exchange on postoperative respiratory function
    in myasthenia gravis. J Thorac Cardiovasc Surg
    1985;89:592-6.

78. Mahalati K, Dawson RB, Collins JO, Mayer RF.
    Predictable recovery from myasthenia gravis
    crisis with plasma exchange: Thirty-six cases
    and review of current management. J Clin
    Apher 1999;14:1-8.

79. Yeh J-H, Chiu H-C. Plasmapheresis in myasthe-
    nia gravis. A comparative study of daily versus
    alternately daily schedule. Acta Neurol Scand
    1999;99:147-51.

80. Rodnitzy RL, Bosch EP. Chronic long-interval
    plasma exchange in myasthenia gravis. Arch
    Neurol 1984;41:715-17.

81. Gajdos P. Intravenous immune globulin in
    myasthenia gravis. Clin Exp Immunol 1994;97
    (Suppl 1):49-51.

82. Gajdos P, Chevret S, Clair B, et al for the Mya-
    sthenia Gravis Clinical Study Group. Clinical
    trial of plasma exchange and high-dose intrave-
    nous immunoglobulin in myasthenia gravis.
    Ann Neurol 1997;41:789-96.

83. Qureshi AI, Choudhry MA, Akbar MS, et al.
    Plasma exchange versus intravenous immuno-
    globulin treatment in myasthenic crisis. Neurol-
    ogy 1999;52:629-52.

84. Jensen P, Bril V. A comparison of the effective-
    ness of intravenous immunoglobulin and
    plasma exchange as preoperative therapy of
    myasthenia gravis. J Clin Neuromusc Dis
    2008;9:352-5.

85. Saunders DB. Lambert-Eaton myasthenic syn-
    drome, diagnosis and treatment. Ann N Y Acad
    Sci 2003;998:500-8.

86. Mahadeva B. Autoimmune disorders of neuro-
    muscular transmission. Semin Neurol 2008;
    28:212-27.

87. Newsom-Davis J. Therapy in myasthenia gravis
    and Lambert-Eaton myasthenic syndrome.
    Semin Neurol 2003;23:191-8.

88. Murinson BB. Stiff-person syndrome. Neurolo-
    gist 2004;10:131-7.

89. Espay AJ, Chen R. Rigidity and spasms for
    autoimmune encephalopathies: Stiff-person
    syndrome. Muscle Nerve 2006;34:677-90.

90. Darnell RB, Posner JB. Paraneoplastic syn-
    dromes involving the nervous system. N Engl J
    Med 2003;349:1543-54.

91. Bataller L, Dalmau JO. Paraneoplastic disorders of the central nervous system: Update on diagnostic criteria and treatments. Semin Neurol 2004;24:461-71.

92. Graus F, Dalmau J. Paraneoplastic neurological syndromes: Diagnosis and treatment. Curr Opin Neurol 2007;20:732-7.

93. Toothaker TB, Rubin M. Paraneoplastic neurological syndromes. Neurologist 2009;15:21-33.

94. Stich O, Jarius S, Kleer B, et al. Specific antibody index in cerebrospinal fluid from patients with central and peripheral paraneoplastic syndromes. J Neuroimmunol 2007;183:220-4.

95. Moll JWB, Vecht CJ. Immune diagnoses of paraneoplastic neurological disease. Clin Neurol Neurosurg 1995;97:71-81.

96. Graus F, Vega F, Delattre JY. Plasmapheresis and antineoplastic treatment in CNS paraneoplastic syndromes with antineuronal autoantibodies. Neurology 1992;42:536-40.

97. David YB, Warner E, Levitan M, et al. Autoimmune paraneoplastic cerebellar degeneration in ovarian carcinoma patients treated with plasmapheresis and immunoglobulin. Cancer 1996;78:2153-6.

98. Murphy MA, Thirkill CE, Hart WM Jr. Paraneoplastic retinopathy: A novel autoantibody reaction associated with small-cell lung carcinoma. J Neurophthalmol 1997;17:77-83.

99. Das A, Hochberg FH, McNelis S. A review of the therapy of paraneoplastic neurologic syndromes. J Neurooncol 1999;41:181-94.

100. Noseworthy JH, Lucchinetti C, Rodriguez M, Weinshenker BG. Multiple sclerosis. N Engl J Med 2000;343:938-52.

101. Compston A, Coles A. Multiple sclerosis. Lancet 2002;359:1221-31

102. Wingerchuk DM. Diagnosis and treatment of neuromyelitis optica. Neurologist 2007;13:2-11.

103. Frohman EM, Racke MK, Raine CS. Multiple sclerosis—the plaque and its pathogenesis. N Engl J Med 2006;354:942-55.

104. Dhib-Jalbut S. Pathogenesis of myelin/oligodendrocyte damage in multiple sclerosis. Neurology 2007;66(Suppl 3):S13-21.

105. Gold R, Linington C, Lassman H. Understanding pathogenesis and therapy of multiple sclerosis via animal models: 70 years of merits and culprits in experimental autoimmune encephalomyelitis research. Brain 2006;129:1953-71.

106. Archelos JJ, Storch MK, Hartung H-P. Neurological progress: The role of B cells and autoantibodies in multiple sclerosis. Ann Neurol 2000;47:694-706.

107. Cross AH. MS: The return of the B cell. Neurology 2000;54:1214-5.

108. Lucchinetti C, Bruck W, Paris J, et al. Heterogeneity of multiple sclerosis lesions: Implications for the pathogenesis of demyelination. Ann Neurol 2000;47:707-17.

109. Wiendl H, Toyka KV, Rieckmann P, et al. Basic and escalating immunomodulatory treatments in multiple sclerosis: Current therapeutic recommendations. J Neurol 2008;255:1449-63

110. Wingerchuk D, Lennon VA, Lucchinetti CF, et al. The spectrum of neuromyelitis optica. Lancet Neurol 2007;6:805-15.

111. Lucchinetti CF, Mandler RN, McGavern D, et al. A role for humoral mechanisms in the pathogenesis of Devic's neuromyelitis optica. Brain 2002;125:1450-61.

112. Galetta SL, Bennett J. Neuromyelitis optica is a variant of multiple sclerosis. Arch Neurol 2007;64:901-3.

113. Frohman EM, Kerr D. Is neuromyelitis optica distinct from multiple sclerosis? Arch Neurol 2007;64:903-5.

114. Noseworthy JH, Ebers GC, Vandervoort MK, et al. The impact of blinding on the results of a randomized, placebo-controlled multiple sclerosis clinical trial. Neurology 1994;44:16-20.

115. Goodin DS, Frohman EM, Garmany GP Jr, et al. Disease modifying therapies in multiple sclerosis. Report of the therapeutics and technology assessment subcommittee of the American Academy of Neurology and the MS Council for Clinical Practice Guidelines. Neurology 2002;58:169-78.

116. Sellebjerg F, Barnes D, Filippini G, et al. EFNS guideline on multiple sclerosis relapses: Report of an EFNS task force on treatment of multiple sclerosis relapses. Eur J Neurol 2005;12:939-46.

117. Dau PC, Petajan JM, Johnson KP, et al. Plasmapheresis and immunosuppressive drug therapy in multiple sclerosis. Neurology 1980;30:1023-8.

118. Weiner HL, Dawson DM. Plasmapheresis in multiple sclerosis: Preliminary study. Neurology 1980;30:1029-33.

119. Khatri BO, McQuillen MP, Hoffman RG, et al. Plasma exchange in chronic progressive multiple sclerosis: A long term study. Neurology 1991;41:409-14.

120. Hauser SL, Dawson DM, Lehrich JR, et al. Intensive immunosuppression in progressive

multiple sclerosis: A randomized three-arm study of high dose intravenous cyclophosphamide, plasma exchange, and ACTH. N Engl J Med 1983;308:173-80.

121. Tindall RSA, Walker JE, Ehle AL, et al. Plasmapheresis in multiple sclerosis: Prospective trial of pheresis and immunosuppression versus immunosuppression alone. Neurology 1982; 32:739-43.

122. Khatri BO, McQuillen MP, Harrington GJ, et al. Chronic progressive multiple sclerosis: Double-blind controlled study of plasmapheresis in patients taking immunosuppressive drugs. Neurology 1985;35:312-9.

123. Goodin DS. The use of immunosuppressive agents in the treatment of multiple sclerosis: A critical review. Neurology 1991;41:980-5.

124. Weiner HL. An assessment of plasma exchange in progressive multiple sclerosis. Neurology 1985;35:320-2.

125. Goodkin DE, Ransohoff RM, Rudick RA. Experimental therapies for multiple sclerosis: Current status. Cleve Clin J Med 1992;59:63-74.

126. Weiner HL, Dau P, Khatri BO, et al. Double-blind study of true versus sham plasma exchange in patients being treated with immunosuppression for acute attacks of multiple sclerosis. Neurology 1989;39:1143-9.

127. Canadian Cooperative Multiple Sclerosis Study Group. The Canadian cooperative trial of cyclophosphamide and plasma exchange in progressive multiple sclerosis. Lancet 1991; 337:441-6.

128. Noseworthy JH, Vandervoort MK, Penman M, et al. Cyclophosphamide and plasma exchange in multiple sclerosis. Lancet 1991;337:1540-1.

129. Myers LW. Immunologic therapy for secondary and primary progressive multiple sclerosis. Curr Neurol Neurosci Rep 2001;1:286-93.

130. Vamvakas EC, Pineda AA, Weinshenker BG. Meta-analysis of clinical studies of the efficacy of plasma exchange in the treatment of chronic progressive multiple sclerosis. J Clin Apher 1995;10:163-70.

131. Matiello M, Jacob A, Wingerchuk DM, Weinshenker BG. Neuromyelitis optica. Curr Opin Neurol 2007;20:255-60.

132. Linker RA, Gold R. Use of intravenous immunoglobulin and plasma exchange in neurological disease. Curr Opin Neurol 2008;21:358-65.

133. Kieseier BC, Wiendl H, Hemmer B, Hartung H-P. Treatment and treatment trials in multiple sclerosis. Curr Opin Neurol 2007;20:28-93.

134. Argyriou AA, Makris N. Neuromyelitis optica: A distinct disease of the central nervous system. Acta Neurol Scand 2008;118:209-17.

135. MacLean HJ, Freedman MS. Immunologic therapy for relapsing-remitting multiple sclerosis. Curr Neurol Neurosci Rep 2001;1:277-85.

136. Weinshenker BG, O'Brien PC, Petterson TM, et al. A randomized trial of plasma exchange in acute central nervous system inflammatory demyelinating disease. Ann Neurol 1999;46:878-86.

137. Jansen GA, Waterham HR, Wanders RJA. Molecular basis of Refsum disease: Sequence variations in phytanoyl-CoA hydroxylase (PHYH) and the PTS2 receptor (PEX7). Hum Mutat 2004;23:209-18.

138. Gibberd FB. Plasma exchange for Refsum's disease. Transfus Sci 1993;14:23-6.

139. Lou J-S, Snyder R, Griggs RC. Refsum's disease: Long term treatment preserves sensory nerve action potentials and motor function. J Neurol Neurosurg Psychiatry 1997;62:671-2.

140. Siegmund JB, Meier H, Hoppmann I, Gutsche H-U. Cascade filtration in Refsum's disease. Nephrol Dial Transplant 1995;10:117-9.

141. Choy EHS, Isenberg DA. Treatment of dermatomyositis and polymyositis. Rheumatology 2002;41:7-13.

142. Dau PC. Plasmapheresis in idiopathic inflammatory myopathy. Arch Neurol 1981;38:544-52.

143. Khatri BO, Luprecht G, Weiss SA. Plasmapheresis and immunosuppressive drug therapy in polymyositis. Muscle Nerve 1982;5:568-9.

144. Cecere FA, Spiva DA. Combination plasmapheresis/leukocytapheresis for the treatment of dermatomyositis/polymyositis. Plasma Ther Transfus Technol 1982;3:401-9.

145. Miller FW, Leitman SF, Cronin ME, et al. Controlled trial of plasma exchange and leukapheresis in polymyositis and dermatomyositis. N Engl J Med 1992;326:1380-4.

146. Bien CG, Granata T, Antozzi C, et al. Pathogenesis, diagnosis and treatment of Rasmussen encephalitis: A European consensus statement. Brain 2005;128:454-71.

147. Rodgers SW, Andrews PI, Gahring LC, et al. Autoantibodies to glutamate receptor Glu R3 in Rasmussen's encephalitis. Science 1994; 265:648-51.

148. Andrews PI, McNamara JO. Rasmussen's encephalitis: An autoimmune disorder? Curr Opin Neurobiol 1996;6:673-8.

149. Andrews PI, Dichter MA, Berkovic SF, et al. Plasmapheresis in Rasmussen's encephalitis. Neurology 1996;46:242-6.

150. Hart YM, Cortez M, Andermann F, et al. Medical treatment of Rasmussen's syndrome (chronic encephalitis and epilepsy): Effect of high dose steroids or immunoglobulins in 19 patients. Neurology 1994:44:1030-6.

151. Watson R, Jiang Y, Bermudez I, et al. Absence of antibodies to glutamate receptor type 3 (GluR3) in Rasmussen encephalitis. Neurology 2004;63:43-50.

152. Alvarez-Baron E, Bien C, Schramm J, et al. Autoantibodies to Munc18, cerebral plasma cells and B-lymphocytes in Rasmussen encephalitis. Epilepsy Res 2008;80:93-7.

153. Snider LA, Swedo SE. PANDAS: Current status and directions for research. Mol Psychiatry 2004;9:900-7.

154. Garvey MA, Swedo SE. Sydenham's chorea. Clinical and therapeutic update. Adv Exp Med Biol 1997;418:115-20.

155. Garvey MA, Snider LA, Leitman SF, et al. Treatment of Sydenham's chorea with intravenous immunoglobulin, plasma exchange, or prednisone. J Child Neurol 2005;20:424-9.

156. Nicolson R, Swedo SE, Bedwell J, et al. An open trial of plasma exchange in childhood-onset obsessive-compulsive disorder without poststreptococcal exacerbations. J Am Acad Child Adolesc Psychiatry 2000;39:1313-15.

157. Maddisson P. Neuromyotonia. Clin Neurophysiol 2006;117:2118-27.

158. van den Berg JSP, van Engelen BGM, Oerman RH, de Baets MH. Acquired neuromyotonia: Superiority of plasma exchange over high-dose intravenous human immunoglobulin. J Neurol 1999;246:623-5.

159. Nakatsuji Y, Kaido M, Sugai F, et al. Isaacs' syndrome successfully treated by immunoadsorption plasmapheresis. Acta Neurol Scand 2000;102:271-3.

160. Hayat GR, Kulkantrakorn K, Campbell WW, Giuliani MJ. Neuromyotonia: Autoimmune pathogenesis and response to immune modulating therapy. J Neurol Sci 2000;181:38-43.

161. Verino S, Geschwind M, Boeve B. Autoimmune encephalopathies. Neurologist 2007;13:140-7.

162. Vincent A, Buckley C, Schott JM, et al. Potassium channel antibody-associated encephalopathy: A potentially immunotherapy-responsive form of limbic encephalitis. Brain 2004;127:701-12.

163. Madrid A, Gil-Peralta A, Gil-Néciga E, et al. Morvan's fibrillary chorea: Remission after plasmapheresis. J Neurol 1996;243:350-3.

164. Monstad I, Petlund CF, Sjaastad D, et al. Plasma exchange in motor neuron disease: A controlled study. J Neurol 1979;221:59-66.

165. Silani V, Scarlato G, Valli G, et al. Plasma exchange ineffective in amyotrophic lateral sclerosis. Arch Neurol 1980;37:511-13.

166. Olarte MR, Schoenfeldt RS, McKiernan G, et al. Plasmapheresis in amyotrophic lateral sclerosis. Ann Neurol 1980;8:644-5.

167. Schulz SC, van Kammen DP, Waters R, et al. Double-blind evaluation of plasmapheresis in schizophrenic patients: A pilot study. Artif Organs 1983;7:317-21.

In: McLeod BC, Szczepiorkowski ZM, Weinstein R, Winters JL, eds.
Apheresis: Principles and Practice, 3rd edition
Bethesda, MD: AABB Press, 2010

16

Therapeutic Plasma Exchange in Hematologic Diseases and Dysproteinemias

Joseph E. Kiss, MD

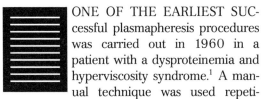 ONE OF THE EARLIEST SUC-cessful plasmapheresis procedures was carried out in 1960 in a patient with a dysproteinemia and hyperviscosity syndrome.[1] A manual technique was used repetitively to withdraw whole blood and centrifuge it "offline" for separation and removal of plasma, followed by dilution of the patient's red cells in saline for reinfusion. Since then, technologic advances described in Chapters 1 and 4 have provided automated centrifugation methods with far greater efficiency and patient safety. The accumulation of experience, publication of cases, and reporting of the results of randomized trials has resulted in a stronger rationale for the application of apheresis in disorders where therapeutic plasma exchange (TPE) has been shown to be of benefit. The American Society for Apheresis (ASFA) has reviewed and summarized the accumulated data and has assigned specific disorders to indication categories to aid in the appropriate use of this therapy.[2]

Hematologic diseases continue to be among the most common indications for TPE. Data from the Canadian Apheresis Study Group (CASG) from 1999 showed that 38.8% of all TPE procedures were performed in patients with the diagnosis of thrombotic thrombocytopenic purpura (TTP), while 7.4% of procedures were performed in patients with Waldenström macroglobulinemia.[3] More recent experience at the Institute for Transfusion Med-

Joseph E. Kiss, MD, Medical Director, Hemapheresis and Blood Services, the Institute for Transfusion Medicine, and Associate Professor of Medicine, University of Pittsburgh, Pittsburgh, Pennsylvania
The author has disclosed no conflicts of interest.

icine in Pittsburgh for the year 2009 indicates that TTP and/or hemolytic uremic syndrome (HUS) accounted for 37% of all procedures in adults, whereas only 1.7% were performed in patients with macroglobulinemia. In aggregate, 44% of TPE procedures in 25% of patients were performed for hematologic disorders or dysproteinemias, reflecting the need for numerous procedures per patient, especially in TTP. TPE is used to acutely replace deficient proteins [eg, ADAMTS13 (a disintegrin and metalloproteinase with a thrombospondin type motif 1, member 13) in TTP], and to reduce levels of specific antibodies or excess immunoglobulins involved in the pathogenesis of hematologic diseases. The therapeutic objective is to restore or reduce the circulating levels of the relevant molecule to ameliorate a disease process. With the exception of its use as primary therapy in TTP, TPE is mainly employed along with pharmacologic therapy on an adjunctive basis to either reduce the time needed for a therapeutic response or provide some improvement when primary pharmacologic therapy is ineffective. This chapter presents hematologic diseases and dysproteinemias for which TPE is considered a primary or important secondary therapy. Several conditions are also discussed for which TPE may be an appropriate adjunctive therapy.

Thrombotic Thrombocytopenic Purpura and other Thrombotic Microangiopathies

In 1924, Moschowitz described a 16-year-old girl with fever, anemia, renal dysfunction, central nervous system impairment, and cardiac failure who died within 2 weeks of presentation.[4] Later descriptions of similar cases suggested a mortality rate of up to 90% and defined the "classic" clinical triad of TTP: 1) thrombocytopenia, 2) hemolytic anemia with schistocytosis, and 3) neurologic symptoms ranging from transitory mental status alterations to seizures and coma. The case reviews also noted the high prevalence of renal impairment and fever in the patients and suggested

that these features be included in a diagnostic "pentad."[5]

TTP belongs to a category of disorders known as thrombotic microangiopathies (TMAs; see Table 16-1), a term coined by Symmers in 1952 to denote the characteristic histologic lesions.[25] The predominant symptoms associated with the various thrombotic microangiopathic syndromes reflect the distribution of microvascular lesions that lead to organ impairment. Characteristic areas of involvement include the central nervous system in TTP, the kidneys in HUS, and the liver in the HELLP syndrome (hemolysis, elevated liver enzymes, low platelet count) associated with pregnancy.

A great deal of knowledge has been gained over the last decade regarding the etiology and pathophysiology of TTP. Molecular defects in, and antibody-mediated deficiency of, ADAMTS13 provide the central pathophysiologic basis for the current understanding of this disorder. This paradigm is beginning to change the clinical approach for patients who have TMAs while also providing the impetus for studies of key issues regarding management, such as the role of TPE in various patient subgroups and identification of which subgroups may benefit from powerful immunosuppressive drugs.

Pathophysiology

The characteristic histopathologic finding in autopsy studies of patients with TTP is the presence of von Willebrand factor (vWF)/platelet thrombi in small vessels of the brain, kidney, heart, abdominal viscera, and other organs. Unlike the microvascular lesions in disseminated intravascular coagulation (DIC), they contain very little fibrin and there is no inflammatory exudate like that seen in patients with vasculitis. In the early 1980s Moake reported finding unusually large multimers of vWF (ULvWF) circulating in the blood between attacks in patients with "chronic-relapsing" TTP, which is now recognized as the congenital form of the disorder.[26] He postulated the absence of a vWF "depolymerase," which

Table 16-1. Classification and Distinguishing Features of Thrombotic Thrombocytopenic Purpura and Other Thrombotic Microangiopathies*

Primary TTP

Congenital

- Caused by mutations in ADAMTS13 gene[6]
- Very rare

Idiopathic

- Diagnosed by exclusion of secondary causes
- Most common form
- IgG autoantibody that binds to ADAMTS13
- ADAMTS13 inhibitor detected in 44%-95%[7-9]

Primary HUS

Congenital

- Acute renal failure
- Defective complement regulatory proteins in large proportion of patients[10]
- ADAMTS13 levels normal

Idiopathic

- Diagnosed by exclusion of secondary causes
- Acute renal failure, renal biopsy differences[†]
- ADAMTS13 levels usually normal, inhibitor absent[11]

Secondary

Human immunodeficiency virus

- High response rate reported to plasma infusion and antiretroviral therapy[12,13]
- ADAMTS13 level usually normal

Collagen vascular diseases (especially SLE)

- Diagnostic confusion between TTP and ITP with vasculitis (similar neurologic changes, renal insufficiency, and schistocytes present on blood smear)
- ADAMTS13 level may aid in diagnosis if severely deficient

Drug-induced immunologic disease

- Ticlopidine (Ticlid[‡]) induces antibody to ADAMTS13[14]
- Treatment is by withdrawing offending drug and performing plasma exchange[15]
- Rapid recovery is typical
- Related drug, clopidogrel (Plavix[§]) also associated, but mechanism uncertain[16]
- Quinine also common—platelet and endothelial antibodies associated
- Must be distinguished from ITP
- ADAMTS13 levels not decreased, and efficacy of plasma exchange questionable[17]

Drug-induced, dose-dependent toxicity

- Associated with cancer chemotherapeutic agents, including mitomycin C (Mutamycin[§]) and gemcitabine (Gemzar[‖])
- Can develop slowly, sometimes after drug is discontinued
- Can also be seen with immunosuppressive agents, including cyclosporin (Neoral[¶]) and tacrolimus (Prograf[#])

(Continued)

Table 16-1. Classification and Distinguishing Features of Thrombotic Thrombocytopenic Purpura and Other Thrombotic Microangiopathies* (Continued)

Drug-induced, dose-dependent toxicity (continued)
- Treated by stopping drug or dose reduction[15]
- Uncertain efficacy of plasma exchange

Pregnancy and postpartum
- May be caused by an IgG inhibitor of ADAMTS13[18]
- Must be distinguished from HELLP syndrome (HELLP usually occurs during the third trimester of pregnancy or immediately postpartum in association with severe preeclampsia)[19,20]

Hematopoietic stem cell transplant-associated disease
- A TTP-like syndrome that may be caused by infection or graft-vs-host disease[21,22]
- Doubtful efficacy of plasma exchange[23]

*Note: If laboratory samples are to be drawn to evaluate a possible secondary cause (eg, SLE), it is important to obtain these before instituting plasma exchange therapy to avoid a dilution effect.
†The typical histologic changes in HUS consist of glomerular and arteriolar fibrin thrombi and subendothelial widening of the glomerular capillaries on electron microscopy. Renal biopsy specimens in TTP generally reveal prominent arterial and capillary thrombosis, and they stain strongly for platelets and von Willebrand factor.[24]
‡Sanofi-Aventis, Paris, France.
§Bristol-Meyers Squibb, New York, NY.
ΙΙEli Lilly, Indianapolis, IN.
¶Novartis AG, Basel, Switzerland.
#Astellas Pharma, Tokyo, Japan.
TTP = thrombotic thrombocytopenic purpura; ADAMTS13 = a disintegrin and metalloproteinase with a thrombospondin type motif 1, member 13; HUS = hemolytic uremic syndrome; SLE = systemic lupus erythematosus; ITP = immune thrombocytopenia; IgG = immunoglobulin G; HELLP = hemolysis with elevated liver enzymes and low platelets.

would normally cleave the larger, highly adhesive vWF multimers secreted by endothelial cells into smaller subunits. Experiments with ULvWF multimers obtained directly from endothelial cell preparations demonstrated increased potency in promoting platelet aggregation, in direct proportion to molecular size.[27] A vWF-cleaving enzyme was identified independently by investigators in the United States[28] and Switzerland[29] as a metalloprotease and was cloned in 2001.[30] Now known as ADAMTS13, the protease cleaves the peptide bond between tyrosine 842 and methionine 843 in the A2 domain when the molecule is bound to the P-selectin receptor on the surface of endothelial cells.[31] After its attachment, the high shear conditions present in small caliber vessels cause ULvWF to stretch out, exposing cleavage sites that are inaccessible in the globular conformation of the protein. The characteristic localization of vWF-platelet thrombi in the capillaries and arterioles of TTP patients, and not in venules or veins, is presumably related to the higher shear stress in the former. In experiments using cultured human endothelial cells, long strings of uncleaved vWF can be seen avidly binding platelets under model conditions of high shear.[32] The platelet-decorated strings break apart when ADAMTS13 is added to the medium, illustrating the key regulatory role played by this enzyme in normal hemostasis.

Some inflammatory cytokines, including tumor necrosis factor and interleukin (IL)-8, have been found to induce vWF secretion from endothelium.[33] Others such as IL-6 appear to inhibit the proteolytic action of ADAMTS13 on the vWF molecule. These observations could suggest a role for inflammatory stimuli and endothelial activation and/or injury in TMAs, especially TTP. This could explain instances in which various infections (eg, central line or urinary tract) or surgery seem to precipitate or exacerbate episodes of TTP. Moreover, endothelial cell activation manifested by very high levels of vWF is a characteristic finding in TMAs, even those not associated with abnormalities in ADAMTS13. Although ADAMTS13 is the only protease demonstrated thus far to regulate vWF multimer size, other plasma proteins in addition to IL-6, such as thrombin and thrombospondin, may also affect ADAMTS13 activity.[34] In addition, free hemoglobin is inhibitory, which may have both diagnostic and pathophysiologic relevance.[35] ADAMTS13 function may also be influenced by its ability to bind to endothelial cells, which is thought to involve an interaction between CD36 and the A1 domain of the enzyme.[36] Shedding or reduced expression of this receptor could also affect the ability of ADAMTS13 to properly cleave vWF, thus providing another potential mechanism for TTP-like conditions to develop without a severe deficiency of ADAMTS13.[32]

Clinical Manifestations and Diagnosis

The full "pentad" of thrombocytopenia, microangiopathic hemolytic anemia, fever, neurologic changes, and renal dysfunction is present in only a minority of patients. A "dyad" of thrombocytopenia and microangiopathic hemolytic anemia, in the absence of another cause, is considered the minimal criterion to consider TTP as a provisional diagnosis. Neurologic manifestations may include headache, confusion, fluctuating sensorimotor deficits (transient ischemic attacks), visual defects, and seizures. The transient nature of some of the early symptoms probably reflects acute formation and breakdown of microthrombi in small cerebral vessels. Coma at the time of presentation is reported to be an adverse prognostic indicator.[37] Renal involvement ranges from mild proteinuria and hematuria to severe azotemia requiring dialysis. Patients who present with severe renal impairment but few neurologic or other systemic findings may be considered to have HUS. It is important to note that TTP is a multisystem disease in which organs other than the brain and kidney are frequently involved. Patients may have diffuse abdominal pain as a symptom of mesenteric ischemia. Cardiac complications consisting of myocardial ischemia and/or infarction, congestive heart failure, and arrhythmia were reported in 18% of patients in one series, leading to a recommendation that patients with TTP have cardiac enzyme screening and cardiac monitoring in the early stages of illness.[38] Interestingly, acute inflammatory conditions have been noted to trigger episodes of TTP. Patients hospitalized with acute pancreatitis (and normal platelet counts) may develop thrombocytopenia and microangiopathic hemolytic anemia a few days later. TTP has also been reported to develop 7 to 10 days after surgical procedures.[39]

Laboratory studies reveal an increase in serum lactate dehydrogenase (LDH) and the presence of schistocytes (red cell fragments) on a peripheral blood smear. Schistocytes reflect an active microangiopathic hemolytic process; fragmentation results from the passage of red cells through partially occluded vessels. Rarely, red cell morphology may appear normal early in the disease course.[24] Tests of coagulation function generally are within normal limits. However, mild elevations of D-dimers and fibrin degradation products may be found.

Classification

Different categories of TMA have been described (Table 16-1), which vary in mechanism, target patient population, and pattern of organ involvement. However, clinical and laboratory features frequently overlap, creating diagnostic uncertainty. TMA may occur on an idiopathic (primary) basis or in association with pregnancy, autoimmune conditions, infections, malignancy, stem cell transplantation, or exposure to certain drugs. Registries have been formed in various countries to better catalog and manage patients with these disorders.[7,34,40-42]

Primary TMA

Hereditary TTP, or Upshaw-Schulman syndrome, arises as a result of a congenital deficiency of ADAMTS13.[34] Over 70 mutations in the ADAMTS13 gene have been identified that can cause this rare autosomal recessive disorder. Only homozygotes or double heterozygotes are affected. Most patients present during the first decade of life with recurrent episodes of microangiopathic hemolysis and thrombocytopenia; early adult onset is seen occasionally. A precipitating event such as infection, surgery, or pregnancy may trigger the full clinical episode of hemolytic anemia and thrombocytopenia. ADAMTS13 activity is undetectable but no inhibitor is present. Low levels of ADAMTS 13, generally 5% to 10%, are sufficient to prevent clinical manifestations, so remission can be maintained by giving 1 or 2 units of Fresh Frozen Plasma (FFP) every 3 weeks. Recombinant ADAMTS13 has also been effective.[43]

The most common form of TMA, idiopathic TTP, is caused by an autoantibody that binds to ADAMTS13, inhibiting its ability to cleave high-molecular-weight vWF multimers. A few cases are reported in which a noninhibitory antibody accelerates the clearance of ADAMTS13.[44] Idiopathic TTP accounts for 40% to 77% of all TMA cases in large series.[40,41] The frequency of severe ADAMTS13 deficiency reported in patients who received this clinical diagnosis varies from 18% to 94% (see Table 16-2). Inhibitory activity in functional assays is reported in 38% to 95% of patients, with a higher prevalence reported in those with severe ADAMTS13 deficiency. Enzyme-linked immunosorbent assays (ELISA) for detection of autoantibodies to ADAMTS13 appear to have greater sensitivity than inhibitor assays; in a group of TTP patients with ADAMTS13 activity <10%, IgG antibodies were found by ELISA

in 97%, whereas the prevalence of inhibitors was only 83%.[48] Of those affected, females predominate by 2:1 to 3:1, and people of African ethnicity outnumber those of European ethnicity in the United States.[40]

In HUS, acute renal failure occurs in conjunction with microangiopathic hemolytic anemia and thrombocytopenia. Table 16-1 lists congenital and idiopathic forms under the heading of primary HUS (also referred to as "atypical" or "sporadic" HUS, in contrast to the "typical," "epidemic," or diarrheal secondary form caused by shigatoxins). In patients with hereditary HUS, TPE may be used to replace missing complement regulatory proteins, such as Factor H, Factor I, or CD46/membrane cofactor protein.[34] ADAMTS13 levels are generally normal or slightly decreased in HUS[11]; severe deficiency is rare.[49] Likewise, ADAMTS13 inhibitors are not found. Considering these data, the rationale for TPE in HUS is uncertain.[24] However, the clinical overlap between some cases of HUS and idiopathic TTP is such that some authorities recommend TPE.[7] Also, in adults with a sporadic bloody diarrhea TTP/HUS presentation, Karpac et al[49] report apparent responses to TPE similar to those in patients with severe ADAMTS13 deficiency (81% vs 89%) after fewer treatments (mean = 10 vs 20). The rate of early exacerbation was lower in bloody diarrhea TTP/HUS (6% vs 47%), and there were no relapses in survivors (vs a 39% relapse rate in idiopathic TTP). However, the mortality rate (33%) was greater compared to patients with severe ADAMTS13 deficiency (13%).[50] Thus, a therapeutic trial of TPE appears reasonable in these patients, despite the lack of severe ADAMTS13 deficiency.

Secondary TMA

Microangiopathic hemolytic anemia and thrombocytopenia are common findings in a number of clinical disease states. Some of these conditions have all the hallmarks of idiopathic TTP, while others appear to have different pathophysiologic mechanisms. The conditions are briefly summarized in Table 16-1. The reader

Table 16-2. Prevalence of ADAMTS13 Deficiency in Patients Clinically Diagnosed With Thrombotic Thrombocytopenic Purpura

Investigators	Year	No. Patients	Percentage of Patients with Severe Deficiency*	Percentage of Patients with Partial Deficiency†
Furlan et al[29]/Tsai[28]	1998	37/30	94	100
Veyradier et al[45] (prospective cohort)	2001	66	71	89
Mori et al[9]	2002	18	72	100
Vesely et al[7] (prospective cohort)	2003	142	18	34
Peyvandi et al[46]	2008	100	48	72
Coppo et al[34]	2004	46	67	80
Zheng et al[8] (prospective cohort)‡	2004	37	43	72
Matsumoto et al[42] (retrospective, "idiopathic TTP")‡	2004	108	52	100
Scully et al[41] (retrospective, "idiopathic TTP")‡	2008	158	73	93
Total		**742**	**56**	**79**

*<10%, except Matsumoto (<3%).
†< the lower limit of the laboratory reference interval (usually 40% to 140%).
‡Adapted from Mannucci et al.[47]
TTP = thrombotic thrombocytopenic purpura.

may consult several reviews that discuss classification, differential diagnosis, and management in more detail.[24,34,51]

Interpretation of ADAMTS13 Measurements

There is a high degree of diagnostic specificity for TTP in patients who have undetectable or very low (<5%-10%) ADAMTS13 levels. However, the overall proportion of patients with clinically diagnosed TTP who have severe deficiency ranges from 18% to 94% (Table 16-2). Several factors have been proposed to account

for this wide variability. Although there are technical differences in assay performance, the most likely reason involves patient selection. For example, studies that included patients with renal failure or HUS reported a lower prevalence of severe deficiency than those that excluded them.[7,52] The same can be said for studies that included patients with secondary causes, because they also have a lower prevalence of ADAMTS13 deficiency. Very low ADAMTS13 levels have rarely been reported in transplant recipients and in patients with cancer or DIC,[34] but their specific clinical circumstances distinguish them from patients with TTP in most cases. Diagnostic uncertainty increases with mild-to-moderate ADAMTS13 deficiency because of overlap with many other clinical disorders, including pregnancy, sepsis multiorgan failure, liver disease, and the post-surgical state.[47] As noted in Table 16-1, some patients with the clinical features of TTP have normal levels of ADAMTS13. The significance of this is not well understood, but many clinicians are, at present, unwilling to rely on a normal value to exclude the diagnosis of TTP when the clinical picture is otherwise compelling. Nevertheless, a number of alternative diagnoses need to be considered in the patient with thrombocytopenia and the many potential causes of red cell fragmentation, including sepsis with or without DIC, malignant hypertension, vasculitis, metastatic malignancy (tumor emboli), severe pulmonary hypertension, and others. The proportion of patients with inhibitors ranges from 44% to 95%, with the highest frequency found in patients with severe ADAMTS13 deficiency.[7-9] As mentioned, ELISA detects autoantibodies in 97% of patients with severe deficiency.[48] ADAMTS13 levels have not been very helpful in deciding when to stop TPE because results may be delayed, because levels obtained during periods of treatment may not represent an endogenous "steady state," and because patients can enter clinical remission despite persistence of severe ADAMTS13 deficiency.[53] Clinical and laboratory parameters—especially the platelet count—remain the best way to assess the status of remission and the decision to discontinue plasma exchange.

Prognosis

The ADAMTS13 level is especially useful as a marker for clinical outcome and potential for relapse. Severely deficient patients, compared to nonseverely deficient patients, experience higher rates of remission (82%-88% vs 20%-75%) and lower mortality (8%-18% vs 18%-80%).[7-9,54] The greater mortality in nonseverely deficient patients may be the result of the higher proportion of secondary causes, with

death from underlying diseases; eg, patients treated with hematopoietic stem cell transplantation for hematologic malignancies. In one study, patients who had persistent ADAMTS13 deficiency and inhibitor at the time of clinical remission had a threefold higher risk of relapse.[46] Another study reported a 38.5% relapse rate at 18 months in patients who had undetectable ADAMTS13 activity in remission, compared to 5% in those with detectable levels.[55]

Treatment

Role of Therapeutic Plasma Exchange

TPE is the only therapy proven to be effective in randomized clinical trials (see Table 16-3). Consequently, TTP is rated as a Category I indication for TPE by ASFA.[2] The Canadian Apheresis Study Group compared plasma infusion (30 mL/kg initially, then 15 mL/kg daily) with TPE (1.5 plasma volumes/day for 3 days, then 1 plasma volume per day). Patients were crossed over to TPE for poor response or inability to tolerate plasma infusion. Survival was significantly higher in the TPE arm (78% vs 63%).[56] TPE not only delivers a greater dose of ADAMTS13 without circulatory overload but also depletes antibodies to ADAMTS13. Both mechanisms appear to be relevant, on the basis of a French study that gave equivalent amounts of plasma to each arm of a randomized trial comparing TPE to plasma infusion and found the complete remission and survival rates were higher in the group that received TPE.[57] Patients with TTP can deteriorate suddenly (as a result of seizures, myocardial infarction, cardiac arrhythmia, etc), so treatment should be initiated as soon as possible after diagnosis. Plasma (15-30 mL/kg) should be infused if TPE cannot be instituted in a timely manner. The treatment approach consists of 1 to 1.5 plasma volume exchanges daily with plasma replacement until clinical symptoms have resolved and the platelet count exceeds 150,000/μL. FFP, 24-hour plasma, thawed plasma, and cryosupernatant plasma are considered equivalent because of compara-

Table 16-3. Randomized Clinical Trials in Acute Thrombotic Thrombocytopenic Purpura

Investigators	Year	Patients	Treament/ Control Groups	Results	Findings
Rock et al[56]	1991	103	TPE vs PI (3× more plasma in TPE arm)	Survival: 78% vs 63% (p = 0.036)	TPE superior; volume overload in PI group
Henon[57]	1991	40	TPE vs PI (plasma dose equal)	Survival: 85% vs 57%	TPE superior
Bobbio-Pallavincini et al[58]	1997	72	ASA + dipyridamole, 15 days vs SOC, then ticlopidine maintenance, 1 year	Survival, day 15: 97.2% vs 86.5% (NS)	No excessive bleeding noted using antiplatelet drugs
Zeigler et al[59]	2001	27	CSP vs FFP	Response comparable; survival: 23% vs 21% (NS)	No difference but underpowered
Rock et al[60]	2005	52	CSP vs FFP	Response: 82% vs 85% (NS)	No difference but underpowered
Mintz et al[61]	2006	35	PCT FFP vs FFP	Response: 89% vs 82% (NS)	No difference but underpowered

TPE = therapeutic plasma exchange; PI = plasma infusion; ASA = acetylsalicylic acid (aspirin); SOC = standard of care; NS = not significant; CSP = cryosupernatant plasma; FFP = Fresh Frozen Plasma; PCT = photochemical-treated.

ble levels of ADAMTS13.[62] A small case series suggested better results with cryosupernatant,[63] but randomized trials showed no difference in outcome (see Table 16-3). Cryosupernatant is relatively low in fibrinogen, so blood fibrinogen should be monitored if it is used.

The platelet count is the most important measure of clinical response. Even with daily TPE it may not rise promptly or may decline unexpectedly. An "inhibitor rebound" phenomenon has been observed in some responding patients after 7 to 10 days, which may be associated with refractoriness despite continuing TPE.[64] One study grouped platelet responses in four patterns: in group I, platelets rose and then declined to <100,000/μL; in group II, platelets declined despite TPE; in group III, platelets rose continuously; and in group IV, platelets decreased slightly to a 100,000-to-150,000/μL plateau after initially rising.[65] The group IV pattern has been termed a "pseudo-refractory state," and the authors suggest that TPE may be safely discontinued in such patients. They also suggest that continued daily TPE in group I and II patients will reverse the decline and eventually achieve remission in most cases.

Although definitions vary, recurrences developing within 30 days after remission are considered exacerbations, while those after 30 days are considered relapses.

The LDH level reflects ongoing tissue ischemia as well as hemolysis.[66] Clinical experience suggests that a normal LDH is not necessary to safely discontinue TPE; a level below 1.5 times the upper limit of normal may be an acceptable endpoint. Persistent schistocytosis alone is not a reason to continue TPE.[67]

Many institutions taper TPE after remission is achieved in an attempt to avoid an early exacerbation. A survey by the US TTP Apheresis Study Group found that eight of 20 responding centers (40%) routinely tapered TPE. Specific schedules were not specified, but there was no significant improvement in outcome from tapering.[68] The Canadian Apheresis Study Group employed a taper consisting of five TPEs over a 2-week period (the typical schedule was every other day × 3, then every third day × 2, then off).[56] However, the efficacy of this schedule in avoiding early exacerbation was not reported. As a result of the lack of evidence-based data, tapering of TPE has not been recommended by any professional association, including the AABB and ASFA. The Society for Hemostasis and Thrombosis (SHT) recommends continuing daily TPE for 2 days after attainment of remission.[24]

In studies reported between 1987 and 2003, mortality in TTP ranged between 10% and 22%, exacerbation within 30 days of remission occurred in 22% to 45%, and late relapses were reported in 13% to 40% of cases.[7,68-70] More recent studies of patients with severe ADAMTS13 deficiency report mortality rates of 5% to 10% and relapse rates of 30% to 50%.[52] TPE does not correct the primary autoimmune defect, and patients may still suffer delayed morbidity or mortality. Furthermore, TPE itself may cause serious adverse effects. The Oklahoma TTP-HUS Registry reported a 26% risk per patient for major complications (primarily catheter-related infections, sepsis, bleeding, and thrombosis) of TPE over 12 years, including a 2.8% fatality rate.[71]

Other Therapies

Antiplatelet Agents. Although the rationale for using antiplatelet therapy in TTP is appealing, platelet inhibitors have not been shown to be beneficial and may increase the risk of hemorrhage, particularly with severe thrombocytopenia. One group[58] reported similar response and survival rates at day 15 between patients treated with antiplatelet therapy and those treated with TPE and corticosteroids, with or without aspirin plus dipyridamole; excessive bleeding was not noted in the antiplatelet-treatment group (see Table 16-3). They also reported a reduced 1-year relapse rate using ticlopidine as a maintenance strategy (6.25% in the ticlopidine-treated group vs 21.4% in controls; p = 0.018%). However, both ticlopidine and clopidogrel have been associated with drug-induced TTP,[15] limiting their usefulness. One consensus group recommends aspirin when the platelet count exceeds 50,000/μL.[24] Novel agents such as antibodies to vWF and peptide aptamers[72] that interfere with vWF-platelet interactions are also being investigated.

Immunosuppressive Treatment. Anecdotal reports, case series, and uncontrolled clinical trials in limited numbers of patients suggest the effectiveness of immunosuppressive therapies in TTP. Improved responses have been attributed to early treatment with corticosteroids[73] or vincristine.[74] These agents are also frequently added as adjunctive therapy after a failure to achieve sustained remission with TPE. The roles of both autoantibody formation and inflammation in idiopathic TTP strengthen the rationale for using corticosteroids in this disorder; however, efficacy remains unclear, with comparable response rates with or without use of corticosteroids reported in the literature.[75] In a retrospective study, seven of eight refractory patients improved after receiving vincristine 1.4 mg/m² intravenously on day 1 followed by 1 mg on days 4 and 7.[76] Vincristine has been reported to rapidly increase platelet count and ADAMTS13 level in patients with TTP before changes in autoantibody levels and ADAMTS13 activity.[53] Interference with vWF/

platelet binding has been proposed as a potential mechanism.

Other immunosuppressive therapies used with reported success include cyclophosphamide, azathioprine, intravenous immunoglobulin (IVIG), cyclosporine A (CSA), staphylococcal protein A immunoadsorption, and splenectomy.[24] Splenectomy has seemed particularly effective in patients with a history of relapses, reducing the frequency from 2.3 ±2 events per year to 0.1 ±0.1 events per year in a retrospective analysis.[77] CSA (2-3 mg/kg/day) has been compared to prednisone in two consecutively treated groups of patients with clinical TTP.[78] Remission was achieved in 10 of 12 patients (83%) in the prednisone group; six of the 10 (60%) developed an exacerbation within 30 days. All eight in the CSA group (100%) achieved remission with no exacerbations noted. The number of TPE treatments needed to induce remission was also decreased in the latter group, from 16 to seven (p = 0.029). The effectiveness of CSA was also suggested when drug treatment alone (without TPE) reversed early recurrences of idiopathic TTP.[79] A direct effect on endothelial cell activation or apoptosis was proposed, because clinical improvement occurred despite persistence of ADAMTS13 deficiency and inhibitor activity.

Rituximab. Confirmation of an immunologic basis for idiopathic TTP has led to interest in rituximab, a chimeric monoclonal antibody directed at the CD20 antigen expressed on the surface of B lymphocytes. B-cell depletion by rituximab occurs by several mechanisms, including complement-mediated cell lysis and antibody-dependent cellular cytotoxicity.[80] In animal experiments, peripheral blood B cells were reduced to undetectable levels by 24 hours after infusion.[81]

Published experience with rituximab treatment of TTP has grown to over 100 patients.[51,52,75] Fakhouri et al[82] studied six patients with acute refractory TTP (unremitting for at least 3 weeks) and five with severe relapsing TTP. All had ADAMTS13 levels less than 5% with an inhibitor. TPE was discontinued so as not to remove rituximab. Clinical responses were noted in all patients, with normalization of the platelet counts between 5 and 14 days after the fourth of four infusions in the acute refractory patients. ADAMTS13 levels recovered to 29% to 75% of normal by 6 months, and inhibitors disappeared between 7 and 24 weeks after rituximab treatment. B-lymphocyte recovery was noted between 6 and 12 months; however, this was accompanied in some patients by the reappearance of inhibitor and decreased levels of ADAMTS13. This salutary experience led to trials using rituximab even earlier after diagnosis. Scully et al[41] treated 14 patients with acute TTP and 11 patients with relapsed TTP. Rituximab was given if the patient's platelet count had not normalized by the seventh day of TPE. TPE was withheld for ~24 hours after each rituximab infusion. They noted complete clinical and laboratory responses at a median of 11 days following rituximab, with disappearance of inhibitors and improvement in ADAMTS13 activity in 23 of 24 patients at 3-months follow-up. They noted no clinical relapses at a median of 10 months later (range = 1 to 33+ months); however, some patients received up to 8 doses of rituximab as maintenance therapy for persisting inhibitor activity.

Mild infusion-related reactions were reported in some cases, consisting of fever, chills, headache, nausea, and hypotension. Serious acute hypotensive reactions such as those reported in patients with B-cell malignancies were cause for initial concern but have not materialized, likely because of the lower B-cell burden in TTP patients. Several serious adverse events have been reported, mainly infectious complications, including herpes zoster transverse myelitis/encephalitis, cytomegalovirus reactivation, and pneumonia.[83] In addition, an episode of acute cardiogenic shock was reported in a 20-year-old TTP patient, who recovered from the episode without residual cardiomyopathy.[84]

Normalization of platelets and LDH has been noted in approximately 95% of patients reported in the literature thus far, usually within 1 to 4 weeks after the first dose. The duration of remission after rituximab treatment has ranged from 9 months to 4 years, with relapses reported in approximately 10%. ADAMTS13 levels have generally increased, though not always to normal levels.[8,85,86] Rituximab treatment alone has also induced remission in patients with early relapse, obviating the need for TPE.[82,85]

ABO-Mismatched Hematopoietic Progenitor Cell Transplantation

ABO-mismatching occurs in 20% to 40% of hematopoietic progenitor cell (HPC) transplantations.[87] This is accepted practice because of the overriding requirement for HLA compatibility and the minimal effects of ABO mismatching on graft rejection, graft-vs-host disease (GVHD), and myeloid or platelet engraftment.[88,89] Depending on the type of ABO mismatch, however, both acute and delayed hemolysis as well as delayed red cell engraftment[90] or pure red cell aplasia (PRCA) may occur. An "ABO-incompatible" donor is one to whom the recipient has an ABO antibody or antibodies (major ABO incompatibility). An "ABO-unmatched" donation is either group O and transplanted to a group A, B, or AB patient, or group A or B and transplanted to a group AB patient (minor ABO incompatibility). "Bidirectional" mismatches involve both major and minor ABO incompatibility.

Pathogenesis

The potential consequences of a major-ABO-incompatible HPC transplantation include acute and delayed hemolysis, delayed red cell engraftment, and PRCA. The risk of acute hemolysis is related to the quantity of donor red cells in the graft and to the recipient's corresponding isoagglutinin titer. The red cell content of marrow products is, at 250 to 450 mL (25% to 30% hematocrit in a 1 to 1.5 L product), much greater than that of peripheral blood progenitor cell (apheresis) products, which averages only 8 mL.[91] Immediate hemolysis may also result from donor isoagglutinins or other red cell alloantibodies in the large amounts of incompatible plasma present in marrow harvests.

Persisting isoagglutinins in the recipient may also result in delayed hemolysis as engraftment occurs. In some cases incomplete chimerism with persisting recipient cells may result in even later onset of "host-vs-graft" hemolytic episodes, necessitating intensive immunosuppressive therapy or donor lymphocyte infusions to achieve full donor chimerism.[92] Persisting or high-titer anti-donor isoagglutinins may also result in delayed red cell recovery or PRCA because of antiproliferative effects on marrow erythroid precursors.[93,94] This appears to occur more in group A- than group B-incompatible transplants.[95,96] Reduced-intensity (nonmyeloablative) conditioning (RIC) regimens rely more on graft-vs-tumor effects and less on chemotherapeutic tumor cell kill. They consequently cause less destruction of normal host cells, including the native immune system. RIC regimens constitute a risk factor for PRCA, as indicated by the slower decline in anti-donor isoagglutinin titers and the delayed appearance of donor red cells in peripheral blood (mean of 114 days vs 40 days seen with myeloablative conditioning).[97] CSA, which blocks the primary T-cell immune response but has limited action on B cells, has also been associated with PRCA following HPC transplantation; its withdrawal has resulted in resolution of PRCA.[98] GVHD prophylaxis including anti-B-cell-proliferative drugs such as mycophenolate mofetil or methotrexate may be protective.[92]

The passenger lymphocyte syndrome (PLS), manifesting as delayed hemolysis, has been reported following ABO-unmatched (but compatible) organ transplantations as well as HPC transplantations. A key risk factor is the lymphoid tissue content of the transplanted organ.[99,100] The corollary in HPC transplantation is the use of peripheral blood HPCs, which have 16-fold more CD3+ T cells and 11-fold more CD19+ B cells than the typical marrow graft.[101] Female donors,[98] RIC regimens, and CSA monotherapy or absence of B-cell immunosuppressive therapy have also been identified as risk factors for PLS.[92,102] Hemolysis, ranging from mild to severe, generally occurs 5 to 15 days after transplantation and is caused by ABO antibodies produced by donor B lymphocytes and plasma cells that proliferate in the immunosuppressed recipient.[102] Hemolysis may ensue when group O HPCs are transplanted into non-group-O patients, or when non-group-AB donors are used for group AB patients. It has also been reported rarely with non-ABO antibodies—including anti-JK[a], anti-Le[a], anti-D, anti-E, and anti-s—when the donor is presensitized to a recipient antigen.[92]

Therapy and Role of Therapeutic Plasma Exchange

Acute hemolysis in HPC marrow grafts with major ABO incompatibility is generally prevented by removal of incompatible red cells from the product. If this is not feasible and the red cell content of the product is expected to be excessive, two to four daily TPEs may be performed to lower the relevant isoagglutinin titer to ≤1:16.[2] A number of strategies have been employed in the therapy of PRCA. In addition to erythropoietin to stimulate red cell production, residual recipient-antibody-producing cells may be targeted by withdrawal of anti-GVHD prophylaxis (eg, CSA) or addition of an anti-B-cell agent (eg, rituximab). Donor lymphocyte infusion has also been used successfully.[103] Intensive TPE may be used to deplete residual anti-donor antibodies. Some institutions would also use donor-type plasma replacement to aid in neutralization of the isoagglutinins. In marrow HPC transplants with minor ABO incompatibility, plasma removal is performed because of the large amount of plasma in marrow grafts. This step is unnecessary with small-volume apheresis HPC products. Finally, careful monitoring of hemoglobin and direct antiglobulin tests may be useful in the 1 to 2 weeks after a transplantation at risk for PLS. If there is evidence of hemolysis, an urgent red cell exchange can remove residual recipient red cells.

ABO-incompatible HPC transplantation is classified by ASFA as a Category II indication for TPE.[2] For further discussion of ABO-unmatched or ABO-incompatible organ transplantation, see Chapter 18.

Acquired Aplastic Anemia and Pure Red Cell Aplasia

Aplastic anemia (AA) and PRCA are stem cell disorders characterized by markedly decreased or absent hematopoietic activity in the marrow. The former involves all cell lines, resulting in a severely hypocellular marrow with pancytopenia; the latter involves selective depletion of erythrocytic precursors, resulting in anemia with minimal effect on white cell and platelet counts. Profound reticulocytopenia helps to distinguish these conditions from other causes of anemia. AA is frequently idiopathic but may result from destruction of hematopoietic precursors by a variety of agents, such as radiation, cytotoxic chemotherapy, chemicals such as benzene, and drugs (historically chloramphenicol and gold, but more commonly anticonvulsants, sulfonamides, and antithyroid medications). It can also occur secondary to viral infections, including Epstein-Barr virus (EBV) and hepatitis viruses (A, B, C, and G)[104,105]; acquired clonal disorders such as paroxysmal nocturnal hemoglobinuria; pregnancy; and autoimmune diseases.

PRCA also has multiple potential causes. Primary PRCA may be idiopathic, autoimmune, or preleukemic. Secondary associations include ABO-incompatible progenitor cell transplants (see above), thymomas, various hematologic and solid malignancies, drugs and chemicals, pregnancy, autoimmune/collagen vascular diseases, and a number of infections including human immunodeficiency virus, EBV, viral hepatitis, and, in immunosuppressed patients, parvovirus B19.[106]

Some evidence suggests that humoral immune mechanisms may be operative in some patients with either of these two conditions. This includes the positive responses of patients with AA to antilymphocyte sera and the finding of cytotoxic T lymphocytes in the marrow that produce the cytokines interferon γ and tumor necrosis factor β, both of which inhibit progenitor cell growth and stem cell analogs in tissue culture.[107,108] In AA, an IgG inhibitor isolated from serum in a case of systemic lupus erythematosus (SLE) and rheumatoid arthritis (RA) has been found to inhibit the growth of erythroid colonies, thus providing a potential rationale for TPE treatment.[106] A novel iatrogenic cause of PRCA has been identified in patients who develop erythropoietin antibodies as a result of treatment with erythropoietic stimulating agents.[2]

Therapy

Recognition and management of an underlying disease process, if present, is the initial step in therapy for both AA and PRCA. Discontinuation of offending drugs, such as recombinant human erythropoietin in PRCA or diphenylhydantoin in AA, or surgical resection of a thymoma in PRCA may be curative. Other approaches to therapy are suggested by the pathophysiology of these disorders: replacement of deficient hematopoietic cells by stem cell transplantation, or suppression of an autoimmune process. HPC transplantation from an HLA-matched donor has been recommended as the first-line therapy in patients 40 years of age or younger with severe AA. In patients who have milder disease or do not have a suitable stem cell donor, immunosuppressive therapy with antithymocyte globulin and/or cyclosporine may be successful. Therapy is generally given until remission is obtained; long-term immunosuppressive therapy may increase the risk of relapse and clonal transformation of marrow precursors.[109] Hematopoietic growth factors and androgens have also been used successfully in some patients.[110,111] Idiopathic or primary acquired PRCA is initially treated with corticosteroids. IVIG is effective in immunosuppressed patients infected with parvovirus B19, who cannot make neutralizing antibodies to this virus.[112] Matched, unrelated peripheral blood, marrow, or cord blood[113] transplantation may be undertaken if a matched, related donor is not available and immunosuppressive therapy has failed.

Role of Therapeutic Plasma Exchange

TPE is not considered primary therapy for AA or PRCA and is rarely used for these conditions. Although TPE has met with some success in isolated reports, no controlled randomized trials have been undertaken. In a few research studies, the finding of a serum inhibitory factor and/or an associated autoimmune disorder appeared to be correlated with response.[107,114] The literature for PRCA is also scant, but TPE has improved this condition in a few cases.[115-117] The absence of published studies since the 1980s indicates the lack of a recognized role of TPE in these disorders, though it might still be considered in patients who have failed to respond to immunosuppressive therapies. Removal of erythropoietin antibodies in patients with refractory anemia resulting from exposure to erythropoietic stimulating agents may also be considered.[2] No defined treatment schedules exist. ASFA has classified AA as a Category III indication for TPE, and PRCA as a Category II indication for TPE.[2]

Autoimmune Hemolytic Anemia

Autoimmune hemolytic anemia is caused by autoantibodies that bind to red cells and decrease their survival in the circulation. The autoantibody is often idiopathic but may also arise in the context of an autoimmune disease, a lymphoproliferative disorder, or an infection. Classification is based on the thermal reactivity of the autoantibody. In warm autoimmune hemolytic anemia (WAIHA), IgG antibodies maximally react with the target antigen at 37 C. Cold agglutinins are IgM antibodies that bind maximally at 4 C. These antibody characteristics lead to distinct pathophysiologic and clinical consequences, including the response to TPE.

Warm Autoimmune Hemolytic Anemia

The target antigen in WAIHA is usually a component of the Rh complex. IgG-coated red cells undergo accelerated destruction by attachment to Fc receptors on macrophages of the reticuloendothelial system (RES), primarily residing in the spleen. As the macrophages progressively remove opsonized portions of the red cell membrane, the red cells assume a spherocytic morphology, a characteristic feature of WAIHA. Spherocytes are less deformable than intact red cells, which increases susceptibility to splenic removal ("extravascular hemolysis"). Idiopathic WAIHA is most commonly seen in young women; the average age range is 20 to 30 and the female-to-male ratio is 3:1.[118] Symptoms may be mild, with the patient complaining of weakness, fatigue, jaundice, and low-grade fever. Alternatively, WAIHA may present as fulminant hemolysis with associated back pain, rapidly decreasing hematocrit, and severe malaise.

Therapy

Initial therapy in WAIHA is directed toward RES blockade and inhibiting antibody production to slow ongoing red cell destruction. Steroids are standard initial therapy. Although responses are seen in the majority of patients, less than 20% will remain in remission during steroid taper or after these drugs are withdrawn. Steroid-refractory patients may be managed with second-line immunomodulating agents such as IVIG; with immunosuppressive agents such as cyclophosphamide, azathioprine, or rituximab; or with splenectomy. Although it is used regularly, IVIG therapy produces transient remissions in only 40% of affected patients. Other therapies attempted in refractory patients or in those for whom splenectomy is contraindicated have included vincristine, danazol, and cyclosporine.[119]

Role of Therapeutic Plasma Exchange

Management of fulminant or treatment-refractory WAIHA with TPE has yielded inconsistent results, and it has been classified as a Category III indication for TPE by ASFA.[2] Apparent stabilization of active hemolysis has been reported in some cases.[120,121] Silberstein reported two patients who received three TPEs and had a decreased red cell transfusion requirement; however, the half-life of chromium-labeled autologous red cells appeared unchanged following the course of TPE.[122] Two studies reported improvement after TPE followed by

either IVIG or cyclophospamide in highly refractory patients.[123,124] More recent experience has been extended to drug-induced immune hemolysis in a report of oxaliplatin-induced hemolytic anemia improving with use of corticosteroids and TPE.[125] Balancing the salutary reports is a negative study in which TPE was not found to reduce the red cell transfusion requirement or improve the hemoglobin level at day 5 after treatment.[126] This study retrospectively analyzed 4 control and 5 TPE patients and found that a single TPE had no effect. However, the study did not test whether more aggressive use of TPE might be effective. TPE is generally reserved for severe cases of WAIHA, especially after failure of immunosuppressive therapy. A reasonable therapeutic trial would be to remove 1.5 plasma volumes every 1 to 2 days until hemolysis improves[2] or for a total of four to six treatments.[127]

Cold Agglutinin Hemolytic Anemia

Cold agglutinin disorders are also subdivided into primary (idiopathic) and secondary forms; the idiopathic form can be a type of paraproteinemia with an IgM monoclonal autoantibody. In idiopathic cold agglutinin syndrome (CAS), the antibody often contains kappa light chains and is present in very high titers, often greater than a million. Secondary CAS can arise from the immune response to certain infections, particularly mycoplasma pneumonia and infectious mononucleosis, and is usually self limited. A cold agglutinin that is reactive in the range of 30 C or higher is described as having a broad thermal amplitude and is more clinically relevant, regardless of the titer at lower temperatures.[128] At temperatures below 37 C, the IgM antibodies reversibly attach to red cells, typically binding to the branched polysaccharide "I" antigen.[118] Bound antibody fixes the early components of the classical complement cascade: C1, C4, and C2, followed by C3b. The antibody may then dissociate from the cell, leaving it coated only with complement. C3b-coated cells may be lysed directly by assembly of the C5-C9 membrane attack complex of complement (intravascular hemolysis) or may attach to a C3b receptor on hepatic RES cells and be phagocytosed (extravascular hemolysis). If C3b is converted to C3d by complement inactivators, the complement-coated cells may have a normal survival in the circulation.

Idiopathic CAS is a disorder of the elderly that displays no gender predilection. Patients frequently report symptoms of cold intolerance, such as acral cyanosis, caused by red cell sludging in the colder portions of the body. It generally results in mild, chronic anemia, with few acute exacerbations as long as cold exposure is avoided.

Therapy

Treatment is largely supportive. Corticosteroids and splenectomy are generally ineffective. Maintaining a warm ambient temperature is essential, particularly if the thermal amplitude of the cold agglutinin is broad. Transfusion therapy should be reserved for patients with marked symptomatic anemia, especially because the transfused red cells may be more susceptible to complement binding and hemolysis than the patient's own C3d-coated cells. Long-term stabilization can be achieved with alkylating agents such as chlorambucil or cyclophosphamide; in patients who are refractory to these agents, fludarabine may be effective.[128] An increasing number of reports describe responses to rituximab. Overall, 45% to 54% of patients treated have shown benefit; however, most have had only partial responses.[128]

Role of Therapeutic Plasma Exchange

Because the causative IgM antibodies are mainly intravascular and bind poorly to red cells at body temperature, TPE may significantly reduce antibody titer. Some studies in patients with severe CAS report improved red cell survival and clinical improvement after TPE.[122,129] Improvement after TPE may be transient, as cold agglutinin levels usually recover within 7 to 10 days without primary therapy.[130] A single report describes sustained improvement in two patients after synchronized therapy with cyclophosphamide following TPE.[124] Effectiveness of

TPE in paroxysmal cold antibody hemolysis ("Donath-Landsteiner" antibody) has also been observed.[131] Extracorporeal blood warming should be employed during TPE to lessen the risk of red cell agglutination in the apheresis circuit and worsening anemia. ASFA has designated CAS a Category II indication for TPE.[2]

Immune Thrombocytopenic Purpura

Immune thrombocytopenic purpura (ITP) is a relatively common autoimmune disorder caused by IgG antibodies to platelet glycoproteins. The IgG-coated platelets are removed by the RES, predominantly in the spleen. The most frequent membrane glycoprotein (GP) antigen targets are GPIIb/IIIa and GPIb/IX, which are expressed on both platelets and megakaryocytes.[132] Although ITP may occur at any age and in both genders, the female-to-male ratio is 3:1 and women aged 20 to 50 account for the majority of cases. The most common presentation is mucocutaneous bleeding, but intracranial hemorrhage is also a risk, particularly in elderly patients.[133,134] Patients typically have isolated thrombocytopenia with normal or increased megakaryocytes.[132]

Therapy

Specific treatment is not indicated for asymptomatic adults with chronic ITP if they only have thrombocytopenia of moderate severity (≥30,000/mL).[135] Corticosteroid treatment, generally prednisone at 1 mg/kg/day, is the first-line therapy for chronic ITP in adults and children. If rapid correction of the platelet count is needed to address serious bleeding or to prepare for surgery, IVIG, 2 g/kg over 2 to 5 days, may be given. In D-positive patients, intravenous Rh Immune Globulin has also been used to induce a "RES blockade" by saturating macrophage Fc receptors with antibody-coated red cells.[135] In steroid-resistant or dependent ITP, "second-line" immunomodulatory therapy consists of either splenectomy or rituximab. Approximately 10% to 15% of adult patients are refractory to both steroids and splenectomy. Licensure of thrombopoietin agonists, such as romiplostim and eltrombopag, has provided a new means to boost platelet production and improve platelet levels in ITP.[132] Other therapies with variable activity in ITP include danazol, vinca alkaloids, cyclophosphamide, azathioprine, and periodic infusion of IVIG or anti-D.

Role of Therapeutic Plasma Exchange

Advances in understanding the pathophysiology of ITP have led to the development of new and more effective pharmacologic agents in this disorder. TPE currently plays a very limited role, if any, in the treatment of ITP. Early reports of success using TPE were anecdotal[121,136] and have not been confirmed in controlled trials. One small controlled trial reported that patients treated with TPE and steroids relapsed less frequently, thus avoiding splenectomy.[137] A beneficial effect was also reported in two uncontrolled studies that combined TPE and IVIG.[138,139] Bussel reported a response in 4 of 8 patients previously refractory to IVIG and prednisone who were treated with TPE on 3 consecutive days followed by IVIG, 1 g/kg/day × 2 days. The response was temporary, however, with platelets dropping to baseline within 2 weeks. ASFA has classified ITP as a Category IV indication for TPE.[2]

Coagulation Factor Inhibitors

IgG inhibitors of specific coagulation factors may develop either as a result of autoimmunity or from alloimmune stimulation by factor replacement therapy in a patient with a congenital factor deficiency, most commonly hemophilia A. Acquired autoantibodies to Factor VIII are typically seen in the elderly, in patients with autoimmune disorders such as SLE, or as a complication of pregnancy. Factor VIII alloantibodies occur in 15% to 20% of patients with severe hemophilia A. Patients with autoantibodies typically present with soft tissue hemorrhage, especially into muscle and skin; hemarthroses are rare.[140] In contrast, patients with congenital hemophilia characteristically bleed into joint spaces. In both acquired and congenital coagulation inhibitor patients, conventional factor replacement therapy for significant bleeding episodes is ineffective, and alternative coagulation products are necessary to obtain hemostasis.

Therapy

A number of approaches have been developed to guide therapy for both types of Factor VIII inhibitors.[141,142] The goals are to achieve hemostasis during bleeding episodes and to suppress production of inhibitor. If the patient is bleeding, therapy depends on the inhibitor titer. High doses of recombinant Factor VIII (•100 IU/kg) are feasible only in the small percentage of cases with low-titer inhibitors [eg, <5 Bethesda units (BU)/mL]. Most patients require products containing activated coagulation factors [eg, FEIBA (Baxter, Vienna, Austria) or NovoSeven (NovoNordisk, Princeton, NJ)] to "bypass" the inhibitor. NovoSeven (recombinant Factor VIIa) has been used successfully for surgical hemostasis in such patients.[143,144] Production of autoimmune inhibitors may be suppressed with high-dose corticosteroids, either alone or in combination with cyclophosphamide, or with other immunosuppressive drugs including CSA.[145,146]

Role of Therapeutic Plasma Exchange

Experience using TPE in patients with clotting factor inhibitors consists of uncontrolled small case series and case reports. Successful management of a congenital hemophiliac who developed postoperative bleeding caused by a new inhibitor has been described.[147] Fourteen daily 4-liter TPEs were performed, resulting in a 90% reduction in inhibitor titer and cessation of bleeding in response to Factor VIII infusion. Transient increases in Factor VIII levels were documented. Another hemophilia A patient with Factor VIII antibodies underwent successful drainage of a psoas muscle abscess despite Factor VIII inhibitor titers as high as 203 BU, though only 15 BU when tested against porcine Factor VIII.[148] TPE on two separate occasions resulted in lowering the porcine inhibitor titer to 4 BU, and therapeutic levels of Factor VIII were achieved using bolus and continuous infusions of porcine Factor VIII.

Case reports also describe TPE for patients with acquired inhibitors in conjunction with immunosuppressive therapy (steroids, cyclophosphamide) plus Factor VIII concentrate, with successful resolution of hemorrhage.[149] In addition, such patients have been treated successfully with daily TPE of 2 to 3 plasma volumes for several days with FFP replacement.[150] Multiple TPEs may be necessary to achieve a reduction in the inhibitor titer. Considering the largely anecdotal evidence of benefit and the availability of increasingly effective and safe bypassing products, the risks associated with placement of a central catheter are difficult to justify in these patients.

TPE has been reported to be useful in other types of coagulation factor inhibitors, including those to Factors V and X, thrombin (as a result of the formation of cross-reactive antibodies from exposure to bovine topical thrombin used during surgery), and vWF (in acquired von Willebrand disease).[121,151] Immunoadsorption columns have also been used to selectively remove coagulation factor inhibitors (see Chapter 20).

Despite these reports, coagulation factor inhibitors are now classified by ASFA as a Category IV indication for TPE.[2]

If volume overload is a concern, TPE may be used in lieu of plasma infusion for rapid correction of factor levels (eg, preoperative treatment) in patients with deficiency of a rare coagulation factor for which a factor concentrate is not available (eg, Factors V, X, XI).

Posttransfusion Purpura

Posttransfusion purpura (PTP) is heralded by sudden, extreme thrombocytopenia occurring 2 to 14 days after transfusion. Most cases have occurred after transfusion of red cells. The condition is most often seen in previously healthy women who have been immunized to a platelet-specific antigen, most often human platelet antigen (HPA)-1a, through pregnancy.[87] Rare cases have been described in men.[152,153] Although PTP is an alloimmune phenomenon, the patient's own platelets are somehow destroyed, and the platelet count may decrease to 10,000/μL or lower. PTP often results in bleeding that may range from purpuric skin lesions to fatal intracranial hemorrhage.

Pathogenesis

In most cases, patients with PTP lack HPA-1a (formerly designated PLA[1]) and have made an alloantibody to it. PTP may also be associated with alloantibodies to other platelet-specific antigens, including HPA-1b, -2b, -3a, -3b, -4a, and -5b.[87,153,154] It is not clear why the patient's own antigen-negative platelets are destroyed. One idea postulates that immune complexes are formed between soluble HPA in donor plasma and platelet antibody in the patient.[155] These complexes bind to Fc receptors on the patient's platelets, thus leading to their destruction. A second explanation invokes the development of a platelet autoantibody after exposure to an incompatible platelet alloantigen.[155,156] The autoantibody binds to both the transfused platelets and the patient's own platelets, resulting in platelet destruction. A third hypothesis is that soluble HPA in donor plasma adsorbs to patient platelets, which then become susceptible to destruction by the alloantibody.[157] Finally, it has been proposed that antigen-positive platelets elicit a "cross-reactive" alloantibody that also binds the patient's antigen-negative platelets, resulting in their destruction.[87]

Therapy

Although the platelet count returns to normal over days to weeks, transfusion is often needed during the period of extreme thrombocytopenia. Random-donor platelets are ineffective in the usual doses; however, a massive transfusion of such platelets may be considered for life-threatening hemorrhage. Platelets negative for

HPA-1a have been reported effective in patients with serious bleeding.[158,159] Reports exist of improvement after high-dose steroids.[160,161] Consistent responses to IVIG have been observed, sometimes within hours of administration, even after failure of steroids and TPE.[162-164] IVIG also avoids the need for central venous catheterization in some patients. As a result, high-dose IVIG has become the primary therapy of choice for PTP patients. A total dose of 2 g/kg divided over 2 to 4 days is generally used.

Role of Therapeutic Plasma Exchange

In the era before IVIG use, both exchange transfusion and TPE appeared to be effective treatment for PTP, on the basis of historical results.[159,165,166] As evidence of a therapeutic response, thrombocytopenia recurred after cessation and improved after resumption of TPE in some cases. At the present time, however, there is little if any role for TPE unless IVIG is not tolerated or is unavailable. TPE given after use of IVIG has the potential to reverse the benefit afforded by IVIG and could theoretically worsen or delay recovery of the platelet count. PTP is classified by ASFA as a Category III indication for TPE.[2]

Therapeutic Plasma Exchange in Dysproteinemias

The dysproteinemias are characterized by excessive or aberrant immunoglobulin production. The abnormal immunoglobulins are usually monoclonal, as in multiple myeloma or Waldenström macroglobulinemia, but may occasionally be polyclonal, as in SLE or RA,[167,168] or a combination of the two, as in mixed cryoglobulinemia. Monoclonal immunoglobulins are referred to informally as paraproteins or M-proteins. An abnormal immunoglobulin may be of any class or subclass. Important clinical manifestations associated with dysproteinemias include hyperviscosity, hypervolemia, bleeding, renal failure, vasculitis, and peripheral neuropathy. This section focuses on disorders associated with hyperviscosity syndrome and cryoglobulinemia. For discussion of "myeloma kidney" (light-chain nephropathy), see Chapter 17; neuropathy associated with monoclonal proteins is discussed in Chapter 15.

Hyperviscosity Syndrome

The hyperviscosity syndrome is occasionally seen in patients with benign polyclonal B-cell proliferations such as SLE and RA; however, the vast majority of cases occur in the context of a clonal B-cell disorder, most commonly Waldenström macroglobulinemia, which is characterized by the production of monoclonal IgM by malignant plasmacytoid lymphocytes in the marrow. The disease occurs mainly in elderly people, with initial symptoms of fatigue and weight loss. Up to 70% of untreated patients may have hyperviscosity, which is responsible for the most serious clinical manifestations, including bleeding, neurologic symptoms, and visual loss. The fully developed hyperviscosity syndrome is characterized by various neurologic symptoms—headache, dizziness, vertigo, and nystagmus—eventually leading to mental status changes—somnolence, stupor, and coma. Retinal hemorrhages with exudates may also lead to visual impairment. A coagulation defect caused by interference with fibrin polymerization by abundant monoclonal protein may occur, resulting in an increased thrombin time.[169] Platelet adhesion and aggregation may also be affected. Anemia may be secondary to gastrointestinal tract bleeding or may be dilutional, resulting from an increase in plasma volume. Bence-Jones proteins (see below) are found in the urine of most patients with Waldenström macroglobulinemia; however, in contrast to multiple myeloma, renal disease in these patients is usually mild. A peripheral neuropathy may also be present.

Medical therapy of Waldenström macroglobulinemia is aimed at controlling B-cell proliferation using alkylating agents such as chlorambucil, either alone or in combination with corticosteroids, nucleoside analogs (fludarabine, 2-chlorodeoxyadenosine), and/or rituximab.[170]

Multiple myeloma is a malignant, monoclonal proliferation of plasma cells that synthesize immunoglobulins. The immunoglobulins may be complete, containing both heavy chains of a single class and light chains of a single type, either kappa or lambda. Most patients produce either gamma or alpha heavy chains. If light chains are produced in excess of heavy chains, free light chains will be excreted in the urine (Bence-Jones proteins). Deposition of light chains in the renal tubules may lead to renal failure. Hyperviscosity syndrome has also been observed in up to 5% of patients with multiple myeloma, predominantly with IgA paraproteins and less commonly with IgG.

Established treatment regimens include alkylating agents such as melphalan and cyclophosphamide, along with dexamethasone, or more intensive regimens such as vincristine, doxorubicin, and dexamethasone. However, myeloma therapy has been transformed in recent years, with immunodulating agents such as thalidomide, lenalidomide, and the proteosome inhibitor bortezomib assuming greater importance in disease control. In addition, autologous and allogeneic stem cell transplantation have resulted in improved patient survival.[170]

Cryoglobulinemia

Cryoglobulins are immunoglobulin proteins or protein complexes that precipitate at refrigerator temperatures. Three main types are recognized. Type I cryoglobulins consist of a single monoclonal protein, most commonly IgG or IgM, and are seen in myeloma, Waldenström macroglobulinemia, and other lymphoproliferative disorders. They may also occur as a chronic, idiopathic entity in older patients. Symptoms in such patients probably result from the cold precipitation characteristics of the cryoglobulin and include acrocyanosis, especially after cold exposure, and cutaneous ulcers resulting from vasocclusion.[118]

Type II cryoglobulins consist of a monoclonal immunoglobulin, usually IgM, which has rheumatoid factor activity, and polyclonal IgG. They are present in about 40% of patients with

chronic hepatitis C virus (HCV) infection[171] and can also occur in IgM lymphoproliferative disorders, autoimmune disease, and other conditions. Type III cryoglobulins are composed entirely of polyclonal immunoglobulins, usually IgM or IgG, and occasionally nonimmunoglobulin substances such as complement or viral antigens. In most of them, one constituent (most often IgM) has anti-IgG activity. Type III cryoglobulins may be associated with an infection such as hepatitis B virus, HCV, or subacute bacterial endocarditis, as well as with autoimmune conditions, but they may also exist without evidence of underlying disease. Symptoms of type II and III cryoglobulins are mainly manifestations of immune complex vasculitis.

Role of Therapeutic Plasma Exchange

TPE can reduce high levels of abnormal immunoglobulins in dysproteinemias and is useful to treat both hyperviscosity and cryoglobulinemia. Although TPE does not alter the course of the primary disease process, it may be used in conjunction with chemotherapy or other treatments that decrease paraprotein synthesis. TPE may also serve as the sole therapy for some patients; for example, elderly macroglobulinemia patients who may not tolerate chemotherapy.[172] Patients who are unresponsive to drug therapy may also be managed by chronic regular TPE.[173]

In hyperviscosity syndrome, high concentrations of immunoglobulin interfere with blood flow in the microcirculation and reduce oxygen delivery to vital organs. The protein level does not necessarily correlate with the blood viscosity and vascular complications.[174] Normal relative serum viscosity ranges from 1.5 to 1.8. Most patients will become symptomatic at relative serum viscosity levels of 4 to 6. The relationship between viscosity and immunoglobulin concentration is nonlinear, such that removal of a relatively small amount of immunoglobulin by TPE will result in a relatively large reduction in viscosity that usually translates into rapid improvement in symptoms.[175] One of the most gratifying experiences in apheresis practice is to witness such a patient "wake up" from a hyperviscosity-induced coma. TPE is also recommended prophylactically before rituximab therapy because of the temporary worsening of IgM levels reported within 4 to 5 weeks of drug administration.[176]

Clinically significant coagulopathies may occur in up to 15%, 40%, and 60% of patients with IgG, IgA, and IgM paraproteins, respectively.[169] TPE can improve coagulation abnormalities and abnormal bleeding in patients with multiple myeloma and other dysproteinemias.

Symptoms of cryoglobulinemia are directly attributable to the presence of the abnormal protein. Therefore, cryoglobulin removal by TPE should result in symptomatic improvement. The clinical evidence for this is presented in detail in Chapter 17. Some cryoglobulins precipitate with only slight decreases in temperature; TPE may therefore require the use of inline or centrifuge blood warmers to avoid precipitation in the apheresis instrument. Rarely, patients may need to have TPE performed at ambient temperatures of 37 C or higher until the concentration of cryoglobulin is reduced.[174]

Colloid replacement fluids used in TPE to treat dysproteinemias are usually either 5% albumin or a mixture of 5% albumin and crystalloid solution (eg, 75:25 ratio). Single-plasma-volume exchanges are most commonly used. It should be noted that the actual plasma volume may exceed the calculated volume in these patients, so the fall in paraprotein level may be less than expected.

The frequency and duration of TPE therapy in the dysproteinemias should be customized to the individual patient. The formation and elimination kinetics of paraproteins depend on their composition and the effects of pharmacologic agents that may be used as primary therapy. In hyperviscosity caused by macroglobulinemia, a single 1.0- to 1.5-plasma-volume TPE with 50% to 80% albumin/50% to 20% normal saline replacement is generally sufficient to lower serum viscosity to a safe range for a number of days. This is because of the predominantly intravascular distribution of IgM. Hyperviscosity syndrome caused by IgG or IgA multiple myeloma or polyclonal proteins may require more frequent treatment. For cryoglobulinemia with skin vasculitis and/or renal insufficiency, TPE should be performed daily or every other day for a total of five or six sessions, followed by clinical and laboratory reassessment. Weekly to monthly maintenance may be valuable to prevent symptom recurrence or worsening renal function. Paraprotein removal is measured by appropriate quantitative immunoglobulin studies, cryoglobulin levels, or serum viscosity, as indicated. Both cryoglobulinemia and the hyperviscosity syndrome are classified as Category I indications for TPE by ASFA.[2]

Summary

TPE serves as the major therapeutic intervention in TTP and has dramatically improved patient outcome. Knowledge accumulated over the past decade regarding ADAMTS13 in the etiology of TTP has further validated the role of TPE. The usefulness of TPE in other forms of thrombotic microangiopathy continues to be the subject of clinical investigations. TPE continues to be the most effective way to manage hyperviscosity syndrome and is often valuable in treatment of cryoglobulinemia. It may be useful in select cases of ABO-mismatched progenitor cell transplantation. Results of TPE in AA and PRCA have been generally disappointing. Other hematologic disorders in which plasma exchange has limited application include autoimmune hemolytic anemia, coagulation factor inhibitors, and ITP.

References

1. Schwab PH, Fahey JL. Treatment of Waldenström's macroglobulinemia by plasmapheresis. N Engl J Med 1960;263:574-9.
2. Szczepiorkowski ZM, Winters JL, Bandarenko N, et al. Guidelines on the use of therapeutic apheresis in clinical practice—evidence-based approach from the Apheresis Applications Committee of the American Society for Apheresis. The fifth special issue. J Clin Apher 2010; 25:83-177.

3. Clark WF, Rock GA, Buskard N, et al. Therapeutic plasma exchange: An update from the Canadian Apheresis Group. Ann Intern Med 1999;131:453-62.
4. Moschcowitz E. Hyaline thrombosis of the terminal arterioles and capillaries: A hitherto undescribed disease. Proc N Y Pathol Soc 1924; 24:21-4.
5. Amorosi EL, Ultmann JE. Thrombotic thrombocytopenic purpura: Report of 16 cases and review of the literature. Medicine 1966;45: 139-59.
6. Uchida T, Wada H, Mizutani M, et al. Identification of novel mutations in ADAMTS13 in an adult patient with congenital thrombotic thrombocytopenic purpura. Blood 2004;104: 2081-3.
7. Vesely SK, George JN, Lammle B, et al. ADAMTS13 activity in thrombotic thrombocytopenic purpura-hemolytic uremic syndrome: Relation to presenting features and clinical outcomes in a prospective cohort of 142 patients. Blood 2003;102:60-8.
8. Zheng XL, Kaufman RM, Goodnough LT, Sadler JE. Effect of plasma exchange on plasma ADAMTS13 metalloprotease activity, inhibitor level, and clinical outcome in patients with idiopathic and nonidiopathic thrombotic thrombocytopenic purpura. Blood 2004;103: 4043-9.
9. Mori Y, Wada H, Gabazza EC, et al. Predicting response to plasma exchange in patients with thrombotic thrombocytopenic purpura with measurement of vWF-cleaving protease activity. Transfusion 2002;42:572-80.
10. Kavanagh D, Goodship THJ, Richards A. Atypical hemolytic uremic syndrome. Br Med Bull 2006;77-78:5-22.
11. Tsai HM. Advances in the pathogenesis, diagnosis, and treatment of thrombotic thrombocytopenic purpura. J Am Soc Nephrol 2003;14: 1072-81.
12. Gruszecki AC, Wehrli G, Ragland BD, et al. Management of a patient with HIV infection-induced anemia and thrombocytopenia who presented with thrombotic thrombocytopenic purpura. Am J Hematol 2002;69:228-31.
13. Becker S, Fusco G, Fusco J, et al. HIV-associated thrombotic microangiopathy in the era of highly active antiretroviral therapy: An observational study. Clin Infect Dis 2004;39(Suppl 5):S267-75.
14. Tsai HM, Rice L, Sarode R, et al. Antibody inhibitors to von Willebrand factor metalloproteinase and increased binding of von Willebrand factor to platelets in ticlopidine-associated thrombotic thrombocytopenic purpura. Ann Intern Med 2000;132:794-9.
15. Zakarija A, Bennett C. Drug-induced thrombotic microangiopathy. Semin Thromb Hemost 2005;31:681-90.
16. Bennett CL, Kim B, Zakarija A, et al; SERF-TTP Research Group. Two mechanistic pathways for thienopyridine-associated thrombotic thrombocytopenic purpura: A report from the SERF-TTP Research Group and the RADAR Project. J Am Coll Cardiol 2007;50:1138-43.
17. Park YA, Hay SN, King KE, et al. Is it quinine TTP/HUS or quinine TMA? ADAMTS13 levels and implications for therapy. J Clin Apher 2009;24:115-19.
18. George JN. The association of pregnancy with thrombotic thrombocytopenic purpura-hemolytic uremic syndrome. Curr Opin Hematol 2003; 10:339-44.
19. Martin JN, Files JC, Blake PG, et al. Pregnancy complicated by preeclampsia-eclampsia with the syndrome of hemolysis, elevated liver enzymes, and low platelet count: How rapid is postpartum recovery? Obstet Gynecol 1990; 76:737-41.
20. Martin JN, Files JC, Blake PG, et al. Postpartum plasma exchange for atypical preeclampsia-eclampsia as HELLP (hemolysis, elevated liver enzymes, and low platelets) syndrome. Am J Obstet Gynecol 1995;172:1107-27.
21. George JN, Li X, McMinn JR, et al. Thrombotic thrombocytopenic purpura-hemolytic uremic syndrome following allogeneic HPC transplantation: A diagnostic dilemma. Transfusion 2004; 44:294-304.
22. Qu L, Kiss JE. Thrombotic microangiopathy in transplantation and malignancy. Semin Thromb Hemost 2005;31:691-9.
23. Ho VT, Cutler C, Carter S, et al. Blood and Marrow Transplant Clinical Trials Network Toxicity Committee consensus summary: Thrombotic microangiopathy after hematopoietic stem cell transplantation. Biol Blood Marrow Transplant 2005;11:571-5.
24. Allford SL, Hunt BJ, Rose P, Machin SJ. Guidelines on the diagnosis and management of the thrombotic microangiopathic haemolytic anaemias. Br J Haematol 2003;120:556-73.
25. Symmers WC. Thrombotic microangiopathic haemolytic anaemia (thrombotic microangiopathy). Br Med J 1952;2:897-903.

26. Moake JL, Rudy CK, Troll JH, et al. Unusually large plasma factor VIII:von Willebrand factor multimers in chronic relapsing thrombotic thrombocytopenic purpura. N Engl J Med 1982;307:1432-5.

27. Moake JL, Turner NA, Stathopoulos NA, et al. Involvement of large plasma von Willebrand factor (vWF) multimers and unusually large vWF forms derived from endothelial cells in shear stress-induced platelet aggregation. J Clin Invest 1986;78:1456-61.

28. Tsai HM, Chun-Yet Lian E. Antibodies to von Willebrand factor-cleaving protease in acute thrombotic thrombocytopenic purpura. N Engl J Med 1998;339:1585-94.

29. Furlan M, Robles R, Galbusera M, et al. Von Willebrand factor-cleaving protease in thrombotic thrombocytopenic purpura and the hemolytic-uremic syndrome. N Engl J Med 1998;339:1578-84.

30. Levy GG, Nichols WC, Lian EC, et al. Mutations in a member of the ADAMTS gene family cause thrombotic thrombocytopenic purpura. Nature 2001;413:488-94.

31. Padilla A, Moake JL, Bernardo A, et al. P-selectin anchors newly released ultralarge von Willebrand factor multimers to the endothelial cell surface. Blood 2004;103:6:2150-6.

32. Dong JF, Moake JL, Nolasco L, et al. ADAMTS-13 rapidly cleaves newly secreted ultra large von Willebrand factor multimers on the endothelial surface under flowing conditions. Blood 2002;100:4033-9.

33. Bernardo A, Ball C, Nolasco L, et al. Effects of inflammatory cytokines on the release and cleavage of the endothelial cell-derived ultralarge von Willebrand factor multimers under flow. Blood 2004;104:100-6.

34. Coppo P, Bengoufa D, Veyradier A, et al. Severe ADAMTS13 deficiency in adult idiopathic thrombotic microangiopathies defines a subset of patients characterized by various autoimmune manifestations, lower platelet count, and mild renal involvement. Medicine 2004;83:233-44.

35. Studt JD, Kremer Hovinga JA, Antoine G, et al. Fatal congenital thrombotic thrombocytopenic purpura with apparent ADAMTS13 inhibitor activity by hemoglobin. Blood 2005;105:542-4.

36. Davis AK, Makar RS, Stowell CP, et al. ADAMTS13 binds to CD36: A potential mechanism for platelet and endothelial localization of ADAMTS13. Transfusion 2009;49:206-13.

37. Pereira A, Mazzara R, Monteagudo J, et al. Thrombotic thrombocytopenic purpura/hemolytic uremic syndrome: A multivariate analysis of factors predicting the response to plasma exhchange. Ann Hematol 1995;70:319-23.

38. Hawkins BM, Abu-Fadel M, Vesely SK, et al. Clinical cardiac involvement in thrombotic thrombocytopenic purpura: A systematic review. Transfusion 2008;48:382-92.

39. Sarode R. Atypical presentations of thrombotic thrombocytopenic purpura: A review. J Clin Apher 2009;24:47-52.

40. George JN, Terrell DR, Swisher KK, Vesely SK. Lessons learned from the Oklahoma thrombotic thrombocytopenic purpura-hemolytic uremic syndrome registry. J Clin Apher 2008;23:129-37.

41. Scully M, Yarranton H, Liesner R, et al. Regional UK TTP registry: Correlation with laboratory ADAMTS 13 analysis and clinical features. Br J Haematol 2008;142:819-26.

42. Matsumoto M, Yagi H, Ishizashi H, et al. The Japanese experience with thrombotic thrombocytopenic purpura-hemolytic uremic syndrome. Semin Hematol 2004;41:68-74.

43. Antoine G, Zimmermann K, Plaimauer B, et al. ADAMTS13 gene defects in two brothers with constitutional thrombotic thrombocytopenic purpura and normalization of von Willebrand factor-cleaving protease activity by recombinant human ADAMTS13. Br J Haematol 2003;120:821-4.

44. Scheiflinger F, Knöbl P, Trattner B, et al. Non-neutralizing IgM and IgG antibodies to von Willebrand factor-cleaving protease (ADAMTS-13) in a patient with thrombotic thrombocytopenic purpura. Blood 2003;102:3241-3.

45. Veyradier A, Obert B, Houllier A, et al. Specific von Willebrand factor-cleaving protease in thrombotic microangiopathies: A study of 111 cases. Blood 2001;98:1765-72.

46. Peyvandi F, Lavoretano S, Palla R, et al. ADAMTS13 and anti-ADAMTS13 antibodies as markers for recurrence of acquired thrombotic thrombocytopenic purpura during remission. Haematologica 2008;93:232-9.

47. Mannucci PM, Peyvandi F. TTP and ADAMTS13: When is testing appropriate? Hematology Am Soc Hematol Educ Program 2007;121-6.

48. Rieger M, Mannucci PM, Hovinga JAK, et al. ADAMTS13 autoantibodies in patients with thrombotic microangiopathies and other

immunomediated diseases. Blood 2005;106: 1262-7.

49. Karpac CA, Li X, Terrell DR, et al. Sporadic bloody diarrhoea-associated thrombotic thrombocytopenic purpura-haemolytic uraemic syndrome: An adult and paediatric comparison. Br J Haematol 2008;141:696-707.

50. Melnyk AMS, Solez K, Kjellstrand CM. Adult hemolytic-uremic syndrome. Arch Intern Med 1995;155:2077-84.

51. Kiss JE. Thrombotic thrombocytopenic purpura: Recognition and management. Int J Hematol 2010;91:36-45.

52. Sadler JE. Von Willebrand factor, ADAMTS13, and thrombotic thrombocytopenic purpura. Blood 2008;112:11-18.

53. Böhm M, Betz C, Miesbach W, et al. The course of ADAMTS-13 activity and inhibitor titre in the treatment of thrombotic thrombocytopenic purpura with plasma exchange and vincristine. Br J Haematol 2005;129:644-52.

54. Raife T, Atkinson B, Montgomery R, et al. Severe deficiency of vWF-cleaving protease (ADAMTS13) activity defines a distinct population of thrombotic microangiopathy patients. Transfusion 2004;44:146-50.

55. Ferrari S, Scheiflinger F, Rieger M, et al. Prognostic value of anti-ADAMTS13 antibody features (Ig isotype, titer, and inhibitory effect) in a cohort of 35 adult French patients undergoing a first episode of thrombotic microangiopathy with undetectable ADAMTS13 activity. Blood 2007;109:2815-22.

56. Rock GA, Shumak KH, Buskard NA, et al. Comparison of plasma exchange with plasma infusion in the treatment of thrombotic thrombocytopenic purpura. The Canadian Apheresis Study Group. N Engl J Med 1991;325:393-7.

57. Henon P. Treatment of thrombotic thrombopenic purpura. Results of a multicenter randomized clinical study. Presse Med 1991;20: 1761-7.

58. Bobbio-Pallavincini E, Gugliotta L, Centurioni R, et al. Antiplatelet agents in thrombotic thrombocytopenic purpura (TTP). Results of a randomized multicenter trial by the Italian Cooperative Group for TTP. Haematologica 1997;82:429-35.

59. Zeigler Z, Shadduck RK, Gryn JF, et al. Cryoprecipitate poor plasma does not improve early response in primary adult thrombotic thrombocytopenic purpura. J Clin Apher 2001;16:19-22.

60. Rock GA, Anderson D, Clark W, et al. Does cryosupernatant plasma improve outcome in thrombotic thrombocytopenic purpura? No answer yet. Br J Haematol 2005;129;79-86.

61. Mintz PD, Neff A, MacKenzie M, et al. A randomized controlled Phase III trial of therapeutic plasma exchange with fresh-frozen plasma (FFP) prepared with amotosalen and ultraviolet A light compared to untreated FFP in thrombotic thrombocytopenic purpura. Transfusion 2006;46:1659-62.

62. Scott EA, Puca KE, Pietz BC, et al. Comparison and stability of ADAMTS13 activity in therapeutic plasma products. Transfusion 2007;47: 120-5.

63. Rock G, Shumak KH, Sutton DM, et al. Cryosupernatant as replacement fluid for plasma exchange in thrombotic thrombocytopenic purpura. Br J Haematol 1996;94:383-6.

64. Fontana S, Kremer Hovinga JA, Lämmle B, Taleghani BM. Treatment of thrombotic thrombocytopenic purpura. Vox Sang 2006;90:245-54.

65. Hay SN, Egan JA, Millward PA, et al. Patterns of platelet response in idiopathic TTP/HUS: Frequency of declining platelet counts with plasma exchange and the recognition and significance of a pseudo-refractory state. Ther Apher Dial 2006;10:237-41.

66. Cohen JA, Brecher ME, Bandarenko N. Cellular source of serum lactate dehydrogenase elevation in patients with thrombotic thrombocytopenic purpura. J Clin Apher 1998;13:16-19.

67. Egan JA, Hay SN, Brecher ME. Frequency and significance of schistocytes in TTP/HUS patients at the discontinuation of plasma exchange therapy. J Clin Apher 2004;19:165-7.

68. Bandarenko N. United States Thrombotic Thrombocytopenic Purpura Apheresis Study Group (US TTP ASG): Multicenter survey and retrospective analysis of current efficacy of therapeutic plasma exchange. J Clin Apher 1998;13:133-41.

69. Rose M, Eldor A. High incidence of relapses in thrombotic thrombocytopenic purpura. Clinical study of 38 subjects. Am J Med 1987;83:437-44.

70. Onundarson PT, Rowe JM, Heal JM, Francis CW. Response to plasma exchange and splenectomy in thrombotic thrombocytopenic purpura. Ann Intern Med 1992;152:791-6.

71. Nguyen L, Terrell DR, Duvall D, et al. Complications of plasma exchange in patients treated for thrombotic thrombocytopenic purpura. Transfusion 2009;49:392-4.

72. Knöbl P, Jilma B, Gilbert JC, et al. Anti-von Willebrand factor aptamer ARC1779 for refractory thrombotic thrombocytopenic purpura. Transfusion 2009;49:2181-5.

73. Bell WR, Braine HG, Ness PM, Kickler TS. Improved survival in thrombotic thrombocytopenic purpura-hemolytic uremic syndrome. Clinical experience in 108 patients. N Engl J Med 1991;325:398-403.

74. Ziman A, Mitri M, Klapper E, et al. Combination vincristine and plasma exchange as initial therapy in subjects with thrombotic thrombocytopenic purpura: One institution's experience and review of the literature. Transfusion 2005;45:41-9.

75. George JN, Woodson RD, Kiss JE, et al. Rituximab therapy for thrombotic thrombocytopenic purpura: A proposed study of the transfusion medicine/hemostasis clinical trials network with a systematic review of rituximab therapy for immune-mediated disorders. J Clin Apher 2006;21:49-56.

76. Ferrara F, Copia C, Annunziata M, et al. Vincristine as salvage treatment for refractory thrombotic thrombocytopenic purpura. Ann Hematol 1999;78:521-3.

77. Crowther MA, Heddle N, Hayward CP, et al. Splenectomy done during hematologic remission to prevent relapse in subjects with thrombotic thrombocytopenic purpura. Ann Intern Med 1996;125:294-6.

78. Cataland SR, Jin M, Ferketich AK, et al. An evaluation of cyclosporine and corticosteroids individually as adjuncts to plasma exchange in the treatment of thrombotic thrombocytopenic purpura. Br J Haematol 2006;132:146-9.

79. Cataland SR, Jin M, Zheng XL, et al. An evaluation of cyclosporine alone for the treatment of early recurrences of thrombotic thrombocytopenic purpura. J Thromb Haemost 2006;4:1162-4.

80. Cartron G, Watier H, Golay J, et al. From the bench to the bedside: Ways to improve rituximab efficacy. Blood 2004;104:2635-42.

81. Reff ME, Carner K, Chambers KS, et al. Depletion of B-cells in vivo by a chimeric mouse human monoclonal antibody to CD20. Blood 1994;83:435-45.

82. Fakhouri F, Vernant JP, Veyradier A, et al. Efficiency of curative and prophylactic treatment with rituximab in ADAMTS13-deficient thrombotic thrombocytopenic purpura: A study of 11 cases. Blood 2005;106:1932-7.

83. Elliott MA, Heit J, Pruthi RK, et al. Rituximab for refractory and or relapsing thrombotic thrombocytopenic purpura related to immune-mediated severe ADAMTS13 deficiency: A report of four cases and a systematic review of the literature. Eur J Haematol 2009;83:365-72.

84. Millward PM, Bandarenko N, Stagg KF, et al. Cardiogenic shock complicates successful treatment of refractory TTP with rituximab. Transfusion 2005;45:1481-6.

85. Tsai HM, Shulman K. Rituximab induces remission of cerebral ischemia caused by thrombotic thrombocytopenic purpura. Eur J Haematol 2003;70:183-5.

86. Yomtovian R, Niklinski W, Silver B, et al. Rituximab for chronic recurring thrombotic thrombocytopenic purpura: A case report and review of the literature. Br J Haematol 2004;124:787-95.

87. Klein HG, Anstee DJ. Some unfavourable effects of transfusion. In: Mollison's blood transfusion in clinical medicine. 11th ed. Malden, MA: Blackwell, 2005:666-700.

88. Rowley SD, Liang PS, Ulz L. Transplantation of ABO-incompatible bone marrow and peripheral blood stem cell components. Bone Marrow Transplant 2000;26:749-57.

89. Seebach JD, Stussi G, Passweg JR, et al. ABO blood group barrier in allogeneic bone marrow transplantation revisited. Biol Blood Marrow Transplant 2005;11:1006-13.

90. Dahl D, Hahn A, Koenecke C, et al. Prolonged isolated red blood cell transfusion requirement after allogeneic blood stem cell transplantation: Identification of patients at risk. Transfusion 2010;50:649-55.

91. Stroncek DF, Caly ME, Smith J, et al. Composition of peripheral blood progenitor cell components collected from healthy donors. Transfusion 1997;37:411-17.

92. Yazer MH, Triulzi DJ. Immune hemolysis following ABO-mismatched stem cell or solid organ transplantation. Curr Opin Hematol 2007;14:664-70.

93. Stussi G, Halter J, Subcheli E, et al. Prevention of pure red cell aplasia after major or bidirectional ABO blood group incompatible hematopoietic stem cell transplantation by pretransplant reduction of host anti-donor isoagglutinins. Haematologica 2008;94:239-48.

94. Griffith LM, McCoy JP Jr, Bolan CD, et al. Persistence of recipient plasma cells and anti-donor isohaemagglutinins in patients with delayed donor erythropoiesis after major ABO incompatible non-myeloablative haematopoietic cell transplantation. Br J Haematol 2005; 128:668-75.

95. Schetelig J, Breitschaft A, Kroger N, et al. After major ABO-mismatched allogeneic hematopoietic progenitor cell transplantation, erythroid engraftment occurs later in patients with donor blood group A than donor blood group B. Transfusion 2005;45:779-87.

96. Malfuson JV, Amor RB, Bonin P, et al. Impact of nonmyeloablative conditioning regimens on the occurrence of pure red cell aplasia after ABO-incompatible allogeneic haematopoietic stem cell transplantation. Vox Sang 2007;92: 85-9.

97. Bolan CD, Childs RW, Procter JL, et al. Massive immune haemolysis after allogeneic peripheral blood stem cell transplantation with minor ABO incompatibility. Br J Haematol 2001;112: 787-95.

98. Bolan CD, Leitman SF, Griffith LM, et al. Delayed donor red cell chimerism and pure red cell aplasia following major ABO-incompatible nonmyeloablative hematopoietic stem cell transplantation. Blood 2001;98:1687-94.

99. Ramsey G, Nusbacker J, Starzl TE, et al. Isohemoagglutinins of graft origin after ABO-unmatched liver transplantation. N Engl J Med 1984;311:1167-70.

100. Cserti-Gazdewich CM, Waddell TK, Singer LG, et al. Passenger lymphocyte syndrome with or without immune hemolytic anemia in all Rh-positive recipients of lungs from rhesus alloimmunized donors: Three new cases and a review of the literature. Transfus Med Rev 2009;23:134-45.

101. Korbling M, Huh YO, Durett A. Allogeneic blood stem cell transplantation: Peripheralization and yield of donor-derived primitive hematopoietic progenitor cells (CD34+ Thy-1dim) and lymphoid subsets, and possible predictors of engraftment and graft-versus-host disease. Blood 1995;86:2842-8.

102. Petz LD. Immune hemolysis associated with transplantation. Semin Hematol 2005;42:145-55.

103. Ebihara Y, Manabe A, Tsuruta T, et al. The effect of donor leukocyte infusion on refractory pure red blood cell aplasia after allogeneic stem cell transplantation in a patient with myelodysplastic syndrome developing from Kostmann Syndrome. Int J Haematol 2007;86: 446-50.

104. Sato S, Fuchinoue S, Abe M, et al. Successful cytokine treatment of aplastic anemia following living-related orthotopic liver transplantation for non-A, non-B, non-C hepatitis. Clin Transplant 1999;13:68-71.

105. Stachel D, Schmid I, Lang T, et al. Double bone marrow transplantation for severe aplastic anemia after orthotopic liver transplantation: Implications for clinical management and immune tolerance. Transplant Int 2002;15:39-44.

106. Dessypris EN. Pure red cell aplasia. In: Hoffman R, Benz EJ, Shattil SJ, eds. Hematology: Basic principles and practice. Philadelphia: Elsevier, 2005:429-39.

107. Young NS, Barrett AJ. The treatment of severe acquired aplastic anemia. Blood 1995;85: 3367-77.

108. Maciejewski JP, Hibbs JR, Anderson S, et al. Bone marrow and peripheral blood lymphocyte type in patients with bone marrow failure. Exp Hematol 1994;22:1102-10.

109. Killick SB, Marsh JC. Aplastic anemia: Management. Blood Rev 2000;14:157-71.

110. Means RT Jr, Dessypris EN, Krantz SB. Treatment of refractory pure red cell aplasia with cyclosporine A: Disappearance of IgG inhibitor associated with clinical response. Br J Haematol 1991;78:114-19.

111. Ball SE. The modern management of aplastic anemia. Br J Haematol 2000;110:41-53.

112. Ballester OF, Saba HI, Moscinski LC, et al. Pure red cell aplasia: Treatment with intravenous immunoglobulin concentrate. Semin Hematol 1992;29(Suppl 2):106-8.

113. Mao P, Liao C, Zhu Z, et al. Umbilical cord blood transplantation from unrelated HLA-matched donor in an adult with severe aplastic anemia. Bone Marrow Transplant 2000;26: 1121-3.

114. Abdou NI. Plasma exchange in the treatment of aplastic anemia. In: Tindall RSA, ed. Therapeutic apheresis and plasma perfusion. New York: Alan R. Liss, 1982:337-46.

115. Messner HA, Fause AA, Curtis JE, et al. Control of antibody-mediated pure red cell aplasia by plasmapheresis. N Engl J Med 1981;304: 1334-8.

116. Freund LG, Hippe E, Strandgaard S, et al. Complete remission in pure red cell aplasia after

plasmapheresis. Scand J Hematol 1985;35: 351-8.

117. Khelif A, Van HV, Tremisi JP, et al. Remission of acquired pure red cell aplasia following plasma exchanges. Scand J Hematol 1985;35: 13-17.

118. Winkelstein A, Kiss JE. Immunohematologic disorders. JAMA 1997;278:1982-92.

119. Cunningham MJ, Silberstein LE. Autoimmune hemolytic anemias. In: Hoffman R, Benz EJ, Shattil SJ, eds. Hematology: Basic principles and practice. Philadelphia: Elsevier, 2005: 693-707.

120. Kutti J, Wadenvik H, Safai-Kutti, et al. Successful treatment of refractory autoimmune haemolytic anemia by plasmapheresis. Scand J Haematol 1984;32:149-52.

121. Isbister JP, Biggs JC, Penny R. Experience with large volume plasmapheresis in malignant paraproteinemia and immune disorders. Aust N Z J Med 1978;8:154-64.

122. Silberstein LE, Berkman EM. Plasma exchange in autoimmune hemolytic anemia. J Clin Apher 1983;1:238-42.

123. Hughes P, Toogood A. Plasma exchange as a necessary prerequisite for the induction of remission by human immunoglobulin in autoimmune haemolytic anemia. Acta Haematol 1994;91:166-9.

124. Silva VA, Seder RH, Weintraub LR. Synchronization of plasma exchange and cyclophosphamide in severe and refractory autoimmune hemolytic anemia. J Clin Apher 1994;9:120-3.

125. Buti S, Ricco M, Chiesa MD, et al. Oxaliplatin-induced hemolytic anemia during adjuvant treatment of a patient with colon cancer: A case report. Anticancer Drugs 2007;18:297-300.

126. Ruivard M, Tournilhac O, Montel S, et al. Plasma exchanges do not increase red blood cell transfusion efficiency in severe autoimmune hemolytic anemia: A retrospective case-control study. J Clin Apher 2006;21:202-6.

127. Therapeutic plasma exchange. In: Winters JL, Gottschal JL, eds. Therapeutic apheresis: A physician's handbook. 2nd ed. Bethesda, MD: AABB, 2008.

128. Petz LD. Cold antibody autoimmune hemolytic anemias. Blood Rev 2008;22:1-15.

129. Valbonesi M, Guzzini D, Zerbi D, et al. Successful plasma exchange for a patient with chronic demyelinating polyneuropathy and cold agglutinin disease due to anti-Pra. J Clin Apher 1986;3:109-10.

130. McLeod B, Strauss RG, Ciavarella D, et al. Clinical applications of therapeutic apheresis; hematological disorders and cancer. J Clin Apher 1993;8:211-30.

131. Roy-Burman A, Glader BE. Resolution of severe Donath-Landsteiner autoimmune hemolytic anemia temporally associated with institution of plasmapheresis. Crit Care Med 2002;30: 931-4.

132. Nugent D, McMillan R, Nichol JL, et al. Pathogenesis of chronic immune thrombocytopenia: Increased platelet destruction and/or decreased platelet production. Br J Haematol 2009;146: 585-96.

133. Cortelazzo S, Finazzi G, Buelli M, et al. High risk of severe bleeding in aged patients with idiopathic thrombocytopenic purpura. Blood 1991;77:31-3.

134. Stasi R, Stipa E, Masi M, et al. Long-term observation of 208 adults with chronic idiopathic thrombocytopenic purpura. Am J Med 1995; 98:436-42.

135. Stasi R, Provan D. Management of immune thrombocytopenic purpura in adults. Mayo Clin Proc 2004;79:504-22.

136. Branda RF, Tate DY, McCullough JJ, et al. Plasma exchange in the treatment of fulminant idiopathic (autoimmune) thrombocytopenic purpura. Lancet 1978;i:688-91.

137. Marder VJ, Nusbacher J, Anderson FW. One-year follow-up of plasma exchange therapy in 14 patients with idiopathic thrombocytopenic purpura. Transfusion 1981;21:291-8.

138. Jungi TW, Nydegger UE. Plasma exchange and intravenous immunoglobulin infusion: Antagonistic effects on mononuclear phagocyte functions with potential implications for therapy. Prog Clin Biol Res 1990;337:429-33.

139. Bussel JB, Saal S, Gordon B. Combined plasma exchange and intravenous gammaglobulin in the treatment of patients with refractory immune thrombocytopenic purpura. Transfusion 1988;28:38-41.

140. Ludlam CA, Morrison AE, Kessler C. Treatment of acquired hemophilia. Semin Hematol 1994;31(Suppl 4):16-19.

141. Garvey MB. Incidence and management of patients with acquired Factor VIII inhibitors: The practical experience of a tertiary care hospital. In: Kessler CM, ed. Acquired hemophilia. Princeton, NJ: Excerpta Medica, 1995:91-111.

142. Kessler CM. Factor VIII inhibitors—an algorithmic approach to treatment. Semin Hematol 1994;31(Suppl 4):33-6.

143. Shapiro AD, Gilchrist GS, Hoots WK, et al. Prospective, randomized trial of two doses of rFVIIa (NovoSeven) in haemophilia patients with inhibitors undergoing surgery. Thromb Haemost 1998;80:773-8.

144. Carr ME, Loughran TP, Cardea JA, et al. Successful use of recombinant factor VIIa for hemostasis during total knee replacement in a severe hemophiliac with high-titer factor VIII inhibitor. Int J Hematol 2002;75:95-9.

145. Lusher JM. Management of patients with Factor VIII inhibitors. Transf Med Rev 1987;1:123-30.

146. Pflieger G, Boda Z, H'arsfalvi J, et al. Cyclosporin treatment of a woman with acquired hemophilia due to factor VIII:C inhibitor. Postgrad Med J 1989;65:400-2.

147. Slocombe GW, Newland AC, Colvin MP, et al. The role of intensive plasma exchange in the prevention and management of haemorrhage in patients with inhibitors to factor VIII. Br J Haematol 1981;47:577-85.

148. Bona RD, Pasquale DN, Kalish RI, et al. Porcine factor VIII and plasmapheresis in the management of hemophiliac patients with inhibitors. Am J Hematol 1986;21:201-7.

149. Pintado T, Taswell HF, Bowie EJW. Treatment of life-threatening hemorrhage due to acquired factor VIII inhibitor. Blood 1975;46:535-41.

150. Pineda AA. Therapeutic applications of plasma exchange and cytapheresis. In: Hamburger HA, Batsakis JG, eds. Clinical laboratory annual. Norwalk, CT: Appleton-Century-Crofts, 1983;145-74.

151. Grima KM. Therapeutic apheresis in hematological and oncological diseases. J Clin Apher 2000;15:28-52.

152. Gabriel A, Lassnigg A, Kurz M, Panser S. Post-transfusion purpura due to HPA-1a immunization in a male patient: Response to subsequent multiple HPA-1a-incompatible red-cell transfusions. Transfus Med 1995;5:131-4.

153. Lucas GF, Pittman SJ, Davies S, et al. Post-transfusion purpura (PTP) associated with anti-HPA-1a, anti-HPA-2b and anti-HPA-3a antibodies. Transfus Med 1997;7:295-9.

154. Simon TL, Collins J, Kunicki TJ, et al. Post-transfusion purpura associated with alloantibody specific for the platelet antigen. Am J Hematol 1988;29:38-40.

155. Taaning E, Skov F. Elution of anti-Zwa (-PI^{A1}) from autologous platelets after normalization of platelet count in post-thrombocytopenic purpura. Vox Sang 1991;60:40-4.

156. Taaning E, Svejgaard A. Post-transfusion purpura: A survey of 12 Danish cases with special reference to immunoglobulin G subclasses of the platelet antibodies. Transfus Med 1994;4:1-8.

157. Kickler TS, Ness PM, Herman JH, Bell WR. Studies on the pathophysiology of post-transfusion purpura. Blood 1986;68:347-50.

158. Win N, Peterkin MA, Watson WH. The therapeutic value of HPA-1a-negative platelet transfusion in post-transfusion purpura complicated by life-threatening hemorrhage. Vox Sang 1995;69:138-9.

159. Brecher ME, Moore SB, Letendre L. Posttransfusion purpura: The therapeutic value of PIA1-negative platelets. Transfusion 1990;30:433-5.

160. Vogelsang G, Kickler TS, Bell WR. Post-transfusion purpura: A report of five patients and a review of the pathogenesis and management. Am J Hematol 1986;21:259-67.

161. Weisberg LJ, Linker CA. Prednisone therapy of post-transfusion purpura. Ann Intern Med 1984;100:76-7.

162. Berney SE, Metcalfe P, Wathen NC, Waters AH. Post-transfusion purpura responding to high dose intravenous IgG: Further observations on pathogenesis. Br J Haematol 1986;61:627-32.

163. Chong BH, Cade J, Smith JA, Taboulis J. An unusual case of post-transfusion purpura: Good transient response to high dose immunoglobulin. Vox Sang 1986;51:182-4.

164. Mueller-Eckhardt C, Kiefel V. High dose IgG for post-transfusion purpura—revisited. Blut 1988;57:163-7.

165. Cimo PL, Aster RH. Post-transfusion purpura: Successful treatment by exchange transfusion. N Engl J Med 1972;287:290-2.

166. Abramson N, Eisenberg PD, Aster RH. Post-transfusion purpura: Immunologic aspects and therapy. N Engl J Med 1974;291:1163-6.

167. Schofield RH, Tardibono G, Ogden SB, et al. Rheumatoid hyperviscosity: Analysis of a patient with intermediate complexes that block other autoantibodies and a review of the literature. Semin Arthritis Rheum 1998;27:382-91.

168. Rezai KA, Patel SC, Eliott D, Becker MA. Rheumatoid hyperviscosity syndrome: Reversibility of microvascular abnormalities after treatment. Am J Ophthalmol 2002;134:130-2.

169. Glaspy JA. Hemostatic abnormalities in multiple myeloma and related disorders. Hematol Oncol Clin North Am 1992;6:1301-14.

170. Tricot G, Fassas A. Multiple myeloma and other plasma cell disorders. In: Hoffman R, Benz EJ, Shattil SJ, eds. Hematology: Basic principles and practice. Philadelphia: Elsevier, 2005:1501-35.
171. Lunel F, Musset L. Hepatitis C infection and cryoglobulinemia. Trends Exp Clin Med 1998; 8:95-103.
172. Kyle RA, Griepp PR, Gertz MA, et al. Waldenström's macroglobulinemia: A prospective study comparing daily with intermittent oral chlorambucil. Br J Haematol 2000;108:737-42.
173. Buskard NA, Glaton DAG, Goldman JM, et al. Plasma exchange in the long-term management of Waldenström's macroglobulinemia. CMAJ 1977;117:135-7.
174. McLeod BC. Therapeutic plasma exchange. In: Simon TL, Snyder EL, Solheim BJ, et al, eds. Rossi's principles of transfusion medicine. 4th ed. Bethesda, MD: AABB Press, 2009:629-51.
175. Bloch KJ, Make DG. Hyperviscosity syndromes associated with immunoglobulin abnormalities. Semin Hematol 1973;10:113-24.
176. Treon SP. How I treat Waldenstrom macroglobulinemia. Blood 2009;114:2375-85.

In: McLeod BC, Szczepiorkowski ZM, Weinstein R, Winters JL, eds.
Apheresis: Principles and Practice, 3rd edition
Bethesda, MD: AABB Press, 2010

17

Therapeutic Plasma Exchange for Renal and Rheumatic Diseases

Andre A. Kaplan, MD, FACP, FASN

MOST GLOMERULONEPHRITIDES are immunologically based with clear evidence of either linear glomerular basement membrane antibody (anti-GBM) deposition or granular immune complex deposition in varying areas of the glomerulus (mesangial, subepithilial, subendothelial, etc) on biopsy. Even those glomerulonephritides that were previously considered to be "pauci-immune," with no obvious immunoglobulin deposition in the glomerulus, are now known to be associated with antineutrophil cytoplasmic antibodies (ANCA). Thus, it is not surprising that many physicians have attempted to treat these disorders with therapeutic plasma exchange (TPE).[1-5] TPE is a particularly appealing technique for treatment of disease caused by pathogenic antibodies. IgG antibodies have a half-life of approximately 21 days and a correspondingly slow synthetic rate that allows a course of TPE to meaningfully lower IgG levels. Furthermore, medication targeting antibody production would not substantially lower circulating antibody levels for weeks, if not months. When there is reason to believe that the pathogenic autoantibodies are acutely toxic, as with anti-GBM disease, TPE is the only treatment that will rapidly remove the antibodies from the plasma. When known, the kinetics of antibody removal can provide a useful guide to the prescription of TPE, as has been recently reviewed.[5]

TPE has also been employed for the removal of nephrotoxic free light chains (FLCs) in the presence of the "cast nephropathy" associated with multiple myeloma, although the far more rapid kinetics of FLC synthesis and catabolism are less favorable to meaningful depletion by this means. The pathogeneses of thrombotic thrombocytopenic purpura (TTP) and hemolytic uremic syndrome (HUS) vary

---

Andre A. Kaplan, MD, FACP, FASN, Professor of Medicine, University of Connecticut Health Center, Farmington, Connecticut
The author has disclosed no conflicts of interest.

with presentation and presumptive inciting factors; TPE is beneficial in some cases by removing antibodies and/or by allowing large volumes of patient plasma to be replaced with normal plasma, thus replenishing a deficient circulating factor. Many favorable case reports and series addressing renal diseases call for more frequent and extensive TPE schedules than those reported effective for some other indications (eg, neurologic diseases). These customary practices are not necessarily supported by measurements of antibody levels.

GBM-Antibody-Mediated Disease (Goodpasture Syndrome)

Goodpasture syndrome is the association of acute glomerulonephritis and pulmonary hemorrhage brought about by an autoantibody directed against the NC1 domain of the alpha-3 chain of type IV collagen, which is enriched in the alveolar and glomerular basement membranes.[6] Although some patients present with relatively mild renal insufficiency, this disorder is typically associated with severe renal injury that, if untreated, progresses quickly to end-stage renal failure. The only randomized controlled study of TPE as an adjunct to imunosuppressive therapy employed a relatively modest TPE schedule (once every 3 days), and its non-TPE group had more severe renal disease (more interstitial fibrosis and tubular atrophy).[7] Nonetheless, the results of this study and of other nonrandomized or case-controlled studies are generally in agreement that TPE is useful in providing a more rapid decline in serum anti-GBM, a lower posttreatment serum creatinine level, and a decreased incidence of end-stage renal disease (ESRD).[2,8-10] TPE has also been found to have a beneficial effect on the course of severe pulmonary hemorrhage.[8,11] It should be noted, however, that the chance of a favorable renal outcome is best when TPE is initiated before the onset of severe renal impairment; avoidance of ESRD is uncommon if treatment is begun after the serum creatinine exceeds 7 mg/dL. Nonetheless, even patients presenting with severe renal impairment have responded to therapy if the presentation is very acute[8,12,13] or if ANCA are present as well as anti-GBM and there are signs of associated vasculitis.[12,14] In a retrospective study of 889 cases of rapidly progressive glomerulonephritis (RPGN), 47 (5%) were positive only for anti-GBM, 246 (28%) were positive only for ANCA, and 20 (2%) had both.[14] Analyzed from a different perspective, of 67 patients positive for anti-GBM, 20 (30%) were also positive for ANCA.

TPE is prescribed to rapidly lower anti-GBM levels. An immunosuppressive regimen with steroids, cyclophosphamide, or azathioprine is also essential to slow the production of anti-GBM and decrease the inflammatory response.[10]

A TPE prescription that has been recommended for Goodpasture syndrome is 14 daily 4-liter exchanges,[15] but the amount exchanged may be modified depending on the patient's plasma volume. The patient should be reassessed at the end of this 2-week regimen. Further TPE may be unnecessary if serum creatinine levels have decreased and there is a marked decline in serum anti-GBM titers. In contrast, continued TPE may be required if antibody levels are still elevated; individual patients have required as many as 25 treatments for successful lowering of the serum antibody titers.[9] Such an intensive replacement of plasma with albumin will cause a depletional coagulopathy with marked elevations of the prothrombin and partial thromboplastin times, as well as a marked reduction of normal serum immunoglobulins. Thus, a patient with a recent renal biopsy or with significant pulmonary hemorrhage may benefit from at least a partial replacement with Fresh Frozen Plasma (FFP).[16]

Immunoadsorption has also been tried in anti-GBM disease. In a single case report,[17] the combination of immunosuppression and immunoadsorption with a sepharose-coupled sheep-antihuman IgG column for 25 cycles was followed by recovery of renal function, with a stable creatinine concentration of 2 mg/dL. This approach, which could eliminate the need for FFP to avoid coagulopathy, is discussed further in Chapter 20.

Anti-GBM disease is listed by the American Society for Apheresis (ASFA) as a Category I indication for TPE.[4]

Rapidly Progressive Glomerulonephritis Not Associated with Anti-GBM

RPGN is a clinical syndrome combining urinary features of glomerular disease with progressive loss of renal function over days, weeks, or months. It is characterized morphologically by extensive crescent formation. With the identification of the ANCA-associated "pauci-immune" glomerulonephritides, the majority of patients with RPGN can be etiologically classified as having either anti-GBM disease, ANCA-associated disease, or one of a variety of well-defined immune complex deposition diseases such as systemic lupus erythematosus (SLE), or IgA- or cryoglobulinemia-associated disease.[18] In the retrospective study by Jayne et al mentioned above, 576 of 889 cases (65%) had neither anti-GBM nor ANCA and probably had one of these systemic diseases.[14]

Given the new-found ability to classify most nephritides, the diagnosis of "idiopathic" RPGN is becoming rare[18] and many previous studies evaluating the potential benefit of TPE for "idiopathic" RPGN are now difficult to interpret. However, because most "pauci-immune" glomerulonephritis is proving to be ANCA-associated, there is a rationale for extrapolating data from older studies accordingly. The use of TPE in ANCA-associated disease is supported by increasing evidence that ANCA is an inciting factor for tissue damage.[19,20] There are three subsets of patients with ANCA-associated vasculitis who may benefit from TPE: those with concurrent anti-GBM disease, those with severe pulmonary hemorrhage, and those who present with severe renal disease.

Concurrent Anti-GBM

Based on benefits observed in anti-GBM disease, TPE is commonly prescribed in combination with immunosuppressive agents for patients with ANCA-associated vasculitis who also have GBM antibodies.[21]

Pulmonary Hemorrhage

Although no controlled studies have been performed, the available evidence suggests that RPGN patients with pulmonary hemorrhage can benefit from TPE.[22,23] This strategy is based on the theoretical benefit of removing ANCA by TPE and the observed efficacy of TPE in patients with pulmonary hemorrhage caused by anti-GBM disease. A retrospective review reported on 20 patients who presented with diffuse alveolar hemorrhage (DAH) and ANCA-associated small vessel vasculitis and received a mean of 6 (range = 4 to 9) TPE treatments. Most received pulse methylprednisolone for 3 days and intravenous cyclophosphamide as well. DAH resolved in all and there were no complications from TPE. One patient died of pulmonary embolism. Among the 13 nondialysis-dependent patients, only one did not achieve disease remission and required chronic therapy.[23]

Patients Who Present with Severe Renal Disease

Despite favorable uncontrolled reports,[24-26] the results of four randomized controlled studies failed to demonstrate a generalized benefit for TPE in the treatment of non-anti-GBM-associated RPGN when added to standard immunosuppressive therapy.[27-30] Nonetheless, in all of these studies, subset analysis suggested that TPE could be beneficial for patients presenting with severe disease or dialysis dependency[31,32] (Table 17-1 lists these four plus another trial). In one study in which this issue was specifically addressed, Pusey et al treated 48 patients having crescentic glomerulonephritis, in whom anti-GBM disease and other well-defined vasculitides (SLE and Henoch-Schonlein purpura, or H-S purpura) were excluded, with prednisolone, cyclophosphamide, and azathioprine.[29] Twenty-five were randomly assigned to receive TPE with five 4-liter exchanges in the first week and a mean total of nine TPEs per patient

Table 17-1. Controlled Trials of TPE for Patients with Severe or Dialysis-Dependent RPGN*

Trial	Index of Severity	TPE	no TPE
Mauri 1985[27]	Creatinine >9		
Initial creatinine (number of patients)		13.5 (6)	13.1 (5)
Creatinine after 3 years		**8.7†**	**13.4**
Glockner 1988[28]	Dialysis dependent		
Initial creatinine (number of patients)		7.4 (8)	9.2 (4)
Creatinine after 6 months		**1.7†**	**5.5**
Pusey 1991[29]	Dialysis dependent		
Initial number of patients on dialysis		11	8
Patients off dialysis at 12 months		**10‡**	**3**
Cole 1992[30]	Dialysis dependent		
Initial number of patients on dialysis		4	7
Patients off dialysis at 12 months		**3**	**2**
Jayne 2007[33]	Creatinine >5.8		
Initial number of patients		70	67
Patients off dialysis at 12 months		**57**	**40**

*Adapted from Kaplan.[32(p184)] All studies had concomitant treatment with steroids and immunosuppressive agents. Subset analysis: creatinine values in mg/dL. (To convert serum creatinine mg/dL to µmol/L, multiply by 88.4.)
†$p < 0.05$ with day 0.
‡$p < 0.05$ TPE vs no TPE.
TPE = therapeutic plasma exchange; RPGN = rapidly progressive glomerulonephritis.

(range = 5-25). Although the patients were not tested for ANCA, the clinical diagnoses were Wegener granulomatosis, microscopic polyarteritis, and idiopathic RPGN. Results revealed no outcome difference when initial serum creatinines were less than 5.8 mg/dL; however, of the patients who were originally dialysis dependent, 10 of 11 receiving TPE recovered renal function, while only 3 of 8 in the non-TPE group recovered to a similar degree ($p = 0.04$). Thus, the results of this study and similar findings in three other controlled trials support the use of TPE in RPGN only in patients presenting with severe renal failure or dialysis dependency.

More recently, a larger study was specifically designed to investigate the role of TPE in ANCA-positive patients with severe renal disease. The Methylprednisolone vs Plasma Exchange (MEPEX) trial[33] enrolled 137 patients with a new diagnosis of Wegener granulomatosis or anti-myeloperoxidase-positive (anti-MPO, a subset of ANCA) pauci-immune glomerulonephritis and a serum creatinine concentration above 5.8 mg/dL. The mean creatinine at presentation was 8.3 mg/dL, and 69% required dialysis. The patients were randomly assigned to receive either seven sessions of TPE over the first 2 weeks after diagnosis (n = 70) or methylprednisolone, 1 g/day for 3 days (n = 67). In addition to these therapies, patients received prednisolone (1 mg/kg per day, tapered over 6 months) and cyclophosphamide (2.5 mg/kg per day for 3 months), followed by azathioprine for remission maintenance. Those treated with TPE had a significantly higher likelihood of survival and having independent renal function at 3 months (69% vs 49% in the methylprednisolone group) and had a significant reduction in the risk of progression to ESRD at 1 year (19% vs 43%). The mortality rate was high in both groups (27% vs 24%). The majority of deaths occurred in the first 3 months of treatment. Of the 35 deaths, 19 were related to infection, six to pulmonary hemorrhage, and four to cardiovascular events.

A major shortcoming of this trial is that the TPE group did not receive the pulse steroid commonly given to patients with severe RPGN. Providing pulse methylprednisolone at the outset of therapy to all patients and randomly assigning them to TPE or no TPE might have been a better design. A disturbing outcome was that mortality in both groups was higher than that reported in other studies, even allowing for the fact that patients in the MEPEX study likely had more severe disease at baseline. Despite these limitations, the results of the MEPEX trial further support the proposition that the addition of TPE to cyclophosphamide and glucocorticoid therapy may enhance the recovery of renal function among patients who present with advanced renal disease (Table 17-1). It is of note that reserving TPE treatment for only those with severe renal disease is in sharp contrast to the general recommendation for treatment of anti-GBM-associated disease, in which there is strong evidence supporting the early initiation of treatment, before severe renal failure is present.

As mentioned above, the schedule of TPE in the MEPEX trial was seven sessions of 60 mL/kg each over 2 weeks.[33,34] Partial replacement with FFP to avoid depletional coagulopathy should be considered after renal biopsy or in the presence of pulmonary hemorrhage.

In general, TPE has been found to be a relatively safe but costly addition to more conventional treatment regimens. This added expense and the risks of vascular access placement should be viewed in the context of the eventual long-term cost and need for vascular or peritoneal access for those patients who develop ESRD and require dialysis. ANCA-associated RPGN with dialysis dependence or DAH has been assigned to indication Category I by ASFA, and dialysis-independent disease is assigned to Category III.[4]

Renal Failure in Multiple Myeloma

Multiple myeloma is a malignant plasma cell dyscrasia that arises from the autonomous growth of a single clone of plasma cells. Uncontrolled immunoglobulin secretion from this single clone produces a monoclonal antibody. Disordered immunoglobulin synthesis is often associated with excess production of light chains (FLCs) that circulate unbound to heavy chains and are believed to be toxic to renal tubules. Renal failure is a relatively common problem in patients with multiple myeloma that may result from a variety of causes, including dehydration, hypercalcemia, radiocontrast media, nonsteroidal anti-inflammatory drugs, hyperuricemia, pyelonephritis, plasma cell infiltration, amyloidosis, light-chain deposition disease[35] (primarily a glomerular disease), and "cast nephropathy," which is the result of the tubular-toxic effect of FLCs and their tendency to obstruct the nephron lumen.[36] The last is the only cause of myeloma-associated renal failure for which there is a target pathogenic substance that might be depleted by TPE, and even in this case there is uncertainty, based on the kinetics of synthesis and catabolism of FLCs, about how effective TPE can be in substance depletion.[37,38]

Cast Nephropathy and Chemotherapy

After a reasonable diagnostic evaluation, including a therapeutic trial of hydration, to rule out other common forms of renal failure in patients with myeloma, the diagnosis of cast nephropathy may be considered in those with elevated serum levels of FLCs. Supportive evidence includes a monoclonal immunoglobulin (M-spike) of similar mobility in both serum and urine that is confirmed to represent FLCs by immunofixation. Quantitative assays specific for FLCs are now available and are also useful.

Once cast nephropathy is identified as the most likely cause for renal failure, rapid lowering of serum FLCs by TPE becomes a therapeutic consideration. One study of TPE in conjunction with an antineoplastic regimen (a combination of steroids with melphalan or cyclophosphamide) in patients with >1 g/day urinary excretion of FLCs suggested an increased likelihood of improved renal function and a better overall survival. Of 29 patients with mean pretreatment serum creatinine levels of 11 mg/dL, 13 of 15 patients randomly assigned to receive TPE (3 to 4 liters on 5 consecutive days) and hemodialysis had substantial return of renal function (to a mean creatinine of 2.6 mg/dL) within 2 months, whereas improvement occurred in only two of 14 managed with peritoneal dialysis and no TPE. The degree of FLC removal and the effect of TPE in serum FLC levels were not measured, and the difference in methods of dialysis support was an unfortunate confounding factor.[39]

These results were not confirmed in a later multicenter trial of 97 patients with newly diagnosed multiple myeloma and acute renal failure who were randomly assigned to receive TPE and chemotherapy or chemotherapy alone.[40] Patients were included if they met the following criteria: progressive worsening of kidney function (serum creatinine >2.3 mg/dL with an increase of >0.6 mg/dL over the preceding 2 weeks) despite correction of hypercalcemia and hypovolemia; monoclonal light chains in urine, plasma, or renal tissue; and no other identifiable cause of acute renal failure. In the control and TPE groups, 14 and 15 patients (36% and 26%), respectively, were on dialysis at baseline, and five and nine patients (13% and 16%), respectively, began dialysis during treatment. At 6 months, mortality was 33% in each group. Further results revealed that the composite outcome [death, dialysis dependence, or glomerular filtration rate (GFR) <30 mL/minute per 1.73 m²] was not significantly different: 58% vs 69% in the TPE and control patients, respectively [95% confidence interval (CI) for difference = −8.3% to 29.1%]. Among 6-month survivors, fewer patients in the TPE group remained dialysis-dependent (13% vs 27%), but the difference was not significant (95% CI = −5.1% to 34.6%). The authors concluded that there was no statistically significant, nor clinically meaningful, difference in outcome, although the wide CI of the difference did not allow excluding the possibility of either benefit or harm. An accompanying editorial suggested that, based on this study, TPE for the treatment of renal failure in multiple myeloma should no longer be routinely recommended.[41]

Notwithstanding its significance as the largest study of TPE in myeloma renal disease, this trial has been criticized by this author.[42] Although all patients had Bence Jones protein, only 76 (78%) of the 97 patients had documented FLCs in their sera. The patients enrolled seemed likely to have cast nephropathy,[43] but relatively few were biopsied for confirmation. Benefits of TPE may also have been obscured by an imbalance in chemotherapy because more patients in the control group received a dexamethasone-containing regimen, which leads to faster reduction in light-chain production than melphalan and prednisone. Finally, TPE was associated with a nonsignificant reduction in dialysis dependency among survivors at 6 months (13% vs 27%).

A subsequent, retrospective study analyzed the efficacy of TPE in patients in whom the diagnosis of cast nephropathy was confirmed by biopsy and in whom serum levels of FLCs were used to guide therapy.[44,45] Fourteen patients had biopsy-proven cast nephropathy and serum FLCs measured before and after a course of TPE and chemotherapy. A renal response, defined as a 50% reduction in serum creatinine and dialysis independence at 180 days, occurred in seven of nine patients (78%) in whom FLCs were reduced by 50% or more. It should be noted, however, that a retrospective study such as this cannot distinguish between a drop in FLCs resulting from renal recovery (via increased excretion) and one causing renal recovery.

Well-established renal failure considered to be caused by cast nephropathy may respond less dramatically, but a combination of TPE and chemotherapy has been successful if treatment is initiated before the onset of oligo-anuria.[46] Johnson et al recommend the use of biopsy to determine the density of cast formation as a guide to the eventual response to TPE.[47]

A cautionary note is that FLCs are rapidly resynthesized and reaccumulate within hours after each TPE.[38] Thus it remains uncertain whether their removal by TPE can be clinically meaningful. Nevertheless, although the evidence for benefit is limited and incomplete, given the possible reduction in dialysis dependency among survivors, TPE is still being recommended for individuals with acute renal failure suspected to be caused by cast nephropathy who have FLCs in the serum.[42] TPE may be requested on the basis of high levels of FLCs in serum or urine, even in the absence of a renal biopsy. A TPE regimen of five to seven procedures within 7 to 10 days is recommended by this author. If FLCs are not substantially reduced by the original course of treatment, the chemotherapy employed must be reconsidered because rapid, unabated light-chain production will overwhelm the removal capabilities of TPE.[38] If renal biopsy is performed and TPE initiated soon after, partial replacement with FFP will prevent any bleeding from dilutional coagulopathy.[48]

If chemotherapy is successful in limiting new FLC synthesis, then a single course of five TPE treatments may be sufficient. Further treatments may be necessary if the chemotherapy employed allows for continued FLC production. Wahlin et al have reported a prophylactic treatment regimen involving chemotherapy plus TPE three times weekly every 5 weeks, with comparison data suggesting substantially improved survival when compared to patients treated with chemotherapy alone.[49] Currently available FLC assays provide an easy, sensitive means to detect recurrent light-chain accumulation.

ASFA rates "myeloma kidney" as a Category I indication for TPE.[4]

Light-Chain Removal by Dialytic Techniques

Removal of FLCs by dialysis would limit the need for albumin replacement. Although light chains are relatively small proteins (approximately 20,000 daltons), standard dialytic techniques are not capable of efficient FLC removal. In one study, net removal in 50 liters of peritoneal dialysate was only 2 grams, in contrast with the 17 grams removed by one 5-liter TPE.[50] Recent reports suggest that significant amounts of FLC may be removed with an alternate hemodialysis approach in which extended daily hemodialysis is performed with a protein-leaking dialyzer with very large pores.[51,52] In a study that included 19 dialysis-dependent patients with multiple myeloma and cast nephropathy, extended dialysis was performed as an adjunct to chemotherapy.[52] Using the Gambro HCO 1100 hemodialysis membrane (CaridianBCT, Lakewood, CO), the dialysis schedule was 8 hours daily for the first 5 days, 8 hours on alternate days for the next 12 days, and then 6 hours three times weekly. Among the 13 patients who completed 6 weeks of uninterrupted chemotherapy and hemodialysis, all had early reductions in FLCs and were dialysis independent at a median of 27 days (range = 13 to 120 days). Interruptions in chemotherapy occurred in all six patients who failed to achieve reduction in FLCs; of these, only one patient had recovery of renal function by 105 days. It is therefore unclear whether the long-term benefits resulted from intensive dialysis or response to chemotherapy or both. Confirmation of these benefits is required in a larger number of patients.

IgA Nephropathy and Henoch-Schonlein Purpura

IgA nephropathy is the most common form of glomerulonephritis and is classified as an immune-complex-mediated disease. Although it was originally considered to be relatively benign, prolonged follow-up suggests that 30% to 35% of patients will progress to ESRD.[53]

The majority of patients will have a relatively indolent course, but about 10% will present with RPGN with exuberant crescent formation and an accelerated decline to ESRD. H-S purpura has, as its renal component, a glomerular involvement that appears to be indistinguishable from the nonsystemic form of primary IgA nephropathy. Mesangial deposition of circulating IgA-containing immune complexes appears to be an integral part of the nephritic process in both IgA nephropathy and H-S purpura, but the underlying pathogenesis is unclear and may involve a dysregulation of IgA synthesis. In some cases, renal deposition of IgA is associated with increased production or decreased excretion (secondary forms).

The removal of circulating IgA complexes by TPE would appear to be an appealing therapeutic approach, and in case reports and uncontrolled trials it has been considered successful in ameliorating both acute and chronically progressive disease.[54-57] Nonetheless, the current availability of alternative treatments such as fish oil and angiotensin-converting enzyme inhibitors[53] have obviated any need for TPE as a treatment option for chronic, progressive IgA nephropathy.

The potential usefulness of TPE as a treatment for acute disease remains unresolved. In one series, Hene and Kater reported a substantial decline in serum creatinine in two patients presenting with rapidly progressive disease in whom TPE was used without steroids or any other immunosuppressive treatment.[54] Indeed, in a review of the literature, Coppo et al list a total of seven case reports in which RPGN caused by IgA nephropathy or H-S purpura resolved after treatment with TPE alone.[55] In another report of acute, fulminant disease, TPE was used in conjunction with cyclophosphamide and low-dose prednisone, which was followed by complete clinical remission.[56] Although it could not be established that TPE played a significant role in the recovery of this patient, it was clear that the TPE treatments rapidly lowered levels of circulating IgA immune complexes. In a rare case of alveolar hemorrhage associated with IgA nephropathy, TPE was followed by rapid improvement in the

steroid-resistant nephritis.[58] Thus, although there is no randomized controlled trial for evaluation, some case reports suggest a possible beneficial effect of TPE in the treatment of IgA-associated RPGN. The authors of these reports have performed TPE thrice weekly for 3 weeks and then once weekly.[54,55] Albumin can be used as the replacement fluid.

Although no formal series is available for assessment, single case reports have suggested that TPE may also be of value in the management of nonrenal morbidities associated with H-S purpura. Thus, TPE has been reported to be of value in the treatment of two patients with H-S purpura and severe intestinal involvement[59,60] and in the management of a pregnant patient with suspected H-S purpura.[61] Neither IgA nephropathy nor H-S purpura has been rated by ASFA.

Systemic Lupus Erythematosus

Despite early, enthusiastic reports suggesting a positive effect of TPE on severe lupus,[62-66] several randomized controlled trials could not document any therapeutic benefit of TPE.[67-69] The largest of these included 86 patients with severe lupus nephritis.[69] All 86 received similar conventional therapy with prednisone and cyclophosphamide, while 40 were randomly assigned to undergo TPE three times weekly for the first 4 weeks of treatment. Despite a more rapid decline in anti-double-stranded DNA titers, 25% in the TPE-treated group developed renal failure as compared to only 17% in those not receiving TPE. Thus, the weight of the currently available evidence suggests that TPE is not beneficial as an adjunct to conventional immunosuppressive therapy for lupus nephritis. Nonetheless, TPE may still be useful for the treatment of TTP associated with SLE[70] and for the treatment of symptoms associated with a lupus anticoagulant (see below). In a single case report, TPE was employed to control disease during pregnancy when cytotoxic agents were undesirable.[71] A retrospective review of 26 patients with SLE and central nervous system (CNS) involvement who were treated with TPE with or without cyclophosphamide revealed that 74% of patients improved, 13% stabilized, and 13% progressed.[72] Anecdotal case reports and small series have suggested beneficial effects of TPE in lupus-associated pulmonary hemorrhage, myasthenia gravis, hyperviscosity, cryoglobulinemia, peripheral neuropathy, hemolytic anemia, ITP, pneumonitis, and rapidly progressive renal disease.[4,73] However, a multinational controlled trial of TPE followed by intravenous cyclophosphamide in a variety of severe manifestations of SLE failed to show any benefit from TPE, either in all patients enrolled[74] or in a subgroup with nephritis.[75] This negative trial was halted early because of an excess of deaths from central line sepsis in the TPE group; the final results, though widely known in the apheresis community, have been published only in abstract form. It has even been suggested that TPE might be detrimental in SLE by inducing a rebound increase in antibody synthesis, but the four cases reported were receiving no concomitant therapy (neither steroids nor immunosuppressives), and the described deterioration occurred up to 6 months after the last TPE treatment.[76]

Several immunoadsorption techniques have been proposed for the treatment of lupus.[77] Despite some encouraging results, there have been, as yet, no randomized, controlled studies to allow formal evaluation of their clinical utility.

ASFA rates lupus nephritis as a Category IV indication for TPE, based on the negative controlled trial. Other severe manifestations are assigned to Category II.[4]

Lupus Anticoagulant, Anticardiolipin Antibodies, and the Antiphospholipid Syndrome

Antibodies directed against negatively-charged phospholipids (antiphospholipid antibodies, or APAs) may be detected as lupus anticoagulants (LAs), anticardiolipin antibodies, and/or antibodies to beta-2 glycoprotein-I, phosphatidylserine, phosphatidylinositol, or prothrombin.

The antiphospholipid syndrome (APS) occurs either as a primary condition or as a condition secondary to an underlying disease, particularly disorders in the spectrum of SLE. APAs are associated with the development of recurrent arterial and venous thromboses, thrombocytopenia, recurrent fetal loss, and, on occasion, renal disease. Systemic coagulation can result in multiple organ involvement and the catastrophic antiphospholipid syndrome (CAPS). An analysis of 29 published series composed of over 1000 patients with SLE found a 34% frequency of LAs and a 44% frequency of anticardiolipin antibodies.[78] However, 65% of patients with APAs do not have SLE. In this group the most common associations are with other autoimmune diseases, certain drugs (chlorpromazine, procainamide, hydralazine), and neoplastic disorders. Standard therapies include heparin, warfarin, aspirin, clopidrogrel, and hydroxychloroquine. Considering that APAs are IgG, IgA, or IgM antibodies, it is not surprising that physicians have employed TPE to treat disorders associated with them.

Renal Disease

Although the majority of patients with SLE-associated nephritis and APA have renal disease compatible with the standard World Health Organization classification of lupus nephritis,[79-81] there is a subset whose glomerular pathology includes intraglomerular thrombi characteristic of a thrombotic microangiopathy. An in-depth study of the different types of APA and lupus nephritis by Frampton et al found no major pathogenetic role for APA but did find an association between IgG APA and the presence of intraglomerular thrombi.[79] Reports of TPE to remove APA in renal disease are scarce. Farrugia et al reported one patient with LA and renal disease who was treated with TPE.[81] Kincaid-Smith et al described 12 patients with LA-associated thrombotic microangiopathy related to pregnancy; complete renal recovery was seen only in the two patients who received TPE.[82] Unfortunately, neither of these reports described the TPE schedule or the resulting changes in LA levels.

Despite the paucity of details regarding the use of TPE for APA-associated renal disease, if APAs are associated with an intraglomerular thrombotic microangiopathy, it might be possible to improve renal outcome by lowering APA levels. Actual prescription of TPE will depend on the individual patient's presentation, but a schedule reported for some manifestations of APS is three to five treatments over a 7-day period.[83] It should be noted that monitoring LA activity by prolongation of the partial thromboplastin time[84] will be invalid once TPE with albumin replacement is initiated, because of the expected dilutional coagulopathy. Under these conditions, APA levels must be monitored with specific antibody testing.[85] Concomitant treatment with anticoagulants, steroids, or immunosuppressive agents should be considered in each individual case.

Catastrophic Antiphospholipid Syndrome

Asherson et al have reported on 31 patients with CAPS, defined as the presence of APA and multiorgan failure.[86] Thirteen suffered from a "primary" APA syndrome, 13 from SLE, 4 from "lupus-like" diseases, and one from rheumatoid arthritis. Precipitating factors were evident in a third of the cases (ie, infections, surgical procedures, oral contraceptives). Mortality was 60%, resulting from myocardial failure, acute respiratory distress syndrome, or CNS causes. Disseminated intravascular coagulation was present in 8 of 31 patients. TPE was followed by improvement in several patients who had not yet responded to conventional therapy with intravenous heparin, steroids, and immunosuppression. Neuwelt et al have reported on the course of a patient with a medical history of the HELLP syndrome (hemolysis, elevated liver enzymes, and low platelets) who developed CAPS.[87] Anticoagulants, corticosteroids, intravenous gamma globulin and cyclophosphamide had all failed to halt the progression of CAPS, but over a 3-year period during which TPE was performed, the patient's condition improved.

Because of the rarity of CAPS, TPE for CAPS has never been investigated in a controlled trial; however, a review of the first 250 patients entered into the CAPS Registry demonstrated that patients who received TPE, anticoagulants, and steroids had an overall survival rate of 78%,[88] leading the authors to suggest that this combination should be the first line of therapy for CAPS patients. Thus TPE can be considered in any patient presenting with CAPS.[4,89] The optimum number of TPE treatments has not been determined, but patients with illness of this severity would likely be treated intensively. ASFA has rated CAPS as a Category II indication for TPE.[4]

Recurrent Fetal Loss

Two reports describe the use of TPE for the removal of APA in order to avoid spontaneous abortion. Frampton et al performed repeated TPE (approximately three or four times per week) starting from the 14th week of pregnancy until successful delivery after 34 weeks gestation,[90] while Fulcher et al performed a total of six TPEs beginning at the 24th week, followed by successful cesarean section in week 29.[91] In both of these reports there was a substantial lowering of the concentration of APA following TPE.

Scleroderma

Progressive systemic sclerosis (scleroderma) is a disease characterized by excessive skin thickening and internal organ fibrosis that can lead to dysphagia, GI hypomotility, pulmonary fibrosis, cardiac abnormalities, hypertension, and renal failure. Over 90% of patients suffer from Raynaud phenomenon. Histologically, there is excessive deposition of collagen and obliteration of capillaries in subcutaneous tissue.[92] The disease may present with evidence of inflammation, and there are overlap syndromes suggesting autoimmunity (CREST: calcinosis, Raynaud phenomenon, esophageal dysmotility, sclerodactyly, and telangiectases syndrome).[93] A variety of autoantibodies may be present, including the scleroderma antibody (SCL-70), which is found in 20% to 60% of patients. Although the presence of these antibodies may aid in diagnosis, the available data have not identified a pathogenic circulating factor that would be a rational target for removal by TPE. Nonetheless, there have been several studies designed to evaluate the utility of TPE.

In an uncontrolled trial, the combination of prednisone, cyclophosphamide, and TPE (weekly for up to 10 weeks and at 1- to 4-week intervals thereafter) was reported to produce substantial clinical improvement in 14 of 15 patients.[94] In a 1987 preliminary report of a controlled trial, 16 patients were randomized to receive no TPE, TPE alone, or TPE with simultaneous lymphocyte depletion (lymphoplasmapheresis).[95] TPE was performed 21 times over 3 months. Statistically significant improvement was found in both treatment groups compared to controls and was manifest in Rodman's skin score, physical therapy assessment, and global assessment. Unfortunately, there seems to be no peer-reviewed publication of the final results of this study. In another controlled trial in which most patients received only one or two TPEs, there was improvement in the frequency of Raynaud attacks and digital ulcer healing but no consistent, objective improvement, and some patients receiving "placebo" TPE had improvement similar to those treated with actual TPE.[96] In another report, a series of TPEs was attempted in seven patients.[97] Treatment was discontinued in three because of poor vascular access. Between eight and 20 TPEs were performed in the remaining four patients. Of these, only one, with an associated progressive myositis, noted any improvement in articular and cutaneous symptoms. In a retrospective study of 28 patients with recent onset or rapidly progressive disease, chronic management including TPE over a mean 33-month period was accompanied by improvement in disease activity markers and a nonsignificant improvement in clinical parameters, while a concurrent group of patients not receiving TPE had a worsening of clinical parameters.[98] The authors suggested that chronic TPEs might help slow the progression of severe disease.

The existence of T-lymphocyte abnormalities has suggested a possible therapeutic role for photopheresis. In a large multicenter con-trolled trial with d-penicillamine, photopheresis was found to yield improved results in terms of skin severity score after 6 months of follow-up.[99] (See also Chapter 28.)

The most prominent renal manifestation of systemic sclerosis is "scleroderma renal crisis," which presents with significant hypertension and acute renal failure. The successful use of angiotensin-converting enzyme inhibitors in treating scleroderma renal crisis strongly suggests a disturbance in the renin-angiotensin-aldosterone axis.[100]

Two separate reports have described the coexistence of scleroderma and a particular type of normotensive, normoreninemic renal disease (ie, not compatible with scleroderma renal crisis), in which the patients were positive for the ANCA commonly associated with vasculitides such as Wegener granulomatosis and periarteritis nodosa.[101,102] In both of these reports, TPE was felt to provide clinical benefit. Endo et al evaluated 100 consecutive patients with scleroderma for the presence of ANCA.[101] They found six patients (6%) to be positive for anti-MPO. All six developed rapidly progressive normotensive renal failure with normal plasma renin levels.[101] Pulmonary hemorrhage, anemia, and thrombocytopenia were associated morbidities. Other autoantibodies found in some of the patients included anti-nRNP, anti-DNA, and anti-Sm. Outcomes were poor except for one patient treated with TPE and cyclophosphamide. A similar patient reported by Omote et al had anti-MPO and a renal biopsy that revealed a necrotizing crescentic glomerulonephritis (pauci-immune type).[102] Pulse methylprednisolone therapy followed by prednisolone and mizoribine did not halt progression of renal failure. Subsequent double-filtration plasmapheresis lowered anti-MPO levels, and the authors suggested that it prevented renal failure despite a relatively low dose of immunosuppressive medication.

Wach et al have reported on three patients with severe, localized scleroderma in whom there were elevated titers of nuclear antibodies.[103] Treatment with TPE (10 to 12 procedures) and systemic steroids was followed by improvement in cutaneous and joint lesions in all three after 2 months of therapy.

ASFA has rated scleroderma as a Category III indication for TPE.[4]

Cryoglobulinemia

Cryoglobulins are immunoglobulins or immunoglobulin-containing complexes that reversibly precipitate on exposure to cold and redissolve on warming. Three types have been defined: type I, composed of a single monoclonal immunoglobulin (usually IgM) and associated with diseases such as Waldenström macroglobulinemia, myeloma, and other lymphoproliferative disorders; type II, composed of mixed cryoglobulins with a monoclonal component (usually IgMκ with anti-IgG specificity) and a polyclonal component (usually IgG) and associated with lymphoproliferative disorders and viral infections, especially HCV; and type III, composed of mixed cryoglobulins with only polyclonal components and associated with autoimmune disorders.[104] Type I cryoglobulins are often associated with impaired microvascular blood flow, which may cause Raynaud phenomenon, acrocyanosis, purpura, and/or gangrene of fingers and toes. Renal disease may arise from cryoglobulin deposition in the glomerular capillaries.[105] Types II and III often present as immune-complex-mediated diseases with hypocomplementemia and vasculitis. Common symptoms include palpable purpura, lymphadenopathy, hepatosplenomegaly, peripheral neuropathy, and glomerulonephritis.

There has never been a randomized controlled study of TPE for cryoglobulinemia. Nonetheless, the clear rationale for its use (ie, removal of pathogenic cryoglobulins) and numerous uncontrolled studies and successful case reports have led to a general consensus that TPE is a useful adjunct for the treatment of severe, active disease, such as progressive renal failure, coalescing purpura, or advanced neuropathy.[4,104-115] There has also been favorable experience with TPE for chronic management of cryoglobulinemia, with one patient receiving

238 treatments over a 12-year period,[115] but given the successful management of HCV-associated disease with interferon, current indications for this approach are less clear.[116]

In the past, TPE was performed in conjunction with the administration of steroids and immunosuppressive agents, but the implication of HCV infection as an etiologic factor in many patients with mixed "essential" cryoglobulinemia[117] is worrisome and suggests that immunosuppressive agents may be detrimental. Indeed, rapid resolution of nephritic renal failure and severe purpuric lesions can be achieved with TPE alone, without the concomitant use of steroids or immunosuppressive agents. Having such an experience, Ferri et al reported on four patients whose renal disease was successfully managed with TPE alone.[112]

A reasonable TPE schedule is one plasma volume three times weekly for 2 to 3 weeks. In one series of 15 patients, D'Amico et al reported that an average of 13 treatments were required to induce clinical improvement (range = 4-39).[110] Frankel et al administered three to 12 daily exchanges for their initial approach.[115] The replacement fluid can be 5% albumin, which must be warmed to body temperature before infusion to prevent precipitation of circulating cryoglobulins.[111,115] An associated peripheral neuropathy is likely to be vasculitic in nature and may require a greater time for reversal of symptoms.

Selective removal techniques can be used to eliminate or minimize the need for replacement fluid (see Chapter 20). Double filtration plasmapheresis employs a "secondary" filter that allows patient plasma to be separated into relatively large proteins (including cryoglobulins), which are retained, and relatively small proteins (albumin, coagulation factors, etc), which are reinfused. Although this technique can substantially reduce the need for replacement fluid, the two-step filtration process is more time consuming and the secondary filter is difficult to obtain in the United States.[118] Cryofiltration selectively removes the circulating cryoglobulins by cooling the plasma in an extracorporeal circuit, but the technique is most efficiently performed by a continuous, on-line process requiring an instrument designed for this purpose.[119] Alternatively, one can perform a two-step procedure in which the patient's own plasma can be reinfused after incubation in the cold to precipitate out the abnormal proteins.[120]

The optimal method for assessing the efficacy of TPE is uncertain. In some cases there is dramatic clinical improvement with a rapid reversal of purpura after two or three treatments, or a substantial improvement in renal function after a recent elevation in serum creatinine. Neuropathy, however, is unlikely to respond during short term therapy and it becomes desirable to follow an objective serologic parameter in order to guide the need for additional treatments.[121,122] Changes in the cryocrit after TPE may not correlate closely with clinical activity, possibly because the cryocrit test is performed at an unphysiologic temperature. It has been suggested that the solubility of cryoglobulins at 37 C, or a decline in the temperature at which their precipitation occurs, might be a better index of the response to therapy,[107,123] but such tests are not commonly performed.

As noted above, treatment with antiviral agents to reduce HCV viremia can lead to a reduction in cryoglobulin levels and clinical remission.[116] A combination of pegylated interferon and ribavirin has also been successful in controlling viremia and improving clinical symptoms in patients with membranoproliferative glomerulonephritis.[124] Unfortunately, viremia and disease activity can recur after discontinuation of antivirals. Considering the delayed onset of clinical response to the reinitiation of antiviral therapy, TPE can be useful as the initial, immediate therapy for these exacerbations. If standard TPE is used (as opposed to the selective techniques described above) and interferon therapy is initiated during a series of TPE treatments, the drug should be administered immediately after TPE in order to minimize its removal. Cryoglobulinemia is considered by ASFA to be a Category I indication for TPE and a Category II indication for immunoadsorption.

Hemolytic Uremic Syndrome

HUS in Adults

HUS is characterized by the triad of microangiopathic hemolytic anemia, thrombocytopenia, and acute renal failure. Two types of HUS have been described: diarrhea-associated (d+ HUS or typical HUS) and non-diarrhea-associated (d− HUS or atypical HUS). Distinguishing between adult HUS, especially the atypical variety, and TTP can sometimes be difficult. In general, however, thrombocytopenia and neurologic manifestations tend to dominate the clinical picture of TTP, while renal failure tends to be prominent in HUS. Nonetheless, some patients may present with severe neurologic abnormalities (eg, seizures, coma) and acute renal failure, while others have neither neurologic abnormalities nor renal failure. Such patients can be subsumed in the comprehensive term TTP-HUS, which connotes the presence of thrombocytopenia and microangiopathic hemolytic anemia without other apparent cause.

Recent studies have attempted to distinguish TTP from HUS based on the presence or absence of abnormalities of the metalloproteinase ADAMTS13 (a disintegrin and metalloproteinase with a thrombospondin type motif 1, member 13).[125,126] Idiopathic TTP is strongly associated with a deficiency of, and often an autoantibody to, ADAMTS13. The deficiency allows accumulation of unusually large von Willebrand factor multimers that promote platelet aggregation and deposition of platelet-rich thrombi in the microvasculature. TPE reverses these processes by removal of the autoantibody to ADAMTS13 when present; TPE with FFP replacement also replenishes the missing ADAMTS13 protease.

Although some have suggested that HUS can be distinguished from TTP by a normal level of ADAMTS13, these levels are not commonly known when treatment decisions must be made. Furthermore, patients without severe ADAMTS13 deficiency have improved on treatment regimens that include TPE.[127] Given the difficulty in distinguishing TTP from HUS on clinical grounds and pathologic features, and given that there is a clear indication for TPE with FFP replacement for TTP,[128] except for some specific conditions (see below), the initial management for any patient presenting with the TTP-HUS entity should include TPE with FFP replacement.[4,129] Further discussion regarding TTP appears in Chapter 16. The following discussion will focus on HUS as an entity in which microangiopathic hemolytic anemia is associated with substantial renal involvement. It should be noted at the outset that the pathogenesis of HUS is unknown and that in most cases there is no particular harmful substance targeted for removal by TPE. The use of TPE for HUS is therefore almost entirely empirical.

Although the clinical and pathologic presentations of HUS and TTP share some features, distinction between them may be possible when a clear etiologic agent can be identified, such as the association of HUS with the verotoxin produced by *Escherichia coli* (*E. coli*) O157:H7[130] or with the presence of certain inciting drugs (eg, ticlodipine, cyclosporine, mitomycin, cisplatinum, quinine, or oral contraceptives)[131-133] or when the syndrome is associated with certain diseases (SLE, carcinoma, etc).[134] In contrast to HUS in children, the prognosis of HUS in adults is poor, with an estimated mortality between 25% and 50% and an incidence of ESRD of up to 40% in the survivors.[135-137] A review combining TTP and HUS found that dialysis was required in 11 of 68 cases.[137] Five of the seven survivors in this group were able to come off dialysis after periods ranging from 4 to 120 days. The authors hypothesized that the better renal outcome was attributable to TPE, which was used on all their patients but was not provided to patients in previous, older studies.

Although there are no randomized controlled studies of TPE in adults with HUS, several observational series suggest benefit. In one study, six of 22 adults with TTP-HUS caused by *E. coli* O157:H7 had contraindications to TPE or died before TPE could be performed.[138] Among the 16 patients who received TPE, there were only five deaths. Another case series of adult patients who presented with overt bloody diarrhea and presumed *E. coli* O157:H7 infection reported that 17 of the 21 improved following TPE treatment.[139] Two patients had severe ADAMTS13 deficiency, indicating that patients with "idiopathic" TTP-HUS may present with bloody diarrhea, possibly because of intestinal ischemia.[140] In two series consisting of 158 cases of TTP-HUS associated with ticlopidine, the mortality rate in patients receiving TPE was significantly lower than in those who did not (24% vs 50% and 18% vs 57%, respectively).[141,142]

Cancer Chemotherapy or Stem-Cell Transplantation

There are only sporadic and anecdotal reports that suggest efficacy of TPE for syndromes that appear similar to TTP and HUS following cancer chemotherapy or hematopoietic progenitor cell transplantation.[143-146] Although commonly prescribed, TPE has not proven to be effective in the latter.[4,146]

An HUS-like syndrome occurring weeks or months after receipt of the chemotherapeutic drug mitomycin has been reported to improve after plasma perfusion over a column containing staphylococcal protein A bound to silica.[147] In an uncontrolled trial of 11 patients, protein A immunoadsorption was followed by improvement in nine, with stabilization of progressive renal failure in six of them.[148] Each treatment consisted of perfusing a mean of 400 mL of plasma over the column and then reinfusing to the patient. The number of treatments ranged from two to 15. In another report, an apparent case of cisplatin-associated HUS did not improve after four TPE treatments, but it did improve after four 2000-mL plasma perfusions over a staphylococcal protein A silica column.[149]

In data obtained by retrospective questionnaire, Snyder et al reported that immunoadsorption with protein A silica was followed by improvement in 25 of 55 patients with chemotherapy-associated TTP-HUS.[150] Although the report attributes substantial benefit to immunoadsorption therapy, four of five nonresponders subsequently improved after alternate treatments including standard TPE using plasma replacement. The mechanism of action of the protein A columns is uncertain; such columns were intended to selectively deplete IgG antibodies (which bind to protein A; see Chapter 20), although the amount of IgG removed by a treatment is less than that removed by standard TPE. In any case, the columns are no longer commercially available. There are also a handful of case reports in which mitomycin or cisplatin-induced HUS was said to improve after treatment with standard TPE.[136,145,151]

In summary, although both a clear rationale and controlled data supporting efficacy are lacking, the available literature would support the use of standard TPE for the initial treatment of adults with TTP-HUS,[137,152-154] even though no benefit has been discerned in clearcut typical HUS.

Recurrent HUS in Renal Transplantation

Recurrent HUS is a well-documented phenomenon in renal transplant recipients who lost function in their native kidneys after an episode of HUS. In an extensive review of the literature, Agarwal et al noted 19 reports describing 68 cases.[154] They concluded that TPE remains an efficacious treatment but that endpoints for terminating the treatments are not well defined. Although improvement or normalization in clinical status, hematocrit, reticulocyte count, peripheral schistocytes, lactate dehydrogenase, and haptoglobin may all be used as criteria for successful treatment, it is not clear if awaiting the return of renal function is reasonable before terminating TPE.

HUS in Children

HUS is a major cause of acute renal failure in the pediatric population and often follows an episode of bloody diarrhea caused by infection with a verotoxin producing *E. coli* (type 0157:H7).[155,156] The prognosis with supportive therapy is generally good, but a small percentage of patients suffer a stroke or develop significant renal failure. Additional patients may have evidence for persistent renal involvement, such as hypertension, proteinuria, and a modest decrease in GFR. There is no target for removal by TPE and no randomized controlled trials of TPE as a therapy for typical diarrhea-associated HUS in childhood; however, controlled trials of plasma infusion have demonstrated only minimal benefit.[157] Retrospective analysis and anecdotal reports suggest that TPE may be beneficial in limiting the incidence of significant renal damage in those children considered to be at particularly high risk of irreversible renal damage, such as those who present without a diarrheal prodrome or those older than 5 years of age.[158-160] Children with significant CNS involvement may also benefit from TPE.[161] Successful TPE prescription for children older than 5 years of age was found to be a median of 4.5 TPE treatments (range = 3-10) with a median of 1 liter of plasma exchanged per session (range = 200-2000 mL).[158]

About 10% of childhood HUS is not associated with a diarrheal illness. Such atypical HUS has a worse prognosis in terms of both short-term mortality and progression to ESRD. Twenty to thirty percent of atypical HUS in children is caused by defective regulation of complement. In most cases there is a congenital defect in, or deficiency of, Factor H, but cases involving Factor I or the membrane cofactor protein have also been described. TPE or plasma infusion as a means of replacement therapy has been reported and has sometimes, though not invariably, seemed worthwhile. Some congenital cases are not detected until adulthood, and a handful of cases have been associated with an antibody to Factor H, which would provide a strong rationale for TPE.[162]

ASFA has rated typical diarrhea-associated HUS as a Category IV indication for TPE, while congenital and autoantibody-mediated defects in complement regulation are rated as Category I indications.[4]

Renal Transplantation

Focal Segmental Glomerulosclerosis: Recurrence After Transplantation

It has been estimated that 15% to 55% of all patients with ESRD secondary to focal segmental glomerulosclerosis will have a rapid recurrence of proteinuria after renal transplantation. Recent studies suggest that some of these patients may have a circulating protein that is capable of increasing glomerular permeability to albumin and may be removable by TPE.[163,164]

Renal Allograft Rejection

The assumed role of cytotoxic antibodies as mediators of acute vascular rejection has prompted several attempts to employ TPE as a means of enhancing antirejection therapy.[165-167]

The Transplant Candidate with Cytotoxic Antibodies

High levels of preformed cytotoxic antibodies against donor ABO, HLA Class I, and perhaps other antigens preclude renal transplantation because of the risk of hyperacute rejection. Despite the theoretical risk of de-novo resynthesis after transplantation, several investigators have attempted to "desensitize" such patients by TPE to remove HLA antibodies.[168,169] Desensitization and renal rejection are covered in detail in Chapter 18.

References

1. Sakellariou G. Plasmapheresis as a therapy in specific forms of acute renal failure. Nephrol Dial Transplant 1994;9(Suppl 4):210-18.
2. Madore F, Lazarus JM, Brady HR. Therapeutic TPE in renal disease. J Am Soc Nephrol 1996;7:367-86.
3. Kaplan AA. Therapeutic TPE for renal disease: Semin Dial 1996;9:61-70.
4. Szczepiorkowski ZM, Winters JL, Bandarenko N, et al. Guidelines on the use of therapeutic apheresis in clinical practice—evidence-based approach from the Apheresis Applications Committee of the American Society for Apheresis. The fifth special issue. J Clin Apher 2010; 25:83-177.
5. Kaplan AA. Therapeutic plasma exchange: Core curriculum 2008. Am J Kidney Dis 2008; 52:1180-96.
6. Kalluri R, Wilson CB, Weber M, et al. Identification of the alpha-3 chain of type IV collagen as the common autoantigen in antibasement membrane disease and Goodpasture syndrome. J Am Soc Nephrol 1995;6:1178-85.
7. Johnson JP, Moore JJ, Austin H III, et al. Therapy of anti-glomerular basement membrane disease: Analysis of prognostic significance of clinical, pathologic and treatment factors. Medicine 1985;64:219-27.
8. Savage CO, Pusey CD, Bowman C, et al. Anti-glomerular basement membrane antibody-mediated disease in the British Isles 1980-4. Br Med J 1986;292:301-4.
9. Simpson IJ, Doak PB, Williams LC, et al. Plasma exchange in Goodpasture's syndrome. Am J Nephrol 1982;2:301-11.
10. Lockwood CM, Rees AJ, Pearson TA, et al. Immunosuppression and TPE in the treatment of Goodpasture's syndrome. Lancet 1976;i: 711-14.
11. McCarthy LJ, Cotton J, Danielson C, et al. Goodpasture's syndrome in childhood: Treatment with plasmapheresis and immunosuppression. J Clin Apher 1994;9:116-19.
12. Maxwell AP, Nelson WE, Hill CM. Reversal of renal failure in nephritis associated with antibodies to glomerular basement membrane. Br Med J 1988;297:333-4.
13. Fort J, Espinel E, Rogriquez JA, et al. Partial recovery of renal function in an oligoanuric patient affected with Goodpasture's syndrome after treatment with steroids, immunosuppressives and plasmapheresis (letter). Clin Nephrol 1984;22:211-12.
14. Jayne DRW, Marshall PD, Jones SJ, Lockwood CM. Autoantibodies to GBM and neutrophil cytoplasm in rapidly progressive glomerulonephritis. Kidney Int 1990;37:965-70.
15. Kaplan AA, Appel GB, Pusey CD. Treatment of anti-GBM antibody mediated disease (Goodpasture's syndrome). In: Rose BD, ed. UpToDate, BDR, version 18.1 (January 2010). Waltham, MA: UpToDate, 2010. [Available at http://www.utdol.com.]

16. Mokrzycki MH, Kaplan AA. Therapeutic TPE: Complications and management. Am J Kidney Dis 1994;23:817-27.

17. Laczika K, Knapp S, Derfler K, et al. Immunoadsorption in Goodpasture's syndrome. Am J Kidney Dis 2000;36:392-5.

18. Angangco R, Thiru S, Esnault VL, et al. Does truly 'idiopathic' crescentic glomerulonephritis exist? Nephrol Dial Transplant 1994;9:630-6.

19. Jennette JC, Xiao H, Falk RJ. Pathogenesis of vascular inflammation by anti-neutrophil cytoplasmic antibodies. J Am Soc Nephrol 2006; 17:1235-42.

20. Lionaki S, Falk RJ. Removing antibody and preserving glomeruli in ANCA small-vessel vasculitis. J Am Soc Nephrol 2007;18:1987-9.

21. Levy JB, Hammad T, Coulthart A, et al. Clinical features and outcome of patients with both ANCA and anti-GBM antibodies. Kidney Int 2004;66:1535-40.

22. Gallagher H, Kwan JT, Jayne DR. Pulmonary renal syndrome: A 4-year, single-center experience. Am J Kidney Dis 2002;39:42-7.

23. Klemmer PJ, Chalermskulrat W, Reif MS, et al. Plasmapheresis therapy for diffuse alveolar hemorrhage in patients with small-vessel vasculitis. Am J Kidney Dis 2003;42:1149-53.

24. Lockwood CM, Rees AJ, Pinching AJ, et al. Plasma exchange and immunosuppression in the treatment of fulminating immune-complex crescentic nephritis. Lancet 1977;i:63-7.

25. Kincaid-Smith P, D'Apice AJF. Plasmapheresis in rapidly progressive glomerulonephritis. Am J Med 1978;65:564-6.

26. Hind CRK, Paraskevakou H, Lockwood CM, et al. Prognosis after immunosuppression of patients with crescentic nephritis requiring dialysis. Lancet 1983;i:263-5.

27. Mauri JM, Gonzales MT, Poveda R, et al. Therapeutic TPE in the treatment of rapidly progressive glomerulonephritis. Plasma Ther Transfus Technol 1985;6:587-91.

28. Glockner WM, Sieberth HG, Wichmann HE, et al. Plasma exchange and immunosuppression in rapidly progressive glomerulonephritis: A controlled multi-center study. Clin Nephrol 1988;29:1-8.

29. Pusey CD, Rees AJ, Evans DJ, et al. Plasma exchange in focal necrotizing glomerulonephritis without anti-GBM antibodies. Kidney Int 1991;40:757-63.

30. Cole E, Cattran D, Magil A, et al. A prospective randomized trial of TPE as additive therapy in idiopathic crescentic glomerulonephritis. Am J Kidney Dis 1992;20:261-9.

31. Kaplan AA. The use of apheresis in immune renal disorders. Therap Apher Dial 2003;7: 165-72.

32. Kaplan AA. A practical guide to therapeutic plasma exchange. Malden, MA: Blackwell Science, 1999.

33. Jayne DR, Gaskin G, Rasmussen N, et al. Randomized trial of TPE or high-dosage methylprednisolone as adjunctive therapy for severe renal vasculitis. J Am Soc Nephrol 2007;18: 2180-8.

34. Stone JH, Kaplan AA, Rose BD. Initial and maintenance therapy of Wegener's granulomatosis and microscopic polyangiitis. In: Rose, BD, ed. UpToDate, BDR, version 18.1 (January 2010). Waltham, MA: UpToDate, 2010. [Available at http://www.utdol.com.]

35. Buxbaum JN, Chuba JV, Hellman GC, et al. Monoclonal immunoglobulin deposition disease: Light chain and light and heavy chain deposition diseases and their relation to light chain amyloidosis. Clinical features, immunopathology, and molecular analysis. Ann Intern Med 1990;112:455-64.

36. Solomon A, Weiss DT, Kattine AA. Nephrotoxic potential of Bence Jones proteins. N Engl J Med 1991;324:1845-51.

37. Kaplan AA. Therapeutic apheresis for the renal complications of multiple myeloma and the dysglobulinemias. Ther Apher 2001;5:171-5.

38. Cserti C, Haspel R, Stowell C, Dzik W. Light chain removal by plasmapheresis in myeloma-associated renal failure. Transfusion 2007;47: 511-14.

39. Zucchelli P, Pasquali S, Cagnoli L, Ferrari G. Controlled TPE trial in acute renal failure due to multiple myeloma. Kidney Int 1988;33: 1175-89.

40. Clark WF, Stewart AK, Rock GA, et al. Plasma exchange when myeloma presents as acute renal failure: A randomized, controlled trial. Ann Intern Med 2005;143:777-84.

41. Gertz MA. Managing myeloma kidney (editorial). Ann Intern Med 2005;143:835-7.

42. Rajkumar SV, Kaplan AA, Leung N. Treatment of renal failure in multiple myeloma. In: Rose BD, ed. UpToDate, BDR, version 18.1 (January 2010). Waltham, MA: UpToDate, 2010. [Available at http://www.utdol.com.]

43. Clark WF. Plasma exchange in multiple myeloma (letter response). Ann Int Med 2006; 144:455.

44. Leung N. Plasma exchange in multiple myeloma (letter). Ann Intern Med 2006;144:455.

45. Leung N, Gertz MA, Zeldenrust SR, et al. Improvement of cast nephropathy with TPE depends on the diagnosis and on reduction of serum free light chains. Kidney Int 2008;73:1282-8.

46. Misiani R, Tiraboschi G, Mingardi G, Mecca G. Management of myeloma kidney: An anti-light chain approach. Am J Kidney Dis 1987;10:28-33.

47. Johnson WJ, Kyle RA, Pineda AA, et al. Treatment of renal failure associated with multiple myeloma. Plasmapheresis, hemodialysis, and chemotherapy. Arch Intern Med 1990;150:863-9.

48. Kaplan AA, Halley SE. Plasma exchange with a rotating filter. Kidney Int 1990;38:160-6.

49. Wahlin A, Lofvenberg E, Holm J. Improved survival in multiple myeloma with renal failure. Acta Med Scand 1987;221:205-9.

50. Russell JA, Fitzharris BM, Corringham R, et al. Plasma exchange v peritoneal dialysis for removing Bence Jones protein. Br Med J 1978;2:1397.

51. Hutchison CA, Cockwell P, Reid S, et al. Efficient removal of immunoglobulin free light chains by hemodialysis for multiple myeloma: In vitro and in vivo studies. J Am Soc Nephrol 2007;18:886-95.

52. Hutchison CA, Bradwell AR, Cook M, et al. Treatment of acute renal failure secondary to multiple myeloma with chemotherapy and extended high cut-off hemodialysis. Clin J Am Soc Nephrol 2009;4:745-54.

53. Galla JH. IgA nephropathy. Kidney Int 1995;47:377-87.

54. Hene RJ, Kater L. Plasmapheresis in nephritis associated with Henoch-Schonlein Purpura and in primary IgA nephropathy. Plasma Ther Transfus Technol 1983;4:165-73.

55. Coppo R, Basolo B, Roccatello D, Piccoli G. Plasma exchange in primary IgA nephropathy and Henoch-Schonlein Syndrome nephritis. Plasma Ther Transfus Technol 1985;6:705-23.

56. Coppo R, Basolo B, Giachino O, et al. Plasmapheresis in a patient with rapidly progressive idiopathic IgA nephropathy: Removal of IgA-containing circulating immune complexes and clinical recovery. Nephron 1985;40:488-90.

57. Nicholls K, Becker G, Walker R, et al. Plasma exchange in progressive IgA nephropathy. J Clin Apher 1990;5:128-32.

58. Afessa B, Cowart RG, Koenig SM. Alveolar hemorrhage in IgA nephropathy treated with plasmapheresis. South Med J 1997;90:237-9.

59. Gaskell H, Searle M, Dathan JR. Henoch-Schonlein purpura with severe ileal involvement responding to plasmapheresis. Int J Artif Organs 1985;8:163-4.

60. Morichau-Beauchant M, Touchard G, Maire P, et al. IgA and C3 deposition in adult Henoch-Schonlein purpura with severe intestinal manifestations. Gastroenterology 1982;82:1438-42.

61. Joseph G, Holtman JS, Kosfeld RE, et al. Pregnancy in Henoch-Schonlein purpura. Am J Obstet Gynecol 1987;157:911-12.

62. Jones JV, Cumming RH, Bucknall RC, et al. Plasmapheresis in the management of acute systemic lupus erythematosus? Lancet 1976;i:709-11.

63. Jones JV, Cumming RH, Bacon PA, et al. Evidence for a therapeutic effect of plasmapheresis in patients with systemic lupus erythematosus. Quart J Med 1979;192:555-76.

64. Jones JV, Robinson MF, Parciany RK, et al. Therapeutic plasmapheresis in systemic lupus erythematosus. Arthritis Rheum 1981;24:1113-20.

65. Abdou NI, Lindsley HB, Pollock A, et al. Plasmapheresis in active lupus erythematosus: Effect on clinical, serum and cellular abnormalities. Case report. Clin Immunol Immunopath 1981;19:44-54.

66. Leaker BR, Becker GJ, Dowling JP, Kincaid-Smith PS. Rapid improvement in severe lupus glomerular lesions following intensive TPE associated with immunosuppression. Clin Nephrol 1986;25:236-44.

67. Wei N, Klippel JH, Huston DP, et al. Randomized trial of TPE in mild systemic lupus erythematosus. Lancet 1983;i;17-21.

68. French Collaborative Group. A randomized trial of TPE in severe acute systemic lupus erythematosus: Methodology and interim analysis. Transfus Technol 1985;6:535-9.

69. Lewis EJ, Hunsicker LG, Lan SP, et al. A controlled trial of plasmapheresis therapy in severe lupus nephritis. N Engl J Med 1992;326:1373-9.

70. Stricker R, Davis JA, Gershow J, et al. Thrombotic thrombocytopenic purpura complicating systemic lupus erythematosus. Case report and

literature review from the plasmapheresis era. J Rheumatol 1992;19:1469-73.

71. Thomson BJ, Watson ML, Liston WA, Lambie AT. Plasmapheresis in a pregnancy complicated by acute systemic lupus erythematosus. Case report. Br J Obstet 1985;92:532-4.

72. Neuwelt CM. The role of plasmapheresis in the treatment of severe central nervous system neuropsychiatric systemic lupus erythematosus. Ther Apher Dial 2003;7:173-83.

73. Kiprov DD, Strauss RG, Ciavarella D, et al. Management of autoimmune disorders. J Clin Apher 1993;8:195-210.

74. Schroeder JO, Schwab U, Zenner R, et al. Plasmapheresis and subsequent pulse cyclophosphamide in severe systemic lupus erythematosus. Preliminary results of the SPSG trial. Arthritis Rheum 1997;40:S325.

75. Wallace DJ, Goldfinger D, Pepkowitz SH, et al. Randomized controlled trial of pulse/synchronization cyclophosphamide/apheresis for proliferative lupus nephritis. J Clin Apher 1998; 13:163-4.

76. Schlansky R, DeHoratius RJ, Pincus T, Tung KSK. Plasmapheresis in systemic lupus erythematosus: A cautionary note. Arthritis Rheum 1981;24:49-53.

77. Gaubitz M, Schneider M. Immunoadsorption in systemic lupus erythematosus: Different techniques and their current role in medical therapy. Ther Apher Dial 2003;7:183-8.

78. Love PE, Santoro SA. Antiphospholipid antibodies: Anticardiolipin and the lupus anticoagulant in systemic lupus erythematosus (SLE) and in non-SLE disorders. Prevalence and clinical significance. Ann Intern Med 1990;112: 682-98.

79. Frampton G, Hicks J, Cameron JS. Significance of anti-phospholipid antibodies in patients with lupus nephritis. Kidney Int 1991;39:1225-31.

80. Kincaid-Smith P, Nicholls K. Renal thrombotic microvascular disease associated with LAC. Nephron 1990;54:285-8.

81. Farrugia E, Torres VE, Gastineau D, et al. Lupus anticoagulant is SLE: A clinical and renal pathological study. Am J Kidney Dis 1992;20:463-71.

82. Kincaid-Smith P, Fairley K, Kloss M. Lupus anticoagulant associated with renal thrombotic microangiopathy and pregnancy related renal failure. Quart J Med 1988;258:795-815.

83. Zar T, Kaplan AA. Predictable removal of anticardiolipin antibody by therapeutic plasma exchange (TPE) in catastrophic antiphospho-

84. Glueck HI, Kant KS, Weiss MA, et al. Thrombosis in systemic lupus erythematosus: Relation to the presence of circulating anticoagulants. Arch Intern Med 1985;145:1389-95.

85. Parke AL, Wilson D, Maier D. The prevalence of antiphospholipid antibodies in women with recurrent spontaneous abortion, women with successful pregnancies and women who have never been pregnant. Arthritis Rheum 1991; 34:1231-5.

86. Asherson RA, Piette JC. The catastrophic antiphospholipid syndrome 1996: Acute multiorgan failure associated with antiphospholipid antibodies: A review of 31 patients. Lupus 1996;5:414-7.

87. Neuwelt CM, Daikh DI, Linfoot JA, et al. Catastrophic antiphospholipid syndrome: Response to repeated plasmapheresis over three years. Arthritis Rheum 1997;40:1534-9.

88. Bucciarelli S, Espinosa G, Cervera R, et al. Mortality in the catastrophic antiphospholipid syndrome: Causes of death and prognostic factors in a series of 250 patients. Arthritis Rheum 2006;54:2568-76.

89. Bermas BL, Schur PH, Kaplan AA. Treatment of the antiphospholipid syndrome. In: Rose BD, ed. UpToDate, BDR, version 18.1 (January 2010). Waltham, MA: UpToDate, 2010. [Available at http://www.utdol.com.]

90. Frampton G, Cameron JS, Thom M, et al. Successful removal of antiphospholipid antibody during pregnancy using TPE and low dose prednisolone. Lancet 1987;ii:1023-4.

91. Fulcher D, Stewart G, Exner T, et al. Plasma exchange and the anticardiolipin syndrome in pregnancy. Lancet 1989;ii:171.

92. Torres J, Sanchez JL. Histopathologic differentiation between localized and systemic scleroderma. Am J Dermatol 1998;20:242-5.

93. Kallenberg CG, Wouda AA, Hoet MH, van Venrooij WJ. Development of connective tissue disease in patients presenting with Raynaud's phenomenon: A six year follow up with emphasis on the predictive value of antinuclear antibodies as detected by immunoblotting. Ann Rheum Dis 1988;47:634-41.

94. Dau PC, Kahaleh MB, Sagebiel RW. Plasmapheresis and immunosuppressive drug therapy in scleroderma. Arthritis Rheum 1981;24: 1128-36.

95. Weiner SR, Kono DH, Osterman HA. Preliminary report on a controlled trial of apheresis in

lipid antibody syndrome (CAPS). Clin Nephrol 2008;70:77-91.

the treatment of scleroderma (abstract). Arthritis Rheum 1987;30:S24.

96. McCune M, Winkelmann RK, Osmundson PJ, Pineda AA. Plasma exchange: A controlled study of the effect in patients with Raynaud's phenomenon and scleroderma. J Clin Apher 1983;1:206-14.

97. Guillevin L, Leon A, Levy Y, et al. Treatment of progressive systemic sclerosis with TPE. Seven cases. Int J Artif Organs 1983;6:315-18.

98. Cozzi F, Marson P, Rosada M, et al. Long-term therapy with TPE in systemic sclerosis: Effects on laboratory markers reflecting disease activity. Transfus Apher Sci 2001;25:25-31.

99. Rook AH, Freundlich B, Jegasothy BV, et al. Treatment of systemic sclerosis with extracorporeal photochemotherapy. Arch Dermatol 1992;128:337-46.

100. Steen VD, Costantino JP, Shapiro AP, Medsger TA Jr. Outcome of renal crisis in systemic sclerosis: Relation to availability of angiotensin converting enzyme (ACE) inhibitors. Ann Intern Med 1990;113:352-7.

101. Endo H, Hosono T, Kondo H. Antineutrophil cytoplasmic autoantibodies in 6 patients with renal failure and systemic sclerosis. J Rheumatol 1994;21:864-70.

102. Omote A, Muramatsu M, Sugimoto Y, et al. Myeloperoxidase-specific anti-neutrophil cytoplasmic autoantibodies-related scleroderma renal crisis treated with double-filtration plasmapheresis. Intern Med 1997;36:508-13.

103. Wach F, Ullrich H, Schmitz G, et al. Treatment of severe localized scleroderma by plasmapheresis—report of three cases. Br J Dermatol 1995;133:605-9.

104. Malchesky PS, Clough JD. Cryoglobulins: Properties, prevalence in disease and removal. Cleve Clin Q 1985;52:175-92.

105. Gilcher RO, Strauss RG, Ciavarella D, et al. Management of renal disorders. J Clin Apher 1993;8:258-69.

106. Solomon A, Fahey JL. Plasmapheresis therapy in macroglobulinemia. Ann Intern Med 1963; 58:789-800.

107. Lockwood CM. Lymphoma, cryoglobulinemia and renal disease. Kidney Int 1979;16:522-30.

108. Berkman EM, Orlin JB. Use of plasmapheresis and partial TPE in the management of patients with cryoglobulinemia. Transfusion 1979;20: 171-8.

109. Geltner D, Kohn RW, Gorevic P, Franklin EC. The effect of combination therapy (steroids, immunosuppressives and plasmapheresis) on 5 mixed cryoglobulinemia patients with renal, neurologic and vascular involvement. Arthritis Rheum 1981;24:1121-7.

110. D'Amico G, Ferrario F, Colasanti G, Bucci A. Glomerulonephritis in essential mixed cryoglobulinemia. In: Davison PJ, Guillon PJ, eds. Proceedings of the XXI Congress of the European Dialysis and Transplant Association. London: Pitman, 1984:527-48.

111. Evans TW, Nicholls AJ, Shortland JR, et al. Acute renal failure in essential mixed cryoglobulinemia: Precipitation and reversal by TPE. Clin Nephrol 1984;21:287-93.

112. Ferri C, Moriconi L, Gremignai G, et al. Treatment of the renal involvement in mixed cryoglobulinemia with prolonged TPE. Nephron 1986;43:246-53.

113. D'Amico G, Colasanti G, Ferrario F, Sinico RA. Renal involvement in essential mixed cryoglobulinemia. Kidney Int 1989;35:1004-14.

114. Flamm S, Chopra S, Kaplan AA, Appel GB. Treatment of essential mixed cryoglobulinemia: In: Rose BD,ed. UpToDate, BDR, version 18.1 (January 2010). Waltham, MA: UpToDate, 2010. [Available at http://www.utdol.com.]

115. Frankel AH, Singer DRJ, Winearls CG, et al. Type II essential mixed cryoglobulinemia: Presentation, treatment and outcome in 13 patients. Q J Med 1992;82:101-24.

116. Misiani R, Bellavita P, Fenili D, et al. Interferon alfa-2a therapy in cryoglobulinemia associated with hepatitis C virus. N Engl J Med 1994; 330:751-6.

117. Misiani R, Bellavita P, Fenili D, et al. Hepatitis C virus infection in patients with essential mixed cryoglobulinemia. Ann Intern Med 1992;117:573-7.

118. Valbonesi M, Garelli S, Montani F, et al. Management of immune-mediated and paraproteinemic diseases by membrane plasma separation and cascade filtration. Vox Sang 1982;43:91-101.

119. Vibert GJ, Wirtz SA, Smith JW, et al. Cryofiltration as an alternative to TPE: Plasma macromolecular solute removal without replacement fluids. In: Nose Y, Malchesky PS, Smith JW, eds. Plasmapheresis. Cleveland, OH: ISAO Press, 1983:281-7.

120. McLeod, BC, Sassetti, RJ. Plasmapheresis with return of cryoglobulin-depleted autologous plasma (cryoglobulinpheresis) in cryoglobulinemia. Blood 1980;55:866-70.

121. Chad D, Oaruser JM, Bradley WG, et al. The pathogenesis of cyroglobulinemic neuropathy. Neurology 1982;32:725-9.

122. Berkman EM, Orlin JB. Use of plasmapheresis and partial TPE in the management of patients with cryoglobulinemia. Transfusion 1980;20:171-8.

123. Valbonesi M, Mosconi L, Montani F, et al. A method for the study of cryoglobulin solubilization curves at 37 degrees Celsius. Preliminary studies and application to TPE in cryoglobulinemic syndromes. Int J Artif Organs 1983;6:87-90.

124. Alric L, Plaisier E, Thebault S, et al. Influence of antiviral therapy in hepatitis C virus-associated cryoglobulinemic MPGN. Am J Kidney Dis 2004;43:617-23.

125. Furlan M, Robles R, Galbusera M, et al. Von Willebrand factor-cleaving protease in thrombotic thrombocytopenic purpura and the hemolytic-uremic syndrome. N Engl J Med 1998;339:1578-84.

126. Tsai HM, Lian EC. Antibodies to von Willebrand factor-cleaving protease in acute thrombotic thrombocytopenic purpura. N Engl J Med 1998;339:1585-94.

127. George JN. ADAMTS13: What it does, how it works, and why it's important (editorial). Transfusion 2009;49:196-8.

128. Rock GA, Shumak KH, Buskard NA, et al. Comparison of TPE with plasma infusion in the treatment of thrombotic thrombocytopenic purpura. N Engl J Med 1991;325:393-7.

129. Rose BD, Kaplan AA, George JN. Treatment of thrombotic thrombocytopenic purpura-hemolytic uremic syndrome in adults In: Rose BD, ed. UpToDate, BDR, version 18.1 (January 2010). Waltham, MA: UpToDate, 2010. [Available at http://www.utdol.com.]

130. Rondeau E, Peraldi MN. *Escherichia coli* and the hemolytic uremic syndrome (editorial). N Engl J Med 1996;335:660-2.

131. Drummond KN. Hemolytic uremic syndrome—then and now (editorial). N Engl J Med 1985;312:116-18.

132. Lyman NW, Michaelson R, Viscuso RL, et al. Mitomycin-induced hemolytic-uremic syndrome: Successful treatment with corticosteroids and intense TPE. Arch Intern Med 1983;143:1617-18.

133. Aster RH. Quinine sensitivity: A new cause of the hemolytic uremic syndrome. Ann Intern Med 1993;119:243-4.

134. Melnyk AMS, Solez K, Kjellstrand CM. Adult hemolytic uremic syndrome: A review of 37 cases. Arch Intern Med 1995;155:2077-84.

135. Morel-Maroger L, Kanfer A, Solez K, et al. Prognostic importance of vascular lesions in acute renal failure with microangiopathic hemolytic anemia (hemolytic uremic syndrome): Clinicopathologic study in 20 adults. Kidney Int 1979;15:548-58.

136. Schieppati A, Ruggenenti P, Cornejo RP, et al. Renal function at hospital admission as a prognostic factor in adult hemolytic uremic syndrome. J Am Soc Nephrol 1992;2:640-4.

137. Conlon PJ, Howell DN, Macik G, et al. The renal manifestations and outcome of thrombotic thrombocytopenic pupura/hemolytic uremic syndrome. Nephrol Dial Transpl 1995;10:1189-93.

138. Dundas S, Murphy J, Soutar RL, et al. Effectiveness of therapeutic TPE in the 1996 Lanarkshire *Escherichia coli* O157:H7 outbreak. Lancet 1999;354:1327-30.

139. Karpac CA, Li X, Terrell DR, et al. Sporadic bloody diarrhoea-associated thrombotic thrombocytopenic purpura-haemolytic uraemic syndrome: An adult and paediatric comparison. Br J Haematol 2008;141:696-707.

140. George JN. Clinical practice. Thrombotic thrombocytopenic purpura. N Engl J Med 2006;354:1927-35.

141. Bennett CL, Weinberg PD, Rozenberg-Ben-Dror K, et al. Thrombotic thrombocytopenic purpura associated with ticlopidine. Ann Intern Med 1998;128:541-4.

142. Bennett Cl, Davidson CJ, Raisch DW, et al. Thrombotic thrombocytopenic purpura associated with ticlopidine in the setting of coronary artery stents and stroke prevention. Arch Intern Med 1999;159:2524-8.

143. Bueno D Jr, Sevigny J, Kaplan AA. Extracorporeal treatment of thrombotic microangiopathy: A ten year experience. Ther Apher 1999;3:294-7.

144. Kaplan AA. Therapeutic apheresis for cancer related hemolytic uremic syndrome. Ther Apher 2000;4:201-6.

145. Palmisano J, Agraharkar M, Kaplan AA. Successful treatment of cisplatin-induced hemolytic uremic syndrome with therapeutic TPE. Am J Kidney Dis 1998;32:314-17.

146. George JN, Li X, McMinn JR, et al. Thrombotic thrombocytopenic purpura-hemolytic uremic syndrome following allogeneic HPC transplan-

tation: A diagnostic dilemma. Transfusion 2004; 44:294-304.

147. Lesesne JB, Rothschild N, Erickson B, et al. Cancer associated hemolytic-uremic syndrome: Analysis of 85 cases from a national registry. J Clin Oncol 1989;7:781.

148. Korec S, Schein PS, Smith FP, et al. Treatment of cancer-associated hemolytic uremic syndrome with staphylococcal protein A immunoperfusion. J Clin Oncol 1986;4:210-15.

149. Watson PR, Guthrie Jr TH, Caruana RJ. Cisplatin-associated hemolytic-uremic syndrome. Cancer 1989;64:1400-3.

150. Snyder HJ, Mittleman A, Oral A, et al. Treatment of cancer chemotherapy-associated thrombotic thrombocytopenic purpura/hemolytic uremic syndrome by protein A immunoadsorption of plasma. Cancer 1993;71:1882-92.

151. Garibotto G, Acquarone N, Saffioti S, et al. Successful treatment of mitomycin C-associated hemolytic uremic syndrome by plasmapheresis. Nephron 1989;51:409-12.

152. Bell WR, Braine HG, Ness PM, Kickler TS. Improved survival of thrombotic thrombocytopenic purpura-hemolytic uremic syndrome: Clinical experience in 108 patients. N Engl J Med 1991;325:398-403.

153. Cattran DC. Adult hemolytic-uremic syndrome: Successful treatment with plasmapheresis. Am J Kidney Dis 1984;3:275-9.

154. Agarwal A, Mauer SM, Matas AJ, Nath KA. Recurrent hemolytic uremic syndrome in an adult renal allograft recipient: Current concepts and management. J Am Soc Nephrol 1995; 6:1160-9.

155. Martin DL, MacDonald KL, White K, et al. The epidemiology and clinical aspects of the hemolytic uremic syndrome in Minnesota. N Engl J Med 1990;323:1161-7.

156. Rondeau E, Peraldi MN. Escherichia coli and the hemolytic uremic syndrome (editorial). N Engl J Med 1996;335:660-2.

157. Rizzoni G, Claris-Appiani A, Edefonti A, et al. Plasma infusion for hemolytic-uremic syndrome in children: Results of a multicenter controlled trial. J Pediatr 1988;112:284-90.

158. Gianviti A, Perna A, Caringella A, et al. Plasma exchange in children with hemolytic-uremic syndrome at risk of poor outcome. Am J Kidney Dis 1993;22:264-6.

159. Robson WLM, Leung AKC. The successful treatment of atypical hemolytic uremic syndrome with plasmapheresis. Clin Nephrol 1991;35:119-22.

160. Denneberg T, Friedberg M, Holmberg L, et al. Combined plasmapheresis and hemodialysis treatment for severe hemolytic-uremic syndrome following Campylobacter colitis. Acta Paediatr Scand 1982;71:243-5.

161. Sheth KJ, Leichter HE, Gill JC, Baumgardt A. Reversal of central nervous system involvement in hemolytic uremic syndrome by use of TPE. Clin Pediat 1987;26:651-6.

162. Noris M, Remuzzi G. Translational minireview series on complement factor H: therapies of renal diseases associated with complement factor H abnormalities: Atypical haemolytic uraemic syndrome and membranoproliferative glomerulonephritis. Clin Exp Immunol 2007;151:199-209.

163. Artero ML, Sharma R, Savin VJ, Vincenti F. Plasmapheresis reduces proteinuria and serum capacity to injure glomeruli in patients with recurrent focal glomerulosclerosis. Am J Kidney Dis 1994;23:574-81.

164. Crosson JT. Focal segmental glomerulosclerosis and renal transplantation. Transplant Proc 2007;39:737-43.

165. Kirubakaran MG, Disney APS, Norman J, et al. A controlled trial of plasmapheresis in the treatment of renal allograft rejection. Transplantation 1981;32:164-5.

166. Allen NH, Dyer P, Geoghegan T, et al. Plasma exchange in acute renal allograft rejection. Transplantation 1983;35:425-8.

167. Bonomini V, Vangelista A, Frasca GM, et al. Effects of plasmapheresis in renal transplant rejection: A controlled study. Trans Am Soc Artif Intern Organs 1985;31:698-701.

168. Charpentier BM, Hiesse C, Kriaa F, et al. How to deal with the hyperimmunized potential recipients. Kidney Int 1992;42(Suppl 38):S-176-81.

169. Ross CN, Gaskin G, Gregor-Macgregor S, et al. Renal transplantation following immunoadsorption in highly sensitized recipients. Transplantation 1993;55:785-9.

In: McLeod BC, Szczepiorkowski ZM, Weinstein R, Winters JL, eds.
Apheresis: Principles and Practice, 3rd edition
Bethesda, MD: AABB Press, 2010

18

Apheresis in Solid Organ Transplantation

Marisa B. Marques, MD

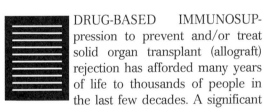DRUG-BASED IMMUNOSUP-pression to prevent and/or treat solid organ transplant (allograft) rejection has afforded many years of life to thousands of people in the last few decades. A significant drawback of the current drugs, however, is the morbidity associated with such regimens in terms of opportunistic infections and the development of malignancies.[1,2] Furthermore, the most commonly used drugs, such as cyclosporine and tacrolimus (calcineurin phosphatase inhibitors), are associated with complications such as nephrotoxicity, neurotoxicity, and thrombotic microangiopathy, among others.[3] In this context, tools to increase allograft tolerance are greatly needed.

Apheresis modalities such as therapeutic plasma exchange (TPE) and extracorporeal photopheresis (ECP) have been extensively used synergistically with drugs to curb and/or avoid solid organ transplant rejection.[4] Overall, apheresis offers a very positive balance between benefits and side effects. At the University of Alabama at Birmingham (UAB) University Hospital, approximately half of all apheresis procedures performed each year are indicated to prevent or treat rejection in patients who have received heart, lung, or kidney transplants.

Before transplantation, TPE is used to remove and/or significantly reduce the titer of preformed antibodies to ABO or HLA antigens to prevent acute rejection. After transplantation, TPE helps avoid or treat acute humoral rejection (antibody-mediated rejection, or AMR). As discussed in this chapter, there is significantly more experience with TPE in renal transplantation than in cardiac, pulmonary, or hepatic transplantation.

Marisa B. Marques, MD, Professor of Pathology, University of Alabama at Birmingham, and Medical Director, University Hospital Transfusion Services, Birmingham, Alabama

The author has disclosed no conflicts of interest.

ECP was developed in the last 25 years to treat cutaneous T-cell lymphoma (CTCL).[5] It has since become an important tool to aid patients with the advanced form of this rare type of malignancy. With the recognition that allograft rejection is characterized by clonal expansion of activated T cells, ECP was also tested in animal models of transplantation. In 1989, two reports described the benefit of ECP when it was used in mice and primates who had received skin and heart allografts, respectively.[6,7] The first patients successfully treated with ECP for allograft rejection had received cardiac transplants and were reported in 1992.[8,9] Since then, many other clinical studies have shown positive results of ECP. In addition to the usefulness of ECP in the management of patients with solid organ transplant rejection, more recent reports have demonstrated improvement in acute and chronic graft-versus-host disease (GVHD).[10,11] GVHD is the major complication of allogeneic stem cell transplantation and poses significant morbidity and mortality. It arises when donor T cells recognize nonself proteins such as HLA expressed by most nucleated cells of the recipient. Acute GVHD affects mainly the skin, gastrointestinal tract, and liver, while chronic GVHD may involve the same organs plus mucous membranes, muscle, lungs, kidneys, heart, and marrow.[10,11] Although the exact mechanism of action of ECP in transplantation is not known, several lines of evidence point to an immunomodulatory effect mediated by the irradiation of lymphocytes ex vivo, reinfusion of these cells into the patient, in-vivo apoptosis, and induction of immune tolerance.[12,13] ECP and GVHD are discussed in detail in Chapter 28.

Renal Transplantation

Thousands of people are listed for a renal transplant in the United States each year.[14] In contrast, the supply of organs is only a fraction of the need, leaving many transplant candidates on chronic dialysis for the rest of their lives. Most patients waiting for a kidney transplant are from blood group O, followed by A, B, and AB. Because group O individuals preferentially receive kidneys from O donors to avoid hyperacute rejection and organ loss, they had a median waiting time of 1454 days in 2003, longer than that of patients of blood groups A or AB. Considering the prevalence of blood groups in the United States, the probability that any two persons will be ABO incompatible is 36%, excluding up to one-third of potential living donors.[15] If ABO incompatibility could be overcome, mathematical models estimate that an additional 1500 transplants could be performed each year in this country.[16] While it is estimated that a renal transplant doubles a person's average life expectancy and improves the quality of life, thousands of people die each year, awaiting renal transplant.

For those who are transplanted, antibody-mediated rejection of the allograft is a threat that may take several forms. Hyperacute rejection, caused by anti-A or anti-B isohemagglutinins, occurs within minutes to hours of transplantation and may present with cyanosis of the allograft, quickly followed by progressive cortical necrosis and urgent need for organ removal.[17] Acute AMR is now widely accepted as a distinct clinicopathologic entity that accounts for approximately 25% of acute rejection episodes.[18] Acute AMR is caused by HLA antibodies and is more likely to occur in patients who are presensitized or in whom immunosuppression is decreased (sometimes because of patient noncompliance with the prescribed regimen). Acute cellular rejection (ACR) is mediated by T cells and has an incidence of approximately 5% to 10% in the first year after transplantation. Patients with ACR present with an abrupt rise in creatinine, fluid retention, and, less commonly, fever and graft tenderness. Chronic rejection may result from AMR, ACR, or both. Histologically, chronic rejection is seen as transplant glomerulopathy, peritubular capillaropathy, transplant arteriopathy, and, less specifically, interstitial fibrosis and tubular atrophy.[18] Understanding of the different types of rejection is essential for optimization of immunosuppression without unnecessarily exposing the patient to the risks associated with the available drugs.[19]

TPE

Apheresis can be used to help overcome the ABO incompatibility barrier by depleting a transplant recipient's isohemagglutinin (A or B) antibodies via TPE before a planned renal transplant from a related or unrelated donor. Furthermore, TPE may be used to remove HLA antibodies in order to allow compatible crossmatches between donor and recipient, treat acute AMR, and combat posttransplant focal segmental glomerulosclerosis (FSGS).[4] (See Table 18-1.)

Desensitization Before and After Transplantation for ABO-Incompatible Transplants

Because A and B antigens are expressed in vascular endothelium, convoluted distal and collecting tubules, kidney allografts may be lost because of hyperacute rejection if transplanted into a recipient with anti-A and/or anti-B. Alexandre and colleagues[20] first reported their experience in 1985 using TPE and splenectomy to reduce anti-A and anti-B titers in ABO-incompatible kidney transplantation. Since then, the indication for TPE has been to decrease the recipient's isohemagglutinin titers (IgM and IgG) before transplantation to <16 by performing as many exchanges as needed to reach this goal. From current experience it is expected, for example, that someone with a titer of 32 will require three TPEs, whereas someone with a titer of 256 may need seven or eight procedures before reaching the pretransplant goal.[21,22] Most centers perform TPE 48 hours apart and replace 1 plasma volume with 5% albumin. Because each laboratory measures isohemagglutinin titers slightly differently, direct comparison between studies is not possible.[21,22] Although most institutions use only the IgG titer, some also test and report the IgM titer in group O recipients.[22] If available, it is preferable that group O individuals receive group A_2 kidneys because of their approximately fivefold lower expression of A antigen compared with A_1 organs.[22] In such cases TPE, used to decrease the recipient anti-A titer, acts synergistically with the presence of fewer antigen sites for the antibody to bind in the allograft.

In addition to preoperative TPE in ABO-incompatible pairs, posttransplant procedures ensure that titers of anti-A and/or anti-B remain low. The number of postoperative procedures is also proportional to the initial titer(s) of A and B antibodies. Posttransplant TPEs are necessary to prevent rebound of anti-A and/or anti-B until tolerance or accommodation occurs. In addition to planned TPE, further treatments may be necessary because of

Table 18-1. Uses of Therapeutic Plasma Exchange in Renal Transplantation

Condition	Indication	ASFA Category[4]
ABO incompatibility	Pretransplant: to lower anti-A and/or anti-B titers Posttransplant: to maintain low titers to allow transplant "accommodation"	II
HLA incompatibility	Pretransplant: to permit compatible crossmatching	II
AMR	To remove DSA to control rejection and protect or restore organ function	I
Posttransplant FSGS	To control proteinuria and preserve renal function	II

ASFA = American Society for Apheresis; AMR = antibody-mediated rejection; DSA = donor-specific antibodies; FSGS = focal segmental glomerulosclerosis.

increases in titers that may be detected during weekly and then monthly posttransplant surveillance, in order to prevent organ damage. Because isohemagglutinin titers cannot predict graft loss, the serum creatinine level is also followed serially along with biopsy results; combined, these data will determine the need for more TPE. Unfortunately, apheresis alone does not ensure successful outcomes, and other immunosuppressive interventions such as intravenous immunoglobulin (IVIG), cytomegalovirus immunoglobulin, antithymocyte globulin, splenectomy, and/or rituximab are used in different combinations in various protocols.

In Japan, double-filtration plasmapheresis in conjunction with TPE have resulted in 90.5% and 95.2% graft and patient survival, respectively, at 3 years, which is comparable to outcomes of patients who received ABO-compatible kidneys.[23] In Stockholm,[24] anti-A and anti-B are removed by immunoadsorption columns with synthetic A or B antigens linked to a Sepharose matrix (GE Healthcare Bio-Sciences AB, Uppsala, Sweden). Their results showed 97% and 98% graft and patient survival, respectively, when immunoadsorption was combined with IVIG, rituximab, and conventional immunosuppression.[24] Although most TPE protocols adjust the number of procedures to the initial isohemagglutinin titer, some patients have been treated with a set number of TPEs with good results.[25] The Mayo Clinic[21] and Johns Hopkins University[22,26] have the most extensive experience with desensitization for ABO-incompatible renal transplants and use similar protocols. Of 26 patients who underwent desensitization at the Mayo Clinic, there were no episodes of hyperacute rejection, and 22 grafts survived.[21] The Johns Hopkins experience with 60 ABO-incompatible renal transplants has been recently reported.[26] Their one-, three-, and five-year graft survival rates were 98.3%, 92.9%, and 88.7%, respectively, which is comparable with the United Network for Organ Sharing data for ABO-compatible living-donor transplants.[27] Furthermore, there were no cases of hyperacute rejection.

It remains to be studied and understood why anti-A and anti-B that rebound after transplantation do not cause renal allograft dysfunction, a phenomenon known as accommodation. A potential yet unproven explanation is that the endothelial cells in the transplanted allograft develop resistance to antibody-mediated injury.[28]

Desensitization Before and After Transplantation for HLA-Mismatched Transplants

As with ABO incompatibility, preformed antibodies to HLA decrease a patient's chance of finding a compatible organ. These antibodies are common in those with previous pregnancy, transplantation, and/or transfusion, especially of nonleukocyte-reduced blood components. Although anti-HLA less often causes hyperacute rejection, it can lead to severe immediate rejection precluding the clinical benefit of transplantation. On kidney transplant waiting lists, between 10% and 20% of people have HLA antibodies to more than 80% of a panel of HLA antigens [panel-reactive antibody (PRA) of 80%], and they are the ones least likely to receive a transplant.[29] Thus, HLA desensitization offers a chance of a better future to thousands of people, and can be accomplished with regimens that incorporate TPE in a fashion similar to ABO desensitization. Indeed, many studies report patients with both types of incompatibility who benefited from TPE-based regimens.[26,30]

Anti-HLA in the recipient's circulation that is specific for antigen present in the potential donor organ is referred as "donor-specific antibody," or DSA. DSA titers may be determined by various techniques, including solid-phase immunoassay and enzyme immunoassay; may be specific for Class I or Class II HLA; and can cause acute or chronic renal allograft rejection.[31] The goal of desensitization may be either total DSA elimination or a significant reduction in its titer.

Several desensitization protocols are currently available and are based on one or more high doses of IVIG (2 g/kg body weight) alone or the combination of TPE and a low dose (100 mg/kg) of IVIG. In addition to determination of the presence and titer of DSA, T- and B-cell crossmatches between the patient's plasma and the donor's lymphocytes are routinely performed either before proceeding with a living-donor transplant or emergently just before surgery if a cadaveric ABO-compatible kidney becomes available. Desensitziation before cadaveric renal transplantation has been less often performed because the suddenness of organ availability generally precludes it.[29] Most studies correlate the use of TPE with DSA titers, crossmatching results, incidence of acute rejection, and/or long-term graft survival. Stegall and colleagues[32] compared the rate of acute rejection among 61 patients with high DSA levels who received one of three different immunosuppression protocols and had negative crossmatching at the time of transplantation. They concluded that regimens containing TPE, low-dose IVIG, and rituximab decreased the number of rejections by more than half compared with high-dose IVIG alone.[32] Akalin et al[33] showed that the percentage of patients with strong pretransplant DSA who developed acute AMR decreased from 44% to 7% with the addition of pretransplant TPE to peritransplant high-dose IVIG. West-Thielke et al[34] studied the outcomes of patients of different races with positive crossmatches who received TPE and low-dose IVIG before and after transplantation with or without rituximab and noted a 3-year graft survival of 65% among 28 patients of non-African ethnicity and 55% among 22 African-American recipients.[34]

Although several other centers have reported good short- or medium-term outcomes with regimens containing TPE,[35,36] a recent report suggests that, despite desensitization protocols, the 5-year survival of organ grafts with positive crossmatching is significantly lower (69.4%) than grafts with negative crossmatching (80.6%).[37] The median survival of positive-crossmatch grafts was 6.8 years. This study highlights the importance of achieving a negative crossmatch during the pretransplant period. Even if the long-term function of organs transplanted into patients with detectable anti-HLA is truly shorter and temporary, the benefit of not requiring dialysis for a few years may justify the continuation of this practice until better methods of desensitization or transplant tolerance induction are developed.

Table 18-2 lists a number of unanswered questions regarding ABO- and HLA-incompatible kidney transplants.

Table 18-2. Unanswered Questions Regarding Immunosuppression in Renal Transplantation

In ABO or HLA Incompatibility:

Which pretransplant immunosuppressive protocol is more effective?

Is daily TPE superior to every-other-day TPE?

Is there a difference in effectiveness between IVIG and CMVIG?

Is splenectomy superior to anti-CD20?

In HLA Incompatibility:

Which test should be used to trigger transplantation?

Does treatment of subclinical AMR prevent organ damage?

Is there a difference in effectiveness between TPE plus IVIG compared with IVIG alone?

TPE = therapeutic plasma exchange; IVIG = intravenous immunoglobulin; CMVIG = cytomegalovirus immunoglobulin; AMR = antibody-mediated rejection.

Posttransplant Antibody-Mediated Rejection

AMR, a new concept in renal transplantation, affects <10% of allografts and is suspected when the serum creatinine increases after transplant. Patients with previously failed transplants as well as those with high PRA are at increased risk of developing AMR. The diagnosis is confirmed by the presence of DSA and an allograft biopsy showing infiltrating neutrophils and circumferential C4d staining in peritubular capillaries (Fig 18-1 and Fig 18-2).[38] ACR may occur simultaneously with AMR and is diagnosed using the Banff 07 classification criteria.[39] In patients with positive crossmatching, the risk of AMR increases with high baseline DSA values, but it does not correlate with T-

and B-cell crossmatching results, and AMR can happen even in patients with a negative T-cell IgG crossmatch.[40] Furthermore, increases in DSA in the first few weeks after transplantation are associated with the development, and the severity, of AMR.[40]

In the Mayo Clinic experience with ABO desensitization[21], AMR developed in 12 of 26 patients and was reversed in 10 using TPE plus increased immunosuppression. Patients with increased serum creatinine required more TPE than those whose AMR was diagnosed by biopsy without evidence of renal dysfunction.[21] AMR occurring in the first 2 weeks after renal transplantation affected close to 50% of 46 patients who underwent desensitization for ABO and/or HLA antibodies at Columbia Uni-

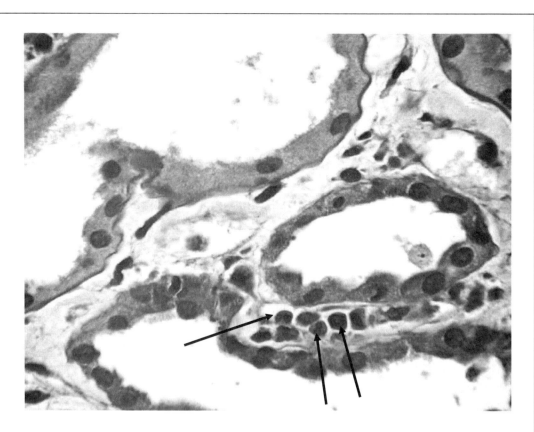

Figure 18-1. Acute antibody-mediated rejection. The earliest finding is neutrophil (arrows) margination in peritubular interstitial capillaries. Associated tubular degenerative changes are also common. (Periodic acid Schiff's biopsy stain. Photo courtesy of Dr. B. Cook, Birmingham, AL.)

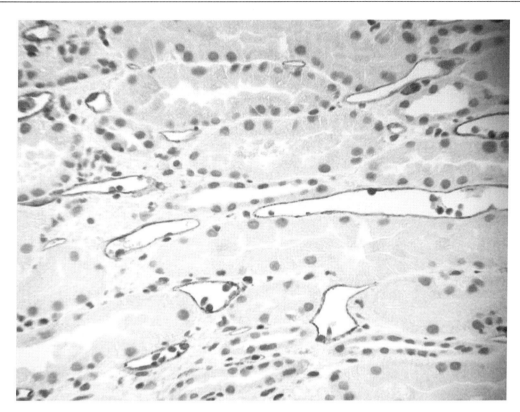

Figure 18-2. Acute antibody-mediated rejection. Antibody to C4d stains the walls of the peritubular capillaries (outlined areas). The intervening cortical tubules show no staining (immunostain for C4d). (Photo courtesy of Dr. B. Cook, Birmingham, AL.)

versity.[30] The authors noted that patients who had required >4 TPEs followed by low-dose IVIG (TPE/IVIG) before transplantation were more likely to develop early AMR despite having achieved negative crossmatching at the time of the transplantation. Based on these findings, they suggested that such patients may benefit from closer monitoring and/or more prophylactic sessions of TPE/IVIG after transplantation.[30] In addition, they reported that patients who received >5 TPE/IVIG procedures because of AMR in the first month after transplantation were at increased risk of developing late ACR (>30 days after transplantation) and of having high serum creatinine at last follow-up, suggesting a lasting damaging effect of the early rejection on the allograft.[30] Lefaucheur and colleagues[41] demonstrated that

a regimen of TPE, IVIG, and rituximab was superior for controlling AMR compared to high-dose IVIG alone, with graft survivals of 92% in the first group compared with 50% in the latter. Because administration of TPE was not the only difference between the groups, the benefit of the TPE-containing regimen is most likely the result of the combination of agents rather than one of the components alone.

Posttransplant Focal Segmental Glomerulosclerosis

Many patients with end-stage renal disease as a result of FSGS are not aware of the cause of their renal failure until the lesion recurs in the transplanted kidney. Posttransplant FSGS occurs in up to one-fourth of allografts and contributes to graft failure in half of the cases.[42] Predictors of recurrence in adults include age, treatment with cyclosporine before transplantation[43] or bilateral nephrectomy, severity of pretransplant FSGS, female gender, and use of living-donor allograft.[42] Recurrent FSGS is suspected when massive proteinuria is noted in the posttransplant period, hours to days postoperatively. If left untreated, FSGS leads to renal dysfunction and eventual graft loss. It has been suggested that prompt initiation of TPE and immunosuppression may halt the progression to end-stage renal disease.[44] Although the cause of FSGS is unknown, there appears to be an ill-defined "permeability factor" in the patient's plasma that is removed by TPE, and plasma concentration correlates with the degree of proteinuria.[45] The reported duration of TPE associated with control of posttransplant FSGS varies widely, with some patients having complete resolution of the proteinuria with <10 sessions and others continuing weekly or monthly TPE to prevent worsening proteinuria.

Much of the experience with TPE in posttransplant FSGS is in children, because FSGS is a common cause of nephrotic syndrome in the young. Garcia and colleagues[46] treated 9 patients with 10 TPE sessions (3 TPEs per week for a total of 10 per patient) combined with high doses of cyclosporine, mycophenolate mofetil, and prednisone, starting <48 hours after diagnosis of proteinuria. A complete remission, defined as proteinuria of <0.2 g/m^2 per day, was obtained in 55%, and a partial response (proteinuria of 1 g/day) was obtained in 12%. None of five children who did not receive TPE achieved remission. Patients remained in remission for an average follow-up period of 2.6 ±1.4 years. The authors suggested that starting TPE early after recurrence is associated with better results because kidney damage is still reversible soon after proteinuria is discovered.[46]

In a French study,[43] eight of nine adult patients achieved partial or complete remission of proteinuria with TPE, but six still lost their grafts. The authors concluded that the benefit of TPE is transient, especially if given as the sole immunosuppression. Valdivia et al treated seven adults with recurrent FSGS.[47] Each patient received 17 sessions of TPE over 10 to 12 weeks, exchanging a fixed volume of 2.5 liters, and the authors reported that all had functioning grafts at an average of 10 months of follow-up.[47] The experience at UAB is that adults whose proteinuria decreased by >50% after a variable number of TPEs had significantly better graft survival than those whose proteinuria did not decrease as much.[44]

ECP

Only a small number of renal transplant patients have been treated with ECP. Between 1995 and 2007, 32 patients were reported to have received ECP in various centers.[48] Lamioni et al[49] showed that the addition of ECP to standard drug immunosuppresion, used prophylactically in two children with cadaveric renal transplants, induced a tolerogenic state mediated by an increase in circulating regulatory T cells (T regs). A recent report from Australia[48] described 10 patients with recurrent biopsy-proven cellular and/or vascular rejection despite corticosteroids and antilymphocyte globulin whose rejection resolved after multiple sessions of ECP. Their ECP methodology was unique: they collected lymphocytes in a Baxter CS 3000 Plus apheresis apparatus (Baxter, Australia) and moved them to an acrylic cell plate designed by one of the authors, where the cells were irradiated in the presence of psoralen.[48] Although they did not use the instrument manufactured by Therakos used for ECP in most centers, their method appears to be similar to conventional ECP, and their results may be able to be generalized.[48] In addition to resolution of rejection, the authors reported that the doses of corticosteroids and antithymocyte globulin could be significantly lowered following ECP, an observation that has important implications in terms of short- and long-term morbidity.

Heart Transplantation

Every year since the first successful operation in 1967, thousands of patients benefit from heart transplantation. Although outcomes have improved over time with the advent of potent immunosuppression, the posttransplant period is still threatened by infection, malignancy, and allograft rejection or vasculopathy. Cellular rejection, the most common type of rejection, is caused by T cells and is diagnosed by biopsy. AMR is less frequent but is associated with increased graft loss, mortality, and vasculopathy.[50] Acute AMR is suspected when the ventricular ejection fraction is found to be decreased but there are no histopathologic signs of T-cell infiltration (Fig 18-3). Estimates of the incidence of AMR in heart transplant recipients vary depending on the employed criteria. When hemodynamic instability is considered essential for the diagnosis, the reported incidence is 8% to 15%; when the presence of C4d in the tissue is required, it is in the range of 3%.[51] Several risk factors have been associated with AMR: young age, female gender, congenital heart disease, positive pretransplant crossmatching, high PRA titer, sensitization to OKT3, and previous exposure to cytomegalovirus.[51] Vasculopathy is an accelerated form of allograft atherosclerosis, with an incidence of

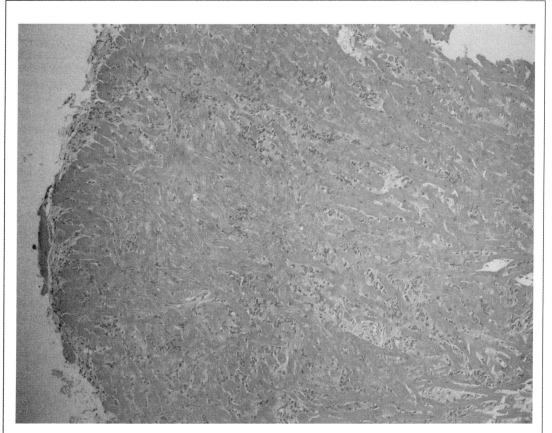

Figure 18-3. Myocardial biopsy demonstrating grade 3A acute cellular rejection. The myocardial interstitium is infiltrated by a cellular inflammatory reaction composed predominantly of T lymphocytes with a minor component of histiocytes. Myocyte dropout and damage is reflected by lymphocytes overlapping the myocyte borders and widening of the interstitium. (Hematoxylin and eosin. Photo courtesy of Dr. T. Winokur, Birmingham, AL.)

approximately 60% within the first 5 years after transplantation.

Drugs used to prevent and/or treat cardiac rejection include cyclosporine, mycophenolate mofetil, and corticosteroids with or without antilymphocyte immunoglobulin. In addition, TPE is useful in acute AMR, and ECP is beneficial to prevent and treat cellular rejection episodes and allograft vasculopathy, as described in more detail in the discussion that follows.

TPE

Although preexisting HLA antibodies may be a significant barrier to heart transplantation, desensitization before transplantation is not practical because of the uncertainty about when an organ will become available. However, because preformed HLA antibodies increase a recipient's chance of rejection and a poor overall outcome after the transplantation, a few investigators have reported their experience with TPE and IVIG in patients with high PRA before transplantation.[52-55] Leech and colleagues[55] showed that 35 patients who had received several sessions of TPE or a single procedure plus IVIG had significantly better overall survival up to 8 years after transplantation compared with historical controls who received only standard immunosuppression after transplantation. Unfortunately their study was retrospective and not all patients received the same TPE and/or immunosuppressive drug protocols, thus compromising the interpretation or application of their results. Overall, current data on desensitization of patients awaiting a cardiac transplant are insufficient to determine its usefulness and/or effectiveness.

Since the late 1980s, TPE has been used in multiple patients to quickly remove DSA during episodes of AMR.[51,56] Although there are no randomized studies of TPE in cardiac AMR, it has been accepted as an effective therapy to curb this type of rejection.[4] On the other hand, TPE does not prevent recurrence of AMR, and immunosuppressive drugs are necessary to prevent further episodes of AMR. UAB performs three daily 1-plasma-volume exchanges as soon as hemodynamic compromise is noted and AMR is suspected. UAB experience suggests that this regimen improves allograft function in most patients as assessed by daily echocardiographic determination of left and right ventricular ejection fraction (Marques, unpublished observation). In UAB experience, patients with cardiac transplant AMR often develop persistent hypofibrinogenemia (<100 mg/dL) during their course of TPE (Marques, unpublished observation). The author speculates that liver congestion brought about by the failing heart is responsible for the inability of the body to replace the fibrinogen removed during apheresis when human serum albumin is the colloid replacement fluid. Thus, fibrinogen monitoring during TPE for AMR is advisable to avoid spontaneous hemorrhage. If the pre-TPE fibrinogen is <100 to 120 mg/dL, plasma or Cryoprecipitated AHF should be included as part of the replacement fluid in order to avoid severe hypofibrinogenemia.

ECP

Rejection prophylaxis after heart transplant is a Category I indication for ECP according to the American Society for Apheresis (see Table 18-3).[4] Category I designation means that ECP is first-line therapy as stand-alone treatment or in conjunction with other modes of treatment.[4]

The largest study to date was a multicenter, international, randomized, double-blind trial published in 1998 that continues to be the most convincing evidence for the role of ECP in heart transplantation.[57] Sixty recently transplanted patients were randomized to standard triple-drug immunosuppression (cyclosporine, azathioprine, and prednisone) alone or with ECP in 12 centers in the United States and Europe.[57] They received two daily ECP treatments per week for the first month followed by every 2 weeks for 2 months and every 4 weeks for 3 months for a total of 24 procedures. Endomyocardial biopsies also followed a standardized protocol and were more often performed in the first month after transplantation, biweekly for 2 months, and once monthly after that. The study's primary end point was the number and frequency of episodes of acute

Table 18-3. Indications for Therapeutic Apheresis in Heart Transplantation[4]

Condition	Therapeutic Plasma Exchange		Extracorporeal Photopheresis	
	Indication	ASFA Category[4]	Indication	ASFA Category[4]
Prophylaxis of rejection	Pretransplant: to decrease DSA titers	III	Posttransplant: to induce tolerance of the organ	I
Treatment of rejection	Acute: to remove DSA and improve hemodynamics	III	To induce tolerance of the transplant and to decrease recurrence of rejection	II

ASFA = American Society for Apheresis; DSA = donor-specific antibody.

rejection as defined histologically in a central laboratory by pathologists blinded to the patient's treatment group.[58] Outcome analysis showed that patients in the ECP group had significantly fewer acute rejection episodes compared with the control group who had received drugs alone.[57] Furthermore, patients treated with ECP were twice as likely to have no rejection, while patients in the standard-therapy group were almost threefold more likely to have two or more occurrences of rejection. On the other hand, ECP did not affect the length of time between transplantation and the first episode of rejection, the incidence of rejection with hemodynamic compromise, or survival at 6 and 12 months.[57]

In 2000, the results of a pilot, prospective, randomized study of prophylactic ECP plus immunossupression to prevent chronic rejection were published.[59] Ten patients had undergone ECP every 4 weeks during the first year, and every 6 or 8 weeks for the first and second halves of the second year, respectively, while 13 patients had received only immunosuppressive drugs. Although the patients in the study arm had a significant reduction (p <0.02) in PRA levels and coronary artery intimal thickness at 2 years, the incidence of atherosclerosis was not different between the groups.[59] As with many other studies with ECP, these results did

not exclude an ECP role in transplant vasculopathy had the schedule of treatments been different. Until more studies are available, the potential benefit of ECP to prevent allograft atherosclerosis remains unknown.

The activity of ECP in decreasing the reoccurrence of rejections (both ACR and AMR) has also been studied. Dall'Amico and colleagues[60] reported in 1995 that when ECP was used as adjuvant treatment, seven of eight patients experienced a reduction in the number and severity of episodes of rejection compared with their history before ECP, as assessed by serial endomyocardial biopsies. Furthermore, immunosuppressive drugs could be successfully tapered in those who received ECP.[60] A few years later, a pilot study of 11 patients who underwent ECP for 6 months showed a reduction (42% vs 18%) in the number of biopsies showing International Society of Heart and Lung Transplantation (ISHLT) grade 3A/3B rejection compared to the pre-ECP period.[61]

UAB performed a retrospective review of the effect of ECP on the likelihood of acute rejection with hemodynamic compromise in 36 patients.[62] Patients referred for ECP procedures were those who had had at least one episode of rejection with hemodynamic compromise and were at high risk for recurrence. Their outcomes were compared with the rejection history of 343 historic controls who were treated at the same time at UAB but were deemed as not requiring ECP because of a lower risk of rejection.[62] After 3 months of ECP, the patients' risk of developing rejection with hemodynamic compromise, or rejection death, decreased markedly (relative risk of 0.29) and approached that of the low-risk patients who did not receive treatment with ECP.[62]

There is yet much to be learned about the mechanism of benefit of ECP in organ transplantation. In 2004, Aubin and Mousson[63] proposed that ECP is able to induce antigen-specific immunomodulation in transplant recipients via T regs. T regs are a subset of lymphocytes that express CD4 and CD25, suppress immune reactions in an antigen-specific mode, and have a central role in the prevention of autoimmunity.[64] Investigators in Germany studied mice that received an intravenous infusion of syngeneic peripheral leukocytes rendered apoptotic after ECP treatment and noticed the induction of antigen-specific T regs.[65] In humans, a group of Italian investigators found that the frequency of T regs with immunosuppressive activity doubled in the peripheral blood of ECP-treated patients with heart and lung allografts compared with healthy controls (p <0.05).[66] In comparison, children treated with immunosuppressive drugs had significantly fewer T regs in their circulation. At 1-year follow-up, two ECP-treated patients still had higher-than-normal numbers of circulating T regs, at which point they started to decrease.[66] The observation that T regs decrease over time suggests that long-term ECP treatments may be needed for the maintenance of the beneficial effect. In a recent mouse model of heart transplantation, George et al[67] also demonstrated a twofold increase in the number of splenic T regs in ECP-treated animals. Furthermore, they showed that ECP extended cardiac allograft survival in two strains of mice and that the effect could be transferred to a non-ECP-treated animal via the infusion of purified T regs.[67] These findings suggest that immunomodulation by ECP has a cellular basis that can be measured and that may be used as a marker to monitor the response to ECP in patients.

Lung Transplantation

Drugs

Approximately 1100 lung transplants are performed each year in the United States for end-stage pulmonary disease resulting from a variety of congenital or acquired conditions such as cystic fibrosis or chronic obstructive pulmonary disease.[4] In order to prevent allograft rejection, immunosuppressive regimens typically employ three drugs, such as a calcineurin inhibitor (cyclosporine or tacrolimus), azathioprine or mycophenolate mofetil, and corticosteroids. Despite the broad immunosuppressive effect of these drugs, around half of transplant recipients develop acute rejection in the first year after surgery.[68] Most lung transplant centers in North America treat uncomplicated acute rejection with a short course of intravenous corticosteroids (methylprednisolone followed by steroid taper over the ensuing weeks).[69] Unfortunately, acute rejection is a risk factor for chronic rejection, which is manifested as bronchiolitis obliterans syndrome (BOS).[70] BOS and infection remain serious threats to long-term survival of lung transplant recipients, currently about 50% at 5 years.[71]

ISHLT developed a staging system for BOS based on the forced expiratory volume in 1 second (FEV_1).[72] In BOS stage 0, the FEV_1 is ≥80% from baseline, and BOS stage 3 refers to severe pulmonary dysfunction with FEV_1 ≤50% from baseline. In addition, each stage is subcategorized to reflect the absence ("a") or presence ("b") of histologic evidence of BOS.

Clinically, BOS is characterized by progressive dyspnea and airflow limitation with declining FEV_1 that cannot be explained by other causes, such as acute rejection or infection. Typically the most precipitous decline in airflow occurs in the first 6 months following a BOS diagnosis, although the time of onset of BOS and rate of decline of FEV_1 are highly variable.[73] A worse course appears to be associated with rapid onset of BOS, female gender, and pretransplant idiopathic pulmonary fibrosis.[73] Furthermore, single lung transplantation carries a higher risk for earlier onset of BOS compared with bilateral transplantation.[74] Successful treatment of BOS is usually defined as "stabilization" or "slowing" of FEV_1 decline instead of true improvement or normalization of airflow.[75] Although the initial treatment of BOS usually consists of repeated pulses of high-dose methylprednisolone, other treatment modalities such as ECP continue to be explored.

ECP

The first successful case of acute lung transplant rejection treated by ECP was published in 1995.[76] In the same year, ECP was shown to stabilize pulmonary function in three lung transplant patients with a deteriorating clinical condition despite high doses of immunosuppressants.[77] Since then, a number of reports have suggested that ECP stabilizes lung function in cases of acute and chronic rejection.[78-80]

Benden and colleagues[81] recently published their results with 12 cycles of ECP performed on 2 consecutive days (one treatment cycle) every 4 to 6 weeks for BOS or recurrent acute rejection. Their primary and secondary outcomes measured rate of decline of FEV_1 and allograft survival after ECP, respectively. Among 12 patients with BOS grades 1 to 3, they saw a significantly decreased monthly decline in FEV_1 (p = 0.011) after ECP compared with the trend before ECP, although there was not a significant effect on the absolute FEV_1 value.[81] Twelve other patients had ECP for recurrent acute rejection (at least two episodes) without evidence of BOS. Among 11 patients who had transbronchial biopsies during ECP, only two patients had one episode of acute rejection, and all experienced clinical stabilization after completing the ECP protocol (12 cycles of ECP on 2 consecutive days).[81] Despite these positive results, two patients had to be retransplanted because of BOS progression after having finished the ECP protocol, and 4 patients died during the 10-year period, all of BOS. On the other hand, as with all other studies of ECP, treatment was well tolerated and no adverse effects were noted. A recent report from Washington University described experi-ence with ECP and confirmed that ECP slowed down the decline in lung function of 60 patients with BOS.[82] Although not directly tested, the accumulated experience suggests that ECP is more beneficial to patients with early-stage BOS (grades 0 or 1).[80,81,83] This assumption is substantiated by the recognition that neither ECP nor any other treatment is likely to reverse fibroblast proliferation in the transplanted lung.

Many questions remain unanswered, however, especially with regard to the schedule, total duration, and immunosuppression used concurrently with ECP treatments. Large multi-center studies are essential to determine the role of ECP and other immunosuppressive regimens in improving the long-term outcome of pulmonary allograft recipients.[84]

Liver Transplantation

In the Scientific Registry of Transplant Recipients database there were more than 16,000 patients awaiting liver transplantation as of December 2008.[85] In 2006, there were <6000 livers donated after brain death and 287 living-donor liver transplantation (LDLT) procedures.[86] Considering that liver transplantation is now highly effective in saving lives and improving the quality of life after end-stage liver disease, the gap between the demand for organs and their availability is unacceptable and has led to a search for alternative sources of organs for transplantation. LDLT is one alternative that has been tried in various countries. Unfortunately LDLT currently accounts for only about 5% of liver transplants in the United States after having peaked at 10% of the total number of organs in 2001.[87] Although LDLT has decreased the mortality of children waiting for a liver transplant to <5%, it has not affected the mortality of adults in the waiting list.[88,89]

TPE

ABO compatibility is not essential for liver transplantation. However, non-ABO-compatible organs increase the recipient's risk of AMR, hepatic artery thrombosis, and biliary stricture, and they compromise recipient and allograft survival.[90] Furthermore, ABO incompatibility may be associated with hyperacute rejection that renders the organ nonfunctional. In the last few years, several groups in various countries have reported their experience using TPE in children and adults receiving ABO-incompatible livers.[91-95]

In 2003, Hanto and colleagues[91] described their results with a protocol that included TPE both before and after transplantation with cadaveric ABO-incompatible organs. Thirteen patients underwent one preoperative TPE exchanging 2 plasma volumes, for plasma compatible with both patient and donor, in order to remove anti-A and/or anti-B.[91] In addition, patients were splenectomized at the time of transplantation, and cyclophosphamide or mycophenolate mofetil plus quadruple immunosuppression were started immediately after transplantation to reduce the risk of cellular rejection. After transplantation, TPEs were performed as needed to maintain anti-A and/or anti-B titers <8 for the first 2 weeks. In the study, 89% of patients had a decrease in IgG titer, and five achieved the goal of a pretransplantation titer of ≤8.[91] In addition, the 1- and 5-year patient and allograft survival rates were 71.4% and 61.2%, respectively.

In the same year, a group from Japan described a protocol that included 2 to 6 TPEs before transplantation and 1 to 6 TPEs after transplantation in conjunction with immunosuppressive drugs for ABO-incompatible LDLT.[92] They followed IgG and IgM titers of anti-A and/or anti-B in the recipient and were able to reach their target IgM of ≤ 16 in all patients and the IgG titer goal of ≤16 in 64% of them. Despite increases in the titers of both immunoglobulin classes in the postoperative period in several patients, survival at 1 year was close to 80%, which is comparable to that of patients who received ABO-compatible organs.[92]

More recent reports involving fewer patients have employed TPE, for ABO-incompatible LDLT,[93] or the combination of TPE with ritux-

imab, IVIG, and splenectomy.[94] Although very preliminary, these results suggest that TPE could contribute to successful liver transplantation across the ABO barrier. A combination of TPE and ECP has also been tried to avoid acute and chronic rejection in adults who received ABO-incompatible organs.[95] In a retrospective comparison study of ABO-incompatible liver transplants, 11 patients (group 1) received a single pretransplantation TPE and posttransplantation TPE for isoagglutinin titers >8, as prophylaxis against humoral rejection. Nine patients (group 2) received IVIG intraoperatively and after every posttransplantation TPE performed for isoagglutinin titers >8, for the first 2 weeks. In addition, group 2 started ECP within the first 7 days after transplantation, beginning with a weekly schedule, followed by monthly procedures depending on liver function tests.[95] Although not all patients were treated using the same ECP method, there was a significant graft survival advantage in group 2 compared with group 1 at 6, 12, and 18 months after surgery.[95] Despite having used two ECP methodologies and variable drug protocols to prevent rejection, this study suggested that ECP potentiates the role of TPE and IVIG in the prophylaxis of AMR. Indeed, none of the 9 patients in group 2 had AMR, compared with 27% in group 1.

ECP

Apart from the above-described study, there are only very preliminary data on the use of ECP in liver transplant recipients. The first case, published in 2000, was a 14-year old who developed refractory acute rejection despite multiple-drug immunosuppression.[96] The child improved after only 4 sessions of two ECPs each. Since then, only a few other cases have been reported in the literature. In 2004, Urbani and colleagues[97] described the outcomes of five patients with allograft rejection with or without steroid-resistance. At a median follow-up of almost 8 months and after undergoing a wide range of ECP schedules, three patients were off ECP (after 20, 51, and 66 courses) with normal liver function and low-dose immunosuppression, and two patients continued to undergo ECP (after 11 and 19 courses) but had started to improve their liver function. A 10-year retrospective study suggested that ECP increased survival of patients who received transplants because of hepatitis-C-induced cirrhosis.[98] However, on multivariate analysis, the benefit of ECP was not confirmed. In summary, ECP in the management of patients with liver transplants has not been widely studied and requires rigorous evaluation of pros and cons.

Conclusion

Therapeutic apheresis for patients with solid organ transplants must undergo the same level of scrutiny and evaluation that is expected of this methodology for any other disease. Its use must be justified by evidence as described by McLeod.[99] The relative dearth of complications associated with TPE and ECP compared with current immunosuppressive drugs provides justification for continued interest in expanding the use of these technologies to improve quality of life and survival of thousands of transplant recipients worldwide.

Acknowledgments

The author thanks Morgan Burke for expert assistance in manuscript preparation and editing and Dr. B. Cook and Dr. T. Winokur for the photomicrographs to illustrate renal and cardiac rejection, respectively.

References

1. Mueller NJ. New immunosuppressive strategies and the risk of infection. Transpl Infect Dis 2008;10:379-84.
2. Zafar SY, Howell DN, Gockerman JP. Malignancy after solid organ transplantation: An overview. Oncologist 2008;13:769-78.
3. Golshayan D, Pascual M. Tolerance-inducing immunosuppressive strategies in clinical transplantation: An overview. Drugs 2008;68: 2113-30.
4. Szczepiorkowski ZM, Winters JL, Bandarenko N, et al. Guidelines on the use of therapeutic apheresis in clinical practice—evidence-based approach from the Apheresis Applications Committee of the American Society for Apheresis. The Fifth Special Issue. J Clin Apher 2010 (in press).
5. Edelson R, Berger C, Gasparro F, et al. Treatment of cutaneous T-cell lymphoma by extracorporeal photochemotherapy. N Engl J Med 1987;316:297-303.
6. Perez M, Edelson R, Laroche L, Berger C. Inhibition of antiskin allograft immunity by infusions with syngeneic photoinactivated effector lymphocytes. J Invest Dermatol 1989;92:669-76.
7. Pepino P, Berger CL, Fuzesi L, et al. Primate cardiac allo- and xeno-transplantation: Modulation of the immune response with photochemotherapy. Eur Surg Res 1989;21:105-13.
8. Rose EA, Barr ML, Xu H, et al. Photochemotherapy in human heart transplant recipients at high risk for fatal rejection. J Heart Lung Transplant 1992;11:746-50.
9. Costanzo-Nordin MR, Hubbell EA, O'Sullivan EJ, et al. Photopheresis versus corticosteroids in the therapy of heart transplant rejection: Preliminary clinical report. Circulation 1992; 86:II242-50.
10. Ferrara JL, Levine JE, Reddy P, Holler E. Graft-versus-host disease. Lancet 2009;373:1550-61.
11. Greinix HT, Knobler RM, Worel N, et al. The effect of intensified extracorporeal photochemotherapy on long-term survival in patients with severe acute graft-versus-host disease. Haematologica 2006;91:405-8.
12. Gatza E, Rogers CE, Clouthier SG, et al. Extracorporeal photopheresis reverses experimental graft-versus-host disease through regulatory T cells. Blood 2008;112:1515-21.
13. Stadler K, Frey B, Munoz LE, et al. Photopheresis with UV-A light and 8-methoxypsoralen leads to cell death and to release of blebs with anti-inflammatory phenotype in activated and non-activated lymphocytes. Biochem Biophys Res Commun 2009;386:71-6.
14. 2007 Annual report of the U.S. Organ Procurement and Transplantation Network and the Scientific Registry of Transplant Recipients: Transplant Data 1997-2006. Rockville, MD: Health Resources and Services Administra-

tion, Healthcare Systems Bureau, Division of Transplantation, 2007.

15. Montgomery RA. ABO incompatible transplantation: To B or not to B. Am J Transplant 2004;4:1011-12.

16. Segev DL, Simpkins CE, Warren DS, et al. ABO incompatible high-titer renal transplantation without splenectomy or anti-CD20 treatment. Am J Transplant 2005;5:2570-5.

17. Racusen LC, Haas M. Antibody-mediated rejection in renal allografts: Lessons from pathology. Clin J Am Soc Nephrol 2006;1:415-20.

18. Cornell LD, Smith RN, Colvin RB. Kidney transplantation: Mechanisms of rejection and acceptance. Annu Rev Pathol 2008;3:189-220.

19. Womer KL, Kaplan B. Recent developments in kidney transplantation—a critical assessment. Am J Transplant 2009;9:1265-71.

20. Alexandre GP, De Bruyere M, Squifflet JP, et al. Human ABO-incompatible living donor renal homografts. Neth J Med 1985;28:231-4.

21. Winters JL, Gloor JM, Pineda AA, et al. Plasma exchange conditioning for ABO-incompatible renal transplantation. J Clin Apher 2004;19:79-85.

22. Tobian AA, Shirey RS, Montgomery RA, et al. The critical role of plasmapheresis in ABO-incompatible renal transplantation. Transfusion 2008;48:2453-60.

23. Kenmochi T, Saigo K, Maruyama M, et al. Results of kidney transplantation from ABO-incompatible living donors in a single institution. Transplant Proc 2008;40:2289-91.

24. Tyden G, Donauer J, Wadstrom J, et al. Implementation of a protocol for ABO-incompatible kidney transplantation—a three-center experience with 60 consecutive transplantations. Transplantation 2007;83:1153-5.

25. Sivakumaran P, Vo AA, Villicana R, et al. Therapeutic plasma exchange for desensitization prior to transplantation in ABO-incompatible renal allografts. J Clin Apher 2009;24:155-60.

26. Montgomery RA, Locke JE, King KE, et al. ABO incompatible renal transplantation: A paradigm ready for broad implementation. Transplantation 2009;87:1246-55.

27. United Network for Organ Sharing. Data: View data reports. Richmond, VA: UNOS, 2010. [Data reports available at http://www.unos.org.]

28. King KE, Warren DS, Samaniego-Picota M, et al. Antibody, complement and accommodation

in ABO-incompatible transplants. Curr Opin Immunol 2004;16:545-9.

29. Faenza A, Fuga G, Bertelli R, et al. Hyperimmunized patients awaiting cadaveric kidney graft: Is there a quick desensitization possible? Transplant Proc 2008;40:1833-8.

30. Padmanabhan A, Ratner LE, Jhang JS, et al. Comparative outcome analysis of ABO-incompatible and positive crossmatch renal transplantation: A single-center experience. Transplantation 2009;87:1889-96.

31. Akalin E, Pascual M. Sensitization after kidney transplantation. Clin J Am Soc Nephrol 2006;1:433-40.

32. Stegall MD, Gloor J, Winters JL, et al. A comparison of plasmapheresis versus high-dose IVIG desensitization in renal allograft recipients with high levels of donor specific alloantibody. Am J Transplant 2006;6:346-51.

33. Akalin E, Dinavahi R, Friedlander R, et al. Addition of plasmapheresis decreases the incidence of acute antibody-mediated rejection in sensitized patients with strong donor-specific antibodies. Clin J Am Soc Nephrol 2008;3:1160-7.

34. West-Thielke P, Herren H, Thielke J, et al. Results of positive crossmatch transplantation in African American renal transplant recipients. Am J Transplant 2008;8:348-54.

35. Magee CC, Felgueiras J, Tinckam K, et al. Renal transplantation in patients with positive lymphocytotoxicity crossmatches: One center's experience. Transplantation 2008;86:96-103.

36. Thielke JJ, West-Thielke PM, Herren HL, et al. Living donor kidney transplantation across positive crossmatch: The University of Illinois at Chicago experience. Transplantation 2009;87:268-73.

37. Haririan A, Nogueira J, Kukuruga D, et al. Positive cross-match living donor kidney transplantation: Longer-term outcomes. Am J Transplant 2009;9:536-42.

38. Takemoto SK, Zeevi A, Feng S, et al. National conference to assess antibody-mediated rejection in solid organ transplantation. Am J Transplant 2004;4:1033-41.

39. Solez K, Colvin RB, Racusen LC, et al. Banff 07 classification of renal allograft pathology: Updates and future directions. Am J Transplant 2008;8:753-60.

40. Burns JM, Cornell LD, Perry DK, et al. Alloantibody levels and acute humoral rejection early after positive crossmatch kidney transplantation. Am J Transplant 2008;8:2684-94.

41. Lefaucheur C, Nochy D, Andrade J, et al. Comparison of combination Plasmapheresis/IVIg/anti-CD20 versus high-dose IVIg in the treatment of antibody-mediated rejection. Am J Transplant 2009;9:1099-107.

42. Sener A, Bella AJ, Nguan C, et al. Focal segmental glomerular sclerosis in renal transplant recipients: Predicting early disease recurrence may prolong allograft function. Clin Transplant 2009;23:96-100.

43. Pardon A, Audard V, Caillard S, et al. Risk factors and outcome of focal and segmental glomerulosclerosis recurrence in adult renal transplant recipients. Nephrol Dial Transplant 2006;21:1053-9.

44. Yang Z, de Mattos AM, Boctor FN, et al. Effect of plasmapheresis on proteinuria and graft survival in focal segmental glomerulosclerosis post renal transplantation (abstract). J Clin Apher 2006;21:7.

45. Savin VJ, Sharma R, Sharma M, et al. Circulating factor associated with increased glomerular permcability to albumin in recurrent focal segmental glomerulosclerosis. N Engl J Med 1996; 334:878-83.

46. Garcia CD, Bittencourt VB, Tumelero A, et al. Plasmapheresis for recurrent posttransplant focal segmental glomerulosclerosis. Transplant Proc 2006;38:1904-5.

47. Valdivia P, Gonzalez Roncero F, Gentil MA, et al. Plasmapheresis for the prophylaxis and treatment of recurrent focal segmental glomerulosclerosis following renal transplant (abstract). Transplant Proc 2005;37:1473-4.

48. Jardine MJ, Bhandari S, Wyburn KR, et al. Photopheresis therapy for problematic renal allograft rejection. J Clin Apher 2009;24:161-9.

49. Lamioni A, Carsetti R, Legato A, et al. Induction of regulatory T cells after prophylactic treatment with photopheresis in renal transplant recipients. Transplantation 2007;83: 1393-6.

50. Taylor DO, Yowell RL, Kfoury AG, et al. Allograft coronary artery disease: Clinical correlations with circulating anti-HLA antibodies and the immunohistopathologic pattern of vascular rejection. J Heart Lung Transplant 2000; 19:518-21.

51. Uber WE, Self SE, Van Bakel AB, Pereira NL. Acute antibody-mediated rejection following heart transplantation. Am J Transplant 2007; 7:2064-74.

52. Pisani BA, Mullen GM, Malinowska K, et al. Plasmapheresis with intravenous immunoglobulin G is effective in patients with elevated panel reactive antibody prior to cardiac transplantation. J Heart Lung Transplant 1999;18: 701-6.

53. Jacobs JP, Quintessenza JA, Boucek RJ, et al. Pediatric cardiac transplantation in children with high panel reactive antibody. Ann Thorac Surg 2004;78:1703-9.

54. Holt DB, Lublin DM, Phelan DL, et al. Mortality and morbidity in pre-sensitized pediatric heart transplant recipients with positive donor crossmatch utilizing peri-operative plasmapheresis and cytolytic therapy. J Heart Lung Transplant 2007;26:876-82.

55. Leech SH, Lopez-Cepero M, LeFor WM, et al. Management of the sensitized cardiac recipient: The use of plasmapheresis and intravenous immunoglobulin. Clin Transplant 2006; 20:476-84.

56. Wang SS, Chou NK, Ko WJ, et al. Effect of plasmapheresis for acute humoral rejection after heart transplantation. Transplant Proc 2006; 38:3692-4.

57. Barr ML, Meiser BM, Eisen HJ, et al. Photopheresis for the prevention of rejection in cardiac transplantation. Photopheresis Transplantation Study Group. N Engl J Med 1998; 339:1744-51.

58. Billingham ME, Cary NRB, Hammond ME, et al. A working formulation for the standardization of nomenclature in the diagnosis of heart and lung rejection: Heart Rejection Study Group. J Heart Transplant 1990;9:587-93.

59. Barr ML, Baker CJ, Schenkel FA, et al. Prophylactic photopheresis and chronic rejection: Effects on graft intimal hyperplasia in cardiac transplantation. Clin Transplant 2000;14:162-6.

60. Dall'Amico R, Livi U, Milano A, et al. Extracorporeal photochemotherapy as adjuvant treatment of heart transplant recipients with recurrent rejection. Transplantation 1995;60: 45-9.

61. Dall'Amico R, Montini G, Murer L, et al. Extracorporeal photochemotherapy after cardiac transplantation: A new therapeutic approach to allograft rejection. Int J Artif Organs 2000;23: 49-54.

62. Kirklin JK, Brown RN, Huang ST, et al. Rejection with hemodynamic compromise: Objective evidence for efficacy of photopheresis. J Heart Lung Transplant 2006;25:283-8.

63. Aubin F, Mousson C. Ultraviolet light-induced regulatory (suppressor) T cells: An approach for promoting induction of operational allograft tolerance? Transplantation 2004;77(Suppl 1): 29-31.

64. Schwarz T. Regulatory T cells induced by ultraviolet radiation. Int Arch Allergy Immunol 2005;137:187-93.

65. Maeda A, Schwarz A, Kernebeck K, et al. Intravenous infusion of syngeneic apoptotic cells by photopheresis induces antigen-specic regulatory T cells. J Immunol 2005;174:5968-76.

66. Lamioni A, Parisi F, Isacchi G, et al. The immunological effects of extracorporeal photopheresis unraveled: Induction of tolerogenic dendritic cells in vitro and regulatory T cells in vivo. Transplantation 2005;79:846-50.

67. George JF, Gooden CW, Guo L, Kirklin JK. Role for CD4(+)CD25(+) T cells in inhibition of graft rejection by extracorporeal photopheresis. J Heart Lung Transplant 2008;27:616-22.

68. Martinu T, Chen DF, Palmer SM. Acute rejection and humoral sensitization in lung transplant recipients. Proc Am Thorac Soc 2009;6: 54-65.

69. Levine SM. A survey of clinical practice of lung transplantation in North America. Chest 2004; 125:1224-38.

70. Burton CM, Iversen M, Carlsen J, et al. Acute cellular rejection is a risk factor for bronchiolitis obliterans syndrome independent of posttransplant baseline FEV1. J Heart Lung Transplant 2009;28:888-93.

71. Corris PA, Christie JD. Update in transplantation. Am J Respir Crit Care Med 2007;175: 432-5.

72. Estenne M, Maurer JR, Boehler A, et al. Bronchiolitis obliterans syndrome 2001: An update of the diagnostic criteria. J Heart Lung Transplant 2002;21:297-310.

73. Nathan SD, Ross DJ, Belman MJ, et al. Bronchiolitis obliterans in single-lung transplant recipients. Chest 1995;107:967-72.

74. Lama VN, Murray S, Lonigro RJ, et al. Course of FEV(1) after onset of bronchiolitis obliterans syndrome in lung transplant recipients. Am J Respir Crit Care Med 2007;175:1192-8.

75. Belperio JA, Lake K, Tazelaar H, et al. Bronchiolitis obliterans syndrome complicating lung or heart-lung transplantation. Semin Respir Crit Care Med 2003;24:499-530.

76. Andreu G, Achkar A, Couetil JP, et al. Extracorporeal photochemotherapy treatment for acute lung rejection episode. J Heart Lung Transplant 1995;14:793-6.

77. Slovis BS, Loyd JE, King LE Jr. Photopheresis for chronic rejection of lung allografts. N Engl J Med 1995;332:962.

78. O'Hagan AR, Stillwell PC, Arroliga A, Koo A. Photopheresis in the treatment of refractory bronchiolitis obliterans complicating lung transplantation. Chest 1999;115:1459-62.

79. Salerno CT, Park SJ, Kreykes NS, et al. Adjuvant treatment of refractory lung transplant rejection with extracorporeal photopheresis. J Thorac Cardiovasc Surg 1999;117:1063-9.

80. Villanueva J, Bhorade SM, Robinson JA, et al. Extracorporeal photopheresis for the treatment of lung allograft rejection. Ann Transplant 2000;5:44-7.

81. Benden C, Speich R, Hofbauer GF, et al. Extracorporeal photopheresis after lung transplantation: A 10-year single-center experience. Transplantation 2008;86:1625-7.

82. Morrell MR, Despotis GJ, Lublin DM, et al. The efficacy of photopheresis for bronchiolitis obliterans syndrome after lung transplantation. J Heart Lung Transplant 2010;29:424-31.

83. Astor TL, Weill D. Extracorporeal photopheresis in lung transplantation. J Cutan Med Surg 2003;7:20-4.

84. Bhorade SM, Stern E. Immunosuppression for lung transplantation. Proc Am Thorac Soc 2009;6:47-53.

85. Grewal HP, Willingham DL, Nguyen J, et al. Liver transplantation using controlled donation after cardiac death donors: An analysis of a large single-center experience. Liver Transpl 2009;15:1028-35.

86. 2008 Annual report of the U.S. Organ Procurement and Transplantation Network and the Scientific Registry of Transplant Recipients. Chapter II: Organ donation and utilization in the United States: 1998-2007. Rockville, MD: US Health Resources and Services Administration, Healthcare Systems Bureau, Division of Transplantation, 2008. [Available at http://www.ustransplant.org/annual_reports/current/chapter_ii_ar_cd.htm?cp_3#3 (accessed April 9, 2010).]

87. Pomfret EA, Fryer JP, Sima CS, et al. Liver and intestine transplantation in the United States, 1996-2005. Am J Transplant 2007;7(Suppl 1):1-14.

88. Renz JF, Emond JC, Yersiz H, et al. Split-liver transplantation in the United States: Outcomes

of a national survey. Ann Surg 2004;239:172-81.

89. Feng S, Si M, Taranto SE, et al. Trends over a decade of pediatric liver transplantation in the United States. Liver Transpl 2006;12:578-84.

90. Yagci G, Cetiner S, Yigitler C, et al. Successful ABO-incompatible liver transplantation with pre- and postoperative plasmapheresis, triple immunosuppression, and splenectomy for fulminant hepatic failure. Exp Clin Transplant 2005;3:390-3.

91. Hanto D, Fecteasu A, Alonso M, et al. ABO-incompatible liver transplantation with no immunological graft losses using total plasma exchange, splenectomy, and quadruple immunosuppression: Evidence for accommodation. Liver Transpl 2003;9:22-30.

92. Ashizawa T, Matsuno N, Yokoyama T, et al. The role of plasmapheresis therapy for perioperative management in ABO-incompatible adult living donor liver transplantation. Transplant Proc 2006;38:3629-32.

93. Testa G, Vidanovic V, Cheifec G, et al. Adult living-donor liver transplantation with ABO-incompatible grafts. Transplantation 2008;85:681-6.

94. Ikegami T, Taketomi A, Soejima Y, et al. Rituximab, IVIG, and plasma exchange without graft local infusion treatment: A new protocol in ABO incompatible living donor liver transplantation. Transplantation 2009;88:303-7.

95. Urbani L, Mazzoni A, Bianco I, et al. The role of immunomodulation in ABO-incompatible adult liver transplant recipients. J Clin Apher 2008;23:55-62.

96. Lehrer MS, Ruchelli E, Olthoff KM, et al. Successful reversal of recalcitrant hepatic allograft rejection by photopheresis. Liver Transpl 2000;6:644-7.

97. Urbani L, Mazzoni A, Catalano G, et al. The use of extracorporeal photopheresis for allograft rejection in liver transplant recipients. Transplant Proc 2004;36:3068-70.

98. Urbani L, Mazzoni A, Colombatto P, et al. A novel immunosuppressive strategy combined with preemptive antiviral therapy improves the eighteen-month mortality in HCV-recipients transplanted with aged livers. Transplantation 2008;86:1666-71.

99. McLeod BC. An approach to evidence-based therapeutic apheresis. J Clin Apher 2002;17:124-32.

In: McLeod BC, Szczepiorkowski ZM, Weinstein R, Winters JL, eds.
Apheresis: Principles and Practice, 3rd edition
Bethesda, MD: AABB Press, 2010

19

Red Cell Exchange and Other Therapeutic Alterations of Red Cell Mass

Beth H. Shaz, MD

RED CELL EXCHANGE (RCE) IS a therapeutic procedure in which the patient's red cells are replaced with donor red cells. This can be performed manually or with an automated system. In manual RCE, whole blood is removed and replaced with allogeneic red cells. In automated systems, whole blood is removed and processed by an apheresis instrument that separates red cells from the other blood components, discards the red cells, and replaces them with allogeneic red cells. RCE is most commonly performed to replace dysfunctional patient red cells with normal donor red cells, as in sickle cell disease (SCD). Red cells can also be replaced with saline and/or albumin to lower the hematocrit

(Hct), as in polycythemia vera; this will be referred to as red cell depletion (RCD).[1,2] Red cells can also be returned to replace plasma removed by an apheresis instrument to raise the Hct; this can be performed to correct anemia at the beginning of a plasma exchange or as a rapid transfusion procedure for patients with chronic anemia.[3]

Techniques for Red Cell Exchange

Manual RCE requires alternately withdrawing and transfusing blood. It is more time consuming, more labor intensive, and less precise than the automated procedure, and it results in larger intravascular volume fluctuations. Auto-

Beth H. Shaz, MD, Associate Professor, Department of Pathology and Laboratory Medicine, Emory University, Atlanta, Georgia

The author has disclosed no conflicts of interest.

mated RCE requires an expensive instrument and appropriate venous access; therefore, it may not be available in some locations.

Total Blood Volume and Red Cell Volume

A patient's total blood volume (TBV) should be known when planning RCE. It can be calculated using the approximate blood volume from Table 19-1 and multiplying it by the patient's weight in kg. Red cell volume is calculated by multiplying the patient's TBV by the patient's Hct.

Manual Red Cell Exchange

Multiple methods for manual RCE in adults are available.[5] One is described in Table 19-2.[5] Manual whole blood exchange transfusion can use a stopcock for removal of blood and infusion of red cells in saline or Fresh Frozen Plasma (FFP), and it can be useful in very small patients or at times of great urgency.

Automated Red Cell Exchange

In automated RCE, the apheresis device will calculate the volume of donor red cells as well as the total replacement volume required for the procedure.[4] Information that must be entered to perform these calculations includes the patient's gender, height, weight, and starting Hct, plus the fraction of cells remaining (FCR), which is the percentage of the patient's red cell volume desired to remain in the circulation at the end of the procedure, and the final patient Hct and fluid balance desired. Finally, the average Hct of the replacement product (generally ~60% for red cell components containing an additive solution and ~80% for those in citrate-phosphate-dextrose-adenine-1) must be entered to determine the required replacement volume of Red Blood Cells (RBCs).[6]

Red Cell Volume Exchanged

The red cell volume to be exchanged depends on the desired FCR for the procedure. When one patient red cell volume is exchanged, approximately 65% of the initial red cells are removed (FCR = 35%), whereas approximately 90% are removed (FCR = 10%) with exchange of two red cell volumes.[4] When treating a patient with sickle cell anemia, if the patient's initial hemoglobin S (HbS) level is 100% and the goal is 30% at the completion of the procedure, the FCR would be set at 30% if Hct is to remain unchanged.[4] The desired postprocedure Hct is also entered (seldom >30% when treating SCD). It should be noted that, in a patient with a starting Hct of 24% or above, a lower FCR can be obtained for a given number of allogeneic units exchanged by replacing removed red cells with saline at the beginning of the exchange and then raising the Hct during or at the end of the procedure.[7]

Table 19-1. Estimating Total Blood Volume[4]

Age Group	Approximate Blood Volume (mL/kg)
Premature infant, at birth	90-105
Term newborn infant	80-90
Children <3 months old	70-75
Children >3 months old and adults	
Male	70
Female	65

Table 19-2. Method for Manual Red Cell Exchange[5]

A. Calculate exchange volume as 1.5 red cell volumes:

    a. Red cell volume = Hct × TBV

    b. Standard unit red cell volume ~200 mL (Hct ~40% × 500 mL)

    c. Number of units = 1.5 × red cell volume (mL)/200

B. Perform adult manual exchange as follows:

    a. Bleed 500 mL and then infuse 500 mL saline/albumin.

    b. Bleed 500 mL and then infuse 2 RBC units.

    c. Repeat Steps a and b until volume of RBC units administered is equal to planned exchange volume.

Hct = hematocrit; TBV = total blood volume; RBC = Red Blood Cell.

Replacement Fluids

Many institutions use leukocyte-reduced red cell components to decrease the risk of febrile reactions.[4] In addition, institutions may have SCD transfusion protocols that provide SCD patients with red cells that are phenotypically matched to some degree (eg, for K, C, and E) and are HbS negative (discussed further in section on SCD).[8,9]

RBC Unit Hematocrit

Each institution should establish the average Hct of the RBC units it receives, as this may vary depending on blood supplier, preservative, and donor population. For small children, the Hct of each RBC unit is usually determined to achieve a precise end Hct for the patient. The Hct of a unit segment is close to that of the unit and therefore can be used, thus obviating the need to obtain a specimen directly from the unit.[10] The patient's Hct should be measured at the completion of all red cell exchange procedures.

Priming the Extracorporeal Circuit

Intraprocedure extracorporeal blood volume (EBV) can be calculated as EBV (%) = (EBV/TBV) × 100, where TBV is the patient's starting TBV. If this parameter would otherwise exceed 15%, or if a given patient cannot tolerate a smaller decrease in EBV, the saline priming fluid can be infused to the patient rather than diverted, thus avoiding initial blood volume loss. Extracorporeal red cell volume (ECRCV) as a percentage of patient red cell volume is given by the formula ECRCV (%) = (ECRCV/red cell volume) × 100, whereas intraprocedure Hct (%) = [(red cell volume − ECRCV)/TBV] × 100. For small (<20 kg) and/or very anemic individuals, who would otherwise have an ECRCV >15% and/or a Hct <20% during the procedure, the apheresis instrument should be primed with red cells.[4] The Spectra (CaridianBCT, Lakewood, CO) has an RCE set volume of 170 mL and an ECRCV of 68 mL.[4] Use of a blood warmer will increase both parameters. When priming fluid has been infused during the initial phase of the procedure, the rinseback step at the end of the procedure may be omitted to avoid fluid overload.

Adverse Effects

Patients receiving RCE are at risk for transfusion reactions, which may include febrile nonhemolytic, allergic, and hemolytic reactions as well as transfusion-related acute lung injury.

There are also risks associated with the procedure itself, such as those related to vascular access and fluid shifts.[1]

Indications for Red Cell Exchange

Indications for RCE and their American Society for Apheresis (ASFA) indication categories are summarized in Table 19-3.

Sickle Cell Disease

SCD is a chronic hemolytic anemia. It is the most prevalent genetic disorder in the African American population, affecting approximately 80,000 individuals in the United States.[11] SCD patients are usually homozygous for HbS, which differs from the normal HbA by the replacement of a glutamic acid with a less polar valine in the β-globin chain,[12] but a similar illness can also be found in patients who carry HbS along with a gene for β-thalassemia, HbC, or another abnormal hemoglobin. One in 400 African Americans express HbSS; such patients now live to an average age of 45 years.[11,13]

Pathophysiology

Under conditions of hypoxia or dehydration, molecules of HbS (and some other abnormal hemoglobins) polymerize within red cells, resulting in cytoplasmic rigidity and changes in the membrane that increase fragility and adherence to vascular endothelium. These changes may lead to vaso-occlusion and hemolysis. In addition, alterations in RBC nitric oxide may compromise hypoxic vasodilation.[12] Factors extrinsic to red cells, such as an elevated whole blood viscosity, a high white cell count, inflammation, and/or reperfusion injury with generation of free radicals after restoration of blood flow, may also contribute to vaso-occlusion and severity of tissue injury. Complications of SCD include pain crisis, infection, aplastic crisis, anemia, and acute and chronic organ damage.[9,14] Red cell transfusion improves or prevents many of these complications. Thus the goals of transfusion therapy in SCD include partial correction of anemia and reduction of the likelihood of sickling by increasing the HbA concentration in the blood, thereby decreasing blood viscosity and improving blood flow.[12,15]

Table 19-3. ASFA Indication Categories for Red Cell Exchange[1]

Disease	Category	Grade of Evidence
Sickle cell disease		
Acute stroke	I	1C
Acute chest syndrome	II	1C
Prophylaxis for primary or secondary stroke to prevent transfusional iron overload	II	1C
Multiorgan failure	III	2C
Malaria		
Severe	II	2B
Babesiosis		
Severe	I	1B
High-risk population	II	2C

ASFA = American Society for Apheresis.

Red Cell Transfusion

Patients with SCD may be challenging to the blood bank because they 1) often require acute and/or chronic simple and/or exchange transfusions, 2) require HbS-negative RBCs, 3) may develop allo- and/or autoantibodies that occur more frequently than in the general hospitalized population and can be challenging to identify, and 4) should be provided phenotypically matched RBCs to prevent alloimmunization.[11]

Simple vs Exchange Transfusion. SCD patients can receive donor red cells via either simple transfusion (ie, without prior removal of the patient's own red cells) or RCE. Disadvantages of simple transfusion include volume overload, increased blood viscosity, and iron accumulation. Advantages of RCE include a more rapid increase in Hct and decrease in HbS level and a lower risk of iron and fluid overload. The disadvantages of maintenance RCE compared to chronic simple transfusion include increased RBC usage, requirements for venous access (automated RCE requires either two large-bore peripheral needles or a dual-lumen central venous catheter), and increased costs for transfusion (which may, however, be offset by avoiding the cost of iron chelation therapy). In any case, all transfusion episodes in SCD should target a final Hct of 30% or less in order to avoid an unsafe increase in blood viscosity.[16]

For the treatment of acute life- or organ-threatening complications of SCD (eg, multiorgan failure and stroke), one RCE that lowers the HbS concentration to below 30% is typically sufficient. For patients receiving chronic transfusion therapy (eg, for stroke prevention), long-term maintenance RCE prevents or mitigates iron accumulation, whereas simple transfusion inevitably results in iron overload.[17] The schedule of maintenance RCE is tailored to maintain the patient's HbS level below 30% or below 50%, depending on the indication.[18] The HbS level should be measured at the conclusion of any RCE performed for treatment of SCD to confirm that the goal was obtained.

Acute vs Chronic Transfusion. Transfusion may be indicated acutely, intermittently,

or chronically, with the latter typically being for purposes of prophylaxis. Acute simple transfusions are used when there is need for an immediate increase in oxygen-carrying capacity.[5] Chronic transfusions not only increase oxygen-carrying capacity but also maintain a lower level of HbS.[5]

Indications for Acute Red Cell Exchange or Simple Transfusion in Sickle Cell Disease

Acute Chest Syndrome. Acute chest syndrome (ACS) is defined by the National Acute Chest Study Group as a new infiltrate, consistent with consolidation and at least segmental in size, accompanied by at least one of the following: chest pain, temperature over 38.5 C, tachypnea, wheezing, or cough.[8] The lifetime incidence of ACS in SCD patients exceeds 30%, and it is a leading cause of death.[16] Red cell transfusions can be used in the treatment of ACS to increase oxygen carrying capacity, especially when there is concomitant hypoxemia. In a prospective study of 671 episodes of ACS in 538 SCD patients, 72% of the patients were transfused, and transfusion was associated with improved oxygenation as determined by an increase in the partial pressure of arterial oxygen (63 mm Hg to 71 mm Hg) and an increase in oxygen saturation (91% to 94%); the latter improvement was greater in patients with pretransfusion hypoxemia (86% to 91%). In this study, no differences were noted in enhancement of oxygenation between RCE and simple transfusion.[8] A retrospective study also failed to show a difference in patient outcome between RCE and simple transfusion; the only significant difference was that RCE patients required more RBC units (mean = 10.3 vs 2.4; p <0.01).[19] A case series associated ACS requiring endotracheal intubation and RCE with reversible posterior leukoencephalopathy syndrome and silent cerebral infarcts; the causes of the neurologic complications are unknown but they are postulated to have resulted from hypoxemia, hypertension, and poor cerebrovascular autoregulation.[20] RCE should be considered in more severe cases, such as those exhibiting a multilobar process or hypoxia not corrected with oxygen therapy, requiring mechanical ventilation, or failing to improve with simple transfusion.[5] The choice between simple transfusion and RCE may also take into account the patient's Hct when prevention of hyperviscosity is an issue.[21]

Acute Multiorgan Failure. Acute multiorgan failure is a life-threatening complication of SCD that is diagnosed when there is acute failure of at least two of the following three organs: lung, liver, or kidney.[22] Aggressive transfusion therapy appears to improve survival. In one retrospective review, dramatic clinical improvement was noted within 24 hours of transfusion (simple or exchange) in 16 of 17 episodes[22]; RCE was used in 8 episodes. In a comparison of outcomes between RCE and simple transfusion, the mean number of RBC units transfused (9 vs 8) and death rates (1/9 vs 0/8) were similar; however, the times to discharge (7 days vs 15 days) and to complete organ recovery (2 months vs 3-6 months) were shorter with RCE. In addition, in patients with a higher Hct (eg, >25%) or more severe organ failure, RCE may be preferable to avoid the risk of unsafe viscosity and volume overload with simple transfusion.[16]

Acute Neurologic Syndrome. Approximately 10% of SCD patients will develop a clinical stroke by the age of 20, with an additional fraction experiencing "silent" strokes.[16] A less frequent, but still severe, neurologic syndrome is acute retinal artery occlusion, which may result in vision loss.[23] In the Cooperative Study of Sickle Cell Disease, which included 4082 patients, a cerebrovascular accident (CVA) occurred in 4% of HbSS patients. The incidence of infarctive CVA was higher in children and older patients, whereas the incidence of hemorrhagic CVA was highest in those aged 20 to 29 years.[24] Urgent RCE targeting an end Hct of 30% and HbS level lower than 30% is the treatment of choice for a patient with an acute ischemic CVA.[23] Primary and secondary prevention of stroke, which require chronic transfusion therapy (see later), decrease morbidity and mortality.

Intrahepatic Cholestasis. Intrahepatic cholestasis is a rare, but often fatal, complication of SCD in which massive sickling and stasis of red cells in hepatic sinusoids lead to severe hepatocellular injury, resulting in a right upper quadrant pain, hepatomegaly, coagulopathy, elevated transaminases, and markedly elevated bilirubin levels.[25] In addition, it is often accompanied by renal failure and encephalopathy.[26] Based on a limited number of case reports, RCE currently seems to be the best treatment option.[5,25-27]

Preoperative for General Anesthesia. Complication rates for SCD patients undergoing general anesthesia have been reported to be as high as 50%, and mortality rates as high as 10%.[28] These events likely resulted from hypoxia, hypoperfusion, and acidosis, causing, in turn, vaso-occlusion and tissue injury. The Preoperative Transfusion in Sickle Cell Disease Study Group randomized 551 HbSS patients undergoing 604 operations to transfusion regimens that were either aggressive (maintaining Hb of 10g/dL and HbS ≤30%) or conservative (maintaining Hb of 10g/dL regardless of HbS level).[28] The nontransfusion-related complication rates were similar (31% and 35%, respectively), while the conservative regimen resulted in 50% fewer transfusion complications. Another report from the same study group described 92 patients with HbSC or other SCD variants who underwent surgical procedures. Analysis of prospectively collected data suggested that preoperative transfusion decreased the risk of SCD-related complications in patients undergoing abdominal procedures (0% vs 35%).[29] Because of high preoperative Hb levels (average = 11 g/dL), the benefits of preoperative transfusion for HbSC patients undergoing intra-abdominal procedures may be best obtained by RCE, which can keep Hb less than 12 g/dL and avoid hyperviscosity. In addition, RCE may be warranted in high-risk patients, such as older patients or patients undergoing high-risk procedures such as retinal surgery, cardiac surgery, or joint-replacement procedures.[5]

Priapism. Priapism is a common complication in males with SCD, 89% of whom will have had one or more episodes by age 20.[9] Priapism results from vaso-occulusion that obstructs the venous drainage of the penis. Prolonged and/or repeated episodes can result in impotence. Urgent RCE to reduce the HbS to less than 30% can be considered in the treatment of priapism that persists for longer than 2 hours, especially if irrigation fails.[9] There is concern regarding the use of RCE for priapism because of reports of neurologic complications in some cases,[5,30,31] termed ASPEN syndrome (association of sickle cell disease, priapism, exchange transfusion, and neurologic events).[31] In these cases, the postprocedure Hb exceeded 12 g/dL, which likely resulted in hyperviscosity that may have contributed to the subsequent neurologic complications.[5] A more recent case series of 10 patients who received 41 whole blood exchanges that maintained the postprocedure Hb below 10g/dL demonstrated no postprocedure neurologic complications; however, no other outcome data were reported.[32] In another series of seven patients who received RCE for priapism 1 to 7 days after onset, only one experienced detumescence, and one experienced a neurologic complication; no information regarding postprocedure Hct or long-term outcome was provided, but postprocedure HbS was less than 30%.[33] Thus the role of RCE in the treatment of priapism remains uncertain.

Indications for Chronic Transfusion Therapy in Sickle Cell Disease

Complicated Pregnancy. Prophylactic transfusion of SCD patients during pregnancy is currently not recommended because of conflicting data.[34] In a randomized controlled trial of 72 pregnancies in HbSS patients, the incidence of ACS and/or preterm labor did not differ between those who received prophylactic vs as-needed simple transfusions.[35] In a retrospective review of 81 pregnancies, women with HbSS or HbSC demonstrated no benefit from prophylactic vs as-needed simple transfusions. In contrast, in a retrospective review comparing 103 SCD patients who received prophylactic RCE to 28 who received only as-needed transfusions, the RCE group demonstrated a decreased incidence of pregnancy complications but also a higher incidence of transfusion reactions, transfusion-transmitted hepatitis, and red cell alloantibody formation.[36] In another report, 18 pregnancies in 14 SCD patients with a history of previous severe maternofetal complication or severe SCD complications were managed with either simple transfusion or RCE to achieve a HbS or HbS plus HbC <50% and total Hb of 9 to 11 g/dL, and all had satisfactory maternal and fetal health outcomes.[37] Thus, prophylactic simple or exchange transfusion throughout pregnancy may be beneficial in women with a history of severe complications, such as preeclampsia.[5,9,34]

Prevention of Stroke. Stroke occurs in over 10% of SCD patients by age 20. The Stroke Prevention Trial in Sickle Cell Anemia (STOP) demonstrated that chronic transfusion therapy to maintain HbS <30% reduced the rate of stroke by 92% in children (age 2-16) who were at increased risk for stroke because of internal carotid or middle cerebral artery flow velocity ≥200 cm/second by transcranial Doppler ultrasound (TCD).[38] A subsequent study (STOP 2)[39] examined whether chronic transfusion therapy could be stopped after at least 30 months in children whose TCD had reverted to normal. The study was halted early when high-risk TCD readings recurred in 14 of 41 children in the transfusion-halted group and when two others in that group had strokes, while neither event occurred in the continuing transfusion group (n = 38).

Chronic transfusion therapy to maintain HbS <30% is also effective in preventing a recurrence in children with SCD who have had a stroke.[9] One study demonstrated a reduction of the secondary stroke rate from 90% to less than 10% with chronic transfusion therapy.[39] Some authors suggest that it may be reasonable to change the HbS target to <50% after 5 years of chronic transfusion therapy for both primary and secondary stroke prevention and/ or to discontinue transfusions after the age of 18, but these approaches have not been systematically studied.[9]

Maintenance RCE can be used instead of chronic simple transfusion to minimize and potentially reverse iron accumulation.[17,18]

Chronic RCE results in higher numbers of RBC units transfused and higher risks of red cell alloimmunization and transfusion complications other than iron overload. Risks and benefits must be weighed for each patient. Alternatives to chronic transfusion, such as hydroxyurea and hematopoietic progenitor cell transplantation, are being investigated.[40] A current randomized clinical trial is studying hydroxyurea plus phlebotomy vs RCE plus iron chelation in children with a history of CVA who have received chronic transfusion for at least 18 months [Stroke with Transfusions Changing to Hydroxyurea (SWiTCH)].

Frequent Pain Episodes. Patients who develop frequent severe pain episodes may benefit from chronic transfusion therapy. In the STOP trial, those who received chronic transfusion had fewer pain episodes (p = 0.014).[41]

Pulmonary Hypertension/Cor Pulmonale. Pulmonary hypertension has recently been shown to be a common cause of mortality in SCD. One study demonstrated that 32% of adult patients had pulmonary hypertension (defined as a tricuspid regurgitant jet velocity exceeding 2.5 m/second on echocardiogram) and had a significant risk of mortality at 30 months.[42] Pulmonary hypertension was associated with chronic hemolysis. Potential treatments include nitric oxide modulators, chronic transfusion, warfarin, oxygen, and vasodilators.[43,44] A pilot trial (n = 6) of chronic transfusion to reverse pulmonary hypertension showed marked improvement in pulmonary artery systemic pressure and room air saturation.[45] Currently, multiple clinical trials are investigating chronic transfusion therapy for pulmonary hypertension.

Prevention of Acute Chest Syndrome. Multiple episodes of ACS may lead to restrictive lung disease, severe pulmonary fibrosis, pulmonary hypertension, and/or cor pulmonale. Patients in STOP who received chronic transfusion therapy had significantly lower rates of ACS compared to controls (p = 0.0027).[41] Another study demonstrated that acute simple transfusion may prevent ACS in SCD patients who are hospitalized for a vaso-occlusive pain episode.[46]

RBC Unit Selection

Patient Phenotype. All SCD patients should have extended red cell antigen phenotype determined (ABO, Rh, Kell, Kidd, Duffy, Lewis, and MNS systems) before the initiation of transfusion therapy. This may help to solve future antibody problems.[9]

Provision of Phenotypically Matched RBCs. Providing partially phenotypically matched RBC units (for C, E, and K) for the treatment of SCD patients has been advocated to lessen the likelihood of red cell alloimmunization and decrease the incidence of delayed hemolytic transfusion reactions.[47,48] Patients who form red cell alloantibodies on this protocol are given RBCs that are also matched for Fy^a, Jk^b, and the antigen to which they made antibody.[16] A study showed a decrease in the red cell alloimmunization rate from 35% to 0% with the exclusive use of RBCs matched for C, c, E, e, K, S, Fy^a, and Fy^b).[49] Despite recommendations to this effect from the National Institutes of Health,[9] many institutions, especially community hospitals, do not routinely provide these products, and phenotypic matching is not standardized among institutions that practice it (73% for E; 70%, K; 68%, C; 41%, c; and 41%, e).[50] The disadvantages of phenotypic matching include increased cost, more difficult inventory management, and occasional inability to procure the desired product at the time of transfusion. In emergencies phenotypic matching may not be possible.

Leukocyte-Reduced Components. In order to prevent HLA immunization and febrile nonhemolytic transfusion reactions, the use of leukocyte-reduced components is warranted.[6]

HbS-Negative Components. Sickle cell trait (HbSA) RBC units are reported to be safe for SCD patients, but they should be avoided if possible because one of the goals of transfusion is to decrease HbS levels.[6]

Adverse Effects of Transfusion Therapy in Sickle Cell Disease

Autoantibody Formation. Autoantibody formation has been reported in 8% of transfused

SCD children, and in 86% these autoantibodies were associated with the presence of alloantibodies.[51,52] These autoantibodies can result in clinically significant hemolysis. The pathogenesis of autoantibody formation, especially in the setting of alloantibody formation, is unknown.

Alloantibody Formation. Alloimmunization occurs in approximately 2% to 6% of all patients who receive RBC transfusions, but the rate may be as high as 36% in patients with SCD.[11] Alloimmunization makes it more difficult to find compatible RBCs and increases the risk of delayed hemolytic transfusion reactions. With no phenotypic matching, studies reported an alloimmunization rate in the range of 19% to 43% in transfused patients with SCD.[53] One study reported alloimmunization in 29% and 47%, respectively, of 78 pediatric and 62 adult SCD patients, with more females than males being immunized. Delayed hemolytic and/or serologic transfusion reactions occurred in 9% and 8%, respectively, and hyperhemolysis occurred in 16% and 5.1%, respectively.[52] In contrast, multiply-transfused, non-SCD, chronic anemia patients not of African ethnicity with either thalassemia major or pure red cell aplasia had an alloimmunization rate of about 5%.[53] In a comprehensive study of the incidence of alloimmunization in SCD patients and risk factors associated with it, Vichinsky and colleagues suggested that the increased alloimmunization rate was likely the result of anti-genic differences between patients, who are mostly of African ethnicity, and the majority of blood donors, who are of European ethnicity (Table 19-4).[53-55] Therefore, provision of RBCs that are phenotypically matched for the high-likelihood antigens (Rh and K) results in decreased alloimmunization.[11]

Hyperhemolytic Transfusion Reactions. A serious complication of RBC transfusion in SCD patients is the hyperhemolytic transfusion reaction, in which both donor and recipient red cells are destroyed and reticulocytopenia may occur.[56] Some patients may have newly detected alloantibodies or autoantibodies, but others have no detectable antibodies to red cell antigens (ie, negative antibody screen and direct antiglobulin test). Possible mechanisms include bystander hemolysis, erythropoietic suppression, and red cell destruction caused by contact lysis via activated macrophages. Bystander hemolysis is hypothesized to result from defective regulation of the membrane attack complex of complement on the patient's own red cells.[55,56] Continued transfusion may exacerbate the hemolysis, and similar reactions may occur after subsequent transfusion, even if the RBCs are extensively phenotypically matched. Treatments for patients with hyper-hemolytic transfusion reactions include erythropoietin, intravenous immunoglobulin, steroids, and plasma exchange.[57] These life-threatening reactions are most often seen in SCD patients

Table 19-4. Red Cell Alloimmunization in Sickle Cell Disease Patients and Phenotypic Racial Differences[53]

Antigen	SCD Antibody Prevalence (%)	Antigen Prevalence	
		African Ethnicity (%)	European Ethnicity (%)
K	18	2	9
E	21	24	35
C	14	28	68
Jk^b	7	39	72

SCD = sickle cell disease.

but have also been reported in patients with thalassemia, myelofibrosis, and anemia of chronic disease.[58]

Iron Overload. Chronic simple transfusion will result in iron overload because the body has no mechanism for excreting excess non-dietary iron. Iron accumulation results in hepatic fibrosis and cardiomyopathy. Liver biopsy is used to quantify hepatic iron content. Noninvasive methods to detect iron overload include serum ferritin measurement, calculation of total transfusion volume, and superconducting quantum interference device magnetic resonance imaging (SQUID MRI).[59] Iron overload is treated with iron chelation therapy. In addition, as mentioned above, RCE in conjunction with chelation therapy can minimize and potentially reverse iron accumulation from ongoing chronic transfusion.

Thalassemia

Thalassemias are hereditary anemias resulting from mutations in the β-globin (β-thalassemia) or α-globin (α-thalassemia) genes that lead to defective Hb synthesis. The disease is clinically heterogeneous because of genotypically diverse mutations or compound heterozygosity with other hemoglobinopathies as well as unknown individual patient factors. Patients with thalassemia may require life-long red cell transfusions to correct anemia and suppress the extramedullary hematopoiesis that would otherwise lead to bone deformities. The only definitive treatment is hematopoietic progenitor cell transplantation.[60]

Chronic transfusion is indicated in homozygous thalassemias and in compound heterozygotes with β-thalassemia major. Patients with β-thalassemia intermedia, β-thalassemia and HbE disease, and HbH disease (3 of 4 mutated α-globulin genes) may require periodic transfusion.[60] The goals of transfusion therapy in thalassemia major are to increase oxygen-carrying capacity, prevent progressive hypersplenism, and suppress erythropoiesis. The latter effect prevents pathologic fractures resulting from osteopenia and extramedullary hematopoiesis

and reduces gastrointestinal iron absorption. The indications for transfusion are growth retardation, failure to thrive, symptomatic anemia, and prevention of progressive hypersplenism and of facial and skull deformities.

Because these patients are transfused from birth, red cell phenotyping should be performed on the initial pretransfusion sample, or genotyping must be used to adequately predict the patient's red cell antigen phenotype.[61] Simple transfusion of leukocyte-reduced red cells is used to maintain a Hb level greater than 9.5 g/dL. RCE has also been used to treat patients with thalassemia, decreasing the transfusion requirement by 30%, increasing the transfusion interval by 43%, and mitigating iron overload.[62]

Malaria

Malaria causes over 1,000,000 deaths annually throughout the world.[63] It is a vector-borne protozoan infection of red cells caused by *Plasmodium vivax, P. ovale, P. malariae,* or *P. falciparum,* which are transmitted by mosquito bites or transfusion. Parasitemia leads to hemolysis and release of inflammatory cytokines, resulting in fever, malaise, chills, headache, myalgia, nausea, vomiting, anemia, jaundice, hepatosplenomegaly, and thrombocytopenia.[64] Severe malaria, as defined by the World Health Organization (WHO; Table 19-5) is usually the result of infection with *P. falciparum.*

Treatment

Antimalarial medications are the recommended treatment for malaria. In severe malaria, treatment ideally includes parenteral medication; supportive care, which usually requires admission to an intensive care unit; and RCE, which replaces parasitized red cells with noninfected red cells, resulting in a rapid reduction of parasitemia.[64] This decreases intravascular hemolysis and consequent cytokine release, and it improves blood flow and oxygen delivery.

Table 19-5. Criteria for Severe Malaria[64]

Manifestation	Features
Cerebral malaria	Unarousable; coma not attributable to any other cause, with a Glasgow coma scale score ≤9, and coma should persist for at least 30 minutes after a generalized convulsion
Severe anemia	Hematocrit <15% or hemoglobin <5 g/dL in the presence of parasite count >10,000/μL
Renal failure	Urine output <400 mL/24 hours in adults (<12 mL/kg/24 hours in children) and a serum creatinine >265 μmol/L (>3.0 mg/dL) despite adequate volume repletion
Pulmonary edema and acute respiratory distress syndrome	Acute lung injury score is calculated on the basis of radiographic densities, severity of distress syndrome hypoxemia, and positive end-expiratory pressure
Hypoglycemia	Whole blood glucose concentration <2.2 mmol/L (<40 mg/dL)
Circulatory collapse	Systolic blood pressure <70 mm Hg in patients >5 years old or <50 mm Hg in children aged 1-5 years, with cold clammy skin or a core-skin temperature difference >10 C
Abnormal bleeding	Spontaneous bleeding from gums, nose, and/or gastrointestinal tract, or laboratory evidence of disseminated intravascular coagulation
Repeated generalized convulsions	≥3 convulsions observed within 24 hours
Acidemia/acidosis	Arterial pH <7.25 or acidosis (plasma bicarbonate <15 mmol/L)
Macroscopic hemoglobinuria	Hemolysis not secondary to glucose-6-phosphate dehydrogenase deficiency
Impaired consciousness	Rousable mental condition, prostration, or weakness
Hyperparasitemia	>5% parasitized erythrocytes or >250,000 parasites/μL (in nonimmune individuals)
Hyperpyrexia	Core body temperature >40 C
Hyperbilirubinemia	Total bilirubin >43 μmol/L (>2.5 mg/dL)

Indications for Red Cell Exchange

RCE may be used in the treatment of severely ill patients with parasitemia >10% and may result in rapid clinical improvement. WHO has suggested indications for RCE in a nonimmune patient (ie, an individual from malaria-free areas with no immunity to malaria); these are presented in Table 19-6.[65] The US Centers for Disease Control and Prevention recommends that exchange transfusion be strongly considered when parasitemia is >10% or when complications such as cerebral malaria, non-volume-overload pulmonary edema, or renal impairment exist.[66] A review of 20 patients with severe malaria [mean parasitemia = 32% ±18% (range = 8% to >70%) and other symptoms] who received RCE demonstrated decreased parasitemia after exchange (mean = 3% ±2%; range <1% to 9%) and uniform survival.[67] A meta-analysis of 8 studies comprising 279 patients with severe malaria compared

Table 19-6. Indications for Red Cell Exchange in Malaria[65]

- Parasitemia >30% in the absence of clinical complications
- Parasitemia >10% in the presence of severe disease, especially cerebral malaria, acute renal failure, adult respiratory distress syndrome, jaundice, and severe anemia
- Parasitemia >10% and failure to respond to optimal chemotherapy after 12-24 hours
- Parasitemia >10% and poor prognostic factors (eg, elderly patient)

survival rates for those who received antimalarial medications alone or with adjunctive RCE and found no survival advantage with adjunctive RCE.[68] A limitation of this analysis was that the RCE patients had higher levels of parasitemia and more severe malaria. In addition, the patients all received manual rather than automated RCE, which is safer and faster.

Whole blood exchange and plasma exchange have been reported as adjuvant treatments for severe malaria to remove circulating factors (eg, tumor necrosis factor α and interferon γ) and parasite toxins.[69,70]

Adverse Effects

Risks of RCE are related to red cell transfusion (eg, transfusion-transmitted disease and hemolytic and allergic transfusion reactions), vascular access (eg, line sepsis), and metabolic disturbances (eg, hypocalcemia).[66] The great majority of cases of severe malaria occur in areas of the world where there may not be adequate resources to perform RCE safely. Therefore, the risk of the procedure should be balanced with the benefits. WHO recommends caution in performing RCE in settings where pathogen-free blood and/or adequate clinical monitoring are not available.[65]

Babesiosis

Babesiosis is caused by the protozoan *Babesia microti*, which can be transmitted from an animal reservoir to humans by tick bite (primarily *Ixodes*) or transfusion. In the United States most cases are in the Northeast plus Wisconsin and Minnesota. Infection can be asymptomatic,

mildly to moderately symptomatic (fever, anorexia, shaking chills, headaches, myalgia, vomiting, and abdominal pain), or severe (hemolytic anemia, acute renal failure, disseminated intravascular coagulation, congestive heart failure, and pulmonary disease).[71,72] Symptoms begin 1 to 6 weeks after a tick bite, with most cases being mild to moderate. Asplenic, immunocompromised (human immunodeficiency virus-infected in particular) and elderly patients are more likely to have a severe course.[73] Twenty percent of patients with severe disease die.[72] In addition, immunocompromised individuals can have relapsing disease. Usually 1% to 10% of circulating red cells are parasitized in normal hosts; parasitemia exceeding 10% is associated with severe disease, and in high-risk individuals, parasitemia can reach 85%. The primary treatment is chemotherapy (atovaquone plus azithromycin, or clindamycin plus quinine) and supportive care as necessary.[74]

Pathophysiology

Babesia species infect red cells and replicate, causing hemolysis and tissue hypoxia.[72] Infection results in a host immune response releasing cytokines, particularly interleukin-12 and interferon-γ.

Indication for Red Cell Exchange

RCE is an effective way to rapidly lower the level of parasitemia and ameliorate the acute hemolytic process because babesia are present only in red cells. RCE is most commonly performed when parasitemia exceeds 10%, depending on the patient's symptoms and comorbidities, and continued until parasitemia is <5%. A recent case series of RCE (n = 4) and literature review of whole blood exchange or RCE (n = 20) in the treatment of babesiosis reported an average patient age of 56 years; mean pre- and postexchange parasitemias of 18% ±14% and 4% ±4%, respectively; and a mortality rate of 16%. Of the patients receiving RCE, 63% were asplenic.[71] Adjunctive treatment with plasma exchange to remove plasma free Hb in severe cases has been reported.[73]

Incompatible Red Cells

RCE to remove Rh-positive red cells from an emergently transfused Rh-negative woman has been reported.[75] The residual Rh-positive red cells could be neutralized by administration of Rh Immune Globulin to avoid Rh sensitization. In addition, red cell removal can be performed prophylactically or as a treatment for immune hemolysis resulting from marrow or solid organ transplantation.[76] The need arises when donor lymphocytes in a minor-ABO-incompatible transplant (eg, group O donor and group A recipient) engraft and produce antibodies against recipient red cells.[76] Other means of preventing or minimizing hemolysis after incompatible transplantation are transfusing group O red cells before and after transplantation, monitoring for delayed hemolytic reactions, and giving immunosuppressive drugs such as methotrexate.[77]

Removal of Toxins

RCE has been used for the removal of red cells carrying toxic compounds. Carbon monoxide results in hypoxia by the formation of carboxy-hemoglobin, which is unable to transport oxygen.[78] Over 30 years ago RCE was used as a treatment for severe carbon monoxide poisoning by replacing the carboxyhemoglobin-carrying red cells with normal red cells.[79,80] Current therapies include 100% oxygen and hyperbaric oxygen chambers.[78] RCE has also been used for the treatment of severe methemoglobinemia in a patient refractory to standard treatment with methylene blue and in patients with G6PD deficiency.[81] Application of RCE followed by plasma exchange to the treatment of cyclosporine A toxicity after solid organ transplantation was based on the fact that 60% of cyclosporine in the blood is bound to red cells, 10% to leukocytes, and 30% to plasma lipoproteins.[82,83] RCE has also been used to treat advanced erythropoietic protoporphyria.[84]

Indications for Red Cell Depletion

Indications for RCD and their ASFA indication categories are summarized in Table 19-7.

Erythrocytosis/Polycythemia

Erythrocytosis and polycythemia are terms that denote an increase in circulating red cell mass. It can be either primary as the result of a myeloproliferative disorder such as polycythemia vera (P. vera) or secondary to a congenital hemoglobin defect, to chronic hypoxia related to a respiratory or cardiac disorder, or to ectopic (eg, produced by a malignancy) or dysregulated (eg, postrenal transplantation) erythropoietin production.[85]

Table 19-7. ASFA Indication Categories for Red Cell Depletion[1]

Disease	Category	Grade of Evidence
Erythrocytosis		
Secondary	III	2B
Polycythemia vera	III	2C
Hemachromatosis	III	2B

P. vera is a myeloproliferative disorder characterized by an absolute increase in red cell mass; it is often associated with leukocytosis, thrombocytosis, and splenomegaly as well.[86]

WHO diagnostic criteria for P. vera include two major and three minor criteria (Table 19-8). The diagnosis of P. vera requires the presence of either both major criteria and 1 minor criterion or the presence of the first major criterion and 2 minor criteria.[87]

Pathophysiology

The increase in Hct results in whole blood hyperviscosity and decreased blood flow.[85] Clinical manifestations of hyperviscosity include headache, dizziness, slow mentation, confusion, fatigue, angina, dyspnea, and thrombosis. Long-term management of secondary erythrocytosis focuses on treating the underlying disorder; however, symptomatic hyperviscosity can be treated as needed by therapeutic phlebotomy. The therapeutic endpoint for phlebotomy varies according to cause of erythrocytosis. In P. vera the usual goal is a Hct <45% in men and <42% in women,[86] whereas in secondary erythrocytosis the goal is individually tailored to the Hct that alleviates the patient's symptoms and decreases the risk of thromboembolism.[85,88]

Indications for Red Cell Depletion

RCD can be performed isovolemically with an apheresis instrument and may be preferable to phlebotomy in hemodynamically unstable patients or in patients who require removal of a large volume of red cells in a short period of time. In a study of 98 patients with erythrocytosis who were treated solely with whole blood phlebotomy of 450 mL (n = 36), RCD only (450-500 mL of red cells removed; n = 30), or phlebotomy followed by RCD (n = 32), RCD was associated with a longer interval between treatments (136 ±50 days vs 52 ±30 days). RCD does cost more than phlebotomy.[75] The volume removed can be either fixed[89] or calculated,[90] but it should be noted that TBV may be expanded in patients with erythrocytosis, and red cell mass may therefore be underestimated by standard weight-based formulas.

Table 19-8. WHO Diagnostic Criteria for Polycythemia Vera[87]

Major Criteria:

1. One of the following applies:
   a. Hb >18.5 g/dL for men or Hb >16.5 g/dL for women
   b. Hb >17 g/dL for men or Hb >15 g/dL for women if associated with a sustained increase of 2 g/dL from baseline that cannot be attributed to correction of iron deficiency
   c. Hb/Hct >99th percentile of reference range
   d. Red cell volume >25% above the mean normal predicted
2. Presence of JAK2 V617F or another functionally similar mutation

Minor Criteria:

1. Marrow biopsy revealing trilineage myeloproliferation
2. Serum erythropoietin level below reference range for normal
3. Endogenous erythroid colony growth in vitro

Hb = hemoglobin; Hct = hematocrit.

Adverse Effects

Adverse effects of RCD may include hypocalcemia, vasovagal reactions, infection, bruising, or hematoma formation at the site of venipuncture. Patients are also at risk of developing iron deficiency.

Hemochromatosis

Iron overload can result from a genetic disorder (hereditary hemochromatosis), or it can be secondary to transfusional iron loading.[91] In the United States the most common cause of iron overload is hereditary hemochromatosis (0.25% of the population), which results from increased iron absorption in the gastrointestinal tract.[92] A variety of mutations are associated with hereditary hemochromatosis; in persons of European ancestry, for example, mutations in the *HFE* gene (C282Y, H63D, or S65C) are the most common.[91] Complications resulting from parenchymal iron deposition include liver disease, diabetes mellitus, gonadal insufficiency, arthropathy, skin pigmentation, and cardiac dysfunction. The severity of liver disease closely reflects the magnitude of hepatic iron deposition. Screening for iron overload is indicated in patients with signs or symptoms of iron overload, a family history of hereditary hemochromatosis, or a history of multiple red cell transfusions. Laboratory evaluation includes serum transferrin saturation and ferritin levels as well as testing for the presence of *HFE* mutations. Therapeutic phlebotomy is the usual first-line therapy. It is typically performed weekly as tolerated, to deplete total body iron, then every 3 to 4 months to maintain serum ferritin <50 ng/mL.[90] Iron depletion through phlebotomy and/or chelation therapy will improve skin pigmentation, hepatic function, and cardiac function, but diabetes, other endocrine abnormalities, and arthropathy usually do not improve.[91]

Pathophysiology

The organs involved in iron overload are predominantly the liver, heart, endocrine glands, and skin. The liver is the major physiologic site for normal iron storage and is the first system to develop pathologic sequelae associated with transfusional iron overload. Hepatomegaly may progress quickly, and cirrhosis may develop. Cardiac symptoms may develop without warning. Cardiac toxicity manifests as congestive heart failure or as a restrictive cardiomyopathy and angina (without coronary occlusion). Pancreatic and pituitary dysfunction, insulin-dependent diabetes, delayed growth, shortened stature, and delayed sexual maturation are all consequences of excess iron accumulation in the endocrine system. Clinical manifestations depend not only on the amount of excess iron but the rate of iron accumulation, the ascorbate level, alcohol use, and viral hepatitis infection.[93]

Indications for Red Cell Depletion

Studies comparing RCD to phlebotomy in the treatment of hereditary hemochromatosis have been performed. One study compared six patients receiving RCD (450-724 mL red cells removed) to six historical controls who had received phlebotomy (500 mL whole blood removed) and reported a decreased number of procedures with RCD.[90] This group then performed a randomized clinical trial (n = 26) comparing RCD (average = 533 mL red cells removed) and phlebotomy (average = 481 mL whole blood removed), which demonstrated a comparatively significant decrease in Hb, ferritin, and side effects with RCD.[94]

Patients with secondary iron overload and chronic anemia usually require iron-chelating agents. As mentioned above, RCE in combination with iron-chelating therapy can deplete iron in patients requiring chronic red cell transfusion.

Adverse Effects

One study reported hypocalcemia and dizziness as complications of RCD for hemochromatosis.[90]

References

1. Szczepiorkowski ZM, Bandarenko N, Kim HC, et al. Guidelines on the use of therapeutic apheresis in clinical practice—evidence-based approach from the Apheresis Applications Committee of the American Society for Apheresis. The fifth special issue. J Clin Apher 2010; 25:83-177.

2. Wayne AS, Kevy SV, Nathan DG. Transfusion management of sickle cell disease. Blood 1993;81:1109-23.

3. McLeod BC, Reed SR, Viernes AV, Valentino L. Rapid red cell transfusion by apheresis. J Clin Apher 1994;9:142-6.

4. Winters J, Gottschall J, eds. Therapeutic apheresis: A physician's handbook. 2nd ed. Bethesda, MD: AABB, 2008.

5. Swerdlow PS. Red cell exchange in sickle cell disease. Hematology Am Soc Hematol Educ Program 2006:48-53.

6. Sarode R, Altuntas F. Blood bank issues associated with red cell exchanges in sickle cell disease. J Clin Apher 2006;21:271-3.

7. Myers L, Paranjape G, Anderson C, et al. Isovolemic hemodilution red blood cell exchange is superior to red blood cell exchange in the management of sickle cell disease patients on hypertransfusion programs following cerebrovascular accident (abstract). Blood 2002; 102:764a.

8. Vichinsky EP, Neumayr LD, Earles AN, et al. Causes and outcomes of the acute chest syndrome in sickle cell disease. National Acute Chest Syndrome Study Group. N Engl J Med 2000;342:1855-65.

9. National Institutes of Health; National Heart, Lung and Blood Insitute; Division of Blood Diseases and Resources. The management of sickle cell disease. NIH Publication No. 02-2117. 4th ed. (Revised, June 2002) Bethesda, MD: 2002.

10. Farrell SB, Shelat SG, Kim HC, Drew C. Alternative method to determine the hematocrit of red blood cell units: A potential use in the apheresis unit. Transfusion 2009;49:1255-8.

11. Shaz BH, Zimring JC, Demmons DG, Hillyer CD. Blood donation and blood transfusion: Special considerations for African Americans. Transfus Med Rev 2008;22:202-14.

12. Wahl S, Quirolo KC. Current issues in blood transfusion for sickle cell disease. Curr Opin Pediatr 2009;21:15-21.

13. Platt OS, Brambilla DJ, Rosse WF, et al. Mortality in sickle cell disease. Life expectancy and risk factors for early death. N Engl J Med 1994;330:1639-44.

14. Ballas SK, Barton FB, Waclawiw MA, et al. Hydroxyurea and sickle cell anemia: Effect on quality of life. Health Qual Life Outcomes 2006;4:59.

15. Lawson SE, Oakley S, Smith NA, Bareford D. Red cell exchange in sickle cell disease. Clin Lab Haematol 1999;21:99-102.

16. Josephson CD, Su LL, Hillyer KL, Hillyer CD. Transfusion in the patient with sickle cell disease: A critical review of the literature and transfusion guidelines. Transfus Med Rev 2007;21:118-33.

17. Kim HC, Dugan NP, Silber JH, et al. Erythrocytapheresis therapy to reduce iron overload in chronically transfused patients with sickle cell disease. Blood 1994;83:1136-42.

18. Singer ST, Quirolo K, Nishi K, et al. Erythrocytapheresis for chronically transfused children with sickle cell disease: An effective method for maintaining a low hemoglobin S level and reducing iron overload. J Clin Apher 1999;14: 122-5.

19. Turner JM, Kaplan JB, Cohen HW, Billett HH. Exchange versus simple transfusion for acute chest syndrome in sickle cell anemia adults. Transfusion 2009;49:863-8.

20. Henderson JN, Noetzel MJ, McKinstry RC, et al. Reversible posterior leukoencephalopathy syndrome and silent cerebral infarcts are associated with severe acute chest syndrome in children with sickle cell disease. Blood 2003; 101:415-19.

21. Maitre B, Habibi A, Roudot-Thoraval F, et al. Acute chest syndrome in adults with sickle cell disease. Chest 2000;117:1386-92.

22. Hassell KL, Eckman JR, Lane PA. Acute multiorgan failure syndrome: A potentially catastrophic complication of severe sickle cell pain episodes. Am J Med 1994;96:155-62.

23. Wanko SO, Telen MJ. Transfusion management in sickle cell disease. Hematol Oncol Clin North Am 2005;19:803-26, v-vi.

24. Ohene-Frempong K, Weiner SJ, Sleeper LA, et al. Cerebrovascular accidents in sickle cell disease: Rates and risk factors. Blood 1998;91: 288-94.

25. Costa DB, Miksad RA, Buff MS, et al. Case of fatal sickle cell intrahepatic cholestasis despite use of exchange transfusion in an African-

American patient. J Natl Med Assoc 2006;98: 1183-7.

26. Ahn H, Li CS, Wang W. Sickle cell hepatopathy: Clinical presentation, treatment, and outcome in pediatric and adult patients. Pediatr Blood Cancer 2005;45:184-90.

27. Irizarry K, Rossbach HC, Ignacio JR, et al. Sickle cell intrahepatic cholestasis with cholelithiasis. Pediatr Hematol Oncol 2006; 23:95-102.

28. Vichinsky EP, Haberkern CM, Neumayr L, et al. A comparison of conservative and aggressive transfusion regimens in the perioperative management of sickle cell disease. The Preoperative Transfusion in Sickle Cell Disease Study Group. N Engl J Med 1995;333:206-13.

29. Neumayr L, Koshy M, Haberkern C, et al. Surgery in patients with hemoglobin SC disease. Preoperative Transfusion in Sickle Cell Disease Study Group. Am J Hematol 1998;57:101-8.

30. Rackoff WR, Ohene-Frempong K, Month S, et al. Neurologic events after partial exchange transfusion for priapism in sickle cell disease. J Pediatr 1992;120:882-5.

31. Siegel JF, Rich MA, Brock WA. Association of sickle cell disease, priapism, exchange transfusion and neurological events: ASPEN syndrome. J Urol 1993;150:1480-2.

32. Ballas SK, Lyon D, Hall N, Kent T. Safety of blood exchange transfusion for priapism complicating sickle cell disease (abstract). J Clin Apher 2006;21:16.

33. McCarthy LJ, Vattuone J, Weidner J, et al. Do automated red cell exchanges relieve priapism in patients with sickle cell anemia? Ther Apher 2000;4:256-8.

34. Hassell K. Pregnancy and sickle cell disease. Hematol Oncol Clin North Am 2005;19:903-16, vii-viii.

35. Koshy M, Burd L, Wallace D, et al. Prophylactic red-cell transfusions in pregnant patients with sickle cell disease. A randomized cooperative study. N Engl J Med 1988;319:1447-52.

36. Morrison JC, Morrison FS, Floyd RC, et al. Use of continuous flow erythrocytapheresis in pregnant patients with sickle cell disease. J Clin Apher 1991;6:224-9.

37. Driss F, Tertian G, Becquemont L, et al. Management of high risk pregnancy in sickle cell disease by a strategy of prophylactic red cell transfusion or automated red cell exchange. Transfus Clin Biol 2007;14:386-92.

38. Adams RJ, McKie VC, Hsu L, et al. Prevention of a first stroke by transfusions in children with sickle cell anemia and abnormal results on transcranial Doppler ultrasonography. N Engl J Med 1998;339:5-11.

39. Russell MO, Goldberg HI, Hodson A, et al. Effect of transfusion therapy on arteriographic abnormalities and on recurrence of stroke in sickle cell disease. Blood 1984;63:162-9.

40. Platt OS. Prevention and management of stroke in sickle cell anemia. Hematology Am Soc Hematol Educ Program 2006:54-7.

41. Miller ST, Wright E, Abboud M, et al. Impact of chronic transfusion on incidence of pain and acute chest syndrome during the Stroke Prevention Trial (STOP) in sickle-cell anemia. J Pediatr 2001;139:785-9.

42. Gladwin MT, Sachdev V, Jison ML, et al. Pulmonary hypertension as a risk factor for death in patients with sickle cell disease. N Engl J Med 2004;350:886-95.

43. Vichinsky EP. Pulmonary hypertension in sickle cell disease. N Engl J Med 2004;350: 857-9.

44. Gladwin MT, Kato GJ. Cardiopulmonary complications of sickle cell disease: Role of nitric oxide and hemolytic anemia. Hematology Am Soc Hematol Educ Program 2005:51-7.

45. Claster S, Hammer M, Hagar W, et al. Treatment of pulmonary hypertension in sickle cell diease with transfusion (abstract). Blood 1999; 94:420a.

46. Styles LA, Abboud M, Larkin S, et al. Transfusion prevents acute chest syndrome predicted by elevated secretory phospholipase A2. Br J Haematol 2007;136:343-4.

47. Vichinsky EP, Luban NL, Wright E, et al. Prospective RBC phenotype matching in a stroke-prevention trial in sickle cell anemia: A multicenter transfusion trial. Transfusion 2001;41: 1086-92.

48. Osby M, Shulman IA. Phenotype matching of donor red blood cell units for nonalloimmunized sickle cell disease patients: A survey of 1182 North American laboratories. Arch Pathol Lab Med 2005;129:190-3.

49. Lau FY, Wong R, Chan NPH, et al. Provision of phenotype-matched blood units: No need for pre-transfusion antibody screening. Haematologica 2001;86:742-8.

50. Afenyi-Annan A, Bandarenko N. Transfusion practices for patients with sickle cell disease at a major academic center. Immunohematology 2006;22:103-7.

51. Castellino SM, Combs MR, Zimmerman SA, et al. Erythrocyte autoantibodies in paediatric

patients with sickle cell disease receiving transfusion therapy: Frequency, characteristics and significance. Br J Haematol 1999;104:189-94.

52. Aygun B, Padmanabhan S, Paley C, Chandrasekaran V. Clinical significance of RBC alloantibodies and autoantibodies in sickle cell patients who received transfusions. Transfusion 2002;42:37-43.

53. Vichinsky EP, Earles A, Johnson RA, et al. Alloimmunization in sickle-cell-anemia and transfusion of racially unmatched blood. N Engl J Med 1990;322:1617-21.

54. Rosse WF, Gallagher D, Kinney TR, et al. Transfusion and alloimmunization in sickle-cell disease. Blood 1990;76:1431-7.

55. Luban NL. Variability in rates of alloimmunization in different groups of children with sickle cell disease: Effect of ethnic background. Am J Pediatr Hematol Oncol 1989;11:314-19.

56. Win N, Doughty H, Telfer P, et al. Hyperhemolytic transfusion reaction in sickle cell disease. Transfusion 2001;41:323-8.

57. Petz LD, Calhoun L, Shulman IA, et al. The sickle cell hemolytic transfusion reaction syndrome. Transfusion 1997;37:382-92.

58. Darabi K, Dzik S. Hyperhemolysis syndrome in anemia of chronic disease. Transfusion 2005;45:1930-3.

59. Brown K, Subramony C, May W, et al. Hepatic iron overload in children with sickle cell anemia on chronic transfusion therapy. J Pediatr Hematol Oncol 2009;31:309-12.

60. Rund D, Rachmilewitz E. Beta-thalassemia. N Engl J Med 2005;353:1135-46.

61. Hillyer CD, Shaz BH, Winkler AM, Reid M. Integrating molecular technologies for RBC typing and compatibility testing into blood centers and transfusion services. Transfus Med Rev 2008;22:117-32.

62. Berdoukas VA, Kwan YL, Sansotta ML. A study on the value of red cell exchange transfusion in transfusion dependent anaemias. Clin Lab Haematol 1986;8:209-20.

63. World Health Organization. Guidelines for the treatment of malaria. 2nd ed. Geneva: WHO, 2010.

64. Trampuz A, Jereb M, Muzlovic I, Prabhu RM. Clinical review: Severe malaria. Crit Care 2003;7:315-23.

65. World Health Organization. Severe falciparum malaria. Trans R Soc Trop Med Hyg 2000;94:S1-S90.

66. Centers for Disease Control and Prevention. CDC treatment guidelines: Treatment of malaria (guidelines for clinicians). (June 2009) Atlanta, GA: CDC, 2009.

67. Nieuwenhuis JA, Meertens JH, Zijlstra JG, et al. Automated erythrocytapheresis in severe falciparum malaria: A critical appraisal. Acta Trop 2006;98:201-6.

68. Riddle MS, Jackson JL, Sanders JW, Blazes DL. Exchange transfusion as an adjunct therapy in severe Plasmodium falciparum malaria: A meta-analysis. Clin Infect Dis 2002;34:1192-8.

69. Ahmed T, Lake D, Feldman E, et al. Factors influencing prognosis after dose-intensive therapy for recurrent or refractory Hodgkin's disease. Results of sequential trials: A case for treating patients with resistant disease. Ann N Y Acad Sci 1995;770:305-14.

70. Phillips P, Nantel S, Benny WB. Exchange transfusion as an adjunct to the treatment of severe falciparum malaria: Case report and review. Rev Infect Dis 1990;12:1100-8.

71. Spaete J, Patrozou E, Rich JD, Sweeney JD. Red cell exchange transfusion for babesiosis in Rhode Island. J Clin Apher 2009;24:97-105.

72. Vannier E, Gewurz BE, Krause PJ. Human babesiosis. Infect Dis Clin N Am 2008;22:469-88.

73. Evenson DA, Perry E, Kloster B, et al. Therapeutic apheresis for babesiosis. J Clin Apher 1998;13:32-6.

74. Centers for Disease Control and Prevention. Babesiosis: Treatment. Atlanta, GA: CDC, 2009. [Available at http://www.cdc.gov/babesiosis/treatment.html (accessed April 5, 2010).]

75. Werch J, Todd C. Resolution by erythrocytapheresis of the exposure of an Rh-negative person to Rh-positive cells: An alternative treatment. Transfusion 1993;33:530-2.

76. Worel N, Greinix HT, Supper V, et al. Prophylactic red blood cell exchange for prevention of severe immune hemolysis in minor ABO-mismatched allogeneic peripheral blood progenitor cell transplantation after reduced-intensity conditioning. Transfusion 2007;47:1494-502.

77. Rowley SD. Hematopoietic stem cell transplantation between red cell incompatible donor-recipient pairs. Bone Marrow Transplant 2001;28:315-21.

78. Weaver LK. Clinical practice. Carbon monoxide poisoning. N Engl J Med 2009;360:1217-25.

79. Samartsiev SI, Leshchiner PI. Exchange blood transfusion in severe poisoning with exhaust gases. Voen Med Zh 1972;10:48-9.

80. Radevich OL. Use of exchange blood transfusion in carbon monoxide poisoning. Vrach Delo 1967;1:139-40.
81. Golden PJ, Weinstein R. Treatment of high-risk, refractory acquired methemoglobinemia with automated red blood cell exchange. J Clin Apher 1998;13:28-31.
82. Kwon SU, Lim SH, Rhee I, et al. Successful whole blood exchange by apheresis in a patient with acute cyclosporine intoxication without long-term sequelae. J Heart Lung Transplant 2006;25:483-5.
83. Leitner GC, Hiesmayr M, Hoecker P, Jilma B. Therapeutic approaches in the management of oral cyclosporine A intoxication. Transplantation 2003;75:1764-5.
84. Eichbaum QG, Dzik WH, Chung RT, Szczepiorkowski ZM. Red blood cell exchange transfusion in two patients with advanced erythropoietic protoporphyria. Transfusion 2005;45:208-13.
85. Vecchio S, Leonardo P, Musuraca V, et al. A comparison of the results obtained with traditional phlebotomy and with therapeutic erythrocytapheresis in patients with erythrocytosis. Blood Transfus 2007;5:20-3.
86. Spivak JL. Polycythemia vera: Myths, mechanisms, and management. Blood 2002;100:4272-90.
87. Tefferi A, Thiele J, Vardiman JW. The 2008 World Health Organization classification system for myeloproliferative neoplasms: Order out of chaos. Cancer 2009;115:3842-7.
88. DeFilippis AP, Law K, Curtin S, Eckman JR. Blood is thicker than water: The management of hyperviscosity in adults with cyanotic heart disease. Cardiol Rev 2007;15:31-4.
89. Wijermans P, van Egmond L, Ypma P, et al. Isovolemic erythrocytapheresis technique as an alternative to conventional phlebotomy in patients with polycythemia vera and hemochromatosis. Transfus Apher Sci 2009;40:137.
90. Rombout-Sestrienkova E, van Noord PA, van Deursen CT, et al. Therapeutic erythrocytapheresis versus phlebotomy in the initial treatment of hereditary hemochromatosis—a pilot study. Transfus Apher Sci 2007;36:261-7.
91. Brittenham GM. Disorders of iron metabolism: Iron deficiency and iron overload. In: Hoffman R, Furie B, McGlave P, et al, eds. Hematology: Basic principles and practice. 5th ed. Philadelphia: Elsevier, 2009:453-69.
92. Leitman SF, Browning JN, Yau YY, et al. Hemochromatosis subjects as allogeneic blood donors: A prospective study. Transfusion 2003;43:1538-44.
93. Josephson CJ. Iron overload. In: Hillyer C, Shaz B, Zimring JC, Abshire T, eds. Transfusion medicine and hemostasis: Clinical and laboratory aspects. Philadelphia: Elsevier, 2009:359-60.
94. Rombout-Sestrienkova E, van Noord PA, Reuser E, et al. Therapeutic erythrocytapheresis (TE) versus phlebotomy (p) in the treatment of hereditary hemochromatosis (HH) patients: Preliminary results from an ongoing clinical trial (NCT 00202436). Transfus Apher Sci 2009;40:135-6.

In: McLeod BC, Szczepiorkowski ZM, Weinstein R, Winters JL, eds.
Apheresis: Principles and Practice, 3rd edition
Bethesda, MD: AABB Press, 2010

20

Selective Extraction of Plasma Constituents

Jeffrey L. Winters, MD

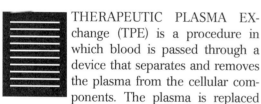THERAPEUTIC PLASMA EX-change (TPE) is a procedure in which blood is passed through a device that separates and removes the plasma from the cellular components. The plasma is replaced with a colloid solution (eg, albumin and/or plasma) or a combination of crystalloid and colloid solutions.[1] TPE is used to remove plasma that may contain harmful substances implicated in a disease, such as monoclonal immunoglobulins (paraproteins), autoantibodies, immune complexes, lipids, and toxins, which are typically present in total amounts of 1 to 2 g.[2] During a 1-volume TPE, 150 g of plasma protein is removed, consisting of 110 g of albumin and 40 g of globulins and other proteins.[2,3]

In TPE, the majority of removed plasma components are substances that have important physiologic functions; thus TPE has the poten-tial to alter normal physiology. This is especially true when the replacement fluid lacks all or most normal plasma constituents. When albumin is used as a replacement fluid, 125 g of albumin will be replaced but other important plasma components (eg, immunoglobulins, coagulation factors, etc.) will not. When hydroxyethyl starch (HES) is used, even albumin is not replaced. Although most physiologically important substances are soon replenished through normal homeostatic mechanisms (4 hours for Factors VIII and IX[4]; 24 hours for almost all other coagulation factors[4] except fibrinogen, which reaches 66% of preapheresis values at 72 hours[5]), they may not be replenished rapidly enough to avoid patient complications, especially when TPE is performed intensively. The potential for bleeding exists,[4,5] and there have been reports of thrombosis caused by the removal of regulators of the coagulation cas-

Jeffrey L. Winters, MD, Medical Director, Therapeutic Apheresis Unit, Division of Transfusion Medicine, Department of Laboratory Medicine and Pathology, Mayo Clinic, and Associate Professor, Mayo Clinic College of Medicine, Rochester, Minnesota
The author has disclosed a financial relationship with Fenwal, Inc.

cade.[6,7] Another frequent concern is that immunoglobulin depletion from TPE may increase susceptibility to infection. In one report, TPE was implicated as a cause of serious infections in patients undergoing TPE while receiving immunosuppressive drugs.[8] Removal of plasma constituents other than those involved in coagulation or humoral immunity may also have adverse effects. There have been reports of a prolonged effect of succinyl choline, a neuromuscular blockade agent, when administered to patients following TPE because of depletion of pseudocholinesterase, which is necessary for its metabolism.[9,10] Medications may also be removed.[11-13]

In addition, the replacement fluids used in TPE may have undesirable effects. When plasma is used, plasma proteins are replaced but complications can occur, including transmission of infectious disease,[14] allergic reactions,[15] anaphylaxis,[16] and transfusion-related acute lung injury.[17-19] The citrate anticoagulant in plasma can cause ionized hypocalcemia if infusion rates are too high. Pharmaceutical albumin, when given as replacement fluid, may not perform all of the normal physiologic functions of plasma albumin. For example, sodium caprylate and other preservatives occupy binding sites for drugs and metabolites.[20] Pharmaceutical albumin has also been "stripped" of bound calcium during the manufacturing process. When used as a replacement fluid, it can bind free calcium and may contribute to ionized hypocalcemia.[21] Finally, reactions to albumin can occur, including hypotensive reactions,[22,23] febrile reactions,[24] and anaphylactic reactions.[25,26] When HES is used, complications can include anaphylactoid reactions[26] and intractable pruritis caused by skin deposition.[27]

Methods have been developed to selectively remove pathologic components from plasma with the "cleansed" plasma returned to the patient in order to avoid these adverse effects of TPE. This approach diminishes removal of desirable substances and avoids complications from replacement fluids. Such techniques vary in their degree of selectivity. They may be extremely selective—removing only antibodies directed toward a specific antigen[28,29]; relatively selective—removing only immunoglobulins[30-32] or lipoproteins[33]; or minimally selective—removing substances above a certain size.[34] The advantages and disadvantages of such selective extraction systems are summarized in Table 20-1.

A number of systems are available worldwide. Only two have been approved by the Food and Drug Administration (FDA) and are available in the United States at the time of this writing: the heparin-induced extracorporeal LDL precipitation (HELP) system and the dextran sulfate LDL removal column. This chapter will include descriptions of several systems available in other countries.

Double Filtration Plasmapheresis

Double filtration plasmapheresis (DFPP), also referred to as membrane differential plasmapheresis or cascade filtration plasmapheresis, is the least selective among the techniques that will be discussed. Plasma is first separated from the cellular components by filtration through the primary membrane plasma separator (MPS). The MPS can be constructed in a number of configurations, including a flat membrane, a bundle of hollow fibers, or a drum-shaped rotating membrane. The separated plasma passes through a second filter, the plasma fractionator (PF). The qualities of the PF determine which plasma constituents are discarded and which are returned to the patient.[34]

The selectivity of DFPP is determined by three factors.[35] The first consists of the size cutoff properties of the PF, determined by the filter pore size. The larger the pore size, the larger the molecule that can pass through the membrane and be retained for return to the patient. As an example, a pore size smaller than the size of IgM would result in the retention of substances the size of IgM and larger while allowing smaller substances to pass and return to the patient. PFs do not have strict cutoffs, and as a result a certain quantity of some smaller substances, such as albumin, will be lost while some large substances, such as IgM, will be returned to the patient.[35] The other fac-

Table 20-1. Advantages and Disadvantages of Selective Removal Systems Compared to Therapeutic Plasma Exchange

Advantages	Disadvantages
Remove only the substance of interest, leaving behind normal and beneficial plasma constituents (eg, HDL) and medications.	May not remove pathologic substance when the pathophysiology of the disease is unknown/uncertain.
Do not require or minimize replacement fluids, avoiding reactions and potential disease transmission.	Expose the patient's blood to biologically active columns and materials that may trigger reactions.
Avoid the expenses associated with replacement fluids.	Some systems are more complex to operate than instruments used to perform TPE.
Some systems can remove more pathologic substance than can TPE.	Limited availability of instrumentation because of government licensure and expense.
Some systems do not require separation of whole blood into plasma and cellular components (eg, hemoperfusion systems).	Expensive to operate, with limited reimbursement.

HDL = high density lipoprotein; TPE = therapeutic plasma exchange.

tors that influence selectivity are the flow rates of plasma entering and leaving the PF. Varying these two parameters can alter the selectivity of the system.[35]

The distribution and synthesis of molecules of interest also influences removal, as is described in Chapter 14 for TPE. A substance limited to the intravascular space, such as IgM or LDL cholesterol, is cleared most effectively by the first two sessions of DFPP, with stable clearance rates during subsequent treatments.[36] Substances with larger volumes of distribution, such as IgG and IgA, are cleared most effectively by the first four or more sessions.[36] In disorders such as familial hypercholesterolemia (FH) or Waldenström macroglobulinemia, treatment with more than two DFPP procedures would not enhance depletion of the pathologic substance but would, because of variable size cutoffs, result in greater losses of smaller plasma components. For the removal of smaller molecules that have a greater extravascular distribution, more treatments are needed.

General Use of DFPP

DFPP has been used to treat a range of disorders similar to those treated with TPE; these are listed in Table 20-2.[37] Studies have reported effective removal of autoantibodies[38,39] and improvement in disease severity[39-42] for some of these disorders. Of note, DFPP has been compared to other apheresis procedures, including immunoadsorption (IA) (discussed later)[39] and TPE,[42] in the treatment of myasthenia gravis and Guillian-Barré syndrome (GBS), respectively. Compared to IA, DFPP was found to produce equivalent clinical results,[39] but with GBS, time to onset of effect was shorter, and change in disability scores, greater with TPE.[40] The authors postulated that unspecified factors other than antibodies, which could be involved in the disease process, may be present in the plasma and might pass through the PF of the DFPP device rather than being removed.[40] Similar comparisons between the use of DFPP

Table 20-2. Autoimmune Disorders that Have Been Treated with Double Filtration Plasmapheresis[37]

Systemic lupus erythematosus

Rheumatoid arthritis

Myasthenia gravis

Guillian-Barré syndrome

Multiple sclerosis

Thrombotic thrombocytopenic purpura

Idiopathic thrombocytopenic purpura

Rapidly progressive glomerulonephritis

Goodpasture syndrome

Pemphigus vulgaris

Bullous pemphigoid

Focal segmental glomerulosclerosis

and TPE in other diseases have not been performed. DFPP has been used in pregnant women to treat hemolytic disease of the fetus and newborn,[43] to remove anti-A and anti-B to allow for ABO incompatible renal transplantation,[44] and to treat hyperviscosity in both Waldenström macroglobulinemia and multiple myeloma.[37]

Finally, DFPP has also been used to treat FH. This disorder is characterized by marked elevations in LDL cholesterol in individuals who are either heterozygous or homozygous for genes encoding abnormal LDL receptors. This results in accelerated atherosclerosis and premature death from cardiac disease.[45] A number of systems are available that can selectively remove LDL cholesterol (LDL-C), a process collectively referred to as LDL apheresis. The other systems are described and compared to DFPP later in this chapter.

DFPP was the first selective removal system used to treat FH following the initial demonstration that TPE could meaningfully reduce LDL-C levels.[46] The 15-nm-pore-size PF used for this application results in greater than 60%

reduction in LDL-C without significant depletion of albumin or immunoglobulins during long-term treatment.[46] One difficulty in using DFPP to remove lipids is the formation of cryogels that clog filter pores in the PF, leading to a decrease in LDL-C selectivity and increased removal of high-density lipoprotein (HDL).[46] To prevent gel formation and enhance separation, DFPP devices include a heating system that maintains the plasma at 38 C as it enters the PF.[46] This process, which employs modified DFPP devices to remove LDL-C and other pathogenic lipids with minimal loss of HDL and immunoglobulins, is referred to as lipidfiltration.[46]

Rheopheresis

The relative lack of selectivity of DFPP might be advantageous in treatment of diseases due not to a single pathologic substance but to aberrant blood flow through the microcirculation. When DFPP is used to alter blood flow, it is referred to as rheopheresis.

Flow through the microcirculation depends on perfusion pressure (generated by the heart), vessel length and diameter, and blood viscosity.[47] In normal vessels, diameter is the most important factor. It is regulated by the smooth muscle of the vessel wall. In diseased vessels, regulation is impaired and viscosity becomes the major determinant of flow. Whole blood viscosity is determined by the shear stress at the interface between the blood stream and the vessel wall as well as hematocrit, red cell deformability, and plasma viscosity.[47] The last is influenced by plasma solutes, with high-molecular-weight proteins such as fibrinogen and α_2-macroglobulin being major determinants of viscosity. In addition to increasing the plasma viscosity, these proteins may also aggregate red cells, which further impedes flow.[47] In rheopheresis, DFPP is performed using a PF, which removes high-molecular-weight plasma components, including fibrinogen, α_2-macroglobulin, LDL-C, and IgM.[47] This reduces plasma viscosity and red cell aggregation and may improve blood flow and tissue oxygenation.

Limited published data are available describing use of rheopheresis to treat diabetic retinopathy,[48] peripheral artery occlusive disease,[49] angina,[50] and acute stroke.[51] It has also been used in dry age-related macular degeneration (AMD), for which a number of case series and randomized trials have been performed.[52-54]

AMD is the leading cause of blindness in those over 60 years old. It is a progressive disorder affecting the macula and leading to loss of central vision. The initial stage, dry AMD, is characterized by the collection of debris (drusen) beneath the retinal pigment epithelium (RTPE). Approximately 10% of dry AMD will progress to wet AMD over 10 years. Wet AMD is characterized by blood vessel growth into the choroid (choroidial neovascularization). AMD risk factors include smoking, hypertension, and elevated body mass index. There is a direct correlation with cholesterol, fibrinogen, and α_2-macroglobulin levels.[55] Finally, inherited risk factors for AMD include mutations in complement factor H, complement factor B, and complement component C2.[56]

AMD pathogenesis has not been completely elucidated. According to one hypothesis, the sclerae become increasingly rigid with age as a result of lipid deposition. This could compromise blood flow in the choroid, diminishing RTPE nutrient and oxygen supply. The hypoxia could lead to loss of RTPE ability to phagocytoze cellular debris and subsequent deposition of extracellular debris as observed in dry AMD. By increasing the distance that oxygen must diffuse to reach the RTPE, such deposits could lead to more hypoxia and greater RTPE dysfunction. Increasing hypoxia could eventually cause RTPE vascular growth factor production and the choroidal neovascularization observed in wet AMD.[55] Dry AMD treatment options are limited to high-dose vitamin C, vitamin E, beta carotene, and zinc. Choroidial neovascularization can be ablated by a variety of methods.[54]

Three randomized controlled trials have examined rheopheresis treatment of dry AMD.[52-54] In the largest of these (MIRA-1) no beneficial effect of DFPP could be discerned in the primary analysis, although an underpowered post hoc analysis was taken to suggest a small improvement in vision in the treated patients. Table 20-3 summarizes these trials.

Based on the MAC-1 and MIRA-1 trials as well as eight published case series, the American Society for Apheresis (ASFA) Clinical Applications Committee evaluated the treatment of AMD with DFPP in the 2007 special applications issue of the *Journal of Clinical Apheresis*.[57] At that time, the use of DFPP to treat AMD was assigned a Category P, indicating strong evidence from Phase III trials suggests efficacy, but the device used in the treatment is not available in the United States.[56] The use of DFPP for the treatment of dry AMD is a Category III, Grade 2B recommendation according to the 2010 special issue, based on post hoc analysis of the MIRA-1 trial and the results of the ART trial.[58]

Yeh et al[59] described reactions among 335 patients undergoing DFPP. In 2502 procedures, 26.3% were complicated by a reaction. The most common reactions directly attributable to DFPP were hemolysis (20%) and hypotension (3.3%). Hemolysis resulted from traumatic damage to the red cells during plasma separation. Although visually identifiable to the instrument operator, the hemolysis was clinically insignificant. The average decrease in hemoglobin was 0.2 g/dL. Klingel et al[47] reported the frequency of reactions in 322 patients undergoing rheopheresis. Reactions occurred in 4.7% of 2021 procedures. The most common were hypotension (2.1%), hematoma/bleeding (0.8%), and dizziness (0.6%). The majority were mild, with only 1.2% requiring intervention.

Rheopheresis is being used to treat dry AMD in Canada and European countries. Although no DFPP devices have been approved for use or are available in the United States, they are the major type of device used to perform plasmapheresis and plasma exchange in many other countries.

Nonspecific Immunoadsorption

IA involves the removal of immunoglobulins from plasma, leaving behind all or the majority

Table 21-3. Summary of Published Controlled Trials of the Use of Rheopheresis in AMD

Trial	Patients	Treatment	Results	Comment
MAC-1[52]	Treatment: 20 Control: 20	10 procedures over 21 weeks vs no treatment	Treated group demonstrated a mean best corrected vision of 1.6 ETDRS lines greater than controls (p <0.01), improved electroretinogram, and improved rheologic parameters. Patients with only dry AMD improved by 2.33 lines (p <0.01).	Enrollment was not limited to patients with dry AMD. Some patients had changes of wet AMD (neovascularization).
MIRA-1[53]	Treatment: 129 Control: 69	8 procedures over 10 weeks vs sham treatment of venipuncture only	Treated group demonstrated logMAR vision improvement of 0.02 ±0.213 vs control improvement of 0.02 ±0.20 (p = 0.977). No significant difference in vision between treated group and controls.	Exclusion criteria included wet AMD and other conditions that could affect visual acuity. Protocol violators, failing to meet inclusion criteria, were 37% of treated and 29% of controls. Analysis excluding violators demonstrated significant improvement in visual acuity (p = 0.001), but the post hoc analysis was underpowered. Overall, the trial was fatally flawed and considered a failure.
ART[54]	Treatment: 22 Control: 21	10 procedures over 17 weeks vs no treatment	Treated group demonstrated improved visual acuity of 0.95 ETDRS lines (p = 0.01) with 9% of patients demonstrating ≥2 lines. No patients in the treated group demonstrated a loss of visual acuity. No controls demonstrated improvement ≥2 lines, and 24% demonstrated visual acuity loss.	Study patients limited to those with dry AMD.

EDTRS = Early Treatment of Diabetic Retinopathy Study; AMD = age-related macular degeneration; logMAR = logarithm of the minimal angle of resolution.

of other plasma components. IA may be specific, removing only a single antibody directed toward a specific antigen, or nonspecific, removing all antibodies. A number of nonspecific IA columns are available. Some columns can be regenerated, meaning that an unlimited amount of plasma can be treated. Others can treat only a fixed plasma volume because of saturation of immunoglobulin binding sites.

Staphylococcal Protein A Columns

Protein A is a cell wall constituent of the Cowan I strain of *Staphylococcus aureus*. The N-terminus contains five homologous regions that bind mammalian IgG.[60] IgG binding to these regions is high affinity and nonimmune. Protein A is stable under a variety of conditions, permitting linkage to various matrices and elution of bound IgG without loss of binding capacity.[61] Protein A binds strongly to IgG1, IgG2, and IgG4 but only to a variable extent with IgG3, IgM, and IgA.[62-65] Because of these characteristics, staphylococcal protein A has been used as a sorbent in IA columns.

Staphylococcal Protein A Silica Column

The Prosorba column (Fresenius Kabi, Redmond, WA) contained protein A immobilized on a silica matrix (protein A silica, or PAS).[30] Up to 2 L of plasma could be treated by a column before it became saturated.[30] It removed both free immunoglobulin and circulating immune complexes (CICs).[66,67]

The PAS column was approved by the FDA for treatment of moderate to severe rheumatoid arthritis based on improvement in measures of disease activity in a randomized, double-blind, sham-controlled trial of patients with active disease refractory to standard therapy.[68] It was also approved for use in immune thrombocytopenic purpura (ITP) with a platelet count <100,000/mL based on a randomized trial in patients refractory to standard therapy.[69] In other countries, the PAS column had been used for indications shown in Table 20-4, for most of which randomized controlled trials are not available.

In December 2006, PAS column production was discontinued with the closure of the US manufacturing plant. These columns are no longer available and are mentioned only for historical interest.

Staphylococcal Protein A Agarose Column

The Immunosorba column (Fresenius Kabi AG, Bad Homburg, Germany) is part of a system that combines two columns with an elution monitor. Each column contains enough protein A—covalently linked to cross-linked beaded Sepharose (GE Healthcare Bio-Sciences AB, Uppsala, Sweden), a brand of agarose (protein A agarose, or PAA)—to bind 1.25 to 1.50 g of IgG. PAA columns have an 18-month refrigerated shelf-life. Plasma produced by an apheresis device is pumped into a microprocessor-controlled elution monitor that directs plasma flow through one of the columns. After one column is saturated, plasma is directed to the other while IgG bound in the saturated column is eluted with an acidic fluid, followed by restoration of physiological pH with a buffer. Treated plasma is combined with the cellular components and returned. Plasma flow is automatically switched between columns every 10 minutes, giving the system almost unlimited capacity for IgG removal. Processing three plasma volumes takes 3 to 5 hours and involves 20 to 30 column regeneration cycles.[70] Treatment of 2.5 plasma volumes results in the following percentage reductions in plasma immunoglobulin concentrations: IgG1, 97%; IgG2, 98%; IgG3, 40%; IgG4, 77%; IgM, 56%; and IgA, 55%.[71] Albumin, fibrinogen, and antithrombin are reduced by less than 20%.[70]

PAA columns have been used in European countries to treat alloimmunized patients awaiting kidney transplantation and patients with inhibitors to Factors VIII or IX.[70,72] They are also used for patients with other diseases listed in Table 20-4. PAA was approved by the FDA for removal of Factor VIII and IX inhibitors. Studies of PAA column efficacy have consisted of case reports and series with no controlled trials.

Table 20-4. Disorders Treated with Staphylococcal Protein A Columns[30,65]

PAS Column (Prosorba*)	PAA Column (Immunosorba†)
Immune thrombocytopenic purpura‡	Factor VIII inhibitors‡
Rheumatoid arthritis‡	Factor IX inhibitors‡
Platelet alloimmunization	Antiglomerular basement membrane disease (Goodpasture syndrome)
Paraneoplastic CNS syndromes	
Papraproteinemic polyneuropathies	Wegner granulomatosis
Chemotherapy-induced thrombotic thrombocytopenic purpura (eg, mitomycin-C)	Focal segmental glomerulosclerosis
	Systemic lupus erythematosus
	Myasthenia gravis
Maligancies unresponsive to conventional therapy	Acute inflammatory demyelinating polyneuropathy (Guillain-Barré syndrome)
	Humoral rejection of solid organ transplants
	Autoimmune hemolytic anemia
	Dilated cardiomyopathy

*Fresenius Kabi, Redmond, WA; PAS = protein A silica.
†Fresenius Kabi AG, Bad Homburg, Germany; PAA = protein A agarose.
‡Uses approved by the US Food and Drug Administration.
CNS = central nervous system.

Preparation for Renal Transplantation. Approximately 10% to 15% of patients awaiting renal transplantation are hypersensitized to HLA, having a panel-reactive antibody score (PRA) >75%. These patients have a reduced chance of obtaining a compatible renal allograft. PAA is used to remove HLA antibodies to produce a negative crossmatch.[70]

Patients undergo an initial course of four to six PAA treatments combined with immunosuppressive therapy and then have HLA antibody titers and PRA monitored. Patients exhibit rapid resynthesis of IgG and the PRA will return to baseline level within a few weeks.[73] Therefore, additional PAA treatments are performed while waiting for a crossmatch-negative donor. In published series, most patients received transplants within 2 months of starting PAA.[73,74]

The success of PAA in removing HLA antibodies depends upon antibody titer. Complete removal of antibodies with a titer as high as 256 has been reported.[75] However, complete removal of high-titer antibodies could not be expected unless there were a 100% reduction in circulating IgG. Hyperimmunized patients may have antibodies with a predominant specificity directed against a single antigen (eg, HLA-A2) as well as cross-reactivity against epitopes shared with other HLA antigens from the same cross-reactive group. Data indicate that if the titer against the predominant antigen is ≥256, PAA is unlikely to have a significant effect on the PRA.[72] Gjörstrup and Watt[70] delineated the rationale for treatment under the assumption that cross-reactive antibody titers can be lower than the predominant antibody titer. If the procedure could eliminate the weaker cross-reactivities, the PRA could be reduced to 40% in a patient with an HLA-A2 predominating antibody. Such a patient could then be transplanted with an allograft that lacks the HLA-A2 antigen, as there would be a negative current crossmatch.[70]

Reductions in HLA antibody titers and PRA were observed in the study of Hakim et al.[76] Significant reductions in PRA occurred although the predominating antibody usually remained detectable. Responses among individual patients varied substantially. Plasma IgG levels were reduced by 90% ±8%. For most patients, the reduction in HLA antibody levels paralleled that in total IgG. Reductions in HLA antibody titers ranged from two- to 64-fold (average = 18-fold). The reductions in PRA before and after treatment ranged from 0 to 87% (average = 39%). The patients were not receiving immunosuppression, and over a 4-week period of follow-up, HLA antibody titers returned to baseline. Antibody rebound with overshoot was noted in only two patients, both of whom had been transfused during follow-up. In a series of patients receiving immunosuppressive drugs, antibody titers returned to baseline either more gradually[74] or as rapidly[77] as those in the series of Hakim et al.[76]

Several studies have reported the clinical outcome of subjects undergoing PAA before kidney transplantation.[74,75,77-84] Gjörstrup[81] reported on 45 treated patients, 32 of whom underwent transplantation. One-year graft survival was 59% in the 22 patients who had a history of positive crossmatches, and 40% in the 10 patients who did not. Overall, eight grafts were lost to acute rejection, three to chronic rejection, and four to nonimmunologic causes. Hiesse et al[83] reported on 15 treated patients, 12 of whom received transplants. Graft survival was 86% in seven patients who did not have a historic positive crossmatch compared with 40% in five patients who had a current negative/historic positive crossmatch. Two grafts failed because of hyperacute rejection, while humoral rejection in a third patient was treated successfully with a second course of PAA, and one patient died with a functional graft. The authors emphasized that patients with a pretreatment titer of ≥64 for a relevant antigen had not benefited from the procedure. In the series of Ross et al,[84] one of five allografts was lost to acute tubular necrosis without evidence of rejection; the other four patients had functional grafts and stable serum creatinine levels 3 to 34 months after transplantation.

It appears that PAA can be an effective means for reducing the alloreactivity of sera in prospective renal allograft recipients with a high PRA. Transplant recipients with a current negative/historic positive crossmatch can expect a chance for graft survival as high as 60%. Variability in response to treatment is substantial, however, and criteria for selecting patients likely to benefit need to be better defined.[83]

ASFA has not specifically categorized the use of PAA or other IA techniques for conditioning in crossmatch-incompatible renal transplant.[58]

Antibody-Mediated Rejection. In addition to preparing sensitized patients for renal transplantation, PAA has been used to treat antibody-mediated rejection (AMR) caused by HLA antibodies. Min et al[85] treated six patients who developed AMR within 5 days of transplantation. AMR was diagnosed based on decreased graft function in the presence of C4d staining and peritubular capillaritis on renal biopsy.[85] Patients were treated with PAA (6.3 ±1.03 treatments), tacrolimus, and mycophenolate mofetil. After a mean of 14 days, serum creatinine improved and the PRA decreased from 50.2% ±6.1% to 8.3% ±2.9%. Four of six patients demonstrated resolution of C4d staining, and all patients and grafts survived with a follow-up of 18.8 ±5.46 months.[85] Böhmig et al performed a randomized controlled trial in acute AMR.[86] Patients were eligible if there was severe graft dysfunction as defined by dialysis dependence or a serum creatinine ≥4 mg/dL plus peritubular C4d deposits on renal biopsy. Ten patients were enrolled; five were treated with PAA (2.5 plasma volumes daily for 3 days and then every 3 days for up to 6 weeks), and five received no PAA treatments. All patients received tacrolimus and anti-cellular-rejection therapy, if appropriate. Patients in the control group were eligible to crossover to PAA treatment after 3 weeks. All PAA-treated patients had resolution of AMR, though one died unrelated to the therapy. None of the controls improved; four were crossed over to PAA treatment, but none improved, and as a result the trial was terminated early because of ethical concerns.[86] Although the trial by Böhmig and the case series by Min have treated only small numbers of patients, they suggest that treatment with PAA may have a role in AMR.

As with the treatment of HLA-sensitized renal transplant candidates, ASFA has not categorized the use of IA techniques in the treatment of AMR.[58]

Coagulation Factor Inhibitors. Patients with alloimmune Factor VIII or IX inhibitors are divided into high responders, who have a strong anamnestic response after exposure to Factor VIII or IX, and low responders, who have little or no anamnestic response.[87] Bleeding episodes in low responders who have an initial inhibitor titer <10 Bethesda units (BU) can be managed by infusion of Factor VIII or IX in sufficiently large doses. High responders with initially low antibody titers should also receive cyclophosphamide to delay the anamnestic response. However, bleeding episodes in patients with initially high antibody titers are difficult to manage, and various treatments have been tried or proposed. These have included inhibitor-bypassing agents (prothrombin complex concentrates, activated prothrombin complex concentrates, and recombinant Factor VIIa), porcine Factor VIII (no longer available in the United States), recombinant porcine Factor VIII (currently in clinical trials), and intensive TPE or PAA for removal of circulating antibodies.[87,88] The rationale for the use of TPE and PAA is that a patient may respond to large doses of Factor VIII or IX after the inhibitor titer has been temporarily reduced.[87]

Another important goal of therapy in these patients is permanent eradication of the inhibitor with induction of tolerance to Factor VIII or IX. Regimens for Factor VIII inhibitors include the administration of very high doses of Factor VIII (Bonn protocol) and the combination of cyclophosphamide, Factor VIII, and very high doses of IVIG (Malmö protocol). PAA is used in the Malmö protocol at the start of treatment if inhibitor levels are >10 BU. The Malmö protocol was successful in eliminating the inhibitor in nine of 11 patients with hemophilia A (nine high responders, one intermediate responder, and one low responder)[89,90] and in two of three high-responding patients with hemophilia B.[91]

Several reports have described the use of PAA to manage inhibitor patients. Gjörstrup and Watt[70] presented experience with 32 patients with congenital (20 cases) or acquired (12 cases) hemophilia reported before 1990. This was followed by additional reports,[92] and Gjörstrup et al[93] reported a series of 10 additional patients in 1991. Uehlinger et al[94] reported the successful treatment of a patient with an acquired von Willebrand factor antibody. PAA should precede the administration of Factor VIII (which should be given only after the inhibitor titer has been reduced below 10 BU). If Factor VIII is administered first, an anamnestic response often results, and the rapid resynthesis of antibody makes the reduction of titers extremely difficult.

In the report of Gjörstrup et al,[93] 10 patients (seven with congenital hemophilia and three with acquired hemophilia) underwent a combined total of 17 courses of PAA: eight for bleeding, two for trauma, five for surgery, and two for the induction of tolerance. In the study, 1.0 to 5.8 plasma volumes were processed per treatment over one to six sessions. Seven courses involved only one session, and six entailed two daily procedures; in only four courses were three to six daily sessions deemed necessary. In six patients with congenital hemophilia and pretreatment inhibitor levels between 1 and 128 BU, the levels were reduced to <10 BU; the seventh patient with congenital hemophilia had a very potent inhibitor (4350 BU), which could only be reduced to 12 BU after five daily sessions. The three patients with acquired hemophilia had levels of 36 to 155 BU before and 4 to 207 BU after treatment. In only one of four courses was the level reduced to <10 BU. In both congenital and acquired hemophilia, antibodies reappeared within 2 to 28 days of treatment.

The authors emphasized the more favorable response of patients with congenital vs acquired hemophilia. In the former, a single 3-plasma-volume PAA may reduce inhibitor levels of 60 to 70 BU to less than 10 BU. With TPE, two or more daily sessions have been required to bring down inhibitor levels initially no higher than 20 to 60 BU.[95-98] In addition, PAA may be safer than the use of prothrombin complex concentrates, whether activated or not.[99,100] Patients with congenital hemophilia and higher inhibitor titers may need two or more daily PAA treatments. In all cases, the need to retreat on the following day because of antibody re-equilibration must also be considered. Patients with exceptionally high inhibitor levels that cannot be reduced to <10 BU have responded to porcine Factor VIII following PAA.[93]

Freedman et al examined the cost effectiveness of PAA treatment in three patients with Factor VIII inhibitors, two with acquired hemophilia and one with congenital hemophilia. The patients with acquired hemophilia failed to respond satisfactorily to treatment with immunosuppression, porcine Factor VIII, recombinant Factor VIIa, and IVIG. They responded rapidly to PAA treatment. The patient with congenital hemophilia with Factor VIII inhibitor was treated with PAA to reduce the inhibitor levels to allow for immune tolerance therapy. Costs of treatment before PAA treatment were substantially greater than after, leading the authors to suggest that PAA may be a cost-effective alternative in Factor VIII inhibitors.[101]

ASFA has assigned IA for treatment of coagulation factor inhibitors as a Category III indication with a recommendation grade of 2B.[57]

Dilated Cardiomyopathy. Dilated cardiomyopathy (DCM) is the most common antecedent to cardiac transplantation worldwide.[102] It is characterized by four-chamber enlargement with impaired ventricular systolic function. A variety of factors may be involved in its pathogenesis, including myocardial viral infection, inherited susceptibility factors, environmental risks such as heavy metal exposure, and autoimmunity.[102] Eighty percent of patients with DCM have one or more autoantibodies directed against myocardial antigens,[102,103] which are listed in Table 20-5. These antibodies have been shown to lyse or impair the contractility of isolated rat cardiac myocytes and to impair calcium transport. When rabbits are immunized to peptides from target antigens, myocar-

Table 20-5. Autoantibodies Implicated in Dilated Cardiomyopathy[102,103]

Myosin heavy chain

β1-adrenergic receptor

Mitochondrial antigens

Adenosine diphosphate carrier protein

Adenosine triphosphate carrier protein

M2 muscarinic receptor

Troponin I

dial changes identical to those seen in DCM are produced.[102,103]

Both specific[28,104] and nonspecific IA[105-114] have been applied to DCM. The initial trial of the PAA column was as an alternative to the antihuman polyclonal immunoglobulin (AHPI) column discussed later in this chapter[105]; results with the PAA column are given in Table 20-6. They suggest that IA with the PAA column can improve cardiac function in DCM patients.

ASFA has assigned IA for chronic DCM with a New York Heart Association (NYHA) functional class of II to IV as a Category III indication with a recommendation grade of 2B.[58]

Adverse Effects of Protein A Columns

Huestis and Morrison presented a comprehensive review of the adverse effects of protein A columns.[115] They concluded that most patients undergoing treatment will experience one or more untoward effects, although most procedures will be completed without a reaction.[115] Among 134 patients in Europe and 54 patients in the United States undergoing 891 and 300 PAA treatments, respectively, 26% and 30% of procedures were complicated by a reaction, and 60% and 37% experienced a complication. Pain was the most frequent side effect in Europe (9.5%), while nausea and vomiting (8.5%) and hypotension (8.5%) were most common in the United States.[115]

Table 20-6. Summary of Trials Treating Dilated Cardiomyopathy with the PAA Column

Study Reference	Study Type	Number of Patients	Results	Comment
Staudt et al[105]	CT	PAA: 9 AHPI: 9	Patients treated with the AHPI column demonstrated improved LVEF, but those treated with PAA did not.	Difference in outcomes was felt to represent the differences in the removal of IgG3 between the two methods, because PAA columns are not as effective at IgG3 removal.
Staudt et al[107]	CT	PAA with standard protocol: 9 PAA with enhanced protocol: 9	Patients treated with the PAA protocol with enhanced IgG3 removal demonstrated significant improvements in cardiac index and LVEF throughout the 3-month follow-up.	Controls consisted of the nine patients treated in the protocol above.
Staudt et al[106]	RCT	Single course of PAA: 11 Single course of PAA each month for four months: 11	Patients in both arms demonstrated an equivalent improvement in LVEF and cardiac index at 6 months	Repeated courses of treatment offered no benefit over a single course.
Staudt et al[108]	CT	Single course of PAA each month for 4 months: 15 Control with no treatment: 15	Treated patients demonstrated a significant increase in LVEF with significant decreases in N-terminal brain natriuretic peptide and N-terminal atrial natriuretic peptide compared to baseline and compared to controls at 3 months.	

CT = controlled trial; RCT = randomized controlled trial; PAA = protein A agarose (column); AHPI = antihuman polyclonal immunoglobulin (column); LVEF = left ventricular ejection fraction.

Patients treated with the PAS column while on angiotensin-converting enzyme (ACE) inhibitors have had severe hypotensive reactions related to bradykinin production.[23,115] Because of this, the manufacturer recommends that ACE inhibitors be held before PAA treatment.

A unique problem reported with the PAA column is mercury poisoning. PAA columns were previously stored in thimerosal, a mercury-containing preservative. Mercury poisoning has occurred when the preservative was not properly rinsed from the columns before use. Recently, cases of elevated mercury levels have been reported in patients undergoing treatments with properly prerinsed columns.[116,117] Because of concern about mercury toxicity, the manufacturer has replaced the thimerosal preservative.

In December 2006, PAA column production in the United States was discontinued. PAA column manufacture continues in Europe, where it remains available, although because columns manufactured in Europe are not approved by the FDA, PAA columns are not currently available in the United States.

Antihuman Polyclonal Immunoglobulin Column (Ig-Therasorb)

Another nonspecific IA system is the Ig-Therasorb (Baxter, Munich, Germany). This system is similar to the PAA system in that it consists of a device containing two parallel columns that are alternately perfused with plasma and then regenerated. In this case the antibody-adsorbing material consists of sheep AHPI bound to a matrix.[118] AHPI columns have been used to treat DCM and a number of disorders, some of which are listed in Table 20-7. Most published experience consists of case series and reports.[109-114] The columns were first used to treat DCM in an uncontrolled pilot series reported by Wallukat et al[121]; subsequent reports are summarized in Table 20-8.

Felix et al[124] reported that AHPI purified cardiodepressant antibodies from the plasma of patients with DCM and demonstrated the effects of these antibodies on isolated rat cardiomyocytes. More recently, Staudt et al[111] similarly purified plasma immunoglobulin from 45

Table 20-7. Disorders Treated with Antihuman Polyclonal Immunoglobulin Columns[119,120]

Dilated cardiomyopathy
Coagulation factor inhibitors
Antiphospholipid antibody syndrome
Systemic lupus erythematosus
Myasthenia gravis
Guillian-Barré syndrome
Idiopathic thrombocytopenic purpura
Pemphigus vulgaris

patients with DCM and demonstrated that material from 29 patients depressed rat cardiomyocyte function. All 45 patients were treated with AHPI, but only the 29 whose serum had cardiac depressant antibody activity showed improvement in LVEF after 3 months of treatment.[111] Mobini et al[115] treated 22 DCM patients with AHPI and then eluted antibody from the columns. Eluates were tested with both an enzyme-linked immunosorbent assay (ELISA) and a bioassay for β1-adrenergic receptor antibodies. ELISA was positive in 32% of the eluates, while 73% were bioassay positive. They found no difference in LVEF response to treatment between patients whose eluates contained β1-adrenergic receptor antibodies or suppressed bioassay function and patients whose eluates did not.[114] Thus it remains to be determined which patients respond to IA and which do not.

As stated above, ASFA has assigned IA in the treatment of chronic DCM with a NYHA functional class II to IV as a Category III indication with a recommendation grade of 2B.[58] The AHPI columns are available in Europe but have not been licensed by the FDA and are not available in the United States.

Dextran Sulfate Column (Selesorb)

The Selesorb system (Kaneka Corporation, Osaka, Japan) consists of two Selesorb dextran

Table 20-8. Summary of Trials Treating Dilated Cardiomyopathy with the AHPI Column

Study Reference	Study Type	Number of Patients	Results	Comment
Wallukat et al[121]	CS	8	Demonstrated reduction in β1-adrenergic receptor antibodies and improvement in NYHA functional class.	Patients had severe heart failure refractory to standard therapy. IVIG was administered after each treatment.
Dorffel et al[122]	CS	9	Improved stroke volume and cardiac index.	Demonstrated persistence of effect for a single 5-day course of therapy.
Dorffel et al[123]	CS	9	Three-year follow-up of the nine patients described above found five alive and four dead from their DCM. Those that were alive demonstrated persistence of the improved LVEF seen initially as well as no increase in β1-adrenergic receptor antibodies. The deceased patients had demonstrated increased antibody titers.	
Felix et al[113]	RCT	Treatment: 9 Control: 9	Treated group demonstrated improvement in cardiac index and systemic vascular resistance compared to controls.	Treatment consisted of AHPI on 3 consecutive days followed by two treatments each month for 3 months. IVIG was administered after each treatment.

Muller et al[109]	CT	Treatment: 17 Control: 17	One year after treatment, significantly improved LVEF and end-diastolic pressures were found in treated group.	Controls consisted of untreated historic controls. All patients had high-titer β1-adrenergic receptor antibodies. No IVIG was administered.
Schimke et al[110]	CT	Treatment: 16 Control: 15	Evaluated markers of oxidative stress from 31 of the 34 patients reported by Muller. Significant changes seen, which correlated with favorable changes in LVEF and NYHA functional class.	Controls consisted of untreated historic controls.
Staudt et al[112]	RCT	Treatment: 12 Control: 13	All patients underwent endomyocardial biopsy. Treated group demonstrated improved LVEF and decreased β1-adrenergic receptor antibodies compared to baseline and controls. Treated group also demonstrated fewer CD3+, CD4+, and CD45+ cells as well as decreased HLA Class II expression compared to baseline and controls.	Treatment consisted of AHPI on 3 consecutive days followed by two treatments each month for 3 months. IVIG was administered after each treatment.

CS = case series; CT = controlled trial; RCT = randomized controlled trial; AHPI = antihuman polyclonal immunoglobulin (column); NYHA = New York Heart Association; LVEF = left ventricular ejection fraction.

sulfate (SDS) cellulose columns mounted in the same device that is used to perform LDL apheresis with the LA-15 dextran sulfate columns (also Kaneka). The difference between the two columns is that the dextran sulfate beads in the SDS column have a much smaller pore size that excludes LDL-C but not antibodies. The columns remove DNA antibodies, cardiolipin antibodies, and immune complexes, all of which bind to the negatively charged dextran sulfate. Plasma separated from whole blood with a hollow fiber plasma separator is pumped through the first column. After 500 mL, flow is switched to the second column while the first column is regenerated. The total volume of plasma treated is determined by the antibody titer and the patient's weight. Adverse events consist predominantly of nausea/vomiting (5.6%) and hypotension (1.2%).[125] Because of the negative charge present on the dextran sulfate cellulose beads, patients on ACE inhibitors must discontinue this medication before treatment.[125,126]

The SDS system is used in Japan to treat severe systemic lupus erythematosus (SLE) complicated by rapidly progressive glomerulonephritis or central nervous system disease and to treat SLE resistant to pharmacologic therapies.[125,126] It has also been used to treat antiphospholipid antibody syndrome[126] and cryoglobulinemia.[127] Randomized controlled trials have not been performed for these indications; the evidence supporting this approach consists of case reports and case series.[125-127]

This system is available in Japan and Europe, but the columns have not been approved by the FDA and are not available in the United States. ASFA has not categorized the use of IA in the treatment of SLE, antiphospholipid antibody syndrome, or cryoglobulinemia.[58]

Tryptophan Polyvinyl Alcohol Gel Column (Immusorba TR) and Phenylalanine Polyvinyl Alcohol Gel Column (Immusorba PH)

Immusorba TR and Immusorba PH (Asahi Medical, Tokyo, Japan) are columns containing the amino acids tryptophan (TR) or phenylalanine (PH) immobilized to a porous polyvinyl

alcohol gel. The columns are not regenerated and are used to treat only a single plasma volume before being discarded. They are available in either 250- or 350-mL sizes to allow for the treatment of more or less plasma, depending upon the patient's plasma volume. Immunoglobulins are removed from the plasma by hydrophobic and ionic interactions with the amino acids. The TR column has a greater removal capacity for acetylcholine receptor antibodies compared to other antibodies. Fibrinogen is also significantly reduced in plasma that has been treated with the columns. Hypotensive reactions can occur in patients on ACE inhibitors, and these must be discontinued before treatment.[128]

Rheumatoid arthritis, myasthenia gravis, GBS, chronic inflammatory demyelinating polyradiculopathy (CIDP), multiple sclerosis, pemphigus vulgaris, and acquired hemophilia A have all been treated with these columns.[128-132] Most reports consist of small case series that report reduction in pathologic antibodies and improvement in symptoms among treated patients.

Rosenow et al[130] randomized 30 GBS patients to either TPE, TR, or symptomatic treatment. In these small groups, TPE and TR were equivalent with regard to time to symptom improvement and duration of hospitalization.[130] Okamiya and colleagues,[131] in a retrospective analysis of 34 GBS patients treated with TR (20 patients), TPE (3 patients), and DFPP (11 patients), also found no significant difference in responses among the three groups but noted fewer side effects in the TR-treated group.[131] Similar small studies have demonstrated no differences in response between patients treated with TPE and TR for myasthenia gravis or TPE and PH for multiple sclerosis.[128] Large randomized trials of the efficacy of the TR and PH columns for the treatment of antibody-mediated diseases are not available.

The TR and PH columns are currently available in Japan and Europe, but they have not been approved by the FDA and are not available in the United States. ASFA has not categorized their use in any disease.

Specific Immunoadsorption: Glycosorb

A truly selective removal system is designed to remove antibodies directed toward a specific antigen. A number of such systems have been described, but only Glycosorb (Glycorex Transplantation AB, Lund, Sweden) has had significant published experience.

The Glycosorb columns contain either a synthetic blood group A or B trisaccharide bound to Sepharose.[133] One single-use column removes >90% of the target isohemagglutinin without lowering levels of albumin, IgG, IgA, IgM, or coagulation factors.[133] When both anti-A and anti-B are to be removed, two columns can be placed in series.[29] In-vitro studies indicate that columns are not saturated during a single use and they are not regenerated.[133]

ABO-Incompatible Renal Transplantation

Case series and reports have described patients undergoing successful ABO-incompatible renal transplantation after preconditioning using the Glycosorb columns to remove ABO antibodies.[29,134-137] The largest series by Tyden and colleagues used columns in 60 consecutive ABO-incompatible renal transplants.[134] Patients underwent four pretransplant treatments of 2 plasma volumes with a goal to reduce titers below 8. In cases where this was not achieved, four additional treatments were performed. Patients also received IVIG. Following transplantation, patients received three additional treatments over 9 days at some centers or only if antibody titers rose.[134] Two grafts were lost, one because of patient noncompliance and one because of patient death with a functioning graft. At 61 months after transplant, graft survival was 97% compared to 95% among 274 concurrent patients who had undergone ABO-compatible transplantation, while patient survival was 98% in both groups.[134]

ABO-Incompatible Liver Transplantation

Troisi et al performed ABO-incompatible living-donor liver transplantation in five patients after preparation with the Glycosorb columns.[138] Patients underwent two to three treatments preoperatively to decrease the isohemagglutinin titer to <16. Postoperatively, patients underwent zero to five procedures. Hyperacute rejection did not occur. Two grafts were lost for technical reasons, and in the remaining three patients, antibody-mediated rejection did not occur.[138]

The columns are available and in use in Europe but have not been approved by the FDA and are not available in the United States. ASFA has not categorized their use for ABO-incompatible solid organ transplantation.[58]

LDL Apheresis

LDL Apheresis in Cardiovascular Disease

FH is a dominantly inherited disorder that causes accelerated atherosclerosis and predisposes to premature death from coronary artery disease (CAD). Patients have underlying apolipoprotein B-100 (apoB100) receptor mutations that result in an inability to clear LDL-C. Age at onset of symptoms, life expectancy, and response to medical and dietary management are related to zygosity. Homozygotes develop soft-tissue cholesterol collections (xanthomas) by age 4 and die from CAD by age 20, while heterozygotes will develop xanthomas by age 20 and atherosclerosis by age 30. All homozygotes and some heterozygotes fail to respond to diet and drug therapy.[45]

TPE was shown to slow the progression of aortic and coronary atherosclerosis[139,140] and to increase survival in homozygotes.[141] Unfortunately, it also depletes cardioprotective HDL.[142] The term LDL apheresis (LDL-A) was coined by Stoffel et al[143] to describe selective removal of apoB100-containing lipoproteins from plasma with an immunoadsorption system. The term is now used for all selective techniques that remove the apoB100-containing lipopro-teins LDL and lipoprotein (a) [Lp(a)].

LDL-A prolongs life in FH homozygotes. It is recommended that it be initiated as early as possible but at least by age 6 or 7,[144] because initiation after age 10 may not prevent aortic stenosis caused by atherosclerosis.[145] The more common FH heterozygotes usually respond to LDL-lowering drugs. LDL-A is used infre-quently, being reserved for the minority who are refractory to, or intolerant of, drugs. LDL-A reduces Lp(a) as well as LDL-C. Lp(a) is appar-ently both atherogenic and thrombogenic.[146] Its levels are under independent genetic control and do not respond to drugs, with the possible exception of high-dose niacin.

Thompson et al[145] performed the first con-trolled trial comparing LDL-A and lipid-lower-ing drugs in FH heterozygotes with CAD. Patients were randomly assigned to receive simvastatin plus LDL-A every 2 weeks or simv-astatin plus colestipol. Significantly greater reductions in mean plasma LDL-C and Lp(a) were seen with LDL-A (3.4 vs 3.2 mmol/L and 21 vs 14 mg/dL, respectively, in the LDL-A vs drug group; p = 0.03), but there were no signif-icant differences in the primary angiographic endpoints. Secondary angiographic endpoints studied favored the drug group. The authors concluded that LDL-A offers no advantage over combination drug therapy in the routine management of drug-responsive FH heterozy-gotes.

The second controlled trial involving LDL-A and lipid lowering drugs was performed by Kroon et al.[147] Patients who had failed dietary management of elevated lipids; were on no lipid-lowering agents; had total cholesterol >8 mmol/L or LDL-C >5.8 mmol/L and fast-ing serum triglycerides <5.0 mmol/L; and had extensive CAD were randomly assigned to receive simvastatin alone or simvastatin plus LDL-A every 2 weeks. After 2 years, mean LDL-C in the LDL-A group decreased from 7.8 to 3.0 mmol/L, while that in the drug-only group decreased from 7.9 to 4.1 mmol/L. In the LDL-A group, mean Lp(a) decreased by 19%, while in the simvastatin-only group it increased by 15%. The angiographic endpoints

of the study were changes in mean segment diameter and minimal obstruction diameter. After 2 years of treatment, there was no differ-ence in these parameters between the LDL-A and medication-only groups, with the mean percentage of stenosis showing a tendency to decrease. In the LDL-A group, more minor lesions disappeared compared to the medica-tion group. In addition, the LDL-A group dem-onstrated an increase of 39% in the time to onset of ST segment depression and a signifi-cantly lower maximal level of ST depression during exercise electrocardiogram testing com-pared to the medication group. The authors interpreted the findings to indicate that both treatments arrested atherosclerosis progression and that LDL-A induced functional improve-ment. They hypothesized that the functional change might precede angiographic changes.

Thompson and the HEART-UK LDL Apher-esis Working Group performed a review of the medical literature published before November 2006.[144] They identified eight published coro-nary angiographic trials of LDL-A. These trials consisted of five uncontrolled trials, one con-trolled trial that did not include randomization, and two randomized controlled trials men-tioned above.[144] Meta-analysis was performed on the results of the six trials that lasted for 2 or more years and in which angiographic changes were expressed on a per patient basis. They also included angiographic data from two drug trials that had a diet-only control arm. Their meta-analysis showed that mean reduc-tions in LDL-C were 7.5% with diet alone, 35% with diet plus drug therapy, and 53% when diet and drug therapy were combined with LDL-A. The percentage of patients show-ing atherosclerotic progression was 46% with diet, 33% with drug therapy added, and 18% with drug therapy plus LDL-A (p = 0.1), while the percentages demonstrating regression were 54%, 67%, and 82%, respectively (p = 0.1).[145] Analysis of variance revealed no difference between drug therapy and LDL-A combined with drug therapy but showed that both were superior to diet alone.[144]

Mabuchi et al[148] assessed the efficacy of two aggressive LDL-lowering strategies in 87 FH heterozygotes with CAD receiving LDL-lowering drugs and 43 similar patients receiving LDL-lowering drugs plus LDL-A. Cholesterol, LDL-C, and clinical outcomes were compared after approximately 6 years of therapy. LDL-C reduction was 28% for drugs alone and 58% for drugs plus LDL-A. Moreover, the rate of coronary events was lower in the LDL-A group (10% vs 36%; p = 0.0088). The authors concluded that LDL-A is an effective treatment for CAD in FH heterozygotes.[148]

Matsuzaki et al[149] assessed whether aggressive lipid lowering, employing LDL-A and lipid-lowering drugs, could induce regression of coronary atherosclerotic plaques in FH heterozygotes. They enrolled 19 patients with CAD who had LDL-C levels of 130 to 230 mg/dL and had been on lipid-lowering drugs and diets for >6 months. All were offered LDL-A, and 12 of 19 received it every 2 weeks in addition to drug therapy for 1 year. Cholesterol and LDL-C did not change in the drug-only group but fell 28.4% and 34.3%, respectively, in the LDL-A group.[147] Coronary angiography and intravascular ultrasound were performed at baseline and again at 1 year of follow-up. Minimum lumen diameter and plaque area improved significantly in the LDL-A group but were unchanged (lumen diameter) or worse (plaque area) in the drug-only group.[149]

Reviewing the findings of Matsuzaki et al,[149] Barter[150] questioned whether LDL-A will have an additional effect when combined with the highest doses of the newest lipid-lowering drugs ("superstatins"). He emphasized that a randomized study allocating patients to receive superstatins plus LDL-A vs superstatins only will have to be conducted before any conclusions are drawn about the role of LDL-A in FH heterozygotes treated with modern lipid-lowering drugs.[150] Such a trial has not yet been performed.

LDL-A has also been used in accelerated CAD following cardiac transplantation, a frequent complication that is refractory to conventional treatment.[151] Criteria for the use of LDL-A in cardiovascular disease have been published[144] and are summarized in Table 20-9. The general treatment goal is to reduce the time-averaged LDL-C by 40% to 60%. Figure 20-1 demonstrates the changes seen and the concept of time-averaged cholesterol. Many patients can be managed with a single treatment every 2 weeks because of the relatively slow recovery of LDL-C. For new patients or for those who fail to respond to this regimen, more frequent procedures may be necessary (eg, weekly). In patients with good response, less frequent treatment may be possible. The total volume of plasma treated with each procedure depends on the type of LDL-A instrument used. Treatment is continued indefinitely.

ASFA has assigned treatment of FH homozygotes as a Category I indication for selective LDL removal techniques with a recommendation grade of 1A. The treatment of FH heterozygotes is a Category II indication for selective LDL removal techniques with a recommendation grade of 1A. Finally, homozygous FH with a blood volume too small to tolerate selective removal techniques is a Category II indication for TPE with a recommendation grade of 1C.[50]

Other Applications of LDL Apheresis

LDL-A has been applied to a number of disorders other than FH. Subjects with steroid-resistant nephrotic syndrome caused by focal segmental glomerulosclerosis (FSGS) have been treated with LDL-A in open trials because the hyperlipidemia in these patients is sometimes associated with the progression of FSGS.[152-154]

The Hearing Loss Study Group used the HELP system (Braun-Melsungen, Melsungen, Germany; see section on instrumentation) to accomplish LDL-A to remove fibrinogen and LDL-C in an attempt to alter blood flow in the microcirculation (conceptually similar to the goal of rheopheresis with DFPP described earlier) to treat sudden sensorineural hearing loss (SSHL).[155] They randomly assigned 201 patients with SSHL to receive a single LDL-A or standard treatment (ie, prednisolone plus infusion of 6% hydroxyethyl starch for 10 days). The primary outcome was recovery of hearing, as measured by audiometry, 48 hours after the start of treatment. This randomized

Table 20-9. Patient Criteria for the Use of LDL Apheresis in Hypercholesterolemia[144]

United States Food and Drug Administration	German Federal Committee of Physicians and Health Insurance Funds	International Panel on Management of FH	HEART-UK
• FH homozygotes with an LDL cholesterol >500 mg/dL (>13 mmol/L) • FH heterozygotes with an LDL cholesterol >300 mg/dL (>7.8 mmol/L) who have failed a 6-month trial of drug therapy in combination with an American Heart Association Step II diet • FH heterozygotes with an LDL cholesterol >200 mg/dL (>5.2 mmol/L) and documented coronary artery disease who have failed a 6-month trial of drug therapy in combination with an American Heart Association Step II diet	• FH homozygotes • Patients with severe hypercholesterolemia in whom maximal dietary and drug therapy for >1 year has failed to lower cholesterol sufficiently	• FH homozygotes • FH heterozygotes with symptomatic coronary artery disease in whom LDL cholesterol is >4.2 mmol/L or decreases by <40% with maximal medical management	• FH homozygotes in whom LDL cholesterol is reduced by <50% and/or is >9 mmol/L with drug therapy • FH heterozygotes or "bad family history" patients in whom there is objective evidence of progression of coronary disease and LDL cholesterol remains >5.0 mmol/L or decreases by <40% despite drug therapy • Individuals with progressive coronary artery disease, severe hypercholesterolemia, and Lp(a) >60 mg/dL in whom LDL cholesterol remains elevated despite drug therapy.

LDL = low-density lipoprotein; FH = familial hypercholesterolemia; UK = United Kingdom.

trial established that LDL-A with HELP reduced plasma fibrinogen, total cholesterol, LDL-C, and Lp(a) by >50%. The mean sound level at which 50% of recorded digits were recognized was significantly lower in the LDL-A group at 48 hours after treatment (21.6 ±20.8 dB vs 29.3 ±29.4 dB; p = 0.034). However, at 6 weeks the difference was not statistically significant. In 49 patients with fibrinogen levels >295 mg/dL, a statistically significant difference was seen (15.3 ±17.3 dB vs 6.1 ±10.4 dB

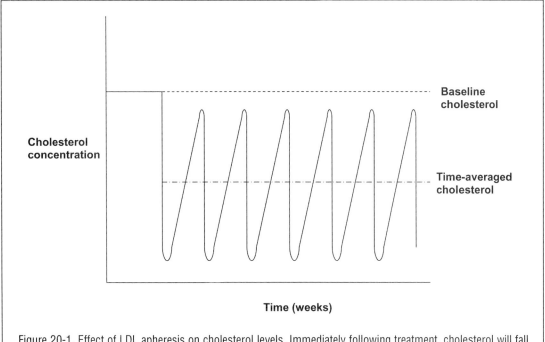

Figure 20-1. Effect of LDL apheresis on cholesterol levels. Immediately following treatment, cholesterol will fall to 25% of baseline. The level will then rise and may reach baseline before the next treatment. Each subsequent procedure will result in a similar reduction so that, over time, the average cholesterol level (time-averaged cholesterol) will be reduced.

at 6 weeks; p = 0.005) compared to 57 patients with lower fibrinogens.[155]

LDL-A has also been evaluated in the treatment of acute stroke, acute myocardial ischemia, and peripheral artery occlusive disease, though randomized controlled trials have not been performed.[156,157] ASFA has not categorized the use of LDL-A in the treatment of FSGS or sudden sensorineural hearing loss.[58]

LDL-A Instrumentation

Six LDL-A systems are in widespread use.[144,158-163] The basic systems are 1) DFPP, 2) dextran sulfate adsorption from plasma [DS-A; Liposorber LA-15 system (Kaneka Pharma America, New York, NY)], 3) HELP, 4) IA, 5) direct removal of lipoproteins from whole blood using polyacrylate-coated polyacrylamide [DALI (Fresenius Kabi AG, Bad Homburg, Germany)], and 6) direct removal from

whole blood using dextran sulfate (Liposorber D, Kaneka). The DS-A and HELP systems have received FDA approval for use in the United States for patients who meet criteria included in Table 20-9. A brief comparison of all of the systems is given in Table 20-10.

Dextran Sulfate (Liposorber LA-15)

The Liposorber LA-15 DS-A system uses dextran sulfate as the ligand and cellulose as the carrier. In this system, plasma is separated by filtration and perfused through the column, where positively charged apoB100 on LDL-C binds electrostatically to negatively charged dextran sulfate moieties. The system has two columns connected in parallel. After one column is perfused with 500 mL, plasma is diverted to the second column while the binding capacity of the first is regenerated by rinsing with 4.1% NaCl, followed by restoration of normal tonicity with lactated Ringer's solution. A salinometer monitors the effluent from the column to prevent the return of the hypertonic saline solution to the patient. The two columns alternate in sequential cycles.[164-168]

Treatment of 3 plasma volumes has been found to reduce LDL-C and Lp(a) levels by 85%.[169] The efficacy of the procedure has been shown in pediatric patients[170-172] and pregnant women.[173,174] There was also a 36% reduction in the concentration of fibrinogen; however, 95% of the baseline HDL level was maintained.[175]

Heparin-Induced Extracorporeal LDL Precipitation System (Plasmat Secura and Plasmat Futura)

The HELP system takes advantage of heparin's ability, at acidic pH (optimal pH = 5.12), to precipitate LDL by forming a complex with apoB100. Plasma separated by a primary filter is mixed with heparin in a sodium acetate buffer of pH 4.84. LDL-C precipitates and is removed by filtration. Lp(a) is also removed. Excess heparin and acetate solution are then removed from the filtered plasma by heparin adsorption and bicarbonate dialysis. Treated plasma is returned to the patient. The system consists of three microprocessor-controlled modules that control the separation, treatment, and dialysis steps. The plasma filter, precipitate filter, heparin adsorber, and dialyzer are discarded after each procedure.[176-182]

Twenty-five weekly treatments with this device were given to 33 high-risk hypercholesterolemic patients (LDL-C 160 mg/dL despite diet and drug therapy). A mean of 2.66 L of plasma was treated per session. LDL-C levels were reduced by ≥30% in 98% of 686 treatments. Mean LDL and HDL cholesterol levels were reduced by 54% and 15%, respectively. Fibrinogen decreased by 58%.[177] In 23 patients, treatment was continued for 6 more

Table 20-10. Comparison of Currently Available LDL Apheresis Systems[156,158,160-163]

System/Commercial Instrument	Method of LDL Removal	Substances Removed*	Advantages	Disadvantages
Dextran Sulfate				
Liposorber LA-15 (Kaneka, Osaka, Japan)	Binding to dextran sulfate on the basis of electrical charge	LDL: 56% to 65% HDL: 9% to 30% Triglycerides: 34% to 40% Lp(a): 52% to 61%	• Column can be regenerated	• System requires plasma separation • High hematocrit may interfere with plasma separation
Heparin-Induced Extracorporeal LDL Precipitation (HELP)				
Plasmat Secura and Plasmat Futura (Braun-Melsungen, Melsungen, Germany)	Precipitation of LDL by heparin at an acidic pH	LDL: 67% HDL: 15% Triglycerides: 41% Lp(a): 62%	• System removes fibrinogen	• High hematocrit may interfere with plasma separation • System is complicated

Table 20-10. Comparison of Currently Available LDL Apheresis Systems[156,158,160-163] (Continued)

System/Commercial Instrument	Method of LDL Removal	Substances Removed*	Advantages	Disadvantages
Double Filtration Plasmapheresis	Separation based on size by filtering plasma with a second filter	LDL: 56% HDL: 25% Triglycerides: 49% Lp(a): 53%	• System removes fibrinogen	• High hematocrit may interfere with plasma separation • System causes loss of some albumin, HDL, and IgG
Immunoadsorption				
Plasmaselect (Plasmaselect, Teterow, Germany)	Immobilized sheep apolipoprotein B-100 antibodies	LDL: 64% HDL: 14% Triglycerides: 42% Lp(a): 64%	• Column can be regenerated	• System causes exposure to animal proteins
Lipoprotein Hemoperfusion				
DALI (Fresenius Kabi AG, Bad Homburg, Germany)	Binding to polyacrylate-coated polyacrylamide beads on the basis of electrical charge	LDL: 61% HDL: 30% Triglycerides: 42% Lp(a): 64%	• Plasma separation is not necessary	• Column cannot be regenerated or reused
Liposorber D (Kaneka)	Binding to dextran sulfate, covalently bonded to cellulose, on the basis of electrical charge	LDL: 62% HDL: 2.5% Triglycerides: 38% to 68% Lp(a): 56% to 72%	• Plasma separation is not necessary • Procedure time is shorter than Liposorber LA-15 • Protocol for reuse of columns has been published	• Column cannot be regenerated

*Percentage removed in a typical treatment.
LDL = low-density lipoprotein; HDL = high-density lipoprotein; Lp(a) = lipoprotein (a); IgG = immunoglobulin G; DALI = direct adsorption of lipoproteins.

months on a biweekly basis.[178] The time-averaged decrease in LDL-C with treatment every 2 weeks was 33% vs 39% with weekly treatment.

Immunoadsorption (Plasmaselect)

The Plasmaselect system (Plasmaselect, Teterow, Germany) also uses two columns in a continuous circuit.[143] Each column contains sheep polyclonal antihuman LDL covalently linked to Sepharose. After the first column becomes saturated, flow switches to the second column while the first is regenerated with a 1-mol/L glycine/HCl buffer (pH = 2.8) followed by a physiologic buffer. Two columns are assigned to each patient and reused in successive treatments. In the report of Stoffel et al,[143] columns had been in use for 9 months at treatment intervals of 1 to 15 weeks without any loss of LDL binding capacity.[143]

Richter et al[183] treated eight patients with FH for 3 years without additional lipid-lowering drug therapy. Mean LDL-C could be maintained at 165 mg/dL between consecutive treatments in patients who were receiving weekly LDL-A. HDL levels increased under regular treatment, and the LDL/HDL ratio decreased from 13.4 to 3.4. The procedure had minimal effects on hemostasis, complement activation, transport proteins, and hematologic parameters.

Polyacrylate-Coated Polyacrylamide Direct Perfusion (DALI)

The four systems described previously can only remove LDL and Lp(a) from plasma and thus require a plasma separation step. Bosch et al[184] first describe the direct adsorption of lipoproteins (DALI) from whole blood with single-use DALI adsorbers (Fresenius Kabi AG) in 1997. In a follow-up report Bosch and colleagues described the efficacy, selectivity, and safety of long-term DALI from whole blood.[185] The DALI adsorbers are made of porous polyacrylamide beads coated by anionic polyacrylate ligands that interact electrostatically with the positively charged apoB100 to retain LDL-C

and Lp(a) in the column. The cellular elements of the blood and molecules larger than lipoproteins cannot diffuse into the interior of the sponge-like structure of the beads. Columns come in 750- and 1000-mL sizes, with the patient's blood volume determining which is used.

Bosch et al[185] enrolled 63 hypercholesterolemic patients with CAD and a starting LDL-C of 238 ±87 mg/dL in an open trial. All patients were receiving maximum tolerated doses of lipid-lowering drugs, and 40 had previously received LDL-A with other systems. DALI was performed every 8.6 ±5.0 days, with 1.5 whole blood volumes processed per treatment. The mean number of treatments was 37. At the end of the study, the mean reduction of LDL-C was 42%, and there was a 4% increase in HDL cholesterol. The column demonstrated good selectivity for LDL-C, with recoveries of albumin, immunoglobulin, and other proteins exceeding 85%.

Ninety-five percent of 2156 treatment sessions were uneventful.[185] The remainder were complicated by hypotension (1.5%), paresthesias (1.1%), venous access problems (1.5%), and technical difficulties (0.5%). The authors concluded that DALI is an effective and safe procedure for removal of LDL-C and Lp(a). Compared with other LDL-A systems, the main advantage of DALI is that an initial plasma separation step is not required.

Dextran Sulfate Direct Perfusion (Liposorber D)

The second whole blood perfusion system for the treatment of hypercholesterolemia was the Liposorber D.[160] This system consists of a single-use column containing dextran sulfate bound to cellulose. These columns, too, come in different sizes. Otto et al[160] described a multicenter open trial that used the Liposorber D in 10 patients with hypercholesterolemia. A total of 93 treatments were performed with mean per treatment reductions of 62 ±11.5% for LDL-C and 55.6 ±16.9% for Lp(a). HDL did not change significantly. Side effects noted included three episodes of mild hypocalcemia and two episodes of mild hypotension. A Japanese multicenter trial involving 33 patients found mean per-treatment reductions of 61.5 ±6.2% for LDL-C and 72.4 ±5.9% for Lp(a).[165]

System Selection

Comparisons of four LDL-A systems have shown similar reductions in LDL-C with all systems.[159,160,186,187] Only the DS-A and HELP systems, however, are approved for use in the United States. Both of these systems require heparinization; in the HELP system it is intrinsic to the LDL-C removal, whereas in the DS-A system the use of citrate anticoagulation would interfere with the charge of the columns, preventing the removal of the LDL-C. Patients who cannot be heparinized safely, as well as patients with hypersensitivity to heparin or ethylene oxide (present in the DS-A columns), cannot undergo LDL-A with these systems. Citrate anticoagulant can be used with some of the other systems not available in the United States (eg, Liposorber D).

In 1994, Matsuda et al[188] compared the specificity, complexity, safety, and cost of the then-available methods for lowering the concentration of LDL (Table 20-11). IA is the most specific, TPE is the least complex, and DFPP is the safest and least expensive. On the basis of their scoring scheme, the performance of different methods was ranked as follows: DFPP, DS-A, TPE, IA, and HELP.[188]

In published studies, all methods appear to be relatively safe. IA received the lowest safety score because sterilization of columns is problematic and the sorbent may leach into treated patient plasma, potentially causing febrile or anaphylactic reactions.[188] The risk from TPE relates to use of replacement solutions other than albumin. DS-A has a somewhat higher risk than secondary filtration because hypotensive events attributed to bradykinin release have been reported.[188] Dextran has also been reported to sensitize some recipients after intravenous injection.[189]

Complexity was included in the scoring system because more complex circuits require more time for preparation.[188] In this regard, the relative simplicity of DALI or Liposorber D (systems not available at the time of the ranking) has already been discussed. Rankings in terms of cost relate to the special reimbursement considerations unique to Japanese apheresis centers that make setup time the most important cost element. In the United States, however, inexpensive disposables are also important.

DS-A and IA procedures do not affect HDL and thus would be expected to be the most

Table 20-11. Comparative Performance of Systems for Lowering the Concentration of LDL in the Circulation*

	Specificity	Complexity	Safety	Cost
Therapeutic plasma exchange	5	1	3	3
Double filtration plasmapheresis	4	2	1	1
HELP	3	5	4	5
Dextran sulfate adsorption	2	3	2	2
Immunoadsorption	1	4	5	4

*Scoring guide: for specificity, 1 = most specific and 5 = least specific; for complexity, 1 = least complex and 5 = most complex; for safety, 1 = safest and 5 = least safe; and for cost, 1 = least expensive and 5 = most expensive. (Modified from Matsuda et al.[188])
LDL = low-density lipoprotein; HELP = heparin-induced extracorporeal LDL precipitation.

effective systems in controlling atherosclerotic disease. IA is more specific than DS-A, which may still lower fibrinogen by one-third of its starting level.[175,190] Despite the ranking of Matsuda et al,[188] DS-A might be preferred in the United States because of its high specificity and safety.

Empen et al[191] demonstrated that HELP, DS-A and IA lower the concentrations of adhesion molecules (E-selectin and vascular cellular adhesion molecule-1). Elevated plasma levels of adhesion molecules are associated with atherosclerotic diseases and major cardiovascular risk factors. However, the levels return to pretreatment values within 2 to 4 days after LDL-A, and the clinical significance of this finding requires further study.

Otto et al[192] directly compared both the DALI and the Liposorber D columns in a group of 6 patients. Patients were randomly assigned to 6 weekly treatments with one column and then switched to the other column for an additional 6 weeks. LDL-C reductions were similar between the two columns (DALI, 68.3% vs Liposorber D, 68.4%). The Liposorber D showed better elimination of C-reactive protein and fibrinogen but also higher interleukin-6 levels, with the latter possibly indicating increased inflammatory activation.[192]

Adverse Effects of LDL Apheresis

Bambauer et al[156] reviewed 4330 LDL-A procedures, which included all the techniques listed in Table 20-11 except the Liposorber D column. They found a reaction rate of 10.9%.[156] The majority of reactions were mild, with no differences between the types and frequencies of reactions among the different systems examined. The most common reactions were posttreatment bleeding (3.5%), vomiting (2.5%), hypoglycemia (2.4%), hypotension (2.2%), allergic reactions (0.2%), and shock (0.1%).[156] Studies of the dextran sulfate cellulose hemoperfusion system revealed similar reaction types and frequencies.[160,163]

The use of ACE inhibitors by patients being treated with dextran sulfate columns is problematic. Concurrent treatment with ACE inhibitors is associated with reactions consisting of flushing, hypotension, bradycardia, and dyspnea. These reactions result from activation of the kinin system, which generates bradykinin. ACE inhibitors also inhibit the enzymes necessary for bradykinin catabolism, allowing high levels of bradykinin to accumulate and cause the symptoms described.[23] Such reactions can be avoided by ensuring that the patient is taking a short-acting ACE inhibitor and withholding the medication before LDL-A. Alternatively, the patient can be switched to another medication, such as an angiotensin II receptor antagonist. If other ACE inhibitors are used, the specified interval after the last dose should be based on the half-life of the agent. In the study by Bambauer et al,[156] patients taking ACE inhibitors were not treated with LDL-A. Similarly, ACE inhibitors were not used in patients undergoing treatment with the dextran sulfate cellulose hemoperfusion system.[160,163]

Conclusion

In summary, a number of selective removal systems are available worldwide and are used to treat a variety of diseases. These systems offer certain advantages over TPE but have disadvantages of their own. The authors of the previous edition of this chapter stated that TPE was a waning technology that would be replaced by selective removal systems, but they also affirmed the need for randomized controlled trials of the use of these devices to prove efficacy. In the ensuing years there has been further development and implementation of selective removal systems elsewhere in the world, but few additional controlled data supporting efficacy have been forthcoming. In the United States, two of the four systems previously available have been withdrawn from the market. In conclusion, selective removal systems hold promise, but further trials are needed. It is the hope of this author that by the time this chapter is next revised, strong evidence from randomized controlled trials will be available to support the use of more devices in the United States.

References

1. Szczepiorkowski ZM, Shaz BH, Bandarenko N, Winters JL. The new approach to assignment of ASFA categories—introduction to the fourth special issue: Clinical applications of therapeutic apheresis. J Clin Apher 2007;22:96-105.
2. Lysaght MJ, Samtleben WS, Schmidt B, Gurland HJ. Closed-loop plasmapheresis. In: MacPherson JL, Kaspirin DO, eds. Therapeutic hemapheresis. Vol 1. Boca Raton, FL: CRC Press, 1985:149-68.
3. Anderson DH, Blumenstein M, Habersetzer R, et al. Mass transfer in membrane plasma exchange. Artif Organs 1982;6:43-9.
4. Flaum MA, Cuneo RA, Appelbaum FR, et al. The hemostatic imbalance of plasma-exchange transfusion. Blood 1979;54:694-702.
5. Orlin JB, Berkman EM. Partial plasma exchange using albumin replacement: Removal and recovery of normal plasma constituents. Blood 1980;56:1055-9.
6. Chirnside A, Urbaniak SJ, Prowse CV, Keller AJ. Coagulation abnormalities following intensive plasma exchange on the cell separator. II. Effects on factors I, II, V, VII, VIII, IX, X and antithrombin III. Br J Haematol 1981;48:627-34.
7. Volkin RL, Starz TW, Winkelstein A, et al. Changes in coagulation factors, complement, immunoglobulins, and immune complex concentrations with plasma exchange. Transfusion 1982;22:54-8.
8. Wing EJ, Bruns FJ, Fraley DS, et al. Infectious complications with plasmapheresis in rapidly progressive glomerulonephritis. JAMA 1980;244:2423-6.
9. Wood GJ, Hall GM. Plasmapheresis and plasma cholinesterase. Br J Anaesth 1978;50:945.
10. Naik B, Hirshhorn S, Dharnidharka VR. Prolonged neuromuscular block due to cholinesterase depletion by plasmapheresis. J Clin Anesth 2002;14:381.
11. Kale-Pradhan PB, Woo MH. A review of the effects of plasmapheresis on drug clearance. Pharmacotherapy 1997;17:684-95.
12. Kintzel TPE, Eastlund T, Calis KA. Extracorporeal removal of antimicrobials during plasmapheresis. J Clin Apher 2003;18:194-205.
13. Ibrahim RB, Liu C, Cronin SM, et al. Drug removal by plasmapheresis: An evidence-based review. Pharmacotherapy 2007;27:1529-49.
14. Boucher CA, de Gans J, van Oers R, et al. Transmission of HIV and AIDS by plasmapheresis for Guillain-Barré syndrome. Clin Neurol Neurosurg 1988;90:235-6.
15. Shemin D, Briggs D, Greenan M. Complications of therapeutic plasma exchange: A prospective study of 1,727 procedures. J Clin Apher 2007;22:270-6.
16. Nguyen L, Terrell DR, Duvall D, et al. Complications of plasma exchange in patients treated for thrombotic thrombocytopenic purpura. IV. An additional study of 43 consecutive patients, 2005 to 2008. Transfusion 2009;49:392-4.
17. Askari S, Nollet K, Debol SM, et al. Transfusion-related acute lung injury during plasma exchange: Suspecting the unexpected. J Clin Apher 2002;17:93-6.
18. Mateen FJ, Gastineau D. Transfusion related acute lung injury (TRALI) after plasma exchange in myasthenic crisis. Neurocrit Care 2008;8:280-2.
19. P'ng SS, Hughes AS, Cooney JP. A case report of transfusion-related acute lung injury during plasma exchange for thrombotic thrombocytopenic purpura. Ther Apher Dial 2008;12:78-81.
20. Koch-Weser J, Sellers EM. Binding of drugs to serum albumin (first of two parts). N Engl J Med 1976;294:311-6.
21. Weinstein R. Prevention of citrate reactions during therapeutic plasma exchange by constant infusion of calcium gluconate with the return fluid. J Clin Apher 1996;11:204-10.
22. Alving BM, Hojima Y, Pisano JJ, et al. Hypotension associated with prekallikrein activator (Hageman-factor fragments) in plasma protein fraction. N Engl J Med 1978;299:66-70.
23. Owen HG, Brecher ME. Atypical reactions associated with use of angiotensin-converting enzyme inhibitors and apheresis. Transfusion 1994;34:891-4.
24. Pool M, McLeod BC. Pyrogen reactions to human serum albumin during plasma exchange. J Clin Apher 1995;10:81-4.
25. Stafford CT, Lobel SA, Fruge BC, et al. Anaphylaxis to human serum albumin. Ann Allergy 1988;61:85-8.
26. Ring J, Messmer K. Incidence and severity of anaphylactoid reactions to colloid volume substitutes. Lancet 1971;1:466-9.
27. Sirtl C, Laubenthal H, Zumtobel V, et al. Tissue deposits of hydroxyethyl starch (HES): Dose-dependent and time-related. Br J Anaesth 1999;82:510-15.
28. Wallukat G, Muller J, Hetzer R. Specific removal of 1-adrenergic autoantibodies from

patients with idiopathic dilated cardiomyopathy. N Engl J Med 2002;347:1806.

29. Kumlien G, Ullstrom L, Losvall A, et al. Clinical experience with a new apheresis filter that specifically depletes ABO blood group antibodies. Transfusion 2006;46:1568-75.

30. Matic G, Bosch T, Ramlow W. Background and indications for protein A-based extracorporeal immunoadsorption. Ther Apher 2001;5:394-403.

31. Hirata N, Kuriyama T, Yamawaki N. Immunosorba TR and PH. Ther Apher Dial 2003;7:85-90.

32. Jansen M, Schmaldienst S, Banyai S, et al. Treatment of coagulation inhibitors with extracorporeal immunoadsorption (Ig-Therasorb). Br J Haematol 2001;112:91-7.

33. Bambauer R, Schiel R, Latza R. Low-density lipoprotein apheresis: An overview. Ther Apher Dial 2003;7:382-90.

34. Siami GA, Siami FS. Membrane plasmapheresis in the United States: A review over the last 20 years. Ther Apher 2001;5:315-20.

35. Mineshima M, Yokoi R, Horibe K, et al. Effects of operating conditions on selectivity of plasma fractionator in double filtration plasmapheresis. Ther Apher 2001;5:444-8.

36. Yeh JH, Chen WH, Chiu HC, Bai CH. Clearance studies during subsequent sessions of double filtration plasmapheresis. Artif Organs 2006;30:111-14.

37. Nakaji S, Yamamoto T. Membranes for therapeutic apheresis. Ther Apher 2002;6:267-70.

38. Yeh JH, Chen WH, Chiu HC, Bai CH. MuSK antibody clearance during serial sessions of plasmapheresis for myasthenia gravis. J Neuro Sci 2007;263:191-3.

39. Yeh JH, Chiu HC. Comparison between double-filtration plasmapheresis and immunoadsorption plasmapheresis in the treatment of patients with myasthenia gravis. J Neurol 2000;247:510-13.

40. Lyu RK, Chen WH, Hsieh ST. Plasma exchange versus double filtration plasmapheresis in the treatment of Guillian-Barré syndrome. Ther Apher 2002;6:163-6.

41. Yu X, Ma J, Tian J, et al. A controlled study of double filtration plasmapheresis in the treatment of active rheumatoid arthritis. J Clin Rheumatol 2007;13:193-8.

42. Otsubo S, Tanabe K, Shinmura H, et al. Effect of post-transplant double filtration plasmapheresis on recurrent focal and segmental glomerulosclerosis in renal transplant patients. Ther Apher and Dial 2004;8:299-304.

43. Hanafusa N, Noiri E, Yamashita T, et al. Successful treatment by double filtration plasmapheresis in a pregnant woman with the rare p blood group and a history of multiple early miscarriages. Ther Apher Dial 2006;10:498-503.

44. Tanabe K. Double-filtration plasmapheresis. Transplant 2007;84:S30S32.

45. Goldstein JL, Hobbs HH, Brown MS. Familial hypercholesterolemia. In: Beuadet AL, Sly WS, Valle D, eds. The metabolic and molecular basis of inherited disease. New York: McGraw-Hill, 1995:1981-2030.

46. Klingel R, Mausfeld P, Fassbender C, Goehlen B. Lipidfiltration—safe and effective methodology to perform lipid-apheresis. Transfus Apher Sci 2004;30:245-54.

47. Klingel R, Fassbender C, Fassbender T, et al. Rheopheresis: Rheologic, functional, and structural aspects. Ther Apher 2000;4:348-57.

48. Luke C, Widder RA, Soudavar F, et al. Improvement of macular function by membrane differential filtration in diabetic retinopathy. J Clin Apher 2001;16:23-8.

49. Kawai T, Agishi T, Yamashita G, et al. The effect of double filtration plasmapheresis on foot ulcers. In: Oda T, ed. Therapeutic plasmapheresis. New York: Schattauer Publishing, 1982:565-7.

50. Tauchert M, Sonntag A, Weidmann B, et al. Extracorporeal hemorheotherapy of refractory angina pectoris. Jpn J Apher 1997;16:35-7.

51. Berrouschot J, Barthel H, Scheel C, et al. Extracorporeal membrane differential filtration—a new and safe method to optimize hemorheology in acute ischemic stroke. Acta Neurol Scand 1998;97:126-30.

52. Brunner R, Widder RA, Walter P, et al. Influence of membrane differential filtration on the natural course of age-related macular degeneration: A randomized trial. Retina 2000;20:483-91.

53. Pulido JS, Winters JL, Boyer D. Preliminary analysis of the final multicenter investigation of Rheopheresis for age-related macular degeneration (AMD) trial (MIRA-1) results. Trans Am Ophthalmol Soc 2006;104:221-31.

54. Koss MJ, Kurz P, Tsobanelis T, et al. Prospective, randomized, controlled clinical study evaluating the efficacy of Rheopheresis for dry age-related macular degeneration. Graefes Arch Clin Exp Ophthalmol 2009;247:1297-306.

55. Pulido J, Sanders D, Winters JL, Klingel R. Clinical outcomes and mechanism of action for

Rheopheresis treatment of age-related macular degeneration (AMD*)*. J Clin Apher 2005;20: 185-94.

56. Lotery A, Trump D. Progress in defining the molecular biology of age related macular degeneration. Hum Genet 2007;122:219-36.

57. Szczepiorkowski ZM, Bandarenko N, Kim HC, et al. Guidelines on the use of therapeutic apheresis in clinical practice—evidence-based approach from the Clinical Applications Committee of the American Society for Apheresis. J Clin Apher 2007;22:106-75.

58. Szczepiorkowski ZM, Winters JL, Bandarenko N, et al. Guidelines on the use of therapeutic apheresis in clinical practice—evidence-based approach from the Apheresis Applications Committee of the American Society for Apheresis. The Fifth Special Issue. J Clin Apher 2010 (in press).

59. Yeh JH, Chen WH, Chiu HC. Complications of double-filtration plasmapheresis. Transfusion 2004;44:1621-5.

60. Hjelm H, Sjödahl J, Sjöquist J. Immunologically active and structurally similar fragments of protein A from *Staphylococcus aureus*. Eur J Biochem 1975;57;395-403.

61. Field PR, Shanker S, Murphy AMJ. The use of protein A-Sepharose affinity chromatography for separation and detection of specific IgM antibody in acquired rubella infection: A comparison with absorption by staphylococci containing protein A and density gradient ultracentrifugation. J Immunol Methods 1980; 32:59-70.

62. Kronvall G, Williams RC. Differences in anti-protein A activity among IgG subgroups. J Immunol 1969;103:828-33.

63. Skvaril F. The question of specificity in binding human IgG subclasses to protein A-Sepharose. Immunochemistry 1976;13:871-2.

64. Harboe M, Folling I. Recognition of two distinct groups of human IgM and IgA based on different binding to staphylococci. Scand J Immunol 1974;3:471-82.

65. Grov A. Human IgM interacting with staphylococcal protein A. Acta Pathol Microbiol Scand 1975;83:173-6.

66. Levy J, Degani N. Correcting immune imbalance: The use of Prosorba column treatment for immune disorders. Ther Apher Dial 2003; 7:197-205.

67. Silverman GJ, Goodyear CS, Siegel DL. On the mechanism of staphylococcal protein A immunomodulation. Transfusion 2005;45:274-80.

68. Felson DT, LaValley MP, Baldassare AR, et al. The Prosorba column for treatment of refractory rheumatoid arthritis: A randomized, double-blind, sham-controlled trial. Arth Rheum 1999;42:2153-9.

69. Snyder HW, Cochran SK, Balint JP, et al. Experience with protein A-immunoadsorption in treatment-resistant adult immune thrombocytopenic purpura. Blood 1992;79:2237-45.

70. Gjörstrup P, Watt RM. Therapeutic protein A immunoadsorption: A review. Transfus Sci 1990;11:281-302.

71. Belak M, Borberg H, Jimenez C, Oette K. Technical and clinical experience with protein A immunoadsorption columns. Transfus Sci 1994;15:419-22.

72. Samuelsson G. Extracorporeal immunoadsorption with Immunosorba protein A. In: Agishi T, Kawamura A, Mineshima M, eds. Therapeutic plasmapheresis: Proceedings of the 4th International Congress of the World Apheresis Association, Sapporo, Japan, 1992. Philadelphia: Coronet Books, 1993:843-5.

73. Kupin W, Venkat KK, Hayaski H, et al. Removal of lymphocytotoxic antibodies by pretreatment immunoadsorption therapy in highly sensitized renal transplant recipients. Transplantation 1991;51:324-9.

74. Palmer A, Welsh K, Gjörstrup P, et al. Removal of anti-HLA antibodies by extracorporeal immunoadsorption to enable renal transplantation. Lancet 1989;1:10-12.

75. Gil-Vernet S, Grino JM, Martorell J, et al. Anti-HLA antibody removal by immunoadsorption (IA). Transplant Proc 1990;22:1904-5.

76. Hakim RM, Milford E, Himmelfarb J, et al. Extracorporeal removal of anti-HLA antibodies in transplant candidates. Am J Kidney Dis 1990;16:423-31.

77. Esnault W, Bignon JD, Testa A, et al. Effect of protein A immunoadsorption on panel lymphocyte reactivity in hyperimmunized patients awaiting kidney graft. Transplantation 1990; 50:449-53.

78. Palmer A, Taube D, Welsh K, et al. Extracorporeal immunoadsorption of anti-HLA antibodies: Preliminary clinical experience. Transplant Proc 1987;19:3750-1.

79. Brocard JF, Farahmand H, Fassi S, et al. Attempt at depletion of anti-HLA antibodies in sensitized patients awaiting transplantation using extracorporeal immunoadsorption, polyclonal IgG, and immunosuppressive drugs. Transplant Proc 1989;21:733-4.

80. Fauchald P, Leivestad T, Albrechtsen D, et al. Plasma exchange and immunoadsorption prior to renal transplantation in allosensitized patients. Transplant Proc 1990;22:149-50.

81. Gjörstrup P. Anti-HLA antibody removal in hyperimmunized ESRF-patients to allow transplantation. Transplant Proc 1991;23:392-5.

82. Fehrman I, Baramy P, Bergstrom J, et al. Measures to decrease HLA antibodies in immunized patients awaiting kidney transplantation. Transplant Proc 1990;22:147-8.

83. Hiesse C, Kriaa F, Rousseau P, et al. Immunoadsorption of anti-HLA antibodies for highly sensitized patients awaiting renal transplantation. Nephrol Dial Transplant 1992;7:944-51.

84. Ross CN, Gaskin G, Gregor-MacGregor S, et al. Renal transplantation following immunoadsorption in highly sensitized patients. Transplantation 1993;55:785-9.

85. Min L, Shuming J, Zheng T, et al. Novel rescue therapy for C4d-positive acute humoral renal allograft rejection. Clin Transplant 2005:19; 51-5.

86. Böhmig GA, Wahrmann M, Regele H, et al. Immunoadsorption in severe C4d-positive acute kidney allograft rejection: A randomized controlled trial. Am J Transplant 2007;7:117-21.

87. Nilsson IM, Berntorp E, Freiburghaus C. Treatment of patients with Factor VIII and IX inhibitors. Thromb Haemost 1993;70:56-9.

88. Ingerslev J. Efficacy and safety of recombinant factor VIIa in the prophylaxis of bleeding in various surgical procedures in hemophiliac patients with factor VIII and factor IX inhibitors. Semin Thromb Hemost 2000;26:425-32.

89. Nilsson IM. The management of hemophilia patients with inhibitors. Transfus Med Rev 1992;6:285-93.

90. Nilsson IM, Berntorp E, Zettervall O. Induction of immune tolerance in patients with hemophilia and antibodies to Factor VIII by combined treatment with intravenous IgG, cyclophosphamide, and Factor VIII. N Engl J Med 1988;318:947-50.

91. Nilsson IM, Berntorp E, Rickard KA. Results in three Australian hemophilia B patients with high-responding inhibitors treated with the Malmö model. Hemophilia 1995;1:59-66.

92. Negrier C, Dechavanne M, Alfonsi F, Tremisi PJ. Successful treatment of acquired Factor VIII antibody by extracorporeal immunoadsorption. Acta Haematol 1991;85:107-10.

93. Gjörstrup P, Berntorp E, Larsson L, Nilsson IM. Kinetic aspects of the removal of IgG and inhibitors in hemophiliacs using protein A immunoadsorption. Vox Sang 1991;61:244-50.

94. Uehlinger J, Rose E, Aledort LM, Lerner R. Successful treatment of an acquired von Willebrand factor antibody by extracorporeal immunoadsorption. N Engl J Med 1989;320:254-5.

95. Edson JR, McArthur JR, Branda RF, et al. Successful management of a subdural hematoma in a hemophiliac with anti-Factor VIII antibody. Blood 1973;41:113-22.

96. Cobcroft R, Tamagnini G, Formandy KM. Serial plasmapheresis in a hemophiliac with antibodies to Factor VIII. J Clin Pathol 1977;30:763-5.

97. Francesconi M, Korninger C, Thaler E, et al. Plasmapheresis: Its value in the management of patients with antibodies to Factor VIII. Hemostasis 1982;11:79-86.

98. Apter B, McCarthy V, Shapiro SS, Ballas SK. Successful preoperative apheresis of Factor VIII antibody using Factor VIII concentrate as a replacement fluid. J Clin Apher 1986;3:140.

99. Kasper CK. Treatment of Factor VIII inhibitors. Prog Hemost Thromb 1989;9:57-86.

100. Lusher JM. Factor VIII inhibitors. Etiology, characterization, natural history and management. Ann N Y Acad Sci 1987;509:89-102.

101. Freedman J, Rand ML, Russell O, et al. Immunoadsorption may provide a cost-effective approach to management of patients with inhibitors to FVIII. Transfusion 2003;43:1508-13.

102. Cooper LT. The natural history and role of immunoadsorption in dilated cardiomyopathy. J Clin Apher 2005;20:256-60.

103. Mobini R, Maschke H, Waagstein F. New insights into the pathogenesis of dilated cardiomyopathy: Possible underlying autoimmune mechanisms and therapy. Autoimmun Rev 2004;3:277-84.

104. Schimke I, Muller J, Dandel M, et al. Reduced oxidative stress in parallel to improved cardiac performance one year after selective removal of anti-beta 1-adrenoreceptor autoantibodies in patients with idiopathic dilated cardiomyopathy: Data of a preliminary study. J Clin Apher 2005;20:137-42.

105. Staudt A, Bohm M, Knebel F, et al. Potential role of autoantibodies belonging to the immunoglobulin G-3 subclass in cardiac dysfunction among patients with dilated cardiomyopathy. Circulation 2002;106:2448-53.

106. Staudt A, Hummel A, Ruppert J, et al. Immunoadsorption in dilated cardiomyopathy: 6-month results from a randomized study. Am Heart J 2006;152:712.e1-e6.

107. Staudt A, Dorr M, Staudt Y, et al. Role of immunoglobulin G3 subclass in dilated cardiomyopathy: Results from protein A immunoadsorption. Am Heart J 2005;150:729-36.

108. Staudt A, Staudt Y, Hummel A, et al. Effects on the nt-BNP and nt-ANP plasma levels of patients suffering from dilated cardiomyopathy. Thera Apher Dial 2006;10:42-8.

109. Muller J, Wallukat G, Dandel M, et al. Immunoglobulin adsorption in patients with idiopathic dilated cardiomyopathy. Circulation 2000;101:385-91.

110. Schimke I, Muller J, Priem F, et al. Decreased oxidative stress in patients with idiopathic dilated cardiomyopathy one year after immunoglobulin adsorption. J Am Coll Cardiol 2001;38:178-83.

111. Staudt A, Staudt Y, Dorr M, et al. Potential role of humoral immunity in cardiac dysfunction of patients suffering from dilated cardiomyopathy. J Am Coll Cardiol 2004;44:829-36.

112. Staudt A, Schaper F, Stangl V, et al. Immunohistochemical changes in dilated cardiomyopathy induced by immunoadsorption therapy and subsequent immunoglobulin substitution. Circulation 2001;103:2681-6.

113. Felix SB, Staudt A, Dorffel WV, et al. Hemodynamic effects of immunoadsorption and subsequent immunoglobulin substitution in dilated cardiomyopathy: Three-month results from a randomized study. J Am Coll Cardiol 2000;35:1590-8.

114. Mobini R, Staudt A, Felix SB, et al. Hemodynamic improvement and removal of autoantibodies against β_1-adrenergic receptor by immunoadsorption therapy in dilated cardiomyopathy. J Autoimmun 2003;20:345-50.

115. Huestis DW, Morrison F. Adverse effects of immune adsorption with staphylococcal protein A columns. Transfus Med Rev 1996;10:62-70.

116. Kramer L, Bauer E, Jansen M, et al. Mercury exposure in protein A immunoadsorption. Nephrol Dial Transplant 2004;19:451-6.

117. Marn-Pernat A, Buturovic-Ponikar J, Logar M, et al. Increased mercury load in protein A immunoadsorption. Ther Apher Dial 2005;9:254-7.

118. Reinke P, Brehme S, Baumann G, et al. Treatment of cardiomyopathy by removal of autoantibodies. International application published under the Patent Cooperation Treaty (PCT). International publication no. WO 97/1798. International application no. PCT/US96/18457.

119. Jansen M, Schmaldienst S, Banyal S, et al. Treatment of coagulation inhibitors with extracorporeal immunoadsorption (Ig-Therasorb). Br J Haematol 2001;112:91-7.

120. Hauser AC, Hauser L, Pabinger-Fasching I, et al. The course of anticardiolipin antibody levels under immunoadsorption therapy. Am J Kid Dis 2005;46:446-54.

121. Wallukat G, Reinke P, Dorffel WV, et al. Removal of autoantibodies in dilated cardiomyopathy by immunoadsorption. Int J Cardiol 1996;54:191-5.

122. Dorffel WV, Wallukat G, Baumann G, Felix SB. Immunoadsorption in dilated cardiomyopathy. Ther Apher 2000;4:235-8.

123. Dorffel WV, Wallukat G, Dorffel Y, et al. Immunoadsorption in idiopathic dilated cardiomyopathy, a 3-year follow-up. Int J Cardiol 2004;97:529-34.

124. Felix SB, Staudt A, Lansberger M, et al. Removal of cardiodepressant antibodies in dilated cardiomyopathy by immunoadsorption. J Am Coll Cardiol 2002;39:646-52.

125. Kutsuki H, Takata S, Yamamoto K, Tani N. Therapuetic selective adsorption of anti-DNA antibody using dextran sulfate cellulose column (Selesorb) for the treatment of systemic lupus erythematosus. Ther Apher 1998;2:18-24.

126. Braun N, Junger M, Klein R, et al. Dextran sulfate (Selesorb) plasma apheresis improves vascular changes in systemic lupus erythematosus. Ther Apher 2002;6:471-7.

127. Stefanutti C, Di Giacomo S, Mareri M, et al. Immunoadsorption apheresis (Selesorb) in the treatment of chronic hepatitis C virus-related type 2 mixed cryoglobulinemia. Transfus Apher Sci 2003;28:207-14.

128. Hirata N, Kuriyama T, Yamawaki N. Immusorba TR and PH. Ther Apher Dial 2003;7:85-90.

129. Luftl M, Stauber A, Mainka A, et al. Successful removal of pathogenic autoantibodies in pemphigus by immunoadsorption with a tryptophan-linked polyvinylalcohol adsorber. Br J Dermatol 2003;149:598-605.

130. Rosenow F, Haupt WF, Grieb P, et al. Plasma exchange and selective adsorption in Guillian-Barré syndrome: A comparison of therapies by

clinical course and side effects. Transfus Sci 1993;14:13-15.

131. Okamiya S, Ogino M, Ogino Y, et al. Tryptophan-immobilized column-based immunoadsorption as the choice method for plasmapheresis in Guillian-Barré syndrome. Ther Apher Dial 2004;8:248-53.

132. Brzoska M, Krause M, Geuiger H, Betz C. Immunoadsorption with single-use columns for the management of bleeding in acquired hemophilia A: A series of nine cases. J Clin Apher 2007;22:233-40.

133. Rydberg L, Bengtsson A, Samuelson O, et al. In vitro assessment of a new ABO immunosorbent with synthetic carbohydrates attached to sepharose. Transpl Int 2005;17:666-72.

134. Tyden G, Donauer J, Wadstrom J, et al. Implementation of a protocol for ABO-incompatible kidney transplantation—a three-center experience with 60 consecutive transplantations. Transplantation 2007;83:1153-5.

135. Genberg H, Kumlien G, Wennberg L, Tyden G. Long-term results of ABO-incompatible kidney transplantation with antigen specific immunoadsorption and Rituximab. Transplantation 2007;84:S44-7.

136. Tyden G, Kumlien G, Fehrman I. Successful ABO-incompatible kidney transplantations without splenectomy using antigen-specific immunoadsorption and Rituximab. Transplantation 2003;76:730-43.

137. Tyden G, Kumlien G, Genberg H, et al. ABO incompatible kidney transplantations without splenectomy, using antigen-specific immunoadsorption and Rituximab. Am J Transplant 2005;5:145-8.

138. Troisi R, Noens L, Montalti R, et al. ABO-mismatch adult living donor liver transplantation using antigen-specific immunoadsorption and quadruple immunosuppression without splenectomy. Liver Transpl 2006;12:1412-17.

139. Thompson GR, Myant NB, Kilpatrick D, et al. Assessment of long-term plasma exchange for familial hypercholesterolaemia. Br Heart J 1980;43:680-8.

140. Tatami R, Inoue N, Itoh H, et al. Regression of coronary atherosclerosis by combined LDL apheresis and lipid-lowering drug therapy in patients with familial hypercholesterolemia: A multicenter study. Atherosclerosis 1992;95:1-13.

141. Thompson GR, Miller JP, Breslow JL. Improved survival of patients with homozy-gous familial hypercholesterolaemia treated by plasma exchange. Br Med J 1985;291:1671-3.

142. Gordon T, Castelli WP, Hjortland MC, et al. High density lipoprotein as a protective factor against coronary heart disease. The Framingham Study. Am J Med 1977;63:707-14.

143. Stoffel W, Borberg H, Greve V. Application of specific extracorporeal removal of low density lipoprotein in familial hypercholesterolaemia. Lancet 1981;2:1005-7.

144. Thompson GR, HEART-UK LDL Apheresis Working Group. Recommendations for the use of LDL apheresis. Atherosclerosis 2008;198:247-55.

145. Thompson GR, Maher VMG, Matthews S, et al. Familial hypercholesterolaemia regression study: A randomized trial of low density lipoprotein apheresis. Lancet 1995;345:811-16.

146. Dahlen GH. Lp(a) lipoprotein in cardiovascular disease. Atherosclerosis 1994;104:111-26.

147. Kroon AA, Aengevaeren WRM, van de Werf T, et al. LDL-Apheresis Atherosclerosis Regression Study (LAARS). Effect of aggressive versus conventional lipid lowering treatment on coronary atherosclerosis. Circulation 1996;93:1826-35.

148. Mabuchi H, Koizumi J, Shimzu M, et al. Long-term efficacy of low-density lipoprotein apheresis on coronary heart disease in familial hypercholesterolemia. Am J Cardiol 1998;82:1489-95.

149. Matsuzaki M, Hiramori K, Imaizumi T, et al. Intravascular ultrasound evaluation of coronary plaque regression by low density lipoprotein-apheresis in familial hypercholesterolemia. J Am Coll Cardiol 2002;40:220-7.

150. Barter PJ. Coronary plaque regression: Role of low density lipoprotein-apheresis. J Am Coll Cardiol 2002;40:228-30.

151. Park JW, Vermeltfoort M, Braun P, et al. Regression of transplant coronary artery disease during chronic HELP therapy: A case study. Atherosclerosis 1995;115:1-8.

152. Tojo K, Sakai S, Miyahara T. Therapeutic trial of low density lipoprotein apheresis (LDL-A) in conjunction with double filtration plasmapheresis (DFPP) in drug-resistant nephrotic syndrome due to focal glomerular sclerosis (FGS). Progr Clin Biol Res 1990;337:193-4.

153. Hattori M, Ito K, Kawaguchi H, et al. Treatment with a combination of low-density lipoprotein apheresis and pravastatin of a patient with drug-resistant nephritic syndrome due to focal

segmental glomerulosclerosis. Pediatr Nephrol 1993;7:196-8.

154. Yokoyama K, Sakai S, Yamaguchi Y, et al. Complete remission of the nephritic syndrome due to focal glomerular sclerosis achieved with low density lipoprotein adsorption alone. Nephron 1996;72:318-20.

155. Suckfull M, for the Hearing Loss Study Group. Fibrinogen and LDL apheresis in treatment of sudden hearing loss: A randomized multicenter trial. Lancet 2002;360:1811-17.

156. Bambauer R, Schiel R, Latza R. Low-density lipoprotein apheresis: An overview. Ther Apher Dial 2003;7:382-90.

157. Thompson J, Thompson PD. A systemic review of LDL apheresis in the treatment of cardiovascular disease. Atherosclerosis 2006;189:31-8.

158. Parhofer KG, Geiss HC, Schwandt P. Efficacy of different low-density lipoprotein apheresis methods. Ther Apher 2000;4:381-5.

159. Bambauer R. Low-density lipoprotein apheresis: Clinical results with different methods. Artif Organs 2002;26:133-9.

160. Otto C, Kern P, Bambauer R, et al. Efficacy and safety of a new whole-blood low-density lipoprotein apheresis system (Liposorber D) in severe hypercholesterolemia. Artif Organs 2003;27:1116-22.

161. Hershcovici T, Schechner V, Orlin J, et al. Effect of different LDL-apheresis methods on parameters involved in atherosclerosis. J Clin Apher 2004;19:90-7.

162. Matsuda Y, Malchesky PS, Nose Y. Assessment of currently available low-density lipoprotein apheresis systems. Artif Organs 1994;18:93-9.

163. Tasaki H, Yamashita K, Saito Y, et al. Low-density lipoprotein apheresis therapy with a direct hemoperfusion column: A Japanese multicenter clinical trial. Ther Apher Dial 2006;10:32-41.

164. Yokoyama S. Treatment of hypercholesterolemia by chemical adsorption of lipoproteins. J Clin Apher 1988;4:66-71.

165. Yamamoto A, Kojima S, Shiba-Harada M, et al. Assessment of the biocompatibility and long-term effect of LDL-apheresis by dextran sulfate-cellulose column. Artif Organs 1992;16:177-81.

166. Riesen WF. Experience with low-density lipoprotein apheresis by polyclonal and monoclonal anti-apolipoprotein B antibodies and by dextran sulfate cellulose. Curr Stud Hematol Blood Transfus 1990;57:208-19.

167. Mabuchi H, Michishita I, Takeda M, et al. A new low-density lipoprotein apheresis system using two dextran sulfate cellulose columns in an automated column regenerating unit (LDL continuous apheresis). Atherosclerosis 1987;68:19-25.

168. Koizumi J, Koizumi I, Uno Y, et al. Reduction of lipoprotein (a) by LDL-apheresis using a dextran sulfate cellulose column in patients with familial hypercholesterolemia. Atherosclerosis 1993;100:65-74.

169. Lasuncion MA, Teruel JL, Alvarez JJ, et al. Changes in lipoprotein (a), LDL-cholesterol and apolipoprotein B in homozygous familial hypercholesterolaemic patients treated with dextran sulfate LDL-apheresis. Eur J Clin Invest 1993;23:819-26.

170. Stefanutti C, Vivenzio A, Colombo C, et al. Treatment of homozygous and double heterozygous familial hypercholesterolemic children with LDL-apheresis. Int J Artif Organs 1995;18:103-10.

171. Zwiener RJ, Uauy R, Petruska ML, Huet BA. Low-density lipoprotein apheresis as long-term treatment for children with homozygous familial hypercholesterolemia. J Pediatr 1995;126:728-35.

172. Uauy R, Zwiener RJ, Phillips MJ, et al. Treatment of children with homozygous familial hypercholesterolemia: Safety and efficacy of low-density lipoprotein apheresis. J Pediatr 1992;120:892-8.

173. Teruel JL, Lasuncion MA, Navarro JF, et al. Pregnancy in a patient with homozygous familial hypercholesterolemia undergoing low-density lipoprotein apheresis by dextran sulfate adsorption. Metabolism 1995;44:929-33.

174. Kroon AA, Swinkles DW, van Dongen PW, Stalenhoef AF. Pregnancy in a patient with homozygous familial hypercholesterolemia treated with long-term low-density lipoprotein apheresis. Metabolism 1994;43:1164-70.

175. Schulzeck P, Olbricht CJ, Koch KM. Long-term experience with extracorporeal low-density lipoprotein cholesterol removal by dextran sulfate cellulose adsorption. Clin Invest 1992;70:99-104.

176. Armstrong VW, Eisenhauer T, Noll D, et al. Extracorporeal plasma therapy: The HELP system for the treatment of hyper-lipoproteinemia. In: Widhalm K, Maito HK, eds. Recent aspects of diagnosis and treatment of lipoprotein disorders: Impact on prevention of

atherosclerotic diseases. New York: AR Liss, 1988:327-35.

177. Lane DM, McConathy WJ, Laughlin LO, et al. Weekly treatment of diet/drug-resistant hypercholesterolemia with the heparin-induced extracorporeal low-density lipoprotein precipitation (HELP) system by selective plasma low-density lipoprotein removal. Am J Cardiol 1993;71:816-22.

178. Lane DM, McConathy WJ, Laughlin LO, et al. Selective removal of plasma low-density lipoprotein with the HELP system: Bi-weekly vs weekly therapy. Atherosclerosis 1995;114: 203-11.

179. Lane DM, Alaupovic P, Knight-Gibson C, et al. Changes in plasma lipid and apolipoprotein levels between heparin-induced extracorporeal low-density lipoprotein precipitation (HELP) treatments. Am J Cardiol 1995;75: 1124-9.

180. Armstrong VW, Schuff-Werner P, Eisenhauer T, et al. Heparin extracorporeal LDL precipitation (HELP): An effective apheresis procedure for lowering Lp(a) levels. Chem Phys Lipids 1994;67-68:315-21.

181. Wieland E, Schettler V, Creutzfeldt C, et al. Lack of plasma lipid peroxidation during LDL-apheresis by heparin-induced extracorporeal LDL precipitation. Eur J Clin Invest 1995;25: 832-42.

182. Fuchs C, Windisch M, Wieland H, et al. Selective continuous extracorporeal elimination of low-density lipoproteins from plasma by heparin precipitation without cations. In: Lysaght MJ, Gurland HJ, eds. Plasma separation and plasma fractionation. Basel, Switzerland: Karger, 1983:272-80.

183. Richter WO, Jacob BG, Ritter MM, et al. Three-year treatment of familial heterozygous hypercholesterolemia by extracorporeal low-density lipoprotein immunoadsorption with polyclonal apolipoprotein B antibodies. Metabolism 1993;42:888-94.

184. Bosch T, Schmidt B, Kleophas W, et al. LDL hemoperfusion—a new procedure for LDL apheresis: First clinical application of an LDL adsorber compatible with human whole blood. Artif Organs 1997;21:977-81.

185. Bosch T, Lennetz A, Schenzle D, Dräger J. Direct adsorption of low-density lipoprotein and lipoprotein(a) from whole blood: Results of the first clinical long-term multicenter study using DALI apheresis. J Clin Apher 2002;17: 161-9.

186. Jovin IS, Taborski U, Muller-Berghaus G. Comparing low-density lipoprotein apheresis procedures: Difficulties and remedies. J Clin Apher 1996;11:168-70.

187. Bambauer R. Low-density lipoprotein apheresis: Clinical results with different methods. Artif Organs 2000;26:133-9.

188. Matsuda Y, Malchesky PS, Nosé Y. Assessment of currently available low-density lipoprotein apheresis systems. Artif Organs 1994;18:93-9.

189. Kottke BA, Pineda AA, Case MT, et al. Hypercholesterolemia and atherosclerosis: Present and future therapy including LDL-apheresis. J Clin Apher 1988;4:35-46.

190. Knisel W, DiNicuolo A, Pfohl M, et al. Different effects of two methods of low-density lipoprotein apheresis on the coagulation and fibrinolytic systems. J Intern Med 1993;234:479-87.

191. Empen K, Otto C, Brodi UI, Parhofer KG. The effects of three different LDL-apheresis methods on the plasma concentrations of E-selectin, VCAM-1, and ICAM-1. J Clin Apher 2002;17: 38-43.

192. Otto C, Berster J, Otto B, Parhofer KG. Effects of two whole blood systems (DALI and Liposorber D) for LDL apheresis on lipids and cardiovascular risk markers in severe hypercholesterolemia. J Clin Apher 2007;22:301-5.

In: McLeod BC, Szczepiorkowski ZM, Weinstein R, Winters JL, eds.
Apheresis: Principles and Practice, 3rd edition
Bethesda, MD: AABB Press, 2010

21

Therapeutic Apheresis in Pediatric Patients

Haewon C. Kim, MD

THE USE OF THERAPEUTIC apheresis in pediatrics is limited by the lack of universally accepted indications in this patient group and by technical challenges in small subjects, including establishment of adequate vascular access. Data from the 2003-2007 World Apheresis Registry showed that of a total of 12,448 procedures in 2013 patients, only 612 procedures were performed in 135 patients under 22 years of age.[1] Furthermore, only 308 procedures were done in children younger than 16 years old, representing only 2.5% of the total. Despite these limitations, therapeutic apheresis in children has been increasing and has been shown to be effective as first-line or adjunctive therapy in children with selected diseases.[2-8] The decision to treat pediatric disease with apheresis is often based on conclusions extrapolated from adult patients; however, there has been reluctance to choose apheresis as a first-line therapy in pediatric patients, even for conditions in which efficacy in adults has been conclusively proven, because pathophysiology, clinical course, and therapeutic responses may differ in children.[9] Nevertheless, improvement in procedural techniques and the availability of various types of central venous catheters and ports have enhanced the safety and encouraged the use of apheresis in children. This chapter discusses special considerations in pediatric apheresis and provide guidelines on modification of standard (adult) operating procedures for pediatric patients.

Haewon C. Kim, MD, Medical Director, Apheresis Service, Departments of Pathology and Laboratory Medicine; Attending Staff, Division of Hematology, Department of Pediatrics, The Children's Hospital of Philadelphia; and Associate Professor of Pediatrics, University of Pennsylvania School of Medicine, Philadelphia, Pennsylvania

The author has disclosed no conflicts of interest.

Special Considerations in Application of Apheresis in Pediatric Patients

Many apheresis centers perform therapeutic apheresis safely in children. However, unforeseen difficulties can still be encountered during a pediatric procedure. To ensure safe and effective treatment of pediatric patients, careful attention should be paid to four areas: technical/procedural, vascular access, anticoagulation, and psychosocial aspects.[10]

Technical/Procedural Considerations

The principles of apheresis are the same in children as in adults; however, available apheresis equipment is designed for adults rather than infants and young children. To perform pediatric procedures safely, one must be familiar with the physical characteristics of apheresis instruments. (See Chapter 4 for detailed descriptions of current instruments.) Because instrumentation affects the physiology of the patient, technical and physiological considerations will be addressed together.

The standard apheresis procedure starts with withdrawal of whole blood into the extracorporeal circuit while diverting the priming saline to the waste bag, which results in a reduction of the patient's total blood volume (TBV). A fixed volume deficit persists throughout the procedure until the content of the centrifuge chamber is rinsed back into the patient at the end of the procedure. The extent of volume depletion is related to the internal volume of the disposable tubing set and is referred to as the extracorporeal volume (ECV). In planning therapeutic apheresis in children, one must know the ECV for the instrument to be used (Table 21-1) and should estimate the effect of ECV on the patient's TBV and circulating red cell volume (RCV).

ECV varies depending on the type of equipment and, even with the same equipment, may depend on the type of procedure. For example, intermittent-flow cell instruments have significantly larger ECV than continuous-flow cell instruments. Even with the same equipment, the ECV of the leukapheresis set may be larger than that of the therapeutic plasma exchange (TPE) or red cell exchange set. For example, the ECV for leukapheresis using the Spectra (CaridianBCT, Lakewood, CO) is 285 mL, whereas it is only 170 mL for a TPE or red cell exchange set. Regardless of the type of instrument, the ECV will represent a larger fraction of TBV in a child than an adult, thus resulting

Table 21-1. Extracorporeal Volume of Continuous-Flow Centrifugal Cell Separators

Cell Separator	Disposable Tubing Set	ECV (mL)	ERCV (mL)
Caridian* Spectra	Plasma/red cell exchange	170	68
Version 4.7	MNC procedure	285	114
Version 6.0	AutoPBSC	165	66
Baxter/Fenwal† CS3000+	Plasma/red cell exchange	393	68
Fresenius‡ AS 104	Plasma/red cell exchange	150	90

*CaridianBCT, Lakewood, CO.
†Fenwal, Lake Zurich, IL.
‡Fresenius Kabi, Redmond, WA.
ECV = extracorporeal volume; ERCV = extracorporeal red cell volume; MNC = mononuclear cell; PBSC = peripheral blood stem cell.

in a greater volume shift in children. To estimate the degree of volume shift, the TBV of the child should also be estimated.

TBV varies with body composition and with other clinical factors. In general, TBV is related to lean body mass and is therefore greater in males than in females of the same weight. Moreover, weight-based calculations overestimate TBV in extremely obese individuals and underestimate it in muscular individuals. Nevertheless, for simplicity, TBV can be calculated by multiplying an age-based estimate of blood volume in mL/kg by the patient's weight in kg. Estimated TBVs for different age groups are as follows: the TBV of a child more than 3 months old is 65 to 75 mL/kg; the TBV is larger in infants younger than 3 months old, ranging from approximately 80 to 100 mL/kg; and in adult males it may be estimated as 75 to 80 mL/kg.[11] Automated apheresis devices may use complex formulae to calculate TBV based on gender, height, and weight; however, a significant discrepancy may be noted in children between TBV derived by the Nadler formula,[12] used by all versions of the Spectra, and TBV calculated from mL/kg. In fact, the TBV calculated by Spectra is inaccurate in children weighing less than 25 kg. (The next-generation Spectra Optia Apheresis System will not calculate TBV for children weighing <25 kg.) In addition, boys under 10 to 12 years of age or weighing less than 30 kg have a TBV smaller than that predicted by the Spectra formula.[13] Consequently, the calculated TBV must be verified against a manual weight-based estimate for children, especially for boys under 10 years or 30 kg. In prepubertal boys, the Spectra TBV may be more accurate if "female" is entered as the gender instead of "male." Simple formulae for estimation of plasma volume (PV) and RCV are shown below, with hematocrit (Hct) expressed as a decimal fraction:

$$PV = TBV \times (1 - Hct) \text{ or } TBV - RCV$$
$$RCV = TBV \times Hct \text{ or } TBV - PV$$

Vascular Access

Adequate vascular access is a prerequisite for a successful procedure. For peripheral access, an antecubital vein adequate for placement of an 18-gauge-or-larger needle should be used for the draw, and a peripheral vein in the opposite arm adequate for placement of a 22-gauge-or-larger device should be used for return. The veins of young children may not accommodate such needles. In this situation, a vascular access device must be placed in a central vein.[14,15] In weighing the risks and benefits of therapeutic apheresis in a child, the risks associated with central venous catheter (CVC) placement, such as thrombosis or infection,[16-19] must be factored into the decision.

When selecting a vascular access device and insertion site, three factors must be considered: 1) the urgency of the need for therapeutic apheresis, 2) the expected frequency and duration of apheresis, and 3) the ease of catheter care. In emergency situations, patients have often not been prepared (ie, by fasting for several hours) to undergo general anesthesia for an invasive procedure. In such cases, a temporary percutaneous dual-lumen catheter can be the best choice.[20] Such a catheter can be inserted into a femoral vein with intravenous sedation and local anesthesia, even at the bedside, without intubation.[21] However, use of a femoral venous catheter should be limited to only a brief period until a CVC can be placed, as it poses a greater risk of infection and thrombosis than an internal jugular or subclavian catheter.[20]

CVCs for short-term use are inserted percutaneously (nontunneled), whereas long-term CVCs (tunneled and cuffed) are usually implanted surgically.[15] Infection rates may be lower with tunneled CVCs,[22,23] although infection rates are higher with multi-lumen as opposed to single-lumen catheters.[24,25] Although infection rates may be higher with internal jugular than with subclavian catheters,[26,27] mechanical complications of insertion and obstruction of flow are less frequent with internal jugular CVCs.[27] Therefore, internal jugular placement is preferable in small children to achieve better flow by reducing mechanical problems associated with agitation or movement. In addition, curved extensions are more comfortable than straight extensions for infants and small children, particularly in the internal jugular vein, because of their short necks.

In children who require chronic apheresis therapy, implantable subcutaneous venous access ports can be used. Of the numerous implantable ports available, Cathlink 20 implanted ports (Bard Access Systems, Salt Lake City, UT)[28] and Vortex ports (AngioDynamics, Queensbury, NY)[29-34] appear to be suitable for long-term apheresis therapy. Several abstracts have reported that single- or dual-lumen Vortex ports have been effectively used in both children and adults who require long-term red cell exchange[29-32] or photopheresis.[33,34] Although one center reported being able to maintain flow rates of up to 60 mL/minute,[32] others reported minor complications including low inlet flow rates, sometimes because of sludge or clots that necessitate installation of tissue plasminogen activator. When ports are accessed infrequently (eg, every 4-6 weeks for red cell exchange in sickle cell disease), a higher concentration of heparin, ranging from 1000 to 5000 U/mL, is instilled into the ports between uses.

Vortex ports have a tangential reservoir outlet that results in less sludge build-up with lower risks of occlusion and infection. In a prospective randomized controlled trial of conventional Celsite (B. Braun Celsa, S.A., Boulogne-Cedex, France) ports vs Vortex ports with a tangential outlet in 200 cancer patients,[35] all functional complications, ranging from sluggish flow to total occlusion, were higher in the Celsite group (16.1% vs 11.4%); however, this difference was not statistically different. In patients weighing 40 kg or more, a dual-lumen Vortex port, size 11.4 French, may be tried. However, a child weighing less than 40 kg may need two ports: one Vortex port for blood withdrawal and another access device such as an Infuse-a-Port (Shiley Infusaid, Norwood, MA) for return, unless a peripheral venous site is available. Arteriovenous shunts or fistulae can be used for vascular access if already in place. Another consideration in selecting an access device is ease of care; in general, ports are easier to care for than CVCs, requiring a heparin flush only every 4 to 8 weeks when not in use.[35]

Catheters for apheresis should be relatively stiff, so as not to collapse under negative pressure when blood is withdrawn at a high flow rate. Large-bore, dual-lumen catheters designed for hemodialysis are suitable for apheresis procedures. These include MedComp (MedComp, Harleysville, PA), Vas-Cath (Vas-Cath, Mississauga, ON, Canada), Quinton-Mahurkar catheter or PermCath catheter (Quinton Instrument Co, Seattle, WA), and Hickman dialysis catheters (Bard Access Systems). Broviac catheters (Bard Access Systems), Infuse-a-Ports, or peripherally inserted CVCs are not suitable for drawing but can be used for returning replacement fluids. Guidelines in use at the author's institution for catheter size according to patient weight are given in Table 21-2.

Anticoagulation

An apheresis procedure requires the use of anticoagulant to prevent clotting in the extracorporeal circuit. Citrate, heparin, or both can be used for this purpose.[1-4,10,36-43] More than 70% of apheresis procedures reported to World Apheresis Registries use citrate anticoagulation, whereas heparin is used in only 18%.[1,39] The Italian Registry of Pediatric Therapeutic Apheresis reported that citrate is used in more than 90% of pediatric apheresis procedures.[38] When heparin is chosen, the patient must be evaluated clinically for a history of

Table 21-2. Recommendations for Central Venous Catheter Size by Patient Weight

Weight (kg)	Size of CVC
<3	Consider two single-lumen CVCs, 5 French (Fr.)
3-10	7 Fr., double-lumen
10-20	8 Fr. or 9 Fr., double-lumen
20-50	9 Fr. or 10 Fr., double-lumen
>50	11.5 Fr., 12 Fr., or 13.5 Fr., double-lumen

hemorrhage or bleeding disorder as well as laboratory evidence for any contraindications. All patients undergoing therapeutic apheresis at the author's institution are screened for an underlying coagulopathy with a complete blood count (CBC), platelet count, prothrombin time (PT), activated partial thromboplastin time (aPTT), and fibrinogen assay.

As noted in Chapter 3, citrate may cause adverse effects related to ionized hypocalcemia. Most adults will report acral and circumoral paresthesias, allowing apheresis operators to reduce the citrate infusion rate while symptoms are mild. In contrast, young or sick children may not be able to inform the operator of symptoms of hypocalcemia. Furthermore, children may not exhibit the symptoms common in adults but often develop abdominal pain, emesis, pallor, and/or hypotension.[2,3,6,36,40] Therefore, monitoring citrate-induced ionized hypocalcemia by clinical observation is more difficult in children than adults.

The risk of citrate toxicity in TPE is higher with Fresh Frozen Plasma (FFP) replacement than with 5% albumin replacement, particularly in subjects with slow citrate metabolism because of hepatic or renal dysfunction. FFP contains approximately four times more citrate than 5% albumin, and the average increase in the plasma citrate level is higher with FFP than albumin (1.1 vs 0.2 mM/L).[44] Both FFP and albumin reduce the ionized calcium level, but with FFP infusion, ionized calcium falls more than total calcium, whereas with albumin infusion, both ionized calcium and total calcium fall in similar amounts because of direct binding of calcium to albumin. Only ionized calcium is physiologically important, and it should be monitored before and frequently during procedures when FFP is used as the replacement fluid in TPE or citrate anticoagulation is used for leukapheresis; intravenous calcium supplementation should be provided when necessary to prevent serious adverse reactions from hypocalcemia.

A combination of heparin with citrate may be preferred in pediatric apheresis, particularly in infants undergoing leukapheresis for hematopoietic progenitor cell (HPC) harvest, unless there is a contraindication to heparin. Methods for citrate and heparin combination are discussed in detail in "Anticoagulation" under "Collection Procedures" later.

Psychological Considerations

Children undergoing therapeutic apheresis exhibit some degree of anxiety, which may result in a lack of cooperation with the apheresis team. A special approach to anxiety is needed in children; however, the approach should be tailored to the age and medical condition of the child. In order to formulate an individual approach, the apheresis operators should respect the patient's interests, learn the psychosocial background of the child, and communicate with the child according to developmental rather than chronological age. Pediatric care cannot be complete or effective without the participation of parents or guardians, who should understand the procedure and its potential benefits and risks and should be aware if their child might experience pain or discomfort.

During a procedure, efforts should be made to divert the child's attention to age-appropriate activities such as watching TV or a favorite video, coloring, or playing games with family members or hospital staff. Infants or small children can be calmed and comforted by the presence of familiar people such as parents or grandparents. Sedation may be medically indicated (eg, for a child who experiences frequent seizures or neuromuscular instability) but should otherwise be reserved as a last resort because it may interfere with recognition of adverse effects.

Procedural Modifications for Pediatric Apheresis

In adults, standard operating procedures can be applied in almost all cases; however, it is imperative to modify each pediatric procedure to fit the individual patient's needs. The key factors for a safe procedure in pediatric patients are adequate venous access, maintenance of adequate intravascular volume and circulating red cell mass, and prevention or prompt recognition of adverse reactions secondary to volume shifts, anticoagulants, and/or replacement fluids. This applies to all types of instrumentation, but continuous-flow equipment is preferred over intermittent-flow equipment for pediatric use because of the smaller ECV.

To perform an apheresis procedure safely, its potential effects on the patient's intravascular volume and RCV must be evaluated. Before the procedure, the predicted volume shifts should be calculated using the ECV and extracorporeal RCV (ERCV) of the disposable tubing set, and the patient's TBV and hematocrit. In addition, results of baseline laboratory tests, including CBC, PT, aPTT, fibrinogen, and ionized calcium should help in selecting the most appropriate types of replacement fluids and evaluating any need for calcium supplementation. Special attention also should be paid to cardiac, renal, and hepatic function, as well as medications and any history of allergy or transfusion reactions.

In children weighing more than 25 kg, the technique is similar to that used in adults. It is in smaller children that significant modifications are required. In this chapter, technical modifications for pediatric patients are described in detail for the Spectra, a continuous-flow instrument with a relatively low ECV that is a common choice for pediatric apheresis in the United States, but the principles can be applied to any continuous-flow device. Readers are referred to a previous publication that provided detailed step-by-step guidelines on procedural modifications and blood priming, with worksheets to calculate fluid and RCV management.[10]

Establishment of Desired Target Limits

Before the procedure, one must compare the expected ECV to the individual's TBV to predict the net volume shift. The expected ECV of the apheresis system should include not only the tubing set but also any ancillary devices, such as a blood warmer or a selective depletion column. The patient's TBV and RCV are estimated on the basis of body weight and hematocrit; the theoretical percentage for volume shifts during the procedure can then be calculated and compared with safe limits for volume shifts based on the patient's size, hematocrit, and medical condition. One can then develop a plan for management of intravascular and RCV shifts during the procedure.

Intravascular Volume Management

A volume deficit or overload, either during or after a procedure, can cause undesirable hemodynamic effects in small children, especially children with anemia, dehydration, or cardiac, renal, or hepatic impairment. With loss of less than 15% of TBV in hemodynamically stable subjects, changes in cardiac output or oxygen consumption are mitigated or prevented primarily by contraction of the great veins.[45] However, when ECV exceeds 15% of TBV, many patients will develop symptoms and signs of hypovolemia. These may range from apprehension, tachycardia, orthostatic hypotension, narrow pulse pressure, weakness, nausea, lightheadedness, pallor, thirst, and cool skin to loss of consciousness with shock. These effects are due more to loss of intravascular fluid volume than to a deficiency of circulating red cells.[46] Hypovolemic reactions are very common, especially in smaller children. Thus, the ECV should not exceed 15% of TBV in any subject, and preferably should not exceed 10% in children.

The operator should monitor fluid balance carefully to help differentiate adverse reactions caused by hypovolemia from those with other causes, such as hypocalcemia, so that the patient can be promptly and appropriately treated. When apheresis is performed on critically ill or hemodynamically unstable patients, it is not easy to differentiate circulatory collapse caused by hypovolemia from circulatory shock arising from other causes, such as cardiac defects, defects in the distribution of blood flow because of sepsis, central nervous system injury, drug intoxication, or vascular obstruction (eg, tamponade, embolism, thrombus, etc). Procedures on such patients should be performed in an intensive-care setting where cardiorespiratory status can be carefully monitored.

To Divert the Priming Saline or Not

With the start of the procedure, withdrawal of whole blood into the apheresis circuit while diverting the priming saline to the waste bag results in a negative fluid balance. This negative volume shift will remain throughout the procedure even with the administration of replacement fluids or red cells until the rinse-back is performed at the end of the procedure. Based on the calculations described above, one should determine whether the volume deficit that would result from diverting saline exceeds the safe limit for the individual patient. The volumes of diverted saline with TPE and red cell exchange are 150 mL and 100 mL, respectively. If the diverted volume exceeds 15% of TBV or the safe limit for the individual patient, the priming saline may be infused to the patient without diverting. If the patient's medical condition warrants, other fluids such as 5% human albumin, FFP, or reconstituted whole blood can be substituted for the priming saline. In this situation, the apheresis set is filled from the inlet to the return line with the desired fluid after first priming with normal saline.

To Rinse Back or Not

The rinse-back process at the end of a typical apheresis procedure recovers red cells that remain in the circuit by first evacuating the channel and then rinsing it with normal saline, thus producing a positive volume shift. With the Spectra, the default rinse-back volume is 345 mL for both TPE and red cell exchange procedures. To decide whether rinse-back can be safely performed, the percent volume shift it represents should be calculated. When the priming saline is diverted, the net volume shift for a procedure is +195 mL with TPE and +245 mL with red cell exchange. If the priming saline volume is not diverted but infused to the patient, the net volume shift is +345 mL with either exchange procedure. If the patient cannot tolerate the positive volume shift that rinse-back would entail, it should be omitted.

Circulating Red Cell Volume Management

Maintenance of a circulating RCV adequate to provide oxygen delivery to tissues is essential. Some deficit in RCV develops as whole blood is withdrawn from the patient into the apheresis circuit and persists until red cells in the instrument are rinsed back to the patient at the end of the procedure. The potential extent of RCV depletion should also be analyzed; it depends on the instrument and the type of procedure performed. ERCV is larger with intermittent-flow than continuous-flow instruments. Because ERCV is fixed for each instrument/procedure combination, a larger fraction of RCV is depleted in children than in adults, and the lower the patient's absolute RCV, the larger the fractional depletion will be. Both patient size and hematocrit influence the degree of RCV shift that is tolerable/allowable. The hemodynamic effects of a given degree of red cell loss may also be influenced by an underlying medical condition. Red cell depletion of any degree may be detrimental to some patients, such as those with cardiovascular or pulmonary impairment or those at risk of developing organ ischemia. Before the procedure, one should establish the lowest hematocrit level that the patient can be expected to tolerate during the procedure.

To Prime with Red Cells or Not

Hematocrit falls from the preapheresis level as red cells enter the extracorporeal circuit. If the anticipated hematocrit level is below the acceptable limit, red cell priming is indicated. Red cell priming to support adequate oxygen delivery to tissues may be warranted in a hemodynamically stable patient with a normal hematocrit in an exchange procedure when the patient's body weight is less than 15 kg (or TBV <1000 mL), or in a peripheral blood HPC collection procedure when body weight is less than 25 kg (or TBV <1700 mL). Red cell priming is also indicated when any degree of reduction in the circulating red cell volume is deemed undesirable; for example, in hemodynamically unstable patients or patients at risk for organ ischemia. Thus it may be indicated for an adult-sized patient with significant anemia. Additional red cells may be needed to compensate for red cell loss during a procedure; for example, in leukocyte depletion procedures, a substantial quantity of red cells is removed with the white cell concentrate, which can be problematic in anemic patients.

Methods for Red Cell Priming

Red cell priming can be achieved in several different ways. Before either of the two methods described below, the entire apheresis system (including the blood warmer, if used) should be primed with normal saline in the usual way. One popular method is to fill the centrifuge chamber and tubing set with donor red cells by connecting a donor unit to the access/draw line via a blood administration set and attaching the return line to an empty transfer pack. Red cells are then pumped into the set until they reach the end of the return line. Another method in use at the author's institution is to prime only the return line of the disposable tubing set with donor red cells, rather than the entire apheresis circuit.[10] With the latter approach, once the patient is connected to the apheresis system, the donor red cells in the return line are infused immediately as whole blood is withdrawn from the patient. The remaining red cell priming volume is infused through the return line by either the replacement pump or an infusion pump running at the same flow rate as the withdrawal pump in the apheresis instrument while saline in the channel is diverted to the waste bag. When patient red cells begin to exit from the separation channel, saline diversion and red cell priming end and the instrument is operated normally. The author prefers the latter approach because 1) it is technically simple; 2) it is less cumbersome if there is a problem with the disposable set (if the system leaks after red cell priming, the entire disposable set has to be replaced and primed again with red cells); and 3) most important, it is easy to achieve the desired target hematocrit level of the patient without volume overload, by infusing a predetermined volume of red cells. An alternative to red cell priming of the system, if intravascular volume expansion is not a concern, is to raise the patient's hematocrit level before the procedure by simple transfusion.

Rinse-Back and Red Cell Balance

The next step is to assess the effect of rinse-back. Although rinse-back will return most of the red cells, it also returns additional saline. A decision should be made after considering whether the patient can tolerate the positive fluid balance associated with rinse-back. If a child cannot tolerate the volume load, then rinse-back should not be performed even though this means that a significant volume of red cells cannot be returned. Partial rinse-back to return some of the red cells in the channel but avoid volume overload may be an option in some cases. When red cell priming is performed, the patient's TBV and RCV will remain at baseline throughout the procedure, and rinse-back is not necessary. With the Spectra, the default (full) rinse-back would return 53 mL of the 68 mL of red cells from the channel for both TPE and red cell exchange, and 90 mL of the 114 mL of red cells from the circuit with leukapheresis.

Pediatric Apheresis Procedures

Apheresis procedures can be classified as either exchange or collection procedures. Exchange procedures are intended to remove abnormal plasma constituents or red cells by exchanging for plasma or a plasma substitute (TPE) or normal donor red cells.[6-9] In practice, collection procedures in pediatrics are limited to leukapheresis, most often performed to collect peripheral blood HPCs for autologous transplantation and, rarely, to deplete leukemic blast cells from patients with hyperleukocytosis.[8,9]

Exchange procedures differ from leukapheresis with respect to replacement fluids and anticoagulation. They require a large volume of plasma replacement fluid or red cells to compensate for the loss of corresponding blood components. Plasma replacement fluids include

5% human serum albumin and FFP. For patients with a coagulopathy or at risk of bleeding, FFP should be considered as a part or all of the replacement fluids. The advantages and disadvantages of various replacement fluids are discussed in Chapter 14.

In pediatric collection procedures, especially therapeutic leukocyte depletion, the volume of leukocyte concentrate removed may represent a significant fraction of the patient's TBV and thus may cause an unacceptable negative volume shift. To minimize or prevent this, additional fluids or donor red cells may be administered during the collection as a form of replacement; the disposable sets for leukapheresis do not provide a replacement line, but such products can be administered via the return access of the disposable set through a Y connector, or through a separate intravenous line. Citrate toxicity is a much greater problem with leukapheresis than with exchange procedures because a much larger amount of citrate is infused to the patient.

Practical guidelines for performing apheresis, using the Spectra, while maintaining adequate intravascular and red cell volumes in pediatric patients of two different sizes are described below. Step-by-step examples of ECV and RCV analysis and procedural modifications for exchange and collection are provided for a 10-kg child with a TBV of about 700 mL. These are compared to a standard apheresis procedure in a 50-kg adolescent boy with a TBV of about 3750 mL. Both boys have a hematocrit of 30%.

Exchange Procedures

Intravascular Volume Management

First, the maximum volume shift that the patient can be expected to tolerate should be established based on size and clinical condition. In general, this should not exceed 10% of TBV for infants and small children. Thus, in a 10-kg infant, the maximum volume shift should never exceed 70 mL (10% of 700 mL). In contrast, the adolescent boy may tolerate an intravascular volume shift of up to 15% of TBV, so the

safe limit would be 563 mL (15% of 3750 mL).

Second, the effect of diverting the priming saline needs to be determined. The volumes of saline diverted to the waste bag in TPE and red cell exchanges are 150 mL and 100 mL, respectively, which would result in blood losses corresponding to 21% and 14% of the infant's TBV. Neither degree of negative volume shift should be allowed in an infant. In contrast, standard exchange procedures with saline diversion should be well tolerated by the adolescent boy, as these diverted volumes represent less than 5% of his TBV. In the infant it is clear that exchange procedures cannot be performed safely without modification. Therefore the standard apheresis procedure would be modified to not divert priming saline and thus to maintain isovolemia throughout the procedure.

Third, the effect of rinse-back on the postapheresis volume shift should be determined. The rinse-back volume for either exchange procedure is 345 mL. In the adolescent boy, this corresponds to only 9% of TBV. Furthermore, because priming saline was diverted in this example, the fluid net gain is actually only 245 mL with red cell exchange (345-100 mL of diverted saline) and 195 mL with TPE (345-150 mL of diverted saline). This degree of volume expansion would be well tolerated in a 50-kg adolescent boy, and there is no need for modification of the procedure. Priming saline was not to be diverted in the infant, who would therefore experience the full 345-mL net fluid gain from rinse-back, corresponding to 49% TBV; therefore, rinse-back should be omitted in the infant to prevent severe volume overload.

Circulating Red Cell Volume Management

With hematocrits of 30%, RCVs of the infant and adolescent boy would be 210 mL (30% of 700 mL) and 1125 mL (30% of 3750 mL), respectively. The ECRV for both TPE and red cell exchange disposables is 68 mL. The steps below should be followed to assess potential changes in RCV during pediatric apheresis.

First, the lowest hematocrit level that the patient can be expected to tolerate should be established based on clinical status. Second, the lowest hematocrit level anticipated during the procedure should be determined. The predicted fall in hematocrit can be calculated by subtracting 68 mL from the patient's total RCV and dividing the difference by TBV times 100. In the 10 kg infant with RCV = 210 mL and TBV = 700 mL, the patient's hematocrit level would drop precipitously to 20% [(210 mL − 68 mL)/700 mL × 100 = 20%] or even lower if a blood warmer or additional blood drawn for laboratory testing must be taken into account. This red cell loss would occur regardless of diversion of priming saline and would persist throughout the procedure until rinse-back is performed.

Third, the effect of rinse-back on the postapheresis hematocrit level must be determined. The rinse-back volume of red cells is 53 mL for both exchange sets. Returning red cells from the instrument to the patient with rinse-back would raise the infant's hematocrit to 28%, which is acceptable; however, the infant's hematocrit should not be allowed to fall to, and remain at, 20% throughout the procedure. This situation therefore necessitates red cell priming to avoid a precipitous drop in hematocrit. It was already recommended that rinse-back should be omitted to avoid volume overload. With red cell priming and omission of rinse-back, both RCV depletion during the procedure and volume overload at the end can be avoided. In the 50-kg boy, the intraprocedural hematocrit should not fall below 28% [(1125 mL − 68 mL/3750 × 100)], which should be well tolerated.

Red Cell Priming. The goal of red cell priming is usually to maintain the patient's initial hematocrit throughout the procedure. Therefore, at least 68 mL of donor red cells should be available during an exchange procedure to compensate for the loss of red cells into the apheresis set. If a unit of donor red cells preserved in anticoagulant-additive solution (AS-RBCs) is presumed to have a volume of approximately 300 mL and a hematocrit of 57%, the volume of donor red cells needed to prime the apheresis circuit for an exchange procedure can be calculated by dividing ERCV by the hematocrit of the donor unit. Using this formula, approximately 120 mL of the AS-RBCs is needed (68 mL/0.57 = 119 mL). Therefore, half a unit of donor red cells must be available for an exchange procedure in the infant. If the donor unit is divided using a sterile connection device, the remainder can be reserved for a subsequent procedure to limit the number of donor exposures. To raise the hematocrit level of the patient without volume overload, the additional volume of donor red cells needed to raise the hematocrit to the desired level can be calculated and infused as a part of the replacement fluid.

Preparation of Reconstituted Blood. A donor RBC unit has a higher hematocrit than the patient but can be reconstituted to a desired hematocrit level by diluting it with an appropriate fluid such as normal saline, 5% albumin, or FFP. Donor red cells may be used without dilution to prime the apheresis circuit when there is a need to raise the patient's hematocrit level, or with a leukapheresis procedure. Instructions for the preparation of reconstituted blood at a desired hematocrit are as follows[10]:

1. Calculate the required volume of reconstituted blood at a desired hematocrit by dividing the ERCV (in mL) by the desired hematocrit of reconstituted blood (68 mL/0.3 = 226 mL).
2. Determine the volume of diluent needed by subtracting the volume of AS-RBCs from the total volume of reconstituted blood (226 mL − 120 mL = 106 mL).
3. Prepare reconstituted blood by adding the diluent to the AS-RBCs (106 mL + 120 mL = 226 mL).

Method for Red Cell Priming. The red cell priming method in use at the author's institution is as follows. After the standard saline prime of the apheresis circuit and before starting the procedure, the return line of the disposable set, including the blood warmer, is primed with either reconstituted blood or donor red cells without dilution. The remainder of the red cell prime is delivered through the return line with the replacement fluid pump while priming saline from the channel is diverted, as described above. When the channel has filled with patient blood, saline diversion ends and the procedure goes on normally.[10] As an alternative, after the apheresis circuit is primed with saline, the circuit is filled with donor red cells as the saline prime is diverted into the waste bag, after which priming saline in the return line is displaced by red cell prime coming from the channel. When the patient is connected to the apheresis system, whole blood is withdrawn from the patient, and donor red cells are immediately returned.

Collection Procedures

Unique problems encountered in pediatric leukapheresis are illustrated by the example of the 10-kg infant described above.[10]

Intravascular Volume Management

After establishing the maximum tolerable volume shift, the effects of diverting the priming saline and rinse-back must be determined. The diverted saline and rinse-back volumes of the Spectra leukapheresis set are 150 mL and 413 mL, respectively. Diversion of priming saline with leukapheresis in the infant described above would result in a 21% negative volume shift during the procedure. Rinse-back of 413 mL would result in a 59% volume overload at the end of the procedure. Therefore, leukapheresis must be modified by omitting diversion and rinse-back.

Circulating Red Cell Volume Management

Hematocrit Determination. After establishing the lowest hematocrit that the patient can tolerate, the lowest anticipated patient hematocrit during the procedure may be calculated. At 114 mL, ERCV for the leukapheresis set exceeds that for the exchange sets because more red cells are retained in the channel to establish a higher interface. The volume of red cells residing in the disposable set would exceed half the RCV of the infant, and the

hematocrit would drop precipitously to 13.7% [(210 mL − 114 mL)/700 mL × 100]. Clearly, leukapheresis will require red cell priming.

Next, the effect of the rinse-back on the post-apheresis hematocrit level should be determined. The rinse-back volume of red cells is 90 mL, which would raise the infant's hematocrit to approximately 27%. Although this would be acceptable, the 13.7% level during the procedure is not. Furthermore, omission of rinse-back was recommended earlier to avoid extreme volume overload. Therefore, red cell priming is indicated in the infant to maintain a constant RCV without rinse-back.

Red Cell Priming. It is more challenging to manage the circulating RCV during leukapheresis for two reasons: First, the ERCV is larger with the leukapheresis set, giving the potential for greater RCV depletion. Second, the disposable set does not include a replacement line; therefore, any products, including donor red cells for priming, must be administered through a separate intravenous line or through a Y connector to the return access of the disposable set. Assuming that a unit of red cells has a volume of 300 mL and a hematocrit of 57%, the volume of donor red cells needed to prime the apheresis circuit is at least 200 mL (114 mL/ 0.57 = 200 mL). As discussed above, red cell priming can be carried out by administering 200 mL of donor red cells to the patient through a Y connector attached to the return access while diverting the priming saline into the waste bag ("off-line prime"). To maintain a constant circulating RCV throughout a procedure, a volume of red cells equal to the ERCV of the leukapheresis set (114 mL) must be administered to the patient during the diversion of saline. This volume of red cells diluted to the patient's hematocrit of 30% would be in a total volume of 380 mL, which exceeds the diverted saline volume by 230 mL (380-150) and would create an undesirable positive fluid shift. Thus dilution of a donor unit for red cell priming is not recommended. The off-line prime with undiluted donor red cells will offset the negative volume shift that would otherwise be created by diverting the priming saline.

Anticoagulation

Citrate toxicity is a greater problem with leukapheresis than with exchange procedures because large amounts are administered to anticoagulate the larger volumes of blood processed (as many as 7-8 blood volumes over a 3- to 7-hour period in an HPC harvest) and because virtually all this citrate is returned to the patient. Heparin may be used alone or in conjunction with citrate to prevent or reduce citrate toxicity.[2,3,37-43] Unless there are patient-specific contraindications to heparin, the combination is preferred over citrate or heparin alone, especially in small children or in pediatric HPC collection, for two reasons. The first is to reduce the amount of citrate infused. The second is to increase the rate of whole blood draw that can be tolerated by children, especially those weighing less than 10 kg, to maintain an inlet/draw pump flow rate of >10 to 12 mL/minute.

Various protocols have been devised for combined use of citrate and heparin with or without monitoring the effect of heparin. One method is to infuse a bolus loading dose of 50 units/kg followed, after a 1-hour interval, by 10 units/kg every 30 minutes. The citrate is provided as acid-citrate-dextrose formula A (ACD-A) at an anticoagulant-to-whole-blood ratio of 20:1 to 30:1 for baseline anticoagulation.[43] The author recommends monitoring aPTT at least hourly with this method. Another method is to add 5000 units of heparin to a 500-mL bag of ACD-A and infuse this mixture at a ratio of 30:1 throughout the procedure.[42] The latter approach obviates the need for additional heparin boluses and monitoring of aPTT.

To further reduce the rate of citrate infusion and still allow a faster draw rate, the author's institution has modified the latter approach by further increasing the anticoagulant-to-whole-blood ratio as more blood is processed (Table 21-3).[10] Under this anticoagulation protocol, the inlet pump flow rate for Spectra is best maintained at 2 mL/kg/minute to ensure that heparinization of the patient continues to be adequate to allow the lower anticoagulant flow rate. If the inlet flow rate falls below 1.5 mL/kg/minute, the anticoagulant/whole blood ratio must be adjusted to increase the anticoagulant flow rate. The dose of heparin administered in an HPC collection procedure is similar to doses used for therapeutic anticoagulation; thus the immediate-postprocedure aPTT is prolonged to about two to three times baseline. None of the patients at the author's institution who have undergone HPC harvest using this guideline have developed symptomatic hypocalcemia or required supplemental calcium. No patient has developed either bleeding or thrombotic complications. However, platelet clumping may be observed in the apheresis system, especially if

Table 21-3. Anticoagulation Guidelines for Peripheral Blood Hematopoietic Progenitor Cell Harvest Using Spectra, Version 4.7*

Blood Volume (BV) Processed	Anticoagulant:Whole Blood[†] Ratio	Inlet Pump Flow Rate (mL/kg/minute)[‡]	Heparin (U/kg/hour)
1st BV	30:1	1.5-2.0	33-44
2nd and 3rd BV	40:1	1.5-2.0	25-33
4th - 7th BV	50:1	1.5-2.0	20-26

*Reprinted with permission from Kim.[10]
[†]Anticoagulant = 5000 units of heparin in a 500-mL bag of acid-citrate-dextrose formula A.
[‡]If inlet pump flow rate is <1.5 mL/kg/minute, anticoagulant:whole blood ratio must be altered to increase anticoagulant flow rate.

the inlet pump flow rate is less than 2 mL/kg/minute or if the platelet count is elevated.

Contraindications for the use of heparin anticoagulation include uncorrected coagulopathy, an underlying bleeding disorder, active and ongoing bleeding, recent (eg, ≤7 days) surgery, brain/spinal cord surgery (<2 weeks of uncomplicated recovery), uncontrolled hypertension, or a history of heparin-induced thrombocytopenia. Again, patients must be screened before the procedure for underlying coagulopathy with a platelet count, PT, aPTT, and fibrinogen assay. Heparin anticoagulation may be safely used in patients with thrombocytopenia and/or hypofibrinogenemia provided that transfusions are given to raise the platelet count to >75,000/µL and/or the fibrinogen level to >100 mg/dL. Anticoagulant therapy should be discontinued before apheresis, if possible. Heparin may be contraindicated for leukocyte depletion in children with hyperleukocytosis, because these patients often present with thrombocytopenia, coagulopathy, or hemorrhage or are at increased risk for bleeding or thrombosis. The ionized calcium level must be monitored frequently and calcium administered as needed to prevent serious hypocalcemic reactions during a therapeutic leukapheresis procedure using citrate anticoagulation.

Pediatric Diseases Treated by Therapeutic Apheresis

The Apheresis Applications Committee of the American Society for Apheresis (ASFA) updated categorization of indications for therapeutic apheresis in 2010.[47] Justifying therapeutic apheresis in a child who has a rare disease or life-threatening condition may be difficult if existing evidence in the literature is insufficient to establish efficacy or clarify the risk/benefit ratio. If the condition is not listed as a Category I or II indication (apheresis is a standard and/or accepted first- or second-line therapy), therapeutic apheresis may sometimes be considered a reasonable option when there is a suggestion of benefit but the available evidence does not establish the specific role of apheresis (Category III). In this situation an overall treatment plan should be developed, including an expected clinical endpoint. Children need not be denied therapeutic apheresis solely because it is technically difficult or because they are very small, severely anemic, or hemodynamically unstable. The apheresis physician should serve as a consultant to evaluate the need for apheresis and assist in developing an overall treatment plan.

Of diseases assigned to Category I or II according to the 2010 ASFA publication,[47] those affecting the pediatric population are listed in Table 21-4. The application of apheresis to each of these disorders is described elsewhere in this book.

Adverse Effects

A prospective, multicenter study reported that adverse effects occur in approximately 4.8% of therapeutic apheresis procedures in adults.[48] Adverse reactions were more common with blood component exchanges than with peripheral blood HPC collections. Performance of apheresis procedures is more challenging and difficult in children than in adults, as set out above.[40,43,49-53] However, there are few data on the frequency of adverse effects in pediatric patients undergoing therapeutic apheresis; reported rates range widely from 4% to 55% of procedures.[38,50-54]

In a retrospective study by Michon et al of 186 children who had undergone a total of 1632 apheresis procedures, adverse reactions occurred in 55% of procedures and in 82% of patients.[53] The most frequent complications were hypotension, symptomatic hypocalcemia, allergic reactions, catheter-related adverse effects, and severe anemia (Hb level <7g/dL). The latter was reported in 2.5% of apheresis procedures and in 17.2% of patients. There were two deaths (1% of patients); attribution to the apheresis procedure was not clear, but both children were hemodynamically unstable before the procedure. Although most complications are benign and transient, severe adverse effects do occur. The incidence of adverse effects in their pediatric cohort was much

Table 21-4. Some ASFA Category I/II Indications for Therapeutic Apheresis Procedures[47]

Procedure	Indication
Plasma exchange	Atypical hemolytic uremic syndrome
	Guillain-Barré syndrome
	Recurrent focal segmental glomerulosclerosis
	Chronic inflammatory demyelinating polyradiculoneuropathy
	Exacerbation of pediatric autoimmune neuropsychiatric disorders associated with streptococcal infections or Sydenham's chorea
	Myasthenia gravis
	Multiple sclerosis with acute central nervous system inflammatory demyelinating disease
	Renal transplantation:
	Antibody-mediated rejection
	Desensitization
	Thrombotic thrombocytopenic purpura
	Goodpasture syndrome (anti-GBM disease)
	ANCA-associated rapidly progressive glomerulonephritis (Wegener's granulomatosis)
	Severe systemic lupus erythematosus (eg, cerebritis, diffuse alveolar hemorrhage)
	ABO incompatible HPC transplantation
	ABO incompatible solid organ transplantation
	Familial hypercholesterolemia
	Neuromyelitis optica (Devic syndrome)
	Catastrophic antiphospholipid syndrome
	Lambert-Eaton myasthenic syndrome
	Rasmussen encephalitis
	Refsum disease
	Fulminant Wilson's disease
	Mushroom poisoning
Red cell manipulations	Red cell exchange for sickle cell disease:
	Acute stroke
	Acute chest syndrome
	Prophylaxis for primary or secondary stroke; prevention of transfusional iron overload
	Multi-organ failure
	Severe malaria
	Severe babesiosis
Leukapheresis	Leukostasis
Plateletpheresis	Symptomatic thrombocytosis
Extracorporeal photochemotherapy	Prophylaxis for, or treatment of, cardiac allograft rejection
	Graft-vs-host disease affecting skin
	Lung allograft rejection
Selective lipoprotein removal	Familial hypercholesterolemia

GBM = glomerular basement membrane; HPC = hematopoietic progenitor cell.

higher than the 4.3% to 28% of procedures in approximately 40% of adult patients reported in the literature.[48,55-60]

The Swedish Apheresis Registry surveyed adverse effects associated with TPE in eight Swedish university hospital centers.[60] There were 620 reports of adverse effects from a total of 12,461 apheresis procedures, with a mean frequency of moderate and severe adverse effects of 5%. Hypotension was the most common adverse reaction. Among the eight centers, there was a fourfold difference in adverse effects rates, which was attributed primarily to differences in indications for therapeutic apheresis, as some centers perform more procedures in critically ill patients, and to the replacement fluids used.

To assess the risks for adverse reactions associated with patients' underlying diseases, Lu et al developed a preprocedure assessment tool with a set of high-risk criteria.[61] Out of a total 3254 procedures, the incidence of overall adverse reactions was 8% for all procedures, but the 36.4% frequency of moderate and severe reactions in the high-risk patients was almost 10 times the 3.7% frequency in the remaining patients.

These studies indicated that hypotension was the most frequent complication reported in both children and adults and that the risk appears to be related to the indications for therapeutic apheresis and the underlying condition of the patient. By identifying a subgroup of patients with a high risk for adverse reactions and by being proactive (eg, careful planning of procedures, maintenance of intravascular volume and circulating red cell mass, prophylactic calcium infusion, and meticulous management of central venous devices), many adverse reactions might be prevented or at least minimized. Needless to say, experienced and knowledgeable apheresis personnel who can recognize the early signs of adverse reactions and effectively manage complications are central to a safe procedure.

Three types of complications are discussed below because they appear to be more common and serious in children than in adults and are sometimes difficult to recognize at an early stage. These are hypovolemia, hypocalcemia, and iron deficiency anemia resulting from chronic iatrogenic blood loss during long-term apheresis.

Hypovolemia

Young children may manifest hypotension secondary to hypovolemia during therapeutic apheresis,[52,54] though this may be difficult to differentiate from hypotension caused by hypocalcemia or a vasovagal reaction. Minor symptoms can be treated by lowering the patient's head below the level of the trunk and legs; however, when a child develops significant hypotension, the procedure should be halted temporarily until the vital signs return to baseline. Significant hypotension, which may occur when more than 25% of TBV is lost, is defined as a systolic blood pressure <65 mmHg in children under age 4, <75 mmHg in children aged 5 to 8, <85 mmHg for those 9 to 12, and <95 mmHg in adolescents and adults.[49] Hypotension from hypovolemia should be treated by administration of a bolus of saline or colloid solution. Hypotension can often be prevented by careful management of intravascular volume shifts. Vasovagal reactions are common in children and are characterized by bradycardia, hypotension, diaphoresis, pallor, nausea, and apprehension. While vasovagal reactions are usually associated with bradycardia, hypovolemia usually results in tachycardia. Vasovagal reactions are managed by interrupting the procedure, elevating the legs, and distracting the child's attention from the procedure; these maneuvers usually allow resumption of the procedure.

Hypocalcemia

Citrate toxicity is a well-recognized complication of apheresis in children. Small infants or children with liver disease, renal disease, or shock may demonstrate impaired citrate metabolism and/or delayed citrate excretion. Citrate chelates calcium, reduces the blood levels of physiologically active ionized calcium (Ca^{++}) and causes ionized hypocalcemia. Hypocalcemia, which may occur when citrate is infused too rapidly or for a prolonged period of time, can cause hemodynamic and myocardial depression with hypotension, arrhythmias, and prolongation of the QTc interval. In adults, the first symptoms of citrate toxicity are perioral numbness and paresthesias of the hands and feet. Children may also report a tingling sensation in the mouth or fingers in response to citrate, but more often manifest acute episodes of abdominal pain and/or vomiting, agitation/irritability, anxiety, pallor, and hypotension. Very young children may not complain of the less obvious symptoms; thus, mild reactions may go undetected and progress to more serious complications. Therefore, careful observation, frequent monitoring of vital signs, and periodic measurements of ionized calcium concentration, especially with the first apheresis procedure, are important to identify hypocalcemia in young children.

Maintaining the ACD-A infusion rate at no higher than 0.8 mL/minute/L of TBV by lowering the inlet pump flow rate of the Spectra can reduce citrate toxicity. Paradoxically, to maintain a minimal inlet pump flow rate of 10 to 12 mL/minute with the Spectra in infants weighing less than 10 kg, it may be necessary to infuse ACD-A at a rate ≥1.2 mL/minute/L of TBV, which is the maximal default value set. Increasing the inlet pump flow rate naturally increases the citrate infusion rate. The risk of citrate toxicity is also increased when a citrated blood product, such as FFP, is infused as replacement fluid. A retrospective study compared citrate-related effects in 35 patients receiving TPE with three different types of replacement solutions.[62] To maintain a targeted ionized calcium level during TPE, significantly more calcium supplementation with 1 M $CaCl_2$ was needed in the group receiving a combination of FFP and human albumin (63 TPEs) than in a comparison group receiving only human albumin (40 TPEs) (7.6 ±1.3 vs 6.2 ±2.7 mL/hour); even more calcium was required in the group (86 TPEs) receiving only FFP (10.8 ±1.7 mL/hour; p <0.001). Furthermore, citrate caused significant metabolic alkalosis in all groups, but the increase in bicarbonate was significantly greater in the FFP group than in the albumin group (4.4 ±3.0 vs 2.6 ±2.1 mmol/L; p = 0.01) because of the additional citrate contained in FFP.

To prevent ionized hypocalcemia during TPE, especially with an ACD-A infusion rate higher than 0.8 mL/minute/L of TBV with the Spectra, 2 to 3 mL of 10% calcium gluconate can be added to each 250-mL bottle of 5% albumin. The same amount can be given, as a bolus over 10 minutes or as a continuous infusion, with each 100 mL of FFP replacement. With the ACD-A infusion rate set higher than 1.2 mL/minute/L of TBV, a proportionately higher prophylactic calcium dose may be required. The ionized calcium concentration should be frequently monitored during the procedure and the dose of intravenous calcium supplementation adjusted as needed.

A plasma ionized calcium concentration <0.75 mmol/L requires immediate correction. Severe symptoms or ionized calcium levels <0.9 mmol/L should also be treated with intravenous calcium at a dose and rate appropriate for the patient's body size. For severe reactions such as tetany in infants and children, 0.5 to 1.0 mL of 10% calcium gluconate/kg, up to a maximum of 10 mL per dose, may be infused over 10 minutes. Ten-percent calcium gluconate can be given via a large peripheral vein with a maximum peripheral concentration of 0.23 mEq/mL at a maximum rate of 0.6 to 1.2 mEq/kg/hour; however, scalp veins and small hand or foot veins should not be used since extravasation can cause skin necrosis and sloughing. In critically ill children, calcium chloride appears to be superior to calcium gluconate because of greater bioavailability.[63] Ten-percent calcium chloride must be given via a central line because of the risk of infiltration with a peripheral venous line. Depending on the ionized calcium level, 20 mg/kg (0.2 mL/kg) of 10% calcium chloride over 10 minutes is a reasonable starting dose. Citrate is also known to chelate ionized magnesium (Mg^{++}) and cause ionized hypomagnesemia,[64] which is also associated with various cardiovascular abnormalities, such as arrhythmia, hypertension, and electrocardiogram changes. Therefore, the Mg^{++} level may also be monitored; magnesium replacement is warranted if cardiac symptoms do not improve with calcium replacement. Of note is that hypomagnesemia can make correction of the hypocalcemia quite difficult, so correction of hypomagnesemia allows better control of the ionized calcium levels.

In April 2009, the Food and Drug Administration updated a previous alert from September 2007 based on postmarketing reports of five neonatal deaths related to the interaction of ceftriaxone with calcium-containing products as follows[65]: Concomitant use of ceftriaxone and intravenous calcium-containing products, such as Ringer's or Hartmann's solution or parenteral nutrition containing calcium, is contraindicated in neonates (<28 days of age) because of particulate formation; in patients >28 days of age, ceftriaxone and intravenous calcium-containing products may be administered sequentially, provided the infusion lines are thoroughly flushed between infusions with a compatible fluid; and ceftriaxone must not be administered simultaneously with intravenous calcium-containing solutions via a Y site in any age group. [See prescribing information from DailyMed (http://dailymed.nlm.nih.gov/dailymed/about.cfm) for details.]

Iron Deficiency Anemia

Despite the use of rinse-back, a small quantity of red cells (15 mL with an exchange and 24 mL with leukapheresis) remains in the disposable set at the completion of a procedure. This loss may not be significant for older children who require only a few procedures, but infants and small children who require long-term apheresis therapy may develop iron deficiency anemia as a result of chronic blood loss. It is therefore advisable to monitor hematocrit regularly and supplement with oral iron—for example, ferrous sulfate at 3 to 4 mg/kg/day—when hematocrit falls more than 5% from baseline in children who require long-term frequent TPE.

Acknowledgment

The author thanks Janet Fithian for her excellent editorial assistance and the Apheresis Unit at Children's Hospital of Philadelphia for their contributions and expert patient care. This chapter is dedicated to my family for their continued encouragement and support, in particular Dr. Young-Nam Kim.

References

1. Witt V, Stegmayr B, Ptak J, et al. World Apheresis Registry data from 2003 to 2007, the pediatric and adolescent side of the registry. Transfus Apher Sci 2008;39:255-60.
2. Fosburg M, Dolan M, Propper R, et al. Intensive plasma exchange in small and critically ill pediatric patients: Techniques and clinical outcome. J Clin Apher 1983;1:215-24.
3. Kevy SV, Fosburg M. Therapeutic apheresis in childhood. J Clin Apher 1990;5:87-90.
4. Strauss RG, Ciavarella D, Gilcher RO, et al. An overview of current management. J Clin Apher 1993;8:189-94.
5. Gorlin JB, Therapeutic plasma exchange and cytapheresis in pediatric patients. Transfus Sci 1999;21:21-39.
6. Eder AF, Kim HC. Pediatric therapeutic apheresis. In: Herman JH, Manno CS, eds. Pediatric transfusion therapy. Bethesda, MD: AABB Press, 2002:471-508.
7. McLeod BC, Kim HC. Therapeutic apheresis. In: Hillyer C, Strauss R, Luban N, eds. Handbook of pediatric transfusion medicine. San Diego, CA: Elsevier Academic Press, 2004: 343-52.
8. Eder AF, Kim HC. Therapeutic cytapheresis. In: Hillyer C, Strauss R, Luban N, eds. Handbook of pediatric transfusion medicine. San Diego, CA: Elsevier Academic Press, 2004: 353-64.
9. Kasprisin DO. Techniques, indications, and toxicity of therapeutic hemapheresis in children. J Clin Apher 1989;5:21-4.
10. Kim HC. Therapeutic pediatric apheresis. J Clin Apher 2000;15:129-57.
11. Stockman JA. Red cell transfusions in pediatrics. In: Rossi EC, Simon TL, Moss GS, Gould SA, eds. Principles of transfusion medicine.

Baltimore, MD: Williams and Wilkins, 1996: 167-76.

12. Nadler SB, Hidalgo JU, Bloct T. Prediction of blood volume in normal human adults. Surgery 1962;51:224.

13. Clough L, Dugan N, Hulitt C, et al. Improved method to estimate total blood volume for erythrocytapheresis using the Cobe Spectra in pediatric sickle cell patients (abstract). J Clin Apher 1998;13:81.

14. Grishaber JE, Cunningham MC, Rohret PA, Strauss RG. Analysis of venous access for therapeutic plasma exchange in patients with neurological disease. J Clin Apher 1992;7:119-23.

15. Thompson L. Central venous catheters for apheresis access. J Clin Apher 1992;7:154-7.

16. Arnow PM, Quimosing EM, Beach M. Consequences of intravascular catheter sepsis. Clin Infect Dis 1993;16:778-84.

17. Pittet D, Tarara D, Wenzel RP. Nosocomial bloodstream infection in critically ill patients. Excess length of stay, extra costs, and attributable mortality. JAMA 1994;271:1598-601.

18. Raad II, Luna M, Khalil SM, et al. The relationship between the thrombotic and infectious complications of central venous catheters. JAMA 1994;271:1014-16.

19. Krafte-Jacobs B, Sivit CJ, Mejia R, Pollack MM. Catheter-related thrombosis in critically ill children: Comparison of catheters with and without heparin bonding. J Pediatr 1995;126:50-4.

20. Skofic N, Buturovic-Ponikvar J, Kovac J, et al. Hemodialysis catheters with citrate locking in critically ill patients with acute kidney injury treated with intermittent online hemofiltration or hemodialysis. Ther Apher Dial 2009;13:327-33.

21. Swerdlow PS. Red cell exchange in sickle cell disease. Hematology Am Soc Hematol Educ Program 2006:48-53.

22. Abrahm JL, Mullen JL. A prospective study of prolonged central venous access in leukemia. JAMA 1982;248:2868-73.

23. Mirro J Jr, Rao BN, Stokes DC, et al. A prospective study of Hickman/Broviac catheters and implantable ports in pediatric oncology patients. J Clin Oncol 1989;7:214-22.

24. Lee RB, Buckner M, Sharp KW. Do multilumen catheters increase central venous catheter sepsis compared to single-lumen catheters? J Trauma 1988;28:1472-5.

25. Gil RT, Kruse JA, Thill-Baharozian MC, Carlson RW. Triple- vs single-lumen central venous catheters. A prospective study in a critically ill population. Arch Intern Med 1989;149:1139-43.

26. Collignon P, Soni N, Pearson I, et al. Sepsis associated with central vein catheters in critically ill patients. Intensive Care Med 1988;14:227-31.

27. Richet H, Hubert B, Nitemberg G, et al. Prospective multicenter study of vascular-catheter-related complications and risk factors for positive central-catheter cultures in intensive care unit patients. J Clin Microbiol 1990;28:2520-5.

28. Raj A, Bertolone S, Bond S, et al. Cathlink 20: A subcutaneous implanted central venous access device used in children with sickle cell disease on long-term erythrocytapheresis—a report of low complication rates. Pediatr Blood Cancer 2005;44:669-72.

29. Just E, Smith S, Saccente SL, Saylors RL. Vascular access with the Triumph 1 port for pediatric apheresis (abstract). J Clin Apher 2001;16:96.

30. Jones R. Use of Vortex MP ports in therapeutic red cell exchanges (abstract). J Clin Apher 2006;21:43.

31. Van Kirk R, Koncsol J, Gutin S, et al. A single-center experience with double and single lumen Vortex ports for chronic erythrocytapheresis in pediatric patients with sickle cell anemia (abstract). J Clin Apher 2006;21:42.

32. Anderson J, Roseff S. Single-center five year experience with successful use of Vortex ports for red cell exchange without infection or need for TPA (abstract). J Clin Apher 2008;23:47.

33. Johnson F, Miller R, Hirner A, et al. Use of an implantable access port, the Vortex port, for extra-corporeal photopheresis (abstract). J Clin Apher 2006;21:25.

34. Shiller D, Simon G, Adams K, Wiltbank TB. Long term use of implanted subcutaneous ports for photopheresis (abstract). J Clin Apher 2009;24:63.

35. Goossens GA, Verbeeck G, Moons P, et al. Functional evaluations of conventional 'Celsite' venous ports versus 'Vortex' ports with a tangential outlet: A prospective randomized pilot study. Support Care Cancer 2008;16:1367-74.

36. Wayne AS, Fosburg MT. Therapeutic plasma exchange and cytapheresis. In: Nathan DG, Oski FA, eds. Hematology of infancy and childhood. 4th ed. Philadelphia: WB Saunders, 1993:1819-31.

37. Sevilla J, Gonzalez-Vicent M, Fernandez-Plaza S, et al. Heparin based anticoagulation during

peripheral blood stem cell collection may increase the CD34+ cell yield. Haematologica 2004;89:249-51.

38. De Silvestro G, Tison T, Vicarioto M, et al. The Italian Registry of Pediatric Therapeutic Apheresis: A report on activity during 2005. J Clin Apher 2009;24:1-5.

39. Stegmayr B, Ptak J, Wikstrom B, et al. World Apheresis Registry 2003-2007 data. Transfus Apher Sci 2008;39:247-54.

40. Galacki DM. An overview of therapeutic apheresis in pediatrics. J Clin Apher 1997;12:1-3.

41. Korbling M, Chan KW, Anderlini P, et al. Allogeneic peripheral blood stem cell transplantation using normal patient-related pediatric donors. Bone Marrow Transplant 1996;18: 885-904.

42. Prather K, Smith M, Bui K, et al. Overview of pediatric peripheral blood stem cell harvests at Fred Hutchinson Cancer Research Center. J Clin Apher 1997;12:33.

43. Bolan CD, Yau YY, Cullis HC, et al. Pediatric large-volume leukapheresis: A single institution experience with heparin versus citrate-based anticoagulant regimens. Transfusion 2004;44: 229-38.

44. Chopek M, McCullough J. Protein and biochemical changes during plasma exchange. In: Berkman EM, Umlas J, eds. Therapeutic hemapheresis. A technical workshop. Washington, DC: AABB, 1980:13-52.

45. Collins JA. Hemorrhage, shock, and burns. In: Petz LD, Swisher SN, eds. Clinical practice of blood transfusion. New York: Churchill Livingstone, 1981:425-53.

46. Hillman RS, Hershko C. Acute blood loss anemia. In: Lichtman MA, Beutler E, Kipps TJ, et al, eds. Williams Hematology. 7th ed. New York: MacGraw-Hill, Inc, 2006:767-71.

47. Szczepiorkowski ZM, Winters JL, Bandarenko N, et al. Guidelines on the use of therapeutic apheresis in clinical practice—Evidence-based approach from the Apheresis Applications Committee of the American Society for Apheresis. The fifth special issue. J Clin Apher 2010; 25:83-177.

48. McLeod BC, Sniecinski I, Ciavarella D, et al. Frequency of immediate adverse effects associated with therapeutic apheresis. Transfusion 1999;39:282-8.

49. Sloan SR, Friedman DF, Kao G, et al. Transfusion medicine. In: Orkin SH, Nathan DG, Ginsberg D, et al, eds. Nathan and Oski's

hematology of infancy and childhood. 7th ed. Philadelphia: Saunders, 2009:1623-75.

50. Stefanutti C, Lanti A, Di Giacomo S, et al. Therapeutic apheresis in low weight patients: Technical feasibility, tolerance, compliance, and risks. Transfus Apher Sci 2004;31:3-10.

51. Pulsipher MA, Levine JE, Hayashi RJ, et al. Safety and efficacy of allogeneic PBSC collection in normal pediatric donors: The Pediatric Blood and Marrow Transplant Consortium experience (PBMTC) 1996-2003. Bone Marrow Transplant 2005;35:361-7.

52. Sevilla J, Plaza SF, Gonzalez-Vicent M, et al. PBSC collection in extremely low weight infants: A single-center experience. Cytotherapy 2007;9:356-61.

53. Michon B, Moghrabi A, Winikoff R, et al. Complications of apheresis in children. Transfusion 2007;47:1837-42.

54. Sevilla J, Gonzalez-Vicent M, Lassaletta A, et al. Peripheral blood progenitor cell collection adverse events for childhood allogeneic donors: Variables related to the collection and safety profile. Br J Haematol 2009;144:909-16.

55. Kiprov DD, Golden P, Rohe R, et al. Adverse reactions associated with mobile therapeutic apheresis: Analysis of 17,940 procedures. J Clin Apher 2001;16:130-3.

56. Rizvi MA, Vesely SK, George JN, et al. Complications of plasma exchange in 71 consecutive patients treated for clinically suspected thrombotic thrombocytopenic purpura-hemolytic-uremic syndrome. Transfusion 2000;40:896-901.

57. Norda R, Stegmayr BG. Therapeutic apheresis in Sweden: Update of epidemiology and adverse events. Transfus Apher Sci 2003;29: 159-66.

58. McMinn JR Jr, Thomas IA, Terrell DR, et al. Complications of plasma exchange in thrombotic thrombocytopenic purpura-hemolytic uremic syndrome: A study of 78 additional patients. Transfusion 2003;43:415-16.

59. Howard MA, Williams LA, Terrell DR, et al. Complications of plasma exchange in patients treated for clinically suspected thrombotic thrombocytopenic purpura-hemolytic uremic syndrome. Transfusion 2006;46:154-6.

60. Norda R, Axelsson CG, Axdorph U, et al. Recognition of intercenter differences may help develop best practice. Ther Apher Dial 2008; 12:347-54.

61. Lu Q, Nedelcu E, Ziman A, et al. Standardized protocol to identify high-risk patients undergoing therapeutic apheresis procedures. J Clin Apher 2008:23111-15.

62. Antonic M, Gubensek J, Buturovic-Ponikvar J, Ponikvar R. Comparison of citrate anticoagulation during plasma exchange with different replacement solutions. Ther Apher 2009;13: 322-6.

63. Broner CW, Stidham GL, Westenkirchner DF, Watson DC. A prospective, randomized, double-blind comparison of calcium chloride and calcium gluconate therapies for hypocalcemia in critically ill children. J Pediatr 1990;117: 986-9.

64. Mercan D, Bastin G, Lambermont M, Dupont E. Importance of ionized magnesium measurement for monitoring of citrate-anticoagulated plateletpheresis. Transfusion 1997;37:418-22.

65. Food and Drug Administration. Information for healthcare professionals: Ceftriaxone (marketed as Rocephin) 9/2007. FDA Alert (9/ 2007). Rockville, MD: FDA, 2007. [Available at http://www.fda.gov/Drugs/DrugSafety/ PostmarketDrugSafetyInformationforPatients andProviders/DrugSafetyInformationforHeath careProfessionals/ucm134328.htm (accessed May 28, 2010).

In: McLeod BC, Szczepiorkowski ZM, Weinstein R, Winters JL, eds.
Apheresis: Principles and Practice, 3rd edition
Bethesda, MD: AABB Press, 2010

22

Hematopoietic Stem Cell Transplantation: An Overview

John R. Wingard, MD; Baldeep Wirk, MD; and Randy Brown, MD

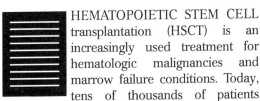HEMATOPOIETIC STEM CELL transplantation (HSCT) is an increasingly used treatment for hematologic malignancies and marrow failure conditions. Today, tens of thousands of patients undergo the procedure annually. Although the stem cells were once collected from the marrow cavity, today often the cells are collected from the blood by apheresis, after "mobilization." This chapter provides a historical perspective, briefly reviews major aspects of the procedure, and describes the various types of donor and stem cell product options.

Historical Perspective

The use of hematopoietic cells for the treatment of hematologic diseases was first described in the late 19th century, and there were sporadic reports subsequently. Interest in hematopoietic cells as a medical therapy accelerated after World War II, following the development of nuclear weapons and power plants. Radiation was noted to suppress hematopoiesis in animals in a dose-dependent fashion such that high doses ablated marrow function. Unirradiated hematopoietic cells, from shielded marrow or spleen of the irradiated animal or from nonirradiated animals, were found to be capable of correcting myeloablative radiation injury.

In the mid-1950s, in a murine model of leukemia, total body irradiation (TBI) followed by administration of marrow cells from homologous animals was found to eradicate an otherwise lethal dose of leukemia cells and restore hematopoiesis.[1] In 1957, patients with advanced leukemia were given TBI followed by marrow

John R. Wingard, MD, Professor of Medicine; Baldeep Wirk, MD, Assistant Professor of Medicine; and Randy Brown, MD, Professor of Medicine, Bone Marrow Transplant Program, Division of Hematology/Oncology, University of Florida College of Medicine, Gainesville, Florida

The authors have disclosed no conflicts of interest.

cells from normal individuals.[2] Transient engraftment was noted in only a single patient and there was no durable benefit in any.

Radiation Sickness

In an unfortunate incident reported in 1959, workers at a nuclear power plant were accidentally exposed to radiation. Marrow cells from healthy individuals were administered in an attempt to reverse the harmful effects.[3] No benefits were noted, but the attempt stirred general interest in HSCT. Three decades later, hematopoietic cell transplants were attempted for victims of the Chernobyl nuclear reactor accident.[4] Transient engraftment occurred in six patients, but endogenous hematopoietic recovery eventually occurred in the majority. Only two of 13 patients survived; however, most deaths were from burns and other nonhematopoietic radiation toxicities. Two patients died of graft-vs-host disease (GVHD), an immunologic attack by donor T cells on host tissues such as the skin, liver, and gastrointestinal tract. These historical examples illustrate some obstacles to HSCT as a remedy for radiation injury, especially damage to nonhematopoietic tissues that would not be reversed by HSCT. It is difficult to know who has received enough radiation to destroy marrow function but not enough to cause irreversible damage to nonhematopoietic tissues and organs; yet only such individuals are reasonable candidates for HSCT. Nevertheless, a potential role for HSCT is still being considered in preparedness for radiation accidents.[5]

Allogeneic Transplantation for Hematologic Disease

Additional attempts were made by multiple investigators to apply HSCT as a treatment for marrow failure or to mitigate the myelosuppressive effects of radiation therapy given to treat hematologic malignancy. Initial attempts to treat leukemia employed TBI, followed by an infusion of marrow cells. Later, cyclophosphamide was added to the treatment regimen. Still later, other agents were employed, including busulfan and antithymocyte globulin (ATG).

The initial outcomes of HSCT were poor. A compilation of human experience up to the early 1970s indicated that few patients benefited. Donor engraftment occurred in fewer than half of transplants, and there were only a few survivors among more than 200 patients so treated.[6] Because of the poor results, interest in clinical HSCT waned during the 1960s, and researchers turned to animal studies to try to resolve the problems.

Based on extensive studies in animals, the failure of early attempts at HSCT was eventually attributed to histocompatibility differences between donors and recipients. In 1960, the Nobel Prize was awarded to Burnet and Medawar for the discovery of acquired immunologic tolerance, establishing the validity of the field of transplantation.[7] Advances in understanding the HLA system and in performing clinical HLA typing led to renewed interest in clinical transplantation in the 1970s. It was recognized that selection of a stringently HLA-matched donor was necessary to ensure reliable donor engraftment in allogeneic HSCT. The short arm of chromosome 6 houses the HLA gene complex, which consists of Class I (HLA-A, HLA-B, and HLA-C) and Class II (HLA-DR and HLA-DP) genes. Because the HLA complex is generally inherited as a complete haplotype, siblings have a 25% probability of being matched.[8]

Advances in ancillary fields also helped to improve outcomes. Platelet transfusion reduced the risk of fatal hemorrhage from thrombocytopenia. More effective antibiotics and better strategies for their use during aplasia reduced the risk of fatal infection. The use of new immunosuppressive regimens after transplant lowered the risk of both graft rejection and GVHD. The first successful HSCT from an unrelated donor was performed in 1979; a patient with acute leukemia engrafted and remained free of leukemia for 2 years without GVHD.[9]

Over subsequent decades further refinements resulted in steadily improving outcomes. Advances in HLA typing led to better donor selection, especially for unrelated donors. New antimicrobials reduced the risk of life-threatening bacterial, viral, and fungal infections. Refinements in pretransplant therapy, called the conditioning regimen, reduced its toxicity. Further improved immunosuppressive drugs and combinations led to lower risks for serious GVHD; for example, in the 1970s either methotrexate or cyclophosphamide was used alone, but by the 1980s it was found that the combination of methotrexate and cyclosporine was superior in preventing GVHD.[10] Transplant outcomes improved incrementally, and with longer follow-up, a plateau was seen in survival curves, suggesting that HSCT offered a cure for some patients.[11]

As results improved, HSCT was considered earlier in the course of diseases in which outcomes of nontransplant treatments were poor. It was shown that results were better when HSCT was performed sooner, with fewer transplant complications and fewer relapses. As a result of these various developments, allogeneic HSCT outcomes reported to registries in the United States and in Europe have shown a 10% increase in survival per decade.[12]

Autologous Transplantation for Cancer

Although the intent of most chemotherapy and radiotherapy regimens is to eradicate cancer cells, collateral destruction of healthy hematopoietic progenitor cells (HPCs) also occurs in a dose-dependent manner. For some cancers, especially the hematologic malignancies, greater malignant cell destruction, accompanied by more frequent and durable responses, can be achieved by dose escalation. However, profound myelosuppression and even lethal myeloablation can occur after such intensive treatment regimens. It was noted, initially in animals and later in patients, that restoration of hematopoiesis could be achieved by infusion of autologous hematopoietic cells collected in advance. Although it had been known since the 1950s that marrow cells could be successfully cryopreserved, it was not until later that this knowledge led to general clinical use. In 1959, three leukemic patients were treated with TBI

followed by thawed autologous marrow that had been collected during remission. One patient survived and attained a remission.[13] In the early 1960s autologous hematopoietic cells from marrow were used to facilitate recovery from myelosuppression caused by high-dose chemotherapy and/or radiotherapy.[14] Unfortunately, whether or not the patients enjoyed any clinical benefit from such early attempts was not easily discerned. It was uncertain whether restoration of hematopoiesis was the result of infused marrow or spontaneous recovery of the residual marrow. Also unknown was whether malignant cells in the infused marrow accounted for relapse. In the late 1970s the benefits of autologous hematopoietic cells in facilitating high-dose chemotherapy were shown more convincingly.[15] In the 1980s advances in cryopreservation and cell processing led to wider clinical application of autologous HSCT. High-dose chemotherapy with autologous HSCT is an ideal therapeutic option for diseases that exhibit a steep dose response to chemotherapy, such as non-Hodgkin lymphoma, Hodgkin lymphoma, and multiple myeloma.

Peripheral Blood Progenitor Cells

Initially, marrow was the source of stem cell grafts for both allogeneic and autologous HSCT. This was sensible because the marrow is the richest source of hematopoietic progenitors, and ordinarily, few hematopoietic progenitors are in the circulation. However, the number of circulating HPCs increases substantially during recovery from conventional-dose chemotherapy and after administration of granulocyte colony-stimulating factor (G-CSF) or G-CSF plus plerixafor (see Chapter 23). Other hematopoietic growth factors, such as granulocyte-macrophage colony-stimulating factor (GM-CSF) or erythropoietin, also cause increases in circulating HPCs but to a lesser degree. Randomized trials comparing HPCs from marrow [HPC, Marrow, or HPC(M)] with peripheral blood progenitor cells (PBPCs) collected by apheresis after growth factor "mobilization" [HPC, Apheresis, or HPC(A)] as sources of autologous progenitors have demonstrated more rapid engraftment with similar treatment outcomes using mobilized peripheral blood grafts.[16,17] Today, autologous HSCT is performed mostly using peripheral blood progenitors as the graft source because of the greater numbers of progenitors collected, the relative ease of collection, and patient convenience.

CD34

The CD34 molecule is expressed on the cell surface of primitive HPCs. A strong correlation between the number of transplanted CD34+ cells and engraftment of HPC(A) has been demonstrated. Enumeration of CD34+ cells by flow cytometry has allowed clinicians to determine the hematopoietic potency of stem cell grafts. Optimization of the graft, achieved by monitoring the CD34+ cell count of apheresis products collected after mobilization, helps to ensure rapid engraftment and minimizes the risk of graft rejection.[18] Refinement of conditioning regimens (to minimize nonhematopoietic toxicities) and optimization of stem cell grafts (to hasten engraftment) have led to reductions in transplant-related mortality after autologous HSCT from 10% or higher in the past to as low as 2% to 4% today.[12,19]

Graft-vs-Host Disease

There has been interest in adopting peripheral blood grafts for allogeneic HSCT as well. However, the greater number of lymphocytes in peripheral blood grafts has raised concern about more GVHD. Trials in matched sibling donor allogeneic HSCTs comparing peripheral blood and marrow grafts have indicated more GVHD (especially chronic GVHD) with peripheral blood grafts.[20-23] For patients treated for advanced leukemia, there appears to be an associated survival advantage that offsets the GVHD risks, while in patients transplanted for early leukemia, there is no survival advantage. In contrast, a retrospective analysis in unrelated donor HSCT noted that peripheral blood grafts are associated with more GVHD but no survival advantage.[24] A prospective randomized

trial is now underway to compare outcomes with the two graft options in donors and recipients.

Matched Unrelated Donors

Matched sibling donors are identified in only one-third of patients in need of an allogeneic HSCT, and with shrinking family size, family donor options will likely continue to decline. Unrelated donor options have been developed to address the shortage of family donors. These include the creation of adult donor registries and the advent of cord blood banking. Volunteer donor registries have been developed in many countries over the years. The number of adult donors listed in various donor registries now exceeds 12 million and continues to grow.[25] The prospects for identifying a suitable match depend on a patient's ethnicity. For example, people of European ethnicity have an 80% chance of finding a donor in these registries. However, because of greater HLA polymorphism and fewer ethnically similar donors, there is a lower likelihood of finding matched unrelated donors in other ethnic groups, such as African Americans and Hispanic Americans.

The outcomes of allogeneic HSCT using unrelated donors were initially poorer than those of matched sibling HSCT. Much of this difference is now recognized to be caused by HLA disparity not detected by older HLA typing methods. Up to half of donor recipient pairs deemed suitable by low-resolution typing methods were found to be mismatched at the allele level using DNA-based high-resolution typing methods.[26] High-resolution DNA matches at HLA-A, HLA-B, HLA-C, and HLA-DRB1 (8/8 match) are the minimum requirement for the highest survival. A mismatch at the allele level is associated with poorer transplant outcomes.[27,28] Today, transplants from unrelated donors matched using high-resolution typing are associated with survival rates similar to those expected after matched sibling transplants. Unfortunately, many registry donors are only partially typed or typed using low-resolution methods. Such donors must often have additional testing to determine their suitability.

This introduces delays; consequently, it may be several months after a search begins before a donation actually occurs.

Umbilical Cord Blood

Umbilical cord blood is rich in hematopoietic progenitors. It can be collected at birth without danger to mother or infant. After testing and cryopreservation, cord blood units [HPC, Cord Blood, or HPC(CB)] are stored at various banks around the world and listed on cord blood registries. Because testing has been completed in advance, suitably matched cryopreserved donor units can be made available for transplant very rapidly. Because the cord's immune cells are immature, greater HLA disparity can be tolerated by recipients, and a unit with up to two antigens mismatched can be a suitable graft.[29] Cord blood has become a preferred option for many children who need a transplant but do not have a suitable sibling donor. In adults, the number of HPCs in a cord blood unit may not be sufficient for reliable engraftment. The use of multiple cord blood units and other investigational strategies are being explored in adults.

Graft-vs-Tumor Effect

When evaluating the quality of a stem cell graft, attention was initially directed exclusively to hematopoietic potency. However, it has become apparent that much of the anti-neoplastic effect of allogeneic HSCT is caused by immune effects of the graft.[30] Lymphoid components mediate potent anti-cancer effects, facilitate engraftment, and are responsible for immune reconstitution that protects against infections and mediates transplant tolerance. Recognition of the importance of graft immune potency has led to two important innovations in transplant practice. First, donor lymphocyte infusions (DLIs) after transplantation can be used to treat relapse[31] or boost immunity to protect against infections or graft rejection (see Chapter 27 for details). Second, the intensive conditioning regimens formulated in the early days of transplantation can sometimes be

replaced by milder regimens. Today, reduced-intensity conditioning regimens (so-called nonablative transplants) emphasize drugs that suppress recipient immunity over those that merely kill cancer cells. After engraftment, donor-derived immunity exerts an anti-cancer effect. Reduced-intensity conditioning has allowed allogeneic HSCT to be offered to older individuals and individuals with comorbid conditions who would not have been considered for transplantation in the past.[32]

With improved outcomes and refinements in transplant practices extending application to patients previously not considered candidates for HSCT, the use of HSCT has grown in clinical practice. Investigations continue to further improve outcomes, to explore adoptive immunotherapy for other neoplastic diseases, to reverse the immune defects in autoimmune diseases, and to explore the use of hematopoietic cells in tissue and organ repair in the incipient field of regenerative medicine.

The Transplant Procedure

From the immunologic standpoint there are three types of HSCT. Allogeneic HSCT uses a person other than the patient as donor. Syngeneic HSCT is a special case in which the donor and recipient are identical twins. Autologous HSCT makes use of a graft collected in advance from the patient. The diseases treated with each type of transplant and the advantages and disadvantages of each type are summarized in Table 22-1.

The transplant procedure can be divided into three basic components: the conditioning regimen, the stem cell infusion, and supportive care measures, including the immunosuppressive regimen for allogeneic HSCT. These are briefly described in Table 22-2.

The Conditioning Regimen

Goals of the conditioning regimen are different in allogeneic and autologous HSCT.[19,33] In autologous transplantation, the goal is to eradicate as many cancer cells as possible. The con-

Table 22-1. Uses, Advantages, and Disadvantages of Different Types of Transplants

	General Uses	Advantages	Disadvantages
Allogeneic	• Correct defective hematopoiesis and/or immunodeficiency • Produce adoptive immunotherapy for cancer • Facilitate high-dose chemoradiotherapy	• Provides GVT effect • Does not require patient to have adequate marrow • Progenitor cells are healthy • May allow use of less intensive cytotoxic agents in conditioning regimen	• Frequent lack of suitable donor • GVHD • Risk of rejection
Autologous	• Facilitate high-dose chemoradiotherapy	• No need for donor • No GVHD	• Tumor may contaminate graft • Previously damaged stem cells may be difficult to collect in adequate numbers or may contribute to risk for myelodysplasia
Syngeneic	• Facilitate high-dose chemoradiotherapy	• No GVHD	• No GVT

GVT = graft-vs-tumor effect; GVHD = graft-vs-host disease.

ditioning regimen consists of agents (drugs and/or radiotherapy) selected to be active against the underlying disease. Desirable attributes of such agents include a steep anti-tumor dose response curve and a lack of severe nonhematopoietic toxicities. A variety of conditioning regimens are suitable for autologous HSCT, depending on the type of underlying cancer. Conditioning regimens have been refined over the years to minimize toxicities such as hepatic veno-occlusive disease, interstitial pneumonitis, mucositis, and hemorrhagic cystitis.

For allogeneic HSCT, the goal of the conditioning regimen is not only an anti-tumor effect but also suppression of recipient immunity to prevent graft rejection. Only a limited number of agents possess both immunosuppressive and anti-tumor activity; thus historically only a few conditioning regimens have been widely used in allogeneic HSCT—cyclophosphamide and TBI being the most common. Busulfan is not immunosuppressive but exhibits potent myeloablative properties; in combination with cyclophosphamide it is useful in allogeneic HSCT conditioning regimens.

Table 22-2. Basic Components of the HSCT Procedure

Component	Purpose (Autologous)	Purpose (Allogeneic)
Conditioning regimen	• Kill tumor	• Suppress host immunity • Kill tumor
Stem cell graft	• Correct myelosuppression and restore hematopoiesis	• Restore hematopoiesis • Correct immunodeficiency or metabolic abnormality caused by abnormal hematopoietically derived cells in congenital metabolic diseases and immunodeficiency diseases • Provide new immune system to give GVT effect
Supportive care, including immunosuppressive regimen	• Prevent/treat infections with antibiotics • Compensate for aplasia with transfusions	• Prevent/treat graft rejection with immunosuppressives • Prevent/treat GVHD with immunosuppressives • Prevent/treat infections with antibiotics • Compensate for anemia and thrombocytopenia with transfusions

GVT = graft-vs-tumor effect; GVHD = graft-vs-host disease.

The introduction of drugs with potent immunosuppressive activity but much less cytotoxicity (eg, the purine analogues, including fludarabine, cladribine, and pentostatin) and potent T-cell antibodies such as antithymocyte globulin and alemtuzumab has increased the number of agents effective in conditioning regimens for allogeneic HSCT.[19,33] In addition, the growing emphasis on reduced-intensity conditioning regimens in allogeneic HSCT, exploiting the adaptive immunotherapeutic properties of the graft while relying less on the anti-tumor properties of the conditioning regimen, has helped to spawn a wide array of new conditioning regimens.

When allogeneic HSCT is performed for a marrow failure state such as aplastic anemia, there is no need for anti-tumor activity, and a conditioning regimen with immunosuppressive properties alone is sufficient. Cyclophosphamide as a single agent is a common choice in this setting.

The Stem Cell Graft

The purpose of the stem cell graft is first and foremost to restore hematopoiesis.[33,34] As noted earlier, hematopoietic potency is related to CD34+ cell content. In the autologous HSCT setting, a CD34+ cell dose of 2 to 2.5 × 10^6/kg of recipient body weight is sufficient to ensure optimal neutrophil recovery. Higher CD34+ cell doses (≥5 × 10^6/kg) are needed to optimize platelet recovery. In the allogeneic setting there has also been interest in the graft's immune potency after clinical observations elucidated the role of immune cells in controlling cancer. Depletion of T lymphocytes was noted to be associated with a higher risk for relapse after allogeneic HSCT. Donor lymphocytes were noted to be capable of re-establishing remission in patients who relapsed after allogeneic HSCT. Immunotherapeutic potency is related to CD3+ cell content, and DLIs containing 10^7 to 10^8 CD3+ cells per kg of recipient body weight generally have potent anti-tumor effects when given to treat relapse after HSCT. However, higher CD3+ cell counts are also associated with greater risk of GVHD. The hope now is to find a CD3+ cell dose that has optimal anti-tumor activity without causing severe GVHD and/or to identify cell subpopulations that will maximize anti-tumor effects while minimizing GVHD.

Three sources of stem cell progenitors have been used for HSCT (Table 22-3). In the past, marrow was the most common source. In the last 2 decades, however, cells from peripheral blood have gradually supplanted marrow. HPC(A) is now used in the majority of allogeneic HSCT cases and in more than 90% of autologous HSCT cases. The third source, cord blood, is increasingly popular for unrelated donor allogeneic HSCT, especially in children.

Marrow

Marrow contains a mixture of mature hematopoietic cells and immature hematopoietic progenitors, including stem cells. Hematopoietic stem cells are characterized by both the capacity for self renewal without differentiation and the ability to differentiate into all hematopoietic lineages. They express the CD34, Thy-1, and c-kit markers and are negative for other markers (ie, lineage negative).[35] Transplantation of a small number of stem cells, possibly only a single cell in some models, restores hematopoiesis in lethally irradiated animals,[36,37] and human marrow contains cells that demonstrate both self renewal and differentiation to all blood cell lineages when serially transplanted in SCID-hu mice (heterochimeric mice with severe combined immunodeficiency transplanted with human fetal thymus, liver, and/or lymph nodes).[35] Long-term colony assays provide an in-vitro assay for stem cells, but they are not useful to assess clinical graft potency because of technical challenges and the need to make clinical decisions quickly. Approximately 1% to 3% of marrow cells are CD34+, and only a small fraction of CD34+ cells bear the more primitive phenotype. However, even though the CD34+ cell fraction contains many non-stem cells and the stem cells make up only a small fraction, the number of CD34+ cells can be quickly quantified, and numerous studies have found it to be a reliable gauge of hematopoietic potency.

Marrow cells are collected by multiple needle aspirations from the posterior iliac crests under general anesthesia to remove a volume of 10 to 20 mL/kg of body weight to achieve a cell count goal of 2 to 5×10^8 white cells/kg of recipient body weight. Between 25% and 75% of this material is contaminating peripheral blood, depending on the quality of the specimen and the collection procedure. The volume of marrow removed represents only 1% to 5% of total marrow volume; marrow harvest results in only transient changes in leukocyte and/or platelet counts and has no known long-term hematopoietic consequences. Donors may become anemic, however, and iron is generally given after a harvest to facilitate red cell recovery. Blood counts normalize within 1 month. Serious complications from marrow harvesting are rare, occurring in less than 1.5% of all donations.[38] However, pain at the marrow extraction sites, throat pain from intubation used to administer general anesthesia, and post-anesthesia headache are frequent occurrences.

Peripheral Blood

Progenitors mobilized into the peripheral blood by chemotherapy or by G-CSF are increasingly being used as a graft source.[12,33,34] As noted earlier, stem cells are infrequent in the circulation. The demonstration that adequate numbers of CD34+ cells can be collected from peripheral blood after mobilization using chemotherapy, growth factors, or a combination of the two, as well as observations that durable multilineage engraftment can regularly be achieved using PBPCs, ushered in the modern

Table 22-3. Stem Cell Sources

Stem Cell Source	Advantages	Disadvantages	Comments
Marrow (HPC, Marrow)	• Rich source of stem cells • Fewer lymphocytes than PBPCs (less GVHD)	• Donor requires general anesthesia • Fewer progenitor cells than PBPCs	• Traditional source of stem cells, so greatest body of experience • Remains the preferred choice for unrelated donor grafts and many sibling transplants
Peripheral blood progenitor cells (HPC, Apheresis)	• Large numbers of stem cells • Large numbers of lymphoid cells (greater GVT effect)	• Donor requires G-CSF and greater time devoted to donation	• Preferred source for autologous HSCT • Preferred source for allogeneic transplants using reduced-intensity conditioning regimens (more stem cells and more lymphoid cells to counter recipient immunity) and probably for advanced leukemia (more GVT effect)
Cord blood (HPC, Cord Blood)	• Can be collected without danger to mother or infant • Less chance of transmission of infectious pathogens • Readily usable (in contrast to time needed to arrange collection with adult donors) • Lymphoid cells are immunologically naive	• Lymphoid cells are immunologically naive (takes longer time to exert GVT effect) • Sufficient numbers of stem cells for engraftment for many children, but insufficient numbers for most adults	• Increasingly the preferred graft for unrelated donor transplants in children

HPC = hematopoietic progenitor cell(s); PBPC = peripheral blood progenitor cell; GVHD = graft-vs-host disease; GVT = graft-vs-tumor; G-CSF = granulocyte colony-stimulating factor.

practice of mobilizing progenitors from the marrow into the circulation for collection by apheresis. Mobilization and collection techniques are described in Chapter 23. Potential advantages of HPC(A) over HPC(M) include more rapid engraftment and potentially better tolerance of collection because there is no need for general anesthesia. In the autologous setting, there may be less tumor contamination of HSCT when tumor is present in the marrow.

Regarding the allogeneic HSCT setting, there are approximately tenfold more mature lymphoid cells; that could be either a disadvantage (causing more GVHD) or an advantage [more lymphoid cells to mediate a graft-vs-tumor (GVT) effect and counter recipient immunity that might mediate graft rejection].

In addition to differences in cell numbers between HPC(M) and HPC(A), other differences have also been noted that have functional significance. CD34+ cells from HPC(A) highly coexpress CD13 but coexpress CD7, CD10, CD19, CD71, and c-kit in only low levels.[39] CD34+ cells from HPC(A) have lower expression of a number of adhesion molecules, including VLA-4.[40] They are more likely to be in G0G1 phase[41] and have self-renewal capacity[42] and greater clonogenic potential in response to growth factors[43] compared to marrow progenitors. The T lymphocytes in HPC(A) also differ from steady-state blood T lymphocytes. They demonstrate a polarization from a Th1 to a Th2 immunophenotype and are thus less apt to cause acute GVHD[44] but more apt to mediate chronic GVHD. HPC(A) contains 50-fold more monocytes and substantially more lymphoid dendritic cells than HPC(M); these cells may contribute to down-regulation of the alloreactive potential of T cells in the HPC(A) graft.[45,46] HPC(A) grafts also contain more natural killer (NK) cells, responsible in part for mediating the anti-tumor effect of the graft.[47] Collectively these differences have important biologic implications for GVHD and GVT effects of HPC(A) in allogeneic HSCT.

Bone pain, a side effect of G-CSF, is the most common complication of HPC(A) collection[38,48]; serious adverse events occur in less than 1% of such collections.[38,39] Concerns have been voiced about long-term hematopoietic toxicities of G-CSF, but to date none have been documented in HPC(A) donors. Donor factors to consider in choosing between marrow harvest and PBPC collection, especially in the allogeneic setting, include adequate peripheral venous access (to avoid placing a central venous catheter), the possibility of homologous blood transfusion (more likely with older persons undergoing marrow harvests), morbid obesity or an orthopedic condition that would make marrow harvesting difficult, and allergy to G-CSF or a history of inflammatory eye disorders or autoimmune diseases that might be exacerbated by G-CSF. From the recipient's perspective, the greater risk for GVHD with HPC(A) noted above[20-24] should be considered, particularly in patients transplanted for nonmalignant diseases such as aplastic anemia, where no GVT effect is needed.

Umbilical Cord Blood

Cord blood is increasingly used for matched unrelated allogeneic HSCT, based on its substantial content of immature progenitors, on the demonstration that it can provide sustained multilineage engraftment after myeloablative conditioning, and on its ability to engraft in recipients differing by two HLA antigens from the donor, with less GVHD. Increasing numbers of cord blood banks around the world offer a graft option that can be made available quickly for allogeneic HSCT when there is no suitable family donor.

HPC(CB) units contain at least 10-fold fewer nucleated cells and CD34+ cells than either HPC(M) or HPC(A) grafts, but they have a much higher percentage of immature progenitor cells[49] compared to HPC(M), although the number of progenitors is limited. Megakaryocytic progenitors may be relatively infrequent[50] and, compared to those from HPC(A), have impaired ability to establish the endomitotic cycles required for maturation.[51] T lymphocytes from cord blood tend to respond to primary allogeneic stimulation as well as those from adult marrow or blood, but they show little responsiveness after rechallenge with alloantigen.[52] Their chemokine responsiveness also differs markedly from that of peripheral blood lymphocytes.[53] Although NK cell activity of cord blood is relatively low, cytokines readily activate cord blood NK activity in vitro.[54] These biologic characteristics of HPC(CB) grafts may account for some of the clinical differences seen in allogeneic HSCT, including slow platelet recovery, greater tolerance of HLA disparity with the recipient, and a lower risk for GVHD with apparent retention of a GVT effect.

From the recipient's perspective, the quick availability and the less stringent HLA matching requirements means that recipients who cannot easily proceed with an unrelated donor transplant, because of delay in donor availability or inability to identify a matched donor, can quickly proceed to a cord blood HSCT. A disadvantage of cord blood is that often numbers of hematopoietic progenitors are not adequate for adult recipients. In addition, engraftment, especially of platelets, may be slower. Graft failure occurs in 10% to 20% of cord blood transplants. The parameter most predictive of failure to engraft has been nucleated cell count (lower count indicates higher likelihood for rejection).[55-57] In general, threshold cell doses of 2.5 to 3.5 $\times$ 10^7/kg of recipient body weight are felt to be required for engraftment.[58] To date, CD34+ cell counts and colony assays have not been predictive of engraftment, though they are likely important and may provide useful information with further study. Greater HLA disparity would be expected to confer an increased risk of graft rejection, but this has been more difficult to demonstrate, at least in individuals in whom the mismatch is two antigens or fewer; again, further study is needed. Immune reconstitution is slower, resulting in a greater risk for early opportunistic infections and later development of an anti-tumor effect. Accordingly, although cord blood is increasingly being used in children, its role in adult transplant recipients has yet to be clarified.

Supportive Care

Supportive care includes measures in HCT that are intended to compensate for transient hematopoietic failure.[33] Platelet and red cell transfusions are provided to prevent severe hemorrhage and the consequences of severe anemia.[59] Typically, platelet transfusions are given when the platelet count falls below 10,000 to 20,000/µL, and red cell transfusions, when the hemoglobin falls below 7 to 8 g/dL. Antibiotics are given to compensate for neutropenia and prevent severe infections.[60]

Because multiple medications must be administered intravenously, a tunneled multilumen central venous catheter is usually placed before transplantation and removed after engraftment and resolution of transplant complications.[61]

For allogeneic HSCT, immunosuppressive drugs are administered to facilitate engraftment and prevent GVHD.[62] The introduction of cyclosporine, a calcineurin inhibitor, in the 1980s dramatically improved the survivability of allogeneic HSCT, with improved engraftment rates and lower risks of serious GVHD. Today a calcineurin inhibitor (either cyclosporine or tacrolimus) is usually given in combination with another immunosuppressive agent, such as methotrexate, mycophenolate mofetil, or sirolimus. Drug levels are monitored and adjusted to provide sufficient immunosuppression but avoid toxicity. In general, immunosuppression is tapered with the goal of eventual discontinuation at 6 months, unless GVHD occurs and necessitates more prolonged immunosuppressive therapy. With reduced-intensity HSCT procedures, immunosuppression is tapered more rapidly to facilitate donor immune reconstitution and the GVT effect, although this increases the risk of GVHD.

Over the years, incremental advances in supportive care and new immunosuppressive regimens have contributed to improvements in transplant outcomes.[33] Indeed, it is often argued that much of the improvement in survival is the result of advances in this area.

Indications for HSCT

Over 800,000 transplants have been performed over the past half century, with 55,000 to 60,000 more being performed each year. Leukemia and the myelodysplastic syndromes account for about two-thirds of allogeneic HSCTs, whereas multiple myeloma and non-Hodgkin lymphoma account for about two-thirds of autologous HSCT.[12]

The decision to consider HSCT in a specific patient involves an evaluation of the likelihood that non-HSCT therapies can achieve durable disease control and evaluation of the physiologic fitness of the patient to tolerate the procedure. A suitably matched donor is also a prerequisite for allogeneic HSCT, while collection of an adequate number of progenitors is a prerequisite for autologous HSCT. Diseases for which HSCT may be considered are listed in Table 22-4.

Allogeneic Transplantation

Allogeneic HSCT is a therapeutic option for patients with acute or chronic leukemias, myelodysplastic syndromes, or aplastic anemia.[33,63] For patients with acute myelogenous or lymphoblastic leukemia, allogeneic HSCT is considered if the leukemia fails to respond to initial induction chemotherapy or relapses after initial response. In patients in first remission, certain cytogenetic abnormalities that indicate a poor prospect for durable control with chemotherapy are considered indications for HSCT. Because durable control of chronic myelogenous leukemia can be achieved with imatinib, allogeneic HSCT is currently considered only in patients who become unresponsive to imatinib or whose disease is in accelerated phase or blast crisis. In patients with myelodysplastic syndrome, allogeneic HSCT is considered if there are excessive numbers of blasts, adverse cytogenetic findings, or multilineage cytopenias. Patients with severe aplastic anemia are considered for allogeneic HSCT if they have a matched sibling donor. Other myeloproliferative diseases, severe sickle cell anemia, thalassemia, and other serious hematologic diseases are occasionally considered for allogeneic HSCT.

Autologous Transplantation

Autologous HSCT is a therapeutic option for patients with multiple myeloma or lymphoma.[12,33,63] For myeloma patients, autologous HSCT has been shown to confer a survival advantage and is therefore considered in patients after a course of initial chemotherapy to reduce disease burden. Autologous HSCT is also beneficial in patients with recurrent myeloma. Clinical trials show that tandem

HSCT can offer an additional survival benefit in patients with multiple myeloma, predominantly in those patients whose response to the first transplant is less than complete. For patients with aggressive lymphoma, autologous HSCT is considered after relapse. In some patients with aggressive forms of lymphoma, autologous HSCT is also considered in first remission. Other diseases, such as advanced neuroblastoma, recurrent or persistent Hodgkin disease, recurrent low-grade non-Hodgkin lymphoma, pediatric central nervous system tumors, and recurrent testicular carcinoma, are also considered for autologous HSCT. For some diseases, such as recurrent lymphoma or Hodgkin disease, cure is frequently achieved with autologous HSCT, while for other diseases such as multiple myeloma, cure is not achievable, but HSCT can provide durable remission and prolongation of survival.

Future Trends

Progress in HSCT in the past can be attributed to advances in supportive care, ease of progenitor cell collection, greater access to suitable donors, and more tolerable conditioning regimens. Improved outcomes in turn led to use of HSCT earlier in the course of disease, in older patients, and for additional diseases. It is anticipated that incremental advances will continue and lead to even better outcomes. A recent State of Science meeting delineated the highest priority trials for the upcoming next 5 to 10 years.[64]

Immunologic Approaches

In particular, if history offers a lesson, improved understanding of immunity is likely to offer keys to improved outcomes. Haploidentical family donors, who share only one set of HLA antigens with the recipient, are almost always available. Outcomes with such donors have been poor in the past because of both GVHD and the inability of recipients to recover robust immunity against opportunistic pathogens. Yet a number of initiatives are underway. Some tri-

Table 22-4. Diseases for Which HSCT Is Often Used

Disease	Disease Status	Type of HSCT
Acute myelogenous leukemia	After relapse	Allogeneic
	In first remission if high-risk cytogenetics	Allogeneic
	Refractory to initial induction	Allogeneic
Acute lymphoblastic leukemia	After relapse	Allogeneic
	In first remission if high-risk cytogenetics	Allogeneic
	Refractory to initial induction	Allogeneic
Myelodysplastic syndromes	Excessive blasts or high-risk cytogenetics or multilineage cytopenias	Allogeneic
Chronic myelogenous leukemia	Imatinib failure	Allogeneic
	Accelerated phase	Allogeneic
	Blast crisis	Allogeneic
Chronic lymphocytic leukemia	After relapse with more aggressive behavior or with high-risk cytogenetics	Allogeneic
Aplastic anemia	Severe category	Allogeneic
Myeloproliferative diseases	"Spent" phase with marrow failure, or high-risk features with impending marrow failure or acceleration to acute leukemia	Allogeneic
Hemoglobinopathies, such as β-thalassemia or sickle cell anemia	Disease state with high-risk prognostic features	Allogeneic
Intermediate- or high-grade non-Hodgkin lymphoma	After relapse	Autologous
	High-risk features in first remission	Autologous
Low-grade non-Hodgkin lymphoma	After relapse with short first remission or aggressive behavior or Richter's transformation	Autologous or allogeneic
Hodgkin disease	After relapse or refractory to initial therapy	Autologous
Multiple myeloma	In first remission	Autologous
	After relapse	Autologous
Neuroblastoma	Advanced stage in first remission	Autologous
Pediatric central nervous system tumors	Aggressive malignancy	Autologous

als are evaluating administration of high-dose cyclophosphamide in the early posttransplant period to abrogate alloreactive donor T cells.[65] Other investigators are rendering donor cells anergic to recipient antigens before transplantation.[66] Additional avenues of research include measures to enhance NK activity after HSCT to enhance the GVT effect.[67] Building on the observations that DLI can reverse relapse, trials are exploring adjuvant DLI to hasten immune reconstitution, enhance donor chimerism, and boost the GVT effect to reduce the chance of relapse.[68] Identification of subpopulations of immune cells, which have anti-infective properties or anti-tumor activity, for expansion ex vivo are under investigation.[69] Such cells could then be administered after transplantation in an adjuvant fashion in patients at high risk for relapse. The use of adoptive immunotherapy in solid tumors is in its infancy, but pilot studies are underway (see Chapters 26 and 27). Vaccine strategies targeting tumors and infectious agents are also being evaluated in the posttransplant setting.[70]

Graft Engineering

Graft engineering was an active area of interest in the past. Much work was done on T-cell depletion; although this is technically feasible and can reduce the risk for severe GVHD, that benefit is offset by greater risks of graft rejection, relapse, and opportunistic infection. Because of negligible net benefit, interest in T-cell depletion has waned. There was also interest in expanding the number of progenitors by incubating the graft ex vivo with mixtures of growth factors. Although several cocktails expanded progenitors, the number of truly primitive stem cells has not been shown to increase, and interest in that approach has also waned, though there has been a recent resurgence of interest focused on cord blood.[71] Using newer expansion strategies, pilot trials are evaluating the utility of "expanded" cord blood units to achieve better engraftment. Molecules that might enhance engraftment by improving the homing of transplanted hemato-poietic cells to the marrow are also under investigation.[72]

Future Applications

As risks recede, HSCT will be offered to yet other individuals not considered candidates at present. Similarly, it is likely that other applications will be explored. The use of hematopoietic stem cells for tissue repair in regenerative medicine is now a field of active research (see Chapter 25), and a number of trials are exploring hematopoietic cells in therapies for cardiovascular diseases, diabetes, degenerative neurologic disorders, and autoimmune diseases.[73-75]

References

1. Barnes DW, Corp MJ, Loutit JF, Neal FE. Treatment of murine leukaemia with X rays and homologous bone marrow; preliminary communication. Br Med J 1956;2:626-7.
2. Thomas ED, Lochte HL Jr, Lu WC, Ferrebee JW. Intravenous infusion of bone marrow in patients receiving radiation and chemotherapy. N Engl J Med 1957;257:491-6.
3. Mathe G, Jammet H, Pendic B, et al. Transfusions and grafts of homologous bone marrow in humans after accidental high dosage irradiation. Rev Fr Etud Clin Biol 1959;4:226-38.
4. Baranov A, Gale RP, Guskova A, et al. Bone marrow transplantation after the Chernobyl nuclear accident. N Engl J Med 1989;321:205-12.
5. Weinstock DM, Case C Jr, Bader JL, et al. Radiologic and nuclear events: Contingency planning for hematologists/oncologists. Blood 2008;111:5440-5.
6. Bortin MM. A compendium of reported human bone marrow transplants. Transplantation 1970;9:571-87.
7. Billingham RE, Brent L, Medawar PB. "Actively acquired tolerance" of foreign cells. Nature 1953;172:603-6.
8. Klein J, Sato A. The HLA system. First of two parts. N Engl J Med 2000;343:702-9.
9. Hansen JA, Clift RA, Thomas ED, et al. Transplantation of marrow from an unrelated donor to a patient with acute leukemia. N Engl J Med 1980;303:165-7.

10. Storb R, Deeg HJ, Whitehead J, et al. Methotrexate and cyclosporine compared with cyclosporine alone for prophylaxis of acute graft-versus-host disease after marrow transplantation for acute leukemia. N Engl J Med 1986;314:729-35.
11. Thomas ED, Storb R, Clift RA, et al. Bone marrow transplantation. N Engl J Med 1975;292:832-43.
12. Horowitz MM. Uses and growth of hematopoietic cell transplantation. In: Appelbaum FR, Forman SJ, Negrin RS, Blume KG, eds. Thomas' hematopoietic cell transplantation. 4th ed. Oxford, UK: Wiley-Blackwell, 2009:15-26.
13. McGovern JJ Jr, Russell PS, Atkins L, Webster EW. Treatment of terminal leukemic relapse by total body irradiation and intravenous infusion of stored autologous bone marrow obtained during remission. N Engl J Med 1959;260:675-83.
14. Kurnick NB. Autologous and isologous bone marrow storage and infusion in the treatment of myelo-suppresson. Transfusion 1962;2:178-87.
15. Appelbaum FR, Deisseroth AB, Graw RG Jr, et al. Prolonged complete remission following high dose chemotherapy of Burkitt's lymphoma in relapse. Cancer 1978;41:1059-63.
16. Kanteti R, Miller K, McCann J, et al. Randomized trial of peripheral blood progenitor cell vs bone marrow as hematopoietic support for high-dose chemotherapy in patients with non-Hodgkin's lymphoma and Hodgkin's disease: A clinical and molecular analysis. Bone Marrow Transplant 1999;24:473-81.
17. Vose JM, Sharp G, Chan WC, et al. Autologous transplantation for aggressive non-Hodgkin's lymphoma: Results of a randomized trial evaluating graft source and minimal residual disease. J Clin Oncol 2002;20:2344-52.
18. Torey CA, Snyder EL. Hematopoietic progenitor cell administration. In: Wingard JR, Gastineau D, Leather H, et al, eds. Hematopoietic stem cell transplantation: A handbook for clinicians. Bethesda, MD: AABB, 2009:151-62.
19. Bolanos-Meade J, Jones RJ. Conditioning regimens. In: Wingard JR, Gastineau D, Leather H, et al, eds. Hematopoietic stem cell transplantation: A handbook for clinicians. Bethesda, MD: AABB, 2009:51-60.
20. Champlin RE, Schmitz N, Horowitz MM, et al. Blood stem cells compared with bone marrow as a source of hematopoietic cells for allogeneic transplantation. IBMTR Histocompatibility and Stem Cell Sources Working Committee and the European Group for Blood and Marrow Transplantation (EBMT). Blood 2000;95:3702-9.
21. Bensinger WI, Martin PJ, Storer B, et al. Transplantation of bone marrow as compared with peripheral-blood cells from HLA-identical relatives in patients with hematologic cancers. N Engl J Med 2001;344:175-81.
22. Schmitz N, Beksac M, Hasenclever D, et al. Transplantation of mobilized peripheral blood cells to HLA-identical siblings with standard-risk leukemia. Blood 2002;100:761-7.
23. Stem Cell Trialists' Collaborative Group. Allogeneic peripheral blood stem-cell compared with bone marrow transplantation in the management of hematologic malignancies: An individual patient data meta-analysis of nine randomized trials. J Clin Oncol 2005;23:5074-87.
24. Eapen M, Logan BR, Confer DL, et al. Peripheral blood grafts from unrelated donors are associated with increased acute and chronic graft versus-host disease without improved survival. Biol Blood Marrow Transplant 2007;13:1461-8.
25. Confer D, Robinett P. The US National Marrow Donor Program role in unrelated donor hematopoietic cell transplantation. Bone Marrow Transplant 2008;42(Suppl 1):S3-S5.
26. Hurley CK, Fernandez-Vina M, Hildebrand WH, et al. A high degree of HLA disparity arises from limited allelic diversity: Analysis of 1775 unrelated bone marrow transplant donor-recipient pairs. Hum Immunol 2007;68:30-40.
27. Lee SJ, Klein J, Haagenson M, et al. High-resolution donor-recipient HLA matching contributes to the success of unrelated donor marrow transplantation. Blood 2007;110:4576-83.
28. Weisdorf D, Spellman S, Haagenson M, et al. Classification of HLA-matching for retrospective analysis of unrelated donor transplantation: Revised definitions to predict survival. Biol Blood Marrow Transplant 2008;14:748-58.
29. Stanevsky A, Goldstein G, Nagler A. Umbilical cord blood transplantation: Pros, cons and beyond. Blood Rev 2009;23:199-204.
30. Weiden PL, Flournoy N, Thomas ED, et al. Antileukemic effect of graft-versus-host disease in human recipients of allogeneic-marrow grafts. N Engl J Med 1979;300:1068-73.

31. Kolb HJ. Graft-versus-leukemia effects of transplantation and donor lymphocytes. Blood 2008;112:4371-83.
32. Valcárcel D, Martino R. Reduced intensity conditioning for allogeneic hematopoietic stem cell transplantation in myelodysplastic syndromes and acute myelogenous leukemia. Curr Opin Oncol 2007;19:660-6.
33. Wingard JR. Overview of hematopoietic stem cell transplantation. In: Wingard JR, Gastineau D, Leather H, et al, eds. Hematopoietic stem cell transplantation: A handbook for clinicians. Bethesda, MD: AABB, 2009:1-8.
34. Korbling M. Stem cell grafts. In: Wingard JR, Gastineau D, Leather H, et al, eds. Hematopoietic stem cell transplantation: A handbook for clinicians. Bethesda, MD: AABB, 2009:105-14.
35. Baum CM, Weissman IL, Tsukamoto AS, et al. Isolation of a candidate human hematopoietic stem-cell population. Proc Natl Acad Sci U S A 1992;89:2804-8.
36. Till JE, McCulloch EA. A direct measurement of the radiation sensitivity of normal mouse bone marrow cells. Radiat Res 1961;14:213-22.
37. Becker AJ, McCulloch EA, Till JE. Cytological demonstration of the clonal nature of spleen colonies derived from transplanted mouse marrow cells. Nature 1963;197:452-4.
38. Miller JP, Perry EH, Price TH, et al. Recovery and safety profiles of marrow and PBSC donors: Experience of the National Marrow Donor Program. Biol Blood Marrow Transplant 2008;14(Suppl 9):29-36.
39. Gyger M, Stuart RK, Perreault C. Immunobiology of allogeneic peripheral blood mononuclear cells mobilized with granulocyte-colony stimulating factor. Bone Marrow Transplant 2000;26:1-16.
40. Mohle R, Murea S, Kirsh M, Haas R. Differential expression of L-selectin, VLA-4 and LFA-1 on CD34+ progenitor cells from the bone marrow and peripheral blood during G-CSF enhanced recovery. Exp Hematol 1995;23:1535-42.
41. Lemoli RM, Tafuri A, Fortuna A, et al. Cycling status of CD34+ cells mobilized into peripheral blood of healthy donors by recombinant human granulocyte colony-stimulating factor. Blood 1997;89:1189-96.
42. Petzer AL, Hogge DE, Landsdorp PM, et al. Self-renewal of primitive human hematopoietic stem cells (long-term-culture initiating cells) *in*

vitro and their expansion in defined medium. Proc Natl Acad Sci U S A 1996;93:1470-4.
43. Brandt JE, Srour EF, van Besien K, et al. Cytokine-dependent long-term culture of highly enriched precursors of hematopoietic progenitor cells from human bone marrow. J Clin Invest 1990;86:932-41.
44. Pan L, Delmonte J, Jalonen CK, Ferrara JLM. Pretreatment of donor mice with granulocyte colony-stimulating factor polarizes donor T lymphocytes toward type-2 cytokine production and reduces the severity of experimental graft-versus-host disease. Blood 1995;86:4422-9.
45. Mielcarek M, Graf L, Johnson G, Torok-Storb B. Production of interleukin-10 by granulocyte colony-stimulating factor mobilized blood products: A mechanism for monocyte mediated suppression of T-cell proliferation. Blood 1998;92:215-22.
46. Arpinati M, Loken M, Anasetti C. G-CSF mobilizes type-2 dendritic cells rather than type 1-dendritic cells (abstract). Blood 1998;92(Suppl 1):111a.
47. Barrett AJ, Malkovska V. Graft-versus-leukemia: Understanding and using the alloimmune response to treat hematological malignancies. Br J Haematol 1996;93:754-61.
48. Pulsipher MA, Chitphakdithai P, Miller JP, et al. Adverse events among 2408 unrelated donors of peripheral blood stem cells: Results of a prospective trial from the National Marrow Donor Program. Blood 2009;113:3604-11.
49. Broxmeyer HE, Hangoc G, Cooper S, et al. Growth characteristics and expansion of human umbilical cord blood and estimation of its potential for transplantation in adults. Proc Natl Acad Sci U S A 1992;89:4109-13.
50. Kanamaru S, Kawano Y, Watanabe T, et al. Low numbers of megakaryocyte progenitors in grafts of cord blood cells may result in delayed platelet recovery after cord blood cell transplant. Stem Cells 2000;18:190-5.
51. Bornstein R, García-Vela J, Gilsanz F, et al. Cord blood megakaryocytes do not complete maturation, as indicated by impaired establishment of endomitosis and low expression of G1/S cyclins upon thrombopoietin-induced differentiation. Br J Haematol 2001;114:458-65.
52. Risdon G, Gaddy J, Horie M, Broxmeyer HE. Alloantigen priming induces a state of unresponsiveness in human umbilical cord blood T cells. Proc Natl Acad Sci U S A 1995;92:2413-17.

53. Sato K, Kawasaki H, Nagayama H, et al. Chemokine receptor expressions and responsiveness of cord blood T cells. J Immunol 2001;166:1659-66.

54. Gaddy J, Risdon G, Broxmeyer HE. Cord blood natural killer cells are functionally and phenotypically immature but readily respond to interleukin-2 and interleukin-12. J Interferon Cytokine Res 1995;15:527-36.

55. Gluckman E, Rocha V, Boyer-Chammard A, et al. Outcome of cord-blood transplantation from related and unrelated donors. Eurocord Transplant Group and the European Blood and Marrow Transplantation Group. N Engl J Med 1997;337:373-81.

56. Rubinstein P, Carrier C, Scaradavou A, et al. Outcomes among 562 recipients of placental-blood transplants from unrelated donors. N Engl J Med 1998;339:1565-77.

57. Rubinstein P, Stevens CE. Placental blood for bone marrow replacement: The New York Blood Center's program and clinical results. Baillieres Best Pract Res Clin Haematol 2000; 13:565-84.

58. Armitage S, Shpall EJ. Cord blood graft collection and processing. In: Wingard JR, Gastineau D, Leather H, et al, eds. Hematopoietic stem cell transplantation: A handbook for clinicians. Bethesda, MD: AABB, 2009:125-35.

59. Meyer ERG, Szczepiorkowski ZM. Transfusion support of HSCT recipients. In: Wingard JR, Gastineau D, Leather H, et al, eds. Hematopoietic stem cell transplantation: A handbook for clinicians. Bethesda, MD: AABB, 2009:207-26.

60. Wingard JR. Infections prior to engraftment. In: Wingard JR, Gastineau D, Leather H, et al, eds. Hematopoietic stem cell transplantation: A handbook for clinicians. Bethesda, MD: AABB, 2009:197-206.

61. Andrews JC. Venous access for hematopoietic stem cell transplant patients. In: Wingard JR, Gastineau D, Leather H, et al, eds. Hematopoietic stem cell transplantation: A handbook for clinicians. Bethesda, MD: AABB, 2009:249-66.

62. Chao NJ, Sullivan KM. Pharmacologic prevention of acute graft-versus-host disease. In: Appelbaum FR, Forman SJ, Negrin RS, Blume KG, eds. Thomas' hematopoietic cell transplantation. 4th ed. Oxford, UK: Wiley-Blackwell, 2009:1257-74.

63. Antin JH. Common uses of hematopoietic stem cell transplantation. In: Wingard JR, Gastineau D, Leather H, et al, eds. Hematopoietic stem cell transplantation: A handbook for clinicians. Bethesda, MD: AABB, 2009:9-26.

64. Ferrara JL, Anasetti C, Stadtmauer E, et al. Blood and Marrow Transplant Clinical Trials Network State of the Science Symposium 2007. Biol Blood Marrow Transplant 2007; 13:1268-85.

65. Kasamon YL, Luznik L, Leffell MS, et al. Non-myeloablative HLA-haploidentical BMT with high-dose posttransplantation cyclophosphamide: Effect of HLA disparity on outcome. Biol Blood Marrow Transplant 2010;16:482-9.

66. Davies JK, Gribben JG, Brennan LL, et al. Outcome of alloanergized haploidentical bone marrow transplantation after ex vivo costimulatory blockade: Results of 2 phase 1 studies. Blood 2008;112:2232-41.

67. Rubnitz JE, Inaba H, Ribeiro RC, et al. NKAML: A pilot study to determine the safety and feasibility of haploidentical natural killer cell transplantation in childhood acute myeloid leukemia. J Clin Oncol 2010;28:955-9.

68. Kolb HJ. Graft-versus-leukemia effects of transplantation and donor lymphocytes. Blood 2008;112:4371-83.

69. Peggs KS. Adoptive T cell immunotherapy for cytomegalovirus. Expert Opin Biol Ther 2009; 9:725-36.

70. Roback JD. Vaccine-enhanced donor lymphocyte infusion (veDLI). Hematology Am Soc Hematol Educ Program 2006:486-91,513.

71. Advani AS, Laughlin MJ. Umbilical cord blood transplantation for acute myeloid leukemia. Curr Opin Hematol 2009;16:124-8.

72. Rocha V, Broxmeyer H. New approaches for improving engraftment after cord blood transplantation. Biol Blood Marrow Transplant 2010;16(1 Suppl):S126-32.

73. George JC. Stem cell therapy in acute myocardial infarction: A review of clinical trials. Transl Res 2010;155:10-19.

74. Haller MJ, Wasserfall CH, McGrail KM, et al. Autologous umbilical cord blood transfusion in very young children with type 1 diabetes. Diabetes Care 2009;32:2041-6.

75. Chang YC, Shyu WC, Lin SZ, Li H. Regenerative therapy for stroke. Cell Transplant 2007; 16:171-81.

In: McLeod BC, Szczepiorkowski ZM, Weinstein R, Winters JL, eds.
Apheresis: Principles and Practice, 3rd edition
Bethesda, MD: AABB Press, 2010

23

Mobilization and Collection of Peripheral Blood Hematopoietic Progenitor Cells

Joseph Schwartz, MD; Anand Padmanabhan, MD, PhD;
Richard O. Francis, MD, PhD; and Michael L. Linenberger, MD, FACP

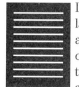 LANDMARK STUDIES IN THE late 1950s demonstrated that autologous or syngeneic marrow cells could successfully reconstitute hematopoiesis after myeloablative treatment.[1] For many years thereafter, marrow was used as the primary graft source for hematopoietic stem cell transplantation (HSCT; see also Chapter 22). Although multipotent hematopoietic stem cells (HSCs) were known to circulate in the blood, their low frequencies in "steady state" (ie, without prior chemotherapy or cytokine prestimulation) precluded routine harvesting from that source. Some patients were successfully transplanted with autologous blood hematopoietic progenitor cells (HPCs), but 6 to 17 daily leukapheresis procedures were required to collect enough cells.[2,3] After 1989, blood HPC products—referred to as HPC, Apheresis or HPC(A)—became increasingly available because mobilization regimens were developed that were safe, reliable, and effective, while mononuclear cell (MNC) collection techniques were

Joseph Schwartz, MD, Associate Professor of Clinical Pathology and Cell Biology, and Director of Transfusion Medicine and Cellular Therapy, Columbia University Medical Center, New York Presbyterian Hospital, New York, New York; Anand Padmanabhan, MD, PhD, Fellow, Transfusion Medicine and Apheresis, The Institute for Transfusion Medicine, University of Pittsburgh Medical Center, Pittsburgh, Pennsylvania; Richard O. Francis, MD, PhD, Chief Resident, Department of Pathology and Cell Biology, Columbia University Medical Center, New York Presbyterian Hospital, New York, New York; and Michael L. Linenberger, MD, FACP, Professor of Medicine, University of Washington, and Medical Director, Apheresis and Cellular Therapy, Seattle Cancer Care Alliance (Associate Member, Fred Hutchinson Cancer Research Center), Seattle, Washington

The authors have disclosed no conflicts of interest.

refined to efficiently and safely collect mobilized HPCs in an outpatient setting.[4-6]

This chapter reviews blood HPC mobilization and procurement, including the rationale and use of this graft source for clinical applications, the relevant physiologic principles, apheresis technical and procedural issues, product safety considerations, regulatory standards, and the potential complications affecting donors and patients. The relative merits and limitations of HPC(A) products vs marrow harvest products—referred to as HPC, Marrow or HPC(M)—are also highlighted in order to provide the apheresis practitioner an appreciation of current practices and future trends.

Clinical Applications of Blood HPCs

Blood HPCs are currently the preferred graft source for most patients undergoing autologous and allogeneic HSCT for malignant hematologic diseases. Compared to standard, unmanipulated marrow harvests, mobilized blood HPC(A) products are relatively small in volume with few contaminating red cells and significantly more multipotent and committed HPCs, lymphocytes, and other MNCs. These enriched cell populations lead to more rapid hematopoietic engraftment and faster immune reconstitution after HSCT. This translates into shorter recovery times [2 vs 3 weeks to reach an absolute neutrophil count of 500/μL and 3 vs 4 weeks to reach a platelet count of 20,000/μL with HPC(A) and HPC(M), respectively] with fewer infectious complications and decreased early morbidity and mortality.[7] Because of these advantages, over 90% of all pediatric and adult autologous HSCTs and two-thirds to three-quarters of adult related and unrelated donor HSCTs in 2007 used HPC(A).[8-10]

Despite the benefits of faster engraftment with HPC(A), limitations and concerns still exist in the allogeneic setting. When the related donor is a child, marrow is often preferred because of uncertainty over the long-term safety of brief cytokine exposure and potential greater risks to the pediatric donor undergoing

apheresis. If the patient has a nonmalignant, acquired marrow failure disorder or a congenital disease, HPC(M) is usually preferred because of concerns about increased risks of graft-vs-host disease (GVHD) complications with HPC(A).

A number of retrospective analyses and nonrandomized trials have observed significantly higher rates of chronic and, in some cases, acute GVHD among adult recipients of sibling and unrelated donor HPC(A) following myeloablative or reduced-intensity HSCT.[11-16] This risk has been linked to higher HPC doses.[17,18] Moreover, the severity, duration, and infectious complications of chronic GVHD among recipients of HPC(A) appear to be worse than in recipients of HPC(M).[19,20] For HPC(A) recipients with more aggressive neoplastic diseases, more GVHD may be associated with a more potent graft-vs-tumor (GVT) effect that translates into lower disease relapse rates.[13,18] Uncertainty remains, however, because some randomized trials observed no differences in GVHD rates and disease outcomes in adult recipients of HPC(M) vs HPC(A) from sibling donors.[21,22] It is also unclear whether pediatric HSCT patients receiving HPC(A) rather than HPC(M) have a higher GVHD risk, a lower relapse rate, and/or different long-term survival.[23-25]

Questions regarding the relative benefits and disadvantages of blood HPCs compared to marrow are currently being addressed in the unrelated donor setting through a large, multicenter, randomized clinical trial sponsored by the Blood and Marrow Transplant Clinical Trials Network and the National Marrow Donor Program (NMDP).[26] This debate has also triggered renewed interest in the potential merits of using exogenous cytokines to "prestimulate" hematopoiesis before standard or large-volume HPC(M) harvest. Administration of recombinant human granulocyte colony-stimulating factor [G-CSF; filgrastim (Neupogen, Amgen Inc, Thousand Oaks, CA)] to healthy individuals at doses of 5 or 10 μg/kg/day for 4 to 6 days can increase the marrow HPC content by 1.5- to 2-fold.[27,28] Neutrophil engraftment rates in nonrandomized trials using "G-primed" (G-CSF-primed) HPC(M) from patients and donors have been significantly faster than those obtained with steady-state marrow alone, and in some cases the speed of engraftment approached that seen with HPC(A).[27,29-32] Ongoing randomized clinical trials are examining the relative engraftment times and clinical benefits of G-primed HPC(M) compared to HPC(A) and whether HPC(M) recipients have lower rates and severity of GVHD and its related complications.

Mobilization of HPCs

Hematopoietic Stem and Progenitor Cells

Multipotent HSCs give rise to all hematopoietic and lymphoid cell types. They can migrate, self-renew, proliferate, and differentiate into a wide range of phenotypic lineages. By comparison, HPCs are a population of functionally and phenotypically heterogenous precursor cells that include HSCs and more committed multipotent, oligopotent, and unipotent progenitors. Short-term engraftment (ranging from weeks to a few months) can be initiated by more committed HPCs, while long-term multilineage hematopoietic reconstitution (years) is carried out by HSCs.[33] The CD34 antigen, a surface glycoprotein present on HPCs, is a very useful molecule in the clinic for identifying, quantitating, and purifying stem and progenitor cells. Multiple studies have shown that the number of transplanted CD34+ cells correlates with engraftment kinetics.[34,35] Although the CD34 antigen is present on approximately 1% to 3 % of MNCs in the marrow, only approximately 0.06% of the circulating nucleated cells in peripheral blood are CD34+.[36,37] Therefore, during steady-state hematopoiesis the concentration of HPCs in peripheral blood is very low. Although blood HPC collection by apheresis has been performed in unstimulated patients and successful HSCT achieved,[2,3] mobilization methods are now universally employed to facilitate procurement.

The Hematopoietic Niche and HPC Homing

The hematopoietic microenvironment plays an important role in the maintenance and proliferation of HSCs and HPCs.[38] Important cellular components of the marrow niche include fibroblasts, endothelial cells, osteoblasts, and mesenchymal stem cells, which are capable of generating osteoblasts, adipocytes, and chondrocytes. HSCs express adhesion molecules, including very late antigen-4 (VLA-4) and Mac-1, chemokine receptors CXCR4 and CXCR2, cell surface glycoproteins CD44 and CD62L, and the tyrosine kinase receptor c-kit.[39] In turn, molecules found on the marrow stromal cells and/or in the extracellular matrix include stromal-cell-derived factor 1 (SDF-1, also designated CXCL12), the CXC chemokine GRO-β, vascular cell adhesion molecule 1 (VCAM-1), kit ligand, P-selectin glycoprotein ligand 1, and hyaluronic acid, which are cognate ligands for stem cell adhesion molecules.[39] In addition to the role of integrins in homing and lodgment, integrin (eg, VLA-4)-mediated binding to extracellular ligands such as fibronectin and VCAM-1 protects HSCs from apoptosis, helps maintain quiescence,[40,41] and preserves the cell in an undifferentiated state.[42] Molecular components of the hematopoietic niche, such as annexin-II,[43] angiopoietin-1, and N-cadherin,[44] have also been implicated in HSC regulation.

Homing is a process by which circulating HPCs actively cross the blood endothelial barrier to lodge in the marrow compartment. Homing is also important in maintaining marrow homeostasis and steady-state hematopoiesis. The most immature HPCs demonstrate several-fold-stronger cytoadhesive properties than more committed lineage-positive cells.[45] SDF-1/CXCL12, which is secreted by marrow stromal cells, binds to the CXCR4 ligand, expressed on CD34+ HPCs.[46] This interaction is thought to be the principal axis that regulates retention, migration, and mobilization of HSCs during steady-state hematopoiesis and microenvironmental injury.[47] Total body irradiation and high-dose chemotherapy used to "condition" a patient before HSCT may aid in passage of cells into and out of the marrow by virtue of the transient physical disruption of the endothelial barrier. This complex process involves different subsets of HPCs with differing homing properties.[48]

Mechanisms of HPC Mobilization

A number of physiologic factors and stressors can affect HPC homing and mobilization, some of which have been evaluated for blood HPC procurement. For example, the sympathetic nervous system transduces circadian information from the suprachiasmatic nucleus of the brain to the marrow microenvironment, directing circadian oscillations in hematopoiesis and HPC migration.[49] Consistent with this finding, a retrospective analysis of G-CSF-mobilized patients has revealed a higher stem cell yield when apheresis occurred later during the day.[50] Parathyroid hormone (PTH) also modulates HSC proliferation and lodgment. Administration of PTH to both humans and mice expands the number of marrow and peripheral blood HPCs.[51,52] Pathologic conditions such as stroke,[53] acute myocardial infarction,[54] and ischemia/reperfusion injury associated with liver transplantation induce mobilization of HPCs from marrow into peripheral blood.

The earliest attempts to specifically mobilize HPCs into the peripheral blood for collection and autologous transplantation employed myelosuppressive chemotherapy.[55] Chemotherapeutic agents that induce transient aplasia, such as high-dose cyclophosphamide, stimulate the egress of HPCs into the blood during hematopoietic recovery. This mobilization effect peaks at 10 to 18 days after administration of chemotherapy.[56] Mobilization with a cytokine in addition to myelosuppressive chemotherapy has a synergistic effect on HPC release from the marrow.

Recombinant human G-CSF, the most commonly used cytokine for HPC mobilization in chemotherapy-treated patients, increases matrix metalloproteinase-9 concentrations and induces the release of other proteolytic enzymes from myeloid cells that cleave cytoadhesive interactions in the marrow microenvironment.[57] Of note, the ability of G-CSF to mobilize HPCs in

protease-deficient mice suggests that both protease-dependent and protease-independent pathways of HPC mobilization exist.[58] When given alone, G-CSF induces a peak in blood HPC concentration at roughly 5 days after administration. This predictable and reproducible effect obviates any need for precollection monitoring of blood CD34+ cell counts when mobilizing healthy donors in steady state. By contrast, G-CSF treatment following myelosuppressive chemotherapy often results in unpredictable HPC mobilization kinetics; therefore, HPC enumeration is necessary to determine the optimal time to start leukapheresis.

Recombinant human granulocyte-macrophage colony-stimulating factor [GM-CSF; sargramostim (Leukine, Bayer Healthcare Pharmaceuticals, Wayne, NJ)] induces mobilization by stimulating proliferation and differentiation of hematopoietic progenitors, monocytes and dendritic cells.[59] GM-CSF is approved by the Food and Drug Administration (FDA) for HPC mobilization in patients but not for allogeneic donors. G-CSF and GM-CSF combinations are sometimes used as a salvage regimen when mobilization with G-CSF alone has been unsuccessful.[60] Other agents, such as the c-kit ligand, stem cell factor (SCF), act as potent synergizing mitogens with other hematopoietic growth factors. Recombinant methionyl human SCF [ancestim (Stemgen, Amgen Inc)] in combination with G-CSF has been shown to enhance HPC mobilization.[61]

Plerixafor (Mozobil, previously AMD3100, Genzyme Corporation, Cambridge, MA) is a selective and reversible antagonist of CXCR4.[62] Plerixafor disrupts the interaction of CXCR4 with SDF-1/CXCL12, causing the release of HPCs into the circulation (Fig 23-1). Initial clinical trials using this drug to investigate activity against human immunodeficiency virus (HIV) showed an unexpected side effect: an increase in white cell (WBC) and blood CD34+ HPC counts.[62] This side effect has been exploited for the purpose of HPC mobilization. Early studies demonstrated that plerixafor augments CD34+ cell mobilization in conjunction with G-CSF, resulting in a median 4.4-fold increase in CD34+ cell mobilization when compared to G-

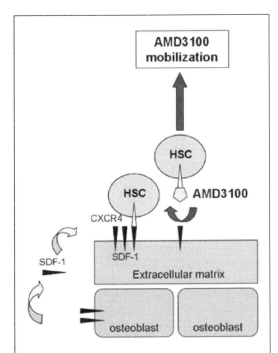

AMD3100
mobilization

HSC

HSC   AMD3100

CXCR4

SDF-1   SDF-1

Extracellular matrix

osteoblast   osteoblast

Figure 23-1. Stromal-cell-derived factor 1 (SDF-1) secreted by marrow stromal cells retains hematopoietic progenitor and stem cells (HSCs) via SDF-1/chemokine receptor 4 (CXCR4) interactions in marrow niches. Plerixafor (AMD3100, now Mozobil) interferes with this interaction by directly binding CXCR4, thereby releasing HSCs into the circulation. (Reproduced with permission from Nervi et al.[39])

CSF alone[63]; more recent trials have confirmed the efficacy and safety of this agent.[64] Plerixafor in combination with G-CSF received FDA approval in 2008 for mobilization of peripheral blood HPCs in patients with non-Hodgkin lymphoma (NHL) and multiple myeloma (MM).

Rapid mobilization with plerixafor alone (without G-CSF) and collection of adequate functional allogeneic donor HPCs for successful myeloablative HSCT has also been reported.[65] In that pilot study, blood CD34+ cell levels increased eightfold following a single dose of plerixafor. Notably, more CD3+ and CD4+ cells but fewer CD34+ cells were mobilized following plerixafor compared with the standard 5-day G-CSF regimen.[65] The incidence of GVHD among recipients was not increased;

however, the follow-up in this small cohort was short. Animal model studies suggest that blood HPCs mobilized with plerixafor are enriched for long-term repopulating cells compared to those mobilized with G-CSF.[66,67] Investigation in a primate model using RNA microarrays also showed that the gene expression pattern of blood CD34+ cells differed based on whether plerixafor and/or G-CSF was used for mobilization.[68] Plerixafor-mobilized CD34+ cells expressed more B-cell, T-cell, and mast-cell genes, while G-CSF-mobilized cells expressed genes typical for neutrophils and mononuclear phagocytes. When both plerixafor and G-CSF were used for mobilization, the up-regulated genes included many that were not up-regulated by either drug alone. The alternative mechanism of action of plerixafor is also reflected by observations that patients who failed prior mobilization attempts with G-CSF and myelosuppressive chemotherapy were often successfully salvaged with the use of plerixafor plus G-CSF.[69,70]

A number of other cytokines and molecularly targeted drugs are in various stages of development as HPC mobilizing agents. Pegylated G-CSF [pegfilgrastim (Neulasta, Amgen Inc)], a variant of G-CSF with a longer plasma half-life compared to G-CSF (33 vs 6 hours) has the obvious advantage of less frequent dosing.[71] Combinations of erythropoietin (EPO) with G-CSF for the purpose of HPC mobilization have produced mixed results,[72,73] whereas recombinant human thrombopoietin (TPO) has been shown to act synergistically with G-CSF to enhance stem cell mobilization.[74] Further trials are required to clarify the role, if any, of EPO or TPO as effective HPC mobilization agents. An analog of GRO-β, a human CXC chemokine involved in directing the movement of stem cells,[75] may be a promising drug for HPC mobilization if efficacy and safety in humans can be proven. Although PTH increases the numbers of circulating stem cells via osteoblast activation in the HPC niche, its clinical efficacy remains to be established.[51,52] Lithium, widely used in psychiatry for decades, causes neutrophilia and increases blood CD34+ cell counts; therefore, its use in HPC mobilization has been suggested.[76] An anti-VLA-4 antibody, natalizumab (Tysabri, Biogen Idec, Cambridge, MA), that disrupts the interaction of VLA-4 with its cognate receptor VCAM-1, is an approved treatment for multiple sclerosis. Patients treated with natalizumab mobilize HPCs into the blood, suggesting that this agent, or other modulators of VLA-4:VCAM-1 binding, could be used as mobilization agents.[77]

HPC Enumeration

The blood CD34+ cell count is the most reliable predictor of the yield of such cells in HPC(A) collections. Blood CD34+ cell enumeration is performed using standard cytofluorometric methods,[78] which may require 1 to 2 hours or more to produce results. An alternative, more rapidly available blood parameter, referred to as the HPC count, has been used to predict the optimal timing of leukapheresis. The blood HPC assay quantifies immature WBCs based on cell size, density, and resistance to osmotic lysis.[79,80] Multiple studies have reported excellent correlations between precollection peripheral blood CD34+ cell counts and HPC levels. In contrast, measurements of WBC and MNC counts are unreliable predictors of CD34+ cell counts and the yield of these cells in the HPC(A) product.

HPC Mobilization for Autologous HPC Donations

For autologous HSCT, blood HPCs are collected and cryopreserved for later use after myeloablative conditioning (see Chapter 22). The indications for autologous HSCT in adult and pediatric patients include certain malignancies, such as MM, lymphomas and some leukemias, and solid tumors. Experimental protocols have also been developed that use autologous HPCs for treatment of autoimmune diseases such as multiple sclerosis and systemic sclerosis, for gene therapy, and for regenerative medicine applications.[81-84] In each case, blood CD34+ cells are collected by MNC leukapheresis after mobilization with myelosuppressive chemotherapy alone, chemotherapy and mobi-

lizing agent(s), or mobilizing agent(s) alone.[81,84] Because the first method has proven inferior to the latter two, it is seldom used at present.

The optimal mobilization strategy can differ among patients with different malignancies. The choice is based on the underlying disease type and duration, the extent of marrow involvement, any comorbidities, the ability of the patient to tolerate the adverse effects of aggressive chemotherapy, any history of prior chemo- and/or radiotherapy, and the costs of treatment.[81] In most cases, maximal blood CD34+ cell numbers are achieved after treatment with marrow-suppressive, but not stem-cell-toxic, cytoreductive agents followed by daily administration of GM-CSF or, more commonly, G-CSF. When used, GM-CSF is commonly given at doses of 5 μg/kg/day or 250 μg/m²/day; G-CSF is usually given at 250 μg/m²/day or 5 to 10 μg/kg/day. The cytokine regimen is usually started within 1 to 5 days after completion of chemotherapy and is continued through the final HPC(A) collection. The elapsed time from chemotherapy completion until successful HPC(A) collection varies based on the disease and the mobilization regimen; however, it is commonly in the range of 10 to 20 days.

Certain chemotherapeutic agents facilitate CD34+ cell mobilization better than others. These include cyclophosphamide, ifosfamide, paclitaxel, and etoposide.[81,85] Because these drugs are highly active against NHL and MM, they are commonly included in conventional front-line or salvage treatment regimens. For these patients, HPC(A) collection is often planned during recovery after one of the regularly scheduled cycles of primary or salvage chemotherapy.

Chemomobilization and HPC(A) collection may also be accomplished as a treatment cycle that is separate from the patient's current regimen. This approach is considered in patients with residual disease who may benefit from further cytoreductive therapy. Regimens designed for this purpose include single agents or combinations using high-dose cyclophosphamide, etoposide, and/or paclitaxel with or without corticosteroids, followed by cytokine administration through recovery and collection.[81,86] For B-cell malignancies, primary and salvage regimens or separate chemomobilization cycles commonly incorporate rituximab because it is highly effective at in-vivo purging of tumor cells from the blood. Moreover, CD34+ cell mobilization and collection are not compromised.[87]

Chemomobilization regimens most commonly incorporate G-CSF rather than GM-CSF.[81,86] Randomized studies have observed higher CD34+ cell yields and/or fewer collections with G-CSF compared to GM-CSF.[88,89] Of note, sequential combinations of G-CSF plus GM-CSF after mobilization chemotherapy have been reported to induce a highly predictable schedule of WBC recovery and CD34+ cell mobilization such that the target blood HPC goal may be successfully collected on days 11 to 13 in the vast majority of patients.[90,91] Protocols with sequential G-CSF plus GM-CSF have therefore been used at some centers to avoid weekend collections. Other variations on the standard schedule for chemomobilization involve delaying the start of G-CSF and using smaller doses (eg, administering 300 or 480 µg/day and starting at 4 or 5 days after completion of chemotherapy) in order to minimize costs without compromising the rate of successful collection.[92]

Mobilization and collection of HPC(A) from steady state (ie, without prior chemotherapy) using G-CSF or GM-CSF alone is appropriate for patients with malignancies who do not require further cytoreductive therapy, for patients undergoing autologous HSCT for nonmalignant disease, and for regenerative medicine or other experimental protocols.[81,84,86] As with chemomobilization, GM-CSF is a less effective single-agent for HPC(A) collection. Compared to G-CSF, GM-CSF is associated with relatively lower CD34+ cell yields and a higher incidence of mild and serious adverse events.[81] When used alone, G-CSF at 10 to 16 µg/kg/day predictably induces maximal blood CD34+ cell concentrations at day 5, when apheresis usually begins. Relatively high circulating CD34+ cell numbers may be sustained for 3 or more days.

One advantage to mobilizing and collecting HPC(A) with single-agent G-CSF is that autologous HSCT can be performed soon thereafter without concern about additional time needed for the patient to recover from chemomobilization. The potential detrimental effects of recent chemomobilization were demonstrated in a comparative study of 716 patients with MM.[93] Significantly longer times for platelet and neutrophil engraftment were seen following HSCT with HPCs mobilized with high-dose cyclophosphamide plus G-CSF compared to those mobilized with G-CSF alone, suggesting that residual chemotherapy-induced marrow injury might impede hematopoietic reconstitution. The major disadvantage of mobilizing with G-CSF alone is that cumulative cell yields are approximately 2.5-fold lower than those after chemomobilization, especially among patients with NHL.[81,86,94]

A number of clinical and treatment-related variables have been linked to poor CD34+ cell mobilization and ultimate failure to collect at least a minimum acceptable number of cells required for autologous HSCT (Table 23-1). Specific anti-tumor drugs associated with poor mobilization include stem-cell-toxic alkylating agents (especially melphalan and carmustine), dacarbazine, platinum analogs, fludarabine, and lenalidomide.[70,86,95-97] Exposure to these agents should be minimized if a patient may undergo autologous HSCT in the future. This issue is particularly relevant for patients with MM, who are routinely considered for autologous HSCT as a part of standard treatment. As a result, the International Myeloma Working Group has published consensus statements and guidelines for the optimal timing and strategies for efficient HPC mobilization and collection during the treatment course.[70,98]

The minimum number of CD34+ cells required for autologous HSCT is usually considered to be 2×10^6 CD34+ cells/kg. Recovery to an absolute neutrophil count (ANC) >500/µL and platelet count >20,000/µL may occur 1 to 2 days sooner with higher doses.[70,81,86,94,99,100] One recent study in patients with NHL reported enhancement of lymphocyte recovery and event-free and overall sur-

---

Table 23-1. Factors Associated with Inadequate Mobilization of CD34+ Cells in Autologous HSCT Candidates

---

Disease type:

- Leukemias and indolent lymphomas (compared to aggressive lymphomas and multiple myeloma)

Marrow involvement with disease

Age >60 years

Prior radiation therapy to marrow-producing areas

Numbers of previous chemotherapy cycles and different cytotoxic regimens, especially previous therapy with particular stem-cell-toxic agents:

- Melphalan, carmustine, dacarbazine, platinum analogs, fludarabine, lenalidomide

Low platelet counts at time of mobilization

Inadequate mobilization regimen:

- Chemotherapy alone (without cytokine)
- Suboptimal chemotherapeutic agents
- Cytokine alone (compared to chemomobilization)

Prior failed chemomobilization attempt

Maximal peripheral blood CD34+ cell count $<5 \times 10^6$/L

---

vival with infusion of $\geq 8.2 \times 10^6$ CD34+ cells/kg.[100] Alternatively, cell doses as low as 1.5×10^6 CD34+ cells/kg are acceptable in some centers, and even 1×10^6 CD34+ cells/kg ideal body weight may be used with the knowledge that posttransplant platelet recovery will be substantially delayed in up to 80% of patients.[86,101,102]

Patients who fail one mobilization attempt may be mobilized and collected again to achieve cumulative CD34+ cell yield adequate for autologous HSCT in a majority of cases. The use of ideal body weight, rather than actual body weight, accurately predicts engraftment response; therefore, this parameter can be used to calculate the minimum required CD34+ cell goal.[103-105] The biologic significance and potential clinical impact of poor HPC mobilization and collection among patients with malignancy who subsequently undergo autologous HSCT are incompletely understood. Early complication rates and supportive care requirements may be adversely affected if engraftment is significantly delayed because of suboptimal cell doses. Moreover, some, but not all, long-term studies have observed shortened overall and progression-free survival among NHL patients who were difficult mobilizers.[106-109] Mobilization efficiency may therefore reflect worse clinicopathologic features of NHL and be an independent predictor of poor prognosis.

A number of salvage options are available for patients who fail a first attempt at HPC mobilization and collection (Table 23-2). When remobilization is not considered feasible, marrow harvest, either after G-CSF prestimulation or in steady state, may provide a total CD34+ cell dose adequate for autologous HSCT.[31] If remobilization is desired, it is most effective if performed after a "wash out" period of 2 to 3 weeks. Salvage approaches reported to be effective in at least some poor mobilizers include the following: high-dose G-CSF alone (ie, 16-32 µg/kg/day or 12-16 µg/kg twice daily); chemomobilization if cytokine alone was used for the first attempt; alternative mobilization chemotherapy regimens if suboptimal agents were used for the first attempt; combinations of G-CSF and GM-CSF following mobilization chemotherapy; or use of plerixafor in combination with G-CSF either in steady state or, less commonly, after mobilization chemotherapy.[81,86,94,102]

Table 23-2. Options for Secondary Mobilization in the Autologous HSCT Candidates who Failed Primary Mobilization

Marrow harvest (with or without prestimulation with G-CSF)

Remobilization with high-dose G-CSF alone

Remobilization with chemotherapy and G-CSF (if first attempt was with cytokine alone)

Remobilization with optimal chemotherapeutic agents (eg, high-dose cyclophosphamide) and G-CSF, if first attempt was with suboptimal regimen

Remobilization with chemotherapy followed by combinations of G-CSF and GM-CSF

Remobilization with plerixafor (CXCR4 antagonist) plus G-CSF

Approaches using experimental agents and/or experimental combinations of agents:

- Pegfilgrastim following chemotherapy
- Erythropoietin with G-CSF
- Interleukin-11 with G-CSF
- Stem cell factor with G-CSF

G-CSF = granulocyte colony-stimulating factor; GM-CSF = granulocyte-macrophage colony-stimulating factor.

Plerixafor mobilizes CD34+ progenitor cells into the peripheral blood within 6 hours after intravenous injection.[110] In the salvage setting with G-CSF and without prior chemotherapy, plerixafor is given at a dose of 240 µg/kg/day on the evening of the fourth day of daily G-CSF (10 µg/kg/day). Apheresis should ideally commence 10 to 11 hours after the plerixafor dose, following a dose of G-CSF on the fifth morning. A total of four daily evening doses of plerixafor can be given, with subsequent morning apheresis collections, to augment the G-CSF effect. This regimen has been shown to successfully salvage 60% to 85% of patients with NHL, MM, or Hodgkin lymphoma who have previously failed mobilization.[69,111] For primary HPC collections, two Phase III randomized, double-blind, placebo-controlled trials have recently been published comparing steady-state mobilization using G-CSF plus placebo vs G-CSF plus plerixafor in patients with MM or NHL.[64,112] For patients with MM (n = 302) the primary goal was 6×10^6 CD34+ cells/kg in ≤2 apheresis collections and for patients with NHL (n = 298) the goal was 5×10^6 CD34+ cells/kg in ≤4 collections. In both studies, plerixafor plus G-CSF achieved the primary endpoint in over twice as many patients as G-CSF plus placebo, and posttransplant engraft-

ment times did not differ between the two regimens.[64,112] At present, plerixafor is recommended as a salvage agent for patients who have failed initial attempts at peripheral blood stem cell mobilization.[70,98] Although the Phase III data on primary mobilization are compelling, cost is a major consideration. Routine use of plerixafor for primary mobilization must await careful pharmacoeconomic analyses that guide the selection of patients most likely to benefit from this expensive drug.

Alternative and more experimental approaches for patients who have failed an initial mobilization attempt include the use of pegfilgrastim (approved by the FDA for febrile neutropenia but not for HPC mobilization). A number of Phase II studies from European centers have documented the effectiveness and safety of pegfilgrastim as a mobilizing agent after chemotherapy for patients with NHL and MM.[113] Other salvage options, based on limited experience, include combinations of G-CSF with either recombinant human EPO[73,114] or recombinant interleukin-11 (oprelvekin).[115] In addition, recombinant SCF, which is not available in the United States, also potentiates the effect of G-CSF and enhances the rate of successful peripheral blood stem cell collections from difficult mobilizers.[61,116] Preclinical studies are investigating the potential roles of a variety of other cytokines, antibodies, chemokines, and receptor modulators as safe and effective alternative clinical mobilizing agents.[117]

HPC Mobilization for Allogeneic HPC Donations

Allogeneic donors include family members who are usually evaluated and mobilized, and undergo collection at the transplant center caring for the recipient, and unrelated adult volunteers who are recruited, evaluated, and mobilized, and undergo collection at centers affiliated with a donor registry. As in autologous HSCT, higher numbers of transplanted CD34+ cells/kg of recipient weight correlate with enhanced parameters of engraftment after allogeneic HSCT. These include somewhat more rapid recovery of neutrophils and platelets after myeloablative conditioning and quicker establishment of full donor CD3+ T-cell and CD3+ myeloid cell chimerisms after nonmyeloablative HSCT. The optimal stem cell dose for allogeneic recipients varies, however, according to the transplant type, conditioning regimen, donor source, HLA disparity, and, in some cases, disease type.

The minimum blood HPC dose for allogeneic HSCT patients undergoing myeloablative conditioning is 2×10^6 CD34+ cells/kg recipient weight, with higher doses up to 8×10^6 CD34+ cells/kg preferred if possible.[17,118] For HLA-matched sibling recipients, controversy exists as to whether high doses of CD34+ cells might be detrimental. Some studies have observed higher rates of chronic GVHD or mortality for patients who received $>8 \times 10^6$ CD34+ cells/kg,[17,118,119] whereas others found no effect of either CD34+ cell dose or numbers of infused CD4+ and CD8+ T cells.[120] By comparison, myeloablated recipients of unrelated donor grafts who receive high cell doses (ie, at >4 to 5×10^6 CD34+ cells/kg) appear to recover blood lymphocytes faster and suffer lower disease relapse (particularly with myeloid malignancies), possibly as a result of more rapid recovery of natural killer (NK) cell activity.[121] Higher numbers of HPC(A) CD34+ cells, T

cells, and NK cells are beneficial in the setting of nonmyeloablative HSCT, in which lower doses of chemotherapy and/or irradiation minimize toxicity but incur a greater risk of graft rejection. High cell doses after nonmyeloablative conditioning are associated with more rapid establishment of full donor T-cell chimerism, which correlates with overall graft stability, without increasing the risk of GVHD.[122]

Before mobilization and collection, healthy blood HPC donors are screened for communicable disease transmission risk and evaluated for medical comorbidities. They also receive counseling on the risks and potential adverse effects of mobilization agents, apheresis, and venous access. Since 1997, formal recommendations have been published and updated regarding the potential safety concerns for donors and appropriate clinical practices.[123-127] These have evolved over time based on retrospective studies and prospective trial data that confirmed the relative safety and efficacy of HPC mobilization with G-CSF and MNC leukapheresis and defined the risk of complications and contraindications.[124,128-135] Ethical implications of exposing family members and healthy volunteer donors to risk are also a consideration, particularly regarding the potential long-term adverse effects of brief G-CSF exposure.[126,127,132] These medical safety and ethical issues must be formally addressed during premobilization evaluations and discussions before obtaining the donor's informed consent. They are particularly important for pediatric donors, who often rely on their parents as surrogate decision makers. Institutions that use minor age children as healthy sibling HPC donors must address these issues in their policies and procedures for obtaining consent.[136-138]

Mobilization and collection of blood HPCs from allogeneic donors routinely involve administration of G-CSF once or twice daily until the prescribed CD34+ cell yield is achieved. The dose and schedule vary according to institutional practice or unrelated donor registry guidelines. The objective is to obtain optimal mobilization and collection efficiency in the context of a specific apheresis instrument and processing schedule. A G-CSF dose of 5 µg/kg/day is inferior to ≥10 µg/kg/day whereas 16 to 20 µg/kg/day maximizes CD34+ cell mobilization; however, higher doses are associated with more side effects.[124,139,140] It is unclear whether twice-daily administration offers any advantage over single dosing.[124,141] Single-dose G-CSF at 10 µg/kg actual body weight per day has been adopted as the standard for many unrelated donor registries, including the NMDP, and many transplant centers.[124,131,138,140,142,143] With this regimen, side effects are minimized, while enough CD34+ cells are mobilized that a single large-volume leukapheresis (LVL) procedure can frequently achieve the goal for HSCT.[135,138,143]

The yield of CD34+ cells from G-CSF-mobilized allogeneic donors may be affected by a number of variables (Table 23-3). Some studies,[144-152] but not others,[153,154] have observed lower yields with increasing age; however, the breakpoints for significant differences in these studies are not consistent, being variously reported as 38, 45, 50, or 55 years of age.[145-149] Female donors in many studies,[130,133,148-153,155] but not others,[145,147,154] mobilized and/or yielded significantly fewer CD34+ cells than males. In turn, greater body weight has been observed as a significant independent factor associated with higher yields,[130,140,150,153,154] although this effect may be more directly related to the higher G-CSF dose.[142,151] Of note, donors of Hispanic, African, and Asian/Pacific ethnicity mobilize and collect significantly greater numbers of CD34+ cells than those of European ethnicity.[151]

Lower baseline blood parameters, including platelet counts, hemoglobin, MNC counts, and preapheresis CD34+ counts, have been associated with significantly fewer CD34+ cells in the HPC(A) product.[142,145,151,152,154] Some of these parameters, along with donor and recipient weights, have been incorporated into a statistical model for predicting the number of collections required for an adequate yield.[152] Because this model was derived from a single-center retrospective analysis, further validation is needed.

The vast majority of healthy allogeneic donors successfully mobilize and collect adequate HPCs for HSCT. However, even with the most efficient modern practices, up to 5% of related donors may require three or more leukapheresis procedures.[129] The recognition that some donors are "difficult" mobilizers, coupled with the preference for higher CD34+ cell doses (particularly for nonmyeloablative HSCT recipients), has led to the search for more effective mobilization strategies.[156]

The sequential combination of GM-CSF, at 10 µg/kg/day for 3 days alone, followed by G-CSF, at 10 µg/kg/day alone for 2 to 3 days, has been reported to mobilize CD34+ cells better than either GM-CSF alone or concurrent combination of G-CSF and GM-CSF (each at 5 µg/kg/day).[157] This regimen has, therefore, been proposed as an alternative to conventional G-CSF mobilization. Long-acting G-CSF, in the form of pegfilgrastim, avoids the need for daily injections, and limited studies in healthy donors suggest that single-dose pegfilgrastim is safe, effective, and equivalent to G-CSF.[158]

Table 23-3. Factors Associated with Suboptimal HPC(A) Collection from Allogeneic Donors

Older age (>38 to 55 years old)
Female gender
Small body weight or body mass index
Lower cumulative G-CSF exposure (related to dose, schedule, and/or body weight)
European ethnicity (compared to Hispanic, African, and Asian/Pacific)
Lower baseline blood platelet count, hemoglobin, and/or mononuclear cell count
Lower preapheresis blood CD34+ cell count

However, well-designed randomized trials are needed to determine whether pegfilgrastim might serve as an alternative or salvage approach in the allogeneic setting.

Plerixafor significantly augments G-CSF-induced mobilization of CD34+ cells in healthy individuals.[159] Plerixafor alone has also been shown to mobilize CD34+ cells safely and efficiently in a pilot study that showed rapid platelet and neutrophil engraftment in 20 out of 20 recipients who underwent myeloablative HSCT using HPC(A) products from healthy HLA-identical siblings.[65] Of note, however, recent primate studies disclosed different expression patterns of myeloid and lymphoid growth-regulating genes in CD34+ cells mobilized by plerixafor alone compared to G-CSF alone or a combination of the two.[68] Additional molecular, biologic, and immunoregulatory studies may be needed to understand the potential influence of plerixafor mobilization on GVHD and graft-vs-malignancy effects in allogeneic HSCT.

HPC Collection by Apheresis

Technical Considerations

The various apheresis instruments used to collect HPC(A) differ somewhat in their hardware specifications, separation technologies, disposable collection kits, extracorporeal volume requirements, and levels of automation (see Chapter 4).[160] The COM.TEC cell separator (Fresenius Kabi, Bad Homburg, Germany), which is used in Europe, is one instrument that has been optimized for HPC(A) collection efficiency (CE) by combining an automated, continuous flow process using single- or dual-stage separation chambers and cyclic MNC collections with a software application that individualizes blood volume processing based on the predicted product yield of CD34+ cells.[161-163]

A number of clinical studies have compared the performance characteristics of different apheresis instruments and systems. Product CD34+ cell yields with the COBE Spectra V4.7 semiautomated system (CaridianBCT, Lakewood, CO) and the Spectra automated V6.0 system are similar.[164-166] However, the relative CEs vary, with some trials reporting a lower mean CD34+ cell CE with the V6.0 system[164] and others reporting a higher CE.[166] The V4.7 system is faster but results in higher product platelet contamination and lower post-procedure platelet counts. A recent randomized controlled trial in patients with MM compared the WBC-kit used with V4.7 to the AUTO-kit used with V6.0. The WBC-kit consistently performed better than the AUTO-kit in this patient group, with fewer procedures per mobilization, superior collection rates, and a decreased incidence of HPC(A) cryoproduct infusion reactions.[167]

The Haemonetics MCS+ cell separator (Haemonetics Corp, Braintree, MA) collects MNCs by discontinuous centrifugation. It processes roughly one-third less blood volume than the COBE Spectra V4.7 and V6.0 systems in comparable procedures and requires a 30% longer run time.[168,169] HPC products collected with the MCS+ instrument contain significantly fewer CD34+ cells, although platelet contamination is similar to products collected with the COBE Spectra V6.0 system.[168,169] The major advantage of the MCS+ system is that single-needle access can be sufficient.

CD34+ cell yields with the CS 3000 Plus system (Fenwal, Lake Zurich, IL) are similar to those obtained with COBE Spectra systems when similar blood volumes are processed.[170-174] The relative CE of the CS 3000 Plus system varies, however, based on preapheresis WBC and blood CD34+ cell counts.[172,173] In one study the CS 3000 Plus had a lower mean CD34+ cell CE than the Spectra V4.7, primarily when WBC counts exceeded $50 \times 10^9/L$ and blood CD34+ cell counts exceeded $50 \times 10^6/L$.[172] Conversely, superior CEs were obtained with the CS 3000 Plus system when preapheresis WBC counts were in a lower range.[173]

A newer apheresis instrument, the Amicus (Fenwal), incorporates a two-stage separation module with intermittent MNC collection cycles as a method to maximize CD34+ cell CE. Two studies comparing the Amicus with the CS 3000 Plus disclosed significantly higher mean CD34+ cell CEs for the Amicus (65% vs 43% and 54.9% vs 46.4%, respectively).[175,176] However, the CE with the Amicus also decreases when the precollection WBC count is >40 to 50 × 10⁹/L. Therefore, modifications to the cycle volumes and whole blood flow rates have been proposed to improve the performance for patients and donors with high WBC counts.[176,177]

Comparison studies of the Amicus and Spectra systems have observed either no difference in CD34+ cell CE (when compared to the Spectra V6.0 system)[178] or a superior CE for Amicus (when compared to the Spectra V6.1 system).[179] The mean CEs for MNC and CD34+ cells are no different between the Amicus and the semiautomated Spectra V4.7 system.[180] Platelet contamination of HPC(A) products is greater with automated Spectra collections, resulting in approximately a 30% decrease in postprocedure platelet counts compared to only a 20% decrease with the Amicus. Similarly, the Spectra V4.7 system collects relatively higher numbers of platelets, resulting in a 30% to 50% decrease in postprocedure platelet count.[180]

Vascular Access for HPC Collections

Apheresis procedures require high blood flow rates. In some cases this can be achieved by peripheral venous access with two large-bore needles, whereas a single venous access site is sufficient for intermittent flow MNC collection. However, up to 20% of healthy female donors and 10% of healthy male donors will require a central venous catheter (CVC) because of poor peripheral access.[135,181]

If a CVC is required, a rigid, dual-lumen, dialysis-type catheter is placed in the subclavian, internal jugular or femoral vein.[182] Femoral CVCs are associated with fewer placement-related complications but pose a greater risk of infection and limit the patient's mobility.[183] Subclavian and internal jugular CVCs have been associated with pneumothorax, hemothorax, cardiac perforation, and tamponade.[184] CVC insertion guided by real-time sonographic visualization is superior to blind puncture,[185] and the Agency for Healthcare Research and Quality has recommended guided catheter placement for better patient care.[186] This practice is expected to become the standard of care in the near future. Patients undergoing HPC(A) collection for autologous HSCT commonly undergo placement of a semipermanent (tunneled) apheresis/dialysis type CVC that will be adequate for both the leukapheresis procedures and for long-term intravenous management throughout the peritransplant period.

Procedural Considerations for HPC(A) Collections

The selection of an anticoagulant for HPC(A) collection is usually based on institutional policies or unrelated donor registry standards. The usual choice is anticoagulant citrate dextrose formula A (ACD-A), at an inlet anticoagulant:blood ratio of 1:12 to 1:15.[135,143,150] Alternatively, some centers use a combination of a citrate solution with unfractionated heparin (eg, 10 units heparin/mL ACD-A) at an inlet ratio of 1:15 to 1:35.[138,155,187,188] Extra anticoagulant can be added to the product collection bag either before or immediately after HPC(A) procurement to prevent clot formation.

Combining heparin with citrate lessens the cumulative citrate dose and thereby reduces the likelihood of hypocalcemic side effects and a need for calcium replacement. Unlike citrate, however, heparin anticoagulates the patient as well as the instrument and therefore confers a risk of bleeding in patients with thrombocytopenia or coagulopathy. In addition, heparin-induced thrombocytopenia (HIT) and associated thrombotic complications could develop in a recently exposed patient/donor.

"Conventional" HPC(A) collection typically involves processing two to three donor blood volumes, or 10 to 12 liters for an adult. LVL, which involves processing 3 to 6 donor blood volumes (up to 20 to 36 liters in an adult), can be performed in pediatric and adult patients to collect proportionally higher numbers of HPCs.[189,190] LVL procedures take longer, entail a greater loss of platelets, and increase the chance of side effects related to the anticoagulant.[143,191,192] Over the past few years, LVL has been more commonly used for HPC(A) collections from allogeneic donors.[143,192] Procedural requirements include good venous access (to support procedures lasting 5 to 7 hours). When ACD-A alone is used for anticoagulation, intravenous calcium supplementation may be desirable.

The blood CD34+ cell count remains relatively constant or may even increase during leukapheresis.[193-199] By contrast, the platelet and granulocyte counts decrease appreciably.[194] This "recruitment" of CD34+ cells into the blood, which is variable,[200] correlates directly with the patient's total blood volume and the amount of blood processed. The mechanism is undefined but may relate to the mobilization kinetics of G-CSF administered before the procedure, to effects of heparin and/or ACD-A on marrow cytoadhesive interactions, and/or to perturbation of feedback signals within the marrow that regulate the egress of CD34+ cells.

The preapheresis blood CD34+ cell count is the most reliable predictor of HPC yield, particularly when the count is $\geq$10 to 20 $\times$ 10^6/L.[143,189,190,192,199] Mid-cycle blood and product CD34+ cell numbers have also been used to assess HPC recruitment during LVL and to predict the procedure time required to achieve a specific goal.[197,199] Yield predictions must also take into account that high circulating leukocyte and/or CD34+ cell counts may alter the CEs of some apheresis instruments.[201-205] The non-CD34+ cell composition of the final product may also vary based on instrument collection methodologies and/or donor characteristics.[206] Differences in HPC(A) lymphocyte content have been reported to affect HSCT outcomes in some settings[206,207]; however, comprehensive studies are needed to better define the influence of specific cell subsets.

Pediatric HPC(A) collections, including LVL and procedures in extremely low-weight infants, can be performed to obtain autologous HSCT.[190,208-211] Similarly, healthy pediatric sibling donors can safely undergo G-CSF mobilization and MNC leukapheresis,[137,212,213] although this is not a standard practice in most centers. Special considerations for pediatric donors include the ethical, legal, and regulatory aspects of informed consent; the frequent need for CVC access; sedation or anesthesia; the potential emotional and psychologic effects; and the risks of exposure to homologous red cells, if needed to prime the instrument. Procedural factors, including blood and extracorporeal volume requirements, anticoagulant choices, calcium supplementation requirements, flow rate adjustments, rinseback criteria, ending fluid balance goals, and effects on blood platelet count and hematocrit must also be anticipated and discussed with the instrument operator to minimize the risk of adverse events.[208,209,211,212,214] In general, the CD34+ cell CEs for children are equivalent to that for adults.[215] Also similar to adults, mid-procedure product CD34+ cell measurements have been used to predict the processed blood volume required to achieve the desired product HPC goal.[216]

Standards and Regulatory Considerations for HPC(A) Products

As blood HPCs have become the preferred graft source for autologous and adult allogeneic HSCT, apheresis collection centers have developed policies and procedures that define their organizational, operational, procedural, and quality management requirements to ensure safe and effective products. The critical role of quality management and regulatory oversight has been recognized by accreditation agencies and, more recently, the FDA, as demonstrated by progressive expansions of the standards and regulations in the field. HPC(A) collection facilities must register with the FDA, and most seek accreditation by an nongovernment agency for the activities performed. Hence, apheresis practitioners need to understand and follow the relevant regulations and standards.

In 1997, the FDA first announced its intention to regulate human cells, tissues, and cellular and tissue-based products (HCT/Ps), which include blood HPCs, therapeutic cells collected by apheresis (TCs; eg, donor T lymphocytes), and umbilical cord blood HPCs. Since that time three rules have been sequentially implemented. The first mandated that all establishments that recover, process, store, label, package, or distribute HCT/Ps, or that screen or test the donor of the HCT/Ps, be registered with the FDA by March 29, 2004 and that their HCT/Ps be listed.[217] All facilities collecting or providing HPC(A) and/or TCs need to be FDA registered and thus must comply with all requirements contained in this rule. Moreover, collection facilities should be aware of and be familiar with the type of products they collect and the specific regulations they need to follow, because a distinction was made between HCT/Ps that are regulated solely under Section 361 of the Public Health Service (PHS) Act and those that are regulated as a drug, device, and/or biological product under Section 351 of the PHS Act. The latter groups are subjected to additional applicable regulations. The second rule from the FDA, finalized on May 25, 2004, outlined requirements for donor screening and eligibility. The third rule, which provided guidance on current good tissue practices, was finalized on November 24, 2004. Both of these rules became effective on May 25, 2005.[218,219]

Donor Screening

The donor eligibility rule, contained in the *Code of Federal Regulations* (CFR; 21 CFR Part 1271 Subpart C), set out the requirements for donor screening and testing to prevent transmission of communicable disease agents.[218,220] Compliance with FDA regulations requires that donor eligibility be determined, with few exceptions, before cells or tissue in HCT/Ps are implanted, transplanted, infused, or transferred. All facilities that perform any function described in the above-mentioned subpart must comply with the requirements that are applicable to that function.

The screening process for donor health and communicable disease transmission risk must occur before the donor is approved to proceed with HPC(A) collection. This screening should include evaluation of medical suitability and eligibility. Evaluation of donor suitability pro-

tects the donor. It usually includes general health history and physical examination relevant to the anticipated donation—eg, assessing risk factors for adverse effects of mobilizing agents, such as hemoglobinopathies, splenic disorders, and autoimmune diseases, as well as evaluating venous access. Testing includes complete blood count and pregnancy testing in female donors with childbearing potential. Additional steps may be needed based on the findings of the history and physical examination.

Evaluation of donor eligibility protects the recipient. It includes a comprehensive health history questionnaire, a review of the donor's relevant medical records for risk factors and/or clinical evidence of potential for infectious disease transmission, and laboratory testing for relevant communicable disease agents and diseases (RCDAD).

The questionnaire is designed to elicit relevant medical history and to identify behaviors associated with risk of communicable disease transmission. Topics include sexual behaviors, nonprescription drug use, skin-breaching procedures (eg, tattooing), and residence in regions where exposure to malaria, Chagas disease, or the agent of bovine spongiform encephalopathy may occur. A uniform donor history questionnaire (DHQ) for allogeneic blood and marrow HPC donors was recently prepared by the interorganizational Cellular Therapies Task Force to include requirements of the FDA and accreditation agencies.[221] Physical examination of the donor should seek signs of risky behaviors, such as recent tattoos, piercings, or signs of intravenous drug use, as well as signs of significant illnesses.

As of mid-year 2009, the required RCDAD screening and testing for all HCT/P donors under 21 CFR 1271.3(r)(1)[218,220] cover HIV types 1 and 2; hepatitis B virus (HBV); hepatitis C virus (HCV); human transmissible spongiform encephalopathy, including Creutzfeldt-Jakob disease (no testing available); and *Treponema pallidum* (syphilis). In addition, donors of viable, leukocyte-rich cells and tissue are also screened and tested for human T-cell lymphotropic virus (HTLV) types I and II and cytomegalovirus (CMV). Although CMV is not considered a RCDAD by the FDA, these donors must be tested for evidence of infection in order to adequately and appropriately address the risk of transmission to the HSCT recipient. Use of CMV-seropositive donors is permissible; however, procedures governing the release of a leukocyte-rich HCT/P product from a CMV-positive donor must be developed by each facility.

Laboratory tests that are currently required for RCDAD screening include HBV surface antigen, antibodies to HBV core antigen, anti-HCV, HCV RNA, anti-HIV-1/2, HIV-1 RNA, anti-HTLV-I/II, and a serologic test for syphilis. Additional RCDAD mentioned for HCT/Ps in the donor eligibility guidance,[220] although not specifically listed under 21 CFR 1271.3(r)(1), include sepsis, vaccinia (the virus used in small-pox vaccine), West Nile virus (WNV), and *Trypanosoma cruzi (T. cruzi,* the agent for Chagas disease). Selection of these RCDAD is based on the risk of transmission, severity of effects, and availability of appropriate screening measures and/or tests. Screening as well as testing for WNV and *T. cruzi* are recommended in the *Circular of Information for the Use of Cellular Therapy Products*[222] (prepared by a multiorganizational task force) but only outlined in draft guidance documents by FDA.

In the donor eligibility guidance,[220] the FDA made specific recommendations for donor screening for WNV but not for donor testing. Once nucleic acid testing (NAT) for WNV became available, the FDA issued an additional draft guidance in April 2008,[223] recommending that blood specimens from all HCT/P donors be tested year-round for WNV using a licensed, individual NAT screening test. As of December 1, 2008, the NMDP requires WNV testing on all blood HPC donors on the first day of collection year-round regardless of geographic location. This is based on the fact that unlike other transfusion-transmitted viruses, WNV is tranmissable only during the viremic phase of the acute infection, while the presence of antibodies usually correlates with clearance of infectious virus from the blood and loss of infectivity.

A March 2009 FDA draft guidance recommended that potential donors be screened for Chagas disease.[224] Furthermore, it was recommended that all HCT/P donors be tested for antibodies to *T. cruzi* using an FDA-licensed donor screening test. In August 2009, the interorganizational DHQ was updated to include a question regarding history of a positive test for Chagas disease.[221] This additional screening step was implemented in advance of final guidance from the FDA. As of December 1, 2008, the NMDP requires that all HPC donors be screened and tested for Chagas disease in order to meet donor eligibility criteria.

The timing of infectious disease testing is clearly defined in the regulations. For donors of HPC(A) products, infectious disease testing may be carried out up to 30 days before collection. For TCs, such as viable-lymphocyte-rich cell products, donor testing must be completed before administration and must be performed on a sample collected within 7 days before or after collection, or in accordance with applicable laws and regulations. The required testing must be performed using an FDA-licensed, -approved, or -cleared donor screening test, in accordance with the manufacturer's instructions [21 CFR 1271.80(c)].

Documentation of the donor's eligibility status must accompany the HPC product at all times. This includes, at a minimum, 1) a distinct identification code affixed to the product (eg, alphanumeric identifier) that relates the product to the donor and to all records pertaining to the product; 2) a statement whether, based on the results of the screening and testing, the donor has been determined to be eligible or ineligible; and 3) a summary of the records used to make the donor eligibility determination.

The summary of records must contain the following information: 1) the name and address of the facility that made the eligibility determination; 2) a listing and interpretation of the results of all communicable disease testing performed; 3) a statement noting the reason for the determination of ineligibility, as applicable; and 4) a statement that the communicable disease testing was performed by a laboratory that is either certified to perform such testing on human specimens under the Clinical Laboratory Improvement Amendments of 1988 (United States Code: 42 USC 263a) and 42 CFR 493 or has met equivalent requirements, as determined by the Centers for Medicare and Medicaid Services.

An HPC product from an ineligible donor can still be collected if its use is justified based on urgent medical need, and the donor, the recipient, and the recipient's physician all approve. "Urgent medical need" means that no comparable HPC product is available, and the recipient is likely to suffer death or serious morbidity without the product.

Labeling

Apheresis facilities are typically accredited by the AABB, the Foundation for the Accreditation of Cellular Therapy (FACT), and/or the College of American Pathologists (CAP), and they can be members of the NMDP network. All of these accreditation organizations follow FDA guidelines on donor eligibility.[225-227] Their standards also include, based on FDA guidelines, requirements for the labeling of the HPC product at the completion of the collection procedure. At a minimum, unique alpha and/or numeric identifiers should be affixed to the product, and the proper name of the product and modifiers can be affixed (FACT) and/or attached (AABB).

As mentioned above, the proper name of a blood HPC product collected by apheresis is "HPC, Apheresis." Other required elements on the label include identification of the collection facility, collection date and end time, identification of donor and recipient, volume of the product, anticoagulant solution used, and recommended storage temperature. There is minimal variation between the organizations for the method of applying these elements to the HPC product.[225,226] In accordance with the FDA donor eligibility rule, appropriate biohazard or warning labels should be attached or affixed to the product when applicable. In an effort to harmonize the different accreditation organizations' requirements and to support the global goal of blood and cell-based product standardization, a US consensus standard for the uniform labeling of cellular therapy products using ISBT 128 was recently published.[228]

Of note, patients donating blood HPC products for autologous HSCT are not required to pass donor eligibility screening determinations, and the FDA does not require testing of cells and tissues for autologous use. However, current AABB and FACT standards do require infectious disease testing for autologous donors. Thus, autologous HPC(A) products require the additional specific labeling including "FOR AUTOLOGOUS USE ONLY" and "NOT EVALUATED FOR INFECTIOUS SUBSTANCES" unless all otherwise applicable screening and testing have been performed. In addition, any abnormal donor screening or testing results require appropriate labeling as applicable. The most recent *Circular of Information for the Use of Cellular Therapy Products* summarizes the labeling requirements.[222]

Microbial Contamination of HPC(A) Products

A well-defined section of the HCT/P regulations deals with microbial contamination of the products. HPC(A) products are routinely tested for bacterial and fungal contaminants. Such testing is required at the completion of processing; however, it is recommended after collection and before processing as well to determine the likely source of contamination should the postprocessing sample test positive. The main sources of microbes in product cultures include donor infections and contamination by operators or handlers during collection, processing, sampling for culture, or thawing.

The incidence of culture-positive HPC(A) products reported in the literature has ranged from 0 to 7.2%, with most between 1% to 2%.[229-233] The most commonly identified organisms are coagulase-negative staphylococci, followed by other common skin flora and environmental microorganisms.[229,230,234,235] If a culture is positive, antimicrobial sensitivities can be determined; furthermore, identification of the organism and strain by techniques such as pulse-field gel electrophoresis can help to pinpoint the source of contamination (eg, recovery of the same strain from multiple products from the same donor suggests donor bacteremia).[236] Analysis of culture results from samples collected at various stages of processing can implicate bacteremic donors as a major source of positivity.[230]

The clinical significance of infusing culture-positive HPC(A) products is unclear; however, the outcomes of most reported cases have been encouraging.[230,234,237,238] In a recent large series, patients receiving culture-positive products did not have a blood culture positive for the same agent, did not develop infections attributable to the contaminated product, and did not experience any clinical sequelae.[235] Hospital admission rates and times to engraftment for recipients of culture-positive products are within the expected range for both autologous and allogeneic transplants.[237,238] No differences in acute infusion-related symptoms, survival, or hematopoietic recovery have been demonstrated between patients receiving culture-positive or culture-negative products.[229,230] Postinfusion blood cultures have been positive for the organism present in the HPC product in some cases, however. Moreover, the use of prophylactic antimicrobial therapy varies among reporting centers (not all patients receive therapy). A correlation between infusion with culture-positive HPC(A) products and longer duration of hospitalization was observed in one study.[235] The potential clinical sequelae of infusion of a culture-positive HPC(A) product depends on pathogenicity and microbial load. In most cases of true contamination, either there is a low inoculum or the organism has low pathogenic potential, or both. The cumulative experience is that use of such products is justified.

The FDA current good tissue practices final rule implemented in 2005 states that a product that is in quarantine, contaminated, or collected from an ineligible donor must not be made available for distribution.[219] However, the product can be released under urgent medical need if no comparable product is available and there is potential severe risk to the recipient without it.

Collection facilities must have standard operating procedures for managing cellular therapy products with positive cultures. These policies and procedures must address, at a minimum, the notification of the recipient's physician, investigation of the cause, follow-up with the donor, and the reporting to regulatory agencies, as appropriate.

Special Considerations for Mobilization and Collection of Autologous HPC(A)

Relapse of malignancy is a major cause of mortality in patients receiving autologous HSCT. Posttransplant recurrence may arise from malignant cells that survive in the patient after high-dose chemotherapy or from malignant cells infused as part of the HPC product.[239] Because HPC(A) product tumor contamination is more likely in patients with refractory or persistent disease,[240] chemo-mobilization (rather than mobilization with cytokine alone) and collection during complete remission may lessen the chance that disease relapse will arise from the graft. This notwithstanding, evidence from a number of studies suggests that, while small numbers of tumor cells are present in HPC products, these may not be ultimately responsible for HSCT failure.[241-247]

Many approaches have been used to minimize the risk of mobilizing, collecting, and transmitting tumorigenic cells in the HPC(A) product. In-vivo purging involves the use of high-dose chemotherapy and, in some cases, tumor antibodies before HPC mobilization.[248] In-vitro purging, on the other hand, involves pharmacologic and/or immunologic manipulation to eradicate malignant cells or purify a population of tumor-free CD34+ cells mixed with tumor cells. Various studies have used B-cell monoclonal antibodies,[249,250] the cytotoxic agent mafosfamide,[251] and CD34+ cell selection.[252] All of these manipulations result in CD34+ cell loss but, disappointingly, confer no significant improvement in patient survival.[253-255]

Indeed, in some studies the incidence of serious infection was significantly higher among patients who received purged or selected products.

Certain disease-related issues must be considered for select patients undergoing HPC mobilization and leukapheresis. Plasma hyperviscosity caused by high levels of monoclonal paraprotein (eg, IgM with lymphoplasmacytoid lymphoma/Waldenstrom macroglobulinemia, or IgG or IgA with MM) can interfere with the establishment of a stable interface in the apheresis instrument; plasma exchange may be required in affected patients before HPC(A) collection.[256] The use of G-CSF to mobilize HPCs in patients (or donors) with sickle cell trait is generally considered to be safe[257]; however, a fatal sickling crisis has been reported in an individual with hemoglobin SC disease with no previous sickling complications.[258]

Patients taking anticoagulants should be carefully monitored, particularly for bleeding at venous access sites. If heparin is used during apheresis, appropriate adjustments should be made to the inlet blood:anticoagulant ratio. Alternatively, consideration should be given to holding the anticoagulant to allow normalization of hemostasis before HPC(A) collection, especially if the risk of thromboembolism when temporarily off therapy is low. Heparin can result in severe bleeding, but its effect can be reversed immediately by protamine. When heparin anticoagulation is being considered, a history of HIT should be ruled out.

Poor HPC mobilization results in lower CD34+ cell yields and a need for multiple collections. Infusion of many cryopreserved HPC(A) products with low numbers of CD34+ cells can be problematic because of the high cumulative product volumes. Dimethylsulfoxide, the cryoprotectant commonly used to maintain cellular viability at low-storage temperatures, can cause mild-to-severe infusion-related adverse reactions.[259] In addition, high numbers of total nucleated cells in cryopreserved HPC(A) are associated with adverse infusion-related events; this effect appears to be directly related to granulocytes, which do not tolerate the freeze-thaw cycle.[260,261] (See also Chapter 24.)

Adverse Events

Complications of HPC Mobilization

The use of chemotherapy for mobilizing HPCs is associated with hematologic and extrahematologic toxicities that can be moderate to severe (Table 23-4). It has been shown that following high-dose cyclophosphamide, a median of 15 days is required for patients to achieve an ANC of 0.5×10^9/L and a platelet count greater than 50×10^9/L. During this period the majority of patients require red cell and platelet transfusions. In a study of 116 MM patients receiving high-dose cyclphosphamide for HPC mobilization, and with the majority also receiving G-CSF or GM-CSF, 110 had fever, 19 had documented septicemia, 2 died from septic shock, and 1 died from cardiac arrest that was possibly related to septic shock. Other toxicities included 101 patients with fluid overload, 32 with severe mucositis, 17 with hemorrhagic cystitis, 2 with cardiac toxicity, 1 with renal insufficiency, and 1 with neurologic toxicity.[262] Similar toxicities of varying severity have also been observed with mobilization regimens using etoposide[263] and ifosfamide.[264]

The short-term adverse events associated with mobilization using G-CSF alone are dose dependent and usually mild (Table 23-4). The most common reactions include bone pain (47%-93.5%), headache (40%-70%), fatigue (14%-70%), nausea/vomiting (10%-26%), myalgias (23%-36%), and fever/chills (0-27%).[128,155,265-268] Oral analgesics are taken by a majority of donors (62%-70%). Less common adverse events include insomnia (4%-48%), injection site reactions (7%), rash (3%), and anorexia (11%-22%).[131,155,268,269] All of these events usually resolve within 2 to 3 days of discontinuing G-CSF.[128,265]

Several rare yet serious adverse events have been documented in healthy donors treated with G-CSF during mobilization. Significant splenic enlargement occurs in the majority of

Table 23-4. Side Effects Caused by Different Mobilization Agents

Mobilization Agent	Complications
Chemotherapy	Fever, mucositis, infection, organ toxicities
G-CSF	Bone pain, fatigue, musculoskeletal pain, headache, nausea/vomiting, fever/chills; rarely, splenic rupture, acute lung injury, flare of rheumatologic/inflammatory disease
GM-CSF	Musculoskeletal pain, headache, fever, hyperuricemia
Plerixafor	Nausea/bloating/flatulence/loose stools, skin reaction at the injection site, headache, paresthesias, lightheadedness

G-CSF = granulocyte colony-stimulating factor; GM-CSF = granulocyte-macrophage CSF.

healthy donors during G-CSF mobilization.[270] The splenomegaly is usually uncomplicated, resolves within 10 days of completing apheresis, and does not significantly correlate with hematologic values.[270,271] Splenic rupture has occurred in both allogeneic donors[272-274] and patients[275,276] undergoing mobilization with G-CSF in the setting of enlarged and normal-sized spleens. Complications possibly related to neutrophil activation following mobilization with G-CSF have been documented, including a case of acute lung injury occurring 4 days after beginning mobilization[277] and capillary leak syndrome occurring after the start of apheresis in a G-CSF-mobilized donor.[278]

Certain patient populations being mobilized with G-CSF may be at increased risk of exacerbation of an underlying disease. Severe sickle cell crises, in some cases leading to multiorgan dysfunction or death, have been precipitated in patients with hemoglobin SC, SS, and S/β+ thalassemia.[258,279,280] G-CSF is currently contraindicated in patients with sickle cell disease; however, in a study of G-CSF mobilization in eight patients with a history of sickle cell trait (hemoglobin AS), none experienced a sickle cell crisis during mobilization.[257] G-CSF has also been associated with disease flares in donors with anti-neutrophilic cytoplasmic antibody-associated vasculitis and arthritis.[137,281]

Several laboratory abnormalities have been attributed to G-CSF in healthy donors and patients. These include increased numbers of neutrophils and lymphocytes, decreased platelets, increased alkaline phosphatase and lactate dehydrogenase, increased uric acid, and minor changes in serum potassium and magnesium.[265,282] Long-term follow-up of hematologic parameters in 94 allogeneic donors for up to 5 to 7 years following G-CSF treatment demonstrated a mild neutropenia or lymphopenia at 4 to 8 months in 30 and 25 donors, respectively. At 5 years all lymphocyte levels were normal, while a reduction in neutrophils persisted in four donors.[282]

G-CSF administration may result in changes in coagulation in HPC donors. Cases of cerebrovascular accident and myocardial infarction following HPC(A) collection with G-CSF mobilization have been documented[123] as well as an increased frequency of angina during mobilization in patients with advanced coronary heart disease.[283] G-CSF administration in healthy donors has been associated with a transient but significant decrease in the activated partial thromboplastin time; with increased levels of Factor VIII, von Willebrand factor antigen, and thrombin generation; and, in some cases, with increased platelet aggregation.[266,284,285] Recently, there have been two incidents of intracerebral bleeding reported to

NMDP. Intracerebral bleeding is now included in the NMDP informed consent as a potential risk of receiving G-CSF.

The long-term safety of brief exposure to G-CSF during HPC mobilization continues to be studied. Several concepts must be kept in mind when evaluating the risk that healthy donors will develop hematologic malignancy as a result of G-CSF treatment. First, the incidence of leukemia in the population is low (3-5 new cases/100,000 people/year), and the latency period for developing leukemia following exposure to a causative agent can be 3 to 8 years. It has been estimated that to detect a 10-fold increase in leukemia, a minimum of 2000 normal donors would need to be followed for 10 years.[286] Second, it is known that siblings (potential donors) of leukemia patients have a two- to fivefold increased risk of leukemia.[287,288] These factors make it difficult to determine the risk solely attributable to G-CSF. A report from the Research on Adverse Drug Events and Reports project identified two out of 200 HPC donors who were mobilized with G-CSF and developed acute myelogenous leukemia (AML) within 4 to 5 years after G-CSF exposure.[289] However, these donors were siblings of AML patients, and the mother of one of the donors also had AML, suggesting the involvement of familial leukemia risk factors.

To address concern that G-CSF may cause hematologic malignancy in healthy donors, laboratory studies have been performed to examine the effects of G-CSF on the genome of hematopoietic cells. Transient genetic and epigenetic changes have been observed. First, the extent of double-stranded DNA relaxation and de-novo synthesis were measured in healthy donors before and at time intervals following G-CSF mobilization to measure DNA destabilization associated with G-CSF. Both parameters were significantly increased after 5 days of G-CSF and then returned to baseline within 1 to 2 months.[290] Second, using fluorescence in-situ hybridization, it was observed that the lymphocytes of G-CSF-mobilized donors had altered replication timing of alleles, an epigenetic alteration, and aneuploidy, a genetic alteration—similar to changes that have been documented in the lymphocytes of cancer patients. The altered replication timing was transient whereas aneuploidy was persistent.[291] In addition, it has been observed that there is a small percentage (0.6%) of tetraploid differentiated myeloid cells in HPC donors following G-CSF mobilization. It is important to note that no numerical chromosomal alterations were detected in the CD34+ cells.[292] The clinical significance of these laboratory findings is unknown at this time.

Available reports from single institutions with follow-up of healthy donors for as long as 7 years have not revealed an increased risk of developing leukemia or myelodysplasia after HPC mobilization. Reviews of 101 donors for 3 to 6 years,[293] 343 donors for a median of 39 months,[294] and 141 donors for up to 7 years[282] did not reveal any cases of hematologic malignancy or myelodysplastic syndrome. Follow-up of 3928 unrelated HPC(A) donors who were mobilized with G-CSF demonstrated an incidence of leukemia among donors that was similar to the expected rate in an age-adjusted control population.[155] Similar results were obtained from a prospective trial including 2408 unrelated HPC(A) donors from the NMDP in which no cases of AML or myelodysplasia were reported.[135] Comparison of the incidence of other malignancies in the donors to expected rates in the Surveillance Epidemiology and End Results database showed no evidence of increased cancer risk in the donors.

The adverse events reported by patients receiving GM-CSF include musculoskeletal pain, headache, and fever, which occur with a frequency similar to that seen with G-CSF mobilization (Table 23-4). However, these symptoms have been rated as more severe with GM-CSF and are more often accompanied by injection-site reactions.[157,295] GM-CSF mobilization is also associated with a transient increase in serum uric acid levels.[295]

Recombinant human SCF has not been approved by FDA for use as a mobilization agent in HPC collection in the United States. It is approved, however, in Canada and New Zealand. Adverse reactions associated with SCF therapy include both local and systemic toxicities. Up to 88% of patients experience mild-to-moderate cutaneous reactions within 24 to 48 hours, predominantly at the SCF injection site, that resolve within an additional 24 to 48 hours[296]; these include erythema, pruritus, urticaria, swelling, and hyperpigmentation. Systemic allergic-type reactions have been documented in up to 10% of patients, who have presented with generalized erythema, urticaria, pruritus, and respiratory symptoms.[61,296,297] These local and systemic reactions are most likely mast-cell-related. Patients receiving SCF have significantly increased numbers of cutaneous mast cells with mast cell degranulation observed on histology, as well as elevated levels of mast cell tryptase in the serum.[298]

The adverse effects associated with plerixafor in both healthy donors and patients undergoing HPC mobilization are generally mild and resolve within a day after administration (Table 23-4). Data concerning long-term effects of this agent are not yet available. No cardiac toxicities have been observed. Among healthy donors the most common adverse effects include injection-site reactions (erythema/pain/burning), gastrointestinal symptoms (nausea/bloating/flatulence/loose stools), headache, paresthesias, and light-headedness.[65,299,300] The severity and type of adverse effects observed in patients were similar to those in healthy donors, with the exception of episodes of anxiety and nightmares.[69,301] No dose-response relationship has been identified for any of these symptoms.

Complications of Central Venous Catheters

Adequate venous access that can sustain blood flow rates of up to 50 to 100 mL/min is required for HPC collection by apheresis. Although the majority of healthy adult donors are able to undergo collection through peripheral veins, some series report that as many as 10% to 30% of allogeneic donors have required a CVC,[129,269,302] with women being more likely to require central access than men.[135]

A CVC is more often required in the autologous setting for several reasons, including unsuitable peripheral veins in these patients, the need for multiple collections, the performance of LVLs that require relatively long time periods at high flow rates, and the concomitant need for central infusion of high-dose chemotherapy or HPCs. Reported rates of CVC placement among patients undergoing autologous collection range from 35% to 100% of patients.[199,303]

CVCs are associated with an overall complication rate of 15%. Arterial puncture is more likely with internal jugular than subclavian insertion, while pneumothorax and hemothorax are more likely at the subclavian site. Femoral vein placement can cause arterial puncture, hematoma, and/or arteriovenous fistula.[304] Image-guidance technology aids in reducing the number of mechanical complications and placement failures.[305]

Catheter thrombosis and/or occlusion may occur in patients undergoing HPC(A) collection. The degree of risk depends on the donor population, the insertion site, the type of catheter, and length of time that it remains in place.[306,307] Catheter-associated clots and fibrin sheaths may be successfully treated with tissue plasminogen activator,[308] and line patency is often maintained with heparin instillation. Because of the risk of heparin-induced thrombocytopenia, however, normal saline flushes may be preferred and have been shown to be as effective as heparin in maintaining patency.[309]

Catheter-related infection can be an early or late complication that can potentially result in a bacterially-contaminated product. Catheters impregnated with antibacterial agents, maximal sterile-barrier precautions during catheter insertion, and strict sterile technique when accessing the catheter hub are critical in prevention of CVC-related nosocomial infections.[304]

Complications of Leukapheresis

Collection of HPC(A) is a relatively safe procedure. An analysis by the NMDP of adverse events among 2408 unrelated donors showed that apheresis-related adverse events on days 1 and 2 of HPC(A) collection were reported by 20% and 10% of female donors and by 7% and 5% of male donors, respectively; serious adverse events occurred in less than 0.6% of donors overall.[135] Complications usually fall into one of three categories: 1) mechanical or technical problems, 2) problems related to the extracorporeal circuit and anticoagulation, and 3) undesired cytopenias caused by cell depletion.

Technical difficulties can include catheter occlusion, obstruction, or leakage in the sets; hemolysis caused by kinks in tubing; inability to return blood to the donor; and the potential for air embolism.[310,311] A review of 554 HPC(A) collections demonstrated that catheter occlusion was the most common complication, occurring in almost 16% of collections performed with a CVC.[306]

Volume shifts may occur as 250 to 300 mL of blood are withdrawn to fill the extracorporeal circuit. Vasovagal reactions—manifest as pallor, diaphoresis, nausea, and bradycardia—or hypovolemic reactions with tachycardia may both lead to hypotension, syncope, and/or seizure-like activity. Treatment for these reactions includes placing the donor into the Trendelenberg position, restoring or expanding blood volume, and if necessary, infusing intravenous pressor agents. (See Chapter 3 for additional details.)

The anticoagulant most commonly used for blood HPC collection is citrate, usually in the form of ACD-A, at an inlet anticoagulant:blood ratio of 1:12 to 1:15. Citrate binds calcium and magnesium. After returning to the donor, citrate is metabolized by the liver to bicarbonate, which in turn increases blood pH and shifts potassium from the extracellular to the intracellular compartment.[191] In vivo, ionized calcium and magnesium levels may decrease by as much as 35% and 56%, respectively, inversely proportional to serum citrate levels.[312] Symptoms of citrate reaction, including paresthesia, headache, lightheadedness, nausea, and chest tightness, account for as many as 50% of apheresis-related adverse events during HPC(A) collection.[135] Such reactions can be treated both by decreasing the infusion rate and by infusing

supplemental calcium. The infusion of a calculated dose of calcium has been shown to reduce the incidence of symptoms related to hypocalcemia from 54% to 20%, especially in small female donors.[312] Use of heparin anticoagulation can also decrease citrate reactions as mentioned above. Cytopenias, typically thrombocytopenia and leukopenia, are well recognized, usually transient effects of leukapheresis. The platelet count has been observed to decrease 30% to 50% after the first HPC(A) collection procedure.[269,302] After completing multiple daily collections, donors may have clinically significant thrombocytopenia for up to 1 week. In the majority of donors, platelet counts return to normal within 1 month and are at predonation baseline by 1 year after donation.[131,282] WBC counts may remain mildly decreased at 1 month following donation, with a return to baseline levels in the majority of donors by 1 year.[131,282]

Psychosocial Considerations and Complications

To ensure optimal donor care, several psychosocial factors should be taken into account, including motivations for donating, donor expectations and attitudes towards the donation process, relationship of the donor to the recipient, donor anxiety, and donor satisfaction with the donation process. Many donors feel that their donation will help to relieve suffering and expect that their lives will have special meaning after they donate.[313] Following donation, donors have reported many psychologic benefits, such as increased self-esteem, pride in the donation, increased sense of personal worth, and a feeling that donating has made their lives more worthwhile.[314,315] Conversely, these feelings may change when outcomes are found to be unfavorable—ie, donors have reported feelings of guilt, grief, and responsibility for the bad outcome.[316,317] Thus it is important to realize that donors may have unrealistic expectations regarding the outcome of a donation.

Related donors have strong motivations for donation, including the feeling that the well-being of one family member is intimately tied to that of another (intrafamilial justification), the belief that one's life is diminished when a family member dies (intimate attachment principle), and the feeling that family members have obligations to each other (duty justification).[318] In a study of HPC donation by siblings, a majority of donors cited the family bond as the main impetus for donation.[319]

Related donors usually do not have the support or advice of an independent advocate and in some cases have reported feeling coerced into donation by family members.[319] To avoid donor coercion, it has been suggested that donors be counseled by and give consent through clinicians who are not directly caring for the patient. Despite such recommendations, a considerable proportion of potential related donors report being approached about donation by family members or the recipient's medical team.[319,320]

Donors of HPC(A) have reported predonation anxiety about pain associated with the donation process, other symptoms that may occur and how they will be managed, and the outcome or other specific aspects of the transplantation experience for the recipient. Anxiety levels reportedly declined following donation, and the majority of donors rated the experience as better than expected, stating that they would donate again.[319,321]

Donor Experiences with Apheresis Collection vs Marrow Collection

The NMDP and the European Group for Blood and Marrow Transplantation estimate that unexpected and severe adverse events occur in 0.1% to 0.6% of HPC(A) donors and in 0.04% to 1.35% of HPC(M) donors, respectively.[131,322] For HPC(M) donors, mechanical injury and anesthesia-related events (eg, postdonation cardiac arrest) are the most frequent cause of prolonged recovery and severe reactions. Severe adverse events in HPC(A) donors are related to mobilizing agents and the collection process, as described above.

Several studies have compared the experiences of HPC(A) donors with HPC(M) donors. Although only HPC(A) donors experienced

pain before the donation procedure, HPC(M) donors were more likely than HPC(A) donors to experience pain at the donation site. Both groups of donors experienced postdonation pain, with HPC(M) donors having more back pain and HPC(A) donors having more skeletal pain. Overall the pain and symptom burden was similar for HPC(A) and HPC(M) donors. In comparison to HPC(A) donors, HPC(M) donors were more likely to develop hemorrhage, anemia, and hypotension; had more discomfort; and were more likely to still have restricted activity at 14 days after donation. HPC(A) donors, however, experienced more difficulty in functioning during the first 7 days of the donation process. In addition, HPC(M) donors required more time away from work and were more likely to require hospitalization. Both groups of donors experienced increased levels of anxiety, psychologic stress and fatigue, and reduced energy related to donation.[181,187,317,321,323]

Complications in Pediatric Patients and Donors

The adverse events encountered during HPC mobilization and collection in pediatric donors and patients are similar to those observed in the adult population; however, their frequencies and manifestations are age related.[137] A study of adverse events during HPC mobilization and collection demonstrated that donors under age 18 had a 41% complication rate whereas adults had a 71% complication rate.[144] Adverse event data of HPC(A) collections from 116 healthy donors (66 pediatric and 50 adult) were examined for age-related adverse events caused by mobilization and apheresis collection.[138] Pediatric donors were further stratified into those who weighed more or less than 20 kg. Adverse events related to G-CSF mobilization occurred in 12% of the smallest donors, 43.3% of the larger pediatric donors, and 79.7% of adults (p = 0.0001). The frequency of adverse events during collection also differed significantly by age and size: 51.7% in the smallest donors, 19.6% in the larger pediatric donors, and 37.3% in adults.[138] Older children required pain medication more often.[212]

Pediatric donors are more likely than adults to require a CVC for collection, and sedation (general, conscious, or local) is required for catheter placement more frequently in younger than in older children. There is no evidence, however, that the overall complication rate related to vascular access differs between pediatric and adult donors.[138,212]

Smaller donors are at increased risk for vasovagal reactions.[211,324,325] When the extracorporeal volume of the collection set exceeds 10% to 15% of the donor's blood volume, or when the donor weighs less than 20 to 25 kg, the collection set is often primed with irradiated, leukocyte-reduced, CMV-negative red cells. This limits volume depletion but exposes the donor to allogeneic blood. An alternative approach for nonanemic patients is to prime the circuit with hydroxyethyl starch or an albumin solution.[326]

The incidence of hypocalcemia during HPC(A) collection in pediatric donors has not been shown to differ significantly from that in adults.[138,212] However, because they may be sedated or unwilling to verbalize, children should be monitored closely for minor clinical symptoms of hypocalcemia, which may be as nonspecific as abdominal pain or dysphoria. Methods for treating and preventing citrate toxicity in pediatric donors include the same measures used in adults.[190,209]

It may be difficult for a child to cooperate with an HPC(A) collection because of young age (eg, as related to restlessness), stress/anxiety, or behavior problems. Strategies to optimize the collection experience include behavioral approaches such as keeping the child in a familiar environment, familiarizing the child with the nursing staff before the procedure, keeping familiar items such as toys and games present, and having a friend or sibling present. As a last resort, the procedure can be performed under anesthesia.[209,214]

References

1. Thomas ED, Blume KG. Historical markers in the development of allogeneic hematopoietic cell transplantation. Biol Blood Marrow Transplant 1999;5:341-6.
2. Kessinger A, Armitage JO, Landmark JD, Weisenburger DD. Reconstitution of human hematopoietic function with autologous cryopreserved circulating stem cells. Exp Hematol 1986;14:192-6.
3. Kessinger A, Armitage JO, Smith DM, et al. High-dose therapy and autologous peripheral blood stem cell transplantation for patients with lymphoma. Blood 1989;74:1260-5.
4. Gianni AM, Siena S, Bregni M, et al. Granulocyte-macrophage colony-stimulating factor to harvest circulating haemopoietic stem cells for autotransplantation. Lancet 1989;2:580-5.
5. Siena S, Bregni M, Brando B, et al. Circulation of CD34+ hematopoietic stem cells in the peripheral blood of high-dose cyclophosphamide-treated patients: Enhancement by intravenous recombinant human granulocyte-macrophage colony-stimulating factor. Blood 1989;74:1905-14.
6. To LB, Shepperd KM, Haylock DN, et al. Single high doses of cyclophosphamide enable the collection of high numbers of hemopoietic stem cells from the peripheral blood. Exp Hematol 1990;18:442-7.
7. Korbling M, Anderlini P. Peripheral blood stem cell versus bone marrow allotransplantation: Does the source of hematopoietic stem cells matter? Blood 2001;98:2900-8.
8. Gratwohl A, Baldomero H, Schwendener A, et al. The EBMT activity survey 2007 with focus on allogeneic HSCT for AML and novel cellular therapies. Bone Marrow Transplant 2009;43:275-91.
9. Ballen KK, King RJ, Chitphakdithai P, et al. The National Marrow Donor Program: 20 years of unrelated donor hematopoietic cell transplantation. Biol Blood Marrow Transplant 2008;14:2-7.
10. Center for International Blood and Marrow Transplant Research. Summary slides—HCT trends and survival data. Milwaukee, WI: CIBMTR, 2010. [Available at http://www.cibmtr.org/ReferenceCenter/SlidesReports/Summary Slides/index.html (accessed April 19, 2010).]
11. Ringden O, Labopin M, Bacigalupo A, et al. Transplantation of peripheral blood stem cells as compared with bone marrow from HLA-identical siblings in adult patients with acute myeloid leukemia and acute lymphoblastic leukemia. J Clin Oncol 2002;20:4655-64.

12. Guardiola P, Runde V, Bacigalupo A, et al. Retrospective comparison of bone marrow and granulocyte colony-stimulating factor-mobilized peripheral blood progenitor cells for allogeneic stem cell transplantation using HLA identical sibling donors in myelodysplastic syndromes. Blood 2002;99:4370-8.

13. Stem Cell Trialists' Collaborative Group. Allogeneic peripheral blood stem-cell compared with bone marrow transplantation in the management of hematologic malignancies: An individual patient data meta-analysis of nine randomized trials. J Clin Oncol 2005;23: 5074-87.

14. Schmitz N, Eapen M, Horowitz MM, et al. Long-term outcome of patients given transplants of mobilized blood or bone marrow: A report from the International Bone Marrow Transplant Registry and the European Group for Blood and Marrow Transplantation. Blood 2006;108:4288-90.

15. Gahrton G, Iacobelli S, Bandini G, et al. Peripheral blood or bone marrow cells in reduced-intensity or myeloablative conditioning allogeneic HLA identical sibling donor transplantation for multiple myeloma. Haematologica 2007;92:1513-18.

16. Eapen M, Logan BR, Confer DL, et al. Peripheral blood grafts from unrelated donors are associated with increased acute and chronic graft-versus-host disease without improved survival. Biol Blood Marrow Transplant 2007;13: 1461-8.

17. Heimfeld S. HLA-identical stem cell transplantation: Is there an optimal CD34 cell dose? Bone Marrow Transplant 2003;31:839-45.

18. Sohn SK, Kim JG, Kim DH, et al. Impact of transplanted CD34+ cell dose in allogeneic unmanipulated peripheral blood stem cell transplantation. Bone Marrow Transplant 2003;31:967-72.

19. Flowers ME, Parker PM, Johnston LJ, et al. Comparison of chronic graft-versus-host disease after transplantation of peripheral blood stem cells versus bone marrow in allogeneic recipients: Long-term follow-up of a randomized trial. Blood 2002;100:415-19.

20. Anderson D, DeFor T, Burns L, et al. A comparison of related donor peripheral blood and bone marrow transplants: Importance of late-onset chronic graft-versus-host disease and infections. Biol Blood Marrow Transplant 2003; 9:52-9.

21. Bensinger WI, Martin PJ, Storer B, et al. Transplantation of bone marrow as compared with peripheral-blood cells from HLA-identical relatives in patients with hematologic cancers. N Engl J Med 2001;344:175-81.

22. Couban S, Simpson DR, Barnett MJ, et al. A randomized multicenter comparison of bone marrow and peripheral blood in recipients of matched sibling allogeneic transplants for myeloid malignancies. Blood 2002;100:1525-31.

23. Eapen M, Horowitz MM, Klein JP, et al. Higher mortality after allogeneic peripheral-blood transplantation compared with bone marrow in children and adolescents: The Histocompatibility and Alternate Stem Cell Source Working Committee of the International Bone Marrow Transplant Registry. J Clin Oncol 2004;22: 4872-80.

24. Remberger M, Ringden O. Similar outcome after unrelated allogeneic peripheral blood stem cell transplantation compared with bone marrow in children and adolescents. Transplantation 2007;84:551-4.

25. Meisel R, Laws HJ, Balzer S, et al. Comparable long-term survival after bone marrow versus peripheral blood progenitor cell transplantation from matched unrelated donors in children with hematologic malignancies. Biol Blood Marrow Transplant 2007;13:1338-45.

26. Comparing peripheral blood stem cell transplantation versus bone marrow transplantation in individuals with hematologic cancers. (BMT CTN 0201). Indentifier:NCT00075816. [Available at http://clinicaltrials.gov/ct2/show/NCT00075816 (accessed April 15, 2010).]

27. Ostronoff M, Ostronoff F, Souto Maior P, et al. Pilot study of allogeneic G-CSF-stimulated bone marrow transplantation: Harvest, engraftment, and graft-versus-host disease. Biol Blood Marrow Transplant 2006;12:729-33.

28. Lowenthal RM, Ragg SJ, Anderson J, et al. A randomized controlled clinical trial to determine the optimum duration of G-CSF priming prior to BM stem cell harvesting. Cytotherapy 2007;9:158-64.

29. Morton J, Hutchins C, Durrant S. Granulocyte-colony-stimulating factor (G-CSF)-primed allogeneic bone marrow: Significantly less graft-versus-host disease and comparable engraftment to G-CSF-mobilized peripheral blood stem cells. Blood 2001;98:3186-91.

30. Frangoul H, Nemecek ER, Billheimer D, et al. A prospective study of G-CSF primed bone marrow as a stem-cell source for allogeneic

bone marrow transplantation in children: A Pediatric Blood and Marrow Transplant Consortium (PBMTC) study. Blood 2007;110:4584-7.

31. Seshadri T, Al-Farsi K, Stakiw J, et al. G-CSF-stimulated BM progenitor cells supplement suboptimal peripheral blood hematopoietic progenitor cell collections for auto transplantation. Bone Marrow Transplant 2008;42:733-7.

32. Kim HJ, Min WS, Cho BS, et al. Overcoming various comorbidities by G-CSF-primed unmanipulated BM SCT in adult patients with AML. Bone Marrow Transplant 2009.

33. Nilsson SK, Simmons PJ. Transplantable stem cells: Home to specific niches. Curr Opin Hematol 2004;11:102-6.

34. Schwartzberg L, Birch R, Blanco R, et al. Rapid and sustained hematopoietic reconstitution by peripheral blood stem cell infusion alone following high-dose chemotherapy. Bone Marrow Transplant 1993;11:369-74.

35. Weaver CH, Hazelton B, Birch R, et al. An analysis of engraftment kinetics as a function of the CD34 content of peripheral blood progenitor cell collections in 692 patients after the administration of myeloablative chemotherapy. Blood 1995;86:3961-9.

36. Krause DS, Fackler MJ, Civin CI, May WS. CD34: Structure, biology, and clinical utility. Blood 1996;87:1-13.

37. Anderlini P, Korbling M. The use of mobilized peripheral blood stem cells from normal donors for allografting. Stem Cells 1997;15:9-17.

38. Raaijmakers MH, Scadden DT. Evolving concepts on the microenvironmental niche for hematopoietic stem cells. Curr Opin Hematol 2008;15:301-6.

39. Nervi B, Link DC, DiPersio JF. Cytokines and hematopoietic stem cell mobilization. J Cell Biochem 2006;99:690-705.

40. Wang MW, Consoli U, Lane CM, et al. Rescue from apoptosis in early (CD34-selected) versus late (non-CD34-selected) human hematopoietic cells by very late antigen 4- and vascular cell adhesion molecule (VCAM) 1-dependent adhesion to bone marrow stromal cells. Cell Growth Differ 1998;9:105-12.

41. Yamaguchi M, Ikebuchi K, Hirayama F, et al. Different adhesive characteristics and VLA-4 expression of CD34(+) progenitors in G0/G1 versus S+G2/M phases of the cell cycle. Blood 1998;92:842-8.

42. Dao MA, Nolta JA. Cytokine and integrin stimulation synergize to promote higher levels of GATA-2, c-myb, and CD34 protein in primary human hematopoietic progenitors from bone marrow. Blood 2007;109:2373-9.

43. Jung Y, Wang J, Song J, et al. Annexin II expressed by osteoblasts and endothelial cells regulates stem cell adhesion, homing, and engraftment following transplantation. Blood 2007;110:82-90.

44. Arai F, Hirao A, Ohmura M, et al. Tie2/angiopoietin-1 signaling regulates hematopoietic stem cell quiescence in the bone marrow niche. Cell 2004;118:149-61.

45. Askenasy N, Farkas DL. Antigen barriers or available space do not restrict in situ adhesion of hemopoietic cells to bone marrow stroma. Stem Cells 2002;20:80-5.

46. Mohle R, Bautz F, Rafii S, et al. The chemokine receptor CXCR-4 is expressed on CD34+ hematopoietic progenitors and leukemic cells and mediates transendothelial migration induced by stromal cell-derived factor-1. Blood 1998;91:4523-30.

47. Cottler-Fox MH, Lapidot T, Petit I, et al. Stem cell mobilization. Hematology Am Soc of Hematol Educ Program 2003:419-37.

48. Lapidot T, Dar A, Kollet O. How do stem cells find their way home? Blood 2005;106:1901-10.

49. Mendez-Ferrer S, Chow A, Merad M, Frenette PS. Circadian rhythms influence hematopoietic stem cells. Curr Opin Hematol 2009;16:235-42.

50. Lucas D, Battista M, Shi PA, et al. Mobilized hematopoietic stem cell yield depends on species-specific circadian timing. Cell Stem Cell 2008;3:364-6.

51. Adams GB, Martin RP, Alley IR, et al. Therapeutic targeting of a stem cell niche. Nature Biotechnol 2007;25:238-43.

52. Ballen KK, Shpall EJ, Avigan D, et al. Phase I trial of parathyroid hormone to facilitate stem cell mobilization. Biol Blood Marrow Transplant 2007;13:838-43.

53. Paczkowska E, Kucia M, Koziarska D, et al. Clinical evidence that very small embryonic-like stem cells are mobilized into peripheral blood in patients after stroke. Stroke 2009;40:1237-44.

54. Wojakowski W, Tendera M, Kucia M, et al. Mobilization of bone marrow-derived Oct-4+ SSEA-4+ very small embryonic-like stem cells in patients with acute myocardial infarction. J Am Coll Cardiol 2009;53:1-9.

55. Stiff PJ, Murgo AJ, Wittes RE, et al. Quantification of the peripheral blood colony forming unit-culture rise following chemotherapy. Could leukocytaphereses replace bone marrow for autologous transplantation? Transfusion 1983;23:500-3.

56. Demirer T, Buckner CD, Bensinger WI. Optimization of peripheral blood stem cell mobilization. Stem Cells 1996;14:106-16.

57. Ford CD, Greenwood J, Anderson J, et al. CD34+ cell adhesion molecule profiles differ between patients mobilized with granulocyte-colony-stimulating factor alone and chemotherapy followed by granulocyte-colony-stimulating factor. Transfusion 2006;46:193-8.

58. Levesque JP, Liu F, Simmons PJ, et al. Characterization of hematopoietic progenitor mobilization in protease-deficient mice. Blood 2004; 104:65-72.

59. Gazitt Y. Comparison between granulocyte colony-stimulating factor and granulocyte-macrophage colony-stimulating factor in the mobilization of peripheral blood stem cells. Curr Opin Hematol 2002;9:190-8.

60. Bashey A, Corringham S, Gilpin E, et al. Simultaneous administration of G-CSF and GM-CSF for re-mobilization in patients with inadequate initial progenitor cell collections for autologous transplantation. Cytotherapy 2000;2:195-200.

61. Glaspy JA, Shpall EJ, LeMaistre CF, et al. Peripheral blood progenitor cell mobilization using stem cell factor in combination with filgrastim in breast cancer patients. Blood 1997;90:2939-51.

62. De Clercq E. The AMD3100 story: The path to the discovery of a stem cell mobilizer (Mozobil). Biochem Pharmacol 2009;77:1655-64.

63. Flomenberg N, Devine SM, Dipersio JF, et al. The use of AMD3100 plus G-CSF for autologous hematopoietic progenitor cell mobilization is superior to G-CSF alone. Blood 2005; 106:1867-74.

64. DiPersio JF, Stadtmauer EA, Nademanee A, et al. Plerixafor and G-CSF versus placebo and G-CSF to mobilize hematopoietic stem cells for autologous stem cell transplantation in patients with multiple myeloma. Blood 2009;113: 5720-6.

65. Devine SM, Vij R, Rettig M, et al. Rapid mobilization of functional donor hematopoietic cells without G-CSF using AMD3100, an antagonist of the CXCR4/SDF-1 interaction. Blood 2008;112:990-8.

66. Larochelle A, Krouse A, Metzger M, et al. AMD3100 mobilizes hematopoietic stem cells with long-term repopulating capacity in nonhuman primates. Blood 2006;107:3772-8.

67. Hess DA, Bonde J, Craft TP, et al. Human progenitor cells rapidly mobilized by AMD3100 repopulate NOD/SCID mice with increased frequency in comparison to cells from the same donor mobilized by granulocyte colony stimulating factor. Biol Blood Marrow Transplant 2007;13:398-411.

68. Donahue RE, Jin P, Bonifacino AC, et al. Plerixafor (AMD3100) and granulocyte colony stimulating factor (G-CSF) mobilize different CD34+ cell populations based on global gene and microRNA expression signatures. Blood 2009;114:2530-41.

69. Calandra G, McCarty J, McGuirk J, et al. AMD3100 plus G-CSF can successfully mobilize CD34+ cells from non-Hodgkin's lymphoma, Hodgkin's disease and multiple myeloma patients previously failing mobilization with chemotherapy and/or cytokine treatment: Compassionate use data. Bone Marrow Transplant 2008;41:331-8.

70. Giralt S, Stadtmauer EA, Harousseau JL, et al. International myeloma working group (IMWG) consensus statement and guidelines regarding the current status of stem cell collection and high-dose therapy for multiple myeloma and the role of plerixafor (AMD 3100). Leukemia 2009;23:1904-12.

71. Fruehauf S, Klaus J, Huesing J, et al. Efficient mobilization of peripheral blood stem cells following CAD chemotherapy and a single dose of pegylated G-CSF in patients with multiple myeloma. Bone Marrow Transplant 2007;39: 743-50.

72. Olivieri A, Offidani M, Cantori I, et al. Addition of erythropoietin to granulocyte colony-stimulating factor after priming chemotherapy enhances hemopoietic progenitor mobilization. Bone Marrow Transplant 1995;16:765-70.

73. Perillo A, Ferrandina G, Pierelli L, et al. Cytokines alone for PBPC collection in patients with advanced gynaecological malignancies: G-CSF vs G-CSF plus EPO. Bone Marrow Transplant 2004;34:743-4.

74. Somlo G, Sniecinski I, ter Veer A, et al. Recombinant human thrombopoietin in combination with granulocyte colony-stimulating factor enhances mobilization of peripheral blood progenitor cells, increases peripheral blood platelet concentration, and accelerates hemato-

poietic recovery following high-dose chemotherapy. Blood 1999;93:2798-806.

75. Pelus LM, Fukuda S. Peripheral blood stem cell mobilization: The CXCR2 ligand GRObeta rapidly mobilizes hematopoietic stem cells with enhanced engraftment properties. Exp Hematol 2006;34:1010-20.

76. Focosi D, Azzara A, Kast RE, et al. Lithium and hematology: Established and proposed uses. J Leukoc Biol 2009;85:20-8.

77. Zohren F, Toutzaris D, Klarner V, et al. The monoclonal anti-VLA-4 antibody natalizumab mobilizes CD34+ hematopoietic progenitor cells in humans. Blood 2008;111:3893-5.

78. Sutherland DR, Anderson L, Keeney M, et al. The ISHAGE guidelines for CD34+ cell determination by flow cytometry. International Society of Hematotherapy and Graft Engineering. J Hematother 1996;5:213-26.

79. Kozuka T, Ikeda K, Teshima T, et al. Predictive value of circulating immature cell counts in peripheral blood for timing of peripheral blood progenitor cell collection after G-CSF plus chemotherapy-induced mobilization. Transfusion 2002;42:1514-22.

80. Padmanabhan A, Reich-Slotky R, Jhang JS, et al. Use of the haematopoietic progenitor cell parameter in optimizing timing of peripheral blood stem cell harvest. Vox Sang 2009;97: 153-9.

81. Bensinger W, DiPersio JF, McCarty JM. Improving stem cell mobilization strategies: Future directions. Bone Marrow Transplant 2009;43:181-95.

82. Banna GL, Simonelli M, Santoro A. High-dose chemotherapy followed by autologous hematopoietic stem-cell transplantation for the treatment of solid tumors in adults: A critical review. Curr Stem Cell Res Ther 2007;2:65-82.

83. Hale GA. Autologous hematopoietic stem cell transplantation for pediatric solid tumors. Expert Rev Anticancer Ther 2005;5:835-46.

84. Burt RK, Loh Y, Pearce W, et al. Clinical applications of blood-derived and marrow-derived stem cells for nonmalignant diseases. JAMA 2008;299:925-36.

85. Nowrousian MR, Waschke S, Bojko P, et al. Impact of chemotherapy regimen and hematopoietic growth factor on mobilization and collection of peripheral blood stem cells in cancer patients. Ann Oncol 2003;14(Suppl 1):i29-36.

86. Fu S, Liesveld J. Mobilization of hematopoietic stem cells. Blood Rev 2000;14:205-18.

87. Copelan E, Pohlman B, Rybicki L, et al. A randomized trial of etoposide and G-CSF with or without rituximab for PBSC mobilization in B-cell non-Hodgkin's lymphoma. Bone Marrow Transplant 2009;43:101-5.

88. Arora M, Burns LJ, Barker JN, et al. Randomized comparison of granulocyte colony-stimulating factor versus granulocyte-macrophage colony-stimulating factor plus intensive chemotherapy for peripheral blood stem cell mobilization and autologous transplantation in multiple myeloma. Biol Blood Marrow Transplant 2004;10:395-404.

89. Kopf B, De Giorgi U, Vertogen B, et al. A randomized study comparing filgrastim versus lenograstim versus molgramostim plus chemotherapy for peripheral blood progenitor cell mobilization. Bone Marrow Transplant 2006; 38:407-12.

90. Hicks ML, Lonial S, Langston A, et al. Optimizing the timing of chemotherapy for mobilizing autologous blood hematopoietic progenitor cells. Transfusion 2007;47:629-35.

91. Bashey A, Donohue M, Liu L, et al. Peripheral blood progenitor cell mobilization with intermediate-dose cyclophosphamide, sequential granulocyte-macrophage-colony-stimulating factor and granulocyte-colony-stimulating factor, and scheduled commencement of leukapheresis in 225 patients undergoing autologous transplantation. Transfusion 2007;47: 2153-60.

92. Jacoub JF, Suryadevara U, Pereyra V, et al. Mobilization strategies for the collection of peripheral blood progenitor cells: Results from a pilot study of delayed addition G-CSF following chemotherapy and review of the literature. Exp Hematol 2006;34:1443-50.

93. Gertz MA, Kumar SK, Lacy MQ, et al. Comparison of high-dose CY and growth factor with growth factor alone for mobilization of stem cells for transplantation in patients with multiple myeloma. Bone Marrow Transplant 2009; 43:619-25.

94. Pusic I, Jiang SY, Landua S, et al. Impact of mobilization and remobilization strategies on achieving sufficient stem cell yields for autologous transplantation. Biol Blood Marrow Transplant 2008;14:1045-56.

95. Ford CD, Green W, Warenski S, Petersen FB. Effect of prior chemotherapy on hematopoietic stem cell mobilization. Bone Marrow Transplant 2004;33:901-5.

96. Tournilhac O, Cazin B, Lepretre S, et al. Impact of frontline fludarabine and cyclophosphamide combined treatment on peripheral blood stem cell mobilization in B-cell chronic lymphocytic leukemia. Blood 2004;103:363-5.

97. Kumar S, Dispenzieri A, Lacy MQ, et al. Impact of lenalidomide therapy on stem cell mobilization and engraftment post-peripheral blood stem cell transplantation in patients with newly diagnosed myeloma. Leukemia 2007;21:2035-42.

98. Kumar S, Giralt S, Stadtmauer EA, et al. Mobilization in myeloma revisited: IMWG consensus perspectives on stem cell collection following initial therapy with thalidomide, lenalidomide or bortezomib-containing regimens. Blood 2009;114:1729-35.

99. Siena S, Schiavo R, Pedrazzoli P, Carlo-Stella C. Therapeutic relevance of CD34 cell dose in blood cell transplantation for cancer therapy. J Clin Oncol 2000;18:1360-77.

100. Yoon DH, Sohn BS, Jang G, et al. Higher infused CD34+ hematopoietic stem cell dose correlates with earlier lymphocyte recovery and better clinical outcome after autologous stem cell transplantation in non-Hodgkin's lymphoma. Transfusion 2009;49:1890-900.

101. Jantunen E, Kuittinen T. Blood stem cell mobilization and collection in patients with lymphoproliferative diseases: Practical issues. Eur J Haematol 2008;80:287-95.

102. Kessinger A, Sharp JG. The whys and hows of hematopoietic progenitor and stem cell mobilization. Bone Marrow Transplant 2003;31:319-29.

103. Maclean PS, Parker AN, McQuaker IG, et al. Ideal body weight correlates better with engraftment after PBSC autograft than actual body weight, but is under-estimated in myeloma patients possibly due to disease-related height loss. Bone Marrow Transplant 2007;40:665-9.

104. Gidron A, Singh V, Egan K, Mehta J. Significance of low peripheral blood CD34+ cell numbers prior to leukapheresis: What should the threshold required for apheresis be? Bone Marrow Transplant 2008;42:439-42.

105. Singh V, Krishnamurthy J, Duffey S, et al. Actual or ideal body weight to calculate CD34+ cell dose in patients undergoing autologous hematopoietic SCT for myeloma? Bone Marrow Transplant 2009;43:301-5.

106. Stockerl-Goldstein KE, Reddy SA, Horning SF, et al. Favorable treatment outcome in non-Hodgkin's lymphoma patients with "poor" mobilization of peripheral blood progenitor cells. Biol Blood Marrow Transplant 2000;6:506-12.

107. Goterris R, Hernandez-Boluda JC, Teruel A, et al. Impact of different strategies of second-line stem cell harvest on the outcome of autologous transplantation in poor peripheral blood stem cell mobilizers. Bone Marrow Transplant 2005;36:847-53.

108. Pavone V, Gaudio F, Console G, et al. Poor mobilization is an independent prognostic factor in patients with malignant lymphomas treated by peripheral blood stem cell transplantation. Bone Marrow Transplant 2006;37:719-24.

109. Tomblyn M, Burns LJ, Blazar B, et al. Difficult stem cell mobilization despite adequate CD34+ cell dose predicts shortened progression free and overall survival after autologous HSCT for lymphoma. Bone Marrow Transplant 2007;40:111-18.

110. Stewart DA, Smith C, MacFarland R, Calandra G. Pharmacokinetics and pharmacodynamics of plerixafor in patients with non-Hodgkin lymphoma and multiple myeloma. Biol Blood Marrow Transplant 2009;15:39-46.

111. Fowler CJ, Dunn A, Hayes-Lattin B, et al. Rescue from failed growth factor and/or chemotherapy HSC mobilization with G-CSF and plerixafor (AMD3100): An institutional experience. Bone Marrow Transplant 2009;43:909-17.

112. DiPersio JF, Micallef IN, Stiff PJ, et al. Phase III prospective randomized double-blind placebo-controlled trial of plerixafor plus granulocyte colony-stimulating factor compared with placebo plus granulocyte colony-stimulating factor for autologous stem-cell mobilization and transplantation for patients with non-Hodgkin's lymphoma. J Clin Oncol 2009;27:4767-73.

113. Kobbe G, Bruns I, Fenk R, et al. Pegfilgrastim for PBSC mobilization and autologous haematopoietic SCT. Bone Marrow Transplant 2009;43:669-77.

114. Hart C, Grassinger J, Andreesen R, Hennemann B. EPO in combination with G-CSF improves mobilization effectiveness after chemotherapy with ifosfamide, epirubicin and etoposide and reduces costs during mobilization and transplantation of autologous hematopoietic progenitor cells. Bone Marrow Transplant 2009;43:197-206.

115. Goldman SC, Bracho F, Davenport V, et al. Feasibility study of IL-11 and granulocyte colony-stimulating factor after myelosuppressive chemotherapy to mobilize peripheral blood stem cells from heavily pretreated patients. J Pediatr Hematol Oncol 2001;23:300-5.

116. Herbert KE, Morgan S, Prince HM, et al. Stem cell factor and high-dose twice daily filgrastim is an effective strategy for peripheral blood stem cell mobilization in patients with indolent lymphoproliferative disorders previously treated with fludarabine: Results of a Phase II study with an historical comparator. Leukemia 2009;23:305-12.

117. Pelus LM. Peripheral blood stem cell mobilization: New regimens, new cells, where do we stand? Curr Opin Hematol 2008;15:285-92.

118. Singh AK, Savani BN, Albert PS, Barrett AJ. Efficacy of CD34+ stem cell dose in patients undergoing allogeneic peripheral blood stem cell transplantation after total body irradiation. Biol Blood Marrow Transplant 2007;13:339-44.

119. Mielcarek M, Martin PJ, Heimfeld S, et al. CD34 cell dose and chronic graft-versus-host disease after human leukocyte antigen-matched sibling hematopoietic stem cell transplantation. Leuk Lymphoma 2004;45:27-34.

120. Cao TM, Wong RM, Sheehan K, et al. CD34, CD4, and CD8 cell doses do not influence engraftment, graft-versus-host disease, or survival following myeloablative human leukocyte antigen-identical peripheral blood allografting for hematologic malignancies. Exp Hematol 2005;33:279-85.

121. Nakamura R, Auayporn N, Smith DD, et al. Impact of graft cell dose on transplant outcomes following unrelated donor allogeneic peripheral blood stem cell transplantation: Higher CD34+ cell doses are associated with decreased relapse rates. Biol Blood Marrow Transplant 2008;14:449-57.

122. Baron F, Maris MB, Storer BE, et al. High doses of transplanted CD34+ cells are associated with rapid T-cell engraftment and lessened risk of graft rejection, but not more graft-versus-host disease after nonmyeloablative conditioning and unrelated hematopoietic cell transplantation. Leukemia 2005;19:822-8.

123. Anderlini P, Korbling M, Dale D, et al. Allogeneic blood stem cell transplantation: Considerations for donors. Blood 1997;90:903-8.

124. Gutierrez-Delgado F, Bensinger W. Safety of granulocyte colony-stimulating factor in normal donors. Curr Opin Hematol 2001;8:155-60.

125. Horowitz MM, Confer DL. Evaluation of hematopoietic stem cell donors. Hematology Am Soc Hematol Educ Program 2005:469-75.

126. Sacchi N, Costeas P, Hartwell L, et al. Haematopoietic stem cell donor registries: World Marrow Donor Association recommendations for evaluation of donor health. Bone Marrow Transplant 2008;42:9-14.

127. Pamphilon D, Nacheva E, Navarrete C, et al. The use of granulocyte-colony-stimulating factor in volunteer unrelated hemopoietic stem cell donors. Transfusion 2008;48:1495-501.

128. Anderlini P, Donato M, Chan KW, et al. Allogeneic blood progenitor cell collection in normal donors after mobilization with filgrastim: The M.D. Anderson Cancer Center experience. Transfusion 1999;39:555-60.

129. Anderlini P, Rizzo JD, Nugent ML, et al. Peripheral blood stem cell donation: An analysis from the International Bone Marrow Transplant Registry (IBMTR) and European Group for Blood and Marrow Transplant (EBMT) databases. Bone Marrow Transplant 2001;27:689-92.

130. Confer DL, Miller JP. Optimal Donor Selection: Beyond HLA. Biol Blood Marrow Transplant 2007;13(Suppl 1):83-6.

131. Miller JP, Perry EH, Price TH, et al. Recovery and safety profiles of marrow and PBSC donors: Experience of the National Marrow Donor Program. Biol Blood Marrow Transplant 2008;14:29-36.

132. McCullough J, Kahn J, Adamson J, et al. Hematopoietic growth factors—use in normal blood and stem cell donors: Clinical and ethical issues. Transfusion 2008;48:2008-25.

133. Leitner GC, Baumgartner K, Kalhs P, et al. Regeneration, health status and quality of life after rhG-CSF-stimulated stem cell collection in healthy donors: A cross-sectional study. Bone Marrow Transplant 2009;43:357-63.

134. Martino M, Console G, Dattola A, et al. Short and long-term safety of lenograstim administration in healthy peripheral haematopoietic progenitor cell donors: A single centre experience. Bone Marrow Transplant 2009;44:163-8.

135. Pulsipher MA, Chitphakdithai P, Miller JP, et al. Adverse events among 2408 unrelated donors of peripheral blood stem cells: Results of a prospective trial from the National Marrow Donor Program. Blood 2009;113:3604-11.

136. Pentz RD. Healthy sibling donation of G-CSF primed stem cells: A call for research. Pediatr Blood Cancer 2006;46:407-8.

137. Pulsipher MA, Nagler A, Iannone R, Nelson RM. Weighing the risks of G-CSF administration, leukopheresis, and standard marrow harvest: Ethical and safety considerations for normal pediatric hematopoietic cell donors. Pediatr Blood Cancer 2006;46:422-33.

138. Sevilla J, Gonzalez-Vicent M, Lassaletta A, et al. Peripheral blood progenitor cell collection adverse events for childhood allogeneic donors: Variables related to the collection and safety profile. Br J Haematol 2009;144:909-16.

139. Kroger N, Renges H, Sonnenberg S, et al. Stem cell mobilisation with 16 microg/kg vs 10 microg/kg of G-CSF for allogeneic transplantation in healthy donors. Bone Marrow Transplant 2002;29:727-30.

140. Beelen DW, Ottinger H, Kolbe K, et al. Filgrastim mobilization and collection of allogeneic blood progenitor cells from adult family donors: First interim report of a prospective German multicenter study. Ann Hematol 2002;81:701-9.

141. Anderlini P, Donato M, Lauppe MJ, et al. A comparative study of once-daily versus twice-daily filgrastim administration for the mobilization and collection of CD34+ peripheral blood progenitor cells in normal donors. Br J Haematol 2000;109:770-2.

142. Bolan CD, Hartzman RJ, Perry EH, et al. Donation activities and product integrity in unrelated donor allogeneic hematopoietic transplantation: Experience of the National Marrow Donor Program. Biol Blood Marrow Transplant 2008;14:23-8.

143. Bolan CD, Carter CS, Wesley RA, et al. Prospective evaluation of cell kinetics, yields and donor experiences during a single large-volume apheresis versus two smaller volume consecutive day collections of allogeneic peripheral blood stem cells. Br J Haematol 2003;120:801-7.

144. de La Rubia J, Diaz MA, Verdeguer A, et al. Donor age-related differences in PBPC mobilization with rHuG-CSF. Transfusion 2001;41:201-5.

145. Anderlini P, Przepiorka D, Seong C, et al. Factors affecting mobilization of CD34+ cells in normal donors treated with filgrastim. Transfusion 1997;37:507-12.

146. Shimizu N, Asai T, Hashimoto S, et al. Mobilization factors of peripheral blood stem cells in healthy donors. Ther Apher 2002;6:413-18.

147. de la Rubia J, Arbona C, de Arriba F, et al. Analysis of factors associated with low peripheral blood progenitor cell collection in normal donors. Transfusion 2002;42:4-9.

148. Ikeda K, Kozuka T, Harada M. Factors for PBPC collection efficiency and collection predictors. Transfus Apher Sci 2004;31:245-59.

149. Martino M, Callea I, Condemi A, et al. Predictive factors that affect the mobilization of CD34(+) cells in healthy donors treated with recombinant granulocyte colony-stimulating factor (G-CSF). J Clin Apher 2006;21:169-75.

150. Ings SJ, Balsa C, Leverett D, et al. Peripheral blood stem cell yield in 400 normal donors mobilised with granulocyte colony-stimulating factor (G-CSF): Impact of age, sex, donor weight and type of G-CSF used. Br J Haematol 2006;134:517-25.

151. Vasu S, Leitman SF, Tisdale JF, et al. Donor demographic and laboratory predictors of allogeneic peripheral blood stem cell mobilization in an ethnically diverse population. Blood 2008;112:2092-100.

152. Namba N, Matsuo K, Kubonishi S, et al. Prediction of number of apheresis procedures necessary in healthy donors to attain minimally required peripheral blood CD34+ cells. Transfusion 2009;49:2384-9.

153. Miflin G, Charley C, Stainer C, et al. Stem cell mobilization in normal donors for allogeneic transplantation: Analysis of safety and factors affecting efficacy. Br J Haematol 1996;95:345-8.

154. Brissot E, Chevallier P, Guillaume T, et al. Factors predicting allogeneic PBSCs yield after G-CSF treatment in healthy donors. Bone Marrow Transplant 2009;49:613-15.

155. Holig K, Kramer M, Kroschinsky F, et al. Safety and efficacy of hematopoietic stem cell collection from mobilized peripheral blood in unrelated volunteers—12 years of single-centre experience in 3928 donors. Blood 2009;114:3757-63.

156. Cashen AF, Lazarus HM, Devine SM. Mobilizing stem cells from normal donors: Is it possible to improve upon G-CSF? Bone Marrow Transplant 2007;39:577-88.

157. Sohn SK, Kim JG, Seo KW, et al. GM-CSF-based mobilization effect in normal healthy donors for allogeneic peripheral blood stem cell transplantation. Bone Marrow Transplant 2002;30:81-6.

158. Kroschinsky F, Holig K, Ehninger G. The role of pegfilgrastim in mobilization of hematopoie-

tic stem cells. Transfus Apher Sci 2008;38: 237-44.

159. Liles WC, Rodger E, Broxmeyer HE, et al. Augmented mobilization and collection of CD34+ hematopoietic cells from normal human volunteers stimulated with granulocyte-colony-stimulating factor by single-dose administration of AMD3100, a CXCR4 antagonist. Transfusion 2005;45:295-300.

160. Moog R. Apheresis techniques for collection of peripheral blood progenitor cells. Transfus Apher Sci 2004;31:207-20.

161. Movassaghi K, Jaques G, Schmitt-Thomssen A, et al. Evaluation of the COM.TEC cell separator in predicting the yield of harvested CD34+ cells. Transfusion 2007;47:824-31.

162. Del Fante C, Perotti C, Viarengo G, et al. Clinical impact of a new automated system employed for peripheral blood stem cell collection. J Clin Apher 2006;21:227-32.

163. Schwella N, Movassaghi K, Scheding S, et al. Comparison of two leukapheresis programs for computerized collection of blood progenitor cells on a new cell separator. Transfusion 2003;43:58-64.

164. Rowley SD, Prather K, Bui KT, et al. Collection of peripheral blood progenitor cells with an automated leukapheresis system. Transfusion 1999;39:1200-6.

165. Wilke R, Brettell M, Prince HM, et al. Comparison of COBE Spectra software version 4.7 PBSC and version 6.0 auto PBSC program. J Clin Apher 1999;14:26-30.

166. Ravagnani F, Siena S, De Reys S, et al. Improved collection of mobilized CD34+ hematopoietic progenitor cells by a novel automated leukapheresis system. Transfusion 1999;39:48-55.

167. Cooling L, Hoffmann S, Herrst M, et al. A prospective randomized trial of two popular mononuclear cell collection sets for autologous peripheral blood stem cell collection in multiple myeloma. Transfusion 2010;50:100-19.

168. Morrison AE, Watson D, Buchanan S, Green RH. Prospective randomised concurrent comparison of the COBE spectra version 4.7, COBE spectra version 6 (Auto PBSC), and Haemonetics MCS+ cell separators for leucapheresis in patients with haematological and non haematological malignancies. J Clin Apher 2000;15:224-9.

169. Abdelkefi A, Maamar M, Torjman L, et al. Prospective randomised comparison of the COBE spectra version 6 and Haemonetics MCS(+)

cell separators for hematopoietic progenitor cells leucapheresis in patients with multiple myeloma. J Clin Apher 2006;21:111-15.

170. Stroncek DF, Clay ME, Smith J, et al. Comparison of two blood cell separators in collecting peripheral blood stem cell components. Transfus Med 1997;7:95-9.

171. Hitzler WE, Wolf S, Runkel S, Kunz-Kostomanolakis M. Comparison of intermittent- and continuous-flow cell separators for the collection of autologous peripheral blood progenitor cells in patients with hematologic malignancies. Transfusion 2001;41:1562-6.

172. Mehta J, Singhal S, Gordon L, et al. Cobe Spectra is superior to Fenwal CS 3000 Plus for collection of hematopoietic stem cells. Bone Marrow Transplant 2002;29:563-7.

173. Ford CD, Lehman C, Strupp A, Kelley L. Comparison of CD34+ cell collection efficiency on the COBE Spectra and Fenwal CS-3000 Plus. J Clin Apher 2002;17:17-20.

174. Padley D, Strauss RG, Wieland M, Randels MJ. Concurrent comparison of the Cobe Spectra and Fenwal CS3000 for the collection of peripheral blood mononuclear cells for autologous peripheral stem cell transplantation. J Clin Apher 1991;6:77-80.

175. Snyder EL, Baril L, Cooper DL, et al. In vitro collection and posttransfusion engraftment characteristics of MNCs obtained by using a new separator for autologous PBPC transplantation. Transfusion 2000;40:961-7.

176. Jeanne M, Bouzgarrou R, Lafarge X, et al. Comparison of CD34+ cell collection on the CS-3000+ and Amicus blood cell separators. Transfusion 2003;43:1423-7.

177. Hartwig D, Dorn I, Kirchner H, Schlenke P. Recommendations for optimized settings of the Amicus Crescendo cell separator for the collection of CD34+ progenitor cells. Transfusion 2004;44:758-63.

178. Adorno G, Del Proposto G, Palombi F, et al. Collection of peripheral progenitor cells: A comparison between Amicus and Cobe-Spectra blood cell separators. Transfus Apher Sci 2004;30:131-6.

179. Ikeda K, Ohto H, Kanno T, et al. Automated programs for collection of mononuclear cells and progenitor cells by two separators for peripheral blood progenitor cell transplantation: Comparison by a randomized crossover study. Transfusion 2007;47:1234-40.

180. Ikeda K, Ohto H, Nemoto K, et al. Collection of MNCs and progenitor cells by two separators

for PBPC transplantation: A randomized cross-over trial. Transfusion 2003;43:814-9.

181. Favre G, Beksac M, Bacigalupo A, et al. Differences between graft product and donor side effects following bone marrow or stem cell donation. Bone Marrow Transplantation 2003; 32:873-80.

182. Stegmayr B, Wikdahl AM. Access in therapeutic apheresis. Ther Apher Dial 2003;7:209-14.

183. Lorente L, Jimenez A, Garcia C, et al. Catheter-related bacteremia from femoral and central internal jugular venous access. Eur J Clin Microbiol Infect Dis 2008;27:867-71.

184. Ruesch S, Walder B, Tramer MR. Complications of central venous catheters: Internal jugular versus subclavian access—a systematic review. Crit Care Med 2002;30:454-60.

185. Froehlich CD, Rigby MR, Rosenberg ES, et al. Ultrasound-guided central venous catheter placement decreases complications and decreases placement attempts compared with the landmark technique in patients in a pediatric intensive care unit. Crit Care Med 2009; 37:1090-6.

186. Feller-Kopman D. Ultrasound-guided internal jugular access: A proposed standardized approach and implications for training and practice. Chest 2007;132:302-9.

187. Rowley SD, Donaldson G, Lilleby K, et al. Experiences of donors enrolled in a randomized study of allogeneic bone marrow or peripheral blood stem cell transplantation. Blood 2001;97:2541-8.

188. Sevilla J, Gonzalez-Vicent M, Fernandez-Plaza S, et al. Heparin based anticoagulation during peripheral blood stem cell collection may increase the CD34+ cell yield. Haematologica 2004;89:249-51.

189. Abrahamsen JF, Stamnesfet S, Liseth K, et al. Large-volume leukapheresis yields more viable CD34+ cells and colony-forming units than normal-volume leukapheresis, especially in patients who mobilize low numbers of CD34+ cells. Transfusion 2005;45:248-53.

190. Bolan CD, Yau YY, Cullis HC, et al. Pediatric large-volume leukapheresis: A single institution experience with heparin versus citrate-based anticoagulant regimens. Transfusion 2004;44:229-38.

191. Humpe A, Riggert J, Munzel U, Kohler M. A prospective, randomized, sequential crossover trial of large-volume versus normal-volume leukapheresis procedures: Effects on serum electrolytes, platelet counts, and other coagulation measures. Transfusion 2000;40:368-74.

192. Gasova Z, Marinov I, Vodvarkova S, et al. PBPC collection techniques: Standard versus large volume leukapheresis (LVL) in donors and in patients. Transfus Apher Sci 2005;32:167-76.

193. Humpe A, Riggert J, Munzel U, et al. A prospective, randomized, sequential, crossover trial of large-volume versus normal-volume leukapheresis procedures: Effect on progenitor cells and engraftment. Transfusion 1999;39:1120-7.

194. Knudsen LM, Nikolaisen K, Gaarsdal E, Johnsen HE. Kinetic studies during peripheral blood stem cell collection show CD34+ cell recruitment intra-apheresis. J Clin Apher 2001;16:114-19.

195. Humpe A, Riggert J, Koch S, et al. Prospective, randomized, sequential, crossover trial of large-volume vs. normal-volume leukapheresis procedures: Effects on subpopulations of CD34(+) cells. J Clin Apher 2001;16:109-13.

196. Rowley SD, Yu J, Gooley T, et al. Trafficking of CD34+ cells into the peripheral circulation during collection of peripheral blood stem cells by apheresis. Bone Marrow Transplant 2001;28:649-56.

197. Ford CD, Greenwood J, Strupp A, Lehman CM. Change in CD34+ cell concentration during peripheral blood progenitor cell collection: Effects on collection efficiency and efficacy. Transfusion 2002;42:904-11.

198. Cull G, Ivey J, Chase P, et al. Collection and recruitment of CD34+ cells during large-volume leukapheresis. J Hematother 1997;6:309-14.

199. Fontana S, Groebli R, Leibundgut K, et al. Progenitor cell recruitment during individualized high-flow, very-large-volume apheresis for autologous transplantation improves collection efficiency. Transfusion 2006;46:1408-16.

200. Cassens U, Momkvist PH, Zuehlsdorf M, et al. Kinetics of standardized large volume leukapheresis (LVL) in patients do not show a recruitment phenomenon of peripheral blood progenitor cells (PBPC). Bone Marrow Transplant 2001;28:13-20.

201. Burgstaler EA, Pineda AA, Winters JL. Hematopoietic progenitor cell large volume leukapheresis (LVL) on the Fenwal Amicus blood separator. J Clin Apher 2004;19:103-11.

202. Sarkodee-Adoo C, Taran I, Guo C, et al. Influence of preapheresis clinical factors on the effi-

ciency of CD34+ cell collection by large-volume apheresis. Bone Marrow Transplant 2003;31:851-5.

203. Ford CD, Pace N, Lehman C. Factors affecting the efficiency of collection of CD34-positive peripheral blood cells by a blood cell separator. Transfusion 1998;38:1046-50.

204. Gidron A, Verma A, Doyle M, et al. Can the stem cell mobilization technique influence CD34+ cell collection efficiency of leukapheresis procedures in patients with hematologic malignancies? Bone Marrow Transplant 2005; 35:243-6.

205. Heuft HG, Dubiel M, Rick O, et al. Inverse relationship between patient peripheral blood CD34+ cell counts and collection efficiency for CD34+ cells in two automated leukapheresis systems. Transfusion 2001;41:1008-13.

206. Katipamula R, Porrata LF, Gastineau DA, et al. Apheresis instrument settings influence infused absolute lymphocyte count affecting survival following autologous peripheral hematopoietic stem cell transplantation in non-Hodgkin's lymphoma: The need to optimize instrument setting and define a lymphocyte collection target. Bone Marrow Transplant 2006;37:811-17.

207. Panse JP, Heimfeld S, Guthrie KA, et al. Allogeneic peripheral blood stem cell graft composition affects early T-cell chimaerism and later clinical outcomes after non-myeloablative conditioning. Br J Haematol 2005;128:659-67.

208. Kim HC. Therapeutic pediatric apheresis. J Clin Apher 2000;15:129-57.

209. Sevilla J, Diaz MA, Fernandez-Plaza S, et al. Risks and methods for peripheral blood progenitor cell collection in small children. Transfus Apher Sci 2004;31:221-31.

210. Cecyn KZ, Seber A, Ginani VC, et al. Large-volume leukapheresis for peripheral blood progenitor cell collection in low body weight pediatric patients: A single center experience. Transfus Apher Sci 2005;32:269-74.

211. Sevilla J, Plaza SF, Gonzalez-Vicent M, et al. PBSC collection in extremely low weight infants: A single-center experience. Cytotherapy 2007;9:356-61.

212. Pulsipher MA, Levine JE, Hayashi RJ, et al. Safety and efficacy of allogeneic PBSC collection in normal pediatric donors: The pediatric blood and marrow transplant consortium experience (PBMTC) 1996-2003. Bone Marrow Transplant 2005;35:361-7.

213. Grupp SA, Frangoul H, Wall D, et al. Use of G-CSF in matched sibling donor pediatric alloge-neic transplantation: A consensus statement from the Children's Oncology Group (COG) Transplant Discipline Committee and Pediatric Blood and Marrow Transplant Consortium (PBMTC) Executive Committee. Pediatr Blood Cancer 2006;46:414-21.

214. Ravagnani F, Coluccia P, Notti P, et al. Peripheral blood stem cell collection in pediatric patients: Feasibility of leukapheresis under anesthesia in uncompliant small children with solid tumors. J Clin Apher 2006;21:85-91.

215. Witt V, Fischmeister G, Scharner D, et al. Collection efficiencies of MNC subpopulations during autologous CD34+ peripheral blood progenitor cell (PBPC) harvests in small children and adolescents. J Clin Apher 2001;16: 161-8.

216. Sidhu RS, Orsini E Jr, Giller R, et al. Midpoint CD34 measurement as a predictor of PBPC product yield in pediatric patients undergoing high-dose chemotherapy. J Clin Apher 2006; 21:165-8.

217. Food and Drug Administraion. 21 CFR Parts 207, 807, and 1271 [Subparts A and B], Human cells, tissues, and cellular and tissue-based products; establishment registration and listing; final rule. [Docket no. 97N-484R.] (January 19, 2001) Fed Regist 2001;66:5447-69. [Available at http://frwebgate.access.gpo. gov/cgi-bin/getdoc.cgi?dbname=2001_regi ster&docid=fr19ja01-4.pdf (accessed April 17, 2010).]

218. Food and Drug Administration. 21 CFR Parts 210, 211, 820, and 1271 [Subpart C]. Eligibility determination for donors of human cells, tissues, and cellular and tissue-based products; final rule. [Docket no. 1997N-0484S.] (May 25, 2004) Fed Regist 2004;69:29786-834.

219. Food and Drug Administration. 21 CFR Parts 16, 1270, and 1271 [Subparts D, E, and F]. Current good tissue practice for human cell, tissue, and cellular and tissue-based product establishments; inspection and enforcement; final rule. (November 24, 2004) Fed Regist 2004;69:68612-88.

220. Food and Drug Administration. Guidance for industry: Eligibility determination for donors of human cells, tissues, and cellular and tissue-based products (HCT/Ps). (August 8, 2007) Rockville, MD: CBER Office of Communication, Outreach, and Development, 2007. [Available at http://www.fda.gov/cber/tissue/ docs.htm (accessed April 17, 2010).]

221. Donor history questionnaire for allogeneic HPC, Apheresis and HPC, Marrow (HPC-DHQ). HPC-DHQ version 1.2. (July 2009) Bethesda, MD: AABB, 2009. [Available at http://www.aabb.org/Content/Donate_Blood/Donor_History_Questionnaires/HPC_Donor_History_Questionnaire (accessed April 17, 2010).]

222. Circular of information for the use of cellular therapy products. (November 2009) Bethesda, MD: AABB, 2009. [Available at http://www.aabb.org/Content/About_Blood/Circulars_of_Information/aabb_coi.htm (accessed April 14, 2010).]

223. Food and Drug Administration. Draft guidance for industry: Use of nucleic acid tests to reduce the risk of transmission of West Nile virus from donors of whole blood and blood components intended for transfusion and donors of human cells, tissues, and cellular and tissue-based products (HCT/Ps). (April 25, 2008) Rockville, MD: CBER Office of Communication, Outreach, and Development, 2008.

224. Food and Drug Administration. Draft guidance for industry: Use of serological tests to reduce the risk of transmission of *Trypanosoma cruzi* infection in whole blood and blood components for transfusion and human cells, tissues, and cellular and tissue-based products. (March 2009) Rockville, MD: CBER Office of Communication, Outreach, and Development, 2009.

225. Padley D, ed. Standards for cellular therapy product services. 4th ed. Bethesda, MD: AABB, 2009.

226. FACT-JACIE international standards for cellular therapy product collection, processing, and administration. 4th ed. Omaha, NE: Foundation for the Accreditation of Cellular Therapy and Joint Accreditation Committee—ISCT and EBMT, 2008. [Available at http://www.factwebsite.org (accessed April 17, 2010).]

227. National Marrow Donor Program 20th edition standards and glossary. (Effective date: March 30, 2009) Minneapolis, MN: NMDP, 2009. [Available at http://www.marrow.org/ABOUT/Who_We_Are/NMDP_Network/Maintaining_NMDP_Standards/index.html (accessed April 17, 2010).]

228. United States consensus standard for the uniform labeling of cellular therapy products using *ISBT 128*. Version 1.1.0. (June 2009) San Bernardino, CA: ICCBBA, 2009. [Available at http://www.iccbba.org/cellular therapy_home.html (accessed April 17, 2010).]

229. Larrea L, de la Rubia J, Soler MA, et al. Quality control of bacterial contamination in autologous peripheral blood stem cells for transplantation. Haematologica 2004;89:1232-7.

230. Padley DJ, Dietz AB, Gastineau DA. Sterility testing of hematopoietic progenitor cell products: A single-institution series of culture-positive rates and successful infusion of culture-positive products. Transfusion 2007;47:636-43.

231. Prince HM, Page SR, Keating A, et al. Microbial contamination of harvested bone marrow and peripheral blood. Bone Marrow Transplant 1995;15:87-91.

232. Schwella N, Zimmermann R, Heuft HG, et al. Microbiologic contamination of peripheral blood stem cell autografts. Vox Sang 1994;67:32-5.

233. Webb IJ, Coral FS, Andersen JW, et al. Sources and sequelae of bacterial contamination of hematopoietic stem cell components: Implications for the safety of hematotherapy and graft engineering. Transfusion 1996;36:782-8.

234. Klein MA, Kadidlo D, McCullough J, et al. Microbial contamination of hematopoietic stem cell products: Incidence and clinical sequelae. Biol Blood Marrow Transplant 2006;12:1142-9.

235. Majado MJ, Garcia-Hernandez A, Morales A, et al. Influence of harvest bacterial contamination on autologous peripheral blood progenitor cells post-transplant. Bone Marrow Transplant 2007;39:121-5.

236. Reich-Slotky R, Wu F, Della-Latta P, et al. Application of pulsed-field gel electrophoresis to identify the source of bacterial contamination of peripheral blood progenitor cell products. Transfusion 2008;48:2409-13.

237. Kamble R, Pant S, Selby GB, et al. Microbial contamination of hematopoietic progenitor cell grafts-incidence, clinical outcome, and cost-effectiveness: An analysis of 735 grafts. Transfusion 2005;45:874-8.

238. Patah PA, Parmar S, McMannis J, et al. Microbial contamination of hematopoietic progenitor cell products: Clinical outcome. Bone Marrow Transplant 2007;40:365-8.

239. Rill DR, Santana VM, Roberts WM, et al. Direct demonstration that autologous bone marrow transplantation for solid tumors can return a multiplicity of tumorigenic cells. Blood 1994;84:380-3.

240. Dreyfus F, Ribrag V, Leblond V, et al. Detection of malignant B cells in peripheral blood

stem cell collections after chemotherapy in patients with multiple myeloma. Bone Marrow Transplant 1995;15:707-11.

241. Gorin NC, Lopez M, Laporte JP, et al. Preparation and successful engraftment of purified CD34+ bone marrow progenitor cells in patients with non-Hodgkin's lymphoma. Blood 1995;85:1647-54.

242. McQuaker IG, Haynes AP, Anderson S, et al. Engraftment and molecular monitoring of CD34+ peripheral-blood stem-cell transplants for follicular lymphoma: A pilot study. J Clin Oncol 1997;15:2288-95.

243. Hohaus S, Pforsich M, Murea S, et al. Immunomagnetic selection of CD34+ peripheral blood stem cells for autografting in patients with breast cancer. Br J Haematol 1997;97:881-8.

244. Mapara MY, Korner IJ, Hildebrandt M, et al. Monitoring of tumor cell purging after highly efficient immunomagnetic selection of CD34 cells from leukapheresis products in breast cancer patients: Comparison of immunocytochemical tumor cell staining and reverse transcriptase-polymerase chain reaction. Blood 1997;89:337-44.

245. Hildebrandt M, Rick O, Salama A, et al. Detection of germ-cell tumor cells in peripheral blood progenitor cell harvests: Impact on clinical outcome. Clin Cancer Res 2000;6:4641-6.

246. McCann JC, Kanteti R, Shilepsky B, et al.. High degree of occult tumor contamination in bone marrow and peripheral blood stem cells of patients undergoing autologous transplantation for non-Hodgkin's lymphoma. Biol Blood Marrow Transplant 1996;2:37-43.

247. Leung W, Chen AR, Klann RC, et al. Frequent detection of tumor cells in hematopoietic grafts in neuroblastoma and Ewing's sarcoma. Bone Marrow Transplant 1998;22:971-9.

248. Gisselbrecht C. In vivo purging and relapse prevention following ASCT. Bone Marrow Transplant 2002;29(Suppl 1):S5-9.

249. Yerly-Motta V, Racadot E, Fest T, et al. Comparative preclinical study of three bone marrow purging methods using PCR evaluation of residual t(14;18) lymphoma cells. Leuk Lymphoma 1996;23:313-21.

250. Martin-Henao GA, Picon M, Limon A, et al. Immunomagnetic bone marrow (BM) and peripheral blood progenitor cell (PBPC) purging in follicular lymphoma (FL). Bone Marrow Transplant 1999;23:579-87.

251. Fouillard L, Laporte JP, Labopin M, et al. Autologous stem-cell transplantation for non-Hodgkin's lymphomas: The role of graft purging and radiotherapy posttransplantation—results of a retrospective analysis on 120 patients autografted in a single institution. J Clin Oncol 1998;16:2803-16.

252. Kawabata Y, Hirokawa M, Komatsuda A, Sawada K. Clinical applications of CD34+ cell-selected peripheral blood stem cells. Ther Apher Dial 2003;7:298-304.

253. Williams CD, Goldstone AH, Pearce RM, et al. Purging of bone marrow in autologous bone marrow transplantation for non-Hodgkin's lymphoma: A case-matched comparison with unpurged cases by the European Blood and Marrow Transplant Lymphoma Registry. J Clin Oncol 1996;14:2454-64.

254. Schouten HC, Kvaloy S, Sydes M, et al. The CUP trial: A randomized study analyzing the efficacy of high dose therapy and purging in low-grade non-Hodgkin's lymphoma (NHL). Ann Oncol 2000;11(Suppl 1):91-4.

255. Bourhis JH, Bouko Y, Koscielny S, et al. Relapse risk after autologous transplantation in patients with newly diagnosed myeloma is not related with infused tumor cell load and the outcome is not improved by CD34+ cell selection: Long term follow-up of an EBMT phase III randomized study. Haematologica 2007;92:1083-90.

256. Alex J, Erickson YO, Schlueter AJ. Improved peripheral blood stem cell collection following plasma exchange in a patient with elevated viscosity and coagulopathy. J Clin Apher 2007;22:339-41.

257. Kang EM, Areman EM, David-Ocampo V, et al. Mobilization, collection, and processing of peripheral blood stem cells in individuals with sickle cell trait. Blood 2002;99:850-5.

258. Adler BK, Salzman DE, Carabasi MH, et al. Fatal sickle cell crisis after granulocyte colony-stimulating factor administration. Blood 2001;97:3313-14.

259. Sauer-Heilborn A, Kadidlo D, McCullough J. Patient care during infusion of hematopoietic progenitor cells. Transfusion 2004;44:907-16.

260. Donmez A, Tombuloglu M, Gungor A, et al. Clinical side effects during peripheral blood progenitor cell infusion. Transfus Apher Sci 2007;36:95-101.

261. Calmels B, Lemarie C, Esterni B, et al. Occurrence and severity of adverse events after autologous hematopoietic progenitor cell infusion are related to the amount of granulocytes

in the apheresis product. Transfusion 2007; 47:1268-75.

262. Marit G, Thiessard F, Faberes C, et al. Factors affecting both peripheral blood progenitor cell mobilization and hematopoietic recovery following autologous blood progenitor cell transplantation in multiple myeloma patients: A monocentric study. Leukemia 1998;12:1447-56.

263. Reiser M, Josting A, Draube A, et al. Successful peripheral blood stem cell mobilization with etoposide (VP-16) in patients with relapsed or resistant lymphoma who failed cyclophosphamide mobilization. Bone Marrow Transplant 1999;23:1223-8.

264. Vela-Ojeda J, Tripp-Villanueva F, Montiel-Cervantes L, et al. Prospective randomized clinical trial comparing high-dose ifosfamide + GM-CSF vs high-dose cyclophosphamide + GM-CSF for blood progenitor cell mobilization. Bone Marrow Transplant 2000;25:1141-6.

265. Anderlini P, Przepiorka D, Seong D, et al. Clinical toxicity and laboratory effects of granulocyte-colony-stimulating factor (filgrastim) mobilization and blood stem cell apheresis from normal donors, and analysis of charges for the procedures. Transfusion 1996;36:590-5.

266. LeBlanc R, Roy J, Demers C, et al. A prospective study of G-CSF effects on hemostasis in allogeneic blood stem cell donors. Bone Marrow Transplant 1999;23:991-6.

267. Martinez C, Urbano-Ispizua A, Marin P, et al. Efficacy and toxicity of a high-dose G-CSF schedule for peripheral blood progenitor cell mobilization in healthy donors. Bone Marrow Transplant 1999;24:1273-8.

268. Stroncek DF, Clay ME, Petzoldt ML, et al. Treatment of normal individuals with granulocyte-colony-stimulating factor: Donor experiences and the effects on peripheral blood CD34+ cell counts and on the collection of peripheral blood stem cells. Transfusion 1996; 36:601-10.

269. Murata M, Harada M, Kato S, et al. Peripheral blood stem cell mobilization and apheresis: Analysis of adverse events in 94 normal donors. Bone Marrow Transplant 1999;24: 1065-71.

270. Stroncek D, Shawker T, Follmann D, Leitman SF. G-CSF-induced spleen size changes in peripheral blood progenitor cell donors. Transfusion 2003;43:609-13.

271. Stroncek DF, Dittmar K, Shawker T, et al. Transient spleen enlargement in peripheral blood progenitor cell donors given G-CSF. J Transl Med 2004;2:25.

272. Becker PS, Wagle M, Matous S, et al. Spontaneous splenic rupture following administration of granulocyte colony-stimulating factor (G-CSF): Occurrence in an allogeneic donor of peripheral blood stem cells. Biol Blood Marrow Transplant 1997;3:45-9.

273. Dincer AP, Gottschall J, Margolis DA. Splenic rupture in a parental donor undergoing peripheral blood progenitor cell mobilization. J Pediatr Hematol Oncol 2004;26:761-3.

274. Falzetti F, Aversa F, Minelli O, Tabilio A. Spontaneous rupture of spleen during peripheral blood stem-cell mobilisation in a healthy donor. Lancet 1999;353:555.

275. Kasper C, Jones L, Fujita Y, et al. Splenic rupture in a patient with acute myeloid leukemia undergoing peripheral blood stem cell transplantation. Ann Hematol 1999;78:91-2.

276. Veerappan R, Morrison M, Williams S, Variakojis D. Splenic rupture in a patient with plasma cell myeloma following G-CSF/GM-CSF administration for stem cell transplantation and review of the literature. Bone Marrow Transplant 2007;40:361-4.

277. Arimura K, Inoue H, Kukita T, et al. Acute lung Injury in a healthy donor during mobilization of peripheral blood stem cells using granulocyte-colony stimulating factor alone. Haematologica 2005;90:ECR10.

278. de Azevedo AM, Goldberg Tabak D. Life-threatening capillary leak syndrome after G-CSF mobilization and collection of peripheral blood progenitor cells for allogeneic transplantation. Bone Marrow Transplant 2001;28:311-12.

279. Abboud M, Laver J, Blau CA. Granulocytosis causing sickle-cell crisis. Lancet 1998;351: 959.

280. Grigg AP. Granulocyte colony-stimulating factor-induced sickle cell crisis and multiorgan dysfunction in a patient with compound heterozygous sickle cell/beta+ thalassemia. Blood 2001;97:3998-9.

281. Iking-Konert C, Ostendorf B, Foede M, et al. Granulocyte colony-stimulating factor induces disease flare in patients with antineutrophil cytoplasmic antibody-associated vasculitis. J Rheumatol 2004;31:1655-8.

282. Tassi C, Tazzari PL, Bonifazi F, et al. Short- and long-term haematological surveillance of

healthy donors of allogeneic peripheral hae-matopoietic progenitors mobilized with G-CSF: A single institution prospective study. Bone Marrow Transplant 2005;36:289-94.

283. Sinha S, Poh KK, Sodano D, et al. Safety and efficacy of peripheral blood progenitor cell mobilization and collection in patients with advanced coronary heart disease. J Clin Apher 2006;21:116-20.

284. Canales MA, Arrieta R, Gomez-Rioja R, et al. Induction of a hypercoagulability state and endothelial cell activation by granulocyte col-ony-stimulating factor in peripheral blood stem cell donors. J Hematother Stem Cell Res 2002; 11:675-81.

285. Harada M, Nagafuji K, Fujisaki T, et al. G-CSF-induced mobilization of peripheral blood stem cells from healthy adults for allogeneic trans-plantation. J Hematother 1996;5:63-71.

286. Hasenclever D, Sextro M. Safety of AlloPBPCT donors: Biometrical considerations on monitor-ing long term risks. Bone Marrow Transplant 1996;17(Suppl 2):S28-30.

287. Rauscher GH, Sandler DP, Poole C, et al. Fam-ily history of cancer and incidence of acute leu-kemia in adults. Am J Epidemiol 2002;156: 517-26.

288. Shpilberg O, Modan M, Modan B, et al. Famil-ial aggregation of haematological neoplasms: A controlled study. Br J Haematol 1994;87:75-80.

289. Bennett CL, Evens AM, Andritsos LA, et al. Haematological malignancies developing in previously healthy individuals who received haematopoietic growth factors: Report from the Research on Adverse Drug Events and Reports (RADAR) project. Br J Haematol 2006;135:642-50.

290. Shapira MY, Kaspler P, Samuel S, et al. Granu-locyte colony stimulating factor does not induce long-term DNA instability in healthy peripheral blood stem cell donors. Am J Hema-tol 2003;73:33-6.

291. Nagler A, Korenstein-Ilan A, Amiel A, Avivi L. Granulocyte colony-stimulating factor gener-ates epigenetic and genetic alterations in lym-phocytes of normal volunteer donors of stem cells. Exp Hematol 2004;32:122-30.

292. Kaplinsky C, Trakhtenbrot L, Hardan I, et al. Tetraploid myeloid cells in donors of peripheral blood stem cells treated with rhG-CSF. Bone Marrow Transplant 2003;32:31-4.

293. Cavallaro AM, Lilleby K, Majolino I, et al. Three to six year follow-up of normal donors

who received recombinant human granulo-cyte colony-stimulating factor. Bone Marrow Transplant 2000;25:85-9.

294. Anderlini P, Chan FA, Champlin RE, et al. Long-term follow-up of normal peripheral blood progenitor cell donors treated with filgrastim: No evidence of increased risk of leu-kemia development. Bone Marrow Transplant 2002;30:661-3.

295. Fischmeister G, Kurz M, Haas OA, et al. G-CSF versus GM-CSF for stimulation of peripheral blood progenitor cells (PBPC) and leukocytes in healthy volunteers: Comparison of efficacy and tolerability. Ann Hematol 1999;78:117-23.

296. Moskowitz CH, Stiff P, Gordon MS, et al. Recombinant methionyl human stem cell fac-tor and filgrastim for peripheral blood progeni-tor cell mobilization and transplantation in non-Hodgkin's lymphoma patients—results of a phase I/II trial. Blood 1997;89:3136-47.

297. Stiff P, Gingrich R, Luger S, et al. A random-ized phase 2 study of PBPC mobilization by stem cell factor and filgrastim in heavily pre-treated patients with Hodgkin's disease or non-Hodgkin's lymphoma. Bone Marrow Trans-plant 2000;26:471-81.

298. Costa JJ, Demetri GD, Harrist TJ, et al. Recom-binant human stem cell factor (kit ligand) pro-motes human mast cell and melanocyte hyperplasia and functional activation in vivo. J Exp Med 1996;183:2681-6.

299. Hubel K, Liles WC, Broxmeyer HE, et al. Leu-kocytosis and mobilization of CD34+ hemato-poietic progenitor cells by AMD3100, a CXCR4 antagonist. Support Cancer Ther 2004; 1:165-72.

300. Liles WC, Broxmeyer HE, Rodger E, et al. Mobilization of hematopoietic progenitor cells in healthy volunteers by AMD3100, a CXCR4 antagonist. Blood 2003;102:2728-30.

301. Dugan MJ, Maziarz RT, Bensinger WI, et al. Safety and preliminary efficacy of plerixafor (Mozobil) in combination with chemotherapy and G-CSF: An open-label, multicenter, explor-atory trial in patients with multiple myeloma and non-Hodgkin's lymphoma undergoing stem cell mobilization. Bone Marrow Trans-plant 2010;45:39-47.

302. Lysak D, Koza V, Jindra P. Factors affecting PBSC mobilization and collection in healthy donors. Transfus Apher Sci 2005;33:275-83.

303. Majado MJ, Minguela A, Gonzalez-Garcia C, et al. Large-volume-apheresis facilitates autolo-

gous transplantation of hematopoietic progenitors in poor mobilizer patients. J Clin Apher 2009;24:12-17.

304. Taylor RW, Palagiri AV. Central venous catheterization. Crit Care Med 2007;35:1390-6.

305. Sadler DJ, Gordon AC, Klassen J, et al. Image-guided central venous catheters for apheresis. Bone Marrow Transplant 1999;23:179-82.

306. Goldberg SL, Mangan KF, Klumpp TR, et al. Complications of peripheral blood stem cell harvesting: Review of 554 PBSC leukaphereses. J Hematother 1995;4:85-90.

307. Moreiras-Plaza M, Albo C, Ares C. Efficacy and safety of femoral vascular access for peripheral blood stem cell (PBSC) collection. Bone Marrow Transplant 2004;33:347-50.

308. Semba CP, Deitcher SR, Li X, et al. Treatment of occluded central venous catheters with alteplase: Results in 1,064 patients. J Vasc Interv Radiol 2002;13:1199-205.

309. Stephens LC, Haire WD, Tarantolo S, et al. Normal saline versus heparin flush for maintaining central venous catheter patency during apheresis collection of peripheral blood stem cells (PBSC). Transfus Sci 1997;18:187-93.

310. Moog R. Adverse events in peripheral progenitor cell collection: A 7-year experience. J Hematother Stem Cell Res 2001;10:675-80.

311. Rhodes B, Anderlini P. Allogeneic peripheral blood stem cell collection as of 2008. Transfus Apher Sci 2008;38:219-27.

312. Bolan CD, Cecco SA, Wesley RA, et al. Controlled study of citrate effects and response to i.v. calcium administration during allogeneic peripheral blood progenitor cell donation. Transfusion 2002;42:935-46.

313. Switzer GE, Dew MA, Magistro CA, et al. The effects of bereavement on adult sibling bone marrow donors' psychological well-being and reactions to donation. Bone Marrow Transplant 1998;21:181-8.

314. Butterworth VA, Simmons RG, Bartsch G, et al. Psychosocial effects of unrelated bone marrow donation: Experiences of the National Marrow Donor Program. Blood 1993;81:1947-59.

315. Simmons RG, Schimmel M, Butterworth VA. The self-image of unrelated bone marrow donors. J Health Soc Behav 1993;34:285-301.

316. Butterworth VA, Simmons RG, Schimmel M. When altruism fails: Reactions of unrelated bone marrow donors when the recipient dies. Omega (Westport) 1992;26:161-73.

317. Heldal D, Brinch L, Tjonnfjord G, et al. Donation of stem cells from blood or bone marrow: Results of a randomised study of safety and complaints. Bone Marrow Transplant 2002; 29:479-86.

318. Pentz RD, Haight AE, Noll RB, et al. The ethical justification for minor sibling bone marrow donation: A case study. Oncologist 2008;13: 148-51.

319. Williams S, Green R, Morrison A, et al. The psychosocial aspects of donating blood stem cells: The sibling donor perspective. J Clin Apher 2003;18:1-9.

320. Clare S, Mank A, Stone R, et al. Management of related donor care: A European survey. Bone Marrow Transplant 2010;45:97-101.

321. Fortanier C, Kuentz M, Sutton L, et al. Healthy sibling donor anxiety and pain during bone marrow or peripheral blood stem cell harvesting for allogeneic transplantation: Results of a randomised study. Bone Marrow Transplant 2002;29:145-9.

322. Halter J, Kodera Y, Ispizua AU, et al. Severe events in donors after allogeneic hematopoietic stem cell donation. Haematologica 2009;94: 94-101.

323. Kennedy GA, Morton J, Western R, et al. Impact of stem cell donation modality on normal donor quality of life: A prospective randomized study. Bone Marrow Transplant 2003;31:1033-5.

324. Michon B, Moghrabi A, Winikoff R, et al. Complications of apheresis in children. Transfusion 2007;47:1837-42.

325. Sevilla J, Gonzalez-Vicent M, Madero L, et al. Large volume leukapheresis in small children: Safety profile and variables affecting peripheral blood progenitor cell collection. Bone Marrow Transplant 2003;31:263-7.

326. Orbach D, Hojjat-Assari S, Doz F, et al. Peripheral blood stem cell collection in 24 low-weight infants: Experience of a single centre. Bone Marrow Transplant 2003;31:171-4.

In: McLeod BC, Szczepiorkowski ZM, Weinstein R, Winters JL, eds.
Apheresis: Principles and Practice, 3rd edition
Bethesda, MD: AABB Press, 2010

24

Receipt, Processing, and Infusion of Hematopoietic Progenitor and Therapeutic Cells

Kathryn M. Bushnell, MT(ASCP), and
Zbigniew M. Szczepiorkowski, MD, PhD, FCAP

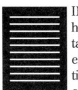

IN THE PAST 60 YEARS, hematopoietic stem cell transplantation (HSCT) has evolved from an experimental therapy for radiation exposure to the standard of care for many malignant and some benign hematologic disorders (see Chapter 22.).[1] Autologous HSCT after high-dose chemotherapy is the standard treatment for diseases such as lymphoma, multiple myeloma, and a few solid tumors.[2] Allogeneic transplants, both myeloablative and nonmyeloablative (the latter also known as reduced intensity), provide cures or prolonged remissions for a variety of hematologic malignancies, including acute and chronic leukemias, myelodysplastic syndrome, and others.[2] The source of an allogeneic product can be a related donor, such as a sibling, parent, or child, or an unrelated donor identified through national and/or international registries.[3] Unrelated donor sources include healthy adults and units of cord blood collected and stored for public use. Both the type of HSCT and the source of the cells affect the extent of involvement of the cell processing facility.

This chapter reviews the types of hematopoietic progenitor cells (HPCs), their collection

Kathryn M. Bushnell, MT(ASCP), Technical Specialist, Cellular Therapy Center, Dartmouth-Hitchcock Medical Center, and Zbigniew M. Szczepiorkowski, MD, PhD, FACP, Associate Professor of Pathology and of Medicine, Dartmouth Medical School, and Director, Transfusion Medicine Service and Director, Cellular Therapy Center, Dartmouth-Hitchcock Medical Center, Lebanon, New Hampshire

The authors have disclosed no conflicts of interest.

and transportation, and both minimal and more-than-minimal processing in the laboratory, including cryopreservation, graft assessment, and administration. ISBT 128 terminology is used throughout.

Types of Hematopoietic Stem Cell Transplantation

Autologous HSCT

The choice between an autologous or allogeneic transplant involves a number of factors, including the patient's age, donor availability, and the type of malignancy.[4] Autologous HSCT recipients must undergo some form of preliminary chemotherapy. Subsequently, when the disease is in complete or, less commonly, partial remission, the patient's autologous HPCs are collected. Autologous transplantation does not require immunosuppression and is generally safer, but it carries the risk of relapse and/or contamination of the graft by tumor cells.[4]

Related Allogeneic HSCT

Allogeneic transplants exploit the potential for a "graft-vs-leukemia" or "graft-vs-tumor" effect—the ability of donor cells to eradicate the malignant cells in the recipient (see Chapter 27).[3] Engraftment time and mortality rates are generally higher than those for autologous transplantation.[4] Some facilities will consider allogeneic transplantation only when 10 out of 10 HLA antigens are matched between the donor and the recipient. Matching in fewer antigenic sites (eg, 6 out of 10) is associated with higher rates of graft-vs-host disease (GVHD; see Chapter 22).

Unrelated Allogeneic HSCT

Unrelated allogeneic HSCTs are often called matched unrelated donor (MUD) transplantations. Approximately 30% of patients requiring allogeneic HSCT will find a donor among siblings or other relatives. Patients without a related donor can seek unrelated donors through national or international registries. In the United States, the National Marrow Donor Program (NMDP) provides the vast majority of such grafts (www.bethematch.org), making possible more than 5000 matches annually. It has more than 8 million registered US donors and has access to approximately 5 million international donors. The ideal donor matches with the recipient in 10 alleles,[5] though it is only fairly recently that donors are really matched at the allele level. Before the late 1990s, matching was based on antigen typings, which in many cases led to transplantation of allele-mismatched donor-recipient pairs. The odds of finding a match depend on the patient's ethnicity. Individuals belonging to ethnic minorities or having a mixed heritage make up only a small percentage of the donor pool and typically present more diverse HLA haplotypes. Patients who cannot find a matched adult donor can sometimes be transplanted using HPCs found in umbilical cord blood (UCB); however, chances of finding an appropriate cord blood unit (or units) are also fairly low for patients with uncommon HLA types.

Characteristics of Hematopoietic Progenitor Cell Products

The "active ingredients" in HPC products are progenitor and stem cells that provide for hematopoietic reconstitution after myeloablation or myelodepletion.[6] HPCs are identified by the presence of the CD34 antigen on their surfaces. Discovery of this antigen in the early 1980s led to the current practice of dosing HPCs based on the content of CD34+ cells/kg of patient body weight. Early studies showed that a purified population of such cells will form colonies of blood precursors and provide immune reconstitution.[7] Stem cells that are negative for both the CD34 antigen and lineage-specific antigens have also been isolated. They give rise to hematopoietic cells, including CD34+ cells, indicating that CD34 lineage-negative cells are probably less differentiated stem cells.[7] Until distinct markers are identified, the CD34 antigen will continue to serve as a marker for the "stemness" of HPCs and also as the most convenient measure of engraftment potential.

The vast majority of HPCs reside in the marrow, which was the source of HPCs in the early days of HSCT. However, marrow harvest is an invasive procedure that typically requires general anesthesia and overnight hospitalization. With the advent of mobilizing agents such as granulocyte colony-stimulating factor (G-CSF) or granulocyte-macrophage colony-stimulating factor (GM-CSF), peripheral blood hematopoietic progenitors and stem cells harvested by leukapheresis have become the most common source of HPCs used for HSCT (see Chapter 23). Mobilizing agents in combination with chemotherapy, so called chemomobilization, are often used to harvest HPCs for autologous HSCT. The nadir leukocyte count after chemotherapy is followed by an increase in the number of CD34+ cells in the circulation that is further enhanced by administration of mobilizing agents.

Hematopoietic Progenitor Cells— Product Types

Hematopoietic Progenitor Cells, Apheresis

HPCs collected by leukapheresis are labeled "HPC, Apheresis," abbreviated as HPC(A).[6] This designation implies that the product was collected after administration of cytokines and/or chemotherapy to the donor/patient to mobilize the HPCs.[3] G-CSF and GM-CSF are still the most commonly used mobilizing agents (see Chapter 23). Both work by down-regulating adhesion molecules that hold the CD34+ cells in the marrow stroma as well as releasing metalloproteinases that remodel the tissue matrix. These actions increase the number of CD34+ cells in peripheral blood in comparison to the steady state.[8] Some patients fail to mobilize with G-CSF, possibly because of prior chemotherapy or radiation or underlying malignancy.[9] A new mobilizing agent, plerixafor (Mozobil, previously AMD3100, Genzyme Corporation,

Cambridge, MA), can be used in combination with G-CSF as a rescue agent, increasing the likelihood of successful collection.[10] Plerixafor reversibly inhibits the binding of stromal-cell-derived factor 1 to the CXCR-4 receptor on HPCs, favoring release of CD34+ cells into the blood.[10]

HPC(A) products can be autologous, allogeneic, or (in the case of identical twins) syngeneic. Regardless of source, their potency is evaluated by the number of CD34+ cells they contain. For most centers, a minimum dose of 1 to 2×10^6 CD34+ cells/kg of patient body weight is considered adequate.[5] HPC(A) are preferred over HPC, Marrow [HPC(M)], not only because the collection process is less invasive but also because engraftment occurs faster than with HPC(M).[11] However, the clinical superiority of HPC(A) has not been definitively established. A randomized controlled trial comparing the two sources of HPCs is underway; accrual of patient-donor pairs was completed in 2009, and a preliminary analysis will be available after 2011 (www.clinicaltrials.gov; NCT00075816).

The most common procedures performed on autologous HPC(A) products are volume reduction before cryopreservation, CD34+ cell selection, and washing before infusion.[6] For allogeneic HPC(A) products, the most common procedures are removal of ABO-incompatible red cells and/or plasma, CD34+ cell selection, and T-cell depletion.[6] Specific procedures are described below in the section on processing.

Therapeutic Cells, Apheresis

Therapeutic cells from apheresis [TC, Apheresis, or TC(A)] are products collected by leukapheresis without mobilization. They are composed primarily of peripheral blood lymphocytes and usually dosed based on the yield of CD3+ cells. All T cells have CD3 present on their membranes. TC(A) products can be further characterized by analysis of additional T-cell antigens, such as CD4 or CD8. After characterization (eg, enumeration, antigen typing) and additional processing, the product name may be changed to reflect the composition of the final product (eg, TC-CTL or TC-DC; see below).

Autologous and allogeneic TC(A) products are collected for very different purposes. Autologous TC(A) may be further processed in the laboratory to generate therapeutic products such as expanded cytotoxic lymphocytes (TC-CTL) or dendritic cells (TC-DC). Allogeneic TC(A) are often collected in tandem with HPC(A) and cryopreserved for future reinfusion. If a patient relapses after allogeneic HSCT, these T cells (TC-T cells) are thawed and reinfused in doses ranging from 1×10^7 to 1×10^8 CD3+ cells/kg in an attempt to induce remission. This product is often referred to as a donor lymphocyte infusion (see Chapter 27).[3]

Hematopoietic Progenitor Cells, Marrow

HPCs obtained by needle aspirations of the iliac crests are designated HPC(M).[6] HPC(M) contain cells of hematopoietic origin admixed with cells of the marrow stroma and peripheral blood.[6] HPC(M) are now mostly used for pediatric patients or in the event of an insufficient HPC(A) collection, though some centers continue to use HPC(M) for a wider population of patients.[9,12,13] The product is collected in the operating room under anesthesia. Marrow is pulled into a syringe and transferred into a collection bag containing anticoagulant, most commonly heparin.[5] A skin site is used repeatedly, but the needle is repositioned to different marrow sites. Using fewer than 8 puncture holes per side, more than a liter of product can be harvested, which provides an adequate yield of HPCs without the need for recombinant growth factors.[13]

Hematopoietic Progenitor Cells, Cord Blood

HPCs are also found in UCB. HPC, Cord Blood [HPC(CB)], can be collected either in utero (ie, the cord blood is collected before delivery of the placenta) or ex utero (ie, after delivery of the placenta and typically outside the delivery room). HPC(CB) has a lower volume and a lower nucleated cell count than HPC(A) and

HPC(M) products. HSCT using a single HPC(CB) unit is feasible for a child or an adult weighing less than 100 pounds.[14,15] For larger adults, the current strategy is to infuse two or more cord blood units (double cord transplant). Recent data from the NMDP indicate that the proportion of unrelated donor allogeneic HSCTs using HPC(CB) is approximately 20%.[12]

The volume of red cells in HPC(CB) is often reduced to standardize volume before cryopreservation. Red cell reduction can be achieved by either differential sedimentation or density gradient centrifugation.[14,16] Because the HPCs in UCB are less mature and have a higher proliferative potential, the cell dose necessary for successful HSCT is lower (minimum of 2×10^5 CD34+ cells/kg).[5] The T lymphocytes in HPC(CB) are more naïve, which decreases the risk of GVHD. Hence, HSCTs using HPC(CB) can be performed between recipients and donors with a higher degree of mismatch than is acceptable for HSCTs using HPC(A) and HPC(M).[5] T-cell naïvety is also likely to increase the time to immunocompetence for the recipient. This and the relatively low number of cells in HPC(CB) translate into an increased time to engraftment, an increased risk of infection, and consequently a longer hospital stay.

Collection, Processing, Issue, and Administration

The progress of a cellular therapy product from the donor/patient through the laboratory to the bedside is outlined in Fig 24-1. This process is overseen by a number of voluntary standard-setting and accrediting organizations [eg, AABB; NMDP; the Foundation for the Accreditation of Cellular Therapy (FACT) and Joint Accreditation Committee—ISCT (International Society for Cellular Therapy) and EBMT (European Group for Blood and Marrow Transplantation), or FACT-JACIE; and The Joint Commission] and regulated by the US Food and Drug Administration (FDA). It is important to see the process as driven as much by patients' clinical outcomes as by the quality of

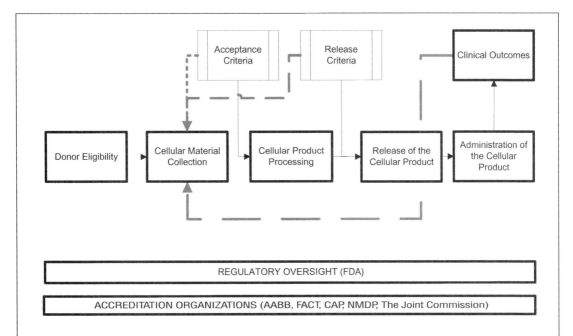

Figure 24-1. General process from collection through processing to administration of cellular therapy products. The figure also illustrates the regulatory oversight of cellular therapy products. The dashed arrows show the interactions between clinical outcomes, release criteria, and acceptance criteria on the collection of cellular material such as apheresis products.
FDA = Food and Drug Administration; FACT = Foundation for the Accreditation of Cellular Therapy; CAP = College of American Pathologists; NMDP = National Marrow Donor Program.

the product before processing (acceptance criteria), after processing (release criteria), and at the time of issue to the patient.

Transportation and Receipt

Cellular therapy products may be collected in an apheresis facility, an operating room, or a delivery room (see Chapters 22 and 23). They must then be transported to the processing laboratory under controlled conditions. Products can be collected and processed at the same institution or transported from the collection facility to another location. The level of control and requirements for transportation depend on the distance, external conditions, and time. When the HPC product reaches the laboratory, properties such as those listed in Table 24-1 are determined to establish its quality. Most products are processed and/or infused within

hours after collection, but unrelated donor products may have a transit time of 48 hours or, rarely, more.[18] Proper transportation of HPC products requires monitoring and control of temperature, transport time, product cellular concentration, and cellular composition.[18]

Most allogeneic HPCs are transported in the liquid state. This approach is dictated not only by the logistics of the collection but also by the fact that cryopreservation and processing may result in loss of up to one-third of the colony-forming units (CFUs; see "Cryopreservation" below).[18] Recent data support transportation of HPC(A) at 4 C, especially if transit time will exceed 24 hours. In products transported at room temperature, only 75% of the initial CD34+ cells are viable at 24 hours, and after 48 hours only 20% remain viable.[19] However, some concerns have been raised about these data, as they were obtained using containers

Table 24-1. Examples of Quality Characteristics (ie, Acceptance Criteria)* of Cellular Therapy Products after Collection[17]

Characteristic	HPC (M)	HPC (A)	HPC (C)	TC (A)
TNC	See comment[†]	See comment[†]	>60 to 100 $\times$ 10^7	See comment[†]
MNC content (%)	As measured	>60	As measured	>80
Viability (%)	>70	>90	>70	>90
Expiration time	24 hours	48 hours	48 hours	48 hours
Bacterial cultures[‡]	No growth	No growth	No growth	No growth
Fungal cultures[‡]	No growth	No growth	No growth	No growth
Potency assays				
Cellular content	Yes	No	Yes	Yes
CD34	No	Yes	Yes	No
CD3	No	No/Yes	No	Yes
CD14	No	No	No	Yes (TC-DC)
CD56	No	No	No	Yes (TC-NK)
CFU-GM	Yes/No	No	Yes	No

*The acceptable content of cells will vary widely according to the weight of the recipient and the expected level of postcollection manipulation.

[†]The acceptance criteria for this product depend on the desired function of the final CT product.

[‡]Microbial contamination needs to be assessed. The culture results are usually not available at the time of distribution from the collection facility to the processing facility.

HPC = hematopoietic progenitor cell; HPC (M) = HPCs from marrow; HPC (A) = HPCs from apheresis; HPC (C) = HPCs from cord blood; TC (A) = therapeutic cells from apheresis; TNC = total nucleated cell(s); MNC = mononuclear cell; DC = dendritic cell; NK = natural killer; CFU-GM = colony-forming unit—granulocyte-macrophage.

that did not allow for gas exchange with the environment. At least two more studies awaiting publication (G. Kao, Dana Farber/NMDP, and D. Pamphilon, BEST Collaborative, personal communication) have shown that the loss of viability at room temperature is not as great as noted by Jansen et al[19]; nevertheless, the conclusion that 4 C is the preferred temperature seems to be valid. The NMDP requires transportation of HPC(A) products in coolers with frozen ice packs, while FACT-JACIE standards state that the cellular therapy products should be transported at the temperature specified by the processing facility.[18]

Cord blood products are shipped for transplantation in the cryopreserved state. Most institutions use a dry shipper, which contains liquid nitrogen in an absorbent material surrounding a central chamber. The space for the product is left "dry" and maintains the temperature of liquid-nitrogen vapor during shipping. Dry shippers can be equipped with a data logger that records temperature at predefined intervals. The data can be downloaded at the transplant center and/or after return to the cord blood bank to verify that the chamber temperature remained within the acceptable range during shipment.

Products must arrive at their destination appropriately labeled and accompanied by all required information.[20(p55)] Standardization of labeling has been critical to allow for transportation of products to other institutions, both domestic and international. The ISBT 128 system of labeling cellular therapy products has gained international acceptance. Recognizing that full implementation of ISBT 128 takes resources and time, voluntary accrediting organizations (eg, AABB, FACT-JACIE, NMDP) require only the use of ISBT 128 product names at this time. However, it is likely that the use of ISBT 128 formats for unique identifiers and labels will be required in the future. Commercial vendors have now produced software and on-demand label printing products that should facilitate the transition.

Table 24-2 summarizes current requirements for warning and biohazard labels on the cellular therapy products collected, processed, and/or administered in the United States.[6]

Acceptance Criteria

Acceptance criteria are product characteristics that should be met by, and records that should be available for, any cellular therapy product entering a laboratory. Some elements are defined by standards and regulations, while others may be determined by individual laboratories. At a minimum, cellular therapy products must be accompanied by infectious disease testing results, ABO and Rh type identification, and a completed label; for products to be used in the United States, a summary of records is also required. The label must identify donor, recipient, collection facility, and product and must specify the date and time of collection. It must include a unique numeric or alphanumeric identifier that will allow the product to be traced from collection to final disposition. This unique identifier will also help track records, results, and deviations for the product. Standards require that this unique identifier be present on the product at all times, unaltered and uncovered.[20(p26)]

Processing

Processing times have increased as a result of advances in the field and the development of more complex processes. Furthermore, large-volume leukapheresis, which may involve processing up to 40 L of blood, increases collec-

tion time and delays the start of processing.[11] Overnight storage before processing was formerly a rare occurrence but is now often essential for laboratory work flow, especially for complex processing.[2,11] However, there are no published guidelines for liquid storage of HPC products. In one study, overnight storage at 4 C before CD34 selection was compared to immediate processing and did not significantly affect engraftment.[21] A study by Antonenas et al showed that CD34 viability decreased in HPC(A) products stored at 4 C; however, such a change was not observed in HPC(M) products stored under the same conditions.[2] Unpublished studies (referenced earlier) have suggested that pH, cell concentration, type of product, and storage temperature may all affect HPC viability.

Laboratory manipulations of cellular therapy products can be divided into two categories: simple and complex. Simple procedures separate different cell types and their components by physical properties such as size and density but retain the natural physiologic function of these cells.[14] Simple processing includes cryopreservation (which is the most common procedure), cell selection, plasma reduction, and other processes described further in this chapter. The FDA defines such procedures as "minimal manipulation" and categorizes the resulting materials as "361 products," which refers to Section 361 of the US Public Health Service Act.[22-26] Complex processing is "more than minimal manipulation"; cells so manipulated are characterized as "351 products" (ie, regulated under Section 351 of the US Public Health Service Act).[22-26] Complex procedures separate cell types by their unique surface markers and biologic characteristics.[14] They include ex-vivo expansion, dendritic cell generation, and other processes described later. Table 24-3 illustrates the difference between the two product types.

ABO Incompatibility

Selection of an allogeneic HSCT donor is primarily based on the degree of HLA match. If the donor and recipient share the same blood type, there is no need for additional processing. However, HLA type is inherited separately

Table 24-2. Biohazard and Warning Labels on Cellular Therapy Products Collected, Processed, and/or Administered in the United States[6]

	Status					Product Labels				
	All Donor Screening and Testing Completed	Abnormal Results of Donor Screening	Abnormal Results of Donor Testing	Other Condition*	Urgent Medical Need	Biohazard Legend [per 21 CFR 1271.3 (h)]	For Autologous Use Only	Not Evaluated for Infectious Substances	WARNING: Advise patient of communicable disease risks	WARNING: Reactive test results for (name of disease agent or disease)
Donor Eligibility Determination Required [21 CFR 1271.45(b)]										
1. Allogeneic donors with incomplete donor eligibility determination[†]	No	No	No		Yes			X	X	
2. Allogeneic donors found ineligible										
A first-degree or second-degree blood relative[‡]	Yes	No/Yes	Yes		NA	X			X	X
A first-degree or second-degree blood relative[‡]	Yes	Yes	No		NA	X			X	
Unrelated donor[§]	Yes	No/Yes	Yes		Yes	X			X	X
Unrelated donor[§]	Yes	Yes	No		Yes	X			X	
Unrelated donor	Yes	No	No	Yes	Yes			X	X	

Table 24-2. Biohazard and Warning Labels on Cellular Therapy Products Collected, Processed, and/or Administered in the United States (Continued)

Donor Eligibility Determination Not Required [21 CFR 1271.90(a)]						
3. Autologous donors‖						
Autologous donor¶	No	No	No	NA	X	X
Autologous donor#	Yes	No/Yes	Yes	NA	X	X	X
Autologous donor#	Yes	Yes	No	NA	X	X

NOTE: Application of biohazard and warning labels extends outside the product described in 21 CFR 1271 based on adherence to professional standards and applies to unmanipulated HPC(M). Alternatively, unmanipulated HPC(M) is not regulated under 21 CFR 1271 but is included based on voluntary adherence to professional standards. Other cellular products which are not described in the 21 CFR 1271 [eg, HPC(A) from unrelated donors; HCP(CB)] are included in this table.

*Testing for infectious disease markers performed in non-CLIA-certified laboratory and/or using non-FDA cleared, approved, or licensed tests.

†The donor eligibility determination must be finalized during or after the use of the cellular therapy product. The results must be communicated to the treating physician [21 CFR 1271.60 (d)(4)]. Abnormal results of any screening or testing requires labeling as in item 2 in this table (21 CFR 1271.65 applies).

‡Notification of the recipient's and donor's physicians of abnormal screening and/or testing results is required. 21 CFR1271.65 (b)(1)(i).

§21 CFR 1271.65 (b)(1)(ii).

‖Any abnormal donor screening or testing results (even though neither screening nor testing is mandated for this group of donors) require appropriate labeling [21 CFR 1271.90(b)]. 21 CFR 1271.90(a)(b).

¶21 CFR 1271.90(a)(1)(2).

#21 CFR 1271.90(b)(1)(3).

CFR = Code of Federal Regulations; CLIA = Clinical Laboratory Improvement Amendments of 1988; FDA = Food and Drug Administration.

Table 24-3. Criteria Determining the HCT/P Regulatory Path[26]

PHS Act Section 361, 21 CFR 1271	PHS Act Section 351, Regulation of Biological Products, Premarket Approval
To be regulated solely under Section 361 of the PHS Act and CFR Title 21 Part 1271, an HCT/P must meet all four criteria:	Sections 351 and 361 of the PHS Act and premarket approval authorities apply to HCT/Ps if they meet at least one of the following criteria:
1. Minimally manipulated. 2. Intended for allogeneic use only. 3. Not combined with a device or drug, except for sterilizing, preserving, or storage agents that do not raise clinical safety concerns. 4. Free of systemic effects and independent of the metabolic activity of living cells for its primary function, *unless* the HCT/P is for (a) autologous use, (b) allogeneic use in a first-degree or second-degree blood relative, or (c) reproductive use.	1. Manipulated such that biological or relevant functional characteristics of the cells or tissues are altered. 2. Genetically modified. 3. Expanded ex vivo. 4. Used for other-than-normal function of the HCT/P, or for structural tissue, used for a structural purpose in a location of the body where such functional purpose does not normally occur (non-allogeneic use). 5. Combined with a drug, device, or biological product that may raise clinical safety concerns. 6. Active systemically or dependent on the metabolic activity of the living cells for their primary function, *unless* minimally manipulated for (a) autologous use, (b) use in a first-degree or second-degree blood relative, or (c) reproductive use.

HCT/P = human cells, tissues, and cellular and tissue-based product; PHS = Public Health Service; CFR = Code of Federal Regulations.

from ABO, and approximately four out of ten HLA-identical donors will have a blood type that differs from their potential recipient's.[27,28] Table 24-4 illustrates all possible combinations between donor and recipient blood types. The management of a mismatched recipient's transfusions of blood components before and after a transplantation can be quite complex, and approaches to the problem vary among transplant centers.[28] If the donor and recipient have incompatible ABO types, appropriate processing can minimize the risk of a transfusion reaction that might otherwise complicate the HPC infusion. In addition, one study by Worel et al showed that ABO-mismatched transplants have an increased risk of transplant-related mortality.[27] Figure 24-2 summarizes some of the problems associated with ABO-incompatible transplants as well as the laboratory processing required to minimize the risk of complications.

Major ABO incompatibility exists when the recipient has antibodies against the donor's red cells.[28,30] Red cells in the HPC product can be reduced by manual gradient centrifugation or by processing on an automated cell washer.[14] Red cell reduction is performed on HPC(A), HPC(M), and HPC(CB) products when necessary, targeting a packed red cell content less than 20 to 25 mL.[30,31] Minor ABO incompatibility exists when the donor has antibodies against the recipient's red cells.[28,30] The amount of incompatible plasma in the HPC product can be reduced by centrifugation and resuspension in saline and albumin[14]; the antibody titer that triggers plasma removal varies widely among institutions. This process can be performed manually or on an automated device. A bidirectional mismatch exists when recipient and donor each have antibodies against the other's blood type. Both manipulations may be necessary in such cases.

Cryopreservation

Cryopreservation is currently the most common procedure performed in a processing laboratory.[32,33] It allows for the graft to be counted, tested, and stored while the patient is being prepared for HSCT. It is necessary for autologous transplantation and may be used for allogeneic transplantation as well, where it is helpful in scheduling the conditioning regimen and coping with unforeseen clinical conditions in the recipient. However, many institutions infuse HPC(A) or HPC(M) without cryopreservation, particularly in the setting of unrelated allogeneic HSCT.

Cryopreservation carries some risks. It reduces the viability of nucleated cells and lowers the number of cells ultimately available for infusion.[34] Nonetheless, CD34+ HPCs seem to be more resistant to the effects of cryopreservation than other nucleated cells and thus have higher viability at the time of infusion.[34]

Cryopreservation of living cells has been possible for many years. It is well known that to recover viable cells, a freezing solution must be used that contains suitable concentrations of

Table 24-4. ABO Compatibility in Hematopoietic Stem Cell Transplantation[29]

		Donor			
		0	**A**	**B**	**AB**
Recipient	0	Compatible	Major	Major	Major
	A	Minor	Compatible	Bidirectional	Major
	B	Minor	Bidirectional	Compatible	Major
	AB	Minor	Minor	Minor	Compatible

See text for an explanation of the terms: major, minor, and bidirectional incompatibilities.

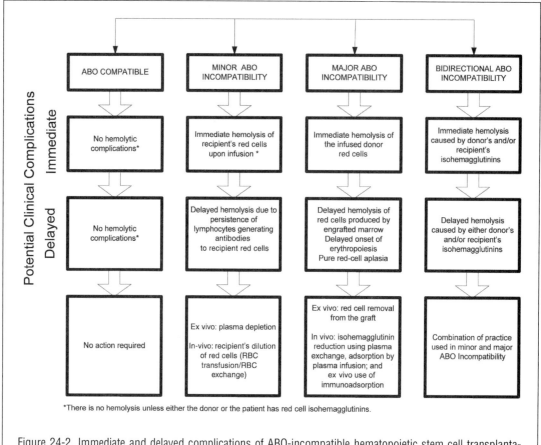

Figure 24-2. Immediate and delayed complications of ABO-incompatible hematopoietic stem cell transplantation.[30]

protein and a cryoprotective agent in an isotonic solution. The source of protein for autologous grafts is usually autologous plasma collected concurrently with HPCs or TCs during apheresis. For allogeneic grafts it can be donor plasma or 5% human serum albumin.[35] The protein helps to stabilize the cell membrane after thawing.[33,36] The isotonic solution can be normal saline or commercially available electrolyte solutions, such as Normosol-R (Abbott Laboratories, Abbott Park, IL) and Plasma-Lyte A (Baxter International, Deerfield, IL).[32,33] Tissue culture media were used in the past, but they are not approved for clinical use and have been replaced to comply with regulatory requirements.[5] Cryoprotectants can be classified as either intracellular or extracellular. The agent almost universally used in freezing

HPCs is the intracellular cryoprotectant dimethylsulfoxide (DMSO).[32,33] When cold, DMSO is relatively nontoxic to cells, even at the final concentrations of 5% to 10% used in freezing solutions; it need not be removed by washing before infusion.[14] Hydroxyethyl starch (HES) is an extracellular cryoprotectant that can be used in combination with DMSO.[33,36] HES does not penetrate the cell membrane; instead it forms an impermeable viscous solution extracellularly that helps maintain viability by preventing cellular dehydration.[14] Use of HES allows the DMSO content of the freezing solution to be decreased.

Current techniques use DMSO as the cryoprotectant, with gradual cooling to the freezing point, rapid freezing, and gradual cooling in the frozen state.[36] The cells experience minor dehydration, forming extracellular and intracellular ice in small amounts. Rapid thawing just before infusion minimizes expansion of ice crystals and dilutes the increased solute concentration within the cell.[33,36]

Most processing laboratories cryopreserve HPCs and TCs in controlled-rate freezers (CRFs), which control the cooling rate in the freezing chamber through preprogrammed steps. There are typically two probes that register the temperature of the chamber and the temperature of the product, respectively.[33,36] The role of the CRF is to transition the product from liquid to solid state through three phases. Figure 24-3 shows the steps in a standard freeze curve, which is the recording of the temperature of the product and the chamber. The

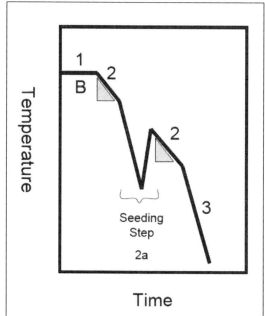

Figure 24-3. Temperature vs time for a typical controlled-rate freezing protocol. Description: 1) equilibration of samples and chamber temperatures; 2) constant cooling rate followed by rapid cooling and warming step, the so-called automatic seeding step (2a), to induce controlled nucleation of ice in the solution; and 3) constant cooling rate to achieve temperature low enough to facilitate transfer to long-term storage. (Reprinted from Hubel.[33])

CRF is pre-cooled to a product- and protocol-specific temperature before freezing solution is added to the cells. HPCs in freezing solution are then placed in the CRF in bags thin enough to allow the entire product to cool at about the same rate and therefore to freeze at the same time, which helps to maintain cellular integrity from freeze to thaw.[14,33] Most products that enter the laboratory for processing are frozen within 24 hours of collection.

Processing–Minimal Manipulation

Positive or Negative Cell Selection

Selection of cells can be accomplished by targeting antigen sites on the cells of interest. Antibodies against antigens expressed on cell surfaces (eg, CD14, CD34) or in the cytoplasm (eg, aldehyde dehydrogenase) are used to characterize different cell populations immunophenotypically.

Cell selection instruments use such antibodies, most often bound to magnetic beads, to enrich or deplete desired cell populations in HPC products.[6] One example is the CliniMACS system (Miltenyi Biotec, Bergisch Gladbach, Germany), in which an HPC product is incubated with a specific antibody conjugated to magnetic iron-dextran particles.[37] The antibodies bind to the corresponding antigen on the target cell, and excess antibody is then washed off. The product is loaded onto the CliniMACS instrument, which performs a series of steps, including loading cells into the chamber in an applied magnetic field to attract cells that have bound the antibody-iron particles, washing off the unbound cells (ie, cells lacking iron-dextran particles), disengaging the magnetic field, and collecting the selected cells in a bag.[37] For positive selection, the desired cells are targeted by antibody. For negative selection, the nontargeted cells become the final product. The CliniMACS does not remove the magnetic beads from targeted cells; therefore, positively selected cells are infused with beads still attached.

In another magnetic separator, the Isolex 300i (Baxter Healthcare, Deerfield, IL), the majority of the processing steps are performed on the instrument, and the larger magnetic beads are removed after collection. The initial steps include a product wash to deplete platelets, an incubation with specific IgG antibody, and another wash to remove unbound antibody.[37] Magnetic beads conjugated to an anti-IgG reagent are then introduced and bind to cells that have bound the specific antibody.[37] Cells that have bound antibody are then separated with a magnet. Before completion of the process, the beads are released from the cells through the action of a specific releasing agent.[37]

Both the CliniMACS and Isolex 300i require an investigational device exemption from the FDA before use on patient-derived material. The most common procedure is positive selection of CD34+ cells, which also helps to deplete a graft of T lymphocytes that might contribute to GVHD and can concentrate a dilute product before a pediatric transplantation. Because most tumor cells do not express the CD34 antigen, CD34 selection also decreases the number of tumor cells in an autologous product.[21] In a small comparison study, the Isolex 300i showed a slightly higher recovery of CD34+ cells, while the CliniMACS showed a slightly higher purity.[37] The CliniMACS CD34 selection is completed in less than 3 hours, whereas the Isolex 300i requires approximately 4 to 5 hours.[37] Magnetic cell separation can also be used to isolate a number of other cell types, including monocytes, lymphocytes, tumor cells, B cells, and natural killer (NK) cells. Positive selection with an antibody such as CD19 can remove immature B cells from the collected material.[36] Positive selection for CD14 can be used to enrich the monocyte fraction in preparation for dendritic cell generation.

Depletion

T cells play an active role in acute and chronic GVHD. T-cell depletion decreases the risk of GVHD but also decreases the beneficial graft-vs-tumor effect and increases the chance of graft rejection.[5] T cells were initially depleted by incubating marrow with T-cell-specific anti-

bodies.[38] Today, T cells are depleted either by positive CD34 selection or by negative selection with specific T-cell antibody (anti-CD3).[3] Growing interest in subclasses of T cells and their role in GVHD has also prompted some to use antibodies other than anti-CD3; examples include anti-CD6, anti-CD2, and anti-CD7. The reader is encouraged to seek more information on relevant new trials at www.clinicaltrials.gov (search term: eg, T-cell selection).

Cell Separation/Enrichment Using Counterflow Centrifugal Elutriation

The Elutriator (Beckman Coulter, Brea, CA) and the Elutra Cell Separation System (CaridianBCT, Lakewood, CO) both use the process of counterflow centrifugal elutriation (CCE) to separate cells by density and size (see Fig 24-4).[39] The cells are loaded into a chamber that spins continuously as medium flows across the cells in a direction opposite to the centrifugal force. The opposing centrifugal and counterflow forces cause cells in the chamber to separate into radial layers, with small or lighter cells closer to the center and heavier or larger cells closer to the outer wall.[39] Distinct fractions can be collected by changing the centrifuge speed and/or the medium flow rate after the chamber is loaded. CCE can be used for T-cell depletion, enrichment of monocytes for DC generation, and lymphocyte collection for expanding T cells.[39] The Elutriator is an open system that requires sterilization of all components between uses as well as a significant amount of operator training; consequently it is used infrequently.[40] The Elutra has a closed system disposable kit; it takes approximately an hour to process the cells and is fairly easy to operate.[39] A closed system is preferred for any clinical process to minimize exposure of a product to environmental contaminants.[40]

Plasma Reduction

A cellular therapy product may undergo plasma removal when the plasma is ABO incompatible (discussed earlier) or when there is a need to reduce product volume before infu-

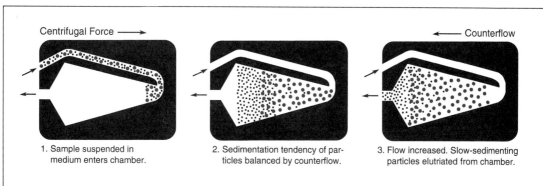

1. Sample suspended in medium enters chamber.

2. Sedimentation tendency of particles balanced by counterflow.

3. Flow increased. Slow-sedimenting particles elutriated from chamber.

Figure 24-4. Schema explaining the principle of counterflow centrifugal elutriation. (Courtesy of Beckman Instruments, Inc.)

sion or cryopreservation.[6] Smaller recipients or those who have cardiac or renal insufficiency or other fluid clearance problems may benefit from plasma reduction.[6] A significant proportion of HPC products are stored in the frozen state with an expiration date of 5 to 20 years after collection. Reducing the volume of HPCs by plasma removal before cryopreservation minimizes the space required for long-term storage. A smaller final volume also reduces the amount of DMSO infused into the recipient. Plasma can be easily removed by simple centrifugation or processing on an instrument such as the COBE 2991 (CaridianBCT). All HPC products can be plasma reduced, but the process can be particularly appropriate for a large-volume HPC(M) product intended for a small recipient.

Buffy-Coat Enrichment

The buffy coat is the leukocyte-rich portion that remains after both plasma and red cells have been depleted from an HPC product.[6] An autologous HPC(M) product is often processed to isolate the buffy coat to decrease its volume before freezing (buffy-coat enrichment). The procedure is semiautomated and can be performed with cell washers or apheresis devices.[14] A buffy coat generally retains 80% to 90% of the starting product's nucleated cells, with less than 15% of its plasma and red cells.[1] Buffy-

coat enrichment may also be used before complex processing to debulk the product.[14]

Mononuclear Cell Separation

A mononuclear cell (MNC) separation is a density-based separation of the MNC layer from red cells and granulocytes.[6] MNCs can be separated manually on a density gradient centrifugation medium [eg, Ficoll-Paque (GE Healthcare, Chalfont St. Giles, United Kingdom)] or a lymphocyte separation medium, both of which have a density similar to lymphocytes. By overlaying harvested cells with media and then spinning them in a centrifuge, the MNC layer can be separated from the rest of the product and isolated for further processing. The apheresis procedure performed to collect an HPC(A) or TC(A) product is actually a form of automated MNC collection, and apheresis instruments can be used in the cell processing laboratory, drawing material from a product bag instead of a patient's bloodstream. MNC separation can be appropriate when there is a bidirectional ABO incompatibility between the patient and the donor; the final product has both plasma and red cells removed and is usually infused fresh.

Cord Blood Processing

HPC(CB) is rich in HPCs, especially the early progenitors. Public cord blood banks are unique in the field of cellular therapy in that they store allogeneic units in advance for subsequent use by an appropriately matched recipient who is unknown at the time of collection. There are many benefits to this scenario, the most important being that a well-matched HPC(CB) product can be identified quickly, as practically all available units are listed by national and international registries, and delivered to the patient within days.

Initially, cord blood products were cryopreserved without any significant processing. Eventually, limitations of storage space prompted many laboratories to process HPC(CB) to decrease the volume of plasma and red cells. HPC(CB) products are typically cryopreserved in a volume of about 20 mL, with integrally attached segments available for further confirmatory testing when necessary. In manual processing, the plasma is depleted by centrifugation and the red cells are depleted by sedimentation with HES.[16] There are also automated instruments available to accomplish MNC enrichment of the HPC(CB). The Optipress (Baxter Healthcare), Sepax (BioSafe, Eysins, Switzerland), and AutoXPress (Thermogenesis, Rancho Cordova, CA) are devices developed for this purpose.[16] Many cord blood banks have adopted automated processing to standardize volume, optimize cell recovery, and maintain sterility.

Processing—More than Minimal Manipulation

Preparation and administration of cellular therapy products characterized as "more than minimally manipulated" are regulated by the FDA and require an investigational new drug (IND) submission. The IND must include information concerning indications for product use, manufacturing, administration, critical reagents, and any toxicities or side effects expected.[6] The following sections outline several examples of more-than-minimally manipulated cellular therapy products.

HPC(CB) Expansion Ex Vivo

The major limitation of HPC(CB) products is the relatively small number of HPCs they contain. The average number of CD34+ cells in HPC(CB) units is one-tenth that in HPC(A) or HPC(M) products.[41] For patients weighing more than 100 lbs, a single unit is frequently insufficient to provide timely engraftment. A potential solution is to expand the number of pluripotent stem cells (rather than committed hematopoietic progenitors) ex vivo without attendant maturation. Several methods have been proposed to accomplish this, and some have been studied in small clinical trials. One option is to split an HPC(CB) unit into two fractions. One fraction is stored unmanipulated until transplantation; the other is processed to isolate either CD34+ or the more primitive CD133+ cells.[15] The selected cells are then cultured for 7 to 14 days in the presence of cytokines and growth factors, increasing the number of HPCs 10-fold. Both fractions are then infused, either together or separated by a few days.[15]

Another method to expand HPCs in cord blood is to culture the product with mesenchymal stem cells (MSCs).[15] MSCs can help simulate the marrow microenvironment by providing some of the nonhematopoietic components present in marrow but missing from liquid culture.[42] (See Chapter 25 for a description of the hematopoietic stem cell niche). MSCs act as a feeder layer and also appear to interact directly with the cord blood cells to increase the number of CD34+ cells by greater than 35-fold.[15,42]

Yet another option is based on the experience with cellular bioreactors. A small number of HPC(CB) have also been expanded in such devices, though the technology is very new and thus far does not seem to provide a better outcome than liquid-cultured or co-cultured units.[42]

Earlier studies on HPC(CB) units achieved up to 100-fold expansion of CD34+ cells over the course of 8 weeks.[41] There are concerns, however, that expansion promotes the growth of shorter-lived or more committed HPCs rather than those desired for lasting engraftment.[42] Attempts to culture HPC(A) under similar conditions yielded only a twofold CD34+ cell expansion and significant cell loss after 2 weeks in culture.[41] On the plus side, expansion of HPC products could eliminate tumor contamination and may be a necessary step to allow for genetic modification of cells before administration.[14,36]

Adoptive T-Cell Therapy

Unlike HPC(A), TC(A) can be expanded ex vivo (see Chapter 26 for more information). The immunosuppression required after allogeneic HSCT is a main cause of morbidity and mortality. Even after it is discontinued, months to years may elapse before a recipient regains full immunocompetence. Patients are therefore at risk for opportunistic infections, including reactivation of latent viral infections such as cytomegalovirus (CMV).[43] Therapeutic cells from the hematopoietic stem cell donor with antigen specificity directed against CMV can be adoptively transferred into the recipient to treat an infection.[43] The process for isolation, expansion, and reinfusion of antigen-specific T cells is time consuming and has significant limitations.[43] However, significant effort is being made to generate therapeutic cells with antiviral specificity, particularly against CMV and Epstein-Barr virus.[44-47]

Dendritic Cell Generation

Dendritic cells (DCs) are antigen-presenting cells of marrow origin that are disseminated throughout the body. Their primary role is to translate a "danger signal" into a host response by engagement of T cells, NK cells, and B cells (see Chapter 26). A strong argument has been made for using DCs expanded ex vivo to enhance patient immune responses against cancer (eg, renal cell carcinoma, glioblastoma multiforme, melanoma) or chronic infection (eg, human immunodeficiency virus). Results from early trials indicate that treatment with DCs alone is insufficient to obtain significant clinical response; however, DCs given in conjunction with in-vivo lymphodepletion or other therapeutic modalities may hold more promise.

DCs are primarily used in the autologous setting, so the starting material is a therapeutic cell product collected from the peripheral blood of the patient. The MNC fraction is further enriched in monocytes by positive selection for CD14, elutriation, or adherence to plastic (monocytes adhere to plastic, while other cell types float in the medium). CD14 selection is an excellent method for enriching monocytes above 95% purity, but it is also time consuming and expensive.[48] Adherence to plastic is labor intensive, and the use of open systems encourages microbial contamination.[48] Elutriation with the Elutra Cell Separation System isolates monocytes in an hour in a closed, single-use system, with a yield above 80% and purity approaching 90%.[48]

Isolated monocytes are then cultured in the presence of interleukin-4 (IL-4) and GM-CSF, cytokines that foster generation of immature DCs. After 4 to 6 days in culture, the DCs are matured with cytokines, the most common being tumor necrosis factor alpha, either alone or in a combination with IL-6, IL-1β, and prostaglandin E_2. Immature cultured DCs can be exposed to an antigen before maturation. The antigen source varies based on the clinical application; it can be as simple as a peptide or as complex as a tumor-cell lysate. Mature and antigen-loaded DCs can be administered fresh or cryopreserved. The site and route of administration vary but regional lymph nodes are becoming the most common site of injection. TC-DC products can be administered in tandem with antigen-specific expanded T cells (see Chapter 26).

Graft Assessment

The introduction of quality programs into the area of cellular therapy began in the early 1990s. Voluntary standards have been developed that encompass all aspects of cellular therapy, from selection of the donor through the collection process to administration. Cell processing laboratories have improved quality control measures to ensure that cellular therapy products meet all required standards and guidelines promulgated by regulatory agencies.[17,36,49] Graft assessment is intended to document safety (eg, bacterial and fungal contamination, donor infectious disease markers), potency (eg, cell count, viability, CD34 count, CFU assay), and efficacy (eg, engraftment, clinical outcome).

Microbial Contamination

Before cryopreservation or at the end of processing, each product is assessed for microbial contamination.[14] Typically the product is cultured upon receipt in the laboratory and again after processing. If either culture is positive, the dual checks will aid in determining when contamination occurred. The absence of microbial contamination in the starting product and prevention of contamination during processing are the primary goals of FDA regulations for cellular therapy products. Many processing laboratories use either the BacT/ALERT system (bioMérieux, Marcy l'Etoile, France) or the BACTEC system (BD, Franklin Lakes, NJ) for automated culture, often both aerobic and anaerobic, to test for bacterial and fungal contaminants. Both systems rely on bacteria-generating carbon dioxide to induce a color change in a disk at the bottom of the bottle, which is continuously monitored. An alarm is activated when a color change is detected; the bottle contents are then Gram-stained and sub-cultured for species identification. According to the College of American Pathologists (CAP) Proficiency Testing Survey, laboratories most commonly incubate the cultures for 5, 7, 10, or 14 days.

Cellular therapy products that test positive for microbial contamination cannot be infused unless there is "urgent medical need"; exceptions require notification of the FDA. A stem cell product is much more difficult to replace than a blood unit and, in some cases, is irreplaceable. The risk to the patient from a microbially contaminated product must be weighed against the risk of not receiving a product at all or having to wait longer for an additional collection.[50] The decision to infuse a microbially contaminated product is made by transplant physicians who evaluate the organism isolated, its antibiotic susceptibility, the amount of product available, the recipient's status, and other factors.[14] The source of contamination, whether of laboratory, donor, or patient origin, is also important to consider.[50] Microbially contaminated products, when used, are generally administered with concomitant antibiotic therapy.

Large transplant centers have published data on outcomes after administration of contaminated products. In the study by Klein et al, 36 of nearly 3000 products infused at one institution between 1990 and 2004 were culture-positive.[51] Only one of these products, which was contaminated during laboratory processing, may have contributed to a patient's death.[51] This is the only report of a patient's demise from receiving a microbially contaminated product. At the University of Texas MD Anderson Cancer Center, just over 3000 patients were infused between 2000 and 2005, with a 1.2% contamination rate.[52] Antibiotic coverage was provided and no deaths were attributable to administration of the products.[52]

More complex processing spread over days and weeks allows multiple opportunities for microbial contamination.[51] Hence, microbial culture is a release criterion for more-than-minimally manipulated products. Additional tests may be performed, including a Gram's stain, an endotoxin assay, and/or a mycoplasma assay. Endotoxin, a toxic component of gram-negative bacteria, can be acquired from a number of sources.[53] Reagents and antibodies for clinical use are all tested for endotoxin by the manufacturer. The processing laboratory, as a manufacturer, must do the same before product infusion. The most common test method is the limulus amebocyte lysate (LAL) assay, which is based on the ability of endotoxin to clot the blood of a horseshoe crab.[53] Several manufacturers market an LAL assay, but all are based on the same principle and most require time-consuming dilutions and positive controls.[53] A newer version of Endosafe PTS (Charles River Laboratories, Wilmington, MA) takes only 15 minutes to perform and is comparable to the standard versions that require 3 to 4 hours.[54]

In a comparison study, the Endosafe PTS was easier to set up and perform and had the advantage of rapid repeatability.[54]

Cell Counts

The easiest and fastest way to quantify a cellular therapy product is to perform a nucleated cell count. Because this information is available immediately and immunophenotyping using flow cytometry takes several hours, most products are cryopreserved based on the total number of nucleated cells per bag. A sample is collected from the product upon receipt and typically tested on a hematology analyzer, located either in the processing laboratory or in the hematology laboratory. Manual cell counts are still performed, most often on products with a smaller number of cells than HPC products, such as TC-DC.

Viability

When processing cellular therapy products, a rapid and reliable measurement of viability is essential.[55] Viability can be assessed with vital dyes such as trypan blue or fluorescent stains such as acridine orange with propidium iodide or fluorescein diacetate with ethidium bromide. Trypan blue, an exclusion dye, stains cells with damaged membranes (ie, dead or apoptotic cells).[56] Red cells and cellular debris tend to affect staining with trypan blue.[55] Acridine orange with propidium iodide is also a stain for membrane integrity but is not affected by the presence of red cells.[56] Acridine orange binds to viable cells and fluoresces green, while propidium iodide will stain only the DNA of necrotic and apoptotic cells and fluoresces orange.[55] Evaluation with both stains is quick and easy and requires only a microscope.[14] Unfortunately, the great majority of cells examined are not HPCs.[14] The CFU assay (described later) is the best method of measuring viable cells with proliferative potential, but it takes 7 to 14 days to perform. Mascotti et al compared a viability assay using trypan blue to an assay based on acridine orange/propidium iodide stain to determine which correlated better with

CFU assays in HPC(M).[55] The acridine orange/propidium iodide method correlated better and was more stable.[55] Fresh products usually have nearly 100% viability. For fresh products transported between centers, viability upon arrival is an important indicator of the products' overall quality.[14]

CD34 Immunophenotyping

It has been long established that transplantation of CD34-expressing cells in the marrow can provide long-term hematopoietic reconstitution after myeloablative therapy. There is a strong correlation between the time to engraftment and the CD34+ cell dose infused.[34] Current data suggest that autologous engraftment occurs promptly when a minimum dose of approximately 2×10^6 CD34+ cells/kg are infused.[49] CD34+ cells are rare in the peripheral blood of healthy individuals but can be mobilized from marrow into the peripheral blood with the use of chemotherapy or cytokines (see Chapter 23).[11]

Measuring the concentration of CD34+ cells in peripheral blood or HPC products requires accurate flow-cytometric quantitation when a single-platform method is used, and a combination of precise flow-cytometric analysis and an accurate nucleated cell count when a dual platform method is used.[57] A number of protocols for CD34+ cell detection exist; they differ in terms of antibody reagents used, gating, calculation, multiple measurements, and other factors. The viability of CD34+ cells can also be specifically assessed by flow cytometry, using 7-amino-actinomycin-D as a second fluorescent marker to identify nonviable cells.[34,58,59]

Most transplant facilities rely on CD34 flow cytometry to assess the HPC product yield and indicate whether additional collections are required because the measurement can be completed within hours of product receipt.[57] Multiple studies have documented significant interlaboratory variations on the same sample.[60] Efforts within the field from academic groups, professional societies, and companies have highlighted the importance of uniform sample preparation, equipment calibration, and standardization of the acquisition and analysis procedures.[60] Despite this progress, the CAP proficiency surveys continue to show significant variability in reported values when the same specimen is sent to multiple laboratories.

Colony-Forming Cell Assays

A more direct ex-vivo measurement of an HPC product's potential to engraft is a CFU assay, which measures the ability of HPCs to form colonies in methylcellulose medium supplemented with specific growth factors. Different committed HPCs give rise to different types of colonies, the most relevant being colony-forming unit–granulocyte-macrophage; colony-forming unit–granulocyte, erythrocyte, macrophage, megakaryocyte; burst-forming unit–erythroid; and colony-forming unit–erythroid. In the routine CFU test, the formation of megakaryocyte colonies is not evaluated. Unfortunately, as a result of the complexity of the assay and individual variability, there is only indirect correlation with engraftment.[61] The standard assay takes up to 2 weeks and requires significant skills to reliably count and classify the colonies formed. The 2-week turnaround time for results limits its use in clinical practice. CFU assays are more frequently used in cord blood banks, where turnaround time is not an issue, and in laboratories generating more-than-minimally manipulated products, because the additional processing could alter progenitor cell function.[14]

Postthaw Quality Control Samples

Reference vials frozen under the same conditions as their associated HPC products can be used to assess a number of factors after thawing without having to sacrifice a large volume of product. They are often used to check sterility or viability.[11]

Postthaw Viability

A recent study showed that postthaw CD34+ cell viability, measured by flow cytometry, was greater than 80% and higher than total nucle-ated cell viability. HPCs are more resistant to damage caused by cryopreservation and subsequent thawing than other nucleated cells. Therefore, a low nucleated-cell viability after thawing need not indicate a high risk of impaired engraftment.[34]

Proficiency Testing

Proficiency tests are required for analytes regulated under the Clinical Laboratory Improvement Amendments regulations. The CAP proficiency program for stem cell processing includes cell counts, viability, sterility assays, CFU assays, and immunophenotyping. Stemcell Technologies (Vancouver, BC, Canada) offers a proficiency program specifically for CFU assays.

Interlaboratory comparisons are difficult to assess for stem cell products because of varied instruments and protocols. Studies have shown interlaboratory variation for CD34+ enumeration of up to a 100-fold difference for nonmobilized cellular therapy products.[60,62] The CAP proficiency testing results from 2009 show three- to fourfold variation (after exclusion of outliers) between institutions for both CD34+ cell content and CFU assays.

Infusion

Cryopreserved cells are thawed for infusion at the patient's bedside or in the laboratory. HPC(A) and HPC(M) are usually thawed rapidly at the patient's bedside in a 37-C water bath and infused immediately. They are transported frozen to the bedside, where bags are individually removed one at a time from the portable freezer, placed in an overwrap bag to contain any spills from breakage, and put directly in the water bath. As the contents of the bag thaw, gentle massage is used to speed the process until nearly all the ice is gone. The bag is removed from the water bath, and contents are infused through a microaggregate filter via gravity or syringe.[14] A second bag is not thawed until the previous one is infused, in case the patient develops side effects requiring temporary discontinuation of the infusion.[14]

The most common side effects are cough, throat tickle, nausea, and vomiting. The majority of these events are mild but a small percentage affect the cardiac and respiratory systems.[63] The most common adverse events are listed in Table 24-5. A larger fluid volume, a higher DMSO dose, a higher percentage of granulocytes, and a higher red cell content all correlate with adverse infusion events.[14,63] Milone et al reported that patient age greater than 50 years

and infusion of more than 0.5×10^8 granulocytes/kg correlated with a higher percentage of noncardiac adverse events.[63] HPC(M) infusions have a lower rate of adverse events compared to HPC(A) products, which might be partially due to the lower granulocyte content of HPC(M) products.

Cardiac adverse events are linked to large infusion volumes, with correspondingly large amounts of DMSO.[63] It is possible to reduce the

Table 24-5. Complications and Management of Adverse Events After HPC Infusion[64]

Complication	Signs and Symptoms	Management
Intravascular red cell hemolysis	Fever, back pain, tachycardia, shock, hemoglobinemia, hemoglobinuria	Stop infusion, IV hydration, intensive monitoring, blood product support (as needed)
Pulmonary complications	Severe hypoxemia (O_2 saturation decreased), fever, chills	Stop infusion, supplemental oxygen, intensive monitoring, intubation (as needed)
Bacterial contamination	High fever, tachycardia, sustained hypotension, nausea, vomiting, shock	Stop infusion, culture patient and HPC unit, broad-spectrum antibiotics, intensive monitoring, cardiac and pulmonary support (as needed)
Volume overload	Dyspnea, hypoxemia, tachycardia, hypertension, jugular-venous distention	Slow infusion rate, elevate the patient's head, diuresis
DMSO toxicity	Pruritis, urticaria, flushing, wheezing, nausea, fever	Antihistamine agents (pre- and post-infusion), HPC washing
Neurologic complications	Muscle spasms, seizures, mental status changes, loss of consciousness	Airway protection, supportive care, imaging, sedative-hypnotics, intensive monitoring (as needed)
Febrile reactions	Fever, rigors, chills, mild dyspnea	Antipyretic agents (pre- and post-infusion), meperidine (severe rigors)
Mild allergic reactions	Urticaria, wheezing, rash, pruritis	Antihistamine agents (pre- and post-infusion)
Severe allergic reactions	Wheezing/bronchospasm, hypoxemia, hypotension	Antihistamine agents, corticosteroids, epinephrine (as needed), cardiac and pulmonary support (as needed)

HPC = hematopoietic progenitor cell; IV = intravenous; DMSO = dimethylsulfoxide.

Table 24-6. Engraftment Terminology[49]

Term	Definition
Neutrophil engraftment	The first of 3 days of neutrophil count above 500/μL
Platelet engraftment	The first day of >20,000 platelets/μL, untransfused (in older literature, the engraftment level was often reported as >50,000 platelets/μL)
Erythroid engraftment	$>30 \times 10^6$ reticulocytes/μL or >1% reticulocytes, untransfused
T-cell engraftment	Mixed donor-host chimerism is the presence of 5% to 95% donor T cells; full donor chimerism is >95% donor T cells
Primary graft failure	Failure to achieve a neutrophil count of ≥500/μL in patients who survive ≥28 days following transplantation and who have not undergone a second transplant procedure (marrow and peripheral blood stem cell grafts; for umbilical cord blood, the time point for primary graft failure is now considered to be 42 days after transplantation)
Secondary graft failure	Decline of neutrophils to <500/μL after having engrafted that is unresponsive to growth factors and unrelated to effects of medications or infection

DMSO content by thawing in the laboratory and washing the product before issuing it for infusion. One study by Calmels et al compared infusion of washed and unwashed HPC products to analyze the effect of DMSO on adverse events.[65] They reported no difference in events, finding that the most significant factor influencing adverse events was the granulocyte content of the infusion product.[65] Nevertheless, HPC(CB) products for pediatric and other small patients are routinely either washed to remove DMSO or diluted to lower the DMSO concentration before infusion to reduce adverse effects.[14]

Engraftment

The true measure of a successful transplantation is engraftment and hematopoietic reconstitution.[66] The indicators of engraftment after transplantation are the times to recovery for each cell type. Table 24-6 summarizes definitions of engraftment for different cell lineages. When a patient's neutrophil count is greater than 0.5×10^6/μL for 3 consecutive days, the first day is considered as the neutrophil engraftment day.[49] Platelet engraftment is defined as day 1 of 3 consecutive days with a platelet count greater than 20×10^6/μL without platelet support.[49] CD34+ cell dose and CFU results correlate with short-term engraftment, but a study of autologous marrow transplants found that the most important indicator of long-term reconstitution is time to neutrophil engraftment.[66] CD34− progenitor or stem cells might contribute more to long-term reconstitution.[66]

References

1. Pazdur R. Medical oncology: A comprehensive review. Huntington, NY: PRR, 1993.
2. Antonenas V, Garvin F, Webb M, et al. Fresh PBSC harvests, but not BM, show temperature-related loss of CD34 viability during storage and transport. Cytotherapy 2006;8:158-65.
3. Abraham J, Gulley JL, Allegra CJ. Bethesda handbook of clinical oncology. 2nd ed. Philadelphia: Lippincott Williams and Wilkins, 2005.
4. Kufe DW, Pollock RE, Weichselbaum RR, et al. Holland-Frei cancer medicine. 6th ed. Hamilton, ON: BC Decker, 2003.

5. Munker R. Modern hematology: Biology and clinical management. 2nd ed. Totowa, NJ: Humana Press, 2006.
6. Circular of information for the use of cellular therapy products. Bethesda, MD: AABB, 2009.
7. Engelhardt M, Lubbert M, Guo Y. CD34(+) or CD34(–): Which is the more primitive? Leukemia 2002;16:1603-8.
8. Gazitt Y. Comparison between granulocyte colony-stimulating factor and granulocyte-macrophage colony-stimulating factor in the mobilization of peripheral blood stem cells. Curr Opin Hematol 2002;9:190-8.
9. Vose JM, Ho AD, Coiffier B, et al. Advances in mobilization for the optimization of autologous stem cell transplantation. Leuk Lymphoma 2009;50:1412-21.
10. Flomenberg N, Devine SM, Dipersio JF, et al. The use of AMD3100 plus G-CSF for autologous hematopoietic progenitor cell mobilization is superior to G-CSF alone. Blood 2005; 106:1867-74.
11. Lane TA. Peripheral blood progenitor cell mobilization and collection. In: Ball ED, Lister JW, Law P, eds. Hematopoietic stem cell therapy. New York: Churchill Livingstone, 2000: 269-86.
12. Ballen KK, King RJ, Chitphakdithai P, et al. The National Marrow Donor Program: 20 years of unrelated donor hematopoietic cell transplantation. Biol Blood Marrow Transplant 2008; 14:2-7.
13. Rutecki B, Lister J. Bone marrow harvesting. In: Ball ED, Lister JW, Law P, eds. Hematopoietic stem cell therapy. New York: Churchill Livingstone, 2000:265-8.
14. Law P. Graft, processing, storage, and infusion. In: Ball ED, Lister JW, Law P, eds. Hematopoietic stem cell therapy. New York: Churchill Livingstone, 2000:312-21.
15. Yang H, Robinson SN, Lu J, et al. CD3(+) and/or CD14(+) depletion from cord blood mononuclear cells before ex vivo expansion culture improves total nucleated cell and CD34(+) cell yields. Bone Marrow Transplant 2009 (in press). doi: 10.1038/bmt.2009.289.
16. Coelho PH, Loper K. Umbilical cord blood processing. In: Areman EM, Loper K, eds. Cellular therapy: Principles, methods, and regulations. Bethesda, MD: AABB, 2009:330-5.
17. Kao GS. Assessment of collection quality. In: Areman EM, Loper K, eds. Cellular therapy: Principles, methods, and regulations. Bethesda, MD: AABB, 2009:291-7.
18. Pamphilon DH, Selogie E, Szczepiorkowski ZM. Transportation of cellular therapy products: Report of a survey by the cellular therapies team of the Biomedical Excellence for Safer Transfusion (BEST) collaborative. Vox Sang 2010 (in press). doi: 10.1111/j.1423-0410.2010.01329.x.
19. Jansen J, Nolan PL, Reeves MI, et al. Transportation of peripheral blood progenitor cell products: Effects of time, temperature, and cell concentration. Cytotherapy 2009;11:79-85.
20. Padley D, ed. Standards for cellular therapy product services. 4th ed. Bethesda, MD: AABB, 2008.
21. Lazarus HM, Pecora AL, Shea TC, et al. CD34+ selection of hematopoietic blood cell collections and autotransplantation in lymphoma: Overnight storage of cells at 4 degrees C does not affect outcome. Bone Marrow Transplant 2000;25:559-66.
22. Food and Drug Administration. Human cells, tissues, and cellular and tissue-based products; establishment registration and listing; final rule. (January 19, 2001) Fed Regist 2001;66:5447-69.
23. Food and Drug Administration. Current good tissue practice for human cell, tissue, and cellular and tissue-based product establishments: Inspection and enforcement. (November 18, 2004) Fed Regist 2004;69:68612-88.
24. Food and Drug Administration. Eligibility determination for donors of human cells, tissues, and cellular and tissue-based products; final rule. (May 25, 2004) Fed Regist 2004; 62:29786-834.
25. Food and Drug Administration. Human cells, tissues, and cellular and tissue-based products; donor screening and testing, and related labeling; interim final rule. (May 24, 2005) Fed Regist 2005;70:29949-52.
26. Harvath L. A brief history of FDA regulation of human cells and tissues. In: Areman EM, Loper K, eds. Cellular therapy: Principles, methods, and regulations. Bethesda, MD: AABB, 2009:2-12.
27. Worel N, Kalhs P, Keil F, et al. ABO mismatch increases transplant-related morbidity and mortality in patients given nonmyeloablative allogeneic HPC transplantation. Transfusion 2003;43:1153-61.
28. Worel N, Panzer S, Reesink HW, et al. Transfusion policy in ABO-incompatible allogeneic stem cell transplantation. Vox Sang 2010;98: 455-67.

29. Szczepiorkowski Z. Transfusion support for hematopoietic transplant recipients. In: Roback JD, Combs MR, Grossman BJ, Hillyer CD, eds. Technical manual. 16th ed. Bethesda, MD: AABB, 2008:679-96.

30. Meyer EKG, Szczepiorkowski ZM. Transfusion support of HSCT recipients. In: Wingard JR, Gastineau D, Leather H, et al, eds. Hematopoietic stem cell transplantation: A handbook for clinicians. Bethesda, MD: AABB; 2009:207-26.

31. Rowley SD, Liang PS, Ulz L. Transplantation of ABO-incompatible bone marrow and peripheral blood stem cell components. Bone Marrow Transplant 2000;26:749-57.

32. Berz D, McCormack EM, Winer ES, et al. Cryopreservation of hematopoietic stem cells. Am J Hematol 2007;82:463-72.

33. Hubel A. Cryopreservation of cellular therapy products. In: Areman EM, Loper K, eds. Cellular therapy: Principles, methods, and regulations. Bethesda, MD: AABB, 2009:342-9.

34. Reich-Slotky R, Colovai AI, Semidei-Pomales M, et al. Determining post-thaw CD34+ cell dose of cryopreserved haematopoietic progenitor cells demonstrates high recovery and confirms their integrity. Vox Sang 2008;94:351-7.

35. Snyder EL, Haley NR, Triulzi DJ, eds. Cellular therapy: A physician's handbook. Bethesda, MD: AABB, 2004.

36. Buchsel PC, Kapustay PM. Stem cell transplantation: A clinical trial textbook. Pittsburgh, PA: Oncology Nursing Society, 2000.

37. O'Donnell PV, Myers B, Edwards J, et al. CD34 selection using three immunoselection devices: Comparison of T-cell depleted allografts. Cytotherapy 2001;3:483-8.

38. de Witte T, Hoogenhout J, de Pauw B, et al. Depletion of donor lymphocytes by counterflow centrifugation successfully prevents acute graft-versus-host disease in matched allogeneic marrow transplantation. Blood 1986;67:1302-8.

39. Edwards J. Cell separation by counterflow centrifugal elutriation. In: Areman EM, Loper K, eds. Cellular therapy: Principles, methods, and regulations. Bethesda, MD: AABB, 2009:410-16.

40. Wong EC, Lee SM, Hines K, et al. Development of a closed-system process for clinical-scale generation of DCs: Evaluation of two monocyte-enrichment methods and two culture containers. Cytotherapy 2002;4:65-76.

41. Gilmore GL, DePasquale DK, Lister J, Shadduck RK. Ex vivo expansion of human umbilical cord blood and peripheral blood CD34(+) hematopoietic stem cells. Exp Hematol 2000; 28:1297-305.

42. Kelly SS, Sola CB, de Lima M, Shpall E. Ex vivo expansion of cord blood. Bone Marrow Transplant 2009;44:673-81.

43. Berger C, Turtle CJ, Jensen MC, Riddell SR. Adoptive transfer of virus-specific and tumor-specific T cell immunity. Curr Opin Immunol 2009;21:224-32.

44. Ahmed N, Heslop HE, Mackall CL. T-cell-based therapies for malignancy and infection in childhood. Pediatr Clin North Am 2010;57:83-96.

45. Brenner MK, Heslop HE. Adoptive T cell therapy of cancer. Curr Opin Immunol 2010;22:251-7.

46. Heslop HE, Slobod KS, Pule MA, et al. Long-term outcome of EBV-specific T-cell infusions to prevent or treat EBV-related lymphoproliferative disease in transplant recipients. Blood 2010;115:925-35.

47. Micklethwaite KP, Savoldo B, Hanley PJ, et al. Derivation of human T lymphocytes from cord blood and peripheral blood with antiviral and antileukemic specificity from a single culture as protection against infection and relapse after stem cell transplantation. Blood 2010;115:2695-703.

48. Rouard H, Leon A, De Reys S, et al. A closed and single-use system for monocyte enrichment: Potential for dendritic cell generation for clinical applications. Transfusion 2003;43:481-7.

49. O'Donnell PV. Engraftment. In: Wingard JR, Gastineau D, Leather H, et al, eds. Hematopoietic stem cell transplantation: A handbook for clinicians. Bethesda, MD: AABB, 2009:163-80.

50. Padley DJ, Dietz AB, Gastineau DA. Sterility testing of hematopoietic progenitor cell products: A single-institution series of culture-positive rates and successful infusion of culture-positive products. Transfusion 2007;47:636-43.

51. Klein MA, Kadidlo D, McCullough J, et al. Microbial contamination of hematopoietic stem cell products: Incidence and clinical sequelae. Biol Blood Marrow Transplant 2006;12:1142-9.

52. Patah PA, Parmar S, McMannis J, et al. Microbial contamination of hematopoietic progenitor

cell products: Clinical outcome. Bone Marrow Transplant 2007;40:365-8.

53. Kadidlo D. Endotoxin testing of cellular therapy products. In: Areman EM, Loper K, eds. Cellular therapy: Principles, methods, and regulations. Bethesda, MD: AABB, 2009:620-1.

54. Gee AP, Sumstad D, Stanson J, et al. A multicenter comparison study between the Endosafe PTS rapid-release testing system and traditional methods for detecting endotoxin in cell-therapy products. Cytotherapy 2008;10: 427-35.

55. Mascotti K, McCullough J, Burger SR. HPC viability measurement: Trypan blue versus acridine orange and propidium iodide. Transfusion 2000;40:693-6.

56. Yang H, Acker JP, Cabuhat M, McGann LE. Effects of incubation temperature and time after thawing on viability assessment of peripheral hematopoietic progenitor cells cryopreserved for transplantation. Bone Marrow Transplant 2003;32:1021-6.

57. Sutherland DR, Keeney M, Pecora A, Chin-Yee I. Stem Cell Quantification: The ISHAGE guidelines for CD34+ determination—applications in autologous and allogeneic hematopoietic stem cell transplantation. In: Ball ED, Lister JW, Law P, eds. Hematopoietic stem cell therapy. New York: Churchill Livingstone, 2000: 298-311.

58. Lopez MC, Lawrence DA. Proficiency testing experience for viable CD34+ stem cell analysis. Transfusion 2008;48:1115-21.

59. Xiao M, Dooley DC. Assessment of cell viability and apoptosis in human umbilical cord blood following storage. J Hematother Stem Cell Res 2003;12:115-22.

60. Brecher ME, Sims L, Schmitz J, et al. North American multicenter study on flow cytometric enumeration of CD34+ hematopoietic stem cells. J Hematother 1996;5:227-36.

61. Clarke E. Colony-forming cell assays for determining potency of cellular therapy products. In: Areman EM, Loper K, eds. Cellular therapy: Principles, methods, and regulations. Bethesda, MD: AABB, 2009:573-80.

62. Rock G, Chin-Yee I, Cantin G, et al. Quality assurance of progenitor cell content of apheresis products: A comparison of clonogenic assays and CD34+ enumeration. The Canadian Apheresis Group and the Transplant Group. Canadian Bone Marrow Group. Transfus Med 2000;10:67-75.

63. Milone G, Mercurio S, Strano A, et al. Adverse events after infusions of cryopreserved hematopoietic stem cells depend on non-mononuclear cells in the infused suspension and patient age. Cytotherapy 2007;9:348-55.

64. Tormey CA, Snyder EL. Hematopoietic progenitor cell administration. In: Wingard JR, Gastineau D, Leather H, et al, eds. Hematopoietic stem cell transplantation: A handbook for clinicians. Bethesda, MD: AABB, 2009:151-62.

65. Calmels B, Lemarie C, Esterni B, et al. Occurrence and severity of adverse events after autologous hematopoietic progenitor cell infusion are related to the amount of granulocytes in the apheresis product. Transfusion 2007; 47:1268-75.

66. Zubair A, Zahrieh D, Daley H, et al. Early neutrophil engraftment following autologous BMT provides a functional predictor of long-term hematopoietic reconstitution. Transfusion 2003; 43:614-21.

In: McLeod BC, Szczepiorkowski ZM, Weinstein R, Winters JL, eds.
Apheresis: Principles and Practice, 3rd edition
Bethesda, MD: AABB Press, 2010

25

Regenerative Medicine

Daniela S. Krause, MD, PhD, and David T. Scadden, MD

Prometheus, a Titan in Greek mythology, was punished by Zeus, the father of all Gods, for stealing fire from Zeus and giving it to the mortals. His punishment was to be bound to a rock while an eagle daily ate at his liver, which regenerated during the night—only to be eaten again the next day.

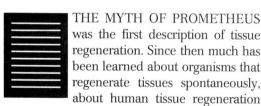 THE MYTH OF PROMETHEUS was the first description of tissue regeneration. Since then much has been learned about organisms that regenerate tissues spontaneously, about human tissue regeneration in utero, and finally about ways to harness tissue regeneration for medical needs. Regenerative medicine is the augmentation or substitution of diseased or injured cells or tissues by one of two means: improvement in the ability of endogenous cells to reform damaged tissue or the use of exogenous cells or tissues to replace cells or tissues that are damaged.

To date, regenerative medicine has been confined mostly to exogenous strategies, using organ transplantation or hematopoietic stem cell (HSC) transplantation (HSCT) to achieve tissue repair, based on the straightforward logic that what is dysfunctional should be removed and replaced with more functional substitutes. It is a familiar model from, for example, the care of automobiles, and one that has succeeded in both solid organ and marrow transplantation because of the pioneering work in immunology that has permitted tissue typing and immunologic matching. It has succeeded in the setting of HSCT because of the remarkable features of stem cells.

Daniela S. Krause, MD, PhD, Research Fellow, Center for Regenerative Medicine, Massachusetts General Hospital, and David T. Scadden, MD, Harvard Stem Cell Institute and Department of Stem Cell and Regenerative Biology, Harvard University, Center for Regenerative Medicine, Massachusetts General Hospital, Boston, Massachusetts

D. Krause has disclosed no conflicts of interest. D. Scadden has disclosed financial relationships with Genzyme, Hospira, and Fate Therapeutics.

Support for this chapter was provided by the National Heart, Lung, and Blood Institute and the National Institute of Diabetes and Digestive and Kidney Diseases.

It is the burgeoning field of stem cell biology that has suggested that regenerative medicine might move beyond its current confines of organ transplantation and HSCT. The last decade has been one of explosive growth in understanding the range of stem cell types, the extent of stem cell plasticity and the potential to use stem-cell-based approaches to diseases well beyond those currently treated with transplantation.

Stem cells, as originally proposed in 1909 by Maximov in considering the blood, are self-replenishing cells capable of forming all blood elements.[1] He was proven correct experimentally by Becker et al some 50 years later, using regeneration of radiation-destroyed marrow in mice as an assay system.[2] They ingeniously demonstrated that this could be accomplished clonally; that is, single cells were the source of regeneration. Nonetheless, blood was thought to be a special case, a liquid tissue with features different from those of other tissue types. Since the 1990s, however, it has been recognized that many tissue types contain stem or progenitor cell populations and that it is possible to generate human cells that have pluripotency—that is, the capacity to form cell types across germ layers.

James Thomson cultured pluripotent stem cells from human blastocysts,[3] and John Gearhart et al did the same with fetal genital ridge.[4] The cells they cultured could generate cell types belonging to each of the three germ layers (pluripotency), resulting in more than could be achieved from any cell derived from later fetal, cord blood, or adult tissues, which are generally restricted to generating cells from a single germ layer (multipotency). The impact of these discoveries on regenerative medicine was immediate and profound as they suggested the possibility of using pluripotent cells, embryonic stem cells (ES) by common parlance, to create essentially any type of cell in the body.

Less heralded contemporaneous discoveries regarding multipotent cells have also fueled optimism about stem-cell-based regenerative medicine. It was recognized that blood was not alone in having true stem cells supporting the maintenance of adult tissue. It was found that the skin, intestine, skeleton, muscle, heart, and brain all possessed multipotent stem cells. Consequently, the profound impact that blood stem cell transplantation had on the treatment of hematologic malignancies was envisioned as a paradigm for what might be possible with other tissues as well.

Finally, in 2006, Takahashi and Yamanaka announced a breathtaking discovery: somatic cells could be reprogrammed back to become pluripotent cells.[5] His group refuted the concept that differentiation was a one-way street and demonstrated that cells can be readily manipulated to rewind back to their most primitive level. Since this initial discovery, it has become clear that cells are far more plastic than was once believed and that reprogramming cells to become a cell type of therapeutic importance is now a real possibility.

This chapter will cover the use of endogenous cells, exogenous cells, and cell reprogramming as approaches to regenerative medicine.

Regeneration from Endogenous Cells

It has long been known that certain vertebrates—prominently, urodele (salamanders and newts) and anuran (frogs and toads) amphibians and teleost fish—are capable of regenerating complex tissues (Table 25-1). Tissue regeneration can be found in injured limbs, tails, jaws, and certain eye tissues of some urodeles and anurans. Completely amputated limbs or tails can be regenerated in newts, fish, and salamanders by recapitulation of ontogenesis of the particular organ, allowing interplay between mesenchymal and epithelial tissues. Two mechanisms of regeneration exist in newts. In one, progenitors of differentiated cell types such as bone, cartilage, muscle, nerve sheath, and connective tissue cells at the amputation site are thought to contribute to a collection of proliferating progenitor cells in a structure called a regeneration blastema.[6] Alternatively, as in freshwater planarians (a family of flatworms), pluripotent, stem-like cells termed "neoblasts" divide and differentiate into approx-

---

Table 25-1. Examples of Endogenous and Exogenous Tissue Regeneration

Endogenous Tissue Regeneration

1. Limb regeneration in urodele and anuran amphibians and teleost fish[6]
2. Replacement of antlers in deer[7]
3. Spontaneous closure of holes in pinnae of ears of rabbits and pikas[7]
4. Scarless restoration of incisional wounds in embryos up to first trimester[8]
5. Regeneration of marrow, epithelia, and muscle in humans[7]
6. Pharmacologic manipulation of the environment of cells with regenerative potential[9,10]

Exogenous Tissue Regeneration

1. Hematopoietic stem cell transplantation[11-13]
2. Reprogramming of adult cells into pluripotent stem cells[5,14-18]

---

imately 40 different cell types essential for regeneration of the planarian body. In salamander limbs, these pluripotent cells may be derived from skeletal muscle satellite (stem) cells. Up-regulation of platelet-derived growth factor (PDGF), fibroblast growth factor (FGF), bone morphogenetic protein 4 (BMP4), the Notch signaling pathway, and metalloproteinases have been implicated as mediators in heart, fin, and limb regeneration in zebrafish and newts.[19]

In mammals, the most obvious case of tissue regeneration is found in the annual replacement of antlers in deer or in the healing of corneal incisions. In rabbits and pikas, full-thickness holes in the pinna of the ear can be spontaneously closed, which is a process involving cartilage regeneration as well as scarless healing of two skin surfaces. Site-specific, complete, and scarless restoration of incisional wounds in human embryos and early fetuses occurs up to the early first trimester. Marrow, epithelia, and muscle in mammals undergo permanent regeneration in order to maintain the integrity of tissues experiencing cell loss as a result of normal cell turnover or injury. In mammals, this is mediated by stem cells, whereas in newts, as mentioned above, this process can be mediated by dedifferentiation of lineage-specified cells.

Murphy Roths Large (MRL) mice, which have been used for modeling autoimmune dis-

eases, harbor the Fas deletion mutant gene lpr, leading to accumulation of CD4–, CD8–, CD3+ T cells in lymphoid tissue caused by altered apoptosis of T cells. The spontaneous closure of ear punches in these mice led to new theories about the role of the immune system in scarless healing and tissue regeneration. Specifically, as the MRL mice also do not form scars after injury of the heart muscle, it was hypothesized that lack of scarring may increase the regenerative capacity of tissues. This hypothesis was supported by the fact that the ability to regenerate limbs in anurans is dependent on the developmental stage of the regenerating organism; thus, maturation of the immune system may underlie the organism's declining regenerative potential.[7]

The Role of the Immune System in Tissue Regeneration and Scarring

In normal wound repair, tissue injury precipitates a cascade of events leading to the formation of scar tissue. Tissue injury disrupts capillaries, resulting in activation of platelets and the clotting cascade. With neutrophils entering injured tissue and releasing proteases, growth factors, and cytokines, inflammation is initiated. Injured epithelia are resealed by keratinocytes, and the cytokines secreted by macrophages activate fibroblasts, which, consequently, secrete hyaluronate and fibronectin.

As a result of the production of proteoglycans and collagen by fibroblasts, granulation tissue is formed and angiogenesis is initiated. Developing myofibroblasts lead to wound contraction. In the next phase, collagen turnover and remodeling of the matrix lead to a decrease in vascularity and the formation of scar tissue. Wound repair is, therefore, marked by profound fibroproliferation leading to a fibrotic scar, with an injured organ being repaired rather than restored.[7]

The difference in the reaction to injury and regenerative capacity between fetal and adult skin is thought to be caused by differing activities of the cells of the immune system that are dependent on the phylogenetic stage and differences in the composition of fetal vs adult skin. Fetal skin contains much more hyaluronic acid in a highly hydrated state that persists longer in wounds. Hyaluronic acid has an influence on the amount and nature of collagen production and forms matrix-binding inhibitors of serine proteases such as plasmin, cathepsin G, and activators of metalloproteinases. Hyaluronan of high molecular weight inhibits angiogenesis and the migration of leukocytes. In adult wounds, collagen type I is predominately produced and aggregates in fibrillar bundles, whereas in fetal wounds, a reticulum of unmodelled collagen of types I, III, IV, and VI is produced.

Tenascin C, a protein of the extracellular matrix more highly expressed in fetal than in adult wounds, consists of a large complex of six similar subunits that allows morphologic and positional changes of cells in the matrix but prevents their apoptosis and differentiation. In closed full-thickness ear punches of MRL mice, as described above, tenascin C is present in regenerating ear tissue. Tenascin C can antagonize the proadhesive effects of collagen and laminin and suppresses proinflammatory effects of cytokines by the inhibition of T-cell activation and secretion of interleukin (IL)-2. These effects induced by tenascin C in fetal wounds, as well as possibly reduced platelet degranulation and a failure to form fibrin clots, lead to changes in the local environment that decrease infiltration of fetal wounds by neutrophils and

macrophages, thereby leading to decreased production of tumor growth factor β (TGFβ). Decreased production of IL-6 and -8 by fetal skin fibroblasts leads to diminished recruitment of neutrophils by IL-8 and diminished recruitment and activation of monocytes/macrophages by IL-6. In addition, gene expression analysis has shown that genes involved in the patterning of embryonic skin are differentially expressed during fetal, but not adult, skin wound healing and are actually inhibited directly by proinflammatory factors in the adult wound microenvironment.[20] If fetal skin is severely injured, however, an immigration of macrophages, inflammation, and scarring can indeed be observed. In addition, the expression of TGFβ3 in regenerating fetal wounds promotes epithelial and mesenchymal migration and changes cell-matrix interactions.[8] The influence of TGFβ and other cytokines on the degree of inflammation and subsequent scarring vs regeneration is corroborated by the finding that in mice deficient for IL-10 (an anti-inflammatory cytokine), infiltration by inflammatory leukocytes in fetal skin is more pronounced, and definite scar formation is seen.

Tissue regeneration in newts and anurans is characterized by rapid closure of the wound by thickened epithelium, accumulation of proliferating mesenchymal cells, the development of a blastema, and proximal redifferentiation of the new limb. Tenascin C is abundant in the epidermis of newts and in dedifferentiating tissues of amputated newt limbs or tails. As in MRL mice, regeneration in anurans is marked by low levels of fibrosis after injury, whereas excess fibrosis can inhibit normal limb regeneration. Abundant fibrosis in the microenvironment is thought to disrupt signaling events originating from FGF-10, which up-regulates genes involved in dedifferentiation and pattern formation, improving the regenerative outcome via the Wnt signaling pathway. From the example of urodeles—which are immunodeficient compared to anurans as they have very restricted diversity within major histocompatibility complex Class II, poor stimulation of T-helper cells, and low cytokine synthesis—it is apparent that advanced immunocompetence is partly responsible for gradual loss of regenerative potential.[7]

In summary, inhibition of proinflammatory cytokines or decreased expression of genes that promote inflammation within the microenvironment of a wound may contribute to improved wound healing or even tissue regeneration by decreasing fibrosis. Although regenerative potential is lost with increased sophistication of the immune system, tissue regeneration depends on a careful balance of pro- and anti-inflammatory cytokines.

Pharmacologic Activation of Endogenous Cells

The presence of stem/progenitor cells in multiple tissue types raises the possibility that these cells could be the source of a regenerative process if provided with the correct microenvironment. As noted above, immunologic responses to injury may impair a regenerative program. Modulating the signals that a stem/progenitor cell receives in the context of injury or disease might therefore be a means of altering the regenerative process. Such signals may be provided by altering the surrounding cells—for example, reducing an inflammatory infiltrate. Additionally, evidence exists that altering the activity of some support cells in the tissue "stroma" may affect regeneration.

Hematopoietic tissue is known to reside primarily in the marrow in adult mammals. In that context, it is in close contact with bone elements, and osteoblastic cells have been documented to be part of the HSC niche. Consequently, it was thought that altering the activity or number of osteoblastic cells with compounds such as analogues of parathyroid hormone might have an impact on HSCs. This was indeed experimentally demonstrated to be the case, and such treatment of animals resulted in improved regeneration of hematopoiesis following irradiation and HSCT.[9] Pharmacologic modification of "stromal" components may then affect the process of repair following injury.

There are also examples of modulating endogenous stem cell populations directly. A population of mesenchymal cells with osteo-

blast or adipocyte potential exists in mammalian bone. It has been found that these cells can be encouraged to form osteoblastic cells in vivo by the administration of certain medications. Specifically, use of bortezomib in a mouse model of postmenopausal bone loss enhanced osteolineage differentiation and improved bone density.[10] Therefore, pharmacologic manipulation of stem/progenitor cells or their microenvironment as a means to enhance regeneration in settings of tissue injury or disease has experimental precedent and may be the basis for future regenerative medicine interventions.

Exogenous Tissue Regeneration by Transplantation

Because intrinsic tissue regeneration and even the activation of the regenerative capacity in mammals are limited, strategies are being developed that should allow the transplantation of cells that harbor regenerative ability (Table 25-1). The transfer of such cells, ideally, will fulfill the goals of regenerative medicine by providing cells to repair or replace damaged tissues.

To this day, the transplantation of cells that have regenerative capacity is only fully realized in HSCT, wherein the cells may be harvested from peripheral blood (by apheresis), marrow, or cord blood (see Chapters 22 and 23). One of the advantages of allogeneic HSCT with cord blood is a lower incidence of graft-versus-host disease. However, the low number of donor HSCs in these products makes them a suboptimal source for transplantation in adults. Methods to expand these HSCs and HSCs from other sources are being investigated. The transplantation of mesenchymal progenitors or other cell types after in-vitro manipulation is still in its infancy and affected by ongoing research as described below.

Transplantation Requires a Niche, Homing, and Engraftment

Successful transplantation of cells with regenerative potential requires an understanding of niche biology and factors that sustain, augment, or impede the survival and proliferation of these cells. As HSCs are the only such cells that are currently being used successfully for transplantation, knowledge of the biology of the microenvironment—the niche—of this cell type is the most advanced. A niche for neural stem cells in close proximity to the basal lamina, the vasculature, and endothelial cells and surrounded by the extracellular matrix has also been described.[21]

The HSC niche (Fig 25-1), which was first proposed by Schofield in 1978, refers to a specialized environment that regulates HSC function.[22] The microenvironment of HSCs in the marrow may include osteoblasts, osteoclasts, mesenchymal stem cells, fibroblasts, macrophages, endothelial cells, adipocytes, and reticular cells.[23] Different cell types may be important in different niches. Most work on the HSC niche to date has focused on the endosteum, the inner surface of the bone that interfaces with the marrow. The intricate relationship between osteoblasts and HSCs has been studied in mice by means of genetic manipulations that increase osteoblasts and, as a consequence, also increase HSC numbers. In one such study, specific manipulation of the osteoblasts of transgenic mice (PPR mice) rendered the parathyroid hormone (PTH) receptor constitutively active, thereby increasing trabecular bone volume and numbers of HSCs (which do not have PTH receptors).[11] Another study revealed that using mice with conditional inactivation of BMP receptor type IA resulted in an increase in the number of spindle-shaped, N-cadherin+, CD45− osteoblasts, correlating with an increase in the number of HSCs.[12] Osteopontin, an extracellular matrix protein, is produced by many different cell types and binds CD44 as well as $\alpha 4$ and $\alpha 5\beta 1$ integrins. From the observation that osteopontin knockout mice have an increased number of HSCs, it was concluded that osteopontin serves as an important constraint on HSC number.[13]

Other stem cell niche supporting factors are angiopoietin-1, thrombopoietin, sonic hedgehog, and stem cell factor. Most HSCs reside in close proximity to sinusoids in vascular niches that are marked by the presence of perivascular reticular cells expressing high amounts of CXCL12 [or stromal-cell-derived factor (SDF-1α)], a chemokine involved in the migration and maintenance of HSCs in the marrow. These CXCL12-abundant reticular cells surround sinusoidal endothelial cells or are located near the endosteum. Induced deletion of CXCL12 leads to reduction of HSCs and an increased sensitivity to myelotoxic injury. The SDF-CXCR4 axis is therefore essential for the maintenance of a quiescent stem cell pool.[24]

Efforts have been made to visualize the marrow microenvironment by both in-vivo and immunohistochemical studies. Marrow contains unique anatomic regions defined by specialized endothelium. This vasculature expresses E-selectin and SDF-1 in discrete discontinuous areas that influence both the localization of transplanted HSCs and hematopoietic progenitor cells (HPCs) and the homing of tumor cell lines, which is most prominent in marrow microvessels where CXCL12 is abundant.[25] In addition, recent research has shown that the localization of transplanted HSCs and HPCs is dynamic and nonrandom. It seems to be influenced by cell-intrinsic and -extrinsic factors in live mice.[26,27]

Homing, defined as the process by which a transplanted stem cell finds its appropriate environmental niche, is a necessary prelude to engraftment.[28] It is also an important consideration in regenerative medicine. Most of our knowledge of the homing of transplanted cells is derived from the homing of normal HSCs to the marrow, which is characterized by three different steps. First, rolling is mediated by the interactions between P-selectin glycoprotein ligand-1 (PSGL-1) and P-/E-selectin,[29] the integrins lymphocyte function-associated antigen-1 (LFA-1) and intercellular adhesion molecule-1 (ICAM-1 or CD54), and the β1 integrins very late antigen-4/5 (VLA-4/5) and vascular cell adhesion molecule-1 (VCAM-1 or CD106).[30] The second step is firm adhesion, which is mediated by the LFA-1/ICAM-1 and VLA-4/5/VCAM-1 axes. Finally, transmigration is mediated by the interaction of SDF-1 with its receptor CXCR4.[31]

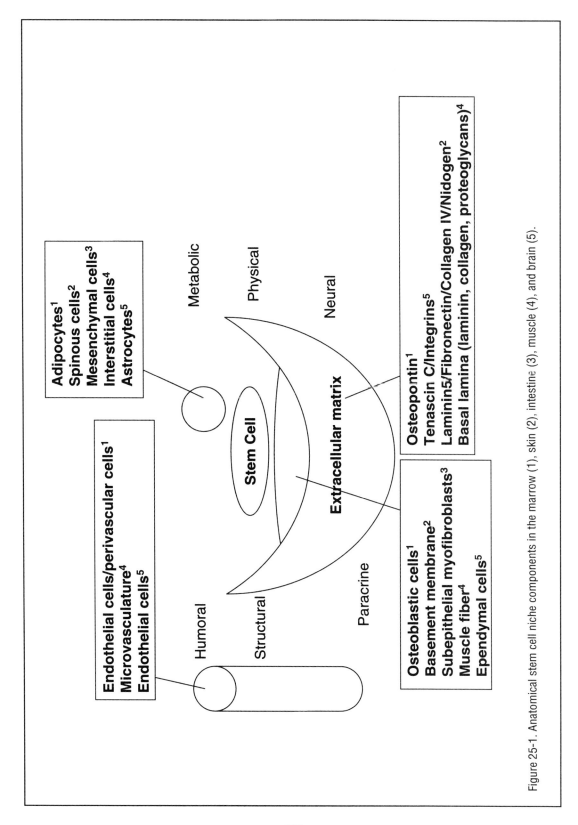

Figure 25-1. Anatomical stem cell niche components in the marrow (1), skin (2), intestine (3), muscle (4), and brain (5).

Mobilization and Isolation of Hematopoietic Stem Cells

Pathways by which HSCs can be mobilized from their microenvironment and subsequently collected for use in transplantation have been identified. The pathways described for HSCs may be important and possibly similar to other cell types with regenerative capacity, for which HSCs may serve as a model.

Granulocyte colony-stimulating factor (G-CSF) is the most commonly used agent for mobilization and collection of HSCs in clinical HSCT (see Chapter 23). Mice treated with G-CSF have higher numbers of active osteoclasts and increased bone resorption. G-CSF modifies niche cells, suppresses osteoblast activity, and leads to decreased production of CXCL12.[32] The mechanism of disengagement from the niche requires the following, among others: activation of neutrophils, causing protease release; cleavage of localizing molecules such as CXCL12; the decrease of osteoblast production of CXCL12; stem cell expression of the dipeptidyl peptidase CD26, which cleaves and inactivates CXCL12; and activation of genes regulating stem cell mobility.[33] The recently approved agent plerixafor (study name, AMD3100), a bicyclam antagonist of the chemokine receptor CXCR4, mobilizes CD34+ hematopoietic cells alone and augments mobilization by G-CSF in humans and other vertebrates.[34,35]

Engineering of Cells with Regenerative Capacity

Following the example of HSCT, a logical next step is the transplantation of cells that have—by in-vitro manipulation—acquired regenerative ability or have differentiated into cell types needed for repair of a specific tissue. This is the goal of research efforts in the field of regenerative medicine. Lessons learned in developmental biology have been crucial for the process of in-vitro stem cell differentiation, as the differentiation of pluripotent stem cells recapitulates key aspects of early embryonic development. The reprogramming of existing adult cells into pluripotent stem cells, from which mature cells of medical importance could be differentiated (eg, neurons, cardiomyocytes, hematopoietic cells, or pancreatic β cells), would provide a permanent supply of fully immunologically matched grafts for a given patient. Different strategies to convert differentiated cells into pluripotent stem cells are described below.

Somatic Cell Nuclear Transfer

The first experiments on nuclear transfer were performed in 1952 by Briggs and King, who generated live xenopus frogs by transplanting nuclei from frog blastula into oocysts.[36] These efforts culminated in the cloning of the sheep "Dolly" in 1997 by Wilmut and colleagues, which was the first evidence that adult mammalian cells retain nuclear plasticity and can be reprogrammed to an embryonic state.[37] In somatic cell nuclear transfer (SCNT), the nucleus of an adult cell is injected into the cytoplasm of an unfertilized egg. Though technically feasible, SCNT in humans has not been performed. It is dependent on the donation of a large number of unfertilized eggs, and is so technically difficult and inefficient that it has not found its way into routine clinical use.[14,19]

Cell Fusion

The fusion of an embryonic stem cell, a pluripotent cell originating from the inner cell mass of a blastocyst, with a somatic cell leads to the generation of a tetraploid pluripotent cell. These cells can be differentiated into various cell types, regenerating all cell types in the body, and can be used for gene therapy.

Direct Reprogramming

In 2006 Takahashi and Yamanaka and colleagues achieved a major breakthrough in the field of regenerative medicine.[5] Genes for the four transcription factors c-Myc, Sox2, Oct4, and Klf4 were inserted via viral vectors into lineage-restricted and, consequently, very stable murine fibroblasts. This made it possible to generate pluripotent cells called induced pluripotent stem (iPS) cells lacking all the epigenetic characteristics that the fibroblasts had acquired during development.[5] Such undifferentiated cells have the ability to proliferate in culture for an extended period of time and to generate derivatives of the three primary germ layers. Murine and human iPS cells have a normal karyotype and are transcriptionally and epigenetically similar to ES cells.[15] However, chromosomal abnormalities occur frequently in human iPS cells, and the risk of insertional mutagenesis is high.[14] Many genes (such as *FGF4* and genes encoding proteins of the polycomb group) expressed in ES cells and linked to self-renewal are reactivated during reprogramming.

Since the original discovery, iPS have been generated by other technologies that use different transcription factors but, more importantly, decrease reliance on integration of the viral genome into the host cell genome. The derivation of iPS cells is easy, rapid, and reproducible. The differentiation of these cells into various functional cell types such as neurons, cardiomyocytes, and pancreatic and hematopoietic cells represents an advance toward the goal of providing large numbers of patient-specific and therefore fully immunologically matched pluripotent cells. Such cells could be used for regenerative and therapeutic purposes in diseases such as Parkinson disease, diabetes mellitus, and potentially many others. In a humanized mouse model of sickle cell disease, for example, the defect was corrected by coupling gene targeting with direct reprogramming.[16]

Disease-specific iPS cell lines have important potential applications. First, they provide an opportunity to generate large numbers of cells with the identical genetic background of the disease. If the cell type associated with the disease can be generated, in-vitro modeling of the disease may be possible. Such strategies are currently underway with multiple neurodegenerative disorders. Second, the availability of large numbers of cells offers the opportunity to create high-throughput, cell-based assays where cells plated in large numbers of replicates can be exposed to compounds of interest to test for response. Such approaches are amenable to screening small molecules for drug discovery.[14]

Although progenitor cells generated by reprogramming may be directly used as cellular therapy, it is possible that they have a much more stringent dependence on their niche after transplantation than mature cells and may undergo differentiation or even apoptosis if these strict niche requirements are not met. Furthermore, the stimulation of cell proliferation during the reprogramming process may facilitate the conversion of different cell types, but increased proliferation over many cycles during the generation of iPS may select for culture-adapted cells with genetic mutations that may result in malignant phenotypes. These potential limitations are important considerations in this quickly growing field.

Dedifferentiation, Transdifferentiation, and Transdetermination

There are other pathways that end in reprogramming by direct conversion of a mature cell into a progenitor cell but without reverting to a pluripotent stage. In salamander limb generation, as mentioned earlier, mature muscle, skin, and cartilage cells dedifferentiate into a progenitor stage, from which the new limb is regenerated. In a process called transdifferentiation, injured pigmented epithelial cells of the iris can form lens cells.[17] A recent study demonstrated that it is possible to convert exocrine pancreatic cells into endocrine pancreatic β cells, which produce insulin, by the expression of three transcription factors.[18] This supports the hypothesis that it may be feasible to convert central nervous system cells into motor neurons as therapy for such intractable diseases as amyotrophic lateral sclerosis. The conversion between different progenitor cells is termed transdetermination.

Clinical Applications of Cells with Regenerative Potential

Hopes are high that the cells generated by the various reprogramming strategies outlined above will serve clinical purposes as frequently and efficiently as HSCs. HSCT, so far still the only modality for transplantation of pluripotent progenitor cells, has been augmented by cord blood transplantation as a stem cell source, as stem cell transplantation from cord blood also leads to full blood reconstitution, is readily available, easy to obtain, and associated with less graft-vs-host disease. Recent studies are aimed at overcoming the low number of HSCs recovered from one cord blood donor, for instance by treatment with prostaglandin E2, which has been shown to regulate HSCs by the Wnt signaling pathway.[38,39]

Cells with stem- or primitive progenitor-like potential have been identified in certain tissues, including brain, marrow, liver, skin, and skeletal muscle, and the cells have been enriched; however, the numbers of these cells are small, and the ability to expand and transplant them is limited. Endogenous stem cells in the central nervous system, for example, are insufficient in their regenerative response, although neural stem cells can engraft in human recipients, can differentiate into cells of a neuronal or astrocytic lineage, and can even deliver therapeutic substances to the brain.[21] With reprogramming technology, abundant human cells such as dermal fibroblasts and adipocytes could, via induction of a pluripotent stage, be converted into other medically important cells, such as neurons, hematopoietic cells, cardiomyocytes, endothelial cells, hepatocytes, or pancreatic β cells, and eventually be transplanted back into the same patient as a fully immunologically matched graft.

The transplantation of iPS cells that have undergone in-vitro differentiation into neural cells could be beneficial in neurologic diseases such as Huntington disease, multiple sclerosis, amyotrophic lateral sclerosis, spinal cord lesions, and many others. Transplantation of autologous neural stem cells seems most appropriate for acute nerve injuries, whereas transplantation of healthy heterologous cells—for instance, dopamine-producing neural cells for the alleviation of the symptoms of Parkinson disease—seems to be the most useful application. In a model of Parkinson disease in primates, the progeny of the transplanted human neural stem cells were located close to the remaining diseased cells and seemed to stop disease progression, probably by modulation of the microenvironment.[21] This could be used to argue that future strategies in regenerative medicine should also be aimed at the interaction of the transplanted stem and/or progenitor cells with their respective environments. In addition, genetically modified neural stem cells have been used to deliver a pro-drug that is subsequently converted to an active chemotherapeutic agent.

In the cardiovascular system, engraftment of transplanted cells has always been problematic, although the generation of cells of the cardiac conduction system and cells that would promote the formation of coronary collaterals is theoretically possible. The difficulty lies in the fact that transplanted myogenic progenitors, for example, would have to align with the ventricular basket-weave formation in order to facilitate contraction and relaxation of the ventricle.[40] In the past, efforts have been made to activate stem cells resident in the heart in situ or to propagate the cardiac stem cells in vitro and subsequently inject them into the heart muscle. Another model has been to transplant adult stem cells capable of differentiating into contractile myocytes into the heart. In other studies, it has been shown that transplantation of progenitor cell populations derived from marrow (possibly by apheresis), skeletal muscle, or endothelium can increase cardiac function in models of cardiac injury. In any case, the transplanted cell type would have to differentiate into a forcefully contractile myocyte. However, it has been hypothesized that the improvement in cardiac function may be the result of a paracrine effect of the injected cells rather than transdifferentiation.[41] Further advancement of the field of cardiology-relevant regenerative medicine may even provide tissue-engineered heart valves and blood vessels.

Mesenchymal stem cells derived from marrow, adipose tissue, or cord blood can form myocytes, osteoblasts, chondrocytes, and adipocytes. They have been used to repair bone defects in genetic diseases of the bone such as osteogenesis imperfecta, for the regeneration of damaged cartilage as in osteoarthritis, and for immunomodulation.[42] Even the healing of wounds, burn injuries, or injured or torn ligaments seems theoretically feasible with transplantation of mesenchymal stem cells, but the medical value and cost-effectiveness of such procedures still need to be established in larger clinical trials.

The transplantation of hepatic stem and progenitor cells is an attractive idea because of the shortage of livers for organ transplantation. Cells in the c-Met$^+$, CD49f$^{+/low}$, c-kit$^-$, CD45$^-$, Ter119−, ie, CD49f, fraction of fetal liver cells have the capacity of self-renewal and bipotential differentiation in vitro, which would seem to argue that this fraction harbors hepatic stem cells. The identification of adult liver stem cells has been difficult, but liver can regenerate after partial hepatectomy and by hyperplasia of the hepatocytes. Liver repopulation after acute liver failure is dependent on hepatic stem or progenitor cells, although, probably because of their low number, these cells are rarely detectable. "Oval cells," located in the terminal bile duct, are one of several liver stem/progenitor cell populations that are activated by liver injury. Studies have shown that liver stem cells derived from murine embryonic stem cells have improved the function of injured livers. Human embryonic stem cells differentiated into hepatocytes have also been shown to engraft in mice and to express human α1 antitrypsin for a certain amount of time. So far, however, there have not been any trials in human patients.[43]

Despite the great promise of regenerative medicine, there are some important limitations and barriers. First, the tissue source of reprogrammable cells should be well defined, as these cells have to be HLA-matched in order to prevent graft rejection. Second, the cell source should be easily and efficiently isolated and engineered into a medically useful biologic product. However, engineered cells may have reduced survival in the host because of an inflammatory response generated after grafting and because of a loss of the interaction between engrafted cells and their environment. Third, the risks of teratoma formation and of acquisition of multiple karyotypic abnormalities that may lead to cancerous phenotypes are not negligible. Finally, ethical and social issues associated with the use of embryonic stem cells should be addressed.

In summary, the potential of regenerative medicine and the provision of unlimited numbers of patient-specific, engineered cells with the capacity to repair or replace damaged human tissues is a daunting and exciting new dimension that may contribute future treatment options for human disease. To date, apheresis has been used only routinely for collection of HSCs and HPCs for use in transplantation. Studies collecting mesenchymal cells for use as disease modifiers in settings of ischemic injury or as immune-suppressing agents are being conducted. Whether other cells types can be mobilized into the blood and harvested by apheresis for regenerative strategies is, at this point, uncertain.

References

1. Maximov A. Der Lymphozyt als gemeinsame Stammzelle der verschiedenen Blutelemente in der embryonalen Entwicklung und postfetalen Leben der Saeugetiere. Folia Haematologica (Leipzig) 1909;8:125-41.

2. Becker AJ, McCullough CE, Till JE. Cytological demonstration of the clonal nature of spleen colonies derived from transplanted mouse marrow cells. Nature 1963;197:452-4.

3. Thomson JA, Itskovitz-Eldor J, Shapiro SS, et al. Embryonic stem cell lines derived from human blastocysts. Science 1998;282:1145-7.

4. Shamblott MJ, Axelman J, Wang S, et al. Derivation of pluripotent stem cells from cultured human primordial germ cells. Proc Natl Acad Sci U S A 1998;95:13726-31.

5. Takahashi K, Yamanaka S. Induction of pluripotent stem cells from mouse embryonic and adult fibroblast cultures by defined factors. Cell 2006;126:663-76.

6. Kragl M, Knapp D, Nacu E, et al. Cells keep a memory of their tissue origin during axolotl limb regeneration. Nature 2009;460:60-5.

7. Harty M, Neff AW, King MW, Mescher AL. Regeneration or scarring: An immunologic perspective. Dev Dyn 2003;226:268-79.

8. Tredget EE, Ding J. Wound healing: From embryos to adults and back again. Lancet 2009;373:1226-8.

9. Adams GB, Martin RP, Alley IR, et al. Therapeutic targeting of a stem cell niche. Nat Biotechnol 2007;25:238-43.

10. Mukherjee S, Raje N, Schoonmaker JA, et al. Pharmacologic targeting of a stem/progenitor population in vivo is associated with enhanced bone regeneration in mice. J Clin Invest 2008; 118:491-504.

11. Calvi LM, Adams GB, Weibrecht KW, et al. Osteoblastic cells regulate the haematopoietic stem cell niche. Nature 2003;425:841-6.

12. Zhang J, Niu C, Ye L, et al. Identification of the haematopoietic stem cell niche and control of the niche size. Nature 2003;425:836-41.

13. Stier S, Ko Y, Forkert R, et al. Osteopontin is a hematopoietic stem cell niche component that negatively regulates stem cell pool size. J Exp Med 2005;201:1781-91.

14. Amabile G, Meissner A. Induced pluripotent stem cells: Current progress and potential for regenerative medicine. Trends Mol Med 2009; 15:59-68.

15. Maherali N, Hochedlinger K. Guidelines and techniques for the generation of induced pluripotent stem cells. Cell Stem Cell 2008;3:595-605.

16. Hanna J, Wernig M, Markoulaki S, et al. Treatment of sickle cell anemia mouse model with iPS cells generated from autologous skin. Science 2007;318:1920-3.

17. Zhou Q, Melton DA. Extreme makeover: Converting one cell into another. Cell Stem Cell 2008;3:382-8.

18. Zhou Q, Brown J, Kanarek A, et al. In vivo reprogramming of adult pancreatic exocrine cells to beta-cells. Nature 2008;455:627-32.

19. Riazi AM, Kwon SY, Stanford WL. Stem cell sources for regenerative medicine. In: Audet J, Stanford W, eds. ed. Stem cells in regenerative medicine. New York: Humana, 2009:55-90.

20. Stelnicki EJ, Chin GS, Gittes GK, Longaker MT. Fetal wound repair: Where do we go from here? Semin Pediatr Surg 1999;8:124-30.

21. Lederer CW, Santama N. Neural stem cells: Mechanisms of fate specification and nuclear reprogramming in regenerative medicine. Biotechnol J 2008;3:1521-38.

22. Schofield R. The relationship between the spleen colony-forming cell and the haemopoietic stem cell. Blood Cells 1978;4:7-25.

23. Morrison SJ, Spradling AC. Stem cells and niches: Mechanisms that promote stem cell maintenance throughout life. Cell 2008;132:598-611.

24. Sugiyama T, Kohara H, Noda M, Nagasawa T. Maintenance of the hematopoietic stem cell pool by CXCL12-CXCR4 chemokine signaling in bone marrow stromal cell niches. Immunity 2006;25:977-88.

25. Sipkins DA, Wei X, Wu JW, et al. In vivo imaging of specialized bone marrow endothelial microdomains for tumour engraftment. Nature 2005;435:969-73.

26. Lo Celso C, Fleming HE, Wu JW, et al. Live-animal tracking of individual haematopoietic stem/progenitor cells in their niche. Nature 2009;457:92-6.

27. Nilsson SK, Johnston HM, Coverdale JA. Spatial localization of transplanted hemopoietic stem cells: Inferences for the localization of stem cell niches. Blood 2001;97:2293-9.

28. Quesenberry PJ, Colvin G, Abedi M. Perspective: Fundamental and clinical concepts on stem cell homing and engraftment: A journey to niches and beyond. Exp Hematol 2005;33:9-19.

29. Mazo IB, Gutierrez-Ramos JC, Frenette PS, et al. Hematopoietic progenitor cell rolling in bone marrow microvessels: Parallel contributions by endothelial selectins and vascular cell adhesion molecule 1. J Exp Med 1998;188:465-74.

30. Papayannopoulou T, Priestley GV, Nakamoto B, et al. Molecular pathways in bone marrow homing: Dominant role of alpha(4)beta(1) over beta(2)-integrins and selectins. Blood 2001; 98:2403-11.

31. Peled A, Kollet O, Ponomaryov T, et al. The chemokine SDF-1 activates the integrins LFA-1, VLA-4, and VLA-5 on immature human CD34(+) cells: Role in transendothelial/stromal migration and engraftment of NOD/SCID mice. Blood 2000;95:3289-96.

32. Kollet O, Dar A, Shivtiel S, et al. Osteoclasts degrade endosteal components and promote mobilization of hematopoietic progenitor cells. Nat Med 2006;12:657-64.

33. Purton LE, Scadden DT. Osteoclasts eat stem cells out of house and home. Nat Med 2006; 12:610-11.

34. Flomenberg N, Devine SM, Dipersio JF, et al. The use of AMD3100 plus G-CSF for autologous hematopoietic progenitor cell mobiliza-

tion is superior to G-CSF alone. Blood 2005; 106:1867-74.

35. Larochelle A, Krouse A, Metzger M, et al. AMD3100 mobilizes hematopoietic stem cells with long-term repopulating capacity in nonhuman primates. Blood 2006;107:3772-8.

36. Briggs R, King TJ. Transplantation of living nuclei from blastula cells into enucleated frogs' eggs. Proc Natl Acad Sci U S A 1952;38:455-63.

37. Wilmut I, Schnieke AE, McWhir J, et al. Viable offspring derived from fetal and adult mammalian cells. Nature 1997;385:810-3.

38. Goessling W, North TE, Loewer S, et al. Genetic interaction of PGE2 and Wnt signaling regulates developmental specification of stem cells and regeneration. Cell 2009;136:1136-47.

39. North TE, Goessling W, Walkley CR, et al. Prostaglandin E2 regulates vertebrate haemato-poietic stem cell homeostasis. Nature 2007; 447:1007-11.

40. Chien KR, Domian IJ, Parker KK. Cardiogenesis and the complex biology of regenerative cardiovascular medicine. Science 2008;322:1494-7.

41. Irion S, Nostro MC, Kattman SJ, Keller GM. Directed differentiation of pluripotent stem cells: From developmental biology to therapeutic applications. Cold Spring Harb Symp Quant Biol 2008;73:101-10.

42. Sensebe L, Bourin P. Mesenchymal stem cells for therapeutic purposes. Transplantation 2009; 87:S49-53.

43. Kakinuma S, Nakauchi H, Watanabe M. Hepatic stem/progenitor cells and stem-cell transplantation for the treatment of liver disease. J Gastroenterol 2009;44:167-72.

In: McLeod BC, Szczepiorkowski ZM, Weinstein R, Winters JL, eds.
Apheresis: Principles and Practice, 3rd edition
Bethesda, MD: AABB Press, 2010

26

Autologous Cellular Immunotherapies

David W. O'Neill, MD

 PROTECTIVE IMMUNITY RESULTS from the coordinated action of innate and adaptive immune systems.[1] The innate immune system, which includes phagocytic cells such as granulocytes and macrophages, certain lymphocytes such as natural killer (NK) cells, and molecular mediators of the complement cascade, functions to respond rapidly to pathogens to protect the host early in infection. The adaptive immune system, which consists of B and T lymphocytes characterized by highly polymorphic antigen receptors that are the product of genetic recombination, functions later in the course of an infection and is required for the eventual clearance of many types of pathogens, as well as for the generation of immunologic memory. In addition to protecting the host from pathogens, both innate and adaptive immunity may act in the surveillance for and elimination of malignant cells.[2,3]

This chapter focuses on cellular therapies derived from autologous apheresis products designed to harness the power of the adaptive immune system to treat disease. We refer to these as "autologous cellular immunotherapies." Allogeneic cellular immunotherapies such as donor lymphocyte infusions (used following hematopoietic stem cell transplantation)[4-6] are discussed in Chapter 27, and granulocyte transfusions[7,8] are covered in Chapter 11.

Autologous cellular immunotherapies have been used experimentally in humans to treat viral infections, virus-induced malignancies, and a number of other types of malignancies such as melanoma, prostate cancer, colon cancer, and even glioblastoma multiforme. They can potentially be used to treat autoimmune diseases or to induce tolerance to transplanted organs, but these applications remain limited to animal models at present. The production and use of cellular immunotherapies are highly

David W. O'Neill, MD, Assistant Professor of Pathology, New York University School of Medicine, and Director, New York University Cancer Institute Vaccine and Cell Therapy Core Facility, New York University School of Medicine, New York, New York

The author has disclosed no conflicts of interest.

complex undertakings that require specialized manufacturing facilities and personnel. Their use has thus been limited to a relatively small number of academic medical centers, or to a few industry-sponsored multi-center trials. To date, no autologous cellular immunotherapy has been approved by the Food and Drug Administration (FDA) as a treatment for any disease or has gained wide use in clinical practice. This may change, however, because there have been some very promising clinical results associated with a number of these treatments, which are discussed below.

Autologous cellular immunotherapies can be divided into two principal types: 1) active cellular immunotherapies [ie, dendritic cell (DC) or antigen-presenting cell (APC) vaccines], which attempt to stimulate the patient's immune system to kill a specific target pathogen or cell, and 2) adoptive cell transfer (ie, adoptive T-cell therapies), in which large numbers of antigen-specific T lymphocytes are propagated ex vivo and then infused back into the patient.[9-13]

Active Cellular Immunotherapies (Dendritic Cell/Antigen-Presenting Cell Vaccines)

Principles Underlying the Use of Dendritic Cells or Other Antigen-Presenting Cells for Immunotherapy

Specialized APCs such as macrophages, B cells, and DCs are marrow-derived cells that form an important link between innate and adaptive immunity. APCs acquire both foreign antigens and autoantigens from their environment, process antigenic proteins into peptides that are presented on cell-surface major histocompatibility complex Class I and II molecules (MHC I and II), and secrete inflammatory mediators on exposure to pathogen components. Antigenic peptides presented on MHC I and II are then recognized by CD8+ and CD4+ T cells, respectively, initiating an adaptive immune response.[14] DCs are particularly specialized to process and present peptide antigens to stimulate T cells and have accordingly generated

great interest as vehicles for immunotherapy.[15-18] In addition to their function in priming adaptive immune responses, DCs also play an important role in the maintenance of immune tolerance.[19-21]

Dendritic Cell Types

DCs are a diverse group of lineage-negative (CD3–, CD14–, CD19–, and CD56–), HLA-DR+ mononuclear cells of hematopoietic origin.[22] In human blood, DCs can be divided into two major subpopulations by staining with antibodies to CD11c and CD123. CD11c+, CD123^{lo} DCs have a monocyte-like appearance and are often referred to as "conventional" or "myeloid" DCs (mDCs), whereas CD11c–, CD123^{hi} DCs have morphologic features reminiscent of plasma cells and are known as "plasmacytoid" DCs (pDCs).[23] pDCs, which are found primarily in blood and lymphoid organs, secrete high amounts of interferon alpha (IFNα) when stimulated with microbial components and play an important role in antiviral immunity.[24,25] There are two principal subtypes of mDCs— 1) so-called interstitial, dermal, or submucosal DCs (variously named according to their anatomic location) and 2) Langerhans cells, which are found in the epidermis and the oral, respiratory, and genital mucosa; express the C-type lectin, langerin (CD207); and have unique intracellular organelles called Birbeck granules.[26,27]

Antigen Uptake and Processing by Dendritic Cells

In tissues, DCs and DC precursors such as monocytes may be infected directly by pathogens or may endocytose antigens from microorganisms, apoptotic cells, necrotic cells, extracellular proteins, or immune complexes.[28,29] DCs have many different antigen uptake receptors for endocytosis, including scavenger receptors,[30] Fc receptors,[31] and C-type lectins.[32] Some of these receptors—such as the Fc receptors—can induce either stimulatory or inhibitory signals on antigen uptake, depending on the receptor type.[31]

DCs process antigenic proteins into peptides that are loaded onto MHC I and II, and these peptide-MHC complexes (pMHC I and II) are transported to the cell surface for recognition by antigen-specific T cells.[14] Antigens acquired endogenously (synthesized by pathogens within the DC cytosol) are processed and loaded onto MHC I, whereas antigens acquired exogenously (through endocytosis) are typically processed onto MHC II.

Processing of endogenous proteins onto MHC I is through a cytosolic pathway that involves ubiquitination, degradation by proteasomes, and transport by TAP molecules (transporters for antigen presentation) into the endoplasmic reticulum. Exogenously acquired proteins are typically taken up in endocytic vesicles and degraded in lysosomes, where the peptides are loaded onto MHC II.[14,16] An alternative pathway also exists whereby DCs can process endocytosed antigens onto MHC I. This pathway, called "cross-presentation," permits DCs to elicit CD8+ T-cell responses to exogenous antigens such as apoptotic or necrotic tumor cells, virus-infected cells, and immune complexes.[14,33,34] Cross-presentation has been linked to a number of specific types of antigen uptake receptors on DCs, including Fc and mannose receptors.[28,34,35]

Other, less polymorphic antigen-presenting molecules structurally similar to MHC I are also found on DCs. For example, CD1 molecules function to present microbial lipids to T cells.[36,37] Different DC subtypes express different CD1 molecules. For example, CD1a is expressed primarily on Langerhans cells.[27]

Dendritic Cell Maturation/Activation

In the steady-state, DCs function to maintain immunologic tolerance to captured antigens, and DCs must be activated before they can become effective stimulators of immunity. This DC activation process—known as "maturation"—transforms DCs from cells specialized for antigen capture into terminally differentiated cells specialized for T-cell stimulation.[38,39] DC maturation is induced by components of pathogens called pathogen-associated molecular patterns (PAMPs) as well as by host molecules associated with inflammation or tissue injury.[39,40] Stimuli from PAMPs are mediated by signaling through germline pattern recognition receptors (PRRs) such as Toll-like receptors (TLRs), Nod proteins, or NALP3.[1,41] PRRs can be found on the DC surface, in endocytic compartments, or in the cytosol, depending on the receptor. Different DC types express different PRRs, which can determine whether the DC will respond to specific inflammatory stimuli. For example, pDCs—important mediators of antiviral immunity—express primarily TLRs 7 and 9, which function in the recognition of viral nucleic acids.[24]

DCs are also matured by inflammatory mediators produced by cells of the host immune system as well as by products of damaged host tissues.[39,40] These host-derived molecules include cytokines such as IFNα, interleukin (IL)-1, or IL-6; tumor necrosis factor (TNF) family members such as TNFα or CD40L; and molecules released by dead or dying cells such as uric acid crystals or heat-shock proteins. Like PAMPs, host-derived mediators also stimulate intracellular signaling pathways through specific receptors on or within the DC.

DC maturation is characterized by a variety of morphologic and functional changes. At maturation, DCs acquire cytoplasmic processes or "veils," giving them their characteristic dendritic appearance. Mature DCs down-regulate expression of chemokine receptors such as CCR1 and CCR5, which are associated with migration to sites of inflammation,[42] and up-regulate CCR7, which is associated with migration to T-cell areas of secondary lymphoid tissue.[43] Mature DCs up-regulate surface expression of adhesion and co-stimulatory molecules that promote further DC activation and T-cell stimulation. Examples include intercellular adhesion molecule (ICAM)-1 (CD54) and members of the TNF receptor family (CD40), TNF family (OX40L, CD27L), and B7 family (CD80, CD86).[44,45] Maturation also stimulates DCs to secrete cytokines and chemokines that promote T-cell proliferation and cytokine production and that recruit other inflammatory cells into the local environment.[39,46] Other markers up-regulated at DC maturation include CD83, a molecule involved in lymphocyte maturation and DC-DC interactions, and DC-LAMP, a DC-specific lysosomal-associated membrane protein.[44,47]

It is important to note that DC antigen processing coordinates with, and is regulated by, maturation[15] and is associated with reduced phagocytic uptake, acidification of endosomes (which activates endosomal proteases), removal of the invariant chain from the antigen-binding pockets of MHC II (providing access for processed antigenic peptides), and exocytosis of pMHC II to the cell surface. Maturation also up-regulates specific proteasome subunits to create the "immunoproteasome," which recognizes new cleavage sites on proteins to enhance the processing of peptides onto MHC I.[48,49]

Cross-presentation of antigens can also be enhanced by certain DC maturation stimuli.[50-52]

Dendritic Cell Interactions with T Lymphocytes

DCs initiate ("prime") T-cell responses in secondary lymphoid organs such as lymph nodes, the spleen, or mucosal lymphoid tissue, where dynamic DC-T-cell interactions occur.[53] Priming of naive T cells is mediated by three types of signal from the DC: 1) through presentation of antigen on pMHC to the T-cell antigen receptor (TCR), 2) through DC-T-cell interactions among a wide range of co-stimulatory molecules (such as CD80 and CD86 on DCs, and CD28 on T cells), and 3) through the effects of proinflammatory cytokines, such as IFNα or IL-12, secreted by DCs (Fig 26-1).[39] Through these signals, mature DCs can induce naive T cells to

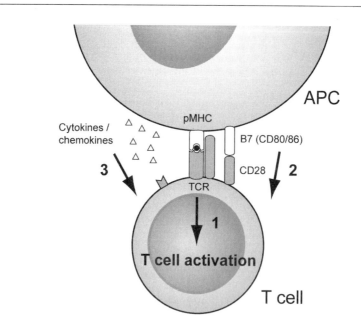

Figure 26-1. Three signals from a specialized APC are required to prime a fully effective T-cell response. This example shows activation of a CD4+ T cell via pMHC II (signal 1), with co-stimulation via B7-CD28 interactions (signal 2) and the effect of secreted cytokines from the APC on the T cell (signal 3).
APC = antigen-presenting cell; MHC = major histocompatibility complex; pMHC = peptide MHC. Adapted from Janeway et al.[54]

expand clonally and to differentiate into antigen-specific memory and effector cells. All three signals are believed to be required for full T-cell effector function, and provision of signal 1 alone can result in immune tolerance through anergy, clonal deletion, or the induction of regulatory T cells (Treg).[39] An effective adaptive immune response is associated with enhanced T-cell survival following priming and the induction of memory T cells, which are characterized by resistance to cell death and by responsiveness to the "homeostatic" cytokines IL-7 and IL-15 in the absence of antigen stimulation.[55-58]

The state of DC maturation and the type of maturation stimulus have direct consequences on the ability of DCs to prime an effective T-cell response. Significantly, it is thought that stimulation of DCs with cytokines alone is insufficient for the generation of a full T-cell effector response, even though such stimulation may result in a DC that appears phenotypically mature.[39] Stimulation of DC PRRs by PAMPs, along with stimulation of DC CD40, appears to be required for the generation of full T-cell effector function and CD8+ T-cell memory.[39,59,60]

Dendritic Cell Vaccine Approaches

Dendritic Cell Isolation and Culture Methods

The most common approach for DC vaccines is to prepare large numbers of autologous mDCs ex vivo, load them with antigens, and mature them with cytokines before injecting them back into the patient.[9,61,62] Although it is possible to enrich circulating pDCs from peripheral blood,[63] this approach has not yet been employed for clinical use in humans. Three general methods have been described for the preparation of mDCs for human vaccines: 1) differentiating DCs from nonproliferating monocyte precursors, 2) differentiating DCs from proliferating CD34+ hematopoietic progenitor cells, or 3) directly isolating DCs or mixed APCs from peripheral blood.

Monocyte-Derived DCs. Cells similar to dermal/interstitial mDCs may be produced by culturing peripheral blood monocytes in the presence of granulocyte-macrophage colony-stimulating factor (GM-CSF) and IL-4 for 2 to 7 days.[64-66] IL-13 may also be used in place of IL-4.[67] These monocyte-derived DCs (Mo-DCs) have been probably the most widely used DC type for active cellular immunotherapy clinical trials to date. To prepare Mo-DCs, CD14+ monocytes are first purified from peripheral blood mononuclear cells (PBMCs) from whole blood or, more commonly, from apheresis mononuclear cells. Monocytes can be isolated from PBMCs using a simple plastic adherence step at the beginning of the culture period (monocytes adhere to the plastic culture vessels, whereas lymphocytes do not). Alternatively, monocytes can be isolated from apheresis mononuclear cells by elutriation or by large-scale cell sorting using immunomagnetic beads.[68-70] IL-4 and GM-CSF induce the monocytes to differentiate into immature (CD14−, CD83−) mDCs, which are then loaded with antigens and matured/activated as described below (see "Dendritic Cell Maturation Methods").

DCs Derived from CD34+ Hematopoietic Progenitor Cells. A mixture of APCs that includes cells phenotypically resembling Langerhans cells and cells similar to dermal/interstitial mDCs can be obtained by culturing CD34+ hematopoietic progenitor cells in the presence of GM-CSF and TNFα for 1 to 2 weeks.[71-74] Flt3 ligand, stem cell factor, and thrombopoietin may be added to the cultures to expand DC progenitors, and differentiation may be skewed towards Langerhans cells by adding transforming growth factor β (TGFβ).[75] For this method, CD34+ progenitor cells must first be mobilized from the marrow by treating patients with granulocyte CSF (G-CSF) before leukapheresis. CD34+ progenitors can then be purified by immunomagnetic selection and cultured. The final cellular therapy product is not as pure as a Mo-DC preparation and contains a fairly large percentage of myeloid cells at varying stages of differentiation, including some CD14+ cells. CD34+ progenitor-cell-derived DCs can be matured and loaded with antigens similarly to Mo-DCs.[74]

DCs or APCs Enriched from Peripheral Blood. In the first clinical trial of DC-based immunotherapy for cancer, DCs were purified directly from PBMCs by a series of density-gradient centrifugation steps.[76] PBMCs were first depleted of monocytes by centrifugation through discontinuous Percoll gradients, then cultured for 24 hours in the presence of antigen without exogenous cytokines. Next, DCs were separated from lymphocytes by sequential centrifugation through two metrizamide gradients, and the low-density fraction containing DCs was cultured overnight in the presence of antigen, then washed and injected back into the patient. This and similar procedures typically yield a final product that is enriched with a mixture of APCs phenotypically similar to mature mDCs, expressing maturation markers such as CD80, CD86, CD83, and CCR7.[77] The yield of DCs can be significantly improved by stimulating the patient with Flt3 ligand before leukapheresis, although pharmaceutical grade Flt3 ligand is not currently commercially available.[77] G-CSF mobilization of progenitor cells before apheresis is not required. APCs prepared by a streamlined version of this method in a commercial closed system are being used in Phase III trials for the immunotherapy of prostate cancer.[78-80]

Choice of Cell Preparation Method. All three of the above methods have been shown to yield a final product that can induce antigen-specific T-cell responses in humans, and all three have been associated with occasional clinical responses in cancer patients. No direct comparisons of the three methods have been performed in clinical trials, so it is not known if any one is superior. To date, only APCs enriched directly from blood have been associated with a clinical benefit compared to a control group in a randomized Phase III clinical trial [see "Cancer" ("Phase III Clinical Trials")].[80]

Dendritic Cell Maturation Methods

Before administration to the patient, DCs are typically matured by culturing for an additional 1 to 2 days in the presence of proinflammatory cytokines. A number of phenotypic markers of maturation are typically analyzed by cell-surface staining with fluorescent antibodies to assess the quality of this maturation stimulus. Among the most commonly tested are HLA-DR, CD40, co-stimulatory molecules such as CD80 and CD86, and the widely used maturation marker CD83.

Before clinical grade cytokines were available, DCs were matured using supernatants from cultured monocytes (monocyte-conditioned medium, or MCM) as the source of cytokines.[64,65,81] MCM has now been largely supplanted by a cocktail of three cytokines (IL-1β, IL-6, and TNFα) plus prostaglandin E$_2$ (PGE$_2$) that mimics its effects.[82] Clinical studies comparing immature DCs to DCs matured with cytokines indicate that ex-vivo matured DCs more effectively stimulate T-cell responses[83,84] and that the use of immature DCs can even lead to immune tolerance.[85,86]

Still, there are a number of concerns with this maturation method. Several groups have observed that cytokine- and PGE$_2$-matured DCs do not secrete detectable, biologically active IL-12p70, although they still express CCR7 and can induce Th1 and CD8+ T-cell responses in vitro.[87,88] However, IL-12 is thought to be of central importance for the induction of Th1 responses in vivo. Removal of PGE$_2$ from the cocktail can lead to the secretion of at least some IL-12, but PGE$_2$ is considered important for inducing DC migratory ability, so it is still typically included.[89] Perhaps most important, evidence in animal models is accumulating that DCs matured with cytokines alone (without the addition of PAMPs), although phenotypically mature, do not induce full T-cell effector responses.[39] Thus, it is likely that the addition of PAMPs to the DC maturation stimulus will be an important component of future DC vaccine studies in humans.

Sources of Antigen and Antigen-Loading Methods

To induce an adaptive immune response to the specified target of interest (typically a pathogen or a malignant cell) DCs are loaded with a source of specific antigen either just before or immediately following maturation. DCs can be loaded with a wide assortment of antigen sources—including whole cells or cell lysates, synthetic peptides, purified or recombinant proteins, or nucleic acids such as RNA, plasmid DNA, or nonreplicating recombinant viral vectors—that encode the antigen of interest.[9] Immunogenicity may be enhanced by using antigens combined or fused with other more immunogenic molecules, including foreign proteins such as keyhole limpet hemocyanin (KLH), cytokines such as GM-CSF, or PAMPs.

Peptides, Proteins, and Immune Complexes. One of the more common methods for loading DCs with antigen is to co-culture them with antigenic peptides.[73,90] This approach has been made possible through the identification of immunodominant peptide epitopes for microbial and tumor-associated antigens that are recognized by T cells.[91-93] Use of peptides requires knowledge of a patient's HLA type and the identification of relevant MHC-restricted antigenic epitopes. HLA-A2-restricted epitopes have been most commonly used because HLA-A2 is a very common HLA type, but other MHC I- and even MHC II-restricted epitopes have been used as well. Altered or enhanced peptides that bind the TCR more tightly or have foreign (xenogeneic) sequences inserted have also been used to boost immunity to less immunogenic autoantigens.[77,94]

Peptides may be loaded onto DCs either before or after maturation. The optimal peptide dose with which to load DCs has not been well examined; lower concentrations may be better because there is evidence in animal models that APCs loaded with very low concentrations of peptide (as little as 0.1 nM) are more effective at inducing high-avidity T-cell clones that kill antigen-expressing target cells in vivo.[94,95] To date, most protocols have pulsed DCs with peptide concentrations in the 1 to 10 μM range.

A major disadvantage of using peptides is that peptide vaccination studies typically need to be restricted to individuals with common HLA types and to MHC-I-presented epitopes only. As an alternative, DCs can be loaded—typically before maturation—with purified or recombinant proteins.[9,78] Using whole protein

antigens allows host HLA molecules to select multiple epitopes from the entire amino acid sequence, regardless of HLA type. The immunogenicity of protein-loaded DCs can be enhanced by using proteins coupled to cytokine (GM-CSF) or carrier (KLH) protein sequences[96,97] or by using proteins of xenogeneic origin.[98]

Protein antigens have the disadvantage that they are typically processed and presented only on MHC II and thus stimulate CD4+ but not CD8+ T-cell responses. However, cross-presentation of protein antigens may be promoted by loading DCs with IgG immune complexes containing those antigens, which are taken up via Fc receptors on the DC, or by linking antigens to antibodies that target DC surface receptors such as DEC-205 or mannose receptor.[99]

Cells and Cell Lysates. For cancer immunotherapy, DCs can also be loaded with killed tumor cells or tumor cell lysates, typically just before DC maturation.[100-102] One advantage of this approach is that it permits vaccination with the complete antigenic content of a tumor. Pulsing DCs with cell lysates may also stimulate cross-priming via the presence of chaperone proteins that target DC heat-shock protein receptors associated with cross-presentation.[103,104]

Microbial Vectors and Nucleic Acids. For vaccines against viral infections, DCs may be loaded with nonreplicating or inactivated forms of the virus.[105] And for both viral infections and cancer, recombinant nonreplicating or attenuated microbial vectors such as adenovirus, pox viruses, or Listeria-encoding antigens from tumors or pathogens may also be used.[106-108] As with loading DCs with proteins, the use of microbial vectors allows vaccines to be generated for patients of any HLA type because the encoded proteins are cleaved and processed onto MHC molecules within the host cell. Some microbial vectors may have the additional advantage of providing PAMPs to induce DC maturation.[108]

DCs may also be loaded by transfecting with nucleic acids, either plasmid DNA or, more commonly, RNA.[9] RNA transfection has been used to successfully load DCs with transcripts encoding specific antigens or even the whole RNA content of a tumor. DCs may be transfected either before or after maturation, although there is evidence that transfecting after maturation is superior.[109,110] The translated protein products are typically processed onto MHC I, but they may be targeted to MHC II by transfecting with chimeric transcripts carrying an endosomal/lysosomal sorting signal.[111]

Storage, Dose, Schedule, and Route of Administration

DC vaccines may be given immediately following preparation or may be stored frozen until needed. In-vitro studies have shown that frozen/thawed DCs have activity comparable to fresh DCs, although the two have never been compared in a clinical trial.[112]

There is little consensus on the optimal dose and route of administration of DC vaccines. DCs have most commonly been injected intradermally, subcutaneously, or intravenously, in numbers ranging from 1 million to 100 million cells per injection. Injection into lymph nodes has also been investigated because approximately 2% or fewer DCs typically migrate to draining nodes following cutaneous injection.[61,99] Intranodal injection can be effective if the node is actually injected, but immunogenicity is very poor if the node is missed.[61] Only a handful of studies have performed dose escalations or compared injection schedules or routes of administration. From dose escalation studies it is not clear that higher numbers of injected DCs translate into improved responses. For Mo-DCs, a dose of 10 to 50 million DCs per injection is most commonly used, and injecting larger numbers is typically not practical. Studies comparing routes of administration have indicated that intradermal injection is probably more effective than subcutaneous injection, whereas intravenous administration may be important for stimulating humoral immunity or targeting visceral sites.[61,113]

Results of Clinical Trials

Clinical trials with healthy volunteers[114,115] as well as studies in patients with cancer or chronic human immunodeficiency virus (HIV) infection have shown that DC vaccines can generate T-cell responses to a variety of antigens. However, these responses are often weak, and clinical efficacy has not been clearly established in randomized clinical trials. It has also not been established whether DC vaccines are more effective than conventional vaccines that are simpler and less expensive to prepare. The results of a few key clinical trials illustrating these points are summarized below.

Chronic Viral Infections

Conventional vaccines against microbial pathogens are traditionally prepared by isolating an attenuated or killed version of the pathogen and mixing it with an adjuvant that serves to boost the immune response. The success of this type of vaccine often depends on its ability to induce neutralizing antibodies.[94] However, for a number of chronic intracellular infections, such as HIV or hepatitis C virus (HCV), this approach has not yet proved sufficient.[116] DC-based vaccine approaches attempt to generate T-cell-mediated responses to chronic infections in the therapeutic, rather than prophylactic, setting, although these efforts have largely been confined to animal models or in-vitro studies with human cells.[117-122]

One exception is HIV infection, for which there have been a number of DC vaccine clinical trials.[105,107,123] In general, these studies have shown that DC vaccination is well tolerated and can generate CD4+ as well as CD8+ T-cell responses to HIV antigens. Reduction in viral load for a year or more was reported in 8 of 18 subjects given Mo-DCs loaded with inactivated whole autologous virus,[105] although in this trial the subjects were not randomized. A randomized study comparing injection of Mo-DCs loaded with a recombinant canarypox virus encoding HIV antigens to injection of the recombinant canarypox virus alone (not loaded onto Mo-DCs) showed no difference in immunogenicity between the two study arms.[107]

Cancer

Early attempts at active cancer immunotherapy used killed tumor cells or whole tumor lysates, often mixed with immunologic adjuvants. To date, however, these approaches have failed to demonstrate a significant therapeutic effect in large randomized trials.[124-127] More recently, through the study of naturally occurring cellular immune responses in cancer patients, a wide variety of tumor-associated antigens (TAAs) have been identified that are recognized by T cells, and these antigens can also be used to vaccinate individuals against their tumors.[128,129] One advantage of this approach is that it is much easier to monitor immune responses generated by the vaccine because the target antigen (and, in the case of peptide vaccines, the precise antigenic epitope) is already known.

There are several different classes of TAAs, summarized in Table 26-1. Classes such as mutated gene products, antigens expressed by oncogenic viruses, or antigens in the cancer-testis group are particularly attractive candidates for vaccines because these represent relatively foreign proteins distinct from host somatic tissues.[130] Vaccines against TAA using reagents ranging from peptides or recombinant proteins mixed with adjuvants to recombinant viruses encoding TAA can clearly induce specific T-cell responses, but it remains to be demonstrated in randomized trials that such vaccines can provide a clinically significant benefit in the form of improved survival.[12,126,130-133]

In mice, DCs loaded ex vivo with TAA by a number of methods have been shown to induce antigen-specific CD8+ T-cell responses that protect the animals from challenge with tumors bearing the target antigen, and they can even cause complete regression of established tumors.[134-137] These promising results have led to the development of protocols for the use of DC vaccines in human subjects with cancer.

Phase I and II Clinical Trials. Numerous Phase I and II clinical trials of DC vaccines for cancer have now been published. In general, these studies have demonstrated that DC vaccines appear safe and can induce specific CD8+ and CD4+ T-cell responses, including cells that secrete IFNγ and kill antigen-bearing targets, a necessary first step toward attaining clinical efficacy.[9,61] T-cell responses can often be weak or undetectable, however, and typically lack durability.

DC vaccines have been associated with occasional tumor regression in a number of small clinical studies. Clinical responses have been reported in patients with metastatic melanoma, renal cell carcinoma, and B-cell lymphoma as well as in patients with prostate, breast, ovarian, colon, and lung cancers.[138] Perhaps the most impressive clinical responses have been associated with the use of whole proteins, killed tumor cells, or tumor lysates.[138] Objective responses tend to be seen in only a small fraction of patients, however, and correlation of immune responses with tumor regression has been variable, at least in part because these smaller studies were not designed to rigorously evaluate clinical efficacy.

Of importance, there have been very few comparative DC vaccine studies, and it has yet to be demonstrated in humans that DC vaccines have improved potency over conventional vaccines. A randomized trial in patients with metastatic melanoma comparing peptide-pulsed immature Mo-DCs to peptides administered with a mineral oil adjuvant (Montanide ISA 51) and GM-CSF demonstrated significantly *lower* immunogenicity in patients receiving the DC vaccine.[139] A more recent study using peptide- and KLH-loaded, cytokine-matured Mo-DCs also demonstrated superior immunogenicity of a conventional vaccine composed of Montanide ISA 51 mixed with the same antigens.[140]

Phase III Clinical Trials. There have been two randomized Phase III studies of DC vaccination to treat cancer. In the first, subcutaneously administered, cytokine-matured Mo-DCs loaded with a mixture of MHC I- and II-restricted peptide antigens were compared to conventional chemotherapy in patients with stage IV melanoma. Designed to compare clinical response rates (as measured by tumor regression) between the two study arms, the study closed at first interim analysis as a result

Table 26-1. Classes of Tumor-Associated Antigens*

Category	Examples	Characteristics
Lineage-specific antigens	Melanocyte antigens: • Tyrosinase (TYR) • Melan-A/MART-1 (MLANA) • gp100/Pmel17 (SILV)	Nonmutated, tissue-specific self proteins. Not restricted to malignant cells.
Tumor-specific altered gene products	HER-2/neu (ERBB2) p53 (TP53) Ras genes (KRAS2, HRAS, NRAS) Mucin 1 (MUC1) BCR-ABL fusion products Survivin (BIRC5) TERT CEA AFP	Examples include genes that are amplified, aberrantly expressed, or mutated and splice variants or gene fusion products. Associated with a wide variety of tumors. Mutated forms represent a type of neoantigen because the mutated region is not present in the germ line. KRAS2 is mutated in 30% to 40% of colorectal cancers, and p53 is mutated in up to 70% of all human cancers. Altered MUC1 glycosylation is seen in a variety of adenocarcinomas.
Cancer-testis (CT) antigens	MAGE-1 (MAGEA1) BAGE GAGE-1 (GAGE1) NY-ESO-1 (CTAG1)	Expressed in germ, trophoblast, and tumor cells. Represent a type of neoantigen because not normally expressed in somatic cells.
Immunoglobulin idiotypes	Multiple myeloma B-cell lymphoma	Unique, tumor-specific idiotypes generated by clonal rearrangements of immunoglobulin genes. Restricted to B-cell malignancies.
Viral antigens	HPV E6 and E7 proteins EBV (HHV4) LMP1 and LMP2 proteins	Foreign antigens expressed by oncogenic viruses. Associated with virus-induced tumors such as cervical cancer or EBV-associated lymphomas.

*A useful Web site with links to current cancer antigen databases may be found at http://www.cancerimmunity.org/statics/databases.htm (accessed March 13, 2010).

of less-than-expected tumor regression for both treatments, at frequencies that were statistically comparable.[141]

The second Phase III study compared intravenously administered, partially enriched blood DCs loaded with a prostatic acid phosphatase-GM-CSF fusion protein to placebo in prostate cancer patients.[79] There was no statistically significant difference in time to progression (the study's primary endpoint) between the two treatment arms. There was, however, improved overall survival on the DC arm, and a follow-up study designed to evaluate overall survival is now in progress.

Adoptive Cell Transfer

Principles

As an alternative to active vaccination, autologous antigen-specific T cells can be derived from tumor tissue or an apheresis mononuclear cell collection, propagated in large numbers ex vivo, and then infused back into the patient. Although still an experimental approach, this passive or "adoptive" cell transfer offers several potential advantages.[10,13] It permits the expansion under controlled conditions of very small numbers of autologous T cells having a desired specificity and avidity to levels that may not be obtainable by active vaccination. Autologous T cells can even be engineered in the laboratory to carry previously characterized antigen receptors of known high avidity. In addition, the patient's immune system can be manipulated before infusion to allow for optimal growth and persistence of the transferred cells in vivo. Overall, the technique can result in a much higher proportion of antigen-specific T cells in the patient's circulation than vaccination approaches, and to date it has been associated with more promising clinical results for the treatment of advanced cancer, although the treatment regimens can be associated with substantial toxicity.

Sources of Antigen-Specific Autologous T Cells

Autologous effector T cells of a desired specificity can be 1) amplified from memory T lymphocytes obtained from autologous peripheral blood or tissue samples, 2) primed ex vivo from naive autologous T lymphocytes or 3) engineered by transfecting autologous T lymphocytes with plasmids or transducing them with virus vectors encoding recombinant antigen receptors.

T Cells Primed in Vivo

To obtain T cells that recognize viral antigens, memory T cells from the blood of patients with a history of exposure to the virus can be expanded.[142,143] This is done by co-culturing the cells with autologous antigen-loaded APCs in the presence of IL-2, sometimes followed by plating the cells at limiting dilution in multi-well plates to obtain clones. For example, HIV gag-specific T-cell clones for adoptive immunotherapy have been obtained following this approach using PBMCs from HIV-infected patients.[144] Cells were first plated in plastic culture vessels to prepare plastic-adherent (monocyte) and nonadherent (lymphocyte) fractions. The adherent cells were infected with an HIV gag-encoding vaccinia virus and then co-cultured with the nonadherent lymphocytes for 1 week in the presence of IL-2. After repeat stimulation with more HIV gag vaccinia-infected adherent cells for another week, antigen-specific T-cell clones were obtained by plating the cells at limiting dilution in 96-well plates and culturing for 2 weeks in the presence of allogeneic irradiated accessory ("feeder") cells [PBMCs and Epstein-Barr virus (EBV)-transformed B cells], anti-CD3 monoclonal antibody, and IL-2. Wells were then screened for reactivity to HIV gag and positive wells further expanded in tissue culture flasks with more accessory cells, anti-CD3 antibody, and IL-2 for 10 days or more. These cells were then frozen for use as a cell bank and could be thawed and re-expanded in culture for 2 weeks when needed for infusion.

For cancer, early adoptive immunotherapy studies used lymphokine-activated killer (LAK) cells in combination with intravenous IL-2.[145] LAK cells are a mixed population of lymphocytes of no particular specificity generated by culturing autologous PBMCs ex vivo in the presence of IL-2. However, randomized studies in patients with metastatic melanoma did not show a clear benefit from the addition of LAK cells to high-dose intravenous IL-2, which alone produces some clinical benefit in a minority of patients, and LAK cells have since been abandoned in favor of tumor-infiltrating lymphocytes (TILs), which were found to be more potent.[146,147] One drawback of TILs is that they are often extremely difficult to isolate from tumors other than melanoma.[10]

To generate TILs, tumors are typically minced and individual pieces are placed in wells of multi-well plates to be cultured for 2 to 4 weeks in the presence of high concentrations (6000 U/mL) of IL-2.[148] Wells can be screened for cytokine secretion in response to autologous tumor cells or HLA haploidentical (usually HLA-A2+) tumor cell lines. Cultures exhibiting the highest cytokine secretion are then further expanded with IL-2 for another 2 to 4 weeks, by which time over 50 million cells are typically obtained. The cells can then be retested for tumor cell recognition before being rapidly expanded using irradiated allogeneic feeder cells, anti-CD3 antibody, and high concentrations of IL-2. This last step can result in a 1000-fold expansion of specific T cells within 2 weeks. Although the use of clones was initially described in these methods, bulk methods that do not rely on limiting dilution and that avoid prolonged culture may turn out to be more clinically effective.[10,149]

Antigen-specific T cells can also be expanded from memory T cells generated in vivo following vaccination with tumor antigens such as gp100 or human telomerase reverse transcriptase peptides.[150,151] The vaccine-primed T cells can be enriched in culture by stimulating autologous PBMCs with the vaccine peptide and IL-2 for up to 2 weeks,[150] or the T cells can be nonspecifically expanded using artificial APCs such as immunomagnetic beads coated with anti-CD3 and anti-CD28 monoclonal antibodies.[151] To generate clones, cells may be plated at limiting dilution (as described above) in the presence of anti-CD3 antibody, IL-2, and accessory cells (irradiated allogeneic PBMCs). After 2 weeks in culture, wells are screened for reactivity to the vaccine peptide (by measuring cytokine secretion or by staining for peptide-MHC tetramer) and positive wells expanded with irradiated accessory cells, anti-CD3 and IL-2. T-cell avidity can be assessed by measuring cytokine secretion in response to nanomolar amounts of peptide, with the clones that demonstrate high cytokine secretion selected for continued expansion and infusion.

Naive T Cells Primed ex Vivo

Although this can be difficult to accomplish reproducibly, CD8+ T cells specific to tumor antigens such as MART-1 and gp100, as well as CD4+ T cells specific to the tumor antigen NY-ESO-1, have been generated ex vivo from naive precursors by stimulating peripheral blood lymphocytes with autologous peptide-pulsed Mo-DCs.[152,153] A typical priming would involve up to three 1-week stimulations with peptide-pulsed DCs (or DCs for the first stimulation and monocytes for the subsequent stimulations[154]), followed by cloning by limiting dilution and expansion with irradiated allogeneic feeder cells (PBMCs and B-lymphoblast cell lines), anti-CD3, and IL-2. After infusion, the clones often do not persist in vivo very long—perhaps up to 3 weeks with the co-administration of low-dose IL-2—but can occasionally persist long term.[153] They have been shown to traffic to tumor sites and can be given in multiple infusions if needed.[152]

Engineered T Cells

Autologous T cells can also be engineered to express recombinant antigen receptors of a desired specificity by transfecting them with specific TCRα and β chain genes or with genes encoding artificial chimeric antigen receptors.[155,156] For example, TCRα and β chain genes recognizing an epitope of the MART-1 tumor antigen have been cloned using a TIL clone from a patient who achieved near complete regression of metastatic melanoma after treatment by adoptive cell transfer.[157] A retroviral vector was constructed that expressed both the α and β chain RNAs, and autologous T cells were transduced with the vector. Transduced T cells could be detected by their staining with a MART-1 peptide-MHC tetramer and by staining for a TCR variable region segment associated with the clone (Vβ12). About 40% of transduced cells expressed the recombinant TCR, and these could be expanded rapidly with IL-2, anti-CD3 antibody, and irradiated allogeneic accessory cells.

As an alternative to TCRs, chimeric antigen receptors (CARs) are recombinant artificial T-cell receptors that take advantage of monoclonal antibody single-chain variable fragments (scFv, single chains containing both light- and heavy-chain variable sequences) to bind a target antigen of interest. By encoding the scFv segment as a fusion protein with extracellular, transmembrane and intracellular signaling domains of T-cell signaling molecules such as CD28, CD3ζ, 41BB, or OX40, the CAR can function in many ways like a real TCR.[156,158-160] Potential advantages of CARs include their versatility (ie, specific receptors can be generated to a wide range of targets) plus their lack of HLA restriction (ie, CARs bind unprocessed antigens on the surface of tumor cells, much as an antibody would).[156] However, brief persistence of the CAR-transfected T cells in vivo is a common problem.[161]

As an example of this method, autologous T cells have been transfected with a CAR specific for CD20 to treat patients with B-cell lymphoma.[162] T cells from apheresis PBMCs were first nonspecifically expanded with anti-CD3 antibody and IL-2. On day 4, cells were electroporated with linearized plasmids encoding a CD20-specific scFvFc-CD3ζ CAR. G418 (a neomycin analogue) was added 3 days later to select for transfectants, which carry a neomycin resistance gene. Cells were selected for 8 days, then subjected to limiting dilution and expanded by culturing in the presence of anti-CD3 antibody, IL-2, irradiated accessory cells, and

G418.[163] After 2 to 3 weeks, wells were analyzed for the CD20-specific CAR by flow cytometry and positive wells expanded with anti-CD3, IL-2, and feeder cells over a course of 5 to 8 stimulations. Cells could be infused either fresh or cryopreserved in Plasma-lyte-A (Baxter Healthcare, Deerfield, IL) containing 5% human albumin and 10% DMSO. Longer in-vivo persistence was observed with T cells obtained from bulk cultures rather than by limiting dilution, and with administration of low-dose subcutaneous IL-2.[162]

Methods to Expand T Cells in Culture ex Vivo

Some of the methods to expand therapeutic T cells in culture ex vivo were touched upon above. Here are outlined the principles underlying these approaches and how they have evolved over time.

Expanding T Cells Using IL-2, Stimulatory Antibodies, and Accessory Cells

In early adoptive immunotherapy studies, therapeutic T cells were expanded in culture to large numbers by using high concentrations of IL-2.[146,164] Subsequently, stimulatory monoclonal antibodies to the CD3 complex (which is associated with the TCR and is involved in antigen stimulation) were added and, to a lesser extent, monoclonal antibodies to CD28 (a stimulatory receptor to the co-stimulatory molecules CD80 and CD86). It was found that these additions combined with the use of irradiated allogeneic leukocytes (accessory or "feeder" cells—typically PBMCs or a mixture of EBV-transformed B lymphocytes and PBMCs) could significantly enhance the degree of cell proliferation in the cultures.[165] This method is still widely used in adoptive immunotherapy trials for cancer.[166,167] For virus-specific T cells, the culture conditions can be simpler. For example, EBV-specific T cells can be expanded by repeated stimulation with antigen-loaded APCs (autologous EBV-infected B-cell lines) and IL-2, with no need for accessory cells or anti-CD3.[143]

Antibody-Conjugated Beads as a Replacement for Accessory Cells

To simplify ex-vivo T-cell expansion, magnetic beads coated with stimulatory antibodies to CD3 and CD28 were designed to take the place of soluble anti-CD3 and irradiated accessory cells. By culturing T cells with anti-CD3/CD28 beads in the presence of low-to-moderate concentrations of IL-2, up to a billion-fold expansion of therapeutic T cells can be achieved in less than 3 weeks without the need for accessory cells.[168-170] Before infusion of the cells, the beads are removed using a magnetic separator.

Expanding T Cells Using Artificial Antigen-Presenting Cells in Place of Anti-CD3/CD28 Beads

As a more complex but potentially more potent method to expand therapeutic T cells, allogeneic hematopoietic cell lines such as K562 cells can be engineered into "artificial APCs" by transducing them with retroviral vectors encoding a specific MHC I (typically HLA-A2) and co-stimulatory molecules such as CD80, CD86, and 4-1BBL.[169] In addition, by transducing the cell lines with the high-affinity Fc receptor (CD64), anti-CD3 and anti-CD28 antibodies may be attached to the cell surface, providing the APCs with additional T-cell stimulatory capacity.[169]

Culture Methods to Obtain Specific Clinically Beneficial T-Cell Subtypes

Methods to Obtain Less Differentiated Memory CD8+ T Cells

One major problem with adoptive transfer is that the infused T cells often persist in vivo for only short periods of time, typically 3 weeks or less. It has become apparent that the more differentiated the T cells, the shorter their survival in vivo.[171] For example, fully differentiated effector T cells do not persist as long as less differentiated, effector memory T cells (T_{EM}), and T_{EM} do not persist as long as even less differen-

tiated, central memory T cells (T_{CM}).[172-175] Methods have now been developed in experimental animal models to sort and then expand T_{CM} for adoptive cell transfer. For example, CD8+ T cells derived from macaques with evidence of prior cytomegalovirus (CMV) infection were sorted into CD62L+ (T_{CM}) and CD62L− (T_{EM}) populations using fluorescence-activated cell sorting (FACS).[176] The two populations were cultured separately for 1 week with CMV peptide-pulsed autologous monocytes in the presence of IL-2 and plated at limiting dilution with irradiated, autologous, CMV peptide-pulsed PBMCs; irradiated allogeneic accessory cells; and IL-2. After 2 weeks, CMV-reactive clones were identified and expanded with anti-CD3 and anti-CD28, irradiated accessory cells, and IL-2. When infused into macaques, the cells of T_{CM} origin persisted much longer in vivo than those derived from T_{EM}, and they established T-cell memory in the host.

Manipulation of CD8+ T cells with cytokines or drugs during antigen stimulation—eg, using IL-21 in place of IL-2[177]—can also favor T-cell populations that have enhanced in-vivo persistence and antitumor activity. In a recent study, pharmacologic manipulation of CD8+ T cells during antigen stimulation to mimic *wnt* signaling—which limits T-cell proliferation and terminal differentiation to effectors—generated $CD62^{hi}$, $CD44^{lo}$ cells that have characteristics of so-called T memory stem cells (T_{SCM}). These T_{SCM} demonstrated enhanced in-vivo persistence, recall responses, and antitumor activity in a mouse melanoma model even superior to T_{CM}.[178]

Use of Virus-Specific CD8+ T Cells as Vehicles for CARs

Another way to enhance the in-vivo persistence and survival of infused therapeutic T cells is to transduce virus-specific memory T cells (which naturally persist well in vivo) with CARs. For example, EBV-specific T cells transduced with a CAR for a neuroblastoma antigen, the diasialoganglioside GD2, remain in circulation longer than anti-CD3-activated T cells that express the same receptor but are not EBV-specific. The

EBV- and GD2-specific T cells showed a 50% tumor response rate in a clinical trial in patients with neuroblastoma.[179]

Use of CD4+ T-Cell Subtypes

The use of CD4+ T cells for adoptive transfer has been less well studied but has a number of potential advantages.[180] In particular, CD8+ T cells can fail to provide long-lasting protection and memory in the absence of CD4+ help.[60] In a recent study of nine patients with metastatic melanoma, an autologous CD4+ T-cell clone specific to the tumor antigen NY-ESO-1 led to a complete regression in one patient and persisted for over 2 years.[153,161] This response was accomplished without the need for administration of IL-2 or lymphodepletion of the host, which are commonly required for adoptive cell transfer using CD8+ T cells.

CD4+ T cells can be divided into several subtypes with distinctly different functions.[181] Although still very experimental, differentiation of therapeutic CD4+ T cells can be skewed into any one of these directions by manipulating the culture conditions during antigen stimulation. For example, adding IL-12 to cultures during antigen stimulation can promote differentiation into T helper 1 (Th1) cells, which are important in antitumor and antiviral immunity.[182] Th2 cells, which support humoral immune responses, can be induced by culturing with IL-4. Recent evidence in an animal model suggests that a third CD4+ T-cell subtype, Th17 cells, may be superior to Th1 or Th2 cells for antitumor immunity.[183] Th17 cells can be induced by culturing antigen-stimulated CD4+ T cells in the presence of a mixture of cytokines that includes TGFβ and IL-6.[169,183]

Treg, a type of CD4+ T cell that has inhibitory properties, can potentially be used to treat autoimmune diseases or to maintain tolerance to organ transplants.[184,185] Thus far, adoptive cell transfer using Treg has been explored primarily for the prevention of graft-vs-host disease after allogeneic hematopoietic stem cell transplantation. Experiments using *autologous* Treg for adoptive cell transfer have been limited to animal models or to preclinical studies

using umbilical cord blood for the treatment of type 1 diabetes.[185-187] Cultures enriched in Treg may be obtained by cell sorting using magnetic beads or FACS, for example by depleting CD8+, CD14+, and CD19+ cells, followed by positive selection for $CD25^{hi}$ cells using subsaturating amounts of anti-CD25.[185] These cells are then expanded with either accessory cells or anti-CD3/CD28 beads in the presence of IL-2 and rapamycin. Rapamycin allows the preferential expansion of Treg by inhibiting the mammalian target of the rapamycin (mTOR) signaling pathway, which is important for the differentiation of effector (Th1, Th2, or Th17) CD4+ T cells.[188] Unlike effector CD4+ T cells, Treg need CD28 co-stimulation for their ex-vivo expansion and function; hence, expansion using anti-CD3 without anti-CD28 is not sufficient.[189]

Results of Clinical Trials

Although still considered an experimental therapy, adoptive cell transfer using autologous antigen-specific T cells has shown promise in clinical trials, primarily for the treatment of metastatic malignant melanoma and EBV-associated malignancies.[161,169]

Adoptive Transfer of Autologous T cells to Treat or Prevent Viral Infections and Virus-Induced Malignancies

For Opportunistic Viral Infections and Virus-Induced Malignancy in the Transplant Setting. Adoptive cell transfer to treat or prevent viral infections and virus-induced malignancies has most commonly been explored in the allogeneic hematopoietic stem cell transplant (HSCT) setting, in which adoptive T-cell infusions have met with some success in subjects having opportunistic CMV infections or EBV-associated malignancies.[10,171] Although a number of reports describe use of adoptively transferred autologous T cells to treat such conditions in patients who have received solid organ transplants, in-vivo persistence and clinical effectiveness tend to be more limited than has been observed in the allogeneic HSCT setting.[190,191] For EBV-associated malignancies following solid organ transplants, a more promising approach may be the use of partially HLA-matched cell banks derived from unrelated donors.[171,192]

For Virus-Induced Malignancy in Immunocompetent Individuals. Adoptive transfer of autologous EBV-specific T cells has been used to treat a number of EBV-associated malignancies, notably EBV+ forms of Hodgkin lymphoma, non-Hodgkin lymphoma and nasopharyngeal carcinoma.[171] For the treatment of EBV+ Hodgkin lymphoma, infused autologous EBV-specific CD8+ T cells can persist in vivo for up to 12 months and appear to have some clinical activity in a majority of patients. Complete remissions were reported in 2 of 14 patients in one study, with a partial response reported for one patient.[193] More promising results using improved T-cell stimulation methods have been recently reported, both for the treatment of EBV+ Hodgkin lymphoma and EBV+ non-Hodgkin lymphoma.[194] Significant anti-tumor activity has also been observed following the infusion of autologous EBV-specific CD8+ T cells for the treatment of nasopharyngeal carcinoma.[143,195,196]

For Chronic Persistent Viral Infections in Immunocompetent Hosts. Studies in animal models and in humans have suggested the feasibility of using adoptively transferred autologous CD8+ or CD4+ T cells to treat chronic persistent viral infections such as HIV and HCV. However, adoptive cell therapy in this setting has thus far not met with any clinical success.[171] Most of the work along these lines in humans has been for the treatment of chronic HIV infection.[142,144,168,197] These have been Phase I studies designed to test safety and feasibility. However, they have not shown any long-term clinical benefit. Potential pitfalls with this approach include short-term persistence of infused CD4+ T cells as a result of destruction by the HIV virus. Furthermore, CD8+ T cells in these patients often exhibit loss of function associated with up-regulation of inhibitory molecules such as PD-1.[171] One strategy to overcome HIV-mediated destruction of CD4+ T cells infused to treat HIV infection is to use engineered autologous CD4+ T cells that lack the HIV co-receptor CCR5.[198]

Adoptive Transfer of Autologous T Cells for the Treatment of Cancer

Significant advances have been made in the past 10 years in the use of adoptively transferred T cells to treat cancer. This is currently the most effective treatment for metastatic melanoma, with up to 70% objective response rates observed.[10,158,171] However, there are still a number of serious drawbacks to the approach. One is the relatively short persistence of the adoptively transferred cells in vivo in patients who do not undergo nonmyeloablative lymphodepleting conditioning regimens that entail substantial toxicity, including myelosuppression, autoimmunity, and a vascular leak syndrome associated with high-dose IL-2.[199] Even with conditioning regimens, the majority of clinical responses are partial responses that tend to be short lived. Still, the results are promising, and the toxicities can be managed by experienced personnel. Below are outlined a few key examples from the recent literature describing results of clinical trials using adoptively transferred T cells prepared by a variety of methods.

Adoptive Transfer of Expanded Tumor-Infiltrating Lymphocytes. To date, naturally-occurring (in-vivo-primed) TILs have been reliably expanded only from patients with malignant melanoma.[200] Before the advent of patient conditioning regimens, the longevity of these cells after infusion was typically quite short, usually no longer than 2 weeks.[10,150,171] However the use of nonmyeloablative lymphodepletion combined with the administration of high-dose IL-2 has substantially improved in-vivo persistence of the transferred cells and has improved clinical outcomes.[10,158]

Animal models of adoptive T-cell transfer initially indicated that nonmyeloablative lymphodepletion of the host through the use of chemotherapy, either with or without total body irradiation (TBI), significantly improves the in-vivo persistence and antitumor efficacy of the therapeutic cells. The beneficial effect of nonmyeloablative lymphodepletion before infusion has now been clearly established in human trials as well.[10,166,169,201] Objective responses have been observed in 50% to 70% of patients with metastatic melanoma who had been refractory to standard therapies.[201] Higher response rates are associated with 12 Gy of TBI used in addition to nonmyeloablative chemotherapy such as cyclophosphamide and fludarabine. Many of these responses have been durable. As might be expected, the treatment regimen is associated with significant hematologic toxicities, especially for patients receiving TBI. However, the marrow typically recovers within 2 to 3 weeks. To support patients receiving TBI, an infusion of autologous CD34+ hematopoietic progenitor cells is given 1 to 2 days following the TIL infusion, and these patients typically need to be supported by red cell and platelet transfusions as well.[201]

The co-administration of high dose IL-2 (720,000 U/kg intravenously every 8 hours to tolerance, typically up to 15 doses) at the time of TIL infusion further improves persistence of the adoptively transferred T cells.[201] The use of high-dose IL-2 is associated with fairly severe toxicities, in particular a vascular leak syndrome associated with fever, chills, hypotension, tachycardia, oliguria, edema, and pulmonary congestion. Although such toxicities are commonly encountered, the infusion of high-dose IL-2 can be safe if patients are monitored by experienced personnel.[202] It appears that low-dose IL-2, although less toxic, is not as effective. In a study that did not include a lymphodepletion step, clinical responses (which were minor) were seen only in patients receiving high-dose IL-2, as opposed to those receiving low-dose (125,000 U/kg/day subcutaneously for 12 days) or no IL-2.[150] It is possible that better-tolerated approaches, such as the use of lymphodepleting monoclonal antibodies or the administration of homeostatic cytokines such as IL-7 and IL-15, can eventually obviate the need for such potentially toxic interventions.[171,196]

Use of ex-Vivo-Primed T-Cell Clones. As in the early studies using TILs, treatment of patients with ex-vivo-primed T-cell clones specific to tumor antigens has in general failed to provide complete clinical responses or long-term persistence of the infused cells.[171] For example, in a study using CD8+ T-cell clones specific to the tumor antigens Melan-1 or gp100 to treat 10 patients with metastatic melanoma, only two partial responses and no complete responses were observed.[152] Infused T cells were detectable in the circulation for a median of only 1 week when no exogenous cytokines were given, although preferential migration to tumor sites was observed. In-vivo persistence was improved to a median of 2 to 3 weeks with co-administration of low-dose IL-2.

It is possible that one problem with the use of CD8+ T-cell clones is that they are composed mostly of terminally differentiated effector T cells that characteristically do not persist well in vivo.[149] To determine if tumor-antigen-specific CD4+ T-cell clones fare better, clones of such cells specific for the tumor antigen NY-ESO-1 were tested in nine patients with metastatic melanoma in a recent study.[153] Complete regression of metastatic disease involving the lung and both hilar and inguinal lymph nodes was observed in one patient 2 months after a single infusion of 5 billion T cells.[153,161] The cells, which were primed ex vivo using NY-ESO-1 peptide-pulsed DCs and then expanded with peptide-pulsed monocytes,[154] persisted in the circulation for over 12 weeks without administration of any exogenous IL-2. The patient was reported to be disease-free at last follow-up, 2 years after receiving the infusion. It should be noted, however, that this was the only complete response noted among the nine patients, and it remains to be established whether the use of CD8+ or CD4+ T-cell clones offers significant advantages over the use of bulk populations of TILs.[161]

Adoptive Immunotherapy Using Engineered T Cells. A major problem with the use of TILs or ex-vivo-primed T-cell clones is that these cells are typically reliably derived only from patients with melanoma.[161,171] As an alternative strategy, autologous peripheral blood T cells can be engineered to carry a recombinant TCR or CAR of known high avidity. Therapies using engineered T cells are only just beginning to be tested in humans. In one study, a high-avidity TCR specific to the tumor antigen MART-1 was transfected into autologous CD8+ T cells, which were expanded ex vivo and infused in conjunction with host chemotherapy-based lymphodepletion and high-dose IL-2.[157] Three initial patients whose cells underwent a prolonged ex-vivo expansion with IL-2 but without anti-CD3 showed poor persistence of the adoptively transferred cells. However, T cells derived from a rapid expansion protocol that included irradiated accessory cells and anti-CD3 showed good persistence (>9% remaining after 4 weeks), and two of the patients demonstrated objective partial tumor regressions with durations of 20 and 21 months, respectively.

The use of T cells transduced with CARs for cancer immunotherapy is still largely confined to in-vitro studies or animal models.[156] However, somewhat promising clinical results have been reported for the treatment of non-Hodgkin lymphoma using autologous T cells transfected with a CAR that recognizes the B-cell antigen CD20, although no complete responses were reported.[162]

Summary

The use of autologous cellular immunotherapies, many of which are derived from apheresis products to treat cancer, chronic or opportunistic viral infections, and virus-associated malignancies is still experimental. None of these therapies has yet been approved by the FDA or gained wide clinical acceptance. But there have been a number of promising clinical trials of these therapies, with particularly impressive results observed in cases of adoptive T-cell transfer. Active immunization using DCs or mixed APCs has yet to show an advantage over more conventional vaccine approaches, although for at least one formulation there have been favorable results in a Phase III clinical trial.[79] For adoptive T-cell therapy, reproducible, long-term objective responses have been observed in a minority of subjects, but only in patients with malignant melanoma or virus-induced lymphomas.[10,169,171] For melanoma, objective responses (albeit mostly partial and short term) have now been observed in up to 70% of patients with refractory metastatic disease when adoptive infusion is combined with prior host lymphodepletion and the administration of high-dose IL-2. Building on this significant accomplishment, it may be possible to design more effective and less toxic regimens, particularly in light of recent insights from animal and preclinical models studying the mechanisms of T-cell survival in vivo.

References

1. Palm NW, Medzhitov R. Pattern recognition receptors and control of adaptive immunity. Immunol Rev 2009;227:221-33.
2. Smyth MJ, Dunn GP, Schreiber RD. Cancer immunosurveillance and immunoediting: The roles of immunity in suppressing tumor development and shaping tumor immunogenicity. Adv Immunol 2006;90:1-50.
3. Pages F, Berger A, Camus M, et al. Effector memory T cells, early metastasis, and survival in colorectal cancer. N Engl J Med 2005;353:2654-66.
4. Cesco-Gaspere M, Morris E, Stauss HJ. Immunomodulation in the treatment of haematological malignancies. Clin Exp Med 2009;9:81-92.
5. Feng X, Hui KM, Younes HM, Brickner AG. Targeting minor histocompatibility antigens in graft versus tumor or graft versus leukemia responses. Trends Immunol 2008;29:624-32.
6. Kolb HJ. Graft-versus-leukemia effects of transplantation and donor lymphocytes. Blood 2008;112:4371-83.
7. Dale DC, Price TH. Granulocyte transfusion therapy: A new era? Curr Opin Hematol 2009;16:1-2.
8. Price TH. Granulocyte transfusion therapy. J Clin Apher 2006;21:65-71.
9. Gilboa E. DC-based cancer vaccines. J Clin Invest 2007;117:1195-203.
10. Rosenberg SA, Restifo NP, Yang JC, et al. Adoptive cell transfer: A clinical path to effective cancer immunotherapy. Nat Rev Cancer 2008;8:299-308.
11. Rosenberg SA. Overcoming obstacles to the effective immunotherapy of human cancer. Proc Natl Acad Sci U S A 2008;105:12643-4.

12. Finn OJ. Cancer immunology. N Engl J Med 2008;358:2704-15.

13. Disis ML, Bernhard H, Jaffee EM. Use of tumour-responsive T cells as cancer treatment. Lancet 2009;373:673-83.

14. Vyas JM, Van der Veen AG, Ploegh HL. The known unknowns of antigen processing and presentation. Nat Rev Immunol 2008;8:607-18.

15. Trombetta ES, Mellman I. Cell biology of antigen processing in vitro and in vivo. Annu Rev Immunol 2005;23:975-1028.

16. Savina A, Amigorena S. Phagocytosis and antigen presentation in dendritic cells. Immunol Rev 2007;219:143-56.

17. Steinman RM. Dendritic cells: Understanding immunogenicity. Eur J Immunol 2007;37 (Suppl 1):S53-60.

18. Steinman RM, Bancherau J. Taking dendritic cells into medicine. Nature 2007;449:419-26.

19. Hugues S, Boissonnas A, Amigorena S, Fetler L. The dynamics of dendritic cell-T cell interactions in priming and tolerance. Curr Opin Immunol 2006;18:491-5.

20. Lutz MB, Kurts C. Induction of peripheral CD4+ T-cell tolerance and CD8+ T-cell cross-tolerance by dendritic cells. Eur J Immunol 2009;39:2325-30.

21. Belkaid Y, Oldenhove G. Tuning microenvironments: Induction of regulatory T cells by dendritic cells. Immunity 2008;29:362-71.

22. Wu L, Liu YJ. Development of dendritic-cell lineages. Immunity 2007;26:741-50.

23. Shortman K, Naik SH. Steady-state and inflammatory dendritic-cell development. Nat Rev Immunol 2007;7:19-30.

24. Gilliet M, Cao W, Liu YJ. Plasmacytoid dendritic cells: Sensing nucleic acids in viral infection and autoimmune diseases. Nat Rev Immunol 2008;8:594-606.

25. Villadangos JA, Young L. Antigen-presentation properties of plasmacytoid dendritic cells. Immunity 2008;29:352-61.

26. Merad M, Ginhoux F, Collin M. Origin, homeostasis and function of Langerhans cells and other langerin-expressing dendritic cells. Nat Rev Immunol 2008;8:935-47.

27. Ueno H, Klechevsky E, Morita R, et al. Dendritic cell subsets in health and disease. Immunol Rev 2007;219:118-42.

28. Burgdorf S, Kurts C. Endocytosis mechanisms and the cell biology of antigen presentation. Curr Opin Immunol 2008;20:89-95.

29. Auffray C, Sieweke MH, Geissmann F. Blood monocytes: Development, heterogeneity, and relationship with dendritic cells. Annu Rev Immunol 2009;27:669-92.

30. Areschoug T, Gordon S. Scavenger receptors: Role in innate immunity and microbial pathogenesis. Cell Microbiol 2009;11:1160-9.

31. Nimmerjahn F, Ravetch JV. Fcgamma receptors as regulators of immune responses. Nat Rev Immunol 2008;8:34-47.

32. van Kooyk Y, Rabinovich GA. Protein-glycan interactions in the control of innate and adaptive immune responses. Nat Immunol 2008;9:593-601.

33. Raghavan M, Del Cid N, Rizvi SM, Peters LR. MHC class I assembly: Out and about. Trends Immunol 2008;29:436-43.

34. Lin ML, Zhan Y, Villadangos JA, Lew AM. The cell biology of cross-presentation and the role of dendritic cell subsets. Immunol Cell Biol 2008;86:353-62.

35. Sancho D, Joffre OP, Keller AM, et al. Identification of a dendritic cell receptor that couples sensing of necrosis to immunity. Nature 2009;458:899-903.

36. Silk JD, Salio M, Brown J, et al. Structural and functional aspects of lipid binding by CD1 molecules. Ann Rev Cell Dev Biol 2008;24:369-95.

37. De Libero G, Mori L. How T cells get grip on lipid antigens. Curr Opin Immunol 2008;20:96-104.

38. Reis e Sousa C. Dendritic cells in a mature age. Nat Rev Immunol 2006;6:476-83.

39. Joffre O, Nolte MA, Sporri R, Reis e Sousa C. Inflammatory signals in dendritic cell activation and the induction of adaptive immunity. Immunol Rev 2009;227:234-47.

40. Kono H, Rock KL. How dying cells alert the immune system to danger. Nat Rev Immunol 2008;8:279-89.

41. Medzhitov R. Recognition of microorganisms and activation of the immune response. Nature 2007;449:819-26.

42. Alvarez D, Vollmann EH, von Andrian UH. Mechanisms and consequences of dendritic cell migration. Immunity 2008;29:325-42.

43. Randolph GJ, Ochando J, Partida-Sanchez S. Migration of dendritic cell subsets and their precursors. Annu Rev Immunol 2008;26:293-316.

44. Bancherau J, Briere F, Caux C, et al. Immunobiology of dendritic cells. Annu Rev Immunol 2000;18:767-811.

45. Croft M. The role of TNF superfamily members in T-cell function and diseases. Nat Rev Immunol 2009;9:271-85.

46. Macagno A, Napolitani G, Lanzavecchia A, Sallusto F. Duration, combination and timing: The signal integration model of dendritic cell activation. Trends Immunol 2007;28:227-33.

47. Breloer M, Fleischer B. CD83 regulates lymphocyte maturation, activation and homeostasis. Trends Immunol 2008;29:186-94.

48. Kloetzel PM, Ossendorp F. Proteasome and peptidase function in MHC-class-I-mediated antigen presentation. Curr Opin Immunol 2004;16:76-81.

49. Borissenko L, Groll M. Diversity of proteasomal missions: Fine tuning of the immune response. Biol Chem 2007;388:947-55.

50. Datta SK, Raz E. Induction of antigen cross-presentation by Toll-like receptors. Springer Semin Immunopathol 2005;26:247-55.

51. Schulz O, Diebold SS, Chen M, et al. Toll-like receptor 3 promotes cross-priming to virus-infected cells. Nature 2005;433:887-92.

52. Lapenta C, Santini SM, Spada M, et al. IFN-alpha-conditioned dendritic cells are highly efficient in inducing cross-priming CD8(+) T cells against exogenous viral antigens. Eur J Immunol 2006.

53. Huang AY, Qi H, Germain RN. Illuminating the landscape of in vivo immunity: Insights from dynamic in situ imaging of secondary lymphoid tissues. Immunity 2004;21:331-9.

54. Janeway C Jr, Travers P, Walport M, Shlomchik M. Immunobiology 5: The immune system in health and disease. 5th ed. New York: Garland Publishing, 2001.

55. Klebanoff CA, Gattinoni L, Restifo NP. CD8+ T-cell memory in tumor immunology and immunotherapy. Immunol Rev 2006;211:214-24.

56. Surh CD, Sprent J. Homeostasis of naive and memory T cells. Immunity 2008;29:848-62.

57. Rochman Y, Spolski R, Leonard WJ. New insights into the regulation of T cells by gamma(c) family cytokines. Nat Rev Immunol 2009;9:480-90.

58. van Leeuwen EM, Sprent J, Surh CD. Generation and maintenance of memory CD4(+) T cells. Curr Opin Immunol 2009;21:167-72.

59. Hernandez MG, Shen L, Rock KL. CD40 on APCs is needed for optimal programming, maintenance, and recall of CD8+ T cell memory even in the absence of CD4+ T cell help. J Immunol 2008;180:4382-90.

60. Bevan MJ. Helping the CD8(+) T-cell response. Nat Rev Immunol 2004;4:595-602.

61. Lesterhuis WJ, Aarntzen EH, De Vries IJ, et al. Dendritic cell vaccines in melanoma: From promise to proof? Crit Rev Oncol Hematol 2008;66:118-34.

62. Melief CJ. Cancer immunotherapy by dendritic cells. Immunity 2008;29:372-83.

63. Campbell JD, Piechaczek C, Winkels G, et al. Isolation and generation of clinical-grade dendritic cells using the CliniMACS system. Methods Mol Med 2005;109:55-70.

64. Thurner B, Roder C, Dieckmann D, et al. Generation of large numbers of fully mature and stable dendritic cells from leukapheresis products for clinical application. J Immunol Methods 1999;223:1-15.

65. Bender A, Sapp M, Schuler G, et al. Improved methods for the generation of dendritic cells from nonproliferating progenitors in human blood. J Immunol Methods 1996;196:121-35.

66. Dauer M, Schad K, Herten J, et al. FastDC derived from human monocytes within 48 h effectively prime tumor antigen-specific cytotoxic T cells. J Immunol Methods 2005;302: 145-55.

67. Salcedo M, Bercovici N, Taylor R, et al. Vaccination of melanoma patients using dendritic cells loaded with an allogeneic tumor cell lysate. Cancer Immunol Immunother 2006; 55:819-29.

68. Berger TG, Strasser E, Smith R, et al. Efficient elutriation of monocytes within a closed system (Elutra) for clinical-scale generation of dendritic cells. J Immunol Methods 2005; 298:61-72.

69. Wong EC, Lee SM, Hines K, et al. Development of a closed-system process for clinical-scale generation of DCs: Evaluation of two monocyte-enrichment methods and two culture containers. Cytotherapy 2002;4:65-76.

70. Adamson L, Palma M, Choudhury A, et al. Generation of a dendritic cell-based vaccine in chronic lymphocytic leukaemia using CliniMACS platform for large-scale production. Scand J Immunol 2009;69:529-36.

71. Caux C, Massacrier C, Dezutter-Dambuyant C, et al. Human dendritic Langerhans cells generated in vitro from CD34+ progenitors can prime naive CD4+ T cells and process soluble antigen. J Immunol 1995;155:5427-35.

72. Caux C, Dezutter-Dambuyant C, Schmitt D, Banchereau J. GM-CSF and TNF-alpha cooper-

ate in the generation of dendritic Langerhans cells. Nature 1992;360:258-61.

73. Banchereau J, Palucka AK, Dhodapkar M, et al. Immune and clinical responses in patients with metastatic melanoma to CD34(+) progenitor-derived dendritic cell vaccine. Cancer Res 2001;61:6451-8.

74. Yuan J, Kendle R, Ireland J, et al. Scalable expansion of potent genetically modified human Langerhans cells in a closed system for clinical applications. J Immunother 2007;30:634-43.

75. Heinz LX, Platzer B, Reisner PM, et al. Differential involvement of PU.1 and Id2 downstream of TGF-beta1 during Langerhans-cell commitment. Blood 2006;107:1445-53.

76. Hsu FJ, Benike C, Fagnoni F, et al. Vaccination of patients with B-cell lymphoma using autologous antigen-pulsed dendritic cells. Nat Med 1996;2:52-8.

77. Fong L, Hou Y, Rivas A, et al. Altered peptide ligand vaccination with Flt3 ligand expanded dendritic cells for tumor immunotherapy. Proc Natl Acad Sci U S A 2001;98:8809-14.

78. Small EJ, Fratesi P, Reese DM, et al. Immunotherapy of hormone-refractory prostate cancer with antigen-loaded dendritic cells. J Clin Oncol 2000;18:3894-903.

79. Small EJ, Schellhammer PF, Higano CS, et al. Placebo-controlled Phase III trial of immunologic therapy with sipuleucel-T (APC8015) in patients with metastatic, asymptomatic hormone refractory prostate cancer. J Clin Oncol 2006;24:3089-94.

80. Higano CS, Schellhammer PF, Small EJ, et al. Integrated data from 2 randomized, double-blind, placebo-controlled, Phase 3 trials of active cellular immunotherapy with sipuleucel-T in advanced prostate cancer. Cancer 2009;115:3670-9.

81. Romani N, Reider D, Heuer M, et al. Generation of mature dendritic cells from human blood. An improved method with special regard to clinical applicability. J Immunol Methods 1996;196:137-51.

82. Jonuleit H, Kuhn U, Muller G, et al. Pro-inflammatory cytokines and prostaglandins induce maturation of potent immunostimulatory dendritic cells under fetal calf serum-free conditions. Eur J Immunol 1997;27:3135-42.

83. Jonuleit H, Giesecke-Tuettenberg A, Tuting T, et al. A comparison of two types of dendritic cell as adjuvants for the induction of melanoma-specific T-cell responses in humans following intranodal injection. Int J Cancer 2001;93:243-51.

84. de Vries IJ, Lesterhuis WJ, Scharenborg NM, et al. Maturation of dendritic cells is a prerequisite for inducing immune responses in advanced melanoma patients. Clin Cancer Res 2003;9:5091-100.

85. Dhodapkar MV, Steinman RM, Krasovsky J, et al. Antigen-specific inhibition of effector T cell function in humans after injection of immature dendritic cells. J Exp Med 2001;193:233-8.

86. Steinman RM, Hawiger D, Nussenzweig MC. Tolerogenic dendritic cells. Annu Rev Immunol 2003;21:685-711.

87. Kalinski P, Vieira PL, Schuitemaker JH, et al. Prostaglandin E(2) is a selective inducer of interleukin-12 p40 (IL-12p40) production and an inhibitor of bioactive IL-12p70 heterodimer. Blood 2001;97:3466-9.

88. Lee AW, Truong T, Bickham K, et al. A clinical grade cocktail of cytokines and PGE(2) results in uniform maturation of human monocyte-derived dendritic cells: Implications for immunotherapy. Vaccine 2002;20(Suppl 4):A8-A22.

89. Scandella E, Men Y, Gillessen S, et al. Prostaglandin E2 is a key factor for CCR7 surface expression and migration of monocyte-derived dendritic cells. Blood 2002;100:1354-61.

90. Schuler-Thurner B, Schultz ES, Berger TG, et al. Rapid induction of tumor-specific type 1 T helper cells in metastatic melanoma patients by vaccination with mature, cryopreserved, peptide-loaded monocyte-derived dendritic cells. J Exp Med 2002;195:1279-88.

91. Boon T, Old LJ. Cancer tumor antigens. Curr Opin Immunol 1997;9:681-3.

92. Stevanovic S. Identification of tumour-associated T-cell epitopes for vaccine development. Nat Rev Cancer 2002;2:514-20.

93. Gotch F, Rothbard J, Howland K, et al. Cytotoxic T lymphocytes recognize a fragment of influenza virus matrix protein in association with HLA-A2. Nature 1987;326:881-2.

94. Berzofsky JA, Ahlers JD, Belyakov IM. Strategies for designing and optimizing new generation vaccines. Nat Rev Immunol 2001;1:209-19.

95. Alexander-Miller MA, Leggatt GR, Berzofsky JA. Selective expansion of high- or low-avidity cytotoxic T lymphocytes and efficacy for adoptive immunotherapy. Proc Natl Acad Sci U S A 1996;93:4102-7.

96. Timmerman JM, Czerwinski DK, Davis TA, et al. Idiotype-pulsed dendritic cell vaccination

for B-cell lymphoma: Clinical and immune responses in 35 patients. Blood 2002;99: 1517-26.

97. Kim DT, Mitchell DJ, Brockstedt DG, et al. Introduction of soluble proteins into the MHC class I pathway by conjugation to an HIV tat peptide. J Immunol 1997;159:1666-8.

98. Fong L, Brockstedt D, Benike C, et al. Dendritic cell-based xenoantigen vaccination for prostate cancer immunotherapy. J Immunol 2001;167: 7150-6.

99. Tacken PJ, de Vries IJ, Torensma R, Figdor CG. Dendritic-cell immunotherapy: From ex vivo loading to in vivo targeting. Nat Rev Immunol 2007;7:790-802.

100. Palucka AK, Ueno H, Connolly J, et al. Dendritic cells loaded with killed allogeneic melanoma cells can induce objective clinical responses and MART-1 specific CD8+ T-cell immunity. J Immunother 2006;29:545-57.

101. O'Rourke MG, Johnson MK, Lanagan CM, et al. Dendritic cell immunotherapy for stage IV melanoma. Melanoma Res 2007;17:316-22.

102. Redman BG, Chang AE, Whitfield J, et al. Phase Ib trial assessing autologous, tumor-pulsed dendritic cells as a vaccine administered with or without IL-2 in patients with metastatic melanoma. J Immunother 2008;31:591-8.

103. Binder RJ, Srivastava PK. Peptides chaperoned by heat-shock proteins are a necessary and sufficient source of antigen in the cross-priming of CD8+ T cells. Nat Immunol 2005;6:593-9.

104. Zeng Y, Graner MW, Katsanis E. Chaperone-rich cell lysates, immune activation and tumor vaccination. Cancer Immunol Immunother 2006;55:329-38.

105. Lu W, Arraes LC, Ferreira WT, Andrieu JM. Therapeutic dendritic-cell vaccine for chronic HIV-1 infection. Nat Med 2004;10:1359-65.

106. Butterfield LH, Comin-Anduix B, Vujanovic L, et al. Adenovirus MART-1-engineered autologous dendritic cell vaccine for metastatic melanoma. J Immunother 2008;31:294-309.

107. Gandhi RT, O'Neill D, Bosch RJ, et al. A randomized therapeutic vaccine trial of canarypox-HIV-pulsed dendritic cells vs canarypox-HIV alone in HIV-1-infected patients on antiretroviral therapy. Vaccine 2009;27:6088-94.

108. Skoberne M, Yewdall A, Bahjat KS, et al. KBMA Listeria monocytogenes is an effective vector for DC-mediated induction of antitumor immunity. J Clin Invest 2008;118:3990-4001.

109. Liao X, Li Y, Bonini C, et al. Transfection of RNA encoding tumor antigens following matu-ration of dendritic cells leads to prolonged presentation of antigen and the generation of high-affinity tumor-reactive cytotoxic T lymphocytes. Mol Ther 2004;9:757-64.

110. Schaft N, Dorrie J, Thumann P, et al. Generation of an optimized polyvalent monocyte-derived dendritic cell vaccine by transfecting defined RNAs after rather than before maturation. J Immunol 2005;174:3087-97.

111. Su Z, Vieweg J, Weizer AZ, et al. Enhanced induction of telomerase-specific CD4(+) T cells using dendritic cells transfected with RNA encoding a chimeric gene product. Cancer Res 2002;62:5041-8.

112. Thumann P, Moc I, Humrich J, et al. Antigen loading of dendritic cells with whole tumor cell preparations. J Immunol Methods 2003;277: 1-16.

113. Mullins DW, Sheasley SL, Ream RM, et al. Route of immunization with peptide-pulsed dendritic cells controls the distribution of memory and effector T cells in lymphoid tissues and determines the pattern of regional tumor control. J Exp Med 2003;198:1023-34.

114. Dhodapkar MV, Krasovsky J, Steinman RM, Bhardwaj N. Mature dendritic cells boost functionally superior CD8(+) T-cell in humans without foreign helper epitopes. J Clin Invest 2000;105:R9-R14.

115. Dhodapkar MV, Steinman RM, Sapp M, et al. Rapid generation of broad T-cell immunity in humans after a single injection of mature dendritic cells. J Clin Invest 1999;104:173-80.

116. Berzofsky JA, Ahlers JD, Janik J, et al. Progress on new vaccine strategies against chronic viral infections. J Clin Invest 2004;114:450-62.

117. Zabaleta A, Llopiz D, Arribillaga L, et al. Vaccination against hepatitis C virus with dendritic cells transduced with an adenovirus encoding NS3 protein. Mol Ther 2008;16:210-17.

118. Li W, Krishnadas DK, Li J, et al. Induction of primary human T cell responses against hepatitis C virus-derived antigens NS3 or core by autologous dendritic cells expressing hepatitis C virus antigens: Potential for vaccine and immunotherapy. J Immunol 2006;176:6065-75.

119. Encke J, Findeklee J, Geib J, et al. Prophylactic and therapeutic vaccination with dendritic cells against hepatitis C virus infection. Clin Exp Immunol 2005;142:362-9.

120. Marzocchetti A, Lima M, Tompkins T, et al. Efficient in vitro expansion of JC virus-specific CD8(+) T-cell responses by JCV peptide-stimu-

lated dendritic cells from patients with progressive multifocal leukoencephalopathy. Virology 2009;383:173-7.

121. Lu W, Wu X, Lu Y, et al. Therapeutic dendritic-cell vaccine for simian AIDS. Nat Med 2003;9:27-32.

122. Melhem NM, Liu XD, Boczkowski D, et al. Robust CD4+ and CD8+ T cell responses to SIV using mRNA-transfected DC expressing autologous viral Ag. Eur J Immunol 2007;37: 2164-73.

123. Connolly NC, Whiteside TL, Wilson C, et al. Therapeutic immunization with human immunodeficiency virus type 1 (HIV-1) peptide-loaded dendritic cells is safe and induces immunogenicity in HIV-1-infected individuals. Clin Vaccine Immunol 2008;15:284-92.

124. Rosenthal R, Viehl CT, Guller U, et al. Active specific immunotherapy phase III trials for malignant melanoma: Systematic analysis and critical appraisal. J Am Coll Surg 2008;207: 95-105.

125. Wallack MK, Sivanandham M, Balch CM, et al. A phase III randomized, double-blind multiinstitutional trial of vaccinia melanoma oncolysate-active specific immunotherapy for patients with stage II melanoma. Cancer 1995;75:34-42.

126. Terando AM, Faries MB, Morton DL. Vaccine therapy for melanoma: Current status and future directions. Vaccine 2007;25(Suppl 2): B4-16.

127. Eggermont AM. Immunotherapy: Vaccine trials in melanoma—time for reflection. Nat Rev Clin Oncol 2009;6:256-8.

128. Boon T, Coulie PG, Van den Eynde BJ, van der Bruggen P. Human T cell responses against melanoma. Annu Rev Immunol 2006;24:175-208.

129. Simpson AJ, Caballero OL, Jungbluth A, et al. Cancer/testis antigens, gametogenesis and cancer. Nat Rev Cancer 2005;5:615-25.

130. Srivastava PK. Therapeutic cancer vaccines. Curr Opin Immunol 2006;18:201-5.

131. Dougan M, Dranoff G. Immune therapy for cancer. Annu Rev Immunol 2009;27:83-117.

132. Berzofsky JA, Terabe M, Oh S, et al. Progress on new vaccine strategies for the immunotherapy and prevention of cancer. J Clin Invest 2004;113:1515-25.

133. Bendandi M. Idiotype vaccines for lymphoma: Proof-of-principles and clinical trial failures. Nat Rev Cancer 2009;9:675-81.

134. Ashley DM, Faiola B, Nair S, et al. Bone marrow-generated dendritic cells pulsed with tumor extracts or tumor RNA induce antitumor immunity against central nervous system tumors. J Exp Med 1997;186:1177-82.

135. Celluzzi CM, Falo LD Jr. Physical interaction between dendritic cells and tumor cells results in an immunogen that induces protective and therapeutic tumor rejection. J Immunol 1998; 160:3081-5.

136. Gilboa E, Nair SK, Lyerly HK. Immunotherapy of cancer with dendritic-cell-based vaccines. Cancer Immunol Immunother 1998;46:82-7.

137. Porgador A, Snyder D, Gilboa E. Induction of antitumor immunity using bone marrow-generated dendritic cells. J Immunol 1996;156: 2918-26.

138. O'Neill DW, Adams S, Bhardwaj N. Manipulating dendritic cell biology for the active immunotherapy of cancer. Blood 2004;104:2235-46.

139. Slingluff CL Jr, Petroni GR, Yamshchikov GV, et al. Clinical and immunologic results of a randomized phase II trial of vaccination using four melanoma peptides either administered in granulocyte-macrophage colony-stimulating factor in adjuvant or pulsed on dendritic cells. J Clin Oncol 2003;21:4016-26.

140. O'Neill DW, Adams S, Goldberg JD, et al. Comparison of the immunogenicity of Montanide ISA 51 adjuvant and cytokine-matured dendritic cells in a randomized controlled clinical trial of melanoma vaccines. J Clin Oncol (Meeting Abstracts) 2009;27:3002.

141. Schadendorf D, Ugurel S, Schuler-Thurner B, et al. Dacarbazine (DTIC) versus vaccination with autologous peptide-pulsed dendritic cells (DC) in first-line treatment of patients with metastatic melanoma: A randomized phase III trial of the DC study group of the DeCOG. Ann Oncol 2006;17:563-70.

142. Brodie SJ, Patterson BK, Lewinsohn DA, et al. HIV-specific cytotoxic T lymphocytes traffic to lymph nodes and localize at sites of HIV replication and cell death. J Clin Invest 2000;105: 1407-17.

143. Straathof KC, Bollard CM, Popat U, et al. Treatment of nasopharyngeal carcinoma with Epstein-Barr virus-specific T lymphocytes. Blood 2005;105:1898-904.

144. Brodie SJ, Lewinsohn DA, Patterson BK, et al. In vivo migration and function of transferred HIV-1-specific cytotoxic T cells. Nat Med 1999;5:34-41.

145. Rosenberg SA, Lotze MT, Muul LM, et al. Observations on the systemic administration of autologous lymphokine-activated killer cells and recombinant interleukin-2 to patients with metastatic cancer. N Engl J Med 1985;313: 1485-92.

146. Rosenberg SA, Packard BS, Aebersold PM, et al. Use of tumor-infiltrating lymphocytes and interleukin-2 in the immunotherapy of patients with metastatic melanoma. A preliminary report. N Engl J Med 1988;319:1676-80.

147. Rosenberg SA. Karnofsky Memorial Lecture. The immunotherapy and gene therapy of cancer. J Clin Oncol 1992;10:180-99.

148. Dudley ME, Wunderlich JR, Robbins PF, et al. Cancer regression and autoimmunity in patients after clonal repopulation with antitumor lymphocytes. Science 2002;298:850-4.

149. Tran KQ, Zhou J, Durflinger KH, et al. Minimally cultured tumor-infiltrating lymphocytes display optimal characteristics for adoptive cell therapy. J Immunother 2008;31:742-51.

150. Dudley ME, Wunderlich J, Nishimura MI, et al. Adoptive transfer of cloned melanoma-reactive T lymphocytes for the treatment of patients with metastatic melanoma. J Immunother 2001;24:363-73.

151. Rapoport AP, Stadtmauer EA, Aqui N, et al. Rapid immune recovery and graft-versus-host disease-like engraftment syndrome following adoptive transfer of Costimulated autologous T cells. Clin Cancer Res 2009;15:4499-507.

152. Yee C, Thompson JA, Byrd D, et al. Adoptive T cell therapy using antigen-specific CD8+ T cell clones for the treatment of patients with metastatic melanoma: In vivo persistence, migration, and antitumor effect of transferred T cells. Proc Natl Acad Sci U S A 2002;99:16168-73.

153. Hunder NN, Wallen H, Cao J, et al. Treatment of metastatic melanoma with autologous CD4+ T cells against NY-ESO-1. N Engl J Med 2008;358:2698-703.

154. Ho WY, Nguyen HN, Wolfl M, et al. In vitro methods for generating CD8+ T-cell clones for immunotherapy from the naive repertoire. J Immunol Methods 2006;310:40-52.

155. Schmitt TM, Ragnarsson GB, Greenberg PD. T cell receptor gene therapy for cancer. Hum Gene Ther 2009;20:1240-8.

156. Sadelain M, Brentjens R, Riviere I. The promise and potential pitfalls of chimeric antigen receptors. Curr Opin Immunol 2009;21:215-23.

157. Morgan RA, Dudley ME, Wunderlich JR, et al. Cancer regression in patients after transfer of genetically engineered lymphocytes. Science 2006;314:126-9.

158. Rosenberg SA, Dudley ME. Adoptive cell therapy for the treatment of patients with metastatic melanoma. Curr Opin Immunol 2009; 21:233-40.

159. Dotti G, Savoldo B, Brenner M. Fifteen years of gene therapy based on chimeric antigen receptors: "Are we nearly there yet?" Hum Gene Ther 2009;20:1229-39.

160. Pule MA, Straathof KC, Dotti G, et al. A chimeric T cell antigen receptor that augments cytokine release and supports clonal expansion of primary human T cells. Mol Ther 2005;12: 933-41.

161. Heslop HE, Brenner MK. The clone ranger? Mol Ther 2008;16:1520-1.

162. Till BG, Jensen MC, Wang J, et al. Adoptive immunotherapy for indolent non-Hodgkin lymphoma and mantle cell lymphoma using genetically modified autologous CD20-specific T cells. Blood 2008;112:2261-71.

163. Wang J, Jensen M, Lin Y, et al. Optimizing adoptive polyclonal T cell immunotherapy of lymphomas, using a chimeric T cell receptor possessing CD28 and CD137 costimulatory domains. Hum Gene Ther 2007;18:712-25.

164. Rosenberg SA, Spiess P, Lafreniere R. A new approach to the adoptive immunotherapy of cancer with tumor-infiltrating lymphocytes. Science 1986;233:1318-21.

165. Riddell SR, Greenberg PD. The use of anti-CD3 and anti-CD28 monoclonal antibodies to clone and expand human antigen-specific T cells. J Immunol Methods 1990;128:189-201.

166. Dudley ME, Wunderlich JR, Yang JC, et al. Adoptive cell transfer therapy following non-myeloablative but lymphodepleting chemotherapy for the treatment of patients with refractory metastatic melanoma. J Clin Oncol 2005;23:2346-57.

167. Klapper JA, Thomasian AA, Smith DM, et al. Single-pass, closed-system rapid expansion of lymphocyte cultures for adoptive cell therapy. J Immunol Methods 2009;345:90-9.

168. Levine BL, Bernstein WB, Aronson NE, et al. Adoptive transfer of costimulated CD4+ T cells induces expansion of peripheral T cells and decreased CCR5 expression in HIV infection. Nat Med 2002;8:47-53.

169. Paulos CM, Suhoski MM, Plesa G, et al. Adoptive immunotherapy: Good habits instilled at

youth have long-term benefits. Immunol Res 2008;42:182-96.

170. Hollyman D, Stefanski J, Przybylowski M, et al. Manufacturing validation of biologically functional T cells targeted to CD19 antigen for autologous adoptive cell therapy. J Immunother 2009;32:169-80.

171. Berger C, Turtle CJ, Jensen MC, Riddell SR. Adoptive transfer of virus-specific and tumor-specific T cell immunity. Curr Opin Immunol 2009;21:224-32.

172. Powell DJ Jr, Dudley ME, Robbins PF, Rosenberg SA. Transition of late-stage effector T cells to CD27+ CD28+ tumor-reactive effector memory T cells in humans after adoptive cell transfer therapy. Blood 2005;105:241-50.

173. Gattinoni L, Klebanoff CA, Palmer DC, et al. Acquisition of full effector function in vitro paradoxically impairs the in vivo antitumor efficacy of adoptively transferred CD8+ T cells. J Clin Invest 2005;115:1616-26.

174. Klebanoff CA, Gattinoni L, Torabi-Parizi P, et al. Central memory self/tumor-reactive CD8+ T cells confer superior antitumor immunity compared with effector memory T cells. Proc Natl Acad Sci U S A 2005;102:9571-6.

175. Appay V, Douek DC, Price DA. CD8+ T cell efficacy in vaccination and disease. Nat Med 2008;14:623-8.

176. Berger C, Jensen MC, Lansdorp PM, et al. Adoptive transfer of effector CD8+ T cells derived from central memory cells establishes persistent T cell memory in primates. J Clin Invest 2008;118:294-305.

177. Hinrichs CS, Spolski R, Paulos CM, et al. IL-2 and IL-21 confer opposing differentiation programs to CD8+ T cells for adoptive immunotherapy. Blood 2008;111:5326-33.

178. Gattinoni L, Zhong XS, Palmer DC, et al. Wnt signaling arrests effector T cell differentiation and generates CD8+ memory stem cells. Nat Med 2009;15:808-13.

179. Pule MA, Savoldo B, Myers GD, et al. Virus-specific T cells engineered to coexpress tumor-specific receptors: Persistence and antitumor activity in individuals with neuroblastoma. Nat Med 2008;14:1264-70.

180. Muranski P, Restifo NP. Adoptive immunotherapy of cancer using CD4(+) T cells. Curr Opin Immunol 2009;21:200-8.

181. Zhu J, Paul WE. CD4 T cells: Fates, functions, and faults. Blood 2008;112:1557-69.

182. Kennedy R, Celis E. Multiple roles for CD4+ T cells in anti-tumor immune responses. Immunol Rev 2008;222:129-44.

183. Muranski P, Boni A, Antony PA, et al. Tumor-specific Th17-polarized cells eradicate large established melanoma. Blood 2008;112:362-73.

184. Sakaguchi S, Yamaguchi T, Nomura T, Ono M. Regulatory T cells and immune tolerance. Cell 2008;133:775-87.

185. Riley JL, June CH, Blazar BR. Human T regulatory cell therapy: Take a billion or so and call me in the morning. Immunity 2009;30:656-65.

186. Putnam AL, Brusko TM, Lee MR, et al. Expansion of human regulatory T-cells from patients with type 1 diabetes. Diabetes 2009;58:652-62.

187. Haller MJ, Viener HL, Wasserfall C, et al. Autologous umbilical cord blood infusion for type 1 diabetes. Exp Hematol 2008;36:710-15.

188. Delgoffe GM, Kole TP, Zheng Y, et al. The mTOR kinase differentially regulates effector and regulatory T cell lineage commitment. Immunity 2009;30:832-44.

189. Golovina TN, Mikheeva T, Suhoski MM, et al. CD28 costimulation is essential for human T regulatory expansion and function. J Immunol 2008;181:2855-68.

190. Gottschalk S, Heslop HE, Rooney CM. Adoptive immunotherapy for EBV-associated malignancies. Leuk Lymphoma 2005;46:1-10.

191. Savoldo B, Goss JA, Hammer MM, et al. Treatment of solid organ transplant recipients with autologous Epstein Barr virus-specific cytotoxic T lymphocytes (CTLs). Blood 2006;108:2942-9.

192. Haque T, Wilkie GM, Jones MM, et al. Allogeneic cytotoxic T-cell therapy for EBV-positive posttransplantation lymphoproliferative disease: Results of a phase 2 multicenter clinical trial. Blood 2007;110:1123-31.

193. Bollard CM, Aguilar L, Straathof KC, et al. Cytotoxic T lymphocyte therapy for Epstein-Barr virus+ Hodgkin's disease. J Exp Med 2004;200:1623-33.

194. Bollard CM, Gottschalk S, Leen AM, et al. Complete responses of relapsed lymphoma following genetic modification of tumor-antigen presenting cells and T-lymphocyte transfer. Blood 2007;110:2838-45.

195. Comoli P, Pedrazzoli P, Maccario R, et al. Cell therapy of stage IV nasopharyngeal carcinoma

with autologous Epstein-Barr virus-targeted cytotoxic T lymphocytes. J Clin Oncol 2005; 23:8942-9.

196. Louis CU, Straathof K, Bollard CM, et al. Enhancing the in vivo expansion of adoptively transferred EBV-specific CTL with lymphodepleting CD45 monoclonal antibodies in NPC patients. Blood 2009;113:2442-50.

197. Levine BL, Humeau LM, Boyer J, et al. Gene transfer in humans using a conditionally replicating lentiviral vector. Proc Natl Acad Sci U S A 2006;103:17372-7.

198. Perez EE, Wang J, Miller JC, et al. Establishment of HIV-1 resistance in CD4+ T cells by genome editing using zinc-finger nucleases. Nat Biotechnol 2008;26:808-16.

199. Palmer DC, Chan CC, Gattinoni L, et al. Effective tumor treatment targeting a melanoma/melanocyte-associated antigen triggers severe ocular autoimmunity. Proc Natl Acad Sci U S A 2008;105:8061-6.

200. Schumacher TN, Restifo NP. Adoptive T cell therapy of cancer. Curr Opin Immunol 2009; 21:187-9.

201. Dudley ME, Yang JC, Sherry R, et al. Adoptive cell therapy for patients with metastatic melanoma: Evaluation of intensive myeloablative chemoradiation preparative regimens. J Clin Oncol 2008;26:5233-9.

202. Schwartzentruber DJ. Guidelines for the safe administration of high-dose interleukin-2. J Immunother 2001;24:287-93.

In: McLeod BC, Szczepiorkowski ZM, Weinstein R, Winters JL, eds.
Apheresis: Principles and Practice, 3rd edition
Bethesda, MD: AABB Press, 2010

27

Allogeneic Adoptive Immunotherapy with Apheresis Products

David L. Porter, MD, and Joseph H. Antin, MD

 FOR MANY PATIENTS WITH hematologic malignancies, transplantation of hematopoietic progenitor cells (HPCs) is the best, if not the only, curative therapy. It is well known that the success of an allogeneic hematopoietic stem cell transplantation (HSCT) is related not only to the intensive conditioning therapy but also to the anti-leukemic properties of the donor graft (see Chapter 22 for an introduction to this topic). This graft-vs-tumor (GVT) effect appears to be mediated, at least in part, by immunocompetent mature donor lymphocytes contained in the HPC product. This is directly supported by evidence that donor lymphocytes can induce a direct GVT reaction and restore complete remissions for patients who relapse after HSCT, independent of any transplant conditioning therapy. T cells collected from the original transplant donor by leukapheresis as donor lymphocyte infusions (DLIs) are widely administered now to induce a potent GVT reaction for many patients with relapsed leukemia after allogeneic HSCT. This has been one of the most dramatic and effective methods of adoptive immunotherapy in the clinical setting. The next phase in the evolution of allogeneic adoptive immunotherapy has come with the use of nonmyeloablative allogeneic HSCT. This strategy takes advantage of the antitumor properties of the donor graft in the setting of reduced regimen-related toxicity and results in consistent engraftment and significant antitumor responses in a variety of malignant and nonmalignant diseases. This chapter reviews the evidence for an allogeneic GVT effect in

David L. Porter, MD, Professor of Medicine, University of Pennsylvania, and Director, Blood and Marrow Transplantation, Bone Marrow and Stem Cell Transplant Program, University of Pennsylvania Medical Center, Philadelphia, Pennsylvania, and Joseph H. Antin, MD, Professor of Medicine, Harvard Medical School, and Chief, Stem Cell Transplantation Program, Department of Medical Oncology, Dana-Farber Cancer Institute/Brigham and Women's Hospital, Boston, Massachusetts
The authors have disclosed no conflicts of interest

the transplant setting and presents recent data on the use of donor apheresis products as a source of cells for allogeneic adoptive immunotherapy. The ability to further harness this powerful GVT effect and improve the safety of immunotherapy will come from novel strategies to collect and manipulate appropriate donor cellular components.

Graft-vs-Tumor Effects in Murine Models of Transplantation

The first suggestion that the donor immune system is critical for successful allogeneic HSCT came from transplantation experiments in mice as early as the mid-1950s. Barnes and colleagues treated leukemic mice with a nonmyeloablative dose of radiation therapy followed by transplantation.[1,2] Mice that received syngeneic marrow died of recurrent leukemia, while those that received allogeneic marrow appeared to be cured of their disease. These authors postulated that the allogeneic recipients were cured of residual leukemia by a "process of immunity" provided by the donor graft, a phenomenon now referred to as the GVT effect. It is notable, however, that although recipients of allogeneic marrow did not relapse, they tended to die of a "wasting syndrome" now recognized as graft-vs-host disease (GVHD). These experiments therefore also provided some of the earliest evidence for the intimate relationship between GVT and GVHD. Since these initial studies, many models have been used to define GVT reactions in great detail in different animals, and these have been critical to understanding the GVT effect in the clinical setting. In mice, it is generally accepted that donor T cells mediate acute GVHD,[3] and, in most models, the donor T cells are also critical for GVT.[4-6]

There are likely to be important effector mechanisms for GVT other than T-cell reactivity. For instance, major histocompatibility complex (MHC)-unrestricted cytotoxicity will also contribute to GVT under certain conditions. It is logical to suspect that various cytokines and natural killer (NK) cells will function to enhance GVT in the appropriate setting. Interleukin (IL)-2 is a potent inducer of NK-cell activity and will potentiate GVT in some murine models.[7,8] Some experimental models confirm the importance of NK cells for GVT activity,[9,10] although, in other systems, NK cells did not contribute to the GVT effects of DLI.[11] IL-2 may also exert its effect through mechanisms other than NK-cell activation, such as selective T-cell inhibition.[12] The cytotoxic pathways important for GVT induction are also being investigated. For instance, both the perforin-dependent pathway and the Fas/Fas ligand pathway have been shown to mediate GVT induction in some cases.[13,14] There are now clinical data showing that donor NK cells are important for GVT activity, at least in the setting of haploidentical HSCT.[15] Several investigators are now exploring the role of NK cell infusions to enhance the anti-tumor properties of the donor graft.[16]

Murine experiments provide unique insight into the mechanism of GVT, but the results must be interpreted with caution. The effector cells, target antigens, and cytotoxic pathways may vary depending on the leukemia model studied, the strain combinations used (which influence the degree of MHC compatibility between donor and host), and other variable experimental conditions. It is also likely that more than one cell population or effector mechanism is responsible for the GVT reaction. In addition, because many murine leukemias are virally induced, there is always the concern that the observed GVT activity is caused by specific antiviral immunity. Ultimately, most murine experiments are performed under conditions that are unlikely to have direct clinical application. Nevertheless, these important models form the basis for many subsequent clinical trials and are necessary guides for the design of future studies.

Evidence for a Graft-vs-Tumor Effect in Clinical Transplantation

Suspicion of an important GVT reaction in humans arose from several important but indirect clinical observations, as outlined in Table

27-1 and diagrammed in Fig 27-1. These observations not only provided circumstantial evidence for GVT in the clinical setting but also demonstrated the close association between GVT and GVHD. Moreover, they highlighted the role of donor T cells for GVT reactivity, in part validating the data from animal models. They also provided the basis for newer and more rational approaches to using allogeneic cellular therapy for clinical benefit.

Remission Is Induced by a Flare of GVHD or Withdrawal of Immune Suppression

Several anecdotal case reports describe patients with relapsed leukemia after HSCT who entered remission associated with a flare of acute GVHD[18] or after discontinuation of immunosuppressive therapy.[19-21] In more recent studies, it is common to report the presence of GVT activity based on observations of response associated with GVHD, and more recent trials of adoptive immunotherapy are often designed to include withdrawal of immunosuppression to enhance GVT activity.

Syngeneic Marrow Grafts Are Associated with Increased Relapse Rates

As with hematopoietic transplantation in animal models, relapse rates after human syngeneic marrow transplantation are higher when compared with transplantation of HLA-matched (though not identical) sibling marrow grafts. This was first noted by the Seattle group in patients with advanced leukemia.[22] The loss of GVT activity after receipt of a syngeneic graft is even more obvious for patients with acute myelogenous leukemia (AML) in first remission, where the probability of relapse was 59% ±20% after syngeneic HSCT compared with 18% ±4% after matched sibling HSCT.[23] Similar data have been reported by the International Bone Marrow Transplant Registry (Fig 27-1).[17,24] It is notable, however, that the magnitude of the GVT activity may depend on both the diagnosis and disease stage at the time of transplantation. For instance, a more recent update reported higher relapse rates after receipt of a synegeneic graft for patients with chronic myelogenous leukemia (CML) and AML, but not for patients with acute lymphocytic leukemia (ALL) in first remission.[24] One explanation for the high relapse rate after syngeneic transplantation often mentioned is that recurrent leukemia arises from donor cells; these cells would be impossible to distinguish from the recipient's original leukemia in syngeneic twins. However, leukemia of donor cell origin is a very rare occurrence and certainly cannot account for most of the relapses after syngeneic HSCT.

GVHD Is Protective Against Relapse

There is considerable evidence that GVHD after allogeneic HSCT is protective against relapse. This observation was first made in

---

Table 27-1. Indirect Evidence for a GVT Reaction in Clinical HSCT

- Some patients with relapsed leukemia after allogeneic HPC transplantation will enter complete remission after abrupt withdrawal of immunosuppression or following a flare of graft-vs-host disease (anecdotal).
- Syngeneic HSCT is associated with a higher risk of relapse than matched sibling transplantation.
- Graft-vs-host disease after allogeneic HSCT is protective against relapse.
- T-cell depletion of the donor HPC graft results in an increased risk of relapse, especially for patients with chronic myelogenous leukemia.

GVT = graft-vs-tumor; HSCT = hematopoietic stem cell transplantation; HPC = hematopoietic progenitor cell.

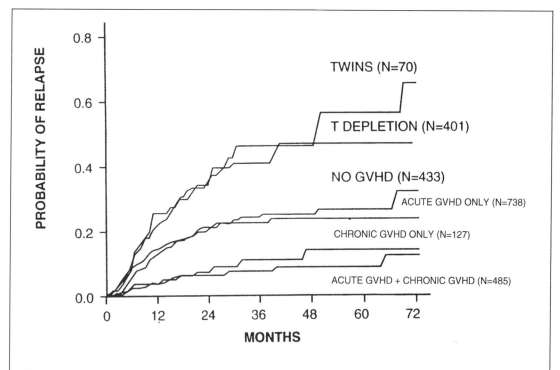

Figure 27-1. Probability of relapse after allogeneic marrow transplantation is a function of the type of graft and the extent of graft-vs-host disease. Reprinted from Horowitz et al.[17]

patients with advanced leukemia (AML or ALL in relapse, CML in accelerated phase or blast crisis, or patients in remission but at high risk of relapse). It was noted in retrospective, observational studies that patients with acute and/or chronic GVHD had lower relapse rates when compared with patients who had no GVHD.[25-27] Similarly, a subsequent analysis showed that GVHD was protective against relapse for patients with early-stage leukemia.[17,28] The risk of relapse after HSCT for over 2200 transplant recipients with "early leukemia" (AML or ALL in first remission or CML in chronic phase) who had acute and chronic GVHD was significantly lower when compared with that of patients who developed no GVHD (Fig 27-1).[17] This report further emphasized that the magnitude of GVT activity is diagnosis dependent. For instance, acute GVHD only was associated with less relapse in ALL, whereas the combination of acute and chronic GVHD was associated with lower relapse rates for patients with ALL, AML, and CML. The association of GVHD with relapse has been confirmed repeatedly over the many years since these early observations.

T-Cell Depletion of the Donor Marrow Graft Results in Increased Relapse Rates

On the basis of animal models and clinical observations, it has generally been accepted that GVHD is mediated by donor T cells in the marrow graft, and many centers began using T-cell depletion of donor marrow before HSCT as a very successful method to prevent GVHD.[29-34] Unfortunately, although T-cell depletion can minimize transplant-related mortality from GVHD, several studies showed that overall survival was not improved by T-cell depletion.[28,32,35-37] This was, in large part, the result of a reciprocal increase in the rates of relapse and graft failure. The higher relapse rate associated with T-cell-depleted grafts was most evident in patients with CML, where the incidence of relapse was up to 50%.[17,35,38] Even when compared with relapse rates of patients who did not develop GVHD after receiving an unmanipulated marrow graft, patients with CML receiving T-cell-depleted marrow had an almost sevenfold increased risk of relapse.[17] These results provide strong, although still indirect, evidence that donor T cells possess important anti-leukemic properties that significantly influence the success of marrow transplantation.

Treatment of Relapsed Leukemia After Allogeneic Transplantation: Graft-vs-Leukemia Induction with Donor Lymphocyte Infusions

The first direct evidence for GVT activity in humans came from the use of DLI to treat relapse after allogeneic HPC transplantation. Effective treatment options for patients who relapse after receiving an allogeneic transplant have been limited. Although second allogeneic HPC grafts may cure a minority of patients, they are associated with extensive morbidity and mortality, and subsequent relapse rates are very high.[39-41] Therefore, there has been a need to develop safer and more effective therapies to treat relapse after allogeneic HSCT.

Adoptive Immunotherapy for Relapsed Chronic Myelogenous Leukemia

On the basis of both animal models and indirect clinical observations that suggested donor leukocytes were responsible for potent GVT activity, trials were initiated to administer DLI to patients with relapsed leukemia after allogeneic HSCT. One of the first published reports to demonstrate that DLI could induce a direct GVT reaction came from Kolb and colleagues.[42] They treated three HSCT recipients who had interferon-resistant, relapsed CML with donor buffy-coat cells obtained by leukapheresis of the original transplant donor. All

three patients entered a complete cytogenetic remission. This report demonstrated the ability of donor leukocytes to induce significant and sustained antitumor responses. The dramatic GVT potential of DLI was rapidly confirmed by several other groups,[43,44] showing that in addition to inducing complete cytogenetic remissions, DLI also resulted in complete molecular remissions with no detectable cells containing *bcr/abl* mRNA transcripts by polymerase chain reaction (PCR) analysis.[44-46] This is significant because PCR analysis can detect 1 CML cell in 10^6 normal cells,[47] and a negative PCR assay in patients with chronic-phase CML represents at least a 6-log reduction in CML,[48] highlighting the potency of the GVT reaction.

In addition to several single-institution trials, results on the use of DLI from larger numbers of patients were compiled in two major registries from both North America and the European Bone Marrow Transplant (EBMT) group; they are summarized in Table 27-2.[49,50] These data are remarkably consistent with single-institution trials and show that 76% to 79% of patients treated with DLI for relapsed chronic-phase CML will achieve complete cytogenetic remission. In addition, the majority of these patients achieved a complete molecular remission by PCR analysis.

The majority of remissions achieved with DLI for chronic-phase CML are sustained. Long-term follow-up after DLI for CML was available for 39 patients reported to the North American registry.[51] Only five patients (13%) relapsed, including two of 32 patients (6%) treated for early-phase relapse and three of seven patients (43%) treated with DLI for advanced-phase (accelerated-phase and blast-crisis) relapse of CML. The probability of event-free survival from the time of remission was 79% at 1 year and 73% at 2 and 3 years. The overall probability of survival in this group was 73% at 3 years. The Hammersmith group reported follow-up from 66 recipients of DLI for relapsed CML.[52] Of the 44 patients who had achieved a molecular remission, four (9%) ultimately had a relapse of CML documented by PCR testing. The probability of molecular remission 3 years after DLI was 68% for the

Table 27-2. Adoptive Immunotherapy with Donor MNC Infusions for Relapsed CML: Complete Cytogenetic Response Rates

CML Phase	North America[49] (n = 55)	EBMT[50] (n = 67)
Chronic phase	76%	79%
Advanced phase	28%	12%
Total	60%	72%

MNC = mononuclear cell; CML = chronic mylelogenous leukemia; EBMT = European Group for Blood and Marrow Transplantation.

entire group. These data also confirmed that patients with advanced-phase CML and a short duration of remission after transplantation were less likely to benefit from DLI. Although complete molecular remissions were durable in the majority of patients, the few late relapses in both long-term follow-up studies raise the concern that GVT effects of the donor T cells might have a limited life span. It is notable that no relapsed patient in the North American analysis received a second course of DLI, whereas the Hammersmith group describes two patients in molecular relapse who had a subsequent molecular remission induced with further DLI.

Adoptive immunotherapy with DLI appears to be less effective for more advanced phases of CML because complete remissions (CRs) occur in only 12% to 28% of patients with accelerated-phase or blast-crisis CML.[49,50] Unfortunately, even those advanced-phase patients who respond to DLI are less likely to enjoy prolonged remissions.[51,52] Relapses after DLI-induced remissions for accelerated or blast-phase CML occurred in up to 43% of patients in one analysis[51] and may be higher with longer follow-up. Given these data, it would seem most appropriate to use DLI early in the course of relapse before disease progression. For instance, low doses of DLI can be given to patients with minimal disease burdens; response rates in this group of patients have been very high, and toxicity from GVHD may

be minimized by using lower doses of T cells.[45,46,53]

Adoptive Immunotherapy for Relapse of Diseases Other than CML

Many HPC graft recipients who relapse with diseases other than CML have also been treated with DLI. However, GVT induced by DLI has disease specificity similar to that seen after allogeneic HSCT and appears to be less effective for diseases other than CML (Table 27-3).

Acute Myelogenous Leukemia and Acute Lymphocytic Leukemia

Responses to DLI for relapsed acute leukemia have been disappointing. Initial reports describe only occasional responses for patients with relapsed AML when DLI is used with or without reinduction chemotherapy.[65-67] In the larger retrospective analyses, complete response rates to DLI were 15% to 29% for relapsed AML without additional chemotherapy (Table 27-3).[49,50] Although complete responses are achieved in only a small number of AML patients, many of these remissions may be durable. Of 10 patients in the North American registry who had achieved a CR from DLI, only two subsequently relapsed at 1 to 3 years. At a median follow-up of 1 year, five patients were alive and in CR. The two who relapsed

Table 27-3. Response Rates to DLI to Treat Relapse After Allogeneic HSCT

Disease	Complete Response Rate*
Acute myelogenous leukemia	15% (6/39)[49]
	29% (5/17)[50]
	47% (27/57)[54†]
	34% (54/158)[55]
Acute lymphoblastic leukemia	18% (2/11)[49]
	0% (0/12)[50]
	13% (2/15)[56]
	70% (7[‡]/10)[57†]
Myelodysplastic syndrome	40% (2/5)[49]
	25% (1/4)[50]
	21% (3/14)[58]
Non-Hodgkin lymphoma	0% (0/6)[49]
	100% (2/2)[59]
	0% (0/3)[60]
Multiple myeloma	50% (2/4)[49]
	31% (4/13)[61]
	22% (6/27)[62]
	9% (2/22)[63§]
	60% (6/10)[64]

*Representative response rates are illustrated from either registry data or, in some cases, larger series of DLI for a specific indication.
†All patients were pretreated with chemotherapy by design of the protocol.
‡Only one patient remained in complete remission.
§A total of 25 patients were treated. An additional 3 patients achieved a complete response after treatment with chemotherapy before DLI.
DLI = donor lymphocyte infusion; HSCT = hematopoietic stem cell transplantation.

died of disease, and three other patients had died of treatment-related causes.[51]

One factor that may limit the success of DLI in AML is the high tumor burden and rapid proliferation of leukemic blasts. Because the effects of DLI may be delayed, disease-related early mortality is significant after DLI but before the anti-leukemia effect is manifest. To minimize this concern, a prospective trial used induction chemotherapy followed by DLI primed with granulocyte colony-stimulating factor (G-CSF) in patients with relapsed AML.[54]

Complete remissions were achieved in 47% (27/57) of patients, but overall survival was only 19% at 2 years. However, several important findings should be highlighted. For patients who were in CR after chemotherapy and DLI, 1- and 2-year survival rates were 51% and 41%, respectively, compared to a 1-year survival of only 5% in nonresponders. Eight patients were not evaluable as a result of early death, and 25 of 30 evaluable patients who did not respond died from progressive disease. It was notable that 10 patients who did not respond initially received additional DLI, and three of them achieved a CR. One of the most important predictors of overall survival was time from transplantation to relapse. In patients who relapsed more than 6 months after receiving a transplant, the overall survival was almost 40% at 2 years compared with almost no patients surviving if they had relapsed within 6 months. These results are comparable to historical controls using DLI where the response rates vary anywhere from 0 to 30% and disease-free survival is 3% to 20%; therefore, the role of initial chemotherapy remains uncertain. A second, smaller trial of 16 patients from Korea also used chemotherapy followed by G-CSF-primed DLI and found a high response rate (63%) with 1- and 2-year survival estimates of 38% and 31%, respectively.[68]

More recently, the EBMT retrospectively analyzed outcomes of almost 400 patients with relapsed AML.[55] For the 171 recipients of DLI, outcomes were improved if DLI was given to patients who achieved remission by other means (such as prior chemotherapy). In a good risk population of patients in remission with a favorable karyotype, 2-year overall survival (OS) was 56%; this is in contrast to patients who received DLI with active disease or during aplasia who had an OS of 9% to 20% (overall,15%) depending on other risk factors. This suggests that inducing remission and a minimal disease state before DLI may either improve outcome with GVT induction or, at the least, select for those patients most likely to benefit from DLI. This report also noted that patients treated with DLI appear to have better outcomes than patients who never receive DLI, with OS of 21% vs 9% at 2 years.[55] Taken together, these data demonstrate a potent GVT effect for patients with relapsed AML. Given the limited treatment options, DLI is a reasonable strategy and will have dramatic benefit for a select group of patients with later relapses and with minimal disease burdens at the time of DLI.

Response rates to DLI for patients with relapsed ALL are even more disappointing (Table 27-3), and many of the remissions that do occur are transient. Initial retrospective studies reported remission rates of 0 and 18%.[49,50] In a subsequent report, the probability of 3-year survival for 44 recipients of DLI for relapsed ALL was 13%.[56] Only 2 of 13 patients had a direct response to DLI, whereas 5 of 25 patients who received DLI after induction chemotherapy achieved a CR. The duration of remission for these 7 patients ranged from 42 to 1112 days, with only 2 of the 44 patients in CR at the time of analysis, approximately 2 years after DLI. It should be emphasized that although response rates are low, durable remissions are possible. One of the first recipients of DLI, who was treated for relapsed ALL, had remained in remission for over 8 years at last report.[66] It is surprising that patients with ALL have poor responses to DLI given the well-documented GVT response seen in analyses of international HSCT registries. The cause of this inconsistency is unknown. However, it does seem that the response rates of ALL to DLI are higher in the setting of minimal residual disease (MRD), such as molecular or cytogenetic relapse.[69] DLI has induced remissions in approximately 30% of children with ALL when given at the time of MRD but before overt relapse.[70,71]

Multiple Myeloma

DLI has also been effective for some patients who relapse with multiple myeloma after receiving an allogeneic HSCT.[72] Complete remissions were noted for 4 of 13 recipients of DLI for relapsed myeloma treated in the Netherlands, and an additional 4 patients had a partial response (overall response rate of 62%).[61] Only 1 patient who achieved a CR had relapsed 14 months later. In an update from this group, 5 of 27 (18%) patients had sustained remission for over 30 months after DLI.[62]

Results were less encouraging from the North American multicenter analysis.[63] Of 22 evaluable recipients of DLI for relapsed myeloma, only 2 achieved a CR and both relapsed, 10 and 26 weeks later. An additional 3 patients were treated with chemotherapy before DLI and achieved CRs lasting 26, 127, and more than 148 weeks; the contribution of chemotherapy compared with DLI could not be determined in these patients. It is notable that 12 of these 25 patients were alive, with a median follow-up of over 1 year, including 2 who were disease free and 3 with continued partial remissions. These data suggest that DLI can generate a meaningful graft-vs-myeloma effect for a minority of patients, but both toxicity and relapse limit the success of DLI for myeloma.

A graft-vs-myeloma effect has also been noted after reduced-intensity-conditioning HSCT. For patients with relapsed or persistent disease in this setting, complete (19%) and partial responses (19%) have been achieved. Unfortunately, many patients will relapse with a median time to progression of 7 months after partial remission and 28 months after CR, highlighting the need for even more definitive therapies.[73] The median time to progression was 7 months for patients with partial remission, and 28 months for patients who achieved CR.

Non-Hodgkin and Hodgkin Lymphoma

Although there are significant data supporting a graft-vs-lymphoma and graft-vs-Hodgkin lymphoma effect in clinical transplantation,[74-76] there are only limited data on the use of DLI for these patients. Most reports of DLI for Hodgkin lymphoma (HL) include only a small number of patients and many received DLI after reduced-intensity-chemotherapy HSCT. Response rates have varied widely, between 15%[77] and 56%.[78] The largest series reported by the EBMT showed an overall response rate of 32% in 41 patients, though an additional 15% of patients had some evidence of at least stable disease. It is nteresting that 18 patients received DLI with no prior chemotherapy for relapse and had a response rate of 44%, again highlighting that in some patients, GVT induction in HL can be quite potent.

Similarly, there is compelling data demonstrating a graft-vs-lymphoma effect in non-Hodgkin lymphoma (NHL) using DLI for relapse, but it is also based on only small numbers of patients. No responses in six patients with NHL were reported to the North American DLI registry,[49] and only minor responses were reported in three additional recipients of DLI for relapse of NHL.[60] In general, patients with indolent histologies seem more likely to respond. Responses may also be durable. Russel et al reported a 65% response rate in 17 patients with relapse NHL or chronic lymphocytic leukemia (CLL) and found a 3-year progression-free survival (PFS) of 52% and 3-year OS of 58%.[79] Other studies have shown response rates of 53% to 76%,[80,81] usually after T-cell depletion of the original graft. Despite the limited data, clinical evidence for a graft-vs-lymphoma reaction in both NHL and HL is compelling, and the administration of DLI for relapse in these patients seems warranted.

Unrelated Donor Lymphocyte Infusions

Relapse is also a major complication after receipt of an unrelated donor HSCT, and available data suggest that unrelated DLI (U-DLI) will also induce an effective GVT reaction with response rates similar to those seen with matched sibling DLI.[49,50] The National Marrow Donor Program collaborated with investigators to retrospectively identify 58 recipients of U-DLI for relapsed leukemia; these data are summarized in Table 27-4.[82] Complete remissions from U-DLI occurred in 46% of patients with CML, 42% of the patients with AML, and two of four evaluable patients with ALL. The incidence of grade II to IV acute GVHD was 25%, and chronic GVHD occurred in 41% of patients. In another report, comparisons were made between 18 recipients of matched sibling DLI and 12 recipients of U-DLI in CML patients and showed similar response rates (64% vs 73% of patients achieved a cytogenetic remission).[83] There was a trend toward more acute GVHD in the U-DLI group, although the incidence of chronic GVHD was similar regardless of donor source. Although direct comparisons are difficult, toxicity from U-DLI is similar to experiences using matched sibling DLI in most studies. However, some data do suggest an increased risk of GVHD at lower T-cell doses with U-DLI compared to

Table 27-4. Clinical Outcomes After Unrelated Donor Lymphocyte Infusion[82]

Outcome	CML (n = 25)	AML (n = 23)	ALL (n = 7)	Other (n = 3)	Total (n = 58)
Response to U-DLI (at risk, n =)*	24	19	4	3	50
CR	11 (46%)	8 (42%)	2 (50%)	0 (0)	21 (42%)
PR/NR	13 (54%)	10 (53%)	1 (14%)	2 (67%)	26 (52%)
		1 (4%)	1 (25%)	1 (33%)	3 (6%)
NE, CR pre-U-DLI	1 (4%)	4 (17%)	3 (43%)		8 (14%)
Alive, in CR	11	4	2	0	17
Acute GVHD (at risk, n =)	25	23	6	2	55
0	17	13	2	2	34
I	1	1	0	0	2
II	2	1	2	0	5
III	2	4	1	0	7
IV	3	3	1	0	7
NE		1			
Chronic GVHD (at risk, n =)	16	10	5	1	30
None	10	4	3	0	17
Limited	1	2	0	0	3
Extensive	3	4	2	1	10
Unknown	2				
Median survival after U-DLI (weeks)	42	11	35	3	34

*Patients in CR at time of U-DLI are excluded from response analysis. Patients who did not survive 28 days for adequate follow-up are shown and are considered nonresponders for this analysis. Patients who received pre-DLI chemotherapy are included in this table as "evaluable" for response.

CML = chronic myelogenous leukemia; AML = acute myelogenous leukemia; ALL = acute lymphoblastic leukemia; DLI = donor lymphocyte infusion; U-DLI = unrelated DLI; CR = complete response; PR = partial response; NR = no response; NE = nonevaluable; GVHD = graft-vs-host disease.

matched sibling DLI, at least after nonmyeloablative allogeneic HSCT.[84]

Response rates are difficult to compare using DLI from unrelated donors vs matched siblings. Responses to U-DLI for patients with CML appear similar to matched sibling DLI. The number of patients treated with U-DLI for acute leukemia is quite small and the reported follow-up has been short, making any comparison to matched sibling DLI more difficult. In addition, many of the patients with AML and ALL underwent chemotherapy before U-DLI, and it is difficult to assess the contribution of chemotherapy independent of U-DLI. For instance, of 15 patients with AML who received U-DLI only, five had a CR but two relapsed quickly, two died of treatment-related complications, and only one was alive and in remission.[82] Two of three patients with ALL responded to U-DLI without prior chemotherapy, and one patient remained in remission for more than 3 years.

Taken together, these studies suggest that the incidence and severity of acute and chronic

GVHD, marrow aplasia, and treatment-related mortality after unrelated donor DLI are comparable to these outcomes after related donor DLI and that response rates are reasonable. Although many clinicians alter the dose of DLI depending on the relationship of the donor to the patients, available data are unclear regarding the need for dosing to be altered for unrelated donors. Unrelated donor DLI is a useful treatment option for patients who relapse after unrelated-donor transplantation, particularly given the anticipated poor outcomes for alternative therapies such as second unrelated donor transplant.

Toxicity of Adoptive Immunotherapy

Although the response rate to DLI is relatively high, especially for patients with CML, the toxicity of adoptive immunotherapy, while acceptable compared with that of alternative therapies, remains significant (see Table 27-5).

Graft-vs-Host Disease

In most initial studies, patients who achieve complete responses typically develop acute and chronic GVHD.[49,50,85] However, it is notable that a relatively high number of donor T cells are administered without the use of GVHD prophylaxis, and GVHD is most often only mild to moderate. Toxicity from GVHD appears to be less than might be anticipated if a similar dose of T cells was administered at the time of transplantation without GVHD prophylaxis. Overall, approximately 36% to 40% of patients treated with DLI experience no acute GVHD, and another 15% to 30% have only grade I acute GVHD. Although 20% to 50% of patients may have grade II to IV acute GVHD, in most patients this has typically responded to immunosuppressive therapy. The North American analysis of 140 patients found a 96% incidence of acute GVHD and a 78% incidence of chronic GVHD in 49 complete responders.[49] In 92 patients who had no response, only 35% had acute GVHD and only 13% had chronic GVHD. It should be noted, however, that many patients who fail to respond to GVT induction will die shortly of progressive disease and may not survive long enough for GVHD to develop. This is particularly important for patients with acute leukemia.

Not all studies found a similar relationship between a GVT effect and GVHD, and there seems to be some threshold dose below which GVHD does not develop. Investigators at the Memorial Sloan Kettering Cancer Center used low-dose DLI with sequential dose escalation for nonresponding patients with relapsed CML and noted a very low incidence of acute GVHD associated with therapy.[45] In this trial, the

Table 27-5. Toxicity After Donor Lymphocyte Infusions

Toxicity	Description
Graft-vs-host disease (GVHD)	Acute Chronic

Infections	Bacterial, fungal, viral
	  Related to neutropenia and marrow aplasia
	  Related to immunosuppression used to treat GVHD

Pancytopenia	Bleeding (thrombocytopenia) Infections Transfusion requirements

development of chronic GVHD correlated with CR, consistent with results from marrow transplant analyses, suggesting that chronic GVHD is most closely associated with the GVT effect.[27] Other studies have confirmed that low-dose DLI followed by dose escalation will induce a similar rate of CRs for patients with CML with minimal complicating GVHD.[53,86] Therefore, dose-escalated DLI is commonly used now for patients with CML. Although a similar number of patients with CML achieve CR, the time to CR is shorter in patients receiving the initial higher cell dose. Therefore, this strategy is very attractive for patients with indolent malignancies such as CML and even Hodgkin lymphoma,[84] but it would not be practical for patients with rapidly proliferating diseases such as AML and ALL, who would be anticipated to die rapidly from disease if the initial DLI attempt was not successful.

Pancytopenia and Marrow Aplasia

The second major complication after DLI has been pancytopenia related to marrow aplasia. Many patients may require transfusions of platelets and red cells, and infectious complications related to transient neutropenia may develop. The phenomenon of marrow aplasia after DLI is reminiscent of transfusion-associated GVHD (TA-GVHD),[87] indicating that HPCs are good targets for T cells. However, TA-GVHD is typically fatal, and marrow aplasia after DLI is usually transient. Possible explanations for this difference are that patients who develop typical TA-GVHD have received HLA-unmatched (and therefore probably dissimilar) leukocytes and are also unlikely to have received adequate numbers of donor HPCs to support donor hematopoiesis. Patients who relapse after allogeneic HSCT and receive DLI may be more likely to recover normal donor hematopoiesis because they may have either adequate numbers of residual donor HPCs persisting from the original transplant or because the infused donor leukocytes contain enough donor HPCs to restore normal hematopoiesis.

Marrow aplasia is presumably related to the destruction of host leukemic hematopoiesis before the recovery of normal donor hematopoiesis. In some cases, persistent marrow aplasia can be successfully reversed with the infusion of additional donor marrow.[43,44] It is unknown why some patients spontaneously recover hematopoiesis and others do not, although it may not be related merely to an absolute lack of normal donor HPCs.[44,88] However, some data argue that patients with residual donor hematopoiesis before DLI are unlikely to experience aplasia.[89] Regardless of the mechanism, in some instances, particularly when chemotherapy is given before DLI for cytoreduction, using G-CSF-stimulated peripheral blood mononuclear cells (MNCs) as the DLI product may at least limit the duration of neutropenia, and persistent aplasia has not developed after such infusions.[54] It is unknown if G-CSF stimulation will alter GVHD or GVT activity, although, in animal models, G-CSF stimulation may polarize donor T cells to a Th-2 phenotype and possibly limit alloreactivity.[13,90]

Mortality

The overall treatment-related mortality after DLI may be as high as 20%. GVHD has been a direct cause of death in 5% to 8% of patients. Another 7% to 12% of patients may die from infectious complications associated with marrow aplasia or immunosuppressive regimens as therapy for GVHD. This toxicity must be taken in context, however, particularly when compared with the anticipated 40% or higher treatment-related mortality associated with second transplantation,[45,46] and the almost certain risk of death without effective therapy.

New Strategies of Adoptive Immunotherapy

Although the induction of a GVT reaction with DLI has provided a safer, more effective treatment for relapsed leukemia after allogeneic HPC transplantation, the toxicity of therapy is still significant, and the responses are highly disease dependent. There is much interest in designing strategies that will limit toxicity from

GVHD and other complications while preserving and maximizing GVT reactivity (see Table 27-6).

Several trials have been performed to limit GVHD after DLI by manipulating the donor leukapheresis product. One approach is the administration of donor leukocytes selectively depleted of effector cells suspected of causing GVHD. In the setting of marrow transplantation, CD8+ T cells have been implicated as potential mediators of GVHD; transplantation of donor grafts depleted of CD8+ cells may result in less GVHD than that associated with transplantation of unmanipulated marrow,[91] and analysis suggests that CD8-depleted marrow grafts may retain GVT reactivity. Some data suggest that CD8-depleted donor leukocyte products used to treat relapsed CML after allogeneic HSCT retain GVT activity but cause minimal GVHD.[92,93] The majority of remissions induced with such products are durable; after a median follow-up of 4.5 years from CD8-depleted DLI for chronic-phase CML, only one of 13 responders ultimately relapsed.[94] CD8-depleted DLI has also been used in a small number of patients with persistent myeloma after allogeneic HSCT, although with a 50% incidence of significant acute or chronic GVHD.[64]

Another approach designed to limit GVHD has been to lower the dose of donor leukocytes. Although it is unclear whether GVT and GVHD are separable, it is possible that a threshold dose of donor cells exists that will induce a GVT reaction without resulting in clinically apparent GVHD. The initial trial from Mackinnon et al showed that an initial dose as low as 10^7 CD3+ cells/kg (up to 1 log fewer cells than administered in many of the earlier trials of DLI) will induce CRs for many patients with relapsed CML, with minimal GVHD.[45] Low-dose DLI is particularly effective for patients with minimal tumor burdens; eight of 16 patients entering molecular remission were

---

Table 27-6. Newer Approaches to Cellular Therapies to Treat Relapse

- Infusion of selected T-cell subsets (ie, after CD8+ cell depletion or CD4+ cell selection)
- Low-dose donor lymphocyte infusions followed by dose escalation
- Inactivation of alloreactive T cells:
  - Transduction of suicide genes into donor T cells
  - Photochemical inactivation
  - Chemotherapy inactivation
  - Irradiation
- Generation and infusion of tumor-specific T cells
- Generation and infusion of minor histocompatibility antigen-specific T cells
- Tumor-specific vaccines (antigen-specific, modified tumor cells, etc) combined with cellular effectors
- Ex-vivo activation and expansion of donor T cells through co-stimulation
- Generation of other cellular effectors such as natural killer and dendritic cells
- Generation and infusion of Th2-type T cells
- Infusion of T-regulatory cells
- Manipulation of antigen-presenting cells to maximize GVT or minimize GVHD
- Recruitment of anti-tumor T cells through use of modified T cells expressing chimeric antigen receptors or using bispecific antibodies

treated at a time of low leukemia cell burden (ie, cytogenetic or molecular relapse) and received the lowest cell doses. This would be anticipated if the GVT reaction was dependent on the effector:target cell ratio. The low numbers of effector cells may be sufficient to eradicate low numbers of leukemic cells but not to induce clinically apparent GVHD. Although patients with more advanced stages of relapse often responded to subsequent dose escalation, they typically required over 10^8 MNC/kg, doses previously reported to be highly associated with GVHD. It is notable, therefore, that very few patients in this study developed clinical GVHD.[45] Subsequent trials have confirmed that for patients with CML, low-dose DLI followed by dose escalation results in response rates similar to high-dose DLI, but with less GVHD.[53] In fact, a dose escalation strategy resulted in less GVHD and in better failure-free and overall survival for patients with CML.[86] This strategy is limited to patients with relapse of indolent diseases and has been applied successfully in relapsed myeloma, HL, and NHL.[84]

It is not completely clear why dose escalation of DLI limits GVHD. It is possible that the initial low dose of donor T cells may be sufficient to induce GVT without causing clinically apparent GVHD. For instance, it may be that low-dose DLI will take a long time to generate a GVT reaction, and the dose escalation technique results in the same outcome as giving low doses and waiting longer. However, it is also possible that the process of dose escalation over time results in generation of anergy and/or suppressor T cells that serve to limit acute GVHD. This is supported by studies that compared recipients of DLI given in large doses with those who received similar doses of T cells given by a process of dose escalation over time; GVHD was still less in patients receiving the same number of cells given by a delayed dose escalation strategy.[53]

An exciting strategy to limit GVHD toxicity from DLI is the use of donor lymphocytes transfected with the herpes simplex virus thymidine kinase (*HSV-TK*) suicide gene. Expression of *HSV-TK* confers sensitivity of these cells to ganciclovir. *HSV-TK*-transfected donor cells have been given to patients with posttransplantation B-cell lymphoproliferative disorders (see section titled "Adoptive Immunotherapy for Nonrelapse Complications after Allogeneic HSCT"), and complete remissions were complicated by acute GVHD, as anticipated. Complete resolution of GVHD occurred after patients were treated with ganciclovir.[95,96] In addition, although ganciclovir significantly decreased the number of circulating cells containing the transduced gene, they were detectable for up to 12 months after infusion.[95] Unfortunately, rapid immune responses against HSV-TK developed often, resulting in disappearance of the gene-modified cells.[97] Undoubtedly, in the future, the use of gene-modified DLI will have broader applications in the treatment of a variety of posttransplantation complications and may provide one of the most effective and safest approaches to limiting the toxicity of therapy. Unfortunately, at the present time, this therapy is cumbersome and time consuming and therefore impractical for the majority of patients.

Other modifications of DLI have also attempted to preserve GVT reactivity while minimizing the potential for GVHD. One trial tested irradiated DLI; preliminary data suggest that these cells may retain GVT activity and may minimize GVHD.[98]

Several groups are exploring the possibility of administering leukemia-specific or tissue-specific T cells generated after selection and in-vitro expansion.[99-101] Minor histocompatibility antigens may be important targets for this approach.[102,103] Preliminary data in small numbers of patients demonstrate that this strategy is feasible and can induce CR for relapsed CML, with minimal toxicity. These experiments also lend further support to the idea that CD4+ T cells are capable of inducing GVT with minimal GVHD.

Vaccinating patients with tumor-specific, tumor-associated, or over-expressed antigens is another potentially powerful method to enhance donor T-cell function. Unfortunately, in most cases, these antigens are poorly defined. In myeloid malignancies, over-expressed proteinase-3 may be an important target antigen, and preliminary studies suggest that vaccination with the PR-1 epitope of proteinase-3 can induce a significant anti-leukemia immune response.[104] Other potentially important antigens that are being explored as targets for vaccination include minor histocompatibility antigens, BCR/ABL (in CML), Wilm's tumor-1 protein, PRAME (preferentially expressed antigen in melanoma), and even the use of gene-modified tumor cells.[104-107]

Given the difficulty generating tumor-specific cellular therapies, the authors have tested the ability of donor T cells activated and expanded ex-vivo through co-stimulation to induce GVT responses in patients with relapse. The hypothesis is that DLI may not be effective because of limited T-cell activation (perhaps because of lack of co-stimulatory molecules on tumor targets, in-vivo suppression of activation, or other mechanisms that can be overcome by ex-vivo activation and co-stimulation). Initial studies showed this approach is safe, with intriguing responses in patients anticipated to have poor responses to conventional DLI.[108]

Other effector cells are likely to be important in GVT induction, at least in some cases. NK cells can lyse tumor cells in vitro and are important effectors for GVT induction after haploidentical transplant.[109] Studies are underway testing adoptive transfer of donor NK cells to treat relapsed leukemia and other cancers after HSCT.[16]

Numerous other strategies are in clinical development to enhance specificity and activity of donor immunotherapy. It is now possible to dissect the immune response and use infusions of regulatory T cells to either enhance activity or limit toxicity.[110] Technology also now allows targeting of cytotoxic T cells to tumor cells through gene modification with chimeric antigen receptors or bifunctional antibodies.[111,112] These and other novel studies will continue to explore methods to improve the specificity, efficacy, and safety of DLI.

Prophylactic DLI

Donor leukapheresis products are clearly important reagents for GVT induction to treat relapse, but they may be as useful, if not more

so, in *preventing* relapsed leukemia after allogeneic HSCT. Because low-dose DLI is effective for minimal residual disease with less complicating toxicity, it is logical to use it before overt relapse. Some patients can be identified whose minimal residual disease puts them at high risk for clinical relapse; for instance, patients with CML who have sequential positive PCR results for *bcr/abl* mRNA transcripts.[113] These patients should be considered appropriate candidates for low-dose donor MNC infusions at the time of PCR positivity for *bcr/abl* mRNA, but before hematologic relapse. DLI given to patients with CML and MRD is quite effective, resulting in 100% responses in some cases[114] and emphasizing the role of DLI with minimal tumor burdens. For ALL, it is possible to use mixed chimerism as a surrogate for impending relapse and use prophylactic DLI presumably at the time of MRD.[71,115] In other settings, prophylactic DLI has been most useful after T-cell depletion of the original donor graft. T-cell depletion may improve the safety of transplantation, and delayed DLI is given in an effort to restore GVT activity. This approach is being increasingly applied in the setting of nonmyeloablative allogeneic HSCT using in-vivo, T-cell-depleting antibodies.[84] It may also be useful for patients at high risk of relapse determined by disease status or chimerism studies after transplantation.[116-118]

The timing and dosing of DLI used as prophylaxis may be critical, at least in terms of safety. The Seattle group attempted to augment GVT activity by either limiting GVHD prophylaxis or by giving donor buffy-coat cells to patients at the time of transplantation.[119,120] Unfortunately, while this increased the incidence of significant GVHD, no improvement in relapse rates or survival was identified. A similar trial designed to enhance GVHD at the time of transplantation by withholding GVHD prophylaxis did show an improvement in relapse rate and survival,[121] although follow-up was short; it is possible that this approach would provide a clinically important GVT effect for a small group of patients, but toxicity is expected to be significant. The lack of apparent GVT activity in trials inducing GVHD at the time of

HSCT may be related, at least in part, to the inclusion of only those patients with advanced leukemia who were at high risk for relapse and toxicity. However, it is also likely that the administration of donor T cells or attenuation of GVHD prophylaxis at the time of transplantation will increase significantly the toxicity associated with the transplant, possibly to unacceptable levels.

There are considerable data to suggest that GVHD may be milder if it is dissociated from other insults associated with transplantation (eg, toxicity related to the conditioning regimen, tissue damage, and infections). In dogs, allogeneic lymphocytes can be administered without undue toxicity only after chimerism has been established.[122] In mice, the administration of donor lymphocytes at the time of transplantation results in severe GVHD, whereas, when given 21 days after conditioning therapy, donor lymphocytes will provide a potent GVT effect without inducing severe GVHD.[123] Similar findings have been noted in other murine models.[124] The lack of significant GVHD in this setting may be the result of the separation of the cytokine phases that occur after transplantation,[125] suggesting that donor T cells may be given safely to patients to prevent relapse if appropriately delayed from the acute transplant setting.

This hypothesis is being tested clinically, and results confirm that delayed DLI is likely to be safer than GVT induction at the time of transplantation. Initial data suggest that prophylactic DLI can be given safely after T-cell-depleted HPCs are given, with reasonable toxicity from GVHD.[64,126,127] Data from the National Institutes of Health[126] showed that 2×10^6 donor T cells per kg given on day 30 and 1×10^7 T cells per kg given on day 45 resulted in acceptable severity of acute GVHD, but 1×10^7 T cells per kg given on day 30 resulted in 100% incidence of acute GVHD. This suggests that the dose and timing of delayed DLI critically affect toxicity. However, of 38 patients treated, only 2 suffered a hematologic relapse of CML, suggesting that delayed DLI will restore GVT activity. Slavin and colleagues have also given incremental T-cell infusions to patients after T-

cell-depleted allogeneic HSCT,[128,129] beginning on either day +1 or day +28 and repeated weekly or monthly. Their initial results showed that T-cell reinfusions resulted in an increase in GVHD but no improvement in event-free survival. Donor T-cell reinfusions resulted in a statistically insignificant trend toward lower relapse rates only in recipients of Campath-1M (anti-CD52 rat IgM)-treated marrow. Delayed DLI has also been used after T-cell-depleted allogeneic transplantations for myeloma; when 1 to 3×10^7 CD4+ cells per kg were given 6 to 9 months after transplantation, 50% of patients developed significant acute or chronic GVHD, an incidence higher than that reported from delayed DLI in other trials.[64] However, significant graft-vs-myeloma therapy was noted as six of 10 patients with residual disease achieved a complete response. Elimination of MRD has been noted in other patients with myeloma, NHL, and HL, who were given prophylactic DLI with encouraging response rates.[84,130]

Unfortunately, in many cases prophylactic DLI cannot be given because of clinical complications of transplantation. In addition, it is often difficult to predict which patients represent the highest risk for relapse. Taken together, the experimental and clinical data indicate that posttransplantation cellular immunotherapy can be performed safely and effectively, but optimization of patient selection, cell dose, and timing of administration may all serve to enhance the potential GVT effects.

Cytokine-Mediated Immunotherapy

The effector mechanisms for GVT are poorly defined, but it is increasingly clear that both GVT and GVHD result from a complex interaction of effector cells and cytokines[125]; therefore, it is logical to expect that qualitative and quantitative changes in cytokine production may influence GVT reactivity. IL-2 is the cytokine studied most extensively in the transplant setting because of its ability to augment the immune system,[131] and there is substantial indirect evidence suggesting that IL-2-activated NK cells may enhance GVT reactivity. The ability of NK cells to lyse tumor cells in vitro can be enhanced by in-vitro exposure to IL-2.[132,133] In addition, NK cell number and activity are increased in the peripheral blood of patients after hematopoietic transplantation,[132,134] and for patients with CML who received T-cell-depleted marrow grafts, the ability of IL-2-stimulated peripheral blood MNCs to lyse leukemic targets may correlate with protection from relapse.[132]

Several trials have shown that IL-2 can be administered safely after either autologous or allogeneic HSCT.[34,123,135-137] After T-cell-depleted allogeneic transplantation, the administration of low-dose IL-2 (200,000 to 500,000 units/m^2) results in up to a 10-fold increase in the number of circulating NK cells,[137] and initial data indicate that relapse rates may be lower in the patients receiving low-dose IL-2 than in similar control patients. This suggests that IL-2 might restore GVT reactivity for recipients of T-cell-depleted allogeneic grafts. It is curious that IL-2 in this setting has not resulted in enhanced GVHD; perhaps it is because at low doses it may activate NK cells selectively without additional T-cell stimulation.

IL-2 has also been used in combination with DLI to enhance GVT activity. In some cases, patients who did not respond to DLI entered CR only after the administration of either in-vitro IL-2-activated donor T cells or DLI and in-vivo administration of IL-2.[66,138] Slavin and coworkers described 11 patients who received IL-2- augmented cellular immunotherapy, and only three developed grade II (n = 2) or III (n = 1) acute GVHD, suggesting that IL-2 will not result in an unacceptable GVHD risk. Five of 11 patients treated previously only with DLI responded after the addition of IL-2, suggesting that it may be possible to enhance GVT activity with cytokine activation.[66]

Adoptive Immunotherapy for Nonrelapse Complications After Allogeneic HSCT

Donor leukocyte products are important new reagents, not only for GVT induction but also for treating other posttransplant complications. The best example is the use of DLI to treat posttransplant, Epstein-Barr virus (EBV)-associated, B-cell lymphoproliferative disorders (BLPD). The incidence of these aggressive lymphomas is particularly high in recipients of T-cell-depleted marrow grafts.[29,139] The lymphomas tend to be of donor origin and presumably arise from uncontrolled proliferation of EBV-infected B cells in the absence of appropriate virus-specific cytotoxic T lymphocytes. In the past, BLPD after allogeneic HSCT has been associated with very high mortality and little effective therapy.[140] DLI consistently induces sustained remissions in patients with these lymphomas.[141-143] It has also been used to reverse life-threatening adenoviral[144] and respiratory syncytial virus[145] infections after receipt of allogeneic grafts and to prevent cytomegalovirus infection.[146] Because unselected DLI may induce significant GVHD, investigators have shown that it is possible to generate EBV-specific T cells from allogeneic marrow donors and that up to 1×10^8 cells/kg can be given safely to control proliferation of EBV-infected B cells and protect against BLPD in high-risk patients.[143,147,148] No doubt, DLI will be useful in treating other posttransplant infectious complications in which it is important to restore cell-mediated immunity.

Conclusion

Fifty years of patient study have revealed substantial insights into the use of allogeneic cells to control both cancers and nonmalignant diseases. The progress from Barnes and Loutit's initial inference based on an experiment in mice to the large-scale adoption in clinical practice is a striking testimony to the insight of these early scientists. The potent allogeneic GVT effects demonstrated so elegantly with the use of DLI are now being rapidly applied clinically to enhance the safety of allogeneic HSCT. Transplantations are now performed with rapidly increasing frequency, using a reduced-intensity but immunosuppressive conditioning regimen. This results in consistent engraftment and relies heavily on graft-vs-leukemia activity to treat the patients with hematologic malignancies. Several excellent reviews on this topic are available.[149-151] On the immediate horizon are new techniques to enhance GVT while avoiding GVHD. The use of cellular vaccines and graft engineering is likely to result in improvements in outcomes for specific malignancies. As the understanding of the immune system and anti-tumor immunoreactivity is rapidly increasing, the ability to select, expand, and infuse cells with increased reactivity or specific regulatory functions will also increase the specificity of GVT induction. Gene-modification of donor cells to redirect targeting also holds great promise to enhance the specificity of GVT activity. Many areas of study using human immune cells collected by apheresis as direct anticancer therapy are rapidly progressing. The greatest challenges are to determine why there is no GVT effect in all cancers and to find ways of harnessing the allogeneic effect for the management of the resistant malignancies.

References

1. Barnes D, Corp M, Loutit J, Neal F. Treatment of murine leukaemia with X rays and homologous bone marrow. Preliminary communication. Br Med J 1956;2:626-30.
2. Barnes D, Loutit J. Treatment of murine leukaemia with X-rays and homologous bone marrow. Br J Haematol 1957;3:241-52.
3. Korngold R, Sprent J. T cell subsets and graft-versus-host disease. Transplant 1987;44:335-9.
4. Sykes M, Romick M, Sachs D. Interleukin 2 prevents graft-versus-host disease while preserving the graft-versus-leukemia effect of allogeneic T cells. Proc Natl Acad Sci U S A 1990; 87:5633-7.
5. Truitt RL, Johnson BD, McCabe CM, Weiler MB. Graft versus leukemia. In: Ferrara JLM, Deeg HJ, Burakoff SJ, eds. Graft-vs-host disease. 2nd ed. New York: Marcel Dekker, 1997:385-424.
6. Truitt R, Shih C, Lefever A, et al. Characterization of alloimmunization-induced T lymphocytes reactive against AKR leukemia in vitro

and correlation with graft-vs-leukemia activity in vivo. J Immunol 1983;131:2050-8.
7. Vourka-Karussis U, Karussis D, Ackerstein A, Slavin S. Enhancement of a GVL effect with rhIL-2 following BMT in a murine model for acute myeloid leukemia. Exp Hematol 1995; 23:196-201.
8. Weiss L, Reich S, Slavin S. Use of recombinant human interleukin-2 in conjunction with bone marrow transplantation as a model for control of minimal residual disease in malignant hematological disorders. Treatment of murine leukemia in conjunction with allogenic bone marrow transplantation and IL2-activated cell-mediated immunotherapy. Cancer Invest 1992;10: 19-26.
9. Johnson B, Truitt R. A decrease in graft-vs-host disease without loss of graft-vs-leukemia reactivity after MHC matched bone marrow transplantation by selective depletion of donor NK cells in vivo. Transplantation 1992;54:104-12.
10. Okunewick J, Kociban D, Machen L, Buffo M. Evidence for a possible role of asialo-GM1-positive cells in the graft-versus-leukemia repression of a murine type-C retroviral leukemia. Bone Marrow Transplant 1995;16:451-6.
11. Johnson BD, Dagher N, Stankowski WC, et al. Donor natural killer (NK1.1+) cells do not play a role in the suppression of GVHD or in the mediation of GVL reactions after DLI. Biol Blood Marrow Transplant 2001;7:589-95.
12. Sykes M, Abraham V, Harty M, Pearson D. IL-2 reduces graft-versus-host disease and preserves a graft-versus-leukemia effect by selectively inhibiting CD4+ T cell activity. J Immunol 1993;150:197-205.
13. Pan L, Teshima T, Hill GR, et al. Granulocyte colony-stimulating factor-mobilized allogeneic stem cell transplantation maintains graft-versus-leukemia effects through a perforin-dependent pathway while preventing graft-versus-host disease. Blood 1999;93:4071-8.
14. Tsukada N, Kobata T, Aizawa Y, et al. Graft-versus-leukemia effect and graft-versus-host disease can be differentiated by cytotoxic mechanisms in a murine model of allogeneic bone marrow transplantation. Blood 1999;93: 2738-47.
15. Ruggeri L, Capanni M, Urbani E, et al. Effectiveness of donor natural killer cell alloreactivity in mismatched hematopoietic transplants (comment). Science 2002;295:2097-100.
16. Miller JS, Soignier Y, Panoskaltsis-Mortari A, et al. Successful adoptive transfer and in vivo

expansion of human haploidentical NK cells in patients with cancer. Blood 2005;105:3051-7.

17. Horowitz M, Gale R, Sondel P, et al. Graft-versus-leukemia reactions after bone marrow transplantation. Blood 1990;75:555-62.

18. Odom L, August C, Githens J, et al. Remission of relapsed leukaemia during a graft-versus-host reaction. A "graft-versus-leukaemia reaction" in man? Lancet 1978;2:537-40.

19. Collins R, Rogers Z, Bennett M, et al. Hematologic relapse of chronic myelogenous leukemia following allogeneic bone marrow transplantation: Apparent graft-versus-leukemia effect following abrupt discontinuation of immunosuppression. Bone Marrow Transplant 1992;10: 391-5.

20. Higano C, Brixey M, Bryant E, et al. Durable complete remission of acute nonlymphocytic leukemia associated with discontinuation of immunosuppression following relapse after allogeneic bone marrow transplantation. A case report of a probable graft-versus-leukemia effect. Transplantation 1990;50:175-7.

21. Sullivan K, Shulman H. Chronic graft-versus-host disease, obliterative bronchiolitis, and graft-versus-leukemia effect: Case histories. Transplant Proc 1989;21:51-62.

22. Fefer A, Sullivan K, Weiden P, et al. Graft versus leukemia effect in man: The relapse rate of acute leukemia is lower after allogeneic than after syngeneic marrow transplantation. In: Truitt R, Gale R, Bortin M, eds. Cellular immunotherapy of cancer. New York: AR Liss, 1987: 401-8.

23. Gale R, Champlin R. How does bone-marrow transplantation cure leukaemia? Lancet 1984; 2:28-30.

24. Gale R, Horowitz M, Ash R, et al. Identical-twin bone marrow transplants for leukemia. Ann Intern Med 1994;120:646-52.

25. Sullivan K, Weiden P, Storb R, et al. Influence of acute and chronic graft-versus-host disease on relapse and survival after bone marrow transplantation from HLA-identical siblings as treatment of acute and chronic leukemia. Blood 1989;73:1720-8.

26. Weiden P, Flournoy N, Thomas ED, et al. Antileukemic effect of graft-versus-host disease in human recipients of allogeneic-marrow grafts. N Engl J Med 1979;300:1068-73.

27. Weiden P, Sullivan K, Flournoy N, et al. Antileukemic effect of chronic graft-versus-host disease. Contribution to improved survival after

allogeneic marrow transplantation. N Engl J Med 1981;304:1529-33.

28. Goldman JM, Gale RP, Horowitz MM, et al. Bone marrow transplantation for chronic myelogenous leukemia in chronic phase. Increased risk for relapse associated with T-cell depletion. Ann Intern Med 1988;108:806-14.

29. Antin J, Bierer B, Smith B, et al. Selective depletion of bone marrow T lymphocytes with anti-CD5 monoclonal antibodies: Effective prophylaxis for graft-versus-host disease in patients with hematologic malignancies. Blood 1991;78:2139-49.

30. Aversa F, Terenzi A, Carotti A, et al. Improved outcome with T-cell-depleted bone marrow transplantation for acute leukemia. J Clin Oncol 1999;17:1545-50.

31. Champlin R. T-cell depletion for allogeneic bone marrow transplantation: Impact on graft-versus-host disease, engraftment, and graft-versus-leukemia. J Hematother 1993;2:27-42.

32. Marmont A, Horowitz M, Gale R, et al. T-cell depletion of HLA-identical transplants in leukemia. Blood 1991;78:2120-30.

33. Papadopoulos EB, Carabasi MH, Castro-Malaspina H, et al. T-cell-depleted allogeneic bone marrow transplantation as postremission therapy for acute myelogenous leukemia: Freedom from relapse in the absence of graft-versus-host disease. Blood 1998;91:1083-90.

34. Soiffer R, Murray C, Mauch P, et al. Prevention of graft-versus-host disease by selective depletion of CD6-positive T lymphocytes from donor bone marrow. J Clin Oncol 1992;10: 1191-200.

35. Apperley J, Mauro F, Goldman J, et al. Bone marrow transplantation for chronic myeloid leukaemia in first chronic phase: Importance of a graft-versus-leukaemia effect. Br J Haematol 1988;69:239-45.

36. Goldman J, Apperley J, Jones L, et al. Bone marrow transplantation for patients with chronic myeloid leukemia. N Engl J Med 1986; 314:202-7.

37. Mitsuyasu R, Champlin R, Gale R, et al. Treatment of donor bone marrow with monoclonal anti-T-cell antibody and complement for the prevention of graft-versus-host disease. Ann Intern Med 1986;105:20-6.

38. Goldman J, Gale R, Horowitz M, et al. Bone marrow transplantation for chronic myelogenous leukemia in chronic phase. Ann Intern Med 1988;108:806-14.

39. Arcese W, Goldman J, D'Arcangelo E, et al. Outcome for patients who relapse after allogeneic bone marrow transplantation for chronic myeloid leukemia. Blood 1993;82:3211-19.

40. Mrsíc M, Horowitz M, Atkinson K, et al. Second HLA-identical sibling transplants for leukemia recurrence. Bone Marrow Transplant 1992;9: 269-75.

41. Radich J, Sanders J, Buckner C, et al. Second allogeneic marrow transplantation for patients with recurrent leukemia after initial transplant with total-body irradiation-containing regimens. J Clin Oncol 1993;11:304-13.

42. Kolb H, Mittermuller J, Clemm C, et al. Donor leukocyte transfusions for treatment of recurrent chronic myelogenous leukemia in marrow transplant patients. Blood 1990;76:2462-5.

43. Drobyski W, Keever C, Roth M, et al. Salvage immunotherapy using donor leukocyte infusions as treatment for relapsed chronic myelogenous leukemia after allogeneic bone marrow transplantation: Efficacy and toxicity of a defined T-cell dose. Blood 1993;82:2310-18.

44. Porter D, Roth M, McGarigle C, et al. Induction of graft-versus-host disease as immunotherapy for relapsed chronic myeloid leukemia. N Engl J Med 1994;330:100-6.

45. Mackinnon S, Papadopoulos E, Carabasi M, et al. Adoptive immunotherapy evaluating escalating doses of donor leukocytes for relapse of chronic myeloid leukemia after bone marrow transplantation: Separation of graft-versus-leukemia responses from graft-versus-host disease. Blood 1995;86:1261-8.

46. van Rhee F, Lin F, Cullis J, et al. Relapse of chronic myeloid leukemia after allogeneic bone marrow transplant: The case for giving donor leukocyte transfusions before the onset of hematologic relapse. Blood 1994;83:3377-83.

47. Roth M, Antin J, Bingham E, Ginsberg D. Detection of Philadelphia chromosome-positive cells by the polymerase chain reaction following bone marrow transpant for chronic myelogenous leukemia. Blood 1989;74:882-5.

48. Antin J. Graft-versus-leukemia: No longer an epiphenomenon. Blood 1993;82:2273-7.

49. Collins R, Shpilberg O, Drobyski W, et al. Donor leukocyte infusions in 140 patients with relapsed malignancy after allogeneic bone marrow transplantation. J Clin Oncol 1997;15: 433-44.

50. Kolb H, Schattenberg A, Goldman J, et al. Graft-versus-leukemia effect of donor lympho-cyte transfusions in marrow grafted patients. Blood 1995;86:2041-50.

51. Porter D, Collins R, Shpilberg O, et al. Long-term follow-up of patients who achieved complete remission after donor leukocyte infusions. Biol Blood Marrow Transplant 1999;5:253-61.

52. Dazzi F, Szydlo RM, Cross NC, et al. Durability of responses following donor lymphocyte infusions for patients who relapse after allogeneic stem cell transplantation for chronic myeloid leukemia. Blood 2000;96:2712-16.

53. Dazzi F, Szydlo RM, Craddock C, et al. Comparison of single-dose and escalating-dose regimens of donor lymphocyte infusion for relapse after allografting for chronic myeloid leukemia. Blood 2000;95:67-71.

54. Levine J, Braun T, Penza S, et al. Prospective trial of chemotherapy and donor leukocyte infusions for relapse of advanced myeloid malignancies after allogeneic stem cell transplantation. J Clin Oncol 2002;20:405-12.

55. Schmid C, Labopin M, Nagler A, et al. Donor lymphocyte infusion in the treatment of first hematological relapse after allogeneic stem-cell transplantation in adults with acute myeloid leukemia: A retrospective risk factors analysis and comparison with other strategies by the EBMT Acute Leukemia Working Party. J Clin Oncol 2007;25:4938-45.

56. Collins RH Jr, Goldstein S, Giralt S, et al. Donor leukocyte infusions in acute lymphocytic leukemia. Bone Marrow Transplant 2000;26:511-16.

57. Choi SJ, Lee JH, Kim S, et al. Treatment of relapsed acute lymphoblastic leukemia after allogeneic bone marrow transplantation with chemotherapy followed by G-CSF-primed donor leukocyte infusion: A prospective study. Bone Marrow Transplant 2005;36:163-9.

58. Campregher PV, Gooley T, Scott BL, et al. Results of donor lymphocyte infusions for relapsed myelodysplastic syndrome after hematopoietic cell transplantation. Bone Marrow Transplant 2007;40:965-71.

59. Mandigers CM, Raemaekers JM, Schattenberg AV, et al. Allogeneic bone marrow transplantation with T-cell-depleted marrow grafts for patients with poor-risk relapsed low-grade non-Hodgkin's lymphoma. Br J Haematol 1998; 100:198-206.

60. van Besien K, de Lima M, Giralt S, et al. Management of lymphoma recurrence after allogeneic transplantation: The relevance of graft-

versus-lymphoma effect. Bone Marrow Transplant 1997;19:977-82.

61. Lokhorst HM, Schattenberg A, Cornelissen JJ, et al. Donor leukocyte infusions are effective in relapsed multiple myeloma after allogeneic bone marrow transplantation. Blood 1997;90: 4206-11.

62. Lokhorst HM, Schattenberg A, Cornelissen JJ, et al. Donor lymphocyte infusions for relapsed multiple myeloma after allogeneic stem-cell transplantation: Predictive factors for response and long-term outcome. J Clin Oncol 2000;18: 3031-7.

63. Salama M, Nevill T, Marcellus D, et al. Donor leukocyte infusions for multiple myeloma. Bone Marrow Transplant 2000;26:1179-84.

64. Alyea E, Weller E, Schlossman R, et al. T-cell-depleted allogeneic bone marrow transplantation followed by donor lymphocyte infusion in patients with multiple myeloma: Induction of graft-versus-myeloma effect. Blood 2001;98: 934-9.

65. Porter D, Roth M, Lee S, et al. Adoptive immunotherapy with donor mononuclear cell infusions to treat relapse of acute leukemia or myelodysplasia after allogeneic bone marrow transplantation. Bone Marrow Transplant 1996; 18:975-80.

66. Slavin S, Naparstek E, Nagler A, et al. Allogeneic cell therapy with donor peripheral blood cells and recombinant human interleukin-2 to treat leukemia relapse after allogeneic bone marrow transplantation. Blood 1996;87:2195-204.

67. Szer J, Grigg A, Phillipos G, Sheridan W. Donor leucocyte infusions after chemotherapy for patients relapsing with acute leukaemia following allogeneic BMT. Bone Marrow Transplant 1993;11:109-11.

68. Choi SJ, Lee JH, Kim S, et al. Treatment of relapsed acute myeloid leukemia after allogeneic bone marrow transplantation with chemotherapy followed by G-CSF-primed donor leukocyte infusion: A high incidence of isolated extramedullary relapse. Leukemia 2004;18: 1789-97.

69. Bader P, Klingebiel T, Schaudt A, et al. Prevention of relapse in pediatric patients with acute leukemias and MDS after allogeneic SCT by early immunotherapy initiated on the basis of increasing mixed chimerism: A single center experience of 12 children. Leukemia 1999;13: 2079-86.

70. Bader P, Beck J, Schlegel PG, et al. Additional immunotherapy on the basis of increasing mixed hematopoietic chimerism after allogeneic BMT in children with acute leukemia: Is there an option to prevent relapse? Bone Marrow Transplant 1997;20:79-81.

71. Bader P, Kreyenberg H, Hoelle W, et al. Increasing mixed chimerism is an important prognostic factor for unfavorable outcome in children with acute lymphoblastic leukemia after allogeneic stem-cell transplantation: Possible role for pre-emptive immunotherapy? J Clin Oncol 2004;22:1696-705.

72. Tricot G, Vesole D, Jagannath S, et al. Graft-versus-myeloma effect: Proof of principle. Blood 1996;87:1196-8.

73. van de Donk NW, Kroger N, Hegenbart U, et al. Prognostic factors for donor lymphocyte infusions following non-myeloablative allogeneic stem cell transplantation in multiple myeloma. Bone Marrow Transplant 2006;37: 1135-41.

74. Jones R, Ambinder R, Piantadosi S, Santos G. Evidence of a graft-versus-lymphoma effect associated with allogeneic bone marrow transplantation. Blood 1991;77:649-53.

75. Ratanatharathorn V, Uberti J, Karanes C, et al. Prospective comparative trial of autologous versus allogeneic bone marrow transplantation in patients with non-Hodgkin's lymphoma. Blood 1994;84:1050-5.

76. Porter D, Stadtmauer EA, Lazarus H. "GVHD": Graft-versus host disease or graft-versus Hodgkin's disease? An old acronym with new meaning. Bone Marrow Transplant 2003;31: 739-46.

77. Armand P, Kim HT, Ho VT, et al. Allogeneic transplantation with reduced-intensity conditioning for Hodgkin and non-Hodgkin lymphoma: Importance of histology for outcome. Biol Blood Marrow Transplant 2008;14:418-25.

78. Peggs KS, Hunter A, Chopra R, et al. Clinical evidence of a graft-versus-Hodgkin's-lymphoma effect after reduced-intensity allogeneic transplantation. Lancet 2005;365:1934-41.

79. Russell L, Jacobsen N, Heilmann C, et al. Treatment of relapse after allogeneic BMT with donor leukocyte infusions in 16 patients. Bone Marrow Transplant 1996;18:411-14.

80. Bloor AJ, Thomson K, Chowdhry N, et al. High response rate to donor lymphocyte infusion after allogeneic stem cell transplantation for

indolent non-Hodgkin lymphoma. Biol Blood Marrow Transplant 2008;14:50-8.

81. Marks DI, Lush R, Cavenagh J, et al. The toxicity and efficacy of donor lymphocyte infusions given after reduced-intensity conditioning allogeneic stem cell transplantation. Blood 2002; 100:3108-14.

82. Porter D, Collins R, Hardy C, et al. Treatment of relapsed leukemia after unrelated donor marrow transplantation with unrelated donor leukocyte infusions. Blood 2000;95:1214-21.

83. van Rhee R, Savage D, Blackwell J, et al. Adoptive immunotherapy for relapse of chronic myeloid leukemia after allogeneic bone marrow transplant: Equal efficacy of lymphocytes from sibling and matched unrelated donors. Bone Marrow Transplant 1998;21:1055-61.

84. Peggs KS, Thomson K, Hart DP, et al. Dose-escalated donor lymphocyte infusions following reduced intensity transplantation: Toxicity, chimerism, and disease responses (comment). Blood 2004;103:1548-56.

85. Porter DL. The graft-versus-tumor potential of allogeneic cell therapy: An update on donor leukocyte infusions and nonmyeloablative allogeneic stem cell transplantation. J Hematother Stem Cell Res 2001;10:465-80.

86. Guglielmi C, Arcese W, Dazzi F, et al. Donor lymphocyte infusion for relapsed chronic myelogenous leukemia: Prognostic relevance of the initial cell dose. Blood 2002;100:397-405.

87. Anderson K, Weinstein H. Transfusion-associated graft-versus-host disease. N Engl J Med 1990;323:315-21.

88. Flowers M, Leisenring W, Beach K, et al. Granulocyte colony-stimulating factor given to donors before apheresis does not prevent aplasia in patients treated with donor leukocyte infusion for recurrent chronic myeloid leukemia after bone marrow transplantation. Biol Blood Marrow Transplant 2000;6:321-6.

89. Keil F, Haas OA, Fritsch G, et al. Donor leukocyte infusion for leukemic relapse after allogeneic marrow transplantation: Lack of residual donor hematopoiesis predicts aplasia. Blood 1997;89:3113-17.

90. Pan L, Delmonte J, Jalonen C, Ferrara L. Pretreatment of donor mice with granulocyte colony-stimulating factor polarizes donor T lymphocytes toward type-2 cytokine production and reduces severity of experimental graft-versus-host disease. Blood 1995;86:4422-9.

91. Nimer S, Giorgi J, Gajewski J, et al. Selective depletion of CD8+ cells for prevention of graft-versus-host disease after bone marrow transplantation. Transplant 1994;57:82-7.

92. Alyea E, Soiffer R, Canning C, et al. Toxicity and efficacy of defined doses of CD4+ donor lymphocytes for treatment of relapse after allogeneic bone marrow transplant. Blood 1998; 91:3671-80.

93. Giralt S, Hester J, Huh Y, et al. CD8-depleted donor lymphocyte infusion as treatment for relapsed chronic myelogenous leukemia after allogeneic bone marrow transplantation. Blood 1995;86:4337-43.

94. Shimoni A, Gajewski J, Donato M, et al. Long-term follow-up of recipients of CD8 depleted donor lymphocyte infusions for the treatment of chronic myelogenous leukemia relapsing after allogeneic progenitor cell transplantation. Biol Blood Marrow Transplant 2001;7:568-75.

95. Bonini C, Ferrari G, Verzeletti S, et al. HSV-TK gene transfer into donor lymphocytes for control of allogeneic graft-versus-leukemia. Science 1997;276:1719-24.

96. Servida P, Rossini S, Traversari C, et al. Gene transfer into peripheral blood lymphocytes for in vivo immunomodulation of donor anti-tumor immunity in a patient affected by EBV-induced lymphoma. Blood 1993;82:214a.

97. Berger C, Flowers ME, Warren EH, et al. Analysis of transgene-specific immune responses that limit the in vivo persistence of adoptively transferred HSV-TK-modified donor T cells after allogeneic hematopoietic cell transplantation. Blood 2006;107:2294-302.

98. Waller EK, Ship AM, Mittelstaedt S, et al. Irradiated donor leukocytes promote engraftment of allogeneic bone marrow in major histocompatibility complex mismatched recipients without causing graft-versus-host disease. Blood 1999;94:3222-33.

99. Falkenburg JH, Heslop HE, Barrett AJ. T cell therapy in allogeneic stem cell transplantation. Biol Blood Marrow Transplant 2008;14:136-41. (Erratum in: Biol Blood Marrow Transplant 2008;14:1317-18.)

100. Falkenburg JH, Wafelman AR, Joosten P, et al. Complete remission of accelerated phase chronic myeloid leukemia by treatment with leukemia-reactive cytotoxic T lymphocytes. Blood 1999;94:1201-8.

101. Mutis T, Verdijk R, Schrama E, et al. Feasibility of immunotherapy of relapsed leukemia with ex vivo-generated cytotoxic T lymphocytes specific for hematopoietic system-restricted

minor histocompatibility antigens. Blood 1999;
93:2336-41.

102. Falkenburg J, Wafelman A, van Bergen C, et al.
Leukemia-reactive cytotoxic T lymphocytes
(CTL) induce complete remission in a patient
with refractory accelerated phase chronic myeloid leukemia (CML). Blood 1997;90:589a.

103. Warren EH, Gavin M, Greenberg PD, Riddell
SR. Minor histocompatibility antigens as targets for T-cell therapy after bone marrow
transplantation. Curr Opin Hematol 1998;5:
429-33.

104. Molldrem JJ. Vaccination for leukemia. Biol
Blood Marrow Transplant 2006;12:13-18.

105. Rezvani K, Yong AS, Mielke S, et al. Leukemia-
associated antigen-specific T-cell responses following combined PR1 and WT1 peptide vaccination in patients with myeloid malignancies.
Blood 2008;111:236-42.

106. Ho V, Vanneman M, Kim H, et al. Biologic
activity of irradiated, autologous, GM-CSF-
secreting leukemia cell vaccines early after
allogeneic stem cell transplantation. Proc Natl
Acad Sci U S A 2009;106:15825-30.

107. Keilholz U, Letsch A, Busse A, et al. A clinical
and immunologic Phase 2 trial of Wilms tumor
gene product 1 (WT1) peptide vaccination in
patients with AML and MDS. Blood
2009;113:6541-8.

108. Porter DL, Levine BL, Bunin N, et al. A Phase
1 trial of donor lymphocyte infusions expanded
and activated ex vivo via CD3/CD28 costimulation. Blood 2006;107:1325-31.

109. Gill S, Olson JA, Negrin RS. Natural killer cells
in allogeneic transplantation: Effect on engraftment, graft- versus-tumor, and graft-versus-host
responses. Biol Blood Marrow Transplant
2009;15:765-76.

110. Fowler DH, Odom J, Steinberg SM, et al. Phase
I clinical trial of costimulated, IL-4 polarized
donor CD4+ T cells as augmentation of allogeneic hematopoietic cell transplantation. Biol
Blood Marrow Transplant 2006;12:1150-60.

111. Milone M, Fish J, Carpentito C, et al. Chimeric
receptors containing CD137 signal transduction domains mediate enhanced survival of T
cells and increased anti-leukemic efficacy in
vivo. Mol Ther 2009;17:1453-64.

112. Buhmann R, Simoes B, Stanglmaier M, et al.
Immunotherapy of recurrent B-cell malignancies after allo-SCT with Bi20 (FBTA05), a tri-
functional anti-CD3 x anti-CD20 antibody and
donor lymphocyte infusion. Bone Marrow
Transplant 2009;43:383-97.

113. Roth M, Antin J, Ash R, et al. Prognostic significance of Philadelphia chromosome-positive
cells detected by the polymerase chain reaction
after allogeneic bone marrow transplant for
chronic myelogenous leukemia. Blood 1992;
79:276-82.

114. Raiola AM, Van Lint MT, Valbonesi M, et al.
Factors predicting response and graft-versus-
host disease after donor lymphocyte infusions:
A study on 593 infusions. Bone Marrow Transplant 2003;31:687-93.

115. Pulsipher MA, Bader P, Klingebiel T, et al.
Allogeneic transplantation for pediatric acute
lymphoblastic leukemia: The emerging role of
peritransplantation minimal residual disease/
chimerism monitoring and novel chemotherapeutic, molecular, and immune approaches
aimed at preventing relapse. Biol Blood Marrow Transplant 2008;15:62-71.

116. Ferra C, Rodriguez-Luaces M, Gallardo D, et al.
Individually adjusted prophylactic donor lymphocyte infusions after CD34-selected allogeneic peripheral blood stem cell transplantation.
Bone Marrow Transplant 2001;28:963-8.

117. Lutz C, Massenkeil G, Nagy M, et al. A pilot
study of prophylactic donor lymphocyte
infusions to prevent relapse in adult acute lymphoblastic leukemias after allogeneic hematopoietic stem cell transplantation. Bone Marrow
Transplant 2008;41:805-12.

118. Schmid C, Schleuning M, Ledderose G, et al.
Sequential regimen of chemotherapy, reduced-
intensity conditioning for allogeneic stem-cell
transplantation, and prophylactic donor lymphocyte transfusion in high-risk acute myeloid
leukemia and myelodysplastic syndrome. J Clin
Oncol 2005;23:5675-87.

119. Sullivan K, Storb R, Buckner D, et al. Graft-versus-host disease as adoptive immunotherapy in
patients with advanced hematologic neoplasms. N Engl J Med 1989;320:828-34.

120. Sullivan K, Storb R, Witherspoon R, et al. Deletion of immunosuppressive prophylaxis after
marrow transplantation increased hyperacute
graft-versus-host disease but does not influence
chronic graft-versus-host disease or relapse in
patients with advanced leukemia. Clin Transplant 1989;3:5-11.

121. Elfenbein G, Graham-Pole J, Weiner R, et al.
Consequences of no prophylaxis for acute
graft-versus-host disease after HLA-identical
bone marrow transplantation (abstract). Blood
1987;70(Suppl 1):305a.

122. Weiden P, Storb R, Tsoi M, et al. Infusion of donor lymphocytes into stable canine radiation chimeras: Implications for mechanism of transplantation tolerance. J Immunol 1978;116: 1212-19.

123. Johnson B, Drobyski W, Truitt R. Delayed infusion of normal donor cells after MHC-matched bone marrow transplantation provides an antileukemia reaction without graft-versus-host disease. Bone Marrow Transplant 1993;11:329-36.

124. Slavin S, Ackerstein A, Weiss L, et al. Immunotherapy of minimal residual disease by immunocompetent lymphocytes and their activation by cytokines. Cancer Invest 1992;10:221-7.

125. Antin J, Ferrara J. Cytokine dysregulation and acute graft-versus-host disease. Blood 1992; 80:2964-8.

126. Barrett AJ, Mavroudis D, Tisdale J, et al. T cell-depleted bone marrow transplantation and delayed T cell add-back to control acute GVHD and conserve a graft-versus-leukemia effect. Bone Marrow Transplant 1998;21:543-51.

127. Ferra C, Rodriguez-Luaces M, Gallardo D, et al. Individually adjusted prophylactic donor lymphocyte infusions after CD34-selected allogeneic peripheral blood stem cell transplantation. Bone Marrow Transplant 2001;28:963-8.

128. Naparsteck E, Or R, Nagler A, et al. T-cell-depleted allogeneic bone marrow transplantation for acute leukaemia using Campath-1 antibodies and post-transplant administration of donor's peripheral blood lymphocytes for prevention of relapse. Br J Haematol 1995;89:506-15.

129. Slavin S, Naparstek E, Nagler A, et al. Graft vs leukemia (GVL) effects with controlled GVHD by cell mediated immunotherapy (CMI) following allogeneic bone marrow transplantation (BMT). Blood 1993;82:423a.

130. Peggs KS, Mackinnon S, Williams CD, et al. Reduced-intensity transplantation with in vivo T-cell depletion and adjuvant dose-escalating donor lymphocyte infusions for chemotherapy-sensitive myeloma: Limited efficacy of graft-versus-tumor activity. Biol Blood Marrow Transplant 2003;9:257-65.

131. Smith K. Lowest dose interleukin-2 immunotherapy. Blood 1993;81:1414-23.

132. Hauch M, Gazzola M, Small T, et al. Anti-leukemia potential of interleukin-2 activated natural killer cells after bone marrow transplantation for chronic myelogenous leukemia. Blood 1990;75:2250-62.

133. Mackinnon S, Hows J, Goldman J. Induction of in vitro graft-versus-leukemia activity following bone marrow transplantation for chronic myeloid leukemia. Blood 1990;76:2037-45.

134. Reittie J, Gottlieb D, Heslop H, et al. Endogenously generated activated killer cells circulate after autologous and allogeneic marrow transplantation but not after chemotherapy. Blood 1989;73:1351-8.

135. Benyunes M, Massumoto C, York A, et al. Interleukin-2 with or without lymphokine-activated killer cells as consolidative immunotherapy after autologous bone marrow transplantation for acute myelogenous leukemia. Bone Marrow Transplant 1993;12:159-63.

136. Hamon M, Prentice H, Gottlieb D, et al. Immunotherapy with interleukin 2 after ABMT in AML. Bone Marrow Transplant 1993;11:399-401.

137. Soiffer R, Murray C, Gonin R, Ritz J. Effect of low-dose interleukin-2 on disease relapse after T-cell-depleted allogeneic bone marrow transplantation. Blood 1994;84:964-71.

138. Varadi G, Ackerstein A, Ben-Neriah S, Nagler A. Adoptive cell-mediated immunotherapy with interleukin-2 (IL-2) for relapsing lymphoblastic crisis following mismatched unrelated bone marrow transplantation in a chronic myelogenous leukemia patient. Bone Marrow Transplant 1998;21:93-6.

139. Zutter M, Maretin P, Sale G, et al. Epstein-Barr virus lymphoproliferation after bone marrow transplantation. Blood 1988;72:520-9.

140. Shapiro R, McClain K, Frizzera G, et al. Epstein-Barr virus associated B cell lymphoproliferative disorders following bone marrow transplantation. Blood 1988;71:1234-43.

141. Papadopoulos E, Ladanyi M, Emanuel D, et al. Infusions of donor leukocytes to treat Epstein-Barr virus-associated lymphoproliferative disorders after allogeneic bone marrow transplantation. N Engl J Med 1994;330:1185-91.

142. Porter D, Orloff G, Antin J. Donor mononuclear cell infusions as therapy for B-cell lymphoproliferative disorder following allogeneic bone marrow transplant. Transplant Sci 1994;4:11-15.

143. Rooney C, Smith C, Ng C, et al. Use of gene-modified virus-specific T lymphocytes to control Epstein-Barr-virus-related lymphoproliferation. Lancet 1995;345:9-13.

144. Hromas R, Cornetta K, Srour E. Donor leuko-cyte infusion as therapy of life-threatening adenoviral infections after T-cell-depleted bone marrow transplantation (letter). Blood 1994; 84:1690-1.

145. Kishi Y, Kami M, Oki Y, et al. Donor lymphocyte infusion for treatment of life-threatening respiratory syncytial virus infection following bone marrow transplantation. Bone Marrow Transplant 2000;26:573-6.

146. Walter E, Greenberg P, Gilbert M, et al. Reconstitution of cellular immunity against cytomegalovirus in recipients of allogeneic bone marrow by transfer of T-cell clones from the donor. N Engl J Med 1995;333:1038-44.

147. Gustafsson A, Levitsky V, Zou JZ, et al. Epstein-Barr virus (EBV) load in bone marrow transplant recipients at risk to develop post-transplant lymphoproliferative disease: Prophylactic infusion of EBV-specific cytotoxic T cells. Blood 2000;95:807-14.

148. Rooney C, Smith C, Ng C, et al. Infusion of cytoxic T cells for the prevention and treatment of Epstein-Barr virus-induced lymphoma in allogeneic transplant recipients. Blood 1998; 92:1549-55.

149. Storb R. Can reduced-intensity allogeneic transplantation cure older adults with AML? Best Pract Res Clin Haematol 2007;20:85-90.

150. Sandmaier BM, Mackinnon S, Childs RW. Reduced intensity conditioning for allogeneic hematopoietic cell transplantation: Current perspectives. Biol Blood Marrow Transplant 2007;13:87-97.

151. Bhatia V, Porter D. Novel approaches to allogeneic stem cell therapy. Exp Opin Biol Ther 2001;1:3-15.

In: McLeod BC, Szczepiorkowski ZM, Weinstein R, Winters JL, eds.
Apheresis: Principles and Practice, 3rd edition
Bethesda, MD: AABB Press, 2010

28

Photopheresis

Jaehyuk Choi, MD, PhD, and Francine M. Foss, MD

 EXTRACORPOREAL PHOTO-chemotherapy (photopheresis, ECP) is a form of apheresis therapy. During an ECP procedure, peripheral blood mononuclear cells (MNCs) are separated by apheresis, exposed extracorporeally in a collection bag to ultraviolet A (UVA) light in the presence of a psoralen compound, and then reinfused to the patient. Unprecedented responses have been demonstrated in patients with cutaneous T-cell lymphoma (CTCL) who were receiving no other antitumor therapy. Improvement after ECP has also been reported in graft-vs-host disease (GVHD), solid organ allograft rejection, and a variety of immune-mediated inflammatory diseases, but mostly in case reports or uncontrolled observational trials in patients who were receiving other treatments as well. Unequivocal confirmation from controlled trials in these settings has not been forthcoming.

Another troubling aspect concerning ECP is that 25 years after its initial use in CTCL, its mechanism(s) of action has not yet been elucidated.

ECP Procedure

Mononuclear Cell Collection Techniques—Intermittent Flow Centrifugation

The most commonly employed ECP device, the UVAR XTS photopheresis system (Therakos, Exton, PA), collects an MNC concentrate by intermittent flow leukapheresis. The fully integrated and process-controlled system is composed of an instrument, control software, single-use procedural kits, lamp assembly, and drug. It has recently replaced the earlier-generation UVAR instrument (Therakos) at most centers conducting ECP. The new system incor-

Jaehyuk Choi, MD, PhD, Dermatology Fellow, Department of Dermatology, and Francine M. Foss, MD, Professor of Medicine (Hematology) and of Dermatology, and Co-Director, Lymphoma, Leukemia, and Myeloma Program, Yale School of Medicine, New Haven, Connecticut

The authors have disclosed no conflicts of interest.

porates technical advances in the separation and fluid control functions that reduce extracorporeal volume and provide an automated and time-efficient procedure, more consistent MNC collection, and a precisely quantitated dose of UVA radiation. The UVAR XTS system uses heparinized saline at a concentration of 10,000 units of heparin per 500 mL of normal saline for both the priming of the instrument and patient anticoagulation throughout the treatment. If heparin is contraindicated, acid-citrate-dextrose solution formula A (ACD-A) can also be used as the anticoagulant. During the collection phase, which takes approximately 90 to 150 minutes, up to 1.5 L of whole blood is processed in three to six cycles. Separation of MNCs from whole blood is accomplished in either a 125-mL or a 225-mL Latham bowl (Haemonetics Corporation, Braintree, MA). The 225-mL bowl allows a shorter collection phase and provides better collection efficiency but requires a higher extracorporeal volume. The 125-mL bowl is reserved for patients with lower body weight, anemia, or hemodynamic instability who may not be able to tolerate larger shifts in intravascular volume. The final collection product contains approximately 90 mL of sterile saline, 80 mL of plasma, and 100 mL of MNC concentrate. Most of the red cells, which would shield MNCs from absorbing UVA energy in the irradiation phase, and excess plasma are returned to the patient. The final suspension has a total volume of approximately 270 mL and a hematocrit of about 4%. Each procedure exposes approximately 10% of the total body peripheral blood MNCs to psoralen and UVA light.

Mononuclear Cell Collection Techniques— Continuous Flow Centrifugation

Continuous flow apheresis instruments, such as the Spectra (CaridianBCT, Lakewood, CO), may also be used to collect MNCs for ECP.[1] The maximum final volume of MNC concentrate is 150 mL. The MNC product is usually diluted with sterile saline to a volume of 300 mL before photoactivation. The hematocrit of the final product is typically less than 5%.

In 2009, a new device, the Therakos Cellex, was approved by the US Food and Drug Administration (FDA). This instrument, which is described in detail in Chapter 4, allows for continuous flow collection of MNCs using either single- or dual-needle configuration. The benefits expected from continuous flow leukapheresis include shorter procedure times, lower sensitivity to hyperlipidemia, and a lower acceptable patient hematocrit; however, clinical experience with this device in the United States is still limited. Bisaccia et al reported a very good safety profile after 155 procedures in a study from the United Kingdom.[2] They also confirmed that the system provides lower extracorporeal volumes, faster treatment times, and flexibility to use either single- or dual-needle access.

Photoactivating Agent

The only photoactivating agent approved for ECP by the FDA is 8-methoxypsoralen (8-MOP), or methoxsalen [9-methoxy-7H-furo(3,2-g)(1)-benzopyran-7-one). It is a naturally occurring substance, found in the seeds of the *Ammi majus* (Umbelliferae) plant and belongs to a class of tricyclic aromatic compounds known as psoralens or furocoumarins. The extended aromatic structure of furocoumarins permits them to absorb UVA light. Methoxsalen is chemically inert until activated by specific wavelengths of UVA light. Upon photoactivation, methoxsalen reversibly intercalated between DNA strands forms covalent bonds with pyrimidine bases that produce both monofunctional (single-strand) and bifunctional (double-strand) photoadducts.[3] Reactions with proteins have also been described. This photoconjugation reaction inhibits proliferation of the treated lymphocytes and leads to the appearance of DNA strand breaks and subsequent apoptosis of treated cells.[4-6] Two formulations of 8-MOP are available for use in ECP: an oral formulation and a sterile solution suitable for injection into the MNC concentrate.

Oral Formulation

The oral formulation is administered 2 hours before beginning leukapheresis at a dose of 0.6 mg/kg to produce a plasma level of approximately 50 ng/mL. Peak blood levels of 8-MOP occur approximately 2 hours after ingestion. Unfortunately, there is substantial inter- and intra-individual variation in drug bioavailability after oral administration of 8-MOP; thus, it is important to measure blood psoralen levels frequently throughout the course of treatment. If the 8-MOP level does not reach 50 ng/mL with the recommended dose, an additional 10 mg may be administered on subsequent procedure days, but not earlier than 24 hours after the previous dose.

Injectable Formulation

Because of erratic absorption and the side effects of the oral formulation, a sterile solution of 8-MOP [UVADEX (Therakos)] has been developed for use with ECP.[7] UVADEX is supplied in 10-mL vials containing 200 μg of 8-MOP at a concentration of 20 μg/mL. This formulation is injected directly into the MNC suspension in the collection bag before UVA exposure. The dosage of 8-MOP is calculated according to the following formula: MNC product volume (mL) × 0.017 = mL of UVADEX to be added. The injected 8-MOP is infused to the patient intravenously along with the photoactivated MNCs.

The advantages of intra-MNC-concentrate administration of 8-MOP include the following: 1) predictable concentrations of 8-MOP that obviate the need to monitor blood levels, 2) elimination of the 2-hour delay associated with the oral formulation, and 3) exposure of the patient to approximately 200 times less 8-MOP, thereby reducing the side effects associated with systemic 8-MOP. When taken orally, methoxsalen is bound reversibly to serum albumin and is metabolized rapidly by humans, and approximately 95% of the drug is excreted as metabolites in the urine within 24 hours.

Plasma levels of 8-MOP obtained during clinical studies have shown no detectable serum level (<10 ng/mL) 30 minutes after reinfusion of treated cell suspensions containing UVADEX.

Side Effects and Contraindications

Oral administration of 8-MOP is associated with a number of side effects, including nausea, vomiting, sunlight sensitivity, nervousness, insomnia, and depression. Administration of psoralen is contraindicated in patients with aphakia (ie, absence or loss of the eye's natural crystalline lens, as after cataract removal), in patients exhibiting idiosyncratic reactions to psoralen compounds, or in patients having a history of a light-sensitive disease such as porphyria cutanea tarda, erythropoietic protoporphyria, variegate porphyria, xeroderma pigmentosa, or albinism. Patients should avoid direct or indirect sunlight for 24 hours following exposure to 8-MOP. If sun exposure is unavoidable, patients should protect their eyes by wearing UVA protective wrap-around eyewear, and their skin, by covering exposed areas or using sunscreen (at least SPF15).

UVA Irradiation

UVAR XTS Apparatus

The irradiation chamber in this device has a volume of 85 mL and a thickness of 1.4 mm. The MNC concentrate containing 8-MOP recirculates through the chamber where UVA energy (320-400 nm) activates the 8-MOP. The instrument automatically calculates and sets the photoactivation time for each treatment based on the remaining lamp life and the volume and hematocrit of the MNC concentrate. A precise dose of UVA energy equivalent to 1.5 Joules/cm^2 is delivered. The photoactivation process typically takes about 35 minutes. After photoactivation, the irradiated MNCs are returned to the patient and the procedure is complete.

UV-matic Irradiator

An alternative device is the UV-matic irradiator (Vilber Lourmat, Marne-La-Vallée, France). This system requires the MNC concentrate to be transferred to a special UVA permeable plastic bag (Macopharma, Tourcoing, France) that is placed between quartz plates.[1] During irradiation with the UV-matic, the MNC concentrate is subjected to continuous horizontal rotation. The energy absorbed at the surface of each quartz plate is monitored to ensure precise energy delivery to the bag. Variations in energy delivered to each cell with this system are not well understood. Slight variations in lamp output, UV transmittance properties of the bag, and MNC concentrate volume and hematocrit may affect the energy delivered.

Side Effects

Side effects observed during ECP procedures are primarily related to volume shifts. Hypotension may occur during any treatment involving extracorporeal circulation. AABB recommends that the intravascular volume deficit be limited to 10.5 mL/kg of the patient's weight.[8(p56)] Patients must be monitored closely during ECP for any signs of hypotension. Hypotensive episodes are generally managed by briefly pausing the procedure and administering fluids. Transient febrile reactions (38-39 C or 100-102 F) have also been observed in some patients within 6 to 8 hours after reinfusion of the photoactivated MNCs. A temporary increase in erythroderma may also accompany febrile reactions in certain of the patient groups discussed below.

Therapeutic Applications of Photopheresis

The first clinical application of ECP was for the treatment of CTCL. Since then, the treatment of scleroderma and other autoimmune diseases has been investigated in pilot studies or observational trials. ECP has also been reported to decrease the clinical manifestations of GVHD and solid organ transplant rejection. More recently, ECP has been tried as prophylaxis to prevent rejection in patients with cardiac allografts and to prevent or decrease the severity of GVHD in the setting of allogeneic hematopoietic stem cell transplantation (HSCT).

Treatment of Cutaneous T-Cell Lymphoma

CTCL is a malignancy of CD4+ helper T lymphocytes that involves the skin in the form of patches, plaques, tumors, or erythroderma, or as the Sézary syndrome, an advanced form of CTCL characterized by generalized erythroderma, lymphadenopathy, and the presence of large numbers of atypical malignant T cells in the blood.[9,10] The prognosis in advanced-stage CTCL or the Sézary syndrome is poor, with median survivals of 2 to 3 years from diagnosis.[11] Further, treatment of Sézary syndrome with conventional cytotoxic chemotherapy has been challenging because of the high incidence of infection related to compromised skin integrity and the underlying T-cell-mediated immunodeficiency.[12-14]

Edelson et al[15] were prompted to explore the implementation of leukapheresis-based therapies in CTCL by 1) an early observation that successive leukapheresis procedures were associated with clinical improvement in patients with the Sézary syndrome and 2) the clinical efficacy of UVA irradiation of skin after psoralen ingestion (PUVA) in CTCL. In the first reports, a favorable response was noted in eight of 11 Sézary patients treated with oral 8-MOP and ECP at Yale[4] and in six of seven patients treated in Vienna.[16] The efficacy of ECP for erythrodermic CTCL was reported subsequently in a multicenter study in which patients were treated on 2 consecutive days every 4 weeks, with clinical evaluation at 6 months of therapy.[17] A skin scoring system that ranged from 0 (entirely uninvolved skin) to 400 (universal involvement, with maximal erythroderma and induration) was used for clinical evaluation. Patients who demonstrated significant improvement were maintained on this treatment schedule until the maximum clearing of skin manifestations was achieved and for an additional 6 months to ensure the stability of the response. Patients were weaned off ECP by gradually increasing the interval between treatments. Twenty-seven of 37 patients with otherwise resistant CTCL responded to ECP, with an average 64% decrease in skin score after a mean of 22 weeks. The responding group included eight of 10 patients with lymph node involvement, 24 of 29 (83%) with exfoliative erythroderma, and 20 of 28 (71%) whose disease was resistant to standard chemotherapy. Response was correlated with a decrease in the number of circulating Sézary cells.

In a follow-up study of the 29 erythrodermic patients, the median survival was 60.3 months from diagnosis and 47.9 months from institution of ECP.[18] Four of the original complete responders remained disease free for 6 to 10 years, without evidence of lymphocytic infiltrates in skin biopsy or clonal tumor cells as measured by T-cell receptor rearrangements in the blood. In prior studies of standard chemotherapies for patients with Sézary syndrome, the median survival was 30 months, suggesting a survival benefit for responders with Sézary syndrome after initiation of ECP.[11]

Other studies[19-30] have confirmed these results (Table 28-1). Among 190 CTCL patients treated at a number of centers, the complete and partial response rates were 23% to 50% and up to 60%, respectively, with most responses seen in patients with erythrodermic CTCL. The time to achieve a partial response in most studies was 4 to 9 months, and the time to achieve a complete response ranged

Table 28-1. Studies of Photopheresis for Treatment of Cutaneous T-Cell Lymphoma

Study	Patients	Response	Comments
Edelson et al[17]	37	27/37	Highest response in Sézary syndrome; median survival = 62 months.
Zic et al[24]	20	11/20	Median survival = 96 months; response by 6-8 months. Predicts better long-term outcome.
Armus et al[19]	8	6/8	Response in 4/5 Sézary syndrome, 1/2 with tumor stage, and 1 with plaque stage disease.
Heald et al[18]	19	15/19	
Duvic et al[20]	34	17/34	Median time to response = 6 months.
Lim et al[27]	41	32/41	Median survival = 70 months; median time to complete response = 12 months.
Suchin et al[28]	16	12/16	Monotherapy with ECP.
	31	26/31	Combination with IFN-α, IFN-γ, sargramostim, or retinoids.
Talpur et al[29]	8	6/8	Combination with systemic bexarotene.
Richardson et al[30]	28	25/28	Combination with two or more adjuvant therapies, including IFN-α, IFN-γ, GM-CSF, PUVA, or retinoids.

ECP = extracorporeal photochemotherapy; IFN = interferon; GM-CSF = granulocyte-macrophage colony-stimulating factor; PUVA = psoralen plus ultraviolet A light.

from 4 to 12 months when ECP was administered for 2 consecutive days each month. Good prognostic factors include short disease course (<2 years), absence of bulky lymphadenopathy or significant internal organ involvement, minimal pretreatment with chemotherapy, and plaque-stage disease limited to 10% to 15% of body surface area. In support of its immunomodulatory mechanism, ECP is also most effective when the white cell count is less than 20,000/mm^3 and there are normal or near-normal levels of natural killer (NK) cells and cytotoxic T lymphocytes.[31]

About 25% of patients with Sézary syndrome fail to respond optimally to ECP.[21] In these cases, ECP may be effective as part of a combination treatment. The addition of interferons (IFNs) or retinoids to ECP has improved response rates and durations in some patients.[32-34] Suchin et al reported an 80% complete response rate in 15 patients who received INF-α-2b at a dose of 5 million units every other day in addition to two consecutive daily ECP treatments every 4 weeks.[28] Vonderheid et al reported on the use of ECP (2 consecutive days every 4 weeks) and 4 million units of INF-α-2b three times a week for the 2 weeks immediately after each ECP treatment.[35] Other agents that have been used as immunomodulators with ECP include IFN-γ, granulocyte-macrophage colony-stimulating factor (GM-CSF), and the retinoic X receptor-retinoid bexarotene [Targretin (Eisai, Woodcliff Lake, NJ)].[31] In particular, combination with bexarotene has been encouraging, with overall response rates of around 75%.[29] Multimodality treatment showed good results in patients with advanced CTCL and multiple poor prognostic factors.[28] In a recent study of 28 patients with Sézary syndrome, there was an overall response rate of 89% and a complete response rate of 29% when ECP was combined with other therapies or combinations of biomodulatory therapies such as IFNs, GM-CSF, or PUVA.[30]

In summary, the activity of ECP in CTCL has been documented in multiple clinical trials. Overall, the responses in these trials correlated with the presence of circulating clonal tumor cells and with an intact immune system capable of generating a CD8-mediated antitumor response. The median time to response is reported to be 4 to 6 months, and the response time may be reduced with the addition of immunomodulatory agents or with shortening of the interval between treatments to every 14 days. The combination of ECP with chemotherapy or total skin irradiation is being explored, as is the use of ECP in patients with less advanced illness. The American Society for Apheresis (ASFA) ranks CTCL (erythrodermic) as Category I (Grade 1B) and CTCL (nonerythrodermic) as Category III (Grade 2C) for ECP treatment.[36-38]

Clinical Efficacy of ECP for Treatment of GVHD

GVHD and its treatment are responsible for considerable morbidity and mortality among patients who have received allogeneic HSCT after standard myeloablative conditioning regimens. Acute GVHD (aGVHD) occurs in up to 40% of patients who receive a graft from a matched sibling donor and up to 70% of those whose graft is from a matched unrelated donor. Several less intensive, nonmyeloablative conditioning regimens have a lower risk of some transplant-related toxicities but no decrease in the incidence of GVHD. In addition, the use of apheresis rather than marrow as a source of hematopoietic progenitor cells (HPCs) has been associated with an increase in GVHD.

Standard therapy for GVHD consists of immunosuppressants. Front-line therapies include high-dose corticosteroids, a calcineurin inhibitor such as cyclosporin A (CSA) or tacrolimus, and sometimes an investigational agent. Despite aggressive therapy, however, mortality in patients with severe aGVHD or extensive chronic GVHD (cGVHD) remains high. Furthermore, the immunosuppressive agents themselves can cause significant morbidity and mortality and may also inhibit donor T cells that mediate the graft-versus-tumor effect, increasing the risk of tumor relapse.[39]

Studies of ECP in Chronic GVHD

Owsianowski et al[40] first reported ECP in a patient with chronic skin GVHD (Table 28-2). They noted improvement in lichenified skin changes, joint contractures, and sicca syndrome, along with normalization of the CD4/CD8 ratio, which had been skewed with an increase in CD8+ cells in this patient. Rossetti et al subsequently reported improvement in skin, liver, and pulmonary GVHD in children, resulting in the ability to taper or discontinue immunosuppressive agents.[41,50] Many subsequent case series have suggested a positive effect of ECP in treatment-resistant cGVHD.

These studies have tended to indicate a positive effect in skin, liver, and mucous membranes. A review of the literature demonstrated overall improvement rates of 72% in skin, 63% in liver, and 74% in oral disease. There also have been reports, albeit fewer, of a positive effect in lung GVHD and thrombocytopenia.[48,51] In one of the largest individual case series, Couriel et al performed a retrospective analysis on the effect of ECP in 71 patients with steroid-refractory cGVHD.[52] In this single-institution study, there was an overall improvement rate of 61%. Improvement was seen in 67% of patients with scleroderma-like skin changes, 71% with liver involvement, 77% with oral mucosal lesions, and 54% with bronchiolitis obliterans. Improvement was sustained in 69% of the surviving patients at 6 months.[52]

Early initiation of ECP appears to be an important predictor of success. In a study by Greinix et al, ECP was initiated at a median of

Table 28-2. Studies of Photopheresis for Treatment of Chronic GVHD

Study	Patients	Response	Comments
Owsianowski et al[40]	1	1	Response in skin, joints, and eye.
Rosetti et al[41]	9	4	Response in skin, lung, GI.
Child et al[42]	11	9	Responses in skin (9/10), lung (2/5), liver (1/5); higher response with ECP every 14 days.
Abhyankar et al[43]	5	3	Response in skin and joints.
Bishop et al[44]	33	14	Responses in skin (14/22), liver (4/4), oral (8/18), eye (4/12), lung (2/7), GI (2/7).
Greinix et al[45]	15	12	Responses in skin (12/15), liver (7/10), oral (11/11), joints (4/4), eye (5/6).
DiVenuti et al[46]	21	15	Responses in skin (14/21), joints (3/6), GI (2/3), lung (2/2).
Couriel et al[47]	63	37	Responses in skin (14/21), liver (5/21), oral mucosa (7/9), eye (4/6), lung (6/11).
Rubegni et al[48]	32	25	Study limited to steroid-refractory patients.
Flowers et al[49]	95	Skin score quantified	No difference between ECP-treated and control patients in this randomized, blinded trial.

ECP = extracorporeal photochemotherapy; GI = gastrointestinal (tract).

178 days after HSCT,[53] whereas in the study by Child et al, ECP was initiated later (median of 510 days).[42] All patients in these two studies had failed first- and second-line therapies, including corticosteroids and CSA. In the group treated early, 12 of 15 patients had improvement in skin score, 11 of 11 in mucocutaneous disease, 7 of 10 in hepatic enzymes, and 5 of 6 in ocular symptoms. In the group treated later, skin improvement was noted in 10 of 10 patients, but only 2 of 4 with oral and 1 of 5 with liver involvement demonstrated improvement in these visceral sites. In this latter group, the greatest improvement in both skin and visceral disease occurred in patients who started ECP less than 10 months after HSCT. After discontinuation of ECP, 14% of patients who had improved experienced a recurrence of symptoms and improved again after retreatment.

Despite the need for semipermanent intravenous access devices for ECP in these immunocompromised patients, there was no increase in infection rate and no increase in reactivation of cytomegalovirus infection. In fact, a potential benefit of ECP might be the ability to taper or discontinue systemic immunosuppressants that carry a higher risk of severe complications. In the Couriel study, 7 of the 63 were able to completely discontinue pharmacologic immunsuppression; 14 were able to discontinue steroids.[52]

Identifying biomarkers that predict responsiveness to ECP could be advantageous. Couriel et al observed that a platelet count less than 100,000/μL predicted a poor response.[52] In a short report, Kuzmina and colleagues suggested that the abundance of immature CD19+ CD21- B lymphocytes could predict improvement after ECP in patients with cGVHD. The proportion of CD19+CD21− B lymphocytes was significantly lower in complete-response patients compared with ECP nonresponders in pretreatment blood samples (mean = 8% vs 22%) and in samples drawn at 6 months (5% vs 25%), 12 months (6% vs 24%), and 21 months (6% vs 26%) after the start of ECP.[54]

A large, randomized, Phase II controlled trial was reported by Flowers et al in 2008.[49] Ninety-five patients were randomly assigned to either standard therapy alone (n = 47) or standard therapy plus ECP (n = 48) over 12 weeks as follows: three treatments in week 1, and two treatments per week for weeks 2 to 12. The primary endpoint of this study was a comparison of percent change from baseline in total skin score (TSS) in 10 body regions at week 12, assessed by a medical professional trained in TSS who was blinded to the patient's treatment arm. The median percent improvements in TSS at week 12 were 14.5% for the ECP arm and 8.5% for the control arm; this modest difference was not statistically significant (p = 0.48). A number of other assessments of clinical improvement and need for immunosuppressive drugs were said to have shown a beneficial effect of ECP; however, these were all made by personnel who were aware of the treatment assignment and were therefore subject to bias. The inconsistent outcomes in this study underscore the challenges faced by investigators who wish to conduct controlled trials in cGVHD. Nevertheless, the primary outcome of this trial, the only one evaluated in a blinded fashion, failed to confirm the conclusions drawn from case reports and uncontrolled series about the efficacy of ECP in cGVHD. There is a need for a Phase III randomized controlled trial of ECP in this setting. At the time of this writing there is a proposal for such a study through the Clinical Transplant Network, sponsored by the National Heart, Lung, and Blood Institute.

Studies of ECP in Acute GVHD

aGVHD, which may affect multiple target organs, including skin, liver, and gastrointestinal (GI) tract, occurs within the first 100 days after infusion of allogeneic HPCs. Early studies suggested a beneficial effect of ECP in steroid-refractory aGVHD.[53,55-58] A pilot study was therefore initiated in 21 patients with steroid-refractory GVHD and subsequently expanded to a Phase II study of 59 patients (37 with steroid-refractory and 22 with steroid-dependent disease). Patients were initially treated on 2 consecutive days at 1- to 2-week intervals until improvement and every 2 to 4 weeks thereafter until maximal improvement.

After a median of 4 cycles of ECP plus continued steroid therapy, 82% of patients with cutaneous involvement, 61% with liver involvement, and 61% with GI involvement experienced a complete resolution of aGVHD. Complete response rates were lower in patients with grade IV disease (30%) than in patients with grade II or III disease (86% and 55%, respectively). As a result of these improvements, tapering and/or discontinuation of corticosteroids was possible in many patients. Survival was higher in patients who improved after ECP compared to those who did not.

Literature reviews revealed mean improvements in ECP-treated patients of 85% with skin involvement, 56% with liver involvement, and 63% with GI involvement.[31] In three of the individual studies, there was better overall survival in those who improved after ECP (38%-69% vs 11%-18%).[31,58]

Subsequent studies in children demonstrated similar results (Table 28-3). In one study, seven of nine children with aGVHD improved, but two with skin, gastrointestinal, and liver GVHD progressed and died.[62] Among the seven children who improved, immunosuppressive treatment was discontinued in three.

In contrast to patients with cGVHD, patients treated early after allogeneic HSCT experienced thrombocytopenia, anemia, and leukopenia associated with ECP. There was no evidence of delayed engraftment in these patients, but this remains an open question because ECP is being more widely implemented in the early posttransplant and pretransplant periods.

Prophylactic ECP to Prevent Acute GVHD

On the basis of observational reports of ECP in patients with cGVHD, an open trial was undertaken using ECP before the infusion of allogeneic HPCs as part of the pretransplant conditioning regimen.[63,64] This study was conducted in a group of patients with hematologic malignancies who were considered at high risk for a standard myeloablative conditioning regimen because of advanced age, lack of a matched sibling donor, or underlying organ dysfunction. Fifty adult patients received 2 days of ECP, followed by intravenous pentostatin (8 mg/m^2 administered by continuous infusion over 48 hours) and reduced-dose total body irradiation (TBI) of 600 cGy as a conditioning regimen. Ten patients received transplants from matched unrelated donors. Eighteen had relapsed or progressive disease at the time of transplantation. Serious aGVHD and extensive cGVHD occurred in 11% and 10% of patients, respectively. Transplant-

Table 28-3. Studies of Photopheresis for Treatment of Acute Graft-vs-Host Disease in Children

Study	Patients	Skin (CR/PR)	Liver (CR/PR)	GI (CR/PR)	Overall Survival
Messina et al[59]	33	27/33	9/14	15/18	19/33
Greinix et al[45]	65	93%	65%	74%	33/65
Smith et al[60]	6	—	0/6	—	0/6
Miller et al[61]	4	3/3	2/4	3/3	2/4
Salvaneschi et al[62]	9	8/9	1/5	3/5	6/9
Perfetti et al[58]	23	66%	27%	40%	NR

CR = complete response; PR = partial response; NR = not reported.

related mortality at day 100 was 18%, and overall survival at a median follow-up of 406 days was 63%. Given the risk factors for aGVHD in this patient population, an incidence of 11% is strikingly low. The role of ECP in reducing acute and chronic GVHD in this regimen has not yet been clarified, and a randomized study comparing ECP with pentostatin and low-dose TBI to pentostatin and TBI alone is under way.

ASFA ranks cGVHD limited to skin as a Category II (Grade 1B) indication, aGVHD limited to skin as a Category II (Grade 2C) indication, and aGVHD and cGVHD with involvement not limited to skin as a Category III (Grade 2C) indication for ECP treatment.[36-38]

Clinical Trials of ECP in Autoimmune Disorders

Progressive Systemic Sclerosis

Systemic sclerosis is an autoimmune disorder characterized by excessive deposition of collagen within the skin and visceral organs, such as the kidneys, heart, lungs, and GI tract. In addition to causing severe morbidity, systemic sclerosis in its severe form is associated with a poor prognosis, with an overall survival of 20% at 10 years. Few treatments have been tested systematically and proven efficacious in treating this disorder.

Small pilot studies have revealed improvement in ECP-treated patients, with normalization of collagen synthesis,[65] reduction in dermal edema,[66] and increased skin elasticity.[67] Case reports in morphea, a variant of scleroderma limited to the skin and the soft tissue, have shown improvement after ECP in patients who had failed corticosteroids, PUVA treatments, and immunosuppressives such as methotrexate and azathioprine.[68,69] In addition, the larger two of three randomized controlled studies of ECP in systemic sclerosis have shown statistically significant improvement in skin severity scores in patients receiving ECP. In the first study, an assessor-blinded comparison published in 1992, 79 patients with recent-onset

systemic sclerosis and progressive skin involvement were randomly assigned to 6 months of treatment with either D-penicillamine or ECP given on 2 consecutive days each month. After 6 months, improvement in skin thickening was noted in eight of 25 (32%) patients in the D-penicillamine group and 21 of 31 patients (68%) in the ECP group (p = 0.02); however, a significant difference was not reported after 10 months. Histopathologic studies demonstrated a decrease in dermal collagen in those who improved, although serologic studies showed no differences in the changes in antinuclear antibody titer among the treated patients.[70] Because the placebo effect could have influenced this study, a subsequent multicenter randomized, double-blind, placebo-controlled study was undertaken. In 64 patients, ECP was compared with a sham procedure. In this study, a statistically significant improvement in skin scores as compared with baseline was observed at 6 and 12 months among those who received ECP but not among those who received the sham treatment. However, comparison of posttransplant skin scores across the two study arms did not achieve statistical significance.[71] A randomized crossover trial of ECP vs no treatment in 19 patients with progressive systemic sclerosis of less than 5 years duration showed a nonsignificant difference in improvement in skin scores in the two groups.[72]

Although observational studies have suggested that ECP may improve systemic sclerosis, the absence of a statistically significant improvement of skin scores over placebo in controlled studies is difficult to explain. Authors of the studies speculated that there were too few patients to achieve the statistical power necessary to recognize an effect, possibly because the effect is modest, though this seems difficult to reconcile with results reported in observational trials; they suggested that ECP might be tested as an element of combination therapy.[69] Alternatively, scleroderma may be a heterogeneous disease with heterogeneous pathogenic factors, only some of which are susceptible to ECP treatment. This possibility is underscored by the impression of a greater impact of ECP in the early stages of scleroderma and by two recent studies that pointed to independent, nonoverlapping genetic and immunopathogenic factors. One study identified circulating antibodies in scleroderma patients that recognize and activate platelet-derived growth factor (PDGF) receptor; similar antibodies are found in patients with cGVHD but not in patients with lupus or other autoimmune diseases.[73,74] The second study explored differences in the activity of a gene that promotes connective tissue growth factor (CTGF) production; a hyperactive CTGF promoter is found in some scleroderma patients and is more common in scleroderma than in controls.[75] Thus, one might speculate that ECP down-regulates PDGF-receptor antibodies, which could have a beneficial effect in both scleroderma and cGVHD. However, ECP may have minimal benefit in scleroderma patients whose disease is driven by dysregulation of prosclerotic genes affecting CTGF. ASFA ranks scleroderma as a Category IV (Grade 1A) indication for ECP treatment.[36-38]

Nephrogenic Systemic Fibrosis

Nephrogenic systemic fibrosis is a multisystem fibrosing disorder characterized by features of scleroderma, scleromyxedema, and eosinophilic fasciitis. Epidemiologic studies have suggested that the disease is iatrogenic; end-stage renal disease and exposure to gadolinium, a magnetic resonance imaging contrast agent, are strong risk factors. The pathogenesis of the disease remains unclear; however, biopsies have revealed increased recruitment of CD34+ fibrocytes to the skin and increased collagen deposition. Pilot studies have suggested limited benefit from ECP. Two recent case series described ECP treatment of eight patients, of whom six had measurable improvement with increased self-ambulation and two had stable disease.[76,77] In one report, patients' skin and joints were further scored based on the Rodnan scoring system and with range of motion, respectively.[77] Based on these objective criteria, there was only a mild improvement in disease. ASFA ranks nephrogenic systemic fibrosis as Category III (Grade 2C) for ECP treatment.[36-38]

Crohn's Disease

Several pilot studies have suggested a benefit of ECP in a subset of patients with Crohn's disease (CD). Currently, standard treatment consists of systemic steroids and salicylate for mild disease, and systemic steroids, immunomodulators, and/or tumor necrosis factor (TNF) inhibitors for moderate to severe disease. A large proportion of patients develop either steroid dependency or resistance, resulting in long-term use of high steroid doses and a high risk of treatment-related complications. Isolated case reports have described ECP treatment of patients with steroid-dependent CD. In an initial study, nine such patients were treated every 2 weeks for 24 weeks; four then had steroid therapy discontinued, and another four had their steroid dose reduced by over 50%.[78] In a larger, open-label study, 28 patients with moderate-to-severe CD activity, who were either refractory to or intolerant of immunosuppressants and/or anti-TNF agents, underwent 12 weeks of ECP (twice weekly in weeks 1 to 4 and twice every other week in weeks 5 to 12). Fourteen (50%) improved, with seven (25%) attaining remission by week 12[79]; three of five patients with open fistulae at baseline had fistula closure. However, patients with the most severe refractory disease will likely be refractory to ECP as well.[79,80]

Studies of ECP in the Treatment of Solid Organ Allograft Rejection

The use of ECP in solid organ allograft rejection originated from studies in animal models demonstrating that UVA exposure was capable of modulating the proliferation of effector T cells. It was demonstrated in 1971 that lymphocytes irradiated with ultraviolet light were unable to stimulate responder cells in mixed lymphocyte cultures.[81] Subsequent experiments in a canine model of transfusion-associated GVHD and in mouse and rat models of allogeneic HPC transplantation have confirmed the usefulness of short-wavelength ultraviolet (UVB) irradiation of transfused lymphocytes in the prevention of GVHD.[82-86] Perez et al[87,88] demonstrated that infusion of syngeneic effector lymphocytes treated extracorporeally with 8-MOP and UVA light could down-regulate the host response to foreign major histocompatibility complex (MHC) antigens in a mouse model. Also, recipients of UVB-irradiated marrow and spleen cell allografts show specific tolerance to transplanted donor skin grafts that were rejected in control animals whose marrow and spleen grafts were not pretreated.[87,88] These results suggested that UVA and psoralen treatment could modulate populations of alloreactive effector cells.[89,90] Similar results were obtained in a primate cardiac xenograft model, in which recipient lymphocytes were treated with ECP immediately following the allograft. The treated animals demonstrated a suppression of responsiveness to donor cells and a prolongation of graft survival.[91]

Treatment of Acute Heart Transplant Rejection

Postoperatively, heart transplant patients routinely receive cyclosporine, azathioprine, and glucocorticoids to prevent rejection, but acute and chronic rejection episodes still occur and remain a major complication of heart transplantation. It is worth noting, however, that rejection of cardiac allografts, unlike other solid organ transplants, is often diagnosed and treated on the basis of mild histologic changes discovered on routine surveillance endomyocardial biopsy (EMB) without evidence of organ dysfunction, even though the need to treat such purely histologic rejection is not universally accepted.[92] Costanzo-Nordin et al[93] reported that addition of ECP to standard immunosuppression was capable of rapidly reversing acute histologic cardiac rejection episodes. Eight of nine episodes were reversed as assessed by EMB performed 7 days after treatment. Histopathologic improvement as measured by degree of inflammatory cell infiltrate in the myocardium was demonstrated after one or two ECP treatments. Lehrer et al reported ECP treatment of four patients at the Hospital of University of Pennsylvania with severe refractory cardiac allograft rejection (International Society of Heart and Lung Transplanta-

tion grades IIIA and IV). Following treatment on 2 consecutive days, three patients demonstrated complete histologic reversal of rejection. The fourth patient improved more gradually but manifested complete cessation of rejection histopathologically following three 2-day treatments.[94]

Based on these experiences, two groups evaluated the benefits of ECP on heart transplant recipients with recurrent rejection. In a report by Dall'Amico et al,[95] eight patients with recurrent histologic rejections (4 to 24 abnormal EMBs) were treated by ECP for consecutive days every 4 weeks. The frequency of recurrent rejections decreased. The proportion of biopsies without findings consistent with rejection went up from 13% (pre-ECP) to 41% (post-ECP). In addition, immunosuppressives could be tapered (prednisone by 44%, cyclosporine by 21%, and azathioprine by 29%). Giunti et al[96] performed a similar study but with a more aggressive treatment protocol. Patients were treated with ECP twice a week for the first month, at weekly intervals for the second month, at 2-week intervals in the following 2 months, and at monthly intervals in the last 2 months for 20 treatments over 6 months. The number of rejection episodes went down from 0.4 rejection/month/patient to 0.07.

The third use of ECP in cardiac rejection is as an adjunct therapy to the standard triple-drug immunosuppressive regimen to prevent allograft rejection. In 1994, Meiser et al reported that patients who received postoperative ECP (either one or two sessions) had more than a 50% reduction in acute rejection episodes. Furthermore, patients who had received ECP had significantly fewer infections.[97] In a larger study, Barr and the Photopheresis Transplantation Study Group[98] randomly assigned 60 patients to standard triple-drug immunosuppressive therapy (cyclosporine, azathioprine, and prednisone) alone or in conjunction with ECP after cardiac allograft surgery (Table 28-4). The ECP group received a total of 24 treatments over the first 6 months after transplantation. After 6 months of follow-up, the mean number of episodes of acute rejection per

Table 28-4. Randomized Study of Photopheresis to Prevent Acute Cardiac Allograft Rejection[98]

	ECP (n = 33)	Standard Therapy (n = 27)	p Value
6-month survival	31/33	25/27	p = NS
Acute rejection episodes	0.91 ±1.0	1.44 ±1.0	p = 0.04
Patients with >2 rejection episodes	18%	48%	p = 0.02
Time to first rejection	38.9 ±42 days	30.4 ±32 days	p = NS
Patients with hemodynamically significant rejection episode	15%	18%	p = NS

ECP = extracorporeal photochemotherapy; NS = not significant.

patient was 1.44 ±1.0 in the standard therapy group, compared with 0.91 ±1.0 in the ECP group (p ‐ 0.04). However, only mild rejection, manifested as minor histologic changes on EMB, was affected; the incidence of rejection associated with hemodynamic compromise did not decline. Also, there was no significant difference in the time to a first episode of rejection or in survival at 6 and 12 months. The investigators concluded that addition of ECP to triple-drug immunosuppressive therapy significantly decreased the incidence of rejection episodes characterized by a mildly abnormal EMB without reducing the risk of severe rejection or increasing the incidence of infection. Subsequently, Barr et al[99] studied 23 patients, 10 of whom were randomly assigned to ECP from 1 month to 2 years after transplantation. There was no difference in survival or in the incidence of any form of acute rejection, but the ECP-treated patients had a significant decrease in coronary artery intimal thickening compared to controls.

ASFA ranks prophylaxis of heart transplant rejection as a Category I (Grade 1A) indication for ECP, and treatment of cellular heart trans-plant cellular rejection as a Category II (Grade 1B) indication for ECP treatment.[36-38]

Acute and Chronic Rejection of Lung Allografts

Several investigators[100-103] have explored the activity of ECP in the treatment of lung allograft rejection (Table 28-5). Andreu et al treated 10 patients who developed bronchiolitis obliterans after lung or heart-lung transplantation.[103] Two ECP procedures were performed weekly for 3 weeks, followed by one per week for 3 weeks, one every 2 weeks for 1 month, and one monthly for a total of 12 months. No acute rejection episodes occurred, and pulmonary function tests improved in four of eight evaluable patients. In a series of eight patients with deteriorating pulmonary allograft function, five improved after a median of six treatments when ECP was added to the anti-rejection regimen, with stabilization of the 1-second forced expiratory volume. Histopathologic reversal of rejection was documented in two patients in this study.[99] In another series of 14 patients with bronchiolitis obliterans related to chronic rejection, seven had improvement with ECP.[102]

Table 28-5. Studies of Photopheresis for Treatment of Lung Allograft Rejection

Study	Patients	Response
Slovis et al[101]	3	3 improved PFTs
Andreu et al[103]	8	4/8 improved PFTs
Salerno et al[100]	8	5 improved PFTs, 2 histopathologic reversals
Villanueva et al[102]	14	3 improved PFTs

PFTs = pulmonary function tests.

ASFA ranks lung transplant rejection as Category II (Grade 1C) for ECP treatment.[36-38]

Renal Allograft Rejection

Several investigators[104-107] have published case reports of improvement in renal allograft rejection after ECP (Table 28-6). Using an accelerated ECP regimen, Wolfe et al[107] observed improvement in a patient who was refractory to T-cell antibody therapy. Sunder-Plassman and colleagues[105] used frequent and long-term ECP in three renal transplant recipients with biopsy-proven rejection. In all patients, graft function improved. Horina et al[104] used monthly ECP to treat one acute and two chronic renal allograft rejections, with improvement in serum creatinine only in one case of chronic rejection. Controlled studies are needed to investigate the role of ECP to prevent and/or reverse acute renal allograft rejection.

Summary of ECP in Allograft Rejection

In summary, uncontrolled studies in small numbers of patients have suggested that ECP may have a beneficial effect in solid organ allograft rejection that is resistant to immunosuppressive therapy. When compared to responses in the setting of CTCL, improvement after ECP in the setting of solid organ allograft rejection is observed more rapidly, sometimes after only one treatment, possibly suggesting a different mechanism of action. Controlled studies of ECP prophylaxis have not shown a decline in functionally significant rejection episodes. Further controlled studies are needed to define the role of ECP in this setting and to explore various treatment schedules.

Table 28-6. Studies of Photopheresis for Treatment of Renal Allograft Rejection

Study	Patients	Time after Transplant	Duration of ECP	Outcome
Horina et al[104]	3	7 weeks, 9 months, 19 months	3 months	1 complete response
Sunder-Plassman et al[105]	3	7 weeks, 5 months, 5 years	4, 9, 34 months	3/3 stable
Dall'Amico et al[106]	4	2-6 weeks (3 patients), 4 months (1 patient)	6 months	3/4 stable
Wolfe et al[107]	1	24 days	2 weeks	complete resolution of rejection episode

Mechanisms of ECP

The mechanism of action of ECP remains unclear. In the case of CTCL, ECP leads to the death of circulating tumor cells by direct photo-destruction and also by subsequent apopto-sis.[108-110] Simultaneously, ECP appears to initiate a cell-mediated immune response,[88] leading to eradication of additional tumor cells. ECP is capable of activating antigen-presenting cells and has been shown to enhance the synthesis of MHC I molecules. Furthermore, Berger et al[111] demonstrated that in the presence of apoptotic Sézary cells, circulating monocytes are induced to undergo maturation to dendritic cells (DCs) with expression of the mature DC marker, CD83. Although immature DCs are incapable of engulfing apoptotic tumor cells, mature DCs avidly phagocytose these cells and can present idiotypic peptides in their Class I grooves.[111] These antigen-MHC complexes are capable of inducing a marked CD8+ T-cell response against CTCL peptides.[112-114]

The putative effects of ECP in GVHD, organ transplant rejection, and autoimmune disease are more difficult to understand, but a number of discrete effects on the immune system have been noted. The reinfusion of syngeneic cells rendered apoptotic by ECP may also induce some tolerogenic effects, which could explain an effect in autoimmune disease. Gorgun et al[115] demonstrated that ECP inhibited antigen-dependent T-cell activation. Mixed lymphocyte reaction assays were markedly decreased after a 2-day cycle of ECP. In a mouse model of contact hypersensitivity, the extracorporeal treatment of splenocytes and lymph node cells with 8-MOP and UVA to mimic ECP led to the induction of tolerance. This tolerance was lost upon depletion of CD11c+ cells during reinfusion, underscoring the importance of DCs in this process. The tolerogenic effects were mediated by regulatory T cells and were antigen specific. Inhibition of contact hypersensitivity could be transferred from primary recipients to naive animals in a manner dependent on CD4+CD25+ cells, a putative regulatory T-cell population.[116] Gatza et al further showed that in murine models of GVHD, ECP increases donor regulatory T cells and indirectly reduces the number of donor effector lymphocytes.[117] In patients with lung transplantation, graft survival was directly correlated with the levels of circulating CD4+CD25+ cells induced by ECP.[118] The importance of T cells in mediating the tolerogenic properties of ECP were under-scored in a study of steroid-refractory cGVHD, which demonstrated that a clinically significant cutaneous response was seen exclusively in patients who developed clonal populations of alloreactive T lymphocytes, presumably regulatory T cells.[114] Immunomodulatory effects reported in ECP-treated patients with cGVHD include normalization of inverted CD4/CD8 ratios, an increase in the number of CD3+CD56+ NK cells, and a decrease in CD80+ and CD123+ circulating DCs.[115,118-120] Furthermore, studies in patients with GVHD demonstrate that there is a cytokine shift away from an inflammatory (Th1) profile.[121]

Summary

ECP has been established as an effective treatment for advanced CTCL, and encouraging results have been obtained in patients with GVHD after allogeneic HSCT as well as in solid organ transplant rejection and in select autoimmune disorders. Investigations into the mechanism of action of ECP have suggested that this modality is a means of actively engaging the immune system to control aberrant T-cell clones, whether malignant or autoreactive. Prophylactic use of ECP to prevent immune-mediated graft failure or GVHD is intuitively promising, and controlled clinical trials are in progress to explore the efficacy of ECP for these indications. Improvements to enhance the efficacy of ECP include the use of biomodulatory agents, such as interferons and retinoids.

References

1. Andreu G, Leon A, Heshmati F, et al. Extracorporeal photochemotherapy: Evaluation of two techniques and use in connective tissue disorders. Transfus Sci 1994;15:443-54.

2. Bisaccia E, Vonderheid EC, Geskin L. Safety of a new, single, integrated, closed photopheresis system in patients with cutaneous T-cell lymphoma. Br J Dermatol 2009;161:167-9.

3. Schmitt IM, Chimenti S, Gasparro FP. Psoralen-protein photochemistry—a forgotten field. J Photochem Photobiol B 1995;27:101-7.

4. Gasparro FP, Chan G, Edelson RL. Phototherapy and photopharmacology. Yale J Biol Med 1985;58:519-34.

5. Gasparro FP, Song J, Knobler RM, Edelson RL. Quantitation of psoralen photoadducts in DNA isolated from lymphocytes treated with 8-methoxypsoralen and ultraviolet A radiation (extracorporeal photopheresis). Curr Probl Dermatol 1986;15:67-84.

6. Yoo EK, Rook AH, Elenitsas R, et al. Apoptosis induction of ultraviolet light A and photochemotherapy in cutaneous T-cell Lymphoma: Relevance to mechanism of therapeutic action. J Invest Dermatol 1996;107:235-42.

7. Knobler RM, Trautinger F, Graninger W, et al. Parenteral administration of 8-methoxypsoralen in photopheresis. J Am Acad Dermatol 1993;28:580-4.

8. Price T, ed. Standards for blood banks and transfusion services. 26th ed. Bethesda, MD: AABB, 2009.

9. Bunn PA Jr, Lamberg SI. Report of the Committee on Staging and Classification of Cutaneous T-Cell Lymphomas. Cancer Treat Rep 1979;63:725-8.

10. Sausville EA, Worsham GF, Matthews MJ, et al. Histologic assessment of lymph nodes in mycosis fungoides/Sézary syndrome (cutaneous T-cell lymphoma): Clinical correlations and prognostic import of a new classification system. Hum Pathol 1985;16:1098-109.

11. Sausville EA, Eddy JL, Makuch RW, et al. Histopathologic staging at initial diagnosis of mycosis fungoides and the Sézary syndrome. Definition of three distinctive prognostic groups. Ann Intern Med 1988;109:372-82.

12. Akpek G, Koh HK, Bogen S, et al. Chemotherapy with etoposide, vincristine, doxorubicin, bolus cyclophosphamide, and oral prednisone in patients with refractory cutaneous T-cell lymphoma. Cancer 1999;86:1368-76.

13. Foss FM, Ihde DC, Linnoila IR, et al. Phase II trial of fludarabine phosphate and interferon alfa-2a in advanced mycosis fungoides/Sézary syndrome. J Clin Oncol 1994;12:2051-9.

14. Kuzel TM, Hurria A, Samuelson E, et al. Phase II trial of 2-chlorodeoxyadenosine for the treatment of cutaneous T-cell lymphoma. Blood 1996;87:906-11.

15. Edelson R, Facktor M, Andrews A, et al. Successful management of the Sézary syndrome. Mobilization and removal of extravascular neoplastic T cells by leukapheresis. N Engl J Med 1974;291:293-4.

16. Knobler RM. Photopheresis—extracorporeal irradiation of 8-MOP containing blood—a new therapeutic modality. Blut 1987;54:247-50.

17. Edelson R, Berger C, Gasparro F, et al. Treatment of cutaneous T-cell lymphoma by extracorporeal photochemotherapy. Preliminary results. N Engl J Med 1987;316:297-303.

18. Heald PW, Perez MI, Christensen I, et al. Photopheresis therapy of cutaneous T-cell lymphoma: The Yale-New Haven Hospital experience. Yale J Biol Med 1989;62:629-38.

19. Armus S, Keyes B, Cahill C, et al. Photopheresis for the treatment of cutaneous T cell lymphoma. J Am Acad Dermatol 1990;23:898-902.

20. Duvic M, Hester JP, Lemak NA. Photopheresis therapy for cutaneous T-cell lymphoma. J Am Acad Dermatol 1996;35:573-9.

21. Gottlieb SL, Wolfe JT, Fox FE, et al. Treatment of cutaneous T-cell lymphoma with extracorporeal photopheresis monotherapy and in combination with recombinant interferon alfa: A 10-year experience at a single institution. J Am Acad Dermatol 1996;35:946-57.

22. Jiang SB, Dietz SB, Kim M, Lim HW. Extracorporeal photochemotherapy for cutaneous T-cell lymphoma: A 9.7-year experience. Photodermatol Photoimmunol Photomed 1999;15:161-5.

23. Lim HW, Edelson RL. Photopheresis for the treatment of cutaneous T-cell lymphoma. Hematol Oncol Clin North Am 1995;9:1117-26.

24. Zic J, Arzubiaga C, Salhany KE, et al. Extracorporeal photopheresis for the treatment of cutaneous T-cell lymphoma. J Am Acad Dermatol 1992;27:729-36.

25. Zic JA, Miller JL, Stricklin GP, King LE Jr. The North American experience with photopheresis. Ther Apher 1999;3:50-62.

26. Zic JA, Stricklin GP, Greer JP, et al. Long-term follow-up of patients with cutaneous T-cell lymphoma treated with extracorporeal photochemotherapy. J Am Acad Dermatol 1996;35:935-45.

27. Lim HW, Edelson RL. Photopheresis for the treatment of cutaneous T-cell lymphoma.

Hematol Oncol Clin North Am 1995;9:1117-26.

28. Suchin KR, Cucchiara AJ, Gottlieb SL, et al. Treatment of cutaneous T-cell lymphoma with combined immunomodulatory therapy: A 14-year experience at a single institution. Arch Dermatol 2002;138:1054-60.

29. Talpur R, Ward S, Apisarnthanarax N, et al. Optimizing bexarotene therapy for cutaneous T-cell lymphoma. J Am Acad Dermatol 2002; 47:672-84.

30. Richardson SK, Lin JH, Vittorio CC, et al. High clinical response rate with multimodality immunomodulatory therapy for Sézary syndrome. Clin Lymphoma Myeloma 2006;7: 226-32.

31. Knobler R, Barr ML, Couriel DR, et al. Extracorporeal photopheresis: Past, present, and future. J Am Acad Dermatol 2009;61:652-65.

32. Bisaccia E, Gonzalez J, Palangio M, et al. Extracorporeal photochemotherapy alone or with adjuvant therapy in the treatment of cutaneous T-cell lymphoma: A 9-year retrospective study at a single institution. J Am Acad Dermatol 2000;43:263-71.

33. Wollina U, Looks A, Meyer J, et al. Treatment of cutaneous T cell lymphoma stage II with interferon-alpha-2a and extracorporeal photochemotherapy: A prospective controlled trial. Ann N Y Acad Sci 2001;941:210-13.

34. Knobler R, Girardi M. Extracorporeal photochemoimmunotherapy in cutaneous T cell lymphomas. Ann N Y Acad Sci 2001;941:123-38.

35. Vonderheid EC, Bigler RD, Greenberg AS, et al. Extracorporeal photopheresis and recombinant interferon alfa 2b in Sézary syndrome. Use of dual marker labeling to monitor therapeutic response. Am J Clin Oncol 1994;17: 255-63.

36. Shaz BH, Linenberger ML, Bandarenko N, et al. Category IV indications for therapeutic apheresis: ASFA fourth special issue. J Clin Apher 2007;22:176-80.

37. Szczepiorkowski ZM, Shaz BH, Bandarenko N, Winters JL. The new approach to assignment of ASFA categories—introduction to the fourth special issue: Clinical applications of therapeutic apheresis. J Clin Apher 2007;22:96-105.

38. Szczepiorkowski ZM, Winters JL, Bandarenko N, et al. Guidelines on the use of therapeutic apheresis in clinical practice—evidence-based approach from the Apheresis Applications Committee of the American Society for Apher-

esis. The Fifth Special Issue. J Clin Apher 2010; 25:83-177.

39. Fefer A. Graft-versus-tumour response. In: Blume KG, Forman SJ, Appelbaum FR, eds. Thomas' hematopoietic stem cell transplantation. 3rd ed. Malden, MA: Blackwell Publishing, 2004:369-79.

40. Owsianowski M, Gollnick H, Siegert W, et al. Successful treatment of chronic graft-versus-host disease with extracorporeal photopheresis. Bone Marrow Transplant 1994;14:845-8.

41. Rossetti F, Dall'Amico R, Crovetti G, et al. Extracorporeal photochemotherapy for the treatment of graft-versus-host disease. Bone Marrow Transplant 1996;2:175-81.

42. Child FJ, Ratnavel R, Watkins P, et al. Extracorporeal photopheresis (ECP) in the treatment of chronic graft-versus-host disease (GVHD). Bone Marrow Transplant 1999;23:881-7.

43. Abhyankar S. Adjunctive treatment of resistant graft-versus-host disease with extracorporeal photopheresis (abstract). Blood 1998;92:454a.

44. Bishop M, Lynch, H, Tarantolo S, et al. Extracorporeal photopheresis permits steroid withdrawal in steroid-resistant chronic graft versus-host disease (abstract). Blood 1998;92:455a.

45. Greinix HT, Volc-Platzer B, Knobler RM. Extracorporeal photochemotherapy in the treatment of severe graft-versus-host disease. Leuk Lymphoma 2000;36:425-34.

46. DiVenuti G, Foss F. Photopheresis as a treatment for chronic graft-versus-host disease after allogeneic bone marrow transplantation (abstract). Blood 2002;100:846a.

47. Couriel D, Hosing C, Saliba R, et al. Extracorporeal photopheresis for acute and chronic graft-versus-host disease: Does it work? Biol Blood Marrow Transplant 2006;12:37-40.

48. Rubegni P, Cuccia A, Sbano P, et al. Role of extracorporeal photochemotherapy in patients with refractory chronic graft-versus-host disease. Br J Haematol 2005;130:271-5.

49. Flowers ME, Apperley JF, van Besien K, et al. A multicenter prospective phase 2 randomized study of extracorporeal photopheresis for treatment of chronic graft-versus-host disease. Blood 2008;112:2667-74.

50. Rossetti F, Zulian F, Dall'Amico R, et al. Extracorporeal photochemotherapy as single therapy for extensive, cutaneous, chronic graft-versus-host disease. Transplantation 1995;59: 149-51.

51. DiVenuti G, Miller DF, Sprague K, et al. Photopheresis as a treatment for chronic graft-vs-host

disease after allogeneic bone marrow transplantation (abstract). Blood 2002;100:846a.

52. Couriel DR, Hosing C, Saliba R, et al. Extracorporeal photochemotherapy for the treatment of steroid-resistant chronic GVHD. Blood 2006; 107:3074-80.

53. Greinix HT, Volc-Platzer B, Rabitsch W, et al. Successful use of extracorporeal photochemotherapy in the treatment of severe acute and chronic graft-versus-host disease. Blood 1998; 92:3098-104.

54. Kuzmina Z, Greinix HT, Knobler R, et al. Proportions of immature CD19+CD21- B lymphocytes predict the response to extracorporeal photopheresis in patients with chronic graft-versus-host disease. Blood 2009;114:744-6.

55. Besnier DP, Chabannes D, Mahe B, et al. Treatment of graft-versus-host disease by extracorporeal photochemotherapy: A pilot study. Transplantation 1997;64:49-54.

56. Dall'Amico R, Zacchello G. Treatment of graft-versus-host disease with photopheresis. Transplantation 1998;65:1283-4.

57. Richter HI, Stege H, Ruzicka T, et al. Extracorporeal photopheresis in the treatment of acute graft-versus-host disease. J Am Acad Dermatol 1997;36:787-9.

58. Perfetti P, Carlier P, Strada P, et al. Extracorporeal photopheresis for the treatment of steroid refractory acute GVHD. Bone Marrow Transplant 2008;42:609-17.

59. Messina C, Locatelli F, Lanino E, et al. Extracorporeal photochemotherapy for paediatric patients with graft-versus-host disease after haematopoietic stem cell transplantation. Br J Haematol 2003;122:118-27.

60. Smith EP, Sniecinski I, Dagis AC, et al. Extracorporeal photochemotherapy for treatment of drug-resistant graft-vs.-host disease. Biol Blood Marrow Transplant 1998;4:27-37.

61. Miller J, Goodman SA, Stricklin GP, Lloyd EK. Extracorporeal photochemotherapy in the treatment of graft-versus-host disease. Paper presented at: International Bone Marrow Transplant Registry Meeting, Keystone Resort, Keystone, Colorado, February 1998.

62. Salvaneschi L, Perotti C, Zecca M, et al. Extracorporeal photochemotherapy for treatment of acute and chronic GVHD in childhood. Transfusion 2001;41:1299-305.

63. Foss F, Roberts T, Miller K. Novel pentostatin/ extracorporeal photopheresis reduced intensity conditioning regimen: Results in relapsed/

refractory NHL (abstract). Blood 2002;100: 112a.

64. Chan G, Foss F, Roberts T, et al. Decreased acute and chronic graft vs host disease with early full donor engraftment following a pentostatin-based preparative regimen for allogeneic bone marrow transplantation in high risk patients (abstract). Blood 2001;98:383a.

65. Ohtsuka T, Okita H, Yamakage A, Yamazaki S. The effect of extracorporeal photochemotherapy on alpha1(I) and alpha1(III) procollagen mRNA expression in systemic sclerosis skin tissue. Arch Dermatol Res 2002;293:642-5.

66. Hashikabe M, Ohtsuka T, Yamazaki S. Quantitative echographic analysis of photochemotherapy on systemic sclerosis skin. Arch Dermatol Res 2005;296:522-7.

67. Fimiani M, Rubegni P, Flori ML, et al. Three cases of progressive systemic sclerosis treated with extracorporeal photochemotherapy. Arch Dermatol Res 1997;289:120-2.

68. Neustadter JH, Samarin F, Carlson KR, Girardi M. Extracorporeal photochemotherapy for generalized deep morphea. Arch Dermatol 2009; 145:127-30.

69. Schlaak M, Friedlein H, Kauer F, et al. Successful therapy of a patient with therapy recalcitrant generalized bullous scleroderma by extracorporeal photopheresis and mycophenolate mofetil. J Eur Acad Dermatol Venereol 2008;22:631-3.

70. Rook AH, Freundlich B, Jegasothy BV, et al. Treatment of systemic sclerosis with extracorporeal photochemotherapy. Results of a multicenter trial. Arch Dermatol 1992;128:337-46.

71. Knobler RM, French LE, Kim Y, et al. A randomized, double-blind, placebo-controlled trial of photopheresis in systemic sclerosis. J Am Acad Dermatol 2006;54:793-9.

72. Enomoto DN, Mekkes JR, Bossuyt PM, et al. Treatment of patients with systemic sclerosis with extracorporeal photochemotherapy (photopheresis). J Am Acad Dermatol 1999;41: 915-22.

73. Lozano E, Segarra M, Cid MC. Stimulatory autoantibodies to the PDGF receptor in scleroderma. N Engl J Med 2006;355:1278-9; author reply, 1279-80.

74. Svegliati S, Olivieri A, Campelli N, et al. Stimulatory autoantibodies to PDGF receptor in patients with extensive chronic graft-versus-host disease. Blood 2007;110:237-41.

75. Fonseca C, Lindahl GE, Ponticos M, et al. A polymorphism in the CTGF promoter region

associated with systemic sclerosis. N Engl J Med 2007;357:1210-20.

76. Mathur K, Morris S, Deighan C, et al. Extracorporeal photopheresis improves nephrogenic fibrosing dermopathy/nephrogenic systemic fibrosis: Three case reports and review of literature. J Clin Apher 2008;23:144-50.

77. Richmond H, Zwerner J, Kim Y, Fiorentino D. Nephrogenic systemic fibrosis: Relationship to gadolinium and response to photopheresis. Arch Dermatol 2007;143:1025-30.

78. Reinisch W, Nahavandi H, Santella R, et al. Extracorporeal photochemotherapy in patients with steroid-dependent Crohn's disease: A prospective pilot study. Aliment Pharmacol Ther 2001;15:1313-22.

79. Abreu MT, von Tirpitz C, Hardi R, et al. Extracorporeal photopheresis for the treatment of refractory Crohn's disease: Results of an open-label pilot study. Inflamm Bowel Dis 2009;15:829-36.

80. Guariso G, D'Inca R, Sturniolo GC, et al. Photopheresis treatment in severe Crohn disease. J Pediatr Gastroenterol Nutr 2003;37:517-20.

81. Lindahl-Kiessling K, Safwenberg J. Inability of UV-irradiated lymphocytes to stimulate allogeneic cells in mixed lymphocyte culture. Int Arch Allergy Appl Immunol 1971;41:670-8.

82. Chabot JA, Pepino P, Wasfie T, et al. UVB pretreatment of rat bone marrow allografts. Prevention of GVHD and induction of allochimerism and donor-specific unresponsiveness. Transplantation 1990;49:886-9.

83. Cohn ML, Cahill RA, Deeg HJ. Hematopoietic reconstitution and prevention of graft-versus-host disease with UVB-irradiated haploidentical murine spleen and marrow cells. Blood 1991;78:3317-22.

84. Deeg HJ, Graham TC, Gerhard-Miller L, et al. Prevention of transfusion-induced graft-versus-host disease in dogs by ultraviolet irradiation. Blood 1989;74:2592-5.

85. Pamphilon DH, Alnaqdy AA, Godwin V, et al. Studies of allogeneic bone marrow and spleen cell transplantation in a murine model using ultraviolet-B light. Blood 1991;77:2072-8.

86. Pamphilon DH, Alnaqdy AA, Wallington TB. Immunomodulation by ultraviolet light: Clinical studies and biological effects. Immunol Today 1991;12:119-23.

87. Perez MI, Edelson RL, John L, et al. Inhibition of antiskin allograft immunity induced by infusions with photoinactivated effector T lympho-

cytes (PET cells). Yale J Biol Med 1989;62:595-609.

88. Perez M, Edelson R, Laroche L, Berger C. Inhibition of antiskin allograft immunity by infusions with syngeneic photoinactivated effector lymphocytes. J Invest Dermatol 1989;92:669-76.

89. Perez MI, Lobo FM, John L, et al. Induction of a cell-transferable suppression of alloreactivity by photodamaged lymphocytes. Transplantation 1992;54:896-903.

90. Yamane Y, Lobo FM, John LA, et al. Suppression of anti-skin-allograft response by photodamaged effector cells—the modulating effects of prednisolone and cyclophosphamide. Transplantation 1992;54:119-24.

91. Pepino P, Hardy MA, Chabot JA, et al. UVB irradiated allogeneic bone marrow transplantation in rats: Prevention of graft versus host disease without immunosuppression. Transplant Proc 1989;21:2995-6.

92. Lloveras JJ, Escourrou G, Delisle MB, et al. Evolution of untreated mild rejection in heart transplant recipients. J Heart Lung Transplant 1992;11:751-6.

93. Costanzo-Nordin MR, McManus BM, Wilson JE, et al. Efficacy of photopheresis in the rescue therapy of acute cellular rejection in human heart allografts: A preliminary clinical and immunopathologic report. Transplant Proc 1993;25:881-3.

94. Lehrer MS, Rook AH, Tomaszewski JE, DeNofrio D. Successful reversal of severe refractory cardiac allograft rejection by photopheresis. J Heart Lung Transplant 2001;20:1233-6.

95. Dall'Amico R, Livi U, Milano A, et al. Extracorporeal photochemotherapy as adjuvant treatment of heart transplant recipients with recurrent rejection. Transplantation 1995;60:45-9.

96. Giunti G, Schurfeld K, Maccherini M, et al. Photopheresis for recurrent acute rejection in cardiac transplantation. Transplant Proc 1999;31:128-9.

97. Meiser BM, Kur F, Reichenspurner H, et al. Reduction of the incidence of rejection by adjunct immunosuppression with photochemotherapy after heart transplantation. Transplantation 1994;57:563-8.

98. Barr ML, Meiser BM, Eisen HJ, et al. Photopheresis for the prevention of rejection in cardiac transplantation. Photopheresis Transplantation Study Group. N Engl J Med 1998;339:1744-51.

99. Barr ML, Baker CJ, Schenkel FA, et al. Prophylactic photopheresis and chronic rejection: Effects on graft intimal hyperplasia in cardiac transplantation. Clin Transplant 2000;14:162-6.

100. Salerno CT, Park SJ, Kreykes NS, et al. Adjuvant treatment of refractory lung transplant rejection with extracorporeal photopheresis. J Thorac Cardiovasc Surg 1999;117:1063-9.

101. Slovis BS, Loyd JE, King LE Jr. Photopheresis for chronic rejection of lung allografts (letter). N Engl J Med 1995;332:962.

102. Villanueva J, Bhorade SM, Robinson JA, et al. Extracorporeal photopheresis for the treatment of lung allograft rejection. Ann Transplant 2000;5:44-7.

103. Andreu G, Achkar A, Couetil JP, et al. Extracorporeal photochemotherapy treatment for acute lung rejection episode. J Heart Lung Transplant 1995;14:793-6.

104. Horina JH, Mullegger RR, Horn S, et al. Photopheresis for renal allograft rejection (letter). Lancet 1995;346:61.

105. Sunder-Plassman G, Druml W, Steininger R, et al. Renal allograft rejection controlled by photopheresis (letter). Lancet 1995;346:506.

106. Dall'Amico R, Murer L, Montini G, et al. Successful treatment of recurrent rejection in renal transplant patients with photopheresis. J Am Soc Nephrol 1998;9:121-7.

107. Wolfe JT, Tomaszewski JE, Grossman RA, et al. Reversal of acute renal allograft rejection by extracorporeal photopheresis: A case presentation and review of the literature. J Clin Apher 1996;11:36-41.

108. Efferth T, Fabry U, Osieka R. Induction of apoptosis, depletion of glutathione, and DNA damage by extracorporeal photochemotherapy and psoralen with exposure to UV light in vitro. Anticancer Res 2001;21:2777-83.

109. Enomoto DN, Schellekens PT, Yong SL, et al. Extracorporeal photochemotherapy (photopheresis) induces apoptosis in lymphocytes: A possible mechanism of action of PUVA therapy. Photochem Photobiol 1997;65:177-80.

110. Song PS, Tapley KJ Jr. Photochemistry and photobiology of psoralens. Photochem Photobiol 1979;29:1177-97.

111. Berger CL, Hanlon D, Kanada D, et al. Transimmunization, a novel approach for tumor immunotherapy. Transfus Apher Sci 2002;26:205-16.

112. Berger CL, Xu AL, Hanlon D, et al. Induction of human tumor-loaded dendritic cells. Int J Cancer 2001;91:438-47.

113. Miracco C, Rubegni P, De Aloe G, et al. Extracorporeal photochemotherapy induces apoptosis of infiltrating lymphoid cells in patients with mycosis fungoides in early stages. A quantitative histological study. Br J Dermatol 1997;137:549-57.

114. Moor AC, Schmitt IM, Beijersbergen van Henegouwen GM, et al. Treatment with 8-MOP and UVA enhances MHC class I synthesis in RMA cells: Preliminary results. J Photochem Photobiol B 1995;29:193-8.

115. Gorgun G, Miller KB, Foss FM. Immunologic mechanisms of extracorporeal photochemotherapy in chronic graft-versus-host disease. Blood 2002;100:941-7.

116. Maeda A, Schwarz A, Kernebeck K, et al. Intravenous infusion of syngeneic apoptotic cells by photopheresis induces antigen-specific regulatory T cells. J Immunol 2005;174:5968-76.

117. Gatza E, Rogers CE, Clouthier SG, et al. Extracorporeal photopheresis reverses experimental graft-versus-host disease through regulatory T cells. Blood 2008;112:1515-21.

118. Meloni F, Cascina A, Miserere S, et al. Peripheral CD4(+)CD25(+) TREG cell counts and the response to extracorporeal photopheresis in lung transplant recipients. Transplant Proc 2007;39:213-17.

119. Alcindor TDM, Baki J, Gorgun G, et al. Increased expression of CD25 antigen in lymphocytes and increased number of NK cells are observed in CTCL patients after photopheresis (abstract). Blood 1999;94:97a.

120. French LE, Alcindor T, Shapiro M, et al. Identification of amplified clonal T cell populations in the blood of patients with chronic graft-versus-host disease: Positive correlation with response to photopheresis. Bone Marrow Transplant 2002;30:509-15.

121. Di Renzo M, Rubegni P, De Aloe G, et al. Extracorporeal photochemotherapy restores Th1/Th2 imbalance in patients with early stage cutaneous T-cell lymphoma. Immunology 1997;92:99-103.

In: McLeod BC, Szczepiorkowski ZM, Weinstein R, Winters JL, eds.
Apheresis: Principles and Practice, 3rd edition
Bethesda, MD: AABB Press, 2010

29

Cellular Gene Therapy

P. Dayanand Borge, Jr, MD, PhD, and Harvey G. Klein, MD

 THE PAST FEW YEARS HAVE witnessed disappointing and tragic results in two well-publicized gene therapy trials. In the first, a young man treated for an inherited metabolic disorder, ornithine transcarbamylase deficiency, developed a fatal episode of hepatitis. The hepatitis was apparently the result of an inflammatory reaction to the adenoviral vector carrying a therapeutic transgene that was injected directly into his hepatic circulation.[1,2] The second instance applies specifically to cellular gene therapy. Five of 20 patients with X-linked severe combined immunodeficiency (SCID-X1) corrected by infusion of gene-modified, marrow-derived hematopoietic progenitor cells (HPCs) in separate studies in Paris and London developed a lymphoproliferative syndrome 2 to 6 years after treatment.[3-5] Although these reports underscore the potential risks of gene therapy, the apparent success of this approach in 17 of the 20 patients in these trials emphasizes the importance of understanding both the science and the promise of cellular gene therapy.[6]

Cellular gene therapy is a strategy whereby a functioning gene is inserted ex vivo into the somatic cells of a patient to correct an inborn genetic error or to provide some new function to the cells. Two concepts in this definition deserve emphasis. First, only somatic cells are modified. The genetic change persists for the life of the cell and, in some cases, for the life of the patient. However, no genetic modification is introduced into the patient's germ-line cells, and therefore none is transmitted to progeny. Second, genes are inserted into harvested cells that are manipulated in the laboratory; the corrected cells, not replication-competent gene vectors, are injected into the patient. The gene-corrected cells may be purified, concentrated, expanded, or infused without further manipulation (see Chapter 24). The skills that apheresis personnel have acquired in mobilizing, collect-

P. Dayanand Borge, Jr, MD, PhD, Transfusion Medicine Fellow, and Harvey G. Klein, MD, Chief, Department of Transfusion Medicine, Warren Grant Magnuson Clinical Center, National Institutes of Health, Bethesda, Maryland

The authors have disclosed no conflicts of interest.

ing, processing, and storing cellular components from patients and healthy donors for transfusion purposes makes them logical partners in developing the field of cellular gene therapy.

Progress in cell biology, molecular genetics, and cell culture methods during the past two decades has moved gene therapy strategies rapidly from the confines of the research laboratory to the bedside, the clinic, and the popular press. Initially, gene transfer technology was applied clinically as a cell marking technique to study lymphocyte traffic and survival in patients with metastatic melanoma.[7] The first therapeutic infusion of gene-corrected cells, autologous lymphocytes transduced with the gene for adenosine deaminase (ADA), was performed on September 14, 1990, for a child with SCID and inherited ADA deficiency.[8] In theory, many inherited disorders could be corrected by the transfer of new genetic information into the appropriate somatic cell. The first unequivocal "cures," targeting marrow-derived HPCs, have been reported.[6,9] However, despite encouraging early results, the achievements still fall short of the expectations, and significant scientific, medical, ethical, and economic issues continue to merit scrutiny and discussion.

Basic Requirements of Gene Transfer Technology

The technical goals of cellular gene therapy appear straightforward: deliver therapeutic genes safely and efficiently to appropriate target cells in a way that ensures sufficiently precise in vivo regulation to provide a beneficial dose of gene product to the appropriate site for the desired period. Achieving these goals, however, is considerably more complicated.[10] The major problems that plague gene therapy include the following:

1. Transient gene expression. The therapeutic transgene must remain functional, and the corrected cells must be long-lived and stable. Difficulties with integrating therapeutic genes into the cell's genome and the rap-

idly dividing nature of many cells limit long-term benefit.

2. Regulation of gene expression. Natural and synthetic enhancer promoters are being investigated to drive gene transcription.[11]

3. Immune response. Both vectors and proteins related to the vector system expressed on the target cell may stimulate an immune response. The immune response may reduce efficacy, prevent repeated treatment, and even harm the recipient.

4. Viral vector systems. Viruses may induce toxicity, immune or inflammatory responses, present gene control and targeting issues, and even recombine to become pathogenic.[12]

5. Multigene disorders. Whereas gene therapy has been directed almost exclusively at single gene mutations, some of the most common disorders are caused by the combined effects of many genes.

For cellular gene therapy to be effective, the appropriate gene must first be identified and isolated; the nucleotide sequence must be determined to ensure that no extraneous sequences are present and to identify potential splice sites; and the laboratory must develop techniques for the stable introduction of the gene into a cellular expression system. Furthermore, the techniques must be suitable for large-scale production sufficient for clinical use, and they must adhere to the principles of current good manufacturing practice required by the Food and Drug Administration (FDA).[13]

The gene must be inserted into the appropriate cell for tissue-specific expression. For example, manipulation of the globin gene to treat hemoglobinopathies must be performed on HPCs, whereas treatment of cystic fibrosis should be directed toward pulmonary and pancreatic cells. The level of gene expression is also important. For certain enzyme deficiencies, loose control of expression is adequate. Genetic studies indicate that persons with as little as 10% of normal ADA levels are immunologically normal, whereas those who have an inherited mutation producing levels 50-fold higher than normal appear to suffer no adverse effects. For other gene products, such as beta globin in thalassemia, precise control of expression is critical. Indiscriminate expression may result in ineffective erythropoiesis and red cell destruction. Finally, the disease under consideration should have a reversible phenotype. Such reversibility may be demonstrated by successful treatment with enzyme replacement or by hematopoietic stem cell transplantation (HSCT).

Desirable Properties of a Gene Delivery Vehicle

Several characteristics define a suitable gene delivery system (ie, a vector). The vehicle must be able to encapsulate the therapeutic gene, regardless of its size. The delivery vehicle should bind efficiently to the target cells and the ideal vector should bind preferentially to a specific cell type. The vehicle should deliver the gene efficiently to the target cell's cytoplasm or nucleus. Transfer of the genetic material into the chromosome of the target cell

(transduction) is desirable for stable expression, although genomic material confined to an extrachromosomal site, for example an episome, may result in high-level expression that proves transient. Gene delivery should result in accurate and stable long-term expression.

Different approaches have been developed for inserting therapeutic genes into somatic cells (Table 29-1). Chemical and physical insertion methods such as electroporation; liposome-mediated, receptor-specific uptake; and direct DNA injection are important in the research laboratory. Their advantages include the ability to transfer large genes to a variety of cell types, regardless of cell cycle status and surface-receptor profile. However, these methods are generally too inefficient and labor intensive for a clinical production facility, and stable integration of DNA is infrequent. Viruses, selected through evolutionary pressures to carry genetic material into a wide variety of mammalian cells, have been readily adapted for therapeutic gene transfer. Certain viruses appear attractive as vectors because of their specific cell tro-

---

Table 29-1. Techniques for Gene Transfer into Mammalian Cells

Technique	Characteristics
Viral Vector-Mediated	
Retrovirus	Stable, efficient, but random integration into genome of dividing cells
Lentivirus	Improved efficiency; nondividing cells
Adenovirus	Transduction of replicating and nonreplicating cells without integration; transient high expression; may lyse target cell or elicit potent immune response
Adeno-associated virus	Requires adenovirus coinfection; potential for site-specific integration
Nonviral	Inefficient; may cause cell damage
Electroporation	Inefficient delivery; stable expression
$CaPO_4$ precipitation	Labor intensive; transient expression
Microinjection	Low cell transfection; transient expression; non-immunogenic
Liposome-mediated fusion	Receptor-mediated endocytosis; degradation within lysosomes
Ligand-DNA conjugates	

---

pisms—for example, herpes viruses for neural cells and adenoviruses for cells in the respiratory tract. However, practical obstacles such as inefficient transduction, cytotoxicity, and immunogenicity render some viruses poorly suited for clinical use. The most successful systems currently use disabled retroviral vectors derived from murine leukemia viruses, although various other viral vectors—including adenoviruses and adeno-associated viruses, parvoviruses, vaccinia viruses, and lentiviruses—are also under study.[14]

For example, the Maloney murine leukemia virus, an enveloped RNA oncoretrovirus, can be readily modified to produce a replication-incompetent vector that can efficiently integrate a therapeutic transgene into dividing cells in vitro.[15] For use as a gene delivery system, the retrovirus is rendered defective by removing functional genes and replacing them with the gene of interest. The vector is thus capable of delivering a therapeutic gene but is incapable of further replication. Producer cell culture systems have been devised to minimize the risk that a recombinational event would yield a replication-competent virus.[16]

Methods for producing a high-titer, clinical-grade, retroviral vector have been described.[17] Retroviral vectors require dividing cells in order to insert their genes into the host genome. Once inserted, however, the integrated provirus is present for the life of the cell and of the cell's progeny. One disadvantage of the retroviral vector is "random integration"; that is, vector insertion of the gene into random sites in the host DNA. The level of gene expression for any given cell may depend on the site of integration. Random integration involves a risk of "insertional mutagenesis" which is defined as malignant transformation by mutagenic activation of nearby oncogenes or by inactivation of tumor-suppressor genes.[18] For this reason, meticulous attention is paid to removal of replication-competent retroviruses from the vector preparation to minimize the number of integration events. A second disadvantage, especially for the delivery of genes to quiescent pluripotent HPCs, is the requirement for active cycling of the target cell. Recent stud-

ies with a lentivirus class of retrovirus may circumvent this problem.[19] One such study employed lentiviral-mediated gene therapy of autologous hematopoietic stem cells to treat X-linked adrenoleukodystrophy in two patients with some success.[20]

Applications of Cellular Gene Therapy

Selection of Diseases

There are several potential general applications for cellular gene therapy. Autologous cells may be used as a "drug-delivery system" in which the product of the inserted gene acts like the drug or activates a prodrug.[21] Almost any kind of cell might be used for this function, from a short-lived circulating cell to a semi-permanent "depot" of fibroblasts engineered to release a clotting factor protein.[22] Autologous cells may also be modified genetically to enhance their function as immune cells in the treatment of infectious or neoplastic disorders or to decrease susceptibility to pathogens such as human immunodeficiency virus (HIV). The lymphocytes—relatively easily collected, expanded in culture, and stored—are one of the likely candidate effector cells, although macrophages and dendritic cells are also being tested in a variety of therapeutic strategies. The challenge is to match the appropriate cell with the right therapeutic gene construct. Autologous HPCs might be gene-corrected for the "permanent" treatment of almost any inherited hematologic disorder that responds to allogeneic HSCT, as well as for the treatment of some acquired disorders. For permanent genetic correction, gene expression must be stable to prevent loss by dilution with each replication cycle, and expression in the relevant hematopoietic cell line must persist at levels sufficient to correct the underlying defect.

Currently, a candidate disease for treatment by cellular gene therapy should meet several of the following criteria:

1. The disease should be associated with high morbidity and mortality.
2. The disease should lack effective or practical treatment but should have a reversible phenotype.
3. The disease process should be stabilized or reversed by a fraction of the gene product ordinarily considered the "normal level."

Strict regulation of gene expression should not be necessary. Candidate diseases for cellular gene therapy are listed in Table 29-2.

Selection of Target Cells for Gene Insertion

Target cells for cellular gene therapy should also meet several criteria. They should be 1)

Table 29-2. Disorders for which Cellular Gene Therapy Is in Development

Disorder	Target Cell (if reported)
Genetic immune deficiency	
ADA-deficient SCID	Lymphocytes, CD34+ marrow, PBPCs, UCB
X-linked SCID	CD34+ marrow, UCB
Wiskott-Aldrich syndrome	
Agammaglobulinemia	
Storage disorders	
Gaucher disease	CD34+ marrow, PBPCs
Mucopolysaccharidoses	Lymphocytes
Leukocyte defects	
Chronic granulomatous disease	CD34+ PBPCs
Leukocyte adhesion defect	CD34+ PBPCs
Chediak-Higashi disease	
Infectious disease	
AIDS	Lymphocytes, CD34+ marrow
Hemoglobinopathies	
Sickling disorders	
Thalassemia	
Neoplastic disorders	
Chronic myelocytic leukemia	
Breast cancer	Marrow
Ovarian cancer	Marrow
Miscellaneous	
Hemophilia A	Fibroblasts
Hemophilia B	
Fanconi anemia	PBPCs
Graft-vs-host disease	Lymphocytes

PBPCs = peripheral blood progenitor cells; UCB = umbilical cord blood; ADA = adenosine deaminase; SCID = severe combined immunodeficiency.

readily harvested from the patient, 2) easily manipulated and expanded, and 3) readily transduced ex vivo and returned to the patient without difficulty. Ideally, the cells should be easily cryopreserved for potential future use and should also be self-renewing so that the transduced gene will persist for the life of the patient.[23]

In practice, several different cell types are used for gene therapy, although few meet all these criteria. Hepatocytes have been used to treat patients with homozygous familial hypercholesterolemia that results from the absence of hepatic receptors for low-density lipoproteins.[24] A segment of the patient's liver is removed surgically, and a single-cell suspension of autologous hepatocytes is transduced in culture with a vector containing the gene for the low-density lipoprotein receptor. Gene-corrected cells are subsequently reinfused through a portal vein catheter. Therapeutic strategies using vascular endothelial cells, keratinocytes, chondrocytes, myoblasts, and fibroblasts have also been initiated.

Two cell types that most closely fit the ideal gene target are peripheral blood lymphocytes (TC, Apheresis) and peripheral blood (hematopoietic) progenitor cells (HPCs from apheresis, or HPC-A).[25,26] Large numbers of TC, Apheresis are easily collected with apheresis instruments and can be expanded in short- or long-term culture systems (see Chapter 24). Stability in culture permits multiple gene insertions as well as comprehensive testing for gene expression and safety purposes. Lymphocytes are mature cells and are less likely than more primitive cells to suppress the expression of inserted genes. They are also hardy cells that can be transported, stored at refrigerator temperatures, or frozen with several cryoprotectant agents and thawed with good recovery of viability and function. Lymphocytes circulate in vivo for months and possibly years after infusion and may persist even longer at tissue sites. Furthermore, they can be expanded in vivo with infusions of the lymphokine interleukin-2 (IL-2).

Finally, lymphocytes express cell-surface markers that may be used to target therapy.

HPCs are easily accessible in marrow, in mobilized peripheral blood (for collection by apheresis; see Chapter 23), and in umbilical cord blood. The most primitive pluripotent stem cell has not been defined using in vitro assays, but stable and efficient gene transfer into early progenitors, as assayed by long-term culture systems, has been achieved.[9,27] Initial attempts at gene transduction of long-lived hematopoietic progenitors were extremely inefficient (0.1 to 1%). The reasons for low levels of gene transfer are unclear but may include a small number of cycling cells, low numbers of receptors for the vectors used, stem cell niche crowding by existing marrow cells (see Chapter 25), and possibly intracellular blocking factors. Recent approaches for improving gene insertion, engraftment, and expression have included altered culture conditions with newly developed cytokine cocktails and molecules to neutralize inhibitors, a recombinant fibronectin support matrix, longer culture times, improved vectors, and, most important, use of modified preinfusion preparatory regimens.[19,28] Low-dose busulfan induces a transient myelosuppression and appears to result in improved, stable engraftment of gene-transduced cells with levels of 1% to 10% gene correction detected in a trial of ADA-corrected cells.[29]

Pluripotent cells compose only 1% to 2% of the total progenitor cell pool. However, it takes only a small pool of these cells to maintain hematopoiesis, perhaps for years. Therefore, correction of a small number of cells could, in theory, provide a patient with a several-log increase in gene-modified cells within each hematopoietic lineage. Large numbers of human HPC-A can be concentrated to high purity using immunologic cell separation techniques; some of the gene-marked HPC-A contribute to long-term engraftment. HPC-A can be cryopreserved in dimethylsulfoxide and subsequently thawed while preserving viability and engraftment potential (see Chapter 24).

Applications of Cellular Gene Therapy in Specific Diseases

SCID Adenosine Deaminase Deficiency

ADA deficiency, which accounts for approximately 20% of SCID syndromes in the United States, was an excellent candidate for the first cellular gene therapy trial. Patients typically present in infancy with failure to thrive and life-threatening infections. Without treatment, most succumb to infection during childhood or adolescence. The disorder results from an autosomal recessive single gene defect. The absence of ADA causes a defect in purine metabolism that leads to intracellular accumulation of deoxyadenosine and other toxic metabolites. Because T lymphocytes contain high levels of kinases that convert adenosine to toxic phosphorylated intermediates, progressive T-cell lymphopenia develops early in the course of the disease and is followed by a decline in B cells with hypogammaglobulinemia. The ADA gene (12 exons spanning 32,040 base pairs) has been cloned. Gene-corrected T cells should have a selective advantage in vivo, thus permitting expansion of therapeutic cells at the expense of the deficient ones. Loose control of gene expression is acceptable because ADA concentrations range widely in immunologically normal subjects. HSCT or T-lymphocyte engraftment alone has been curative.

In 1990, a 4-year-old child with ADA-deficient SCID was entered into a clinical protocol in which autologous T cells were transduced using retrovirus-mediated transfer of the ADA gene.[8] Peripheral leukocytes were collected by apheresis; lymphocytes isolated by gradient separation were cultured with the LASN (long terminal repeat, adenosine deaminase, SV40, Neo$_r$) retroviral vector. Culture for 9 to 12 days resulted in T-cell expansions of 17- to 135-fold and gene transfer efficiency of 0.1% to 10%. This child received 11 lymphocyte infusions, and 4 months later, a second child was begun on a course of 12 lymphocyte infusions, with at least 1 month between successive infusions over a 2-year period. During the first 6 months of therapy, peripheral blood T-cell counts rose rapidly and remained in the normal range. Ten years after the last infusion, approximately 20% of the first patient's polyclonal T cells still carry and express the retroviral transgene, although the number of T cells has fallen below the lower limit of the normal range.[30]

Both patients have shown laboratory and clinical evidence of partial immune reconstitution, and both developed reactivity to a battery of skin tests involving common environmental and vaccine antigens. Each patient's T cells demonstrated production of IL-2 and cytolytic activity that was not present before cellular gene therapy treatment. Each patient developed significant elevations in isohemagglutinin titers and in antibodies to vaccine. In the first patient, these changes have persisted since early in the course of treatment. Both children have grown and gained weight normally, and both are attending school. In the second patient, few (<0.1%) of the gene-corrected cells persist and no evidence of gene expression can be detected. This patient developed antibodies to both the retroviral vector and to fetal calf serum used in preparation of the cells. A patient in Japan developed similar antibodies.[31] Nevertheless, no safety hazards associated with this therapy have been encountered to date in more than a dozen children with this disease entered into various cellular gene therapy protocols. In a recent study of 10 patients with median follow-up of 4 years, engraftment and differentiation in both lymphoid and myeloid cells containing ADA was achieved, with 90% demonstrating stable reconstitution of T cells and normalized T-cell function.[32] Significant adverse effects were minimal and were not attributed to the engraftment of transduced cells. Variations of this method have been used to insert the *ADA* gene into HPCs from different sources. The clinical results, while promising, have been variable.[29,33,34] These patients illustrate the potential of, and some of the obstacles to, successful cellular gene therapy.

X-Linked SCID

The most common cause of SCID, accounting for approximately 40% of cases in the United

States, is SCID-X1, caused by the X-linked inheritance of a defective gene coding the common gamma chain, an essential component of the receptors for IL-2, IL-4, IL-7, IL-9, IL-15, and IL-21 that is critical in the development of T lymphocytes and natural killer cells. Hemizygous males usually die of severe infection during the first year of life, but survival can approach 90% after HSCT. Sustained correction of this defect using HPCs from marrow (HPC-M) for ex-vivo gene therapy has been reported in five patients.[9] This report has been hailed rightfully as the first cure effected by cellular gene therapy. Investigators in London and Paris have now treated 20 patients with various mutations. However, as mentioned in the opening paragraph of this chapter, five of these children have now developed a leukemia-like illness in which the T-cell clone with the transgene has it inserted into an intron of the *LMO2* gene [LIM domain only 2 (rhombotin-like 1)], the product of which serves a regulatory function in normal hematopoiesis.[35] *LMO2* has previously been reported as an oncogene in T-cell acute lymphoblastic leukemia. It seems clear that these cases represent instances of insertional mutagenesis, although further investigation will be necessary to determine whether these unfortunate events are somehow related to this specific illness or to some variable in the treatment protocol.

Other Inherited Disorders

Chronic granulomatous disease is an inherited disorder of neutrophil and monocyte oxidative metabolism that is characterized by granuloma formation and recurrent life-threatening infections. Neutrophils, eosinophils, monocytes, and macrophages lack the oxidative burst required for microbicidal activity against bacteria, fungi, and parasites. The disease is heterogeneous and involves a mutation of one of four genes controlling the membrane superoxide-generation complex.[36] These genes have been cloned and sequenced. The most common autosomal form of chronic granulomatous disease results from a failure to produce the p47[phox] subunit of NADPH oxidase. CD34+ progenitors from patients with this variant, selected by immunologic methods from HPC-A, have been gene-corrected with a replication-defective retrovirus encoding p47[phox].[18] Mature neutrophils and monocytes derived from gene-corrected progenitors by in-vitro differentiation demonstrated significant correction of superoxide generation. Five patients have received autologous, gene-corrected progenitors and demonstrated low-level and transient circulation of gene-corrected cells without definite evidence of clinical improvement.[37] Although prevention of recurrent infections should be achievable with low levels of corrected cells, neither the HPCs nor the granulocytes enjoy the selective advantage seen in the corrected cells of SCID patients. Employing an alternative strategy, two young adults with gp91[phox] mutations who underwent nonmyeloablative marrow conditioning followed by infusion of gene-corrected HPC-A demonstrated initial increases in gene-transduced cells of up to 21%. These levels increased in the subsequent months resulting from clonal expansion of genetically corrected cells with activating insertions in proto-oncogenes *MDS1-EVI1*, *PRDM 16*, or *SETBP1*.[38] These patients showed clearance of significant infections and general clinical improvement as a result.

Gaucher disease, a hereditary disorder of glycosphingolipid metabolism caused by a deficiency of lysosomal glucocerebrosidase, is another candidate for cellular gene therapy. Disease manifestations are related to the accumulation of glucocerebroside in macrophages of the reticuloendothelial system. The type I variant, the most common form, has a reversible phenotype and is manageable by enzyme replacement at a cost of $150,000 to $300,000 per year.[39] The corrective gene has been cloned and is well characterized. Transduction of HPCs could repopulate the reticuloendothelial system with functional macrophages. The gene has now been transferred into autologous HPC-A, and successful engraftment and expression have been reported by two groups.[40,41] Once again, without an obvious selective growth advantage for the corrected cells and without myeloablative therapy, expression proved to be transient and few corrected cells could be detected.

Fanconi anemia, an autosomal recessive inherited form of marrow failure, results from a cellular defect that causes DNA instability and cell death. The disease is characterized by progressive pancytopenia, various physical deformities, and a predisposition to malignancy. Four genetic complementation groups for Fanconi anemia have been identified, and the gene for the complementation group C (*FACC*) has been cloned. Gene-corrected cells have a selective growth advantage in a mouse model, providing the possibility that engraftment of a few corrected HPCs might result in clinical improvement. Human HPC-A have been transduced with retroviral and adeno-associated viral vectors containing *FACC*.[42,43] Three patients have now received autologous gene-corrected HPC-A. Hematopoietic colony growth has increased in vitro, and circulating cells demonstrate the presence of the transgene. In one patient, a transient rise in hemoglobin concentration has been observed.

Great interest continues for several other inherited diseases that are potential candidates for cellular gene therapy. Successful in-vitro gene correction of autologous lymphocytes has been achieved for Hunter syndrome, one of the family of mucopolysaccharidoses,[44-46] and a clinical trial has recently been initiated. Neither hemophilia A nor hemophilia B requires cell-specific gene expression, and expression at a level of 10% to 25% of normal should be sufficient for effective therapy. Recent experience with Factor VIII gene insertion into dermal fibroblasts followed by selection, expansion, and administration of the corrected clone to six patients with hemophilia A suggests this is a promising approach.[22]

The hemoglobinopathies, particularly β-thalassemia and sickle cell anemia, excited early enthusiasm for cellular gene therapy, but complex regulatory mechanisms may make these diseases more difficult to approach by gene-insertion techniques.[47] Several recent studies have investigated the feasibility of correcting hemoglobinopathies in murine models using lentiviral vectors.[48-52] Infusion and engraftment of hematopoietic stem cells transduced with human β-globin in a severe β-thalassemia model and an anti-sickling variant of human β-globin in a sickle cell disease model resulted in incorporation of the transgene-derived human β-globin at levels of 21% and 20% of total chimeric hemoglobin, respectively.[48,52] Important limiting factors were the need for a high percentage of transduced cells expressing the transgene and the effect of the site of genomic integration on the level of transgene expression. In a clinical trial of two patients conducted by Leboulch and colleagues,[53] one patient stably expressed the β-globin transgene but also curiously began expressing enough fetal hemoglobin (HbF) to comprise about one-third of the total hemoglobin. A possibly related but poorly understood phenomenon involves increased expression of HbF that has also been observed after failure of marrow engraftment in patients with hemoglobinopathies.[54,55] Although these results are encouraging, further studies are needed to elucidate implications of transgene expression in human disease.

AIDS

Although the early application of cellular gene therapy focused on genetic disorders, molecular strategies have been directed toward a number of acquired disorders as well. Some of the most provocative examples are aimed at treatment of AIDS. The pathogenesis of AIDS is extremely complex, involving T cells, macrophages, lymph nodes, and the thymus. However, viral progression clearly involves selective reduction of the T-cell compartment, reduction of CD4+ cells, and an aberrant oligoclonal expansion of reactive T cells. One of the initial approaches to restoring normal immune function involved the use of adoptive immune cells collected by apheresis to provide partial and transient immune reconstitution in AIDS.[56] Although syngeneic lymphocytes expanded ex vivo provided cellular replacement, efforts to render these cells resistant to infection by HIV or to suppress or interfere with viral production in already infected CD4+ lymphocytes provide both intellectual and technical challenges. Gene therapy may be directed toward both circulating cell populations and their progenitors. Experience with gene strategies directed against HIV may serve as a model for the role of cellular gene therapy in infectious diseases.[57]

The cell cycle of HIV has been carefully studied and dissected. The virus infects cells by attaching to the CD4 membrane antigen and to other, secondary receptors. Following penetration, the retrovirus is uncoated, generates double-stranded DNA by means of a reverse transcriptase, and inserts provirus into the cellular DNA by means of a viral integrase. The provirus may remain dormant, or it may be activated as a result of constitutive host transcription factors. Sequential production of viral mRNA, regulatory proteins, and structural proteins leads to viral assembly, replication, and release. Several of the genes and gene products involved in the HIV cell cycle have been isolated and studied. The candidate antiviral transgenes, directed against either proteins or RNA in the HIV replication cycle, have been reviewed recently.[58]

Various approaches have been undertaken to prevent HIV from infecting CD4+ lymphocytes and producing free infectious virus from cells that are already infected. One approach has been to transduce cells with a gene to produce soluble CD4 antigen to compete with the cellular receptor for free virus.[59] Genetic constructs have also been proposed to inhibit two viral regulatory genes, *tat* and *rev*, in both lymphocytes and progenitor cells, and to produce HIV-specific cytotoxic T lymphocytes by insertion of a gene coding the hybrid molecule CD4zeta.[60,61] Genes to produce ribozymes, small RNA molecules that cleave specific RNA sequences, have been inserted into infected cells to interfere with the transcription of viral structural genes. Several such approaches are in early clinical trials.[58] Many of these strategies are directed toward transduction of lymphocytes, which may travel to and persist at cellular sites for years.[62] However, transduction of HPCs may be needed to provide more durable therapy once a successful strategy has been identified.

Cancer

The first approved human gene transfer experiment involved retroviral marking of tumor-infiltrating lymphocytes in patients with advanced melanoma.[7] Subsequently, tumor-infiltrating lymphocytes were transduced with the tumor necrosis factor gene in an effort to enhance their cytotoxic activity.[63] Should such studies suggest that cellular therapy can be used effectively to deliver high concentrations of cytokines to local areas of neoplastic proliferation, genes that express gamma interferon, T-cell receptors (TCR), IL-10, and IL-6 might be among the other candidates to examine.[64] Recent studies have evaluated the efficacy of TCR gene transfer to develop lasting tumor-specific immunity. In one mouse model, TCR-transduced splenocytes were able to expand and survive in vivo and eradicate tumors expressing a virally derived peptide.[65] Human peripheral blood lymphocytes transduced with MART-1 (melanoma antigen recognized by T cells)-specific TCR, an antigen expressed in some cases of malignant melanoma, were capable of secreting cytokines upon antigen stimulation and even lysing cultured melanoma cells.[66] Adoptive transfer of MART-1 TCR cells in 15 patients showed sustained levels of circulating transduced cells for up to 2 months after infusion, but only 13% of the patients maintained this level at 1 year and exhibited regression of their metastatic lesions.[67] The application of TCR gene transfer adoptive immunotherapy in ovarian and renal cell carcinomas underscores the inability of transduced cells to persist at high levels in patients, even if they are capable of cytokine secretion.[68,69] However, even when large doses of gene-modified T-cells can be safely administered to patients, expression of the immune target in other tissues could result in unexpected toxicity.[69] Alternatively, genes that express cytokines have been transferred ex vivo into tumor cells to increase their immunogenicity. Suspensions of these autologous gene-modified tumor cells have been injected intravenously into the patient as a cellular vaccine.[70] Subcutaneous and intradermal injections of transduced tumor cells have been used as well.

Cellular gene therapy may be used in the treatment of cancer either to make cells more resistant to chemotherapy or to render them sensitive to a drug. Hematopoietic tissue can be modified ex vivo by insertion of the multidrug-resistance gene so that the patient can, in theory, tolerate more chemotherapy before marrow toxicity becomes a limiting factor. Several studies are exploring the clinical usefulness of this approach.[71] The opposite approach has been taken with the "suicide" gene for thymidine kinase, which phosphorylates nucleoside analogues, such as the drug ganciclovir, into toxic molecules. Effector T cells from a marrow donor, transduced with the thymidine kinase gene, have been used to treat an Epstein-Barr-virus-associated B-cell lymphoma. In these trials, intravenous ganciclovir was administered when there was no evidence of tumor and the patient began to develop graft-vs-host disease from the allogeneic lymphocytes. The drug reduced circulating marked lymphocytes from 13.4% to 3.1%, resulting in dramatic clinical improvement. This technology is being used to mediate graft-vs-leukemia and other graft-vs-tumor treatments in a stem cell transplantation setting.[72]

Regulatory and Safety Issues

The safety issues surrounding gene therapy can no longer be prefaced with the term "theoretical." Vector-induced inflammation has been reported with the in-vivo infusion of vector, as has transient shedding of viral vector; neither has been reported with cellular gene therapy.[35] Complementation of defective vector has been sought because in-vivo propagation of a helper virus and lymphoma have been reported in three of 10 immunosuppressed nonhuman primates.[18] Neither overwhelming viral infection nor novel infectious agents resulting from a recombination of the transferred genome have been observed. However, as mentioned above, insertional mutagenesis has been reported in two children, and a third is under observation. The possibility of environmental contamination with laboratory-generated agents and modification of the human germ line continue to stimulate widespread discussion.

Because of high public visibility in addition to the medical, scientific, and ethical issues, gene therapy has become one of the most highly regulated areas of medicine. In addition to the requirement for approval by an institutional review board and biosafety committee, each protocol must be submitted to the Recombinant DNA Advisory Committee (RAC) of the National Institutes of Health (NIH) and must be approved by the FDA. The FDA regularly updates its "Points to Consider" regarding production of biologics, especially those prepared with recombinant DNA technology, activated mononuclear cells, and gene-modified cells. The most recent update to the NIH guidelines was published in the *Federal Register* in 2009.[73,74] The multiple levels of review and approval are designed to ensure adequate safety and public discussion.

Future Prospects

The previous edition of this book stated that no disease had yet been cured by cellular gene therapy. That is no longer the case. Numerous technical obstacles have been overcome to increase gene insertion efficiency and the stability and expression of the transgene. Numerous challenges remain, however, and some seem almost insurmountable. Nevertheless, with more than 100 clinical protocols now submitted to the RAC, cellular gene therapy will likely undergo rigorous investigation during the next several years. As the Human Genome Project identifies some 30,000 genes and 3 billion chemical base pairs, the urge to find methods to use this technology in novel therapeutic strategies becomes compelling. Problems with the efficiency of gene transfer and the stability of expression will have to be addressed, possibly by the development of improved vectors, new methods of activating quiescent cells, and/or suppression of factors that inhibit cell cycling and proliferation. The availability of sufficient volumes of clinical-grade vector has been a problem; however, commercial and university-based production facilities are moving to fill this gap. As with many new technologies, the costs involved in vector production, cell culture, clinical trials, and regulatory submissions dwarf the costs of developing most new drugs. Costs should moderate as investigators develop experience with this technology.

The ability to collect large numbers of selected cells and to manipulate them ex vivo promises a role for apheresis technology in the development of this discipline. Apheresis facilities that have experience in preparing today's cellular therapy products should play a central role in placing new cellular therapies within the rigorous quality assurance framework required for cellular biologic treatment. These services should continue to participate in the development of cellular gene therapy.

References

1. Smaglik P. Tighter watch urged on adenoviral vectors ... with proposal to report all "adverse events." Nature 1999;402:707.
2. Smaglik P. Gene therapy death: Investigators ponder what went wrong. The Scientist 1999; 12:1.
3. Hacein-Bey-Abina S, von Kalle C, Schmidt M, et al. A serious adverse event after successful gene therapy for X-linked severe combined immunodeficiency. N Engl J Med 2003;348: 255-6.
4. Hacein-Bey-Abina S, Garrigue A, Wang GP, et al. Insertional oncogenesis in 4 patients after retrovirus-mediated gene therapy of SCID-X1. J Clin Invest 2008;118:3132-42.
5. Howe SJ, Mansour MR, Schwarzwaelder K, et al. Insertional mutagenesis combined with acquired somatic mutations causes leukemogenesis following gene therapy of SCID-X1 patients. J Clin Invest 2008;118:3143-50.
6. Fischer A, Cavazzana-Calvo M. Gene therapy of inherited diseases. Lancet 2008;371:2044-7.
7. Rosenberg SA, Aebersold P, Cornetta K, et al. Gene transfer into humans—immunotherapy of patients with advanced melanoma, using tumor-infiltrating lymphocytes modified by retroviral gene transduction. N Engl J Med 1990; 323:570-8.
8. Blaese RM, Culver KW, Miller AD, et al. T lymphocyte-directed gene therapy for ADA-SCID: Initial trial results after 4 years. Science 1995;270:475-80.
9. Hacein-Bey-Abina S, Le Deist F, Carlier F, et al. Sustained correction of X-linked severe combined immunodeficiency by ex vivo gene therapy. N Engl J Med 2002;346:1185-93.
10. Mulligan RC. The basic science of gene therapy. Science 1993;260:926-32.
11. Guo ZS, Li Q, Bartlett DL, et al. Gene transfer: The challenge of regulated gene expression. Trends Mol Med 2008;14:410-18.
12. Nayak S, Herzog RW. Progress and prospects: Immune responses to viral vectors. Gene Ther 2010;17:295-304.
13. Kessler DA, Siegel JP, Noguchi PD, et al. Regulation of somatic-cell therapy and gene therapy by the food and drug administration. N Engl J Med 1993;329:1169-73.
14. Bouard D, Alazard-Dany D, Cosset FL. Viral vectors: From virology to transgene expression. Br J Pharmacol 2009;157:153-65.
15. Hu J, Dunbar CE. Update on hematopoietic stem cell gene transfer using non-human primate models. Curr Opin Mol Ther 2002;4: 482-90.
16. Markowitz D, Goff S, Bank A. A safe packaging line for gene transfer: Separating viral genes on two different plasmids. J Virol 1988;62:1120-4.
17. Kotani H, Newton PB 3rd, Zhang S, et al. Improved methods of retroviral vector transduction and production for gene therapy. Hum Gene Ther 1994;5:19-28.
18. Donahue RE, Kessler SW, Bodine D, et al. Helper virus induced T cell lymphoma in non-human primates after retroviral mediated gene transfer. J Exp Med 1992;176:1125-35.
19. D'Costa J, Mansfield SG, Humeau LM. Lentiviral vectors in clinical trials: Current status. Curr Opin Mol Ther 2009;11:554-64.
20. Cartier N, Hacein-Bey-Abina S, Bartholomae CC, et al. Hematopoietic stem cell gene therapy with a lentiviral vector in X-linked adrenoleukodystrophy. Science 2009;326:818-23.
21. Rigg A, Sikora K. Genetic prodrug activation therapy. Mol Med Today 1997;3:359-66.
22. Roth DA, Tawa NE Jr, O'Brien JM, et al. Nonviral transfer of the gene encoding coagulation Factor VIII in patients with severe hemophilia A. N Engl J Med 2001;344:1735-42.

23. Clapp DW. Somatic gene therapy into hematopoietic cells. Current status and future implications. Clin Perinatol 1993;20:155-68.

24. Raper SE, Grossman M, Rader DJ, et al. Safety and feasibility of liver-directed ex vivo gene therapy for homozygous familial hypercholesterolemia. Ann Surg 1996;223:116-26.

25. Culver K, Cornetta K, Morgan R, et al. Lymphocytes as cellular vehicles for gene therapy in mouse and man. Proc Natl Acad Sci U S A 1991;88:3155-9.

26. Bienzle D, Abrams-Ogg AC, Kruth SA, et al. Gene transfer into hematopoietic stem cells: Long-term maintenance of in vitro activated progenitors without marrow ablation. Proc Natl Acad Sci U S A 1994;91:350-4.

27. Dunbar CE, Cottler-Fox M, O'Shaughnessy JA, et al. Retrovirally marked CD34-enriched peripheral blood and bone marrow cells contribute to long-term engraftment after autologous transplantation. Blood 1995;85:3048-57.

28. Wu T, Kim HJ, Sellers SE, et al. Prolonged high-level detection of retrovirally marked hematopoietic cells in nonhuman primates after transduction of CD34+ progenitors using clinically feasible methods. Mol Ther 2000;1:285-93.

29. Aiuti A, Slavin S, Aker M, et al. Correction of ADA-SCID by stem cell gene therapy combined with nonmyeloablative conditioning. Science 2002;296:2410-13.

30. Muul LM, Tuschong LM, Soenen SL, et al. Persistence and expression of the adenosine deaminase gene for 12 years and immune reaction to gene transfer components: Long-term results of the first clinical gene therapy trial. Blood 2003;101:2563-9.

31. Onodera M, Ariga T, Kawamura N, et al. Successful peripheral T-lymphocyte-directed gene transfer for a patient with severe combined immune deficiency caused by adenosine deaminase deficiency. Blood 1998;91:30-6.

32. Aiuti A, Cattaneo F, Galimberti S, et al. Gene therapy for immunodeficiency due to adenosine deaminase deficiency. N Engl J Med 2009;360:447-58.

33. Bordignon C, Notarangelo LD, Nobili N, et al. Gene therapy in peripheral blood lymphocytes and bone marrow for ADA-immunodeficient patients. Science 1995;270:470-5.

34. Kohn DB, Hershfield MS, Carbonaro D, et al. T lymphocytes with a normal ADA gene accumulate after transplantation of transduced autologous umbilical cord blood CD34+ cells in ADA-deficient SCID neonates. Nat Med 1998;4:775-80.

35. Buckley RH. Gene therapy for SCID—a complication after remarkable progress. Lancet 2002;360:1185-6.

36. Segal BH, Leto TL, Gallin JI, et al. Genetic, biochemical, and clinical features of chronic granulomatous disease. Medicine (Baltimore) 2000;79:170-200.

37. Malech HL, Maples PB, Whiting-Theobald N, et al. Prolonged production of NADPH oxidase-corrected granulocytes after gene therapy of chronic granulomatous disease. Proc Natl Acad Sci U S A 1997;94:12133-8.

38. Ott MG, Schmidt M, Schwarzwaelder K, et al. Correction of X-linked chronic granulomatous disease by gene therapy, augmented by insertional activation of MDS1-EVI1, PRDM16 or SETBP1. Nat Med 2006;12:401-9.

39. Correll PH, Karlsson S. Towards therapy of Gaucher's disease by gene transfer into hematopoietic cells. Eur J Haematol 1994;53:253-64.

40. Schiffmann R, Medin JA, Ward JM, et al. Transfer of the human glucocerebrosidase gene into hematopoietic stem cells of nonablated recipients: Successful engraftment and long-term expression of the transgene. Blood 1995;86:1218-27.

41. Dunbar CE, Kohn DB, Schiffmann R, et al. Retroviral transfer of the glucocerebrosidase gene into CD34+ cells from patients with Gaucher disease: In vivo detection of transduced cells without myeloablation. Hum Gene Ther 1998;9:2629-40.

42. Liu JM, Kim S, Read EJ, et al. Engraftment of hematopoietic progenitor cells transduced with the Fanconi anemia group C gene (FANCC). Hum Gene Ther 1999;10:2337-46.

43. Walsh CE, Nienhuis AW, Samulski RJ, et al. Phenotypic correction of Fanconi anemia in human hematopoietic cells with a recombinant adeno-associated virus vector. J Clin Invest 1994;94:1440-8.

44. Braun SE, Pan D, Aronovich EL, et al. Preclinical studies of lymphocyte gene therapy for mild Hunter syndrome (mucopolysaccharidosis type II). Hum Gene Ther 1996;7:283-90.

45. Pan D, Jonsson JJ, Braun SE, et al. "Supercharged cells" for delivery of recombinant human iduronate-2-sulfatase. Mol Genet Metab 2000;70:170-8.

46. Whitley CB, McIvor RS, Aronovich EL, et al. Retroviral-mediated transfer of the iduronate-2-sulfatase gene into lymphocytes for treatment of mild Hunter syndrome (mucopolysaccharidosis type II). Hum Gene Ther 1996;7: 537-49.

47. Takekoshi KJ, Oh YH, Westerman KW, et al. Retroviral transfer of a human beta-globin/delta-globin hybrid gene linked to beta locus control region hypersensitive site 2 aimed at the gene therapy of sickle cell disease. Proc Natl Acad Sci U S A 1995;92:3014-18.

48. May C, Rivella S, Chadburn A, Sadelain M. Successful treatment of murine beta-thalassemia intermedia by transfer of the human beta-globin gene. Blood 2002;99:1902-8.

49. Imren S, Payen E, Westerman KA, et al. Permanent and panerythroid correction of murine beta thalassemia by multiple lentiviral integration in hematopoietic stem cells. Proc Natl Acad Sci U S A 2002;99:14380-5.

50. Rivella S, May C, Chadburn A, et al. A novel murine model of Cooley anemia and its rescue by lentiviral-mediated human beta-globin gene transfer. Blood 2003;101:2932-9.

51. Pawliuk R, Westerman KA, Fabry ME, et al. Correction of sickle cell disease in transgenic mouse models by gene therapy. Science 2001;294:2368-71.

52. Levasseur DN, Ryan TM, Pawlik KM, Townes TM. Correction of a mouse model of sickle cell disease: Lentiviral/antisickling beta-globin gene transduction of unmobilized, purified hematopoietic stem cells. Blood 2003;102:4312-19.

53. Bank A, Dorazio R, Leboulch P. A phase I/II clinical trial of beta-globin gene therapy for beta-thalassemia. Ann N Y Acad Sci 2005; 1054:308-16.

54. Ferster A, Corazza F, Vertongen F, et al. Transplanted sickle-cell disease patients with autologous bone marrow recovery after graft failure develop increased levels of fetal haemoglobin which corrects disease severity. Br J Haematol 1995;90:804-8.

55. Paciaroni K, Gallucci C, De Angelis G, et al. Sustained and full fetal hemoglobin production after failure of bone marrow transplant in a patient homozygous for beta 0-thalassemia: A clinical remission despite genetic disease and transplant rejection. Am J Hematol 2009;84: 372-3.

56. Lane HC, Zunich KM, Wilson W, et al. Syngeneic bone marrow transplantation and adoptive transfer of peripheral blood lymphocytes

57. combined with zidovudine in human immunodeficiency virus (HIV) infection. Ann Intern Med 1990;113:512-19.

57. Gilboa E, Smith C. Gene therapy for infectious diseases: The AIDS model. Trends Genet 1994;10:139-44.

58. Strayer DS, Akkina R, Bunnell BA, et al. Current status of gene therapy strategies to treat HIV/AIDS. Mol Ther 2005;11:823-42.

59. Morgan RA, Looney DJ, Muenchau DD, et al. Retroviral vectors expressing soluble CD4: A potential gene therapy for AIDS. AIDS Res Hum Retroviruses 1990;6:183-91.

60. Kohn DB, Bauer G, Rice CR, et al. A clinical trial of retroviral-mediated transfer of a rev-responsive element decoy gene into CD34(+) cells from the bone marrow of human immunodeficiency virus-1-infected children. Blood 1999;94:368-71.

61. Mitsuyasu RT, Anton PA, Deeks SG, et al. Prolonged survival and tissue trafficking following adoptive transfer of CD4zeta gene-modified autologous CD4(+) and CD8(+) T cells in human immunodeficiency virus-infected subjects. Blood 2000;96:785-93.

62. Walker RE, Carter CS, Muul L, et al. Peripheral expansion of pre-existing mature T cells is an important means of CD4+ T-cell regeneration HIV-infected adults. Nat Med 1998;4:852-6.

63. Hwu P, Rosenberg SA. The genetic modification of T cells for cancer therapy: An overview of laboratory and clinical trials. Cancer Detect Prev 1994;18:43-50.

64. Fujiwara T, Grimm EA, Roth JA. Gene therapeutics and gene therapy for cancer. Curr Opin Oncol 1994;6:96-105.

65. Kessels HW, Wolkers MC, van den Boom MD, et al. Immunotherapy through TCR gene transfer. Nat Immunol 2001;2:957-61.

66. Clay TM, Custer MC, Sachs J, et al. Efficient transfer of a tumor antigen-reactive TCR to human peripheral blood lymphocytes confers anti-tumor reactivity. J Immunol 1999;163: 507-13.

67. Morgan RA, Dudley ME, Wunderlich JR, et al. Cancer regression in patients after transfer of genetically engineered lymphocytes. Science 2006;314:126-9.

68. Kershaw MH, Westwood JA, Parker LL, et al. A Phase I study on adoptive immunotherapy using gene-modified T cells for ovarian cancer. Clin Cancer Res 2006;12:6106-15.

69. Lamers CH, Langeveld SC, Groot-van Ruijven CM, et al. Gene-modified T cells for adoptive

immunotherapy of renal cell cancer maintain transgene-specific immune functions in vivo. Cancer Immunol Immunother 2007;56:1875-83.

70. Fearon ER, Pardoll DM, Itaya T, et al. Interleukin-2 production by tumor cells bypasses T helper function in the generation of an antitumor response. Cell 1990;60:397-403.

71. Hesdorffer C, Antman K, Bank A, et al. Human MDR gene transfer in patients with advanced cancer. Hum Gene Ther 1994;5:1151-60.

72. Marktel S, Magnani Z, Ciceri F, et al. Immunologic potential of donor lymphocytes expressing a suicide gene for early immune reconstitution after hematopoietic T-cell-depleted stem cell transplantation. Blood 2003;101:1290-8.

73. National Institutes of Health. Office of Biotechnology Activities; Recombinant DNA research: Actions under the NIH guidelines for research involving recombinant DNA molecules (NIH guidelines); notice of changes (September 22, 2009). Fed Regist 2009;74:48275-80.

74. National Institutes of Health. Recombinant DNA research: Notice of intent to propose amendments to the NIH guidelines for research involving recombinant DNA molecules (NIH guidelines) regarding enhanced mechanisms for NIH oversight of recombinant DNA activities. Fed Regist 1996;61:35774-7.

In: McLeod BC, Szczepiorkowski ZM, Weinstein R, Winters JL, eds.
Apheresis: Principles and Practice, 3rd edition
Bethesda, MD: AABB Press, 2010

30

Regulatory Environment for Apheresis Facilities and Personnel

Michelle A. Vauthrin, MT(ASCP)SBB, and Jillian Ferschke, BS

 BOTH DONOR AND THERA-peutic apheresis are regulated by federal legislation and guidance documents as well as by standards developed by professional societies and organizations. This chapter discusses the major regulatory agencies, federal legislation, and professional organizations that promulgate requirements for apheresis activities.

Regulatory Agencies

The Department of Health and Human Services (HHS) is the United States government's principal agency for protecting the health of all Americans and providing essential human services, especially for those who are least able to help themselves. Within HHS, the agencies and offices that regulate blood products and patient care activities include the Food and Drug Administration (FDA), the Centers for Medicare and Medicaid Services (CMS), and the Office for Civil Rights (OCR). The Center for Biologics Evaluation and Research (CBER) is the body within the FDA that regulates biological products for human use under applicable federal laws, including the Public Health Service (PHS) Act and the Federal Food, Drug, and Cosmetic Act.

The Occupational Safety and Health Administration (OSHA) is the agency within the Department of Labor (DOL) that is responsible for ensuring safe and healthful working conditions for working men and women through enforcement of standards developed under the Occupational Safety and Health Act of 1970.[1]

Michelle A. Vauthrin, MT(ASCP)SBB, Senior Project Manager, and Jillian Ferschke, BS, Systems and Validation Specialist, Transfusion Medicine, UMass Memorial Medical Center, Worcester, Massachusetts

The authors have disclosed no conflicts of interest.

Food and Drug Administration

Human blood components and products are regulated by the US government as both drugs and biologics. Title 21 of the *Code of Federal Regulations* (CFR), Part 640, includes specific requirements for human blood, components, and products.[2] Under these regulations, any hospital blood bank or apheresis department collecting blood for transfusion must be registered with the FDA and is subject to inspections every two years even if products are not shipped over state lines.

Current good manufacturing practice (cGMP) regulations for human blood, blood components, and products are listed in 21 CFR 606.[3] A cGMP document for drugs, 21 CFR 210-211, is also applicable to blood product manufacturing.[4] In regulating how blood is collected, processed, and handled, the FDA applies the same manufacturing standards to blood establishments that it does to the pharmaceutical industry.

If a facility collects human cells, tissues, and cellular and tissue-based products (HCT/Ps), the regulations contained in 21 CFR 1270 and 1271 apply. This part of the CFR requires tissue establishments to screen and test donors to prevent the spread of communicable disease in accordance with current good tissue practice (cGTP).[5] Some HCT/Ps may be subject to these regulations and to Section 361 of the PHS Act, whereas others would be regulated as drugs, devices, and/or biological products under Section 351 of the PHS Act and the Federal Food, Drug, and Cosmetic Act.[6]

Other resources include guidance documents, which represent the FDA's current thinking on a subject, and the *Federal Register*, which is the official daily publication for rules, proposed rules, and notices of federal agencies and organizations.

Registration

The type of registration required depends upon the type of product collected. Registration Form FDA 2830, Blood Establishment Registration and Product Listing, must be completed by facilities collecting blood and blood components.[7] Facilities that collect cellular therapy products by apheresis (eg, hematopoietic progenitor cells from apheresis) must use Form FDA 3356, Establishment Registration and Listing for Human Cells, Tissues, and Cellular and Tissue-Based Products (HCT/Ps).[8]

All apheresis collection facilities must register with the FDA within 5 days of beginning operations and annually in December by submitting the proper form. Updates to a product list, if necessary, may be made every June and December. Facilities are encouraged to submit their registration and product list information electronically by following the instructions available on the FDA Web site. Registered, nonlicensed facilities are issued a 7- to 10-digit registration number, which must appear on the facility identification portion of component labels. Registered facilities must comply with cGMP regulations, cGTP regulations, and any additional guidelines and standards promulgated by the FDA.

Licensure

To engage in interstate commerce of biological products, manufacturers must apply for a US biologics license. To obtain a license, a facility must complete Form FDA 356h (Application to Market a New Drug, Biologic, or an Antibiotic Drug for Human Use) and indicate the application type as biologics license application (BLA).[9] The completed form and supporting documentation are submitted to the FDA. The supporting documentation may consist of the following:

- Cover letter that describes the product; lists any devices used in collection, processing, or testing; and includes the name, address, and registration number of the requesting facility.
- Standard Operating Procedures for donor suitability, donor deferral, collection, donor history, product manufacturing, adverse events, failure investigation, quarantine, and disposition of unsuitable products.
- Records and forms, including the donor history questionnaire, informed consent,

product collection and processing records, quality control logs, and results of product validation.

- Labeling information, including FDA Form 2567, Transmittal of Labels and Circulars, and examples of labels.
- Data establishing the stability of the product through the dating period.[10]

Approval of the BLA indicates that both the establishment and the product meet applicable requirements that include, but are not limited to, the cGMP requirements in 21 CFR 210, 211, 600, 606, and 820.

Changes to a licensed product must be reported to the FDA.[11] The three categories of change as defined by the FDA include the following:

1. Major changes: those with substantial potential to have an adverse effect on the safety or effectiveness of the product. These require submission of a supplement and approval by the FDA before distribution of product made under the change.
2. Moderate changes: those with a moderate potential to have an adverse effect on the safety or effectiveness of the product. These require submission of a supplement to the FDA at least 30 days before distribution of product made under the change.
3. Minor changes: those with minimal potential to have an adverse effect on the safety or effectiveness of the product. These changes are described in an annual report to the FDA.

Inspections

Both licensed and registered apheresis facilities are subject to FDA inspections to ensure the safety of the blood supply through compliance with cGMP requirements. The FDA uses a systems-based approach to conduct the inspections. The systems include quality assurance, donor suitability/eligibility, product testing, quarantine/inventory management, and production and processing. A Level I inspection is a comprehensive evaluation of the establishment's compliance and includes the review of all systems. A Level II inspection employs a streamlined evaluation of an establishment's compliance when the facility has met a defined standard of performance during past FDA inspections. A Level II inspection includes review of three systems. Prelicense and preapproval inspections that are part of the review process related to a BLA are conducted by CBER and the Office of Regulatory Affairs. The scope and content of the prelicense and preapproval inspections are established by CBER.[12] Newly licensed or registered blood establishments are inspected within the first year of operation, and cGMP inspections are generally conducted on a biennial schedule.[13]

Deficiencies identified during the inspection are discussed with the manufacturer and documented on FDA Form 483. Additional regulatory actions that may be taken by CBER in an effort to stop practices of biological product manufacturers that are found to be in violation of the regulations include, but are not limited to, issuance of warning letters, suspension, or revocation of licensure.[12]

Mandatory Reporting of Errors and Fatalities

A biologic product deviation (BPD) is any event associated with the testing, processing, packing, labeling, storage, holding, or distribution of blood or a blood component, through which the safety, purity, or potency of the distributed product may be adversely affected. Any establishment that collects, tests, or distributes products prepared by apheresis is required to report these events to CBER's Office of Compliance and Biologics Quality as soon as possible.[14] The report may be submitted by mail or electronically (see the FDA Web site[15]) using Form FDA 3486. The report must be submitted within 45 days of the discovery of the event.[16]

Upon confirmation of a fatality caused by blood collection or transfusion, the facility must notify the Division of Inspections and Surveillance and submit a written report of the investigation within 7 days to the Director of the Office of Compliance and Biologics Quality at CBER.[17,18]

Medical Devices

The FDA has regulatory authority over medical devices. Medical devices are categorized as Class I, II, or III. Manufacturers of all classes are subject to general controls as defined in 21 CFR 807, including establishment registration, medical device listing, GMP requirements, labeling regulations, and submission of a pre-market notification, as applicable. Class II and III devices may also be subject to special controls, premarket notification 510(k) as defined in 21 CRF 807, and premarket approval defined in 21 CFR 814.[19] It is important for purchasers and users of medical devices to verify that the manufacturer has obtained the appropriate clearance before purchasing the device or placing it into service. Devices may be approved to treat certain patient conditions. A listing of approved devices is available on the FDA Web site.[20]

Adverse events involving medical devices must be reported to the FDA by the manufacturer and may be reported by the device user as defined in 21 CFR 803.[21] An adverse event is described as one that caused or contributed to the serious injury or death of a person. The user is required to report the event to the manufacturer and, in the case of death, directly to the FDA as well.

Centers for Medicare and Medicaid Services

CMS regulates all medical laboratory testing performed on humans through the Clinical Laboratory Improvement Amendments (CLIA). These regulations are codified in 42 CFR 493.[22] Clinical laboratories must be properly certified to receive Medicare or Medicaid payments. The CLIA application for certification must be submitted to apply for CMS approval. CMS assesses fees on the basis of the type and number of tests performed by the laboratory. The laboratory must submit evidence of accreditation by an approved accreditation organization for CLIA purposes. The list of approved accreditation organizations includes the AABB, the American Osteopathic Association, the American Society for Histocompatibil-ity and Immunogenetics, the College of American Pathologists (CAP), COLA (formerly, the Commission on Office Laboratory Accreditation) and The Joint Commission.

CMS or its designee conducts biennial inspections using Form CMS 282, Blood Bank Inspection Checklist and Report, and Appendix C, Survey Procedures and Interpretive Guidelines for Laboratories and Laboratory Services.[23] Consequences of noncompliance or failure to permit inspection include suspension of Medicare and Medicaid reimbursements, revocation of the certificate, sanctions, and fines. CMS can bar a noncompliant owner from owning or operating a laboratory for up to 2 years.

A state license suffices in states that have federally approved licensure programs deemed equivalent to CLIA requirements by DHHS; laboratories in other states are licensed directly by CMS.

CLIA defines three categories of test complexity: 1) waived, 2) moderately complex, and 3) highly complex. Laboratories may perform any combination of these tests. The regulations also specify the qualifications required of personnel who perform, supervise, direct, and provide consultation in laboratory testing, based on the complexity of the tests performed in the laboratory. The laboratory is required to participate in an approved proficiency testing program and must have standard operating procedures written in accordance with manufacturers' instructions, appropriate staff training, and competency assessments.

The Health Insurance Portability and Accountability Act of 1996 (HIPAA) required CMS to adopt standards for coding systems that are used for reporting health-care transactions.[24] A standardized coding system is used by Medicare and other health insurance programs to ensure that claims are processed in an orderly and consistent manner. The Healthcare Common Procedure Coding System (HCPCS) is divided into two subsystems referred to as Level I and Level II. HCPCS Level I consists of current procedural terminology (CPT) coding, a numeric coding system maintained by the American Medical Association. CPT codes are used to identify medical services and procedures furnished by physicians and other health-care professionals. HCPCS Level II is used to identify products, supplies, and services not included in the CPT codes. CMS maintains and distributes HCPCS Level II codes.

Office for Civil Rights

The OCR is responsible for enforcing HIPAA standards. The OCR enforces the "Standards for Privacy of Individually Identifiable Health Information" ("Privacy Rule") and administers the regulations that compose the "Security Standards for the Protection of Electronic Protected Health Information" ("Security Rule").[25]

The goal of the Privacy Rule is to ensure that individual health information is properly protected while allowing the flow of health information needed to provide high-quality health care. Health-care institutions, referred to as covered entities, are required to develop and implement policies and procedures that control access to, use of, and transmission of protected health information (PHI). PHI includes the patient's identity, age, social security number, address, medical history, diagnosis, treatment, and billing information.[26]

The Security Rule pertains specifically to securing electronic PHI (ePHI). Health-care institutions must implement security safeguards to ensure the confidentially, integrity, and availability of ePHI. In addition, the facility must protect against threats and hazards to security or integrity, protect against disclosures not permitted, and ensure compliance by its workforce.[27]

Outside agencies with which hospitals contract for the provision of services such as therapeutic apheresis may need access to patients' medical records for treatment purposes. The outside agency may fall into the category of a business associate (a third party acting on behalf of the health-care provider). In such cases, the contracting hospital may be required to obtain a business associate agreement signed by both parties, the substance of which is the securing of the privacy and confidentiality of PHI that must be shared. Some other examples of business associates are transcription services, billing services, record storage or destruction services, laboratories, and certain vendors.[26]

Department of Labor

The DOL is responsible for enforcing the insurance portability requirements of HIPAA. HIPPA protections for coverage under group health plans limit exclusions for preexisting conditions, prohibit discrimination against employees and dependents on the basis of their health status, and provide opportunities to enroll in group health plans.[28]

Occupational Safety and Health Administration

The mission of OSHA is to ensure safe and healthful working conditions for working men and women through the enforcement of standards developed under the Occupational Safety and Health Act of 1970[29] and by assisting and encouraging the state governments in their efforts to ensure safe and healthful working conditions. OSHA standards, codified in 29 CFR 1910,[30] that apply to health-care employers include, but are not limited to, hazard communication, blood-borne pathogens, and personal protective equipment (PPE).[31]

The hazard communication standard requires that employers prepare and implement a written hazard communication program to inform employees about hazardous chemicals in the workplace, to maintain material safety data sheets, and to train employees to safely use the chemicals.[32]

The blood-borne pathogens standard details what employers must do to establish an exposure control plan for the protection of workers whose jobs put them at a reasonable risk of coming into contact with blood or other potentially infectious materials.[33] The plan must include training protocols, training records, exposure records, employer-supplied hepatitis B vaccination for those at risk, and warning signs and labels. Postexposure evaluations with follow-up are required. The plan must also include procedures for implementing universal precautions and the safe handling of sharps, hazardous specimens, and contaminated waste and laundry. The plan must be reviewed annually and upgraded as necessary. A hospital, blood center, or apheresis agency with 11 or more employees must also keep a log of occupational injuries and illnesses.

The PPE standard is designed to protect employees from serious workplace injuries or illnesses resulting from contact with hazardous materials. Employers must select the appropriate equipment and provide training to staff to properly don, adjust, wear, and doff PPE.[34]

Work-related accidents that result in death or hospitalization must be evaluated to determine if the incident is reportable to OSHA.[35]

OSHA guidelines are federal regulations; they must be followed and may be enforced by inspections. OSHA prioritizes its inspections because not all workplaces covered by the Act can be inspected. The top priorities are situations of imminent danger and investigation of fatalities and accidents resulting in a death or hospitalization of three or more employees. Inspections may also be conducted when OSHA receives a complaint or when a workplace has a history of high injury rates. Nonconformance discovered during the inspection is discussed with the organization's compliance officer and may be corrected immediately. Failure to correct deficiencies may result in fines.[36]

States and territories with their own OSHA-approved occupational safety and health plan must adopt and enforce standards identical to the federal standards. Individual companies may develop their own safety programs. Self-audits are recommended for obtaining a satisfactory outcome at inspection. Copies of the safety section of the inspection checklists of The Joint Commission and CAP can be used to conduct self-audits, assess internal compliance, and help ensure a successful inspection outcome.

State and Local Regulations

Each facility should review applicable state and local regulations, which may be different from federal laws. In addition, there may be additional licensure requirements for facilities and/or personnel.

Professional Organizations

Professional organizations and societies in many instances provide training and educational tools for apheresis staff and a communication portal to develop and share ideas for compliance with regulations. In some cases, these organizations have developed standards that meet or exceed federal and local regulations. Apheresis facilities that seek accreditation from these organizations must follow the organizations' standards and may be subject to inspection for compliance. Apheresis facilities and individual members may be assessed fees associated with membership, inspections, and accreditation.

AABB

The AABB, formerly known as the American Association of Blood Banks, is an association that focuses its efforts on activities related to blood transfusion and cellular therapies. It supports medical, technical, and administrative performance by setting standards and providing accreditation as well as through education, advocacy, and other efforts. The AABB publishes standards for voluntary compliance that combine internationally accepted quality management system requirements with technical requirements incorporated for each discipline. Standards that relate to apheresis activities are found in both the *Standards for Blood Banks and Transfusion Services*[37] and *Standards for Cellular Therapy Product Services.*[38] Each set of standards is revised and published on an 18-month cycle. AABB awards a 2-year accreditation following assessment of quality and operational systems to ensure compliance with AABB standards, CFRs, and CLIA. CMS granted AABB deemed status as an accrediting organization under CLIA.[39]

AABB provides resources to assist facilities in understanding compliance requirements. Among those that cover apheresis are the

AABB *Technical Manual,*[40] *Regulations A to Z for Blood and HCT/Ps*[41] and the *AABB Billing Guide for Transfusion and Cellular Therapy Services.*[42] In addition to publications, AABB offers seminars and workshops to educate professionals on regulatory, technical, and operational topics. It also hosts an annual meeting that provides a national forum for presenting new scientific, technical, management, and operational information as well as training in blood banking and transfusion medicine, which includes topics related to apheresis.

Foundation for the Accreditation of Cellular Therapy

The Foundation for the Accreditation of Cellular Therapy (FACT) provides voluntary inspection and accreditation in the field of cellular therapy. FACT has established standards for all areas of cellular therapy treatments: clinical care, donor management, and cell collection, processing, storage, transportation, and administration. These standards are published in the *FACT-JACIE International Standards for Cellular Therapy Product Collection, Processing, and Administration* manual.[43] FACT has also published the *Cellular Therapy Accreditation Manual,*[44] which explains the intent and rationale for specific standards. Apheresis facilities may seek FACT accreditation of cellular therapy activities for reasons including, but not limited to, the following[45]:

- Many health insurance plans and managed care organizations rely on FACT accreditation for designating "centers of excellence."
- Standards are developed by experts and are regularly updated to ensure compliance.
- FACT is the only accrediting agency that focuses on all aspects of cellular therapy.
- FACT standards meet or exceed government regulations.
- Government agencies and health-care insurance companies are increasingly recognizing or requiring FACT accreditation for patient-care reimbursement.

- Patients are researching and evaluating treatment programs that are FACT accredited to find the highest quality care.

FACT offers accreditation after an initial inspection, with reinspection every 3 years. To maintain accreditation, facilities must comply with the program expectations in addition to the inspections. Expectations include, but are not limited to, maintaining FDA registration; notifying FACT regarding changes in key personnel, facilities, and/or services; submitting an interim accreditation report; and performing a defined number of patient treatments and/or cellular therapy collections.[46]

ICCBBA

ICCBBA, formerly known as the International Council for Commonality in Blood Banking Automation, is the organization responsible for managing, developing, and licensing ISBT 128, the global standard for the identification, labeling, and information processing of human blood, tissue, and organ products. ISBT 128 was developed in collaboration with the International Society of Blood Transfusion (ISBT) and designed to ensure the highest level of accuracy, safety, and efficiency for donors, patients, and facilities worldwide. ICCBBA maintains the international databases for ISBT 128 facility identification and product codes. Apheresis collection facilities that use ISBT 128 labels are required to register as licensees with ICCBBA. Registered facilities are responsible for an initial one-time registration fee and an annual license fee and, in return, are assigned a facility identification number. Registered facilities are allowed access to restricted areas of the ICCBBA Web site and have the right to use ISBT 128 data structures and ISBT 128 numbers on blood, cellular, and tissue products.

ICCBBA has published the *United States Industry Consensus Standards for the Uniform Labeling of Blood and Blood Components Using ISBT 128*[47] and the *United States Consensus Standards for the Uniform Labeling of Cellular Therapy Products Using ISBT 128,*[48] which are standards intended for use by facilities implementing ISBT 128, generating labeling protocols, and training staff.

Facilities accredited by AABB are required to use the ISBT 128 labeling standard.[37,38] FACT-accredited facilities are required to use product names, attributes, and modifiers according to ISBT 128.[43] The FDA recognizes the blood and blood component standards, except when inconsistent with regulations. The CFR specifies that the anticoagulant must appear immediately preceding the proper name of the product [21 CFR 606.121(e)(1)]; facilities using ISBT 128 must request a variance from the FDA because this is inconsistent with ICCBBA's standards.[49]

The Joint Commission

The Joint Commission, formerly the Joint Commission on Accreditation of Healthcare Organizations, provides voluntary accreditation nationwide to health-care organizations that meet standards for safety and quality of care. These standards address the facility's level of performance in areas such as patient rights, patient treatment, and infection control. Health-care organizations seek Joint-Commission accreditation for reasons including, but not limited to, the following[50]:

- Accreditation strengthens community confidence in the quality and safety of care, treatment, and services.
- It improves risk management and risk reduction.
- It helps organize and strengthen patient safety efforts.
- It is recognized by insurers and other third parties for medical billing.
- It may reduce liability insurance costs.
- It may fulfill regulatory requirements in select states.

Health-care organizations requesting Medicare and Medicaid approval may choose to be surveyed by an accrediting body such as The Joint Commission as an alternative to state inspections on behalf of CMS. The Joint Commission conducts unannounced surveys within 18 to 39 months from the organization's previous full survey. This assessment is performed by evaluating an organization's compliance with applicable standards on the basis of tracing the care delivered to patients and verbal information and documents provided to The Joint Commission.[51]

Apheresis facilities providing therapeutic services are surveyed according to the current version of the *Comprehensive Accreditation Manual for Laboratory and Point-of-Care Testing*.[52] The manual contains sections related to apheresis activities that include safety, electronic requirements, equipment, staffing, medical and technical supervision, and adverse reactions to transfusion of blood or blood components. In addition to patient safety standards, The Joint Commission requires donor facilities to conform to current AABB standards.[52]

American Society for Apheresis

The American Society for Apheresis (ASFA) focuses its efforts on patient and donor care, research, education, and advocacy in the field of apheresis. ASFA membership is available to any professional actively involved in the field of apheresis medicine. Members of ASFA are entitled to an electronic subscription to the *Journal of Clinical Apheresis*, a subscription to the *ASFA Newsflash,* and access to restricted Web resources. Members may also participate in ASFA Committees, educational seminars, and webinars. ASFA organizes an annual meeting providing educational and networking events. The meetings provide educational content in donor and therapeutic apheresis and presentations of submitted abstracts that cover original work in the field.

Although ASFA does not offer inspections, its committees publish helpful guidelines. *Guidelines for Documentation of Therapeutic Apheresis Procedures in the Medical Record by Apheresis Physicians*[53] and *Guidelines for Therapeutic Apheresis Clinical Privileges*[54] were developed by ASFA and may be used by apheresis facilities in meeting the standards of regulatory and accrediting agencies. ASFA regularly publishes a critical review of indications for therapeutic apheresis and groups the reviewed indications into categories based on evidence supporting therapeutic efficiency.[55,56]

American Society of Clinical Pathology

The American Society of Clinical Pathology (ASCP) is an organization of pathologists, residents, physicians, laboratory professionals, and students. Within the ASCP is the Board of Registry (BOR) which provides certifications to laboratory professionals worldwide. The BOR previously provided certifications that were specific to apheresis professionals. However, on December 31, 2008, the apheresis technician (AT) and hemapheresis practitioner (HP) certification exams were retired.[57] ASCP continues to support AT- and HP-certified individuals and encourages the use of the "HP(ASCP)" or "AT(ASCP)" designations.[58]

College of American Pathologists

CAP is a medical society of pathologists focusing its efforts on laboratory quality assurance and is an advocate for high-quality and cost-effective medical care. CAP has developed laboratory accreditation standards that are translated into checklist questions. CAP offers a 2-year accreditation following an on-site inspection.

CMS granted CAP deemed status as an accrediting organization under CLIA. In addition, CAP's proficiency testing program is recognized by the FDA as conforming to the CLIA statute that requires all laboratories to test for proficiency, when applicable. Apheresis facilities that perform laboratory testing that falls under CLIA may choose to use CAP accreditation and may subscribe to the CAP proficiency testing program.[59]

World Apheresis Association

The World Apheresis Association (WAA) is an association of national and international societies that are committed to research and/or clinical practice in the field of apheresis. Goals of WAA include the following[60]:

- Dissemination of knowledge about safe and effective apheresis techniques for collection of donor cells and plasma or for the treatment of diseases.
- Collaboration in scientific investigation, research, clinical application, education, and exchange of information relating to apheresis.
- Management of a worldwide registry of apheresis treatments and related information.

To accomplish these goals, WAA publishes a newsletter and holds a biennial congress, the proceedings of which are published in its official journal, *Transfusion and Apheresis Science*. In North America, ASFA, the Canadian Apheresis Group (CAG), and the Mexican Asociación Nacional de Medicina Transfusional (ANMT) are member societies of WAA.

Summary

Apheresis blood products are regulated as biologics and pharmaceutical agents. Compliance with federal and state regulations is mandatory. Compliance with standards and guidelines of professional organizations and societies such as the AABB, FACT, and ASFA is desirable but not mandatory. The goal of these organizations is public safety, which includes safety of patients, the blood supply, and health-care workers.

References

1. US Department of Labor. Occupational Safety and Health Administration. OSHA's role. Washington, DC: OSHA, 2010. [Available at http://www.osha.gov/oshinfo/mission.html (accessed January 29, 2010).]
2. Code of federal regulations. Title 21 CFR Part 640. Additional standards for human blood and blood products. Washington, DC: US Government Printing Office, 2010 (revised annually).
3. Code of federal regulations. Title 21 CFR Part 606. Current good manufacturing practice for blood and blood components. Washington,

DC: US Government Printing Office, 2010 (revised annually).

4. Code of federal regulations. Title 21 CFR Parts 200-211. Washington, DC: US Government Printing Office, 2010 (revised annually).

5. Code of federal regulations. Title 21 CFR Parts 1270-1271. Washington, DC: US Government Printing Office, 2010 (revised annually).

6. Food and Drug Administration. Guidance for industry: Regulation of human cells, tissues, and cellular and tissue-based products (HCT/Ps)—small entity compliance guide. (August 2007) Rockville, MD: CBER Office of Communication, Training, and Manufacturers Assistance, 2007. [Available at http://www.fda.gov/BiologicsBloodVaccines / GuidanceCompliance RegulatoryInformation/Guidances/Tissue/ucm 073366.htm (accessed January 29, 2010).]

7. Code of federal regulations. Title 21 CFR Part 607 Subpart B. Procedures for domestic blood product establishments. Washington, DC: US Government Printing Office, 2010 (revised annually).

8. Code of federal regulations. Title 21 CFR Part 1271 Subpart B. Procedures for registration and listing. Washington, DC: US Government Printing Office, 2010 (revised annually).

9. Code of federal regulations. Title 21 CFR Part 601 Subpart A. Licensing: General provisions. Washington, DC: US Government Printing Office, 2010 (revised annually).

10. Coalition for Blood Safety. Biologics license applications checklists. Bethesda, MD: AABB, 2008 [Available at http://www.aabb.org/Con tent/Programs_and_Services/Government_Re gulatory_Issues/blachecklists.htm (accessed January 29, 2010).]

11. Food and Drug Administration. Guidance for industry: Changes to an approved application: Biological products: Human blood and blood components intended for transfusion or for further manufacture. (July 2001) Rockville, MD: CBER Office of Communication, Training, and Manufacturers Assistance, 2001. [Available at http://www.fda.gov/BiologicsBloodVaccines/GuidanceComplianceRegulatoryInformation/Guidances/Blood/ucm076729.htm (accessed January 29, 2010).]

12. Food and Drug Administration. 7342.001—Inspection of licensed and unlicensed blood banks, brokers, reference laboratories, and contractors. Chapter 42. In: Compliance program guidance manual. (October 2006) Rockville, MD: CBER Office of Compliance and Biologics Quality, 2009. [Available at http://www.fda.gov/BiologicsBloodVaccines/GuidanceComplianceRegulatoryInformation/ComplianceActivities/Enforcement/CompliancePrograms/ucm095226.htm (accessed January 29, 2010).]

13. Code of federal regulations. Title 21 CFR Part 600 Subpart C. Establishment inspection. Washington, DC: US Government Printing Office, 2010 (revised annually).

14. Code of federal regulations. Title 21 CFR Part 606.171. Reporting of product deviations by licensed manufacturers, unlicensed registered blood establishments, and transfusion services. Washington, DC: US Government Printing Office, 2010 (revised annually).

15. Food and Drug Administration. Biological product deviations. Rockville, MD: CBER, 2010. [Available at http://www.fda.gov/Bio logicsBloodVaccines/SafetyAvailability/Reporta Problem/BiologicalProductDeviations/default. htm (accessed January 29, 2010).]

16. Food and Drug Administration. Guidance for industry: Biological product deviation reporting for blood and plasma establishments. (October 2006) Rockville, MD: CBER Office of Communication, Training, and Manufacturers Assistance, 2006. [Available at http://www.fda.gov/downloads/BiologicsBloodVac cines/GuidanceComplianceRegulatoryInforma tion/Guidances/Blood/UCM062918.pdf (accessed January 29, 2010).]

17. Code of federal regulations. Title 21 CFR Part 606.170. Adverse reaction file. Washington, DC: US Government Printing Office, 2010 (revised annually).

18. Food and Drug Administration. Guidance for industry: Notifying FDA of fatalities related to blood collection or transfusion. (September 2003) Rockville, MD: CBER Office of Communication, Training, and Manufacturers Assistance, 2003. [Available at http://www.fda.gov/downloads/BiologicsBloodVaccines/GuidanceComplianceRegulatoryInformation/Guidances/Blood/ucm062897.pdf (accessed January 29, 2010).]

19. Food and Drug Administration. Overview of device regulation. Rockville, MD: FDA, 2010. [Available at http://www.fda.gov/MedicalDe vices/DeviceRegulationandGuidance/Overview/default.htm (accessed January 29, 2010).]

20. Food and Drug Administration. Medical devices databases. Rockville, MD: FDA, 2010. [Available at http://www.fda.gov/MedicalDevices/

DeviceRegulationandGuidance/Databases/default. htm (accessed January 29, 2010).]

21. Code of federal regulations. Title 21 CFR Part 803. Medical device reporting. Washington, DC: US Government Printing Office, 2010 (revised annually).

22. Code of federal regulations. Title 42 CFR Part493. Laboratory requirements. Washington, DC: US Government Printing Office, 2010 (revised annually).

23. Centers for Medicare and Medicaid Services. Interpretive guidelines for laboratories. Appendix C: Survey procedures and interpretive guidelines for laboratories and laboratory services. (January 24, 2003) Baltimore, MD: CMS, 2010. [Available at http://www.cms.hhs. gov/clia/03_Interpretive_Guidelines_for_Lab oratories. asp (accessed January 29, 2010).]

24. Centers for Medicare and Medicaid Services. HCPCS—general information. Overview. Baltimore, MD: CMS, 2010. [Available at http:// www.cms.hhs.gov/MedHCPCSGeninfo/ (accessed January 29, 2010).]

25. US Department of Health and Human Services. Health information privacy. Washington, DC: Office for Civil Rights, 2010. [Available at: http://www.hhs.gov/ocr/office/index.html (accessed January 29, 2010).]

26. US Department of Health and Human Services. OCR privacy brief: Summary of the HIPPA privacy rule. Washington, DC: Office for Civil Rights, HIPPA Compliance Assistance, 2003. [Available at http://www.hhs.gov/ocr/ privacy/hipaa/understanding/summary/priva cysummary.pdf (accessed January 29, 2010).]

27. Code of federal regulations. Title 45 CFR Parts 160, 162, and 164. Health insurance reform: Security standards; final rule. Fed Regist 2003;68:8334-81.

28. US Department of Labor. Health plans and benefits. Portability of health coverage (HIPPA). Washington, DC: DOL, 2010. [Available at http://www.dol.gov/dol/topic/health-plans/portability.htm (accessed January 29, 2010).]

29. United States code. Title 29 USC Parts 651-678. Occupational Safety and Health Act. Washington, DC: US Government Printing Office, 1998. [Available at http://www.osha. gov/Other_Docs/USPS/USPS.pdf (accessed January 29, 2010).]

30. Code of federal regulations. Title 29 CFR Part 1910. Occupational safety and health standards. Washington, DC: US Government Printing Office, 2010 (revised annually).

31. Occupational Safety and Health Administration. Compliance assistance quick start: Health care industry. Washington, DC: OSHA, 2010. [Available at http://www.osha.gov/dcsp/com pliance_assistance/quickstarts/health_care/ index_hc.html (accessed January 29, 2010).]

32. Code of federal regulations. Title 29 CFR Part 1910.1200. Hazard communication. Washington, DC: US Government Printing Office, 2010 (revised annually).

33. Code of federal regulations. Title 29 CFR Part 1910.1030. Bloodborne pathogens. Washington, DC: US Government Printing Office, 2010 (revised annually).

34. Code of federal regulations. Title 29 CFR Part 1910 Subpart I. Personal protective equipment. Washington, DC: US Government Printing Office, 2010 (revised annually).

35. Code of federal regulations. Title 29 CFR Part 1904. Recording and reporting occupational injuries and illnesses. Washington, DC: US Government Printing Office, 2010 (revised annually).

36. Occupational Safety and Health Administration. OSHA Inspections. OSHA 2098 (2002 revised). Washington, DC: OSHA, 2002. [Available at http://www.osha.gov/Publica tions/osha2098.pdf (accessed January 29, 2010).]

37. Price T, ed. Standards for blood banks and transfusion services. 26th ed. Bethesda, MD: AABB, 2009.

38. Padley D, ed. Standards for cellular therapy product services. 4th ed. Bethesda, MD: AABB, 2009.

39. Centers for Medicare and Medicaid Services. Medicare, Medicaid, and CLIA Programs; continuing approval of AABB (formerly the American Association of Blood Banks) as a CLIA accreditation organization. Fed Regist 2008; 73:30109-11.

40. Roback JD, Combs MR, Grossman, BJ, Hillyer CD, eds. Technical manual. 16th ed. Bethesda, MD: AABB, 2008.

41. Nunes E, Motschman T. Regulations A to Z for blood and HCT/Ps. 9th ed. Bethesda, MD: AABB Press, 2009.

42. AABB billing guide for transfusion and cellular therapy services, 4.0. Bethesda, MD: AABB, 2007.

43. FACT-JACIE international standards for cellular therapy product collection, processing, and

administration. 4th ed. Omaha, NE: Foundation for the Accreditation of Cellular Therapy and Joint Accreditation Committee—ISCT and EBMT, 2008.

44. Cellular therapy accreditation manual. 4th ed. Omaha, NE: Foundation for the Accreditation of Cellular Therapy, 2008.

45. Benefits of FACT accreditation. Omaha, NE: Foundation for the Accreditation of Cellular Therapy, 2006. [Available at http://www.fact website.org/main.aspx?id=62 (accessed January 29, 2010).]

46. Maintaining accreditation. Omaha, NE: The Foundation for the Accreditation of Cellular Therapy, 2006. [Available at http://www.factwebsite.org/main.aspx?id=63 (accessed January 29, 2010).]

47. Distler P, ed. United States industry consensus standards for the uniform labeling of blood and blood components using ISBT 128. Version 2.0.0. York, PA: ICCBBA, Inc, 2005.

48. Distler P, ed. United States industry consensus standards for the uniform labeling of cellular therapy products using ISBT 128. Version 1.1.0. San Bernardino, CA: ICCBBA, 2009.

49. Food and Drug Administration. Guidance for industry: Recognition and use of a standard for uniform blood and blood component container labels. (September 2006) Rockville, MD: CBER Office of Communication, Training, and Manufacturers Assistance, 2006. [Available at http://www.fda.gov/BiologicsBloodVaccines/GuidanceComplianceRegulatoryInformation/Guidances/Blood/ucm073362.htm (accessed January 29, 2010).]

50. Facts about hospital accreditation: Benefits of accreditation. (January 7, 2009) Oakbrook Terrace, IL: The Joint Commission, 2010 (updated). [Available at http://www.jointcommission.org/AccreditationPrograms/Hospitals/hospital_facts.htm (accessed January 29, 2010).]

51. Accreditation process overview. (November 20, 2008) Oakbrook Terrace, IL: The Joint Commission, 2010 (updated). [Available at http://www.jointcommission.org/AboutUs/Fact_Sheets/overview_qa.htm (accessed January 29, 2010).]

52. The Joint Commission. 2010 comprehensive accreditation manual for laboratory and point-of-care testing. Oakbrook Terrace, IL: The Joint Commission, 2010.

53. American Society for Apheresis. Guidelines for documentation of therapeutic apheresis procedures in the medical record by apheresis physicians. (September 14, 2005) Vancouver, BC, Canada: ASFA, 2005. [Available at http://apheresis.org/~ASSETS/DOCUMENT/PDF/Resources/Guidelines%20for%20Documentation%20of%20TA%20Procedures.pdf (accessed January 29, 2010).]

54. American Society for Apheresis. Guidelines for therapeutic apheresis clinical privileges. (September 14, 2005) Vancouver, BC, Canada: ASFA, 2005. [Available at http://www.apheresis.org/~ASSETS/DOCUMENT/PDF/Resources/Guidelines%20for%20TA%20Clinical%20Privileges.pdf (accessed January 29, 2010).]

55. Szczepiorkowski ZM, Shaz BH, Bandarenko N, Winters JL. The new approach to assignment of ASFA categories—introduction to the fourth special issue: Clinical application of therapeutic apheresis. J Clin Apher 2007:22:96-105.

56. Winters JL, Gottschall JL, eds. Therapeutic apheresis: A physician's handbook. 2nd ed. Bethesda MD: AABB/ASFA, 2008.

57. American Society for Clinical Pathology. Board of Registry. Updates from the October 2007 and the March 2008 Board of Governors' meetings. BOR Newsletter (Spring/Summer) 2008:6. [Available at http://www.ascp.org/FunctionalNavigation/certification/BORNewsletter.aspx (accessed January 29, 2010).]

58. American Society for Clinical Pathology. Board of Registry. Retired certifications. BOR Newsletter (Fall) 2008:2. [Available at http://www.ascp.org/FunctionalNavigation/certification/Fall2008BORNewsletter.aspx (accessed January 29, 2010).]

59. Centers for Medicare and Medicaid Services. Medicare, Medicaid, and CLIA Programs; deeming notice for the College of American Pathologists (CAP) as an accrediting organization under the Clinical Laboratory Improvement Amendments of 1988. Fed Regist 2009; 74:13436-9.

60. World Apheresis Association. General description. Paris, France, WAA, 2010. [Available at http://www.worldapheresis.org/about/index.html (accessed January 29, 2010).]

In: McLeod BC, Szczepiorkowski ZM, Weinstein R, Winters JL, eds.
Apheresis: Principles and Practice, 3rd edition
Bethesda, MD: AABB Press, 2010

31

Principles of Quality Management for Apheresis Facilities

Christopher Chun, MT(ASCP)HP

 IN TODAY'S WORLD, QUALITY is a major priority in every business or organization. The quality of a product or service dictates its success or failure. In the last three decades, no other industry has experienced a greater demand for quality than the drug manufacturing field. Included in this industry are products and services related to the collection and manufacturing of blood and cellular therapy components by apheresis. Quality is also important for therapeutic apheresis services, although they do not receive the same regulatory attention. The goal of apheresis facilities, similar to that of blood collection facilities, is the provision of the highest quality blood and/or cellular therapy products and the highest level of service for their customers. Customers include hospitals (including transfusion and/or cellular therapy transplant services and medical care units) or manufacturers who derive other products from the original product.

Many apheresis facilities consider the development of a quality management program as a daunting task; implementation of a highly effective and comprehensive program that meets all regulatory standards can seem overwhelming. However, such a program is the foundation for the day-to-day work that occurs in an establishment and, once created and documented, should be viewed as critical guidance to be easily maintained for years to follow. Quality management should encompass the organization as a whole to ensure that all aspects of the operation of the apheresis unit meet the expectations and standards outlined by agencies involved in its regulation.

Regulations for blood component and cellular therapy product collections and apheresis facilities come from several agencies, including the Food and Drug Administration (FDA), the

Christopher Chun, MT(ASCP)HP, Clinical Services Manager, American Red Cross Biomedical Services, Salt Lake City, Utah
The author has disclosed no conflicts of interest.

Occupational Safety and Health Administration (OSHA), and the Centers for Medicare and Medicaid Services (CMS). [CMS, formerly the Health Care Financing Administration, is responsible for implementation of the 1988 Clinical Laboratory Improvement Amendments (CLIA '88) to the 1967 Clinical Laboratory Improvement Act.] Professional organizations that promote voluntary accreditation standards include the AABB, the College of American Pathologists (CAP), The Joint Commission (formerly the Joint Commission on Accreditation of Healthcare Organizations), the Clinical and Laboratory Standards Institute (CLSI, formerly the National Committee for Clinical Laboratory Standards), and the Foundation for the Accreditation of Cellular Therapy (FACT). These agencies and organizations, which are discussed in greater detail in Chapter 30, require apheresis facilities to have a quality management program in place to ensure the manufacture of a safe product for distribution as well as to ensure the safety of donors, patients, and staff. Many of the regulations and standards that these agencies and organizations have developed intertwine. In particular, the FDA and the AABB incorporate many of the same requirements into the publications, guidance documents, and correspondence they issue for blood component collection, and the FDA, AABB, and FACT observe the same requirements for cellular therapy collection. Nevertheless, all requirements should be considered to ensure full compliance.

This chapter focuses on the minimal quality system elements that support the basic principles of quality management in the apheresis unit. These quality system elements must comply with current good manufacturing practice (cGMP) and/or current good tissue practice (cGTP). The AABB has defined these minimal elements in its Quality System Essentials (QSEs) for blood banks and transfusion services,[1] which have also been adapted for cellular therapy product services.[2] In addition, FACT recently published minimal quality system elements in its international standards for cellular therapy.[3] These elements were developed to be compatible with International Standardization Organization (ISO) 9001 standards,[4] the FDA "Guideline for Quality Assurance in Blood Establishments,"[5] and other FDA quality system approaches. Many of the regulations and standards focus on blood collection and cellular therapy processing facilities, hospital blood banks, and transfusion services and do not refer directly to apheresis. Nonetheless, all of the regulations and standards discussed here apply to the collection of blood and cellular components by apheresis. Over the past 5 years, greater attention has been devoted to the development of apheresis-focused standards by the FDA, AABB, and FACT and to their application to cellular therapy products.

FDA Criteria

In the context of apheresis, regulations mandated by FDA follow two pathways. The first, which holds the longer tenure in the industry, consists of criteria focusing on cGMP. These regulations are defined under Title 21 of the *Code of Federal Regulations* (CFR), Part 211, "Good Manufacturing Practice for Drug Manufacturers,"[6] and Part 606, "Current Good Manufacturing Practice for Blood and Blood Components."[7] The second pathway was more recently implemented (in May 2005) and consists of the criteria on cGTP, defined under Title 21, Part 1271, "Human Cells, Tissue, and Cellular and Tissue-Based Products."[8]

On June 17, 1993, the FDA published a draft document titled "Guidance for Quality Assurance in Blood Establishments," which was finalized on July 11, 1995.[5] The guideline reviews the regulations that apply to blood establishments and recommends that a systems approach be undertaken to quality management—that is, evaluating an entire process from beginning to end and identifying systems within the process. In Appendix B of the FDA guideline, eight major systems of blood manufacturing are identified:
1. Quality assurance.
2. Donor suitability.
3. Blood collection.
4. Component manufacturing.

5. Product testing.
6. Storage and distribution.
7. Lot release.
8. Computers.

The appendix further identifies several critical control points within each system. Each critical control point is subdivided into key elements which, if not controlled, could affect the safety, purity, potency, and quality of the product. Other aspects that factor into product quality, such as facilities and equipment, are not specifically identified as systems but are incorporated within each of the eight major systems.

Furthermore, on January 15, 2009, the FDA published a draft document titled "Guidance for Industry: Current Good Tissue Practice and Additional Requirements for Manufacturers of Human Cells, Tissues, and Cellular and Tissue-Based Products (HCT/Ps)."[9] The guideline provides recommendations for establishments that manufacture HCT/Ps regulated under Section 361 of the Public Health Service (PHS) Act and the regulations in 21 CFR 1271.[8] cGTP requirements also apply to HCT/Ps regulated under Section 351 of the PHS Act as well as cGMP requirements (21 CFR 210, 211, and 820).[10,6,11] The discussion of products under Sections 361 and 351 of the PHS Act is outside of the scope of this chapter, but suffice it to say that these products are frequently collected by apheresis. Section III of the guidance lists 10 core areas of cGTP requirements, which are essential control points because they directly relate to preventing the introduction, transmission, or spread of communicable disease by HCT/Ps:

1. Facilities.
2. Environmental monitoring.
3. Equipment.
4. Supplies and reagents.
5. Recovery.
6. Process and processing controls.
7. Labeling controls.
8. Storage.
9. Receipt, predistribution shipment, and distribution.
10. Donor eligibility determinations, donor screening, and donor testing.

AABB Criteria

The AABB is an organization that accredits blood banks, transfusion services, and cellular therapy product services. Membership, assessment, and accreditation are voluntary. The AABB has developed and published standards for blood component transfusion and cellular therapy product services that incorporate FDA regulations and guidance as well as the regulations of other agencies: *Standards for Blood Banks and Transfusion Services (BBTS Standards)*[12] and *Standards for Cellular Therapy Product Services (CT Standards)*.[13]

Up until the 19th edition of the *BBTS Standards*, quality management was not the central focus. "Quality assurance" and "quality control" were addressed, but a systems approach to quality management was not the root of the standards. The 19th edition introduced the QSEs, which set forth the minimal standards required of participating organizations for a quality management program and laid the foundation for a systems approach to quality management. The AABB standards, in their current format, include quality in all aspects of the process from the time the donor enters the collection facility to the transfusion or infusion of the prepared blood component or cellular therapy product, respectively. Another AABB publication, the *Technical Manual*,[14] provides methods that satisfy the quality standards for many common tasks and procedures, including apheresis collections, at blood banks, transfusion services, and cellular therapy product services.

On August 1, 1997, the AABB issued Association Bulletin #97-4, titled "Quality Program Implementation,"[1] which explained the purpose and intent of the QSEs and further defined them. The AABB defines the intent of a quality program as "to ensure that quality principles are applied consistently throughout the various operational areas within an organization." The purposes of the QSEs are specified as "1) to define for facilities the generic elements that must exist in any quality program if that program is to comply with AABB *Standards for Blood Banks and Transfusion Services...* and 2) for facilities wanting to maintain AABB accreditation, identifying the minimum quality program requirements." In 2005, the AABB expanded its concept of QSEs to the cellular therapy field and described the step-by-step process to implement these QSEs in the publication *Quality Manual Preparation Workbook for Cellular Therapy Product Services.*[2] These QSEs align with the requirements outlined in the AABB *CT Standards.*[13]

The AABB QSEs for blood banks and transfusion services consist of the following[12]:
1. Organization.
2. Resources.
3. Equipment.
4. Supplier and customer issues.
5. Process control.
6. Documents and records.
7. Deviations, nonconformances, and adverse events.
8. Assessments: internal and external.
9. Process improvement through corrective and preventive action.
10. Facilities and safety.

QSEs for cellular therapy product services consist of the following[13]:
1. Organization.
2. Resources.
3. Equipment.
4. Agreements.
5. Process control.
6. Documents and records.
7. Deviations and nonconforming products or services.
8. Internal and external assessments.
9. Process improvement.
10. Safety and facilities.

Appendix 1-2 of the AABB *Technical Manual* provides a helpful "crosswalk" of CFR Title 21 citations for biologics (Parts 606, 610, and 640), drugs (211), and HCT/Ps (1271) as relevant to various topics covered by the QSEs.[14(p34)]

FACT Criteria

FACT is an international organization that accredits facilities directly involved in collection, processing, and/or infusion (transplantation) of cellular therapy products. This accreditation, similar to that of AABB, is voluntary; however, obtaining insurance reimbursement for services directly involving collection, processing, or transplantation of a cellular therapy product may be a challenge if a facility cannot show proof of this accreditation. FACT has developed and published standards which, like the AABB standards, incorporate FDA regulations and guidance as well as the regulations of other agencies discussed previously. The fourth edition of *FACT-JACIE International Standards For Cellular Therapy Product Collection, Processing, and Administration*[3] focuses on new requirements for quality elements such as donor screening, testing, and eligibility determination; labeling; and cGTP. The quality system elements described in "Part C: Cellular Therapy Collection Standards" include the following:
1. Quality management plan.
2. Organizational chart.
3. Personnel.
4. Processes, policies, and procedures.
5. Document control.
6. Written agreements.
7. Outcome analysis and product efficacy.
8. Audits.
9. Management of products with positive microbial culture results.
10. Detecting, evaluating, and reporting errors, accidents, adverse events, biological product deviations, and complaints.
11. Product tracking and tracing.
12. Continuous operation and electronic record system backup plan.
13. Qualification and validation of critical reagents, supplies, equipment, procedures, and facilities.

Minimal Quality System Elements

The following quality elements found to be common to all agencies and organizations may be considered "minimal quality system elements" that provide the foundation for the apheresis unit's quality management plan. Organizations may stipulate different monitors and controls within each element, but the intention of all standards is to meet all the regulatory requirements mandated by the FDA. The goal of this section is to discuss each element in greater detail in order to give the reader a better perspective on what each quality element consists of and, in most cases, why it is important in the apheresis setting.

Organization

This first quality system element addresses the organization as a whole. The structure of the organization must be defined, either in an organizational chart or by some other mechanism that demonstrates a chain of responsibility. AABB Standard 1.0 states[12(p1)]:

> The blood bank or transfusion service shall have a structure that clearly defines and documents the parties responsible for the provision of blood, components, tissue, derivatives, and services and the relationship of individuals responsible for key quality functions.

In addition to the above requirements, the cellular therapy product service needs to define and document the parties responsible for the provision of services for receipt, storage, and dispensing of autologous and allogeneic tissue, when performed.[13(p1)] Furthermore, the cellular therapy service defines the responsibility, authority, and relationship of personnel who perform, verify, or manage the work in the facility.[13(p1)] As described in the FACT standards, the organizational chart or equivalent should include the reporting structure for the facility's quality management program and reflect the sphere of influence an individual has when reporting to different people for different duties, rather than simply demonstrate the lines of legal authority.[3(pp78-79)] Executive management as a whole has ultimate responsibility and authority for facility operations and the quality management system. Specific functions and responsibilities may be delegated to specific individuals (eg, the medical director may be delegated the responsibility for ensuring the quality management plan is effectively established and maintained).

This element also describes the requirements and responsibility of the laboratory director (of cellular therapy facilities) and medical director. The facility may have a nonphysician laboratory director who may be delegated the responsibility of the technical operations, but the facility should also have a medical director who is a licensed physician qualified by training and/or experience and who is responsible for all medical and technical policies, processes, and procedures. In addition, the medical director should retain ultimate responsibility for medical director duties.

This first quality element also covers the requirements of the FDA, CAP, The Joint Commission, and FACT that a quality management program must be in place. The CFR (21 CFR 211.22) states, "There shall be a quality control unit that shall have the responsibility and authority to approve or reject components … and the authority to review production records to assure that no errors have occurred or, if errors have occurred, that they have been fully investigated."[6]

Finally, this element includes the requirement for a quality representative who reports to executive management and other staff, as appropriate, at least quarterly on the overall performance of the quality system and the quality management plan. All of these requirements help to ensure that the facility or program as a whole has a basic, but solid, foundation in its pursuit of a highly effective quality management process.

Resources and Personnel

The AABB *CT Standards* state, "The facility shall identify and provide adequate staffing, materials, equipment, and facility infrastructure…"[13(p5)] and the *BBTS Standards* state, "The blood bank or transfusion service shall have policies, processes, and procedures that ensure the provision of adequate resources to perform, verify, and manage all activities in the blood bank or transfusion service,"[12(p3)] These two excerpts also apply to cellular therapy facilities and are intended to cover the requirements for the provision of resources mandated by cGMP and cGTP requirements.

Resources include human resources to ensure that a process for the selection (qualification requirements based on the job description), hiring, training, and competency assessment of personnel is established. The CFR[6] [211.25(a)] states, "Each person engaged in the manufacture, processing, packing, and holding of a drug shall have education, training, and experience, or any combination thereof, to enable that person to perform the assigned functions." Part 606.40 requires that any person involved in blood collection, processing, etc have an adequate educational background and receive training particular to the area in which they are employed.[7] Similar language on resources and personnel can be found in the requirements outlined in CLIA '88, CAP, Joint Commission, and FACT standards.

The provision of adequate resources and personnel to the facility or program helps to ensure that job functions are continuously performed in a safe and effective manner. The topic of "personnel" is covered in greater detail in Chapter 32.

Agreements

Agreements should define the needs, expectations, and responsibilities of each party engaged in a facility-customer relationship throughout its duration. Customer needs and expectations may be evaluated against those processes critical to the quality or effectiveness of the product and/or services provided by the facility. An agreement or contract is the most appropriate way to ensure that customer needs and expectations are met. Once agreements have been established, there should be a means to obtain feedback from the customer to ensure that the facility is meeting the customer's expectations (eg, satisfaction surveys, periodic review of agreement).[14(pp8-9)] It may also be valuable to have a plan to deal with complaints and apparent breaches of contract.

AABB standards require that cellular therapy facilities establish, implement, and maintain policies and procedures for developing, approving, and reviewing agreements.[13(p 11)] The cGTP regulations and FACT standards also discuss the need for agreements, which should include the responsibilities of each party, especially in cases of divided responsibilities between facilities. Agreements in the cellular therapy facility (and the other services discussed in this chapter) should include, but not be limited to, the provision of the following:

- Physician orders.
- Collection orders (therapeutic apheresis and HCT/P collections).
- Data reporting.
- Transport.
- Disposition.
- Informed consent.
- Testing services.
- Suppliers, supplies, and materials.
- Donor eligibility determination.
- Notification of deviations and nonconforming products or services.

Apheresis facilities should also consider incorporating these provisions, among other necessary provisions, in their agreements.

Equipment

Discussion of equipment includes selection, qualification, appropriate use, unique identification, control and tracking, monitoring, and maintenance. "Critical" equipment items are those that must operate within defined specifications to ensure the highest level of quality when collecting, processing, or manufacturing blood, components, and tissues and when providing additional services (eg, therapeutic apheresis). Equipment items include blood cell separating devices, measuring devices, and computer systems (hardware and software). Critical equipment must be operated according to the manufacturer's written instructions.

Activities designed to ensure that equipment performs as intended include selection, qualification, validation, calibration, maintenance, and monitoring. Before purchase, equipment should be researched to ensure that it possesses the attributes that best meet the needs of the facility. Prepurchase research on a piece of equipment is useful in that it may reveal methods for qualification and validation and provide field knowledge of performance based on experiences by others.

Qualification is a process of confirming that a piece of equipment performs appropriately and consistently according to the manufacturer's specification in the environment where it will reside. Validation provides documented evidence that a specific process or function will consistently produce a product or result that meets its predetermined specifications and quality attributes.[15] Validation involves testing or stressing the system to ensure the reproducibility of results. The FDA has provided some guidance concerning validation in the May 1987 "Guideline on General Principles of Process Validation."[16] In addition, 21 CFR 211.68(a)(b)[6] and "Guidelines for Industry: General Principles of Software Validation"[17] address validation of computer systems. Validation protocols should be written and should be approved by management and the quality unit before instituting them. Qualification and validation must occur upon receipt and after major repair or upgrades but can occur at other points deemed necessary by the quality management team. Maintenance and monitoring includes performing regular function checks (preventive maintenance), calibration by qualified technicians, and regular cleaning. These activities must be performed according to manufacturer's recommendation and specifications and, of course, must be documented.

Quality control (QC) is verification that equipment is operating within acceptable ranges during daily use. A comprehensive quality management program should entail monitoring the activities and controls used to determine the accuracy and reliability of the facility's equipment in the manufacturing of products, including procurement, testing, and product release. QC involves the comparison of a manufacturing system to a known standard. QC testing is required in 21 CFR Part 211 and Part 606.[6,7]

Each facility must have a mechanism in place to uniquely identify and track all critical equipment. This can be done using the manufacturer's serial number or, in a larger facility,

there may be a mechanism in place that is facility-wide. Possessing a list of critical equipment with unique identifiers can help to facilitate ongoing quality control. Uniquely identifying each piece of critical equipment is important in tracking and trending the activities of each one and identifying equipment associated with problems and adverse events. A table of suggested equipment and reagent QC performance intervals can be found in Appendix 1-4 of the AABB *Technical Manual.*[14(pp37-39)]

Supplier and Customer Issues

Discussion of supplier and customer issues begins with the concept of "critical" supplies and materials. Supplies and materials are considered critical if they affect the quality (safety, purity, and potency) of the product being produced or manufactured. The facility must define acceptance criteria for critical supplies (see 21 CFR 210.3).[10] Another important topic is the quality of "critical services" involved in product manufacture. Examples of critical services include infectious disease testing, transportation, equipment calibration, and preventive maintenance services.[14(p9)] Testing services, in particular, must meet FDA requirements by being performed in a laboratory that is certified by CMS and registered with the FDA, if indicated by 21 CFR 610.40(f).[18] Whether a service is internal (eg, another department within an organization) or external (eg, an outside vendor), it should be held to the same standards, as required by the facility's quality management plan. All inspection agencies stipulate that policies, processes, and procedures must exist to evaluate the ability of suppliers of critical materials and services to meet qualification requirements. The evaluation should include three elements: 1) supplier qualification, 2) agreements, and 3) inspection and testing of incoming supplies.[14(p9)] The first two factors are discussed in this section, and the last factor will be discussed in the next section.

Facilities should maintain a list of suppliers and their materials and services and should periodically review this list to ensure that it is current and accurate. Most collection facilities have agreements or contracts with some kind of supplier, whether it is for the provision of collection supplies, laboratory testing, or other services that are a critical part of the manufacturing process. Agreements and contracts should be designed to meet the needs of the supplier and the collection facility and should ensure the production of a quality product. Furthermore, they should be reviewed, evaluated, and revised as needed.

Finally, the handling of supplier and customer issues, such as concerns or complaints, is an extremely important matter in the client-customer relationship. A process should be defined by the facility to manage such issues and should cover communication of the issue, action taken, follow-up with the affected party, documentation, tracking, and trending. A mechanism for handling client-customer issues may be included in the agreement or contract.

Qualification and Validation (of Supplies, Reagents, and Processes)

Qualification and validation are necessities in the blood bank and cellular therapy service. Qualification is defined as a process for verifying that a supply or reagent functions consistently within established limits.[3(p13)] The FDA allows qualification to occur by means of specification sheets or certificates of analysis, and when qualification by verification of these items cannot be achieved, it is the responsibility of the facility to establish a qualification strategy to ensure the supply or reagent meets criteria to ensure safety, purity, and potency of the product.

Critical supplies and reagents (defined previously) include alcohol swabs, cleaning agents (for sanitizing equipment and instruments), anticoagulants, saline, blood component transfer bags, test kits, and reagents. As mentioned in the previous section, facilities should maintain a list of suppliers and their materials and should periodically review this list to ensure that it is current and accurate. Facilities should ensure that materials are qualified on the basis of defined requirements by the facility. Before

use, incoming critical materials, (ie, supplies and reagents) must be verified and inspected and their acceptability determined. All critical materials used in the collection, processing, storage, distribution, and transfusion or infusion of blood components or cellular therapy products must meet FDA regulations. For example, 21 CFR 606.65(b) states, "Each blood collecting container and its satellite container(s), if any, shall be examined visually for damage or evidence of contamination prior to its use and immediately after filling. Such examination shall include inspection for breakage of seals, when indicated, and abnormal discoloration. Where any defect is observed, the container shall not be used, or, if detected after filling, shall be properly discarded."[7] In addition, AABB Standard 4.3.2.1 states, "All containers and solutions used for collection, preservation, and storage and all reagents used for required tests on blood samples shall meet or exceed applicable FDA criteria."[12(p9)] This also applies to tubing set kits and intravenous solutions that are used in the apheresis collection. Supplies should be logged in and inspected and the acceptability of critical materials documented.

Whereas qualification focuses on components (equipment, supplies, reagents) within a process, "validation" focuses on the entire process with all its components. In this context, validation establishes how supplies and reagents perform within a given process with respect to its predetermined specifications. It is critical to validate processes when it is not feasible to measure or inspect each finished product for conformance to specifications, and validation must be performed according to established procedures. Validation can be classified into three different types. Prospective validation is used for new and revised procedures and should be used for most procedures that undergo validation. Concurrent validation is used when required data cannot be obtained without performance of a "live" process and is usually employed in conjunction with prospective, non-live validation. Retrospective validation is employed when processes are already in operation but were not adequately validated before implementation. This mode of validation should be used only as a last resort.

An effective validation should be planned and documented. In fact, development of a validation plan is required by FACT and AABB standards. A validation plan should consist of the following elements[14(p12)]:

- System description.
- Purpose or objective.
- Risk assessment.
- Responsibilities.
- Validation procedures.
- Acceptance criteria.
- Approval signatures.
- Supporting documentation.

Validation plans should be reviewed and approved by the facility medical director and quality oversight personnel. It is important to refer to the standards of each organization because the different organizations may require approval of one or the other, or both.

Revalidation is often required when a change to a process occurs that has the potential of affecting the safety, purity, or potency of the product. The revalidation plan, which may not have to be as extensive as the original plan, should be approved by the medical director and quality oversight personnel, and staff responsible for carrying out the activities should be trained in the process before the plan is executed.[14(pp12-15)]

Policies and Procedures

Policies and procedures are documents that are fundamentally different from each other. Policies communicate the highest level goals, objectives, and intent of the organization.[14(p17)] Thus facilities should indicate in their institutional policies their intent to meet the standards mandated by the regulatory agencies and organizations they are inspected by. Procedures, on the other hand, are step-by-step directions on how to perform job tasks and functions. Procedures may also be referred to as work instructions. They should include enough detail to allow the task to be performed correctly but not so much detail that they are difficult or cumbersome to read.

It should be realized that in writing policies and procedures, facilities are creating their own set of regulatory requirements, so the documents must incorporate existing regulations and guidelines set forth by official regulating agencies and accrediting organizations. Formats for writing standard operating procedures (SOPs) are generally facility-dependent. At a minimum, an SOP should include the purpose or intent of the procedure, a list of supplies or critical materials needed for that process or procedure, and step-by-step instructions on how to accomplish the process or procedure. Including references helps to ensure that all aspects of the regulations have been considered and can also allow policies and procedures to serve as educational tools for technical personnel. The content and format of policies and procedures are up to the individual facility, as long as they are consistent. The CLSI provides excellent guidance on how to write policies and procedures.[19] FACT standards use this guidance to define the elements required in their standards for policies and procedures, which include the following[3(pp45-46)]:

- A clearly written description of the objective(s).
- A description of the equipment and supplies used.
- Acceptable endpoints and the range of expected results, where applicable.
- A stepwise description of the procedure, including diagrams and tables, as needed.
- References to other SOPs or policies required to perform the procedure.
- A reference section listing appropriate literature, if applicable.
- Documented approval of each procedure by the program director or designated physician before implementation and every 2 years thereafter.
- Documented approval of each procedural modification by the the program director or designated physician before implementation.
- A copy of current versions of orders, worksheets, reports, labels, and forms associated with the procedure, where applicable.

All agencies and organizations require that either an electronic or a hard copy of the most current version of each policy and procedure be available to the facility staff for quick reference at all times. In addition, new and revised policies and procedures must be reviewed by the staff before implementation. When a staff member returns from extended leave, the review and necessary training must be completed before the staff member performs the procedure. Of course, review and training must be documented. The points mentioned above are general elements required for policies and procedures; for additional requirements made by a particular organization, refer to that organization's standards and regulations.

Process Control

Process control is the most comprehensive quality element discussed in this chapter. To begin with, it is important to understand the meaning of "process" in the blood bank and transfusion and cellular therapy services. A process describes a sequence of actions and identifies responsibilities, decision points, requirements, and acceptance criteria. Flow charts and diagrams are very useful tools in describing and documenting processes.[14(p17)] Process control is meant to ensure that practices in the areas of collection, processing, final inspection, testing, handling, storage, distribution, and transport ensure the safety, purity, potency, and quality of the product. AABB Standard 5.0 (which applies to cellular therapy services also) states[12(p10)]:

The blood bank or transfusion service shall have policies and validated processes and procedures that ensure the quality of blood, components, tissue, derivatives, and services. The blood bank or transfusion service shall ensure that these policies, processes, and procedures are carried out under controlled conditions.

In a very simplified form, process control means that every part of the process, including collecting, producing, storing, transporting, and distributing blood and tissue products, must be controlled. Key elements to establishing this control include the following:
* The development and use of procedures (ie, SOPs).
* A process to control change in processes and procedures.
* Acceptance testing and process validation of new or changed processes and procedures.
* Monitoring of all production processes.
* Proficiency testing for each testing system in place.
* An established quality control system.
* A method to ensure that process and product specifications are met as well as a method for dealing with nonconforming processes and products (which will be discussed in a later section).

Written SOPs, as described in the discussion of the previous quality element, are key to the success of process control. The FDA regulations concerning the existence of SOPs are found in 21 CFR 211.100,[6] which states:

(a) There shall be written procedures for production and process control designed to ensure that the drug products have the identity, strength, quality, and purity they purport or are represented to possess.

(b) Written production and process control procedures shall be followed in the execution of the various production and process control functions and shall be documented at the time of performance. Any deviations from the written procedure should be recorded and justified.

21 CFR 211.22(c) further states, "The quality control unit shall have the responsibility for approving or rejecting all procedures or specifications impacting on the identity, strength, quality, and purity of the drug product."[6] A first step in developing a quality program that encompasses process control is to determine whether policies and SOPs exist for all processes and procedures performed. Apheresis facilities are required to have and follow all of their own processes, policies, and procedures. Written validation plans and procedures should exist for quality control, labeling, proficiency testing, and documentation of quality control

performed on reagents, equipment, and all products manufactured. The AABB *Standards*,[12,13] AABB *Technical Manual*,[14] and the FACT accreditation manual[20] offer more detailed guidance on documentation.

For final inspection and testing, a process must be in place to ensure that the finished product is found to be acceptable according to established criteria. There should be documentation of those criteria and evidence of a review of the preparation, testing, and acceptability of the blood component or tissue product. Requirements for handling, storage, distribution, and transport are that critical materials used in production of the blood and tissue itself must be traceable and their dispositions documented.

Documents and Records

Documentation provides a framework for understanding and communication throughout the organization. Documents relating to processes and SOPs should describe how processes are intended to work, how they interact, where they must be controlled, and how to implement them, revise them, make them obsolete, and archive them. Records provide evidence that the process was performed as intended and provide information needed to assess the quality of products or services. Together, documents and records provide useful information to the oversight personnel who evaluate the effectiveness of a facility's policies, processes, and procedures.[14(p16)]

According to AABB standards, policies, processes, and procedures are needed "to ensure that documents are identified, reviewed, approved, and retained and that records are created, stored, and archived in accordance with record retention policies."[12(p62)] Moreover, 21 CFR 606.160(a)(1) states, "Records shall be maintained concurrently with the performance of each significant step in the collection, processing, compatibility testing, storage and distribution of each unit of blood and blood components so that all steps can be clearly traced."[7] The preceding standards apply to cellular therapy services as well.[3,13(p77)]

Document and record control is an integral part of maintaining process control. A system for identifying, creating, implementing, reviewing, changing, and retaining documents and records must be in place. The FDA, AABB, and FACT stipulate information that must be present in the record and the length of time documents and records must be maintained. AABB Reference Standards 6.2A through E (*BBTS Standards*) illustrate retention timetables for donor/unit, patient, and other facility documents, some of which are apheresis specific.[12(pp64-76)] Procedures for document control should be in writing and should include a procedure for review of donor records before a product becomes available for transfusion, infusion, or further manufacturing. Donation records should be reviewed for completeness of demographic information, donor eligibility, legibility, and thoroughness. In addition, quality control records on equipment and reagents used in the production of a blood and tissue product should be reviewed to ensure the safety, purity, and potency of the product. Errors or omissions in the records should be investigated and corrective actions recorded. An annual review of policies, processes, and procedures should be carried out by an authorized person, and this action should be documented.

In addition, investigational documents and records are important to maintain in that they provide evidence that problems, adverse events, and complaints have been addressed (see "Deviations, Nonconformances, and Adverse Events" section).

Personnel records are vital documents that must not be overlooked. Personnel records should include the names, signatures, identification codes, initials, and dates of employment of staff members performing or reviewing critical tasks, as well as training and competency, performance evaluation, and appraisal records. Investigational and personnel records must be maintained in a confidential manner, as required by applicable laws and regulations.

Finally, with respect to records in cases of divided responsibility among facilities, the records of each facility should show plainly the extent of its responsibility.[3(p54)]

Labels and Labeling Controls

A great amount of emphasis has been placed on labels and labeling controls because 1) improper identification or representation of the product or product samples may lead to mix-ups, and 2) improper testing of samples may lead to inaccurate or inappropriate results. Either situation may ultimately cause severe morbidity and/or death from transfusion-related reactions, graft rejection, or transmission of disease. Mislabeling of a product is classified as a major nonconformance that is subject to FDA reporting, product recall, and other severe actions.

AABB and FACT have similar standards based on FDA requirements (under cGTP and cGMP) to address these nonconformances. For example, labels must be clear, legible, and complete and use indelible ink capable of withstanding all appropriate storage conditions. In addition, labels should be applied to containers in such a way that a portion of the container remains uncovered to permit inspection of the contents. The information required to be on labels varies depending on the stage of product manufacture. Additional guidance on label content may be found in FACT standards[3] (cellular therapy products) and AABB standards[12,13] (blood and cellular therapy products).

- Labeling control is a major component of process control and includes the following:
- Verification of labels, upon receipt, against an approved master label template.
- Validation of print-on-demand labeling systems, if used.
- Validation of labels for storage under the conditions for their use.
- Version control of labels.
- A system for storage of labels of different products and modifiers.
- A system for removing and discarding obsolete or unusable labels.
- A system of checks and verification throughout the labeling process (in process,

after collection, and at the time of distribution).
- Verification of proper information on shipping containers.
- Verification of accompanying documentation at the time of distribution (specifically for cellular therapy products).

Deviations, Nonconformances, and Adverse Events

The facility must have a process for detecting, investigating, and responding to events that deviate from accepted policies, processes, and procedures or that fail to meet specified criteria or requirements, as defined by the facility and AABB and FACT standards or applicable regulations.[7,8]

The FDA has established criteria for reporting product deviations in 21 CFR 606.171[7] and in guidance documents.[21,22] This comprehensive process includes the discovery of nonconforming products and services as well as adverse events such as adverse reactions from donations, transfusions, or tissues. The facility should define how to perform the following[14(p20)]:

- Document and classify occurrences.
- Determine the effect, if any, on the quality of the product or services.
- Evaluate the effect on interrelated activities.
- Analyze the event to understand root causes.
- Implement corrective action, including notification and recall, as appropriate on the basis of investigation and root cause analysis.
- Implement preventive actions as appropriate on the basis of analysis of aggregate data about events and their causes.
- Report to external agencies when required (ie, fatality or severe morbidity related to a transfused or infused product).
- Evaluate the effectiveness of the corrective actions and preventive actions taken.

In basic terms, this course of action answers the questions related to who, what, where, when, why, and how. Reporting must occur as soon as possible after detection to prompt an immediate investigation. The cGMP regulations require investigation and documentation of an occurrence that adversely affects patient safety or the safety, purity, or potency of blood components, whereas the cGTP regulations require investigation and documentation of occurrences that expose the product to increase risk of contamination or transmission of a communicable disease.[14(p21)]

Additional requirements outlined in applicable standards are also worth mentioning. Facility personnel should be trained to recognize and report occurrences. "Qualified" personnel (ie, medical director, laboratory director, and/or the patient's physician) must evaluate and approve deviations before final release of a product. The facility should maintain policies, processes, and procedures to prevent unintended release of nonconforming products or services. The facility should report to the customer, as early as possible, products that are lost or damaged, or released products or delivered services that are determined to be nonconforming. In addition, the facility should establish a process to detect, evaluate, and report adverse reactions resulting from collection.

Nonconformance and adverse event management is the key to quality management and should be viewed as an opportunity to improve as facilities continually strive for perfection in safety and quality. Facility personnel should be made aware of the possible consequences of improper performance of their activities[9]; however, adverse event management should not be a mechanism for punishment.

Complaints

The element of management of complaints is sometimes overlooked. The FDA cGTP regulations pay particular attention to complaints in 21 CFR 1271.320,[8] but it is important that all facility types take an interest in this element because, like the management of nonconforming events, investigation of complaints can reveal more deeply rooted system problems. Facilities should establish and maintain proce-

dures for the review, evaluation, and documentation of complaints relating to core cGTP requirements (if applicable); the safety, purity, and potency of the product; and quality of service.

Audits and Assessments (External and Internal)

Although all industry-related accrediting bodies (AABB, CAP, The Joint Commission, and FACT) define standards for audits and assessments, the AABB provides a detailed discussion of these elements in its standards and is thus highlighted in this section.

Quality assessments are performed to verify whether the quality system complies with specified requirements. Assessment activities should include proficiency testing and outcome analysis. For CLIA-regulated testing, proficiency testing should be administered by a CMS-approved proficiency testing program. Outcome analysis involves the collection, evaluation, and distribution of outcome data.[3(p85)] For example, the quality of hematopoietic progenitor cell (HPC) products is assessed by monitoring the number of days after HPC infusion required to achieve neutrophil and platelet engraftment. Patient data is collated and statistically analyzed to determine data point outliers. The statistical analysis is shared with any partnering facilities for review and further investigation, if necessary.

AABB BBTS Standard 8.0[12(p82)] and CT Standard 8.1[13(p93)] require that facilities (blood banks, transfusion services, and cellular therapy services) have policies, processes, and procedures to ensure that external and internal assessments of operations and the quality system are scheduled and conducted.

External assessments are those performed by an organization or a regulating agency not affiliated with the facility, such as the AABB, CAP, The Joint Commission, FACT, the FDA, or OSHA. Facilities should have in place policies and/or procedures on managing external assessments. These should define who is responsible for meeting with the assessor(s). It is helpful to set up a time frame for the assessor to meet with the various personnel involved. If the assessment is scheduled in advance, it is also helpful to anticipate information the assessor(s) will want to review and to make it available in one convenient location. Undergoing external assessments can be very stressful. It is helpful to realize that virtually no one completes an external assessment without receiving at least some recommendations from the assessor. It is important to keep in mind that the purpose of the assessment is to improve on an already seemingly good operation, resulting in an even higher level of quality for the product or service. Apheresis facilities need to be aware that they are held to the same regulations and standards as other types of blood collection facilities.

Internal audits are those performed by personnel within the facility, company, or organization. The audit process should be written and should have a defined scope and purpose. Audits for each of the operational and quality systems should be planned on a defined schedule that can realistically be accomplished. Audits should be detailed enough to identify problem areas but not so detailed that they are too complex to complete. Individuals knowledgeable about the process being reviewed and the process of auditing should conduct the audits. Even for internal audits, the auditors must have the authority to stop the process or initiate a recall if they detect an error in the system that may compromise product quality. A written summary of the audit should be prepared and, if necessary, corrective actions defined. Follow-up audits should be completed to assess the effectiveness of any corrective actions implemented. Results of internal audits should be reported to the quality assurance unit, the facility's management, and the medical director of the facility. To be effective, internal audits should be taken as seriously as external audits. One example of the effective performance of internal audits would be to take each of the quality system elements and write an audit plan based on the criteria outlined for it in the AABB standards.[1,2] The preparer of the audit should also incorporate pertinent requirements set forth by other agencies or organizations. With the combination of external and internal assessments, facilities should be audited and/or assessed on a regular basis that will ensure a comprehensive operational and quality systems review of compliance with current standards of practice.

Process Improvement Through Corrective and Preventive Action

The quality element of process improvement stresses the importance of identifying, investigating, correcting, and preventing errors or deviations that affect product quality. Collecting and reviewing data regarding customer complaints; incidents, errors, and accident reports; and the results of internal and external audits can help to identify opportunities for improvements. Use of a statistical tool for numerical data can be helpful. The practice of root cause analysis is recommended as an approach to problem-solving. The root cause of the problem must be identified in order to implement effective corrective action. FDA, CAP, The Joint Commission, and FACT requirements stress the importance of process improvement by taking action as described above.

Safety and Facilities

Chapter 10 in both sets of AABB *Standards*[12,13] and FACT Part C2[3] outline requirements for safety and facilities, which include, but are not limited to, the following:

- Ensuring the facility is of appropriate design and size to adequately perform all functions (eg, storage of supplies/reagents, donor evaluation, collection).
- Developing and maintaining policies, processes, and procedures to ensure the provision of safe and adequate environmental conditions in the workplace.
- Meeting local, state, and federal regulations, where applicable.
- Developing and maintaining procedures that cover general safety, disaster preparedness, biologic safety, chemical safety, radiation safety, and the disposal of blood, components, and tissues.

- Handling and discarding chemical and bio-hazardous materials in a manner that minimizes the potential for human exposure.
- Defining and monitoring environmental conditions (temperature, humidity, ventilation, air quality) that optimize the safety, purity, potency, and integrity of products.
- Limiting access to collection facilities to authorized personnel.

An apheresis facility should be clean and inviting for potential customers and should be designed in a way that is consonant with tasks, safety, and workflow. Poorly designed facilities, such as those with inadequate space, can contribute to errors and accidents, which in turn can affect the quality of the products and services provided. The FDA addresses blood establishment facilities in 21 CFR Part 211, "Good Manufacturing Practice for Drug Manufacturers," and Part 606, "Current Good Manufacturing Practice for Blood and Blood Components." Accessibility is important to the success of an apheresis facility dependent on volunteer donors. Part 211.42(a) of the CFR states, "Any building or buildings used in the manufacture, processing, packing, or holding of a drug product shall be of a suitable size, construction, and location to facilitate cleaning, maintenance, and proper operations."[6] Part 606 of the CFR is more specific with regard to whole blood and apheresis operations. The regulations outlined in 21 CFR 606.40 require adequate space for private and accurate examinations to determine donor eligibility and many other aspects of donating, processing, testing, storage, and distribution processes.

Apheresis facilities should also be designed to minimize the risks of contamination of products. The FDA's cGTP requirements in Section 1271.195 state[8]:

Where environmental conditions could reasonably be expected to cause contamination or cross contamination of equipment or accidental exposure of products to communicable disease agents, you must adequately control environmental conditions and provide proper conditions for operations.

This would include cleaning and disinfecting of rooms and equipment. Within the collection area, there should be hazardous waste containers for the disposal of materials contaminated with biologic waste. The containers should be located to allow for the easy disposal of sharps and other high-risk material. Lighting, power, and ventilation should be adequate for the equipment in use. Of course, policies and procedures must be developed and maintained to include the requirements and activities related to facility maintenance and safety.

Conclusion

Because of their association with blood banks and transfusion services, apheresis activities are subject to the scrutiny of regulatory agencies. In addition, new standards implemented for cellular therapy services under the cGTP guidelines also apply to the apheresis field. This chapter has examined the principles of a sound quality management system, starting with a solid understanding of the quality system elements that support an apheresis program's quality plan. It has emphasized that many of the requirements of different regulatory agencies and accrediting organizations are very similar. The intent of the chapter was not to cover all the minimal quality elements in detail, but, rather, to provide an understanding of quality management principles and the major elements that make up a comprehensive quality program that will meet the requirements mandated by the various agencies and organizations. A logical approach to building a quality program is to make it comprehensive and to use language that covers all types of products and services, whether or not the establishment provides all or just a few of the services (ie, blood component, cellular therapy, or therapeutic). The more comprehensive a program's quality system or plan is, the fewer the modifications that will be required in the future if new products or services are added. No process or plan is perfect, but a robust and well-organized quality program can instill a high level of confidence in customers, donors, patients, and regulatory agencies that an apheresis program is "in control" of its processes and services.

References

1. Quality program implementation. Association bulletin #97-4. Bethesda, MD: AABB, 1997.
2. Berte LM. Quality manual preparation workbook for cellular therapy product services. Bethesda, MD: AABB Press, 2005.
3. FACT-JACIE international standards for cellular therapy product collection, processing, and administration. 4th ed. Omaha, NE: Foundation for the Accreditation of Cellular Therapy and Joint Accreditation Committee—ISCT and EBMT, 2008.
4. ANSI/ISO/ASQ Q9000-2000 series: Quality management standards. Milwaukee, WI: ASQ Quality Press, 2000.
5. Food and Drug Administration. Guideline for quality assurance in blood establishments. (July 11, 1995) Rockville, MD: CBER Office of Communication, Training, and Manufacturers Assistance, 1995.
6. Code of federal regulations. Title 21 CFR Part 211. Washington, DC: US Government Printing Office, 2010 (revised annually).
7. Code of federal regulations. Title 21 CFR Part 606. Washington, DC: US Government Printing Office, 2010 (revised annually).
8. Code of federal regulations. Title 21 CFR Part 1271. Washington, DC: US Government Printing Office, 2010 (revised annually).
9. Food and Drug Administration. Draft guidance for industry: Current good tissue practice (cGTP) and additional requirements for manufacturers of human cells, tissues, and cellular and tissue-based products (HCT/Ps). (January 15, 2009) Rockville, MD: CBER Office of Communication, Outreach, and Development, 2009.
10. Code of federal regulations. Title 21 CFR Part 210. Washington, DC: US Government Printing Office, 2010 (revised annually).
11. Code of federal regulations. Title 21 CFR Part 820. Washington, DC: US Government Printing Office, 2010 (revised annually).
12. Price TH, ed. Standards for blood banks and transfusion services. 26th ed. Bethesda, MD: AABB, 2009.
13. Padley D, ed. Standards for cellular therapy product services. 3rd ed. Bethesda, MD: AABB, 2008.
14. Roback JD, Combs MR, Grossman BJ, Hillyer CD, eds. Technical manual. 16th ed. Bethesda, MD: AABB, 2008.
15. Zuck TF. Current good manufacturing practices review. Transfusion 1995;35:955-66.
16. Food and Drug Administration. Guideline on general principles of process validation. (May 1987) Rockville, MD: Division of Communications Management, 1987.
17. Food and Drug Administration. Guidance for industry: General principles of software validation: Final guidance for industry and FDA staff. (January 11, 2002) Rockville, MD: CBER Office of Communication, Training, and Manufacturers Assistance, 2002.
18. Code of federal regulations. Title 21 CFR Part 610. Washington, DC: US Government Printing Office, 2010 (revised annually).
19. A quality system model for health care; NCCLS approved guideline (HS1-A2). Wayne, PA: National Committee for Clinical Laboratory Standards, 2004.
20. Cellular therapy accreditation manual. 4th ed. Omaha, NE: Foundation for the Accreditation of Cellular Therapy, 2008.
21. Food and Drug Administration. Guidance for industry: Biological product deviation reporting for blood and plasma establishments. (October 18, 2006) Rockville, MD: CBER Office of Communication, Training, and Manufacturers Assistance, 2006.
22. Food and Drug Administration. Guidance for industry: Certain human cells, tissues, and cellular and tissue-based products recovered from donors who were tested for communicable diseases using pooled specimens or diagnostic tests. (April 2008) Rockville, MD: CBER Office of Communication, Training, and Manufacturers Assistance, 2008.

Suggested Reading

Baldrige National Quality Program. Health care criteria for performance excellence. Gaithersburg, MD: National Institute of Standards and Technology, 2007 (revised annually).

Berte LM. Quality manual preparation workbook for blood banking. 2nd ed. Bethesda, MD: AABB, 2005.

Juran JM, Godfrey AB. Juran's quality handbook. 5th ed. New York: McGraw-Hill, 1999.

Nunes E, Motschman T. Regulations A to Z for blood and HCT/Ps. 9th ed. Bethesda, MD: AABB Press, 2009.

Wagner J, AuBuchon JP, Saxena S, Shulman IA for the Clinical Transfusion Medicine Committee. Guidelines for the quality assessment of transfusion. Bethesda, MD: AABB, 2006.

Walters LM, ed. Introducing the big Q: A practical quality primer. Bethesda, MD: AABB Press, 2004.

Walters LM, Carpenter Badley JK, eds. S[3]: Simple six sigma for blood banking, transfusion, and cellular therapy. Bethesda, MD: AABB Press, 2007.

In: McLeod BC, Szczepiorkowski ZM, Weinstein R, Winters JL, eds.
Apheresis: Principles and Practice, 3rd edition
Bethesda, MD: AABB Press, 2010

32

Quality Management of Apheresis Personnel

Wanda B. Koetz, RN, HP(ASCP)

IT IS OFTEN SAID THAT AN organization is only as good as the people who do the work. The provision of apheresis services is no different. In apheresis donor collections, hematopoietic progenitor cell (HPC) collections, therapeutic apheresis procedures, or any combination of these activities, success depends on having well-trained staff performing clearly described tasks. This chapter looks at some of the issues involved in staffing and directing an apheresis unit from a quality management perspective.

Background

Assessment

Providing apheresis services is an expensive and complex undertaking that requires careful assessment of the institutional or community needs for such services. Such an assessment will provide answers to the questions: "What types of services are needed at what frequency?" and "Do we have the resources and expertise to provide the needed services?" Because different services may require different numbers of staff and different skill levels on the part of each employee, these factors will determine the type of employee resources needed. For example, performing therapeutic procedures requires knowledge and skills in patient assessment, management of fluid and electrolyte balances, vascular access, and administration of medications as well as familiarity with operating and troubleshooting the apheresis instrument and ancillary equipment. Performing donor collection procedures, in contrast, requires knowledge and skills in donor assessment and treatment of donor reactions and injuries as well as familiarity with

Wanda B. Koetz, RN, HP(ASCP), Principal Associate, American Red Cross Biomedical Services, Washington, District of Columbia
The author has disclosed no conflicts of interest.

apheresis instrument operation and trouble-shooting.

Requirements

When decisions have been made regarding the types of apheresis services to be offered, employee requirements—federal, state, and local[1]—must be assessed carefully. There are specific licensing requirements for physicians, nurses, and technologists who are practicing as professionals in an apheresis service; these requirements may vary from state to state. Many states also have nurse practice acts that may affect apheresis services. For example, many state nurse practice acts forbid the administration of intravenous medication by anyone other than a registered nurse (RN), thus significantly limiting the use of unlicensed staff for such services as therapeutic apheresis and HPC collections. Until recently, California law required all phlebotomies for donor collections to be performed by RNs.

The Occupational Safety and Health Administration and the Clinical Laboratory Improvement Amendments of 1988 (CLIA) regulations discussed in Chapter 30 should also be reviewed carefully. The human resources staff in an organization or institution should assist in this assessment of laws and requirements. Job descriptions should then be developed and should reflect employment requirements by job title.

As emphasized in Chapter 30, the Food and Drug Administration (FDA) is the branch of the federal government responsible for licensing and inspecting blood collection facilities. The *Code of Federal Regulations* (CFR), which is published annually by the federal government, outlines federal requirements concerning the activities of blood collection facilities, of which apheresis donor collection facilities are a subset. The CFR does not specify the qualifications of employees; rather, it requires a "qualified, trained individual to be the responsible head" and states that those responsible for "collection, processing, compatibility testing, storage, or distribution of blood or blood components shall be adequate in number, educational back-ground, training, and experience."[2] It is up to facilities providing apheresis services to define in their policies and procedures how they will meet CFR requirements pertaining to employees.

The AABB does not regulate blood collection activities, but it has published voluntary standards for member blood banks and transfusion services to follow. The AABB *Standards for Blood Banks and Transfusion Services (Standards)* states that "the blood bank or transfusion service shall have a medical director who is a licensed physician and qualified by education, training, and/or experience."[3(p1)] In addition, "the blood bank or transfusion service shall have a process to ensure the employment of an adequate number of individuals qualified by education, training, and/or experience."[3(p3)]

The American Society for Apheresis (ASFA) has published voluntary guidelines for therapeutic apheresis facilities. These guidelines state that "each TA [Therapeutic Apheresis] Service should be led by a licensed physician, qualified by training and/or by experience, who will be called the Director" and that the "remainder of the TA Service staff should consist of medical personnel qualified to perform TA procedures."[4]

In addition to the previously described requirements, organizational contracts with individual hospitals may include specific requirements for staff who perform apheresis services.

Handling Inspections

Compliance with personnel requirements in the CFR can be a focus of FDA inspections as problems and deficiencies are identified. To avoid citations for deficiencies, all personnel files must be current and complete. An inspector may ask to see an employee's job description, job qualifications, and regular periodic competency determinations. Each file must also contain supporting documentation that the employee has been properly trained and updated on procedural changes, as necessary, and has maintained current licensure status when working in a professional capacity (eg, RN).

Employee Categories and Roles

Physicians

Medical directors of donor collection facilities should be licensed physicians who have knowledge and experience in hematology and transfusion medicine. These physicians must also be familiar with blood banking principles, appropriate FDA regulations, AABB standards, current good manufacturing practice (cGMP) requirements, and employee safety regulations.

According to the CFR,[2] although the "responsible head" is not required to be a physician, that individual is responsible for the following:

1. Monitoring compliance with all requirements in the CFR for manufacturing blood components.
2. Representing the facility in all matters to the Center for Biologics Evaluation and Research.
3. Enforcing discipline and performance of assigned functions by employees engaged in manufacturing blood products.
4. Training employees in manufacturing methods and appropriate sections of the CFR.

AABB *Standards*[3(pp1-2)] requires that the medical director have responsibility and authority for the following:

1. All medical and technical policies, processes, and procedures, including those that pertain to laboratory personnel and test performance.
2. Approval for the above.
3. The consultative and support services that relate to the care and safety of donors and/or transfusion recipients.

For physicians who will be in charge of therapeutic apheresis services, the following guidelines have been established by ASFA as recommended requirements for medical directors:

1. Knowledge of immunology, of transfusion medicine, and of the principles of apheresis separation and its effects on the body after removal or exchange.
2. Familiarity with various apheresis instruments currently in use.
3. Knowledge of diseases treated by therapeutic apheresis and the clinical indications for it.
4. Expertise in the planning and performance of all modalities of apheresis therapy.
5. Expertise in the management of adverse effects of therapeutic apheresis.
6. Expertise in the logistical, financial, and personnel management of the therapeutic apheresis service.

According to ASFA guidelines, therapeutic apheresis service medical directors are responsible for the following:

1. Medical and technical policies and procedures.
2. Support services related to the safety of patients, including compliance with the published guidelines.
3. Assurance of the safety and adequacy of the place of treatment.
4. Selection, maintenance, and proper use of apheresis devices and other equipment and materials used for therapeutic apheresis.
5. Assurance of adequate training and performance of members of the therapeutic apheresis service staff.

Technical Staff

Under the medical director's supervision, the technical staff members of an apheresis program collect apheresis components and perform therapeutic apheresis and HPC collection procedures. The technical staff in any apheresis unit ordinarily evaluate donor eligibility, obtain consent, establish vascular access, perform the procedures, care for donors and/or patients, and perform maintenance and quality control of supplies and equipment used during apheresis procedures. At a management level, some members of the technical staff may supervise the daily operations of the unit; interact with physicians and other medical professionals; write procedures; train apheresis staff; and enforce compliance with applicable procedures, standards, and requirements.

The technical staff can consist of RNs, medical technologists (MTs), licensed practical nurses (LPNs), medical technicians, trained phlebotomists, those with a bachelor's degree in a science such as biology, or some combination of these categories. Historically, centers that perform therapeutic apheresis or HPC procedures have tended to rely on RNs or MTs. In centers performing apheresis donor collections only, individuals with less formal education, such as LPNs, medical technicians, or trained phlebotomists, have worked successfully. For centers offering a combination of services, a mixture of all levels has worked well. Wright[5] has detailed the differences in educational background, technical skills, and work experience for the various types of technical staff employed in the therapeutic apheresis service. She suggests that the education and training of the employees be used to establish performance standards, that the standards be reviewed periodically, and that changes be made as necessary. The following discussion identifies the different types of technical staff participating in apheresis and examines their unique contributions to apheresis services.

Registered Nurses

The education of nurses includes human anatomy and physiology, basic concepts of human disease, and practical training in patient care. An RN's skills and qualifications usually include patient/donor physical assessment, expertise in interpersonal relationships, interview skills, first aid, training in cardiopulmonary resuscitation, and a license to administer medications and fluids under a physician's prescription. Local and state requirements may dictate that certain tasks be performed by or under the supervision of an RN. These requirements should be kept in mind when decisions are being made about whether nurses are a necessary part of the staffing matrix for a particular apheresis unit. Background and experience in hemodialysis can be especially beneficial when nurses new to the field of apheresis are being hired.

Medical Technologists

Because the education of medical technologists emphasizes laboratory concepts, the contribution of these individuals to the apheresis unit can include knowledge of hematology and blood banking, experience in instrumentation and equipment quality control, skill in problem-solving, and attention to detail. CLIA regulations must be assessed to determine if any tasks to be performed by apheresis staff require the educational background and certification of medical technologists.[1]

Other Technical Staff

Experienced medical technicians, LPNs, emergency medical technicians, and others with some technical/medical training bring some of the clinical and technical skills of RNs and MTs, but their limitations must be recognized. Individual state nurse practice acts will determine at what level LPNs can function compared with RNs. Many centers use staff at this level because they can perform many, but certainly not all, of the same duties at a lower salary than that of an RN or MT.

Employees with a 4-year degree in one of the sciences such as biology can be trained successfully to operate apheresis instruments and to care for donors and patients. They possess good decision-making skills and can use their knowledge of science to better understand the concepts of anatomy and physiology, disease processes, and disease treatment.

Trained phlebotomists have also been used in donor collection facilities, usually at a lower salary. However, phlebotomists are generally not required to have the strong skills in decision-making that are expected in an employee with a degree. For phlebotomists, procedural training may need to be repeated more frequently. Supervision of these individuals may also require more time and involvement.

Nontechnical staff

Donor Recruiters and Schedulers

The success of any donor collection facility depends on the people who recruit new donors into the program, schedule their donation appointments, and assist in donor recognition activities. These people need to demonstrate excellent communication skills along with an ability to generate enthusiasm about the program in potential donors. Extensive education may not be required to perform these tasks successfully, but a basic knowledge of the process of apheresis donations and of the requirements that donors must meet is critical to offer clear explanations to donors and answer their questions.

Other Nontechnical Staff

Whether the apheresis unit operates independently or as a department within a larger organization, certain ancillary functions must be provided to ensure that the unit meets regulatory and legal requirements. One function is legal counsel, which might be required for such activities as the development and review of contracts or informed consent documents. In addition, a lawyer might be necessary during negotiations with employees, particularly if the employee group is part of a union.

Larger organizations often have regulatory affairs staff. These individuals are responsible for keeping abreast of the regulations established by federal and state governments and for interpreting those regulations for the organization. They may also function as the liaison between the government and the organization.

As emphasized in Chapter 31, no organization is complete today without a quality assurance program. If it is large enough, the organization may have dedicated quality assurance staff. If not, systems must be in place to ensure that a quality assurance program is carried out by the regular staff. The quality assurance staff are part of the organization's quality system, which consists of "the organizational structure, responsibilities, policies, processes, procedures, and resources established by executive management to achieve quality."[3(p92)]

Human resource experts are a final element of desirable support staff. No organization can hire staff and manage operations successfully without knowledge in the area of human resource management. With expertise in employment requirements and legal issues surrounding employment, human resource experts can provide input into developing clear and concise job descriptions, establishing salary ranges, and developing a work performance review program. In addition, they can assist in progressive disciplinary actions that meet all legal requirements, thereby helping to protect the organization from employment litigation.

Management of Individuals

Training

If one of the key components of quality management and quality improvement is the staff performing the procedure, then a key component of staff performance is training. To do the job and do it well, staff must be trained to perform the appropriate tasks correctly. A good training program consists of written objectives, written training plans that are consistent with the unit's standard operating procedures (SOPs), and tests or assessments to verify the effectiveness of training.[6] SOP training should include training in the actual steps of the procedure, the rationale for performing the steps in a particular order, and the consequences that can occur if the process is not followed.[7] For all employees, records must be maintained that document the type of training provided, the methods used for training, and the methods used to assess the employee's competency to perform independently. Systems must be in place to ensure that the employee's ongoing training in procedural changes is documented. According to Callery, "The generally accepted industry standard for preparing employees to perform job skills is that of competency-based training."[8]

This means that the training is designed to reflect the job responsibilities and is measured by direct observation of performance. Callery identifies four components of competency-based training: "outcome-based learning objectives, identified content, specific methods of instruction, and a structure for evaluating learning and readiness for the job."[8] She describes in detail how to write objectives that are specific, measurable, and observable as well as how to develop the content, methods of instruction, and methods for evaluation.

Specific training needs may vary, depending on job descriptions. Training for medical directors of donor collection facilities should include hematology; transfusion medicine; cGMP regulations; and working knowledge of the facility's SOPs, of appropriate FDA requirements and AABB standards, and of requirements for employee safety. Medical directors involved in therapeutic apheresis procedures should have the qualifications listed previously in this chapter. They must also be able to determine the suitability of blood and components for transfusion. Training should cover the SOPs, as well as the operational details of the apheresis unit and should provide a basic knowledge of the particular apheresis equipment used. For technical staff, training in such basics as physiology, diseases, physical assessment, fluid and electrolyte balances, and interpersonal skills should be provided in addition to procedure-based training.

Certification and Credentialing

Currently, there is no certification available in the apheresis specialty. The American Society for Clinical Pathology (ASCP) had offered a certification as a hemapheresis practitioner (HP), but as a result of recent organizational changes, the certification is no longer available.

Competency Testing

Staff performing apheresis procedures should be observed and assessed regularly to confirm their competency to perform the procedures.[6] Assessment is usually made after the initial training and annually thereafter. Documentation of these assessments must be maintained in the individual employee's file.

In conjunction with periodic competency testing, an employee's job performance is also documented by means of a performance review or performance appraisal system. This regular written assessment is a result of ongoing review and observation by the supervisor. The performance review is based on the specific job tasks outlined in the job description and assesses the employee's ability to perform each of the identified job tasks successfully. It is often used as a basis for promotion or salary increases.[9]

Continuing Education

Staff should be encouraged and provided opportunities to attend continuing education seminars on topics in apheresis and related fields. In many states, continuing education is mandatory for the renewal of licenses for RNs.

Management of the Apheresis Unit

Once a staffing pattern has been determined and the staff are trained adequately and proven competent to perform their specific tasks, it remains necessary to manage the unit on a daily basis to accomplish the goals and fulfill the purposes of the organization. This is not an easy task, however, as there is no one "right formula" that will work equally well in all apheresis units. Even in large corporate networks such as Blood Systems, Inc, and the American Red Cross, what works well in one area of the country does not necessarily work well in others. Table 32-1 identifies some of the key factors that will determine how best to manage an apheresis unit. It is hoped that the needs for apheresis services in a community have been assessed carefully before a unit is opened. Once the unit is operating, mechanisms should be in place to evaluate the program periodically and implement the changes that are needed to meet the changing demands of the institution or community.[9-11]

Table 32-1. Key Factors Influencing Apheresis Units

- Type of apheresis procedures performed (donor collections, therapeutic procedures, hematopoietic progenitor cell collections)
- Qualifications and skill levels of staff
- Total number of procedures of each type to be performed daily/monthly/yearly
- Size and commitment of donor base
- Hours and days of operation
- Additional services offered/components collected
  - HLA-matched components
  - Platelet crossmatched components
  - Granulocyte components
  - Autologous apheresis Red Blood Cell components
- Miscellaneous issues
  - Distance from facility to clients
  - Distance from collection facility to processing and testing locations

Many decisions about who performs what tasks are determined to some extent by the type of staff hired. Those roles and responsibilities may change daily, depending on the activities and needs of a particular day. However, mechanisms must be in place to ensure adequate coverage so that staff members are not called on to perform tasks for which they have not been trained and tested adequately. The balance between ensuring adequate coverage and avoiding overstaffing becomes difficult to achieve in these days of limited resources.

The job of supervisor or group leader is usually assigned to a person who has a higher level of education as well as advanced technical and management skills. (For purposes of this chapter, the terms *management* and *supervision* are used synonymously.) Table 32-2 summarizes the responsibilities of an apheresis supervisor as well as the tasks that may be reasonably divided among various nonsupervisory staff members. The levels of performance and responsibility for tasks listed in the second column may be influenced by state requirements regarding various tasks. Many apheresis activities can be performed by non-RN, non-MT staff, but written procedures must be compre-

hensive and must clearly delineate responsibilities and limits.

Donor Centers

Procedural load requirements depend in part on the types of instruments. With automated apheresis instruments, it is possible for a single person to be responsible for two or more donors with the appropriate ancillary support to ensure that donor safety is never at risk.

The optimal approach to scheduling donors has been a topic of considerable debate. The type and length of procedures to be performed should be taken into consideration when determining the interval between donations for each instrument. Perhaps there is no single "best" way, and each center must choose a method that works well in its own specific context. Any successful approach, however, must address the following issues regarding donor preference:

- Are there times available before or after the potential donor's usual work hours?
- Are weekend appointment times available?
- Is the scheduling system flexible enough to allow for seasonal and holiday-associated fluctuations in donor availability?

Table 32-2. Tasks in an Apheresis Unit

Supervisor	Staff
• Interviewing, selecting, and training staff • Assessing staff performance • Appraising staff performance • Implementing new policies and procedures • Writing new procedures and revising current procedures • Investigating errors and accidents and determining corrective action • Scheduling staff and assignments • Monitoring component and equipment quality control • Monitoring and tracking instrument validation • Coordinating apheresis services with other departments • Coordinating apheresis services with hospitals and physicians • Functioning as staff person when needed	Donor collection facilities • Conducting donor registration, interview, and assessment • Performing phlebotomy • Performing apheresis collection procedures • Mixing and administering anticoagulants and fluids • Assessing and treating donor reactions and injuries • Providing postdonation care • Troubleshooting apheresis instrument problems • Calibrating equipment Therapeutic services • Assessing patient condition • Performing patient chart review • Performing therapeutic apheresis procedures • Administering medications and/or blood components • Handling patient emergencies • Troubleshooting apheresis instrument problems • Calibrating equipment

- Is the donor center convenient to most donors?
- Are satellite facilities a possibility?

To ensure the success of an apheresis program, methods should be in place to assess the responses to these questions and their effect on the program. Management should also assess productivity and efficiency of individual staff, including recruiters. Many software programs are available on the market today that can assist facilities in tracking and reporting productivity information. This information is critical in determining the financial aspects of apheresis services and ensuring that operations are managed in an effective manner.

Therapeutic Apheresis Services

Scheduling and staffing for therapeutic apheresis can be even more challenging. Initial thera-

peutic procedures are often performed on an emergency basis, usually within 24 hours of notification. The frequency and duration of subsequent treatments are difficult to predict, as they will depend on the disease being treated and the patient's response to successive treatments. Instruments may need to be moved to multiple locations. Periods when there are more procedures requested than staff can perform may alternate with periods when staff have no procedures to perform. Cross-training of therapeutic staff to donor apheresis or whole blood collections can make more efficient use of staff during times of low demand for therapeutic procedures. Independent therapeutic apheresis services may consider cross-training staff to perform dialysis procedures if both services are offered by the facility.

Multiple Services

Scheduling is probably most complex in centers where the same staff are cross-trained to perform donor collections as well as therapeutic procedures. When demand exceeds staffing capacity, therapeutic procedures for cases with well-documented need will usually take priority over donor procedures. Part of the rationale is that there is no substitute therapy for patients who need therapeutic apheresis, while needed blood components can be obtained from units of Whole Blood rather than donor apheresis.

Summary

The operation of an apheresis unit depends on the quality of staff performing the work. With careful attention to selecting the appropriate people, providing comprehensive training that is well documented, and managing the unit in an effective manner that meets all appropriate requirements and regulations, apheresis units can meet the needs of the community successfully.

References

1. Davis B. Governmental regulations. In: Karni KR, Viskochil KR, Amos PA, eds. Clinical laboratory management: A guide for clinical laboratory scientists. Boston: Little, Brown, 1982: 497-516.
2. Code of federal regulations. Title 21 CFR Parts 600-799. Washington, DC: US Government Printing Office, 2010 (revised annually).
3. Price TH, ed. Standards for blood banks and transfusion services. 26th ed. Bethesda, MD: AABB, 2009.
4. American Society for Apheresis, Standards and Education Committee. Organizational guidelines for therapeutic apheresis facilities. J Clin Apher 1996;11:42-5.
5. Wright SK. Standards for personnel performing hemapheresis therapies. In: MacPherson JL, Kasprisin DO, eds. Therapeutic hemapheresis. Boca Raton, FL: CRC Press, Inc, 1985:103-19.
6. Abruzzese RA. Nursing staff development. Garden City, NY: Mosby-Year Book, 1992: 203-14, 249-69.
7. Motscham TL, Moore SB. Error detection and reduction in blood banking. Clin Lab Med 1996;16:961-73.
8. Callery MF. Employee selection and training. In: Kasprisin CA, Laird-Fryer B, eds. Blood donor collection practices. Bethesda, MD: AABB, 1993:41-68.
9. Silver GA. Introduction to management. St. Paul, MN: West Publishing Company, 1981: 80-97, 266-89.
10. Hodgetts RM. Management fundamentals. Hinsdale, IL: Dryden Press, 1981:48-65, 258-77.
11. Sisk HL, Williams JC. Management and organization. 4th ed. Cincinnati: South-Western Publishing Co, 1981:61-82, 127-47.

Index

Table of Contents

Table of Contents

Table of Contents

Table of Contents